Fifth Edition

Core Curriculum for Nephrology Nursing

Editor

Caroline S. Counts, MSN, RN, CNN

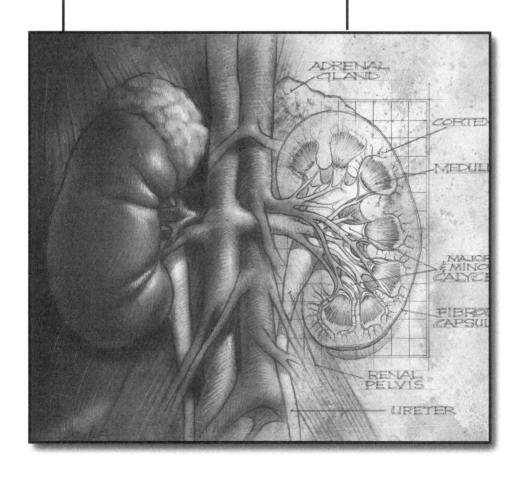

American Nephrology Nurses' Association

www.annanurse.org

Core Curriculum for Nephrology Nursing, 5th Edition

Copyright © 2008 American Nephrology Nurses' Association

Editor
Caroline S. Counts, MSN, RN, CNN
Research Coordinator, Division of Nephrology
Medical University of South Carolina
Charleston, South Carolina

Publication Management
Anthony J. Jannetti, Inc.
East Holly Avenue/Box 56
Pitman, New Jersey 08071-0056

Managing Editor: Claudia Cuddy
Assistant Managing Editor: Katie R. Brownlow
Layout Design and Production: Claudia Cuddy
Design Consultants: Darin Peters, Melody Edwards
Copy Editor: Katie R. Brownlow
Proofreaders: Katie R. Brownlow, Gus Ostrum
Cover Design: Melody Edwards
Cover Illustration: Scott M. Holladay © 2006
Photographer: Sannie Cook (*All photos by Sannie Cook unless otherwise credited.*)

ANNA National Office Staff
Executive Director: Michael Cunningham
Executive Assistant & Marketing Manager, Advertising: Susan Iannelli
Director of Education Services: Sally S. Russell
Director, Membership Services: Lou Ann Leary
Manager, Chapter Services: Janet Betts
Manager, Education Services: Celess Tyrell
Membership Services Coordinator: Pamela M. Monaghan
Director, Jannetti Publications, Inc.: Kenneth J. Thomas
Director of Editorial Services: Carol Ford
Managing Editor, *Nephrology Nursing Journal*: Gus Ostrum
Managing Editor, *ANNA Update* & *ANNA E-News*: Kathleen Thomas
Editorial Coordinator, *Nephrology Nursing Journal*: Laura Douglas
Editorial Assistant, Special Projects: Katie R. Brownlow
Director of Creative Design & Production: Jack M. Bryant
Layout and Design Specialist: Darin Peters
Creative Designers: Melody Edwards, Bob Taylor
Director of Electronic Publishing Services: Todd Lockhart
Director of Information Services: Rae Ann Cummings
Director of Fulfillment: Robert McIlvaine
Fulfillment Coordinator: Laura A. Loges
Director of Public Relations: Janet D'Alesandro
Public Relations Specialist: Linda Alexander
Director of Marketing: Tom Greene

FIFTH EDITION
Copyright © 2008 American Nephrology Nurses' Association

ISBN 978-0-9795029-2-7

American Nephrology Nurses' Association, East Holly Avenue/Box 56, Pitman, New Jersey 08071-0056
Web site: www.annanurse.org ■ E-mail: anna@ajj.com ■ Phone: 888-600-2662

Foreword

Continuing a Long-Standing Tradition!

ANNA members have traditionally awaited each revision of the *Core Curriculum for Nephrology Nursing* with eagerness, enthusiasm, and passion. (And, may I add, with good reason!) This Fifth Edition, which was edited by Caroline Counts – who has a long history of editorial excellence in nephrology nursing publications – presents a new look and new content, as well as updates on the very essentials of our practice.

A changing world

Ever since the previous edition was published in the Spring of 2001, the health care arenas in the United States and the world have transformed our nephrology nursing practice in ways that none of us could have ever imagined.

In just the past 7 years alone, we have seen tragedies and disasters such as September 11th and Hurricane Katrina that have tested our skills, our wills, and yes, our compassion. We have also seen new technologies, new medications, and new ways of providing patient care, all of which are designed to improve patient care outcomes.

Indeed the first four editions, edited by Dr. Larry Lancaster, and all of which were highly respected within our specialty, laid out a solid foundation for our practice. This Fifth Edition builds upon that tradition and presents some new wrinkles of its own.

Content essential to our practice

Of course, the very core modalities of our nephrology nursing practice are covered in this publication, and they are covered well: hemodialysis, peritoneal dialysis, transplantation, vascular access, and home therapies. The same is true for the disease processes themselves, including chronic kidney disease and acute renal failure, as well as the roles of nurses in such areas as advanced practice nursing, pediatrics, and geriatrics.

In addition, the introductory section outlines the normal anatomy and physiology of the renal system and serves as a foundation for understanding the kidney, while other sections examine areas crucial to our clinical practice such as pharmacology, infection control, and nutrition. This publication does not forget such important professional topics as public policy and the political process, evidence-based practice, emergency and disaster preparedness, and more!

Thanks to the contributors!

Finally, the ANNA Board of Directors and I would like to commend Editor and Project Director Caroline Counts, along with the many talented section editors, authors, and reviewers for their efforts in updating this Fifth Edition. Ms. Counts has assembled an impressive group of experts from within nephrology nursing who have covered every important topic within our specialty.

Because of these efforts, the *Core Curriculum* will once again serve as a solid study guide for the Nephrology Nursing Certification Commission's various examinations. Simultaneously, this Fifth Edition adds to the long list of highly regarded ANNA resources, which include *Contemporary Nephrology Nursing: Principles and Practice* and *Career Fulfillment in Nephrology Nursing: Your Guide to Professional Development.*

We hope you will enjoy this important contribution to the nephrology nursing and health care literature!

Sandra Bodin, MA, RN, CNN
ANNA President, 2007-2008

Section Editors and Authors

Kim Alleman, MS, RN, FNP-C, APRN, CNN
Nurse Practitioner
Hartford Hospital Transplant Program
Hartford, Connecticut
Editor & Author, Section 10; Author, Section 5

Rebecca L. Amato, BSN, RN
Staff Nurse, Highline Medical Center
Seattle, Washington
Author, Section 11

Connie Anderson, MBA, BSN
Vice President of Clinical Services
Northwest Kidney Centers
Seattle, Washington
Author, Section 14

Matthew J. Arduino, DrPH, MS
Lead Microbiologist
Centers for Disease Control and Prevention
Atlanta, Georgia
Author, Section 17

Emily Arnold, BSN, RN, CNN, CPHQ
Post-Kidney Transplant Coordinator
UNC Hospitals, University of North Carolina
Chapel Hill, North Carolina
Author, Section 17

Kay Atkins, MS, RD
Transplant Nutrition Specialist
Banner Good Samaritan Transplant Services
Phoenix, Arizona
Author, Section 8

Billie Axley, BSN, RN, CNN
Director of Quality Initiatives
Fresenius-North America (FMC-NA)
Nashville, Tennessee
Author, Section 17

Donna Bednarski, MSN, ANP,BC, CNN, CNP
Nurse Practitioner and Clinical Nurse
    Specialist – Nephrology
Harper University Hospital
Detroit, Michigan
Editor & Author, Sections 4 & 7

Gladys S. Benavente, MSN, ANP-C, CNN-NP
Renal Nurse Practitioner
Primary Care Provider
Southern Arizona V.A. Healthcare Systems
Tucson, Arizona
Author, Section 2

Laurie Biel, BSN, RN, CNN
Staff Nurse, Peritoneal Dialysis Unit
Co-Coordinator, Center for Renal Education
Massachusetts General Hospital
Boston, Massachusetts
Author, Section 3

Jina L. Bogle, MSN, APRN, NP-C, CNN
Nurse, DCI Acute Dialysis Services
University of Nebraska Medical Center
Kidney and Pancreas Transplant Surgery
Omaha, Nebraska
Author, Section 3

Deborah Brommage, MS, RD, CSR, CDN
Renal Clinical Consultant
Genzyme Renal
Long Island, New York
Editor, Section 8

Deborah H. Brooks, MSN, RN, ANP, CNN-NP
Nurse Practitioner
Research Coordinator
Medical University of South Carolina
Charleston, South Carolina
Author, Section 5

Sally Burrows-Hudson, MSN, RN, CNN
President
Nephrology Management Group
Sunnyvale, California
Author, Section 6

Evelyn Butera, MS, RN, CNN
Education/QI Specialist
Mills-Pennisula Health Services
Burlingame, California
Author, Section 17

Molly Lillis Cahill, MSN, RN, ANP-C, APRN, BC, CNN
Nurse Practitioner
Arms, Dodge, Robinson, Wilber, & Crouch
Kansas City, Missouri
Author, Section 4

Sally Campoy, MS, APRN, BC, CNN
Nurse Practitioner
Denver VA Medical Center, Renal Section
Denver, Colorado
Author, Section 5

Debra Castner, MSN, RN, APRN-C, CNN
Supervisor in the CKD Health and
    Wellness Education Program
Horizon Blue Cross Blue Shield of New Jersey
Farmingdale, New Jersey
Author, Section 4

Elizabeth Cincotta, PharmD, BCPS
Clinical Pharmacy Specialist in Nephrology
    and Solid Organ Transplant
Harper University Hospital/Detroit
    Medical Center
Detroit, Michigan
Editor & Author, Section 9

Louise Clement, MS, RD, CSR, LD
Renal Dietitian
South Plains Kidney Disease Center
Lubbock, Texas
Author, Section 8

Ann Beemer Cotton, MS, RD, CNSD
Clinical Dietitian Specialist
Critical Care and Transplant
Methodist Hospital
Indianapolis, Indiana
Author, Section 8

Caroline S. Counts, MSN, RN, CNN
Research Coordinator
Division of Nephrology
Medical University of South Carolina
Charleston, South Carolina
*Editor, Book; Editor & Author, Section 2;
    Author, Section 4*

Maureen Craig, MSN, RN, CNN, CCNS
Clinical Nurse Specialist – Nephrology
University of California Davis Medical Center
Sacramento, California
Editor & Author, Section 3

Susan C. Cronin, MS, RN
Vice President of Clinical Operations
Liberty Dialysis
Old Hickory, Tennessee
Editor & Author, Section 16

Geraldine Curry, BSN, RN, CNN, CPHQ
Corporate Clinical Quality Manager
Fresenius-North America (FMC-NA)
Lexington, Massachusetts
Author, Section 17

Terrence L. Dalton, RN
Nurse Manager, Acute Dialysis Services
Dialysis Clinic, Inc.
Omaha, Nebraska
Author, Section 3

Jaquelyn Davey-Tresemer, BSN, RN
Registered Nurse
Trauma Intensive Care Unit
Creighton University Medical Center
Omaha, Nebraska
Author, Section 3

M. Kay Deck, BS, RN
Director of Nursing and Education
NxStage Medical, Inc.
Lawrence, Massachusetts
Author, Section 14

Lesley C. Dinwiddie, MSN, RN, FNP, CNN
Nephrology Nurse Consultant
Vascular Access Education and Research
Cary, North Carolina
Executive Director
Institute of Excellence, Education and
    Research (ICEER)
Editor & Author, Section 12; Author, Section 5

Andrea Easom, MA, MNSc, APN, BC, CNN-NP
Instructor, College of Medicine
Nephrology Division
University of Arkansas for Medical Sciences
Little Rock, Arkansas
Author, Section 5

Patricia L. Garrigan, BSN, RN
Acute Hemodialysis Registered Nurse
Dialysis Clinic, Inc.
Omaha, Nebraska
Author, Section 3

Norma Gomez, MBA, BSN, RN, CNN
Director of Education
DaVita, Inc.
Homestead, Florida
Editor & Author, Section 18

Cheryl L. Groenhoff, MSN, MBA, RN, CNN
Kidney Patient Educator
Baxter Health Care
Plantation, Florida
Author, Section 4

Lisa M. Hall, MSSW, LCSW
Community Services Coordinator
FMQAI: The Florida ESRD Network
    (Network 7)
Tampa, Florida
Author, Section 4

Glenda F. Harbert, ADN, RN, CNN, CPHQ
Executive Director
ESRD Network of Texas, Inc.
Dallas, Texas
Author, Section 4

Anne E. Harty, MS, APRN, FNP, CNN
Nephrology Nurse Practitioner
Carmichael, California
Editor, Section 3

Diana Hlebovy, BSN, RN, CHN, CNN
Director of Clinical Affairs
Hema Metrics
Kaysville, Utah
Author, Section 11

Katherine Healy Houle, MSN, C-FNP, CNN-NP
Nephrology Nurse Practitioner
Marquette General Health Systems
Marquette, Michigan
Author, Section 5

Margie A. Hull, MEd, MSN, RN, APRN-BC, CDE
Visiting Lecturer
Indiana University School of Nursing
Indianapolis, Indiana
Author, Section 6

Maria Karalis, MBA, RD, LDN
Regional Scientific Manager
Abbott Renal Care
Abbott Park, Illinois
Author, Section 8

Betsy King, MSN, RN, CNN
Clinical Services Specialist
DaVita, Inc.
White Plains, New York
Author, Section 11

Carol L. Kinzner, MSN, ARNP, GNP, CNN-NP
Nurse Practitioner
Evergreen Nephrology Associates
Tacoma, Washington
Author, Section 5

Marjorie J. Kurt, MSN, RN
Assistant Clinical Professor
Indiana University School of Nursing
Indianapolis, Indiana
Author, Section 6

Kristin Larson, MSN, RN, ANP, GNP, CNN
Nurse Practitioner
Nephrology Associates
Salt Lake City, Utah
Author, Section 7

Anita Lipman, MS, BSN, RN, CNN
Anemia Specialist
Roche Labs
Toms River, New Jersey
Author, Section 18

Sharon Longton, BSN, RN, CNN, CCTC
Kidney/Pancreas Transplant Coordinator
Harper University Hospital
Detroit, Michigan
Author, Section 10

Maria Luongo, MSN, BA, RN
CAPD Nurse Manager
Peritoneal Dialysis Unit
Massachusetts General Hospital
Boston, Massachusetts
Author, Sections 3, 14

Donna Mapes, DNSc, MS, RN
Adjunct Senior Researcher
University Renal Research & Education
    Association
President, Donna L. Mapes & Associates
Assistant Clinical Professor (Adjunct)
USCF School of Nursing
Moorpark, California
Author, Section 6

Terran R. Mathers, DNS, RN
Associate Professor
Spring Hill College
Mobile, Alabama
Author, Sections 6, 16

Carrie N. May, MS, RN, ANP, CNN
Adult Nurse Practitioner
Nephrology Care Manager
Lutheran General Hospital
Park Ridge, Illinois
Author, Section 5

Nancy G. McAfee, MN, RN, CNN
Dialysis Clinical Nurse Specialist
Children's Hospital & Regional Medical Center
Seattle, Washington
Editor & Author, Section 15

Patricia Bargo McCarley, MSN, RN, NP, CNN
Nurse Practitioner
Diablo Nephrology Medical Group
Walnut Creek, California
Author, Section 2

Debra McDillon, MSN, RN, CNN
Director of Clinical Education
DaVita, Inc.
Munster, Indiana
Author, Section 18

**Mildred Sue McManus, MSN, RN, APRN
    (FNP)-BC, CNN**
Nephrology Nurse Practitioner
Kidney Transplant Coordinator
Richard L. Roudebush Medical Center
Indianapolis, Indiana
Author, Section 6

Patricia Merenda, MN, ARNP, CNN-NP, CCTC
Nurse Practitioner
Polyclinic Swedish Medical Center
Seattle, Washington
Author, Section 5

Patricia Painter, PhD
Associate Professor
Department of Medicine/Division of
    Renal Medicine
University of Minnesota
Minneapolis, Minnesota
Author, Section 4

Chhaya Patel, MA, RD, CSR
Area 1 Divisional Dietitian
DaVita, Inc.
Walnut Creek, California
Author, Section 8

Eileen J. Peacock, MSN, RN, CNN, CIC, CPHQ
Research Assistant
DaVita, Inc.
Berwyn, Pennsylvania
Author, Section 17

Nancy J. Pelfrey, MSN, RN, ACNP-C, CNN-NP
Nurse Practitioner
DaVita, Inc.
Fairview, North Carolina
Author, Section 2

Suanne Petroff, APRN, BC, CNN
Disease Management Consultant
CKD Consults
South Deerfield, Massachusetts
Author, Section 2

Leonor P. Ponferrada, BSN, BSHSM, RN, CNN
Quality Management Coordinator
Dialysis Clinic, Inc.
Columbia, Missouri
Author, Section 13

Barbara F. Prowant, MS, RN, CNN
Research Associate
Division of Nephrology
Department of Internal Medicine
University of Missouri
Columbia, Missouri
Editor & Author, Section 13

Cindy Richards, BSN, RN, CNN
Pediatric Transplant Coordinator
Children's Hospital
Birmingham, Alabama
Author, Section 15

Karen C. Robbins, MS, RN, CNN
Nurse Educator for Dialysis Services and
     Transplant
Hartford Hospital
Hartford, Connecticut
Associate Editor, *Nephrology Nursing Journal*
Editor, Section 11

Regina M. Rohe, RN, HP(ASCP)
Vice President of Operations
Apheresis Care Group, Inc.
San Francisco, California
Author, Section 3

Troy A. Russell, MSN, RN, APRN, BC, CNN-NP
Nephrology Nurse Practitioner
VA-TN Valley Healthcare System
Nashville, Tennessee
Editor, Section 5

Patricia Baltz Salai, MSN, RN, CRNP, CNN
Nephrology Nurse Practitioner
Veterans Affairs Pittsburgh Healthcare System
Pittsburgh, Pennsylvania
Author, Section 11

Roberta J. Satalowich, BS, RN, CNN
Staff Nurse, Home Dialysis Department
Dialysis Clinic, Inc.
Columbia, Missouri
Author, Section 13

Karen E. Schardin, BSN, RN, CNN
Director of Clinical Field Services
NxStage Medical, Inc.
Carson City, Nevada
Editor & Author, Section 14

Mary Schira, PhD, APRN, BC, ACNP, CNN-NP
Associate Clinical Professor
Director of the ACNP and ENP Programs
School of Nursing
University of Texas at Arlington
Arlington, Texas
Editor & Author, Section 1

Kristine S. Schonder, PharmD
Assistant Professor
University of Pittsburgh School of Pharmacy
Pittsburgh, Pennsylvania
Author, Section 9

Jodi M. Smith, MD, MPH
Assistant Professor of Pediatrics
Division of Nephrology
University of Washington Children's
     Hospital and Regional Medical Center
Seattle, Washington
Author, Section 15

Sheila J. Smith, BSN, RN, HP(ASCP)
Director of Operations
Apheresis Care Group, Inc.
San Francisco, California
Author, Section 3

Lucy Stackiewicz, MSN, CNN, CRNP
Nurse Practitioner, Nephrology & Transplant
University Physicians, Inc.
University of Maryland Medical System
Baltimore, Maryland
Author, Section 2

Jean Stover, RD, LDN
Renal Dietitian
DaVita, Inc.
Philadelphia, Pennsylvania
Author, Section 8

Cynthia J. Terrill, RD, CSR, CD
Pediatric Renal Dietitian
University Healthcare/University Hospitals
     and Clinics
Salt Lake City, Utah
Author, Section 8

Charlotte Thomas-Hawkins, PhD, RN
Assistant Professor
College of Nursing, Rutgers University
Newark, New Jersey
Author, Section 6

Janet L. Welch, DNS, RN, CNS
Associate Professor & Chair, Adult Health
Indiana University School of Nursing
Indianapolis, Indiana.
Editor & Author, Section 6

Gail Wick, MHSA, BSN, RN, CNN
Consultant
Atlanta, Georgia
Author, Section 7

Helen F. Williams, BSN, RN, CNN
Staff Nurse in Acute Dialysis
Western Nephrology
Denver, Colorado
Editor & Author, Section 3

JoAnn Wilson, RN, HP(ASCP)
Apheresis Registered Nurse
Apheresis Care Group, Inc.
San Francisco, California
Author, Section 3

Karen C. Wiseman, MSN, RN, CNN
Director of Policy & Regulatory Affairs
Renal Advantage, Inc.
Brentwood, Tennessee
Editor, Section 17

Beth Witten, MSW, ACSW, LSCSW
Resource and Policy Associate
Medical Education Institute, Inc.
Madison, Wisconsin
Author, Section 4

AUTHOR DISCLOSURES

Deborah Brommage disclosed that she is employed by Genzyme.

Lesley C. Dinwiddie disclosed that she is on the Bureau for Graftcath, Inc., Excelsior Medical, Arrow International, and Hoffman-LaRoche.

Andrea Easom disclosed that she is on the Bureau for Amgen, Abbott, Watson, and Genzyme. She is also on the Advisory Board for Amgen and Abbott.

Diana Hlebovy disclosed that she is Director of Clinical Affairs for Hema Metrics.

Patricia Bargo McCarley disclosed that she is on the Bureau for Amgen, Genzyme, and Ortho Biotech.

Suanne Petroff disclosed that she is a speaker and slide developer for Watson, Ortho Biotech, and Medscape.

All other authors of the *Core Curriculum for Nephrology Nursing* (5th ed.) reported no actual or potential conflict of interest in relation to this continuing nursing education activity.

Reviewers

Lynda K. Ball, BS, BSN, RN, CNN
Quality Improvement Coordinator
Northwest Renal Network
Seattle, Washington

Jenny Bell, BSN, CNN, CCTC
Clinical Transplant Coordinator
Kidney and Kidney/Pancreas Program
Banner Good Samaritan Transplant Services
Phoenix, Arizona

Laurie Biel, BSN, RN, CNN
Staff Nurse, Peritoneal Dialysis Unit
Co-Coordinator, Center for Renal Education
Massachusetts General Hospital
Boston, Massachusetts

Sally Campoy, MS, APRN, BC, CNN
Nurse Practitioner
Denver VA Medical Center, Renal Section
Denver, Colorado

Sue Preuett Cary, MN, RN, APRN, NP, CNN
Nurse Practitioner
Nephrology
Ochsner Health Care Systems Baton Rouge
Baton Rouge, Louisiana

Christine Ceccarelli, MS, MBA, RN, MCNN
Staff Nurse
Hartford Hospital Dialysis Unit and
Central CT Dialysis Unit
Meriden, Connecticut
Adjunct Faculty
Fairfield University School of Nursing
Fairfield, Connecticut

Jean Colaneri, ACNP, CNN
Nurse Practitioner/Clinical Nurse Specialist
Renal/Pancreas Transplant Unit and
Chronic Kidney Disease Clinic
Albany Medical Center Hospital
Albany, New York

Sheila Doss, RN, CNN, CCRA
Nursing Director of Research
Satellite Healthcare, Inc.
Mountain View, California

Sue Fallone, MS, RN, CNN
Clinical Nurse Specialist
Adult and Pediatric Dialysis
Albany Medical Center
Albany, New York

Jon Farlow, BSN, RN
Fresenius Medical Care
Hartford Dialysis
Hartford, Connecticut

Wanda Flynn, BS, RN, CNN
Director
Emergency Care
CVPH Medical Center
Plattsburgh, New York

Margaret Nusser Gerlach, MSN, APRN, CNN
Nephrology Nurse Practitioner, Adult
University of Nebraska Medical Center
Internal Medicine/Section of Nephrology
Omaha, Nebraska

Cyrena M. Gilman, MN, RN, CNN
Manager, Kidney Medical Service Area
Pediatric Dialysis
Riley Hospital for Children
Clarian Health Partners
Indianapolis, Indiana

Debra Hain, DNS, GNP, APRN, BC
Assistant Professor of Nursing
Florida Atlantic University
Christine E. Lynn College of Nursing
Boca Raton, Florida
Nurse Practitioner in Nephrology
Cleveland Clinic Florida
Weston, Florida

Carol M. Headley, DNSc, RN, CNN
Advanced Practice Nurse
Veterans Affairs Medical Center
Memphis, Tennessee

Judy Kauffman, RN, CNN
Clinical Director
Acute Dialysis and Apheresis Unit
University of Virginia Health System
Charlottesville, Virginia

Sara K. Kennedy, BSN, RN, CNN
Facility Administrator & CKD Educator
DaVita Birmingham Home Training Unit
Birmingham, Alabama

MaryRose Kott, MS, RN, ANP, CNN
Clinical Nurse Specialist
Medicine/Nurse Practitioner Palliative Care
St. Joseph Hospital Health Center
Syracuse, New York

Tricia Littig, MSN, APRN-BC, CNN
Nurse Practitioner
Southwest Nephrology Associates
Orland Park, Illinois

Holly Fadness McFarland, MSN, RN, CNN
Facility Administrator
DaVita of Edgecombe County
Tarboro, North Carolina

Mary E. McGraw, MSN, APRN, BC, ACNP, CNN
Nurse Practitioner
Dallas Nephrology Associates
Dallas, Texas

Mildred Sue McManus, MSN, RN, APRN (FNP)-BC, CNN
Nephrology Nurse Practitioner
Kidney Transplant Coordinator
Richard L. Roudebush Medical Center
Indianapolis, Indiana

Anita Molzahn, PhD, MN, RN
Professor
School of Nursing
University of Victoria
Victoria, B.C., Canada

Christine Mudge, MS, RN, PNPc/CNS, CNN, FAAN
Pediatric Nurse Practitioner
CNS Pediatric Transplant
University of California – San Francisco
San Francisco, California

Sheila M. O'Day, MSN, APRN, CNN
Adult Nurse Practitioner, Section of
Nephrology
University of Nebraska Medical Center
Omaha, Nebraska

Sara Otterness, RN, APRN-BC, CNN
Nephrology Nurse Practitioner
Veterans Affairs Medical Center
Minneapolis, Minnesota

Glenda Payne, MS, RN, CNN
ESRD Technical Advisor
Centers for Medicare and Medicaid Services
Dallas, Texas

Jennifer E. Payton, MHCA, BSN, RN, CNN
Home Program Coordinator
Dialysis Clinic, Inc.
Charleston, South Carolina

Sally S. Russell, MN, CMSRN
Director of Education Services
American Nephrology Nurses' Association
Pitman, New Jersey

Caroline Steward, MSN, RN, APN-C, CCRN, CNN
Care Manager for Renaissance Health Care
Fresenius Medical Care, North America
Ewing, New Jersey

Glinda Stricklin, BSN, RN, CNN
Clinical Educator
NxStage Medical, Inc.
Charleston, South Carolina

Charlotte Szromba, MSN, CNN, APRN-BC, NP
Consultant
Nephrology Clinical Solutions
Lisle, Illinois

Nancy Szymanski, RN, CNN
Home Training Coordinator
DCA of Chevy Chase and Rockville
Bethesda, Maryland

Annie W. Tu, MS, ARNP, CNN
Nephrology Clinical Nurse Specialist
University of Washington Medical Center
Seattle, Washington

Joni Walton, PhD, APRN, BC
Faculty
Carroll College
Helena, Montana

REVIEWER DISCLOSURES
Sue Preuett Cary disclosed that she is on Amgen's Speaker's Bureau for anemia.

All other reviewers of the *Core Curriculum for Nephrology Nursing* (5th ed.) reported no actual or potential conflict of interest in relation to this continuing nursing education activity.

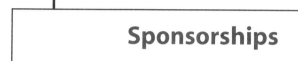

Sponsorships

ANNA thanks the following companies for their sponsorship of this book.

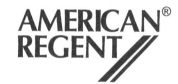

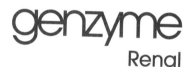

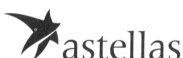

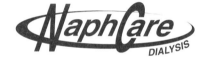

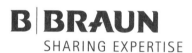

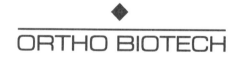

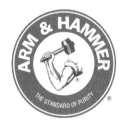

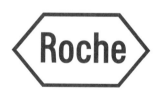

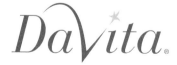

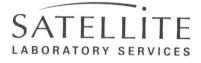

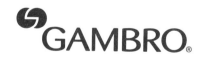

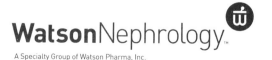

See pages 1093–1099 for profiles of our Corporate Sponsors.

Contents

Preface

From the Editor

It will always be a vivid memory in my mind, the day I received the phone call from Suzann VanBuskirk (ANNA President 2005–2006) and Mike Cunningham (ANNA Executive Director) telling me I had been selected as the next Editor for the *Core Curriculum for Nephrology Nursing*. The news was met with shock, excitement, enthusiasm, and a lot of joy. However, as soon as the call ended, reality set in!

I was going to be the Editor of the Fifth Edition of ANNA's *Core Curriculum*. I was going to be the first person to take on that role since Larry E. Lancaster, EdD, ACNP, created and edited all previous editions. How was I ever going to follow in the footsteps of a person who is held in such high esteem and who had done such a magnificent job with the first four editions? How would I ever assemble a team of qualified authors as he had done? The work was cut out for me as a new journey began!

To all the people who paved the way for the evolution of the Fifth Edition, you have my admiration and humble thanks. I also thank the 2005–2006 ANNA Board of Directors for their vote of confidence in allowing me this privilege and the subsequent ANNA Boards who were so supportive.

Assembling a team to produce a textbook of this magnitude is no easy task. As the reader will see, in this edition there are more than 100 section editors and authors, as well as more than 30 reviewers who provided careful scrutiny and great suggestions. I thank each of these individuals for their efforts and contributions to this text.

The writing team began their own journeys and faced their own challenges. As the core information was being gathered and the text written, changes were occurring in terminology, technology, pharmaceutical agents, clinical practice, etc.

In this fast-paced world, it is challenging to keep current. That is why I suggest that the reader use this book as a foundation for nephrology nursing knowledge, but not by itself. The reader is also advised to use additional reliable sources of new up-to-date knowledge, such as ANNA's *Nephrology Nursing Journal.*

This publication would not exist without the hard work of Managing Editor Claudia Cuddy and Assistant Managing Editor Katie Brownlow. They were always professional, knowledgeable, organized, and ever patient. They were great to work with, and I will miss them in my daily life.

And, speaking of daily life, my thanks go to those persons whom I love the most and who have given me more support than I could ever deserve – my family and friends. To my son Chris (and Christina!) and my daughter Kim, thank you for all your words of support and encouragement. To my husband, Henry, thank you for your patience, understanding, and willingness to support me as I followed my professional aspirations. You are the best!

To the reader, it is hoped that you will enjoy the Fifth Edition of the *Core Curriculum for Nephrology Nursing*. New sections have been added to reflect today's nursing practice in nephrology. Pictures have been added to enhance the textbook's appearance and show real-life situations. (The pictures are of real people – patients and caregivers; they are not models.)

If you are using the *Core* as a means to prepare for one of the certification exams offered by the Nephrology Nursing Certification Commission, you have made a good choice. But please do not make it your only resource. ANNA offers other publications and educational products that complement each other and provide a more global review of nephrology nursing.

The self-assessment questions in this text do not reflect the questions on the exams, but offer a means to judge oneself and to identify areas where further review may be needed.

The journey of bringing the Fifth Edition of the *Core Curriculum for Nephrology Nursing* to fruition has ended. It has been a wonderful learning experience for me. May it now be a good learning experience for many others!

Caroline S. Counts
Project Director and Editor

Section 1

The Kidney

Mary Schira, PhD, APRN, BC, ACNP, CNN-NP

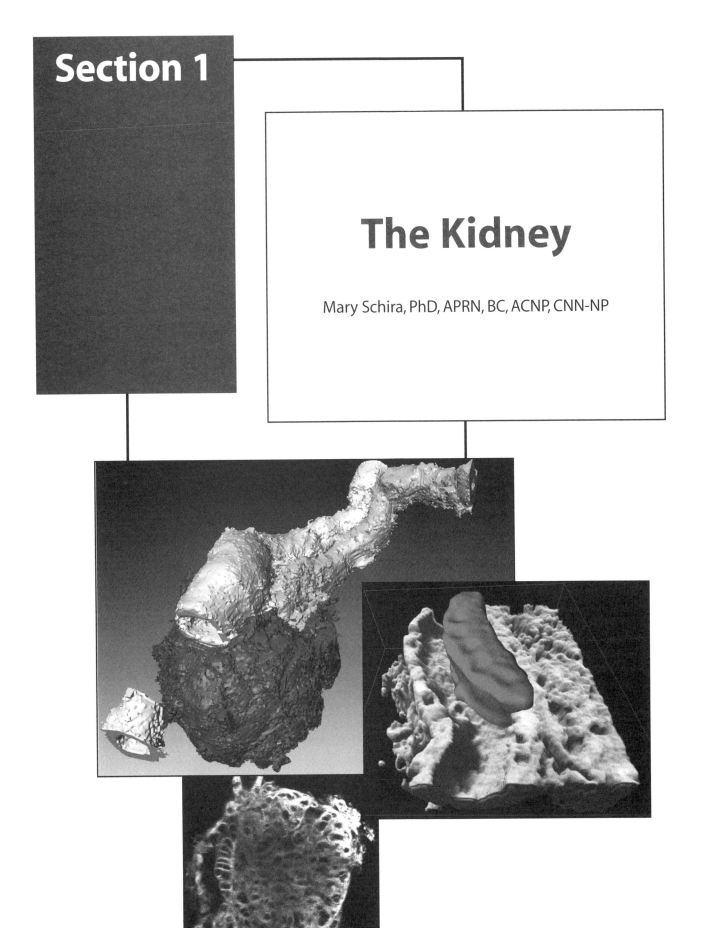

About the Author

Mary Schira, PhD, APRN, BC, ACNP, CNN-NP, Section Editor and Author, is an Associate Clinical Professor and the Director of the ACNP and ENP Programs at the School of Nursing, University of Texas at Arlington, in Arlington, Texas.

Acknowledgment

Thanks to Larry E. Lancaster and Cleo J. Richard, editors and authors of the fourth edition of the *Core Curriculum*, for their contributions to this section.

From page 1:

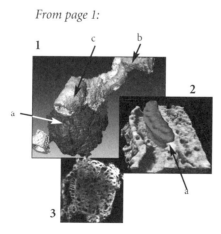

1. Segmented three-dimensional image of the living glomerulus (a). The supplying afferent arteriole (b) and the attached thick ascending limb (c) are also shown.
2. Three-dimensional volume-rendered image of the living juxtaglomerular apparatus with the macula densa (a).
3. Multiphoton confocal micrograph of living glomerulus.

Photos courtesy of P. Darwin Bell, PhD, DCI Professor of Medicine; Director, Renal Biology Research, Division of Nephrology, Medical University of South Carolina, Charleston, SC.

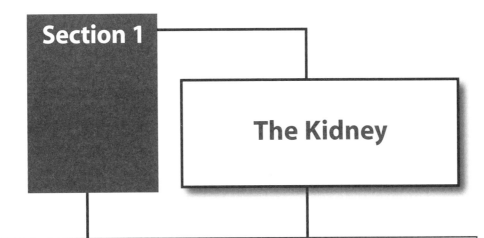

Section 1

The Kidney

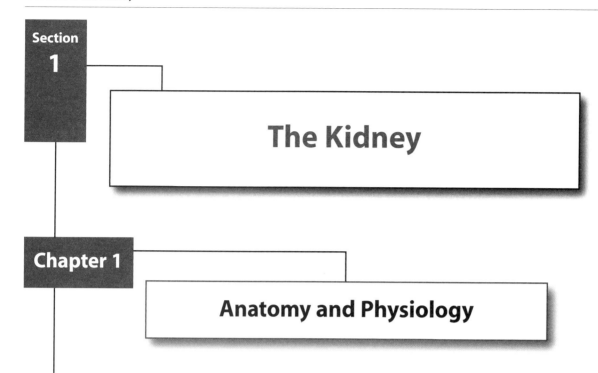

Section 1

The Kidney

Chapter 1

Anatomy and Physiology

Purpose

The purpose of this chapter is to outline the normal anatomy and physiology of the renal system to serve as a foundation for understanding the assessment of kidney function, kidney abnormalities, and how kidney and other diseases affect kidney function.

Objectives

Upon completion of this chapter, the learner will be able to:

1. Given an unlabeled drawing, label the following anatomic structures:
   a. Left and right kidneys.
   b. Ureters.
   c. Urinary bladder.
   d. Urethra.
   e. Renal artery.
   f. Renal vein.
   g. Adrenal glands.
2. Given a bisected mammalian kidney or a model of the kidney, locate the following structures:
   a. Renal cortex.
   b. Renal medulla.
   c. Hilum.
   d. Pelvis.
   e. Pyramid.
   f. Capsule.
3. Describe the anatomic location and protection of the kidneys.
4. Trace the blood supply from the left ventricle to the glomerulus and back to the right atrium.
5. Describe the microscopic anatomy of the vascular and tubular components of the nephron.
6. Describe the anatomy of the juxtaglomerular apparatus/complex.
7. Outline the embryologic development of the kidney.

8. Define the following concepts:
   a. Glomerular filtration rate.
   b. Net (effective) glomerular filtration pressure.
   c. Renal clearance.
   d. Tubular reabsorption.
   e. Tubular secretion.
   f. Tubular transport maximum.
9. Describe renal regulation of water balance.
10. Discuss renal regulation of solutes: electrolytes and metabolic wastes.
11. Outline renal regulation of acid-base balance.
12. List hormones secreted by the kidney and the function(s) of the hormones.

Anatomy of the Renal System

I. Kidneys: Gross anatomy.

A. Location.
   1. Posterior abdominal wall in the retroperitoneal space in front of and on both sides of the vertebral column between twelfth thoracic and third lumbar vertebrae.
   2. Right kidney is slightly lower than the left because the liver is above the right kidney (see Figure 1.1).

B. Protection.
   1. Anteriorly by abdominal muscles, fascia, fat, and intestines.
   2. Posteriorly by large back muscles and ribs.
   3. Right kidney protected superiorly by liver and left kidney by the spleen.

C. Gross structure.
   1. Weight of adult kidney: 120–160 g.
   2. Size of adult kidney: 5–7 cm wide, 11–13 cm long, about 2.5 cm thick.
   3. Covered by a tough, thin fibrous capsule composed of connective tissue, blood vessels, and lymphatics. Around the renal capsule is a large deposit of fat, which provides additional protection from jarring. Kidneys and surrounding fat are suspended from abdominal wall by renal fascia, which is a layer of connective tissue.
   4. Adrenal gland is located on top of each kidney. Function of adrenal glands is separate from renal function; they also have separate blood and nerve supplies.
   5. Renal blood vessels, lymphatics, nerves, and ureter enter or exit through hilum of each kidney.

6. Internal structure of the kidney (see Figure 1.2).
   a. Cortex.
      (1) Outer part of the kidney.
      (2) Approximately 1 cm wide.
      (3) Located immediately below the capsule.
      (4) About 80–85% of the nephrons (called cortical nephrons) and their blood vessels are located in the outer portion of the cortex.
      (5) The remaining 15–20% of nephrons (juxtamedullary nephrons) also have structures located deep in the cortex.
   b. Medulla.
      (1) Approximately 5 cm wide.
      (2) In the inner portion of the kidney.
      (3) Contains pyramids and renal columns (Bertin's columns), loops of Henle, vasa recta, and medullary collecting ducts of juxtamedullary nephrons.

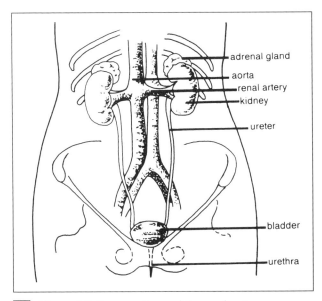

Figure 1.1. Gross anatomy of the renal system.

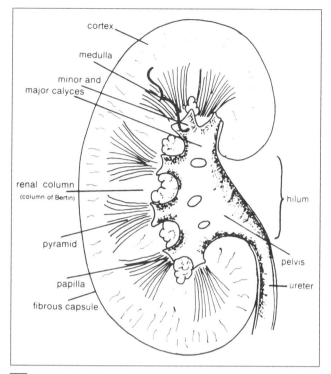

Figure 1.2. Internal structure of the kidney.

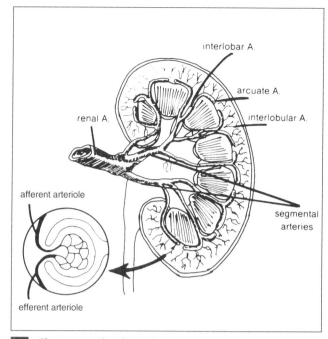

Figure 1.3. Blood supply to the kidney. Renal artery branches from the abdominal aorta. The microscopic circulation is shown in Figure 1.4.

(4) Divided into outer (adjacent to the cortex) and inner (between the outer cortex and the renal pelvis) zones.

(5) Pyramids are triangular-shaped structures composed of nephrons and their blood vessels. Renal columns are cortical tissue between the pyramids.

  c. Calyx.

(1) The tip (apex) of each pyramid, called the papilla, opens into a minor calyx.

(2) Several minor calyces form a major calyx. The major calyces form the common ureter, which exits the renal pelvis and transports urine to the bladder.

  d. Collecting system.

(1) Composed of structures that collect and transport urine, but do not alter its composition or volume.

(2) Once urine flows through the papilla at the tip of the pyramid, the urine composition is unchanged.

II. Blood supply, lymphatic drainage, and innervation.

A. The kidneys receive approximately 20–25% (about 1200 mL/min) of the cardiac output under normal physiologic conditions. This is called the renal fraction.

B. The body's total blood supply circulates through the kidneys approximately 12 times per hour.

C. Approximately 90% of the renal blood supply circulates through the cortex at a rate of about 4.5 mL/min, and 10% circulates through the medulla at about 1 mL/min.

D. Each kidney has one renal artery that branches from the abdominal aorta and enters the kidney at the hilum.

E. Renal artery divides into segmental arteries that further divide into interlobar arteries that travel alongside the pyramids into the cortex (see Figure 1.3).

1. At the junction of the cortex and medulla, the interlobar arteries bend at right angles.

2. Arcuate arteries begin at this point. The arcuate arteries branch into interlobular arteries, which travel further into the cortex.

3. In the cortex, the interlobular arteries divide into afferent arterioles.

4. Each afferent arteriole divides into a tuft of about 12 capillaries called the glomerulus.

5. The glomerular capillaries rejoin to form the efferent arteriole, which then becomes the peritubular capillary network (and vasa recta for the juxtamedullary nephrons).

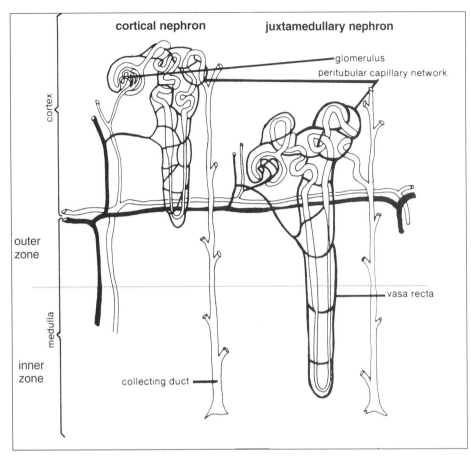

Figure 1.4. Arrangement of a cortical and juxtamedullary nephron. Note the relationship between vascular and tubular components.

6. The microscopic circulation begins with the afferent arteriole and is described later in this chapter.

F. Venous vessels accompany the arterial system and are named similarly.
1. The interlobular veins join the segmental veins which empty into the renal vein.
2. Renal vein exits through hilum and joins inferior vena cava, which returns blood to the right atrium.

G. Lymphatic drainage from the kidneys and upper ureters flows into the aortic and paraaortic lymph nodes and then into the thoracic lymph duct.

H. Kidneys are innervated by sympathetic branches from the celiac plexus, upper lumbar splanchnic and thoracic nerves, and intermesenteric and superior hypogastric plexus. These join to form a surrounding renal nerve plexus.

III. Microscopic anatomy of the nephron.

A. Nephron: structural and functional unit of the kidney.
1. Each nephron consists of two components.
   a. Vascular component, which includes the afferent arteriole, glomerulus, efferent arteriole, peritubular capillary network, and vasa recta (for juxtamedullary nephrons only).
   b. Tubular component, which includes Bowman's capsule, proximal tubule (PT), descending and ascending limbs of the loop of Henle, distal tubule (DT), cortical collecting tubule, and medullary collecting duct.
2. Each kidney has approximately 1 million nephrons.
   a. 80–85% are cortical nephrons with short, thin loops of Henle. Except for the tips of some loops of Henle and the medullary collecting duct, the entire nephron lies in the renal cortex (see Figure 1.4).

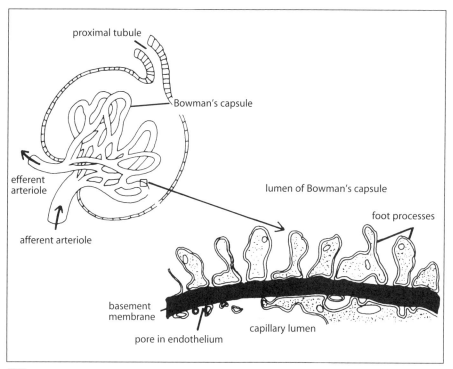

proximal tubule

Bowman's capsule

efferent arteriole

afferent arteriole

lumen of Bowman's capsule

foot processes

basement membrane

capillary lumen

pore in endothelium

Figure 1.5. Structure of the glomerular capillary membrane.

b. 15–20% are juxtamedullary nephrons in which the glomerulus, Bowman's capsule, PT, DT, and cortical collecting tubule lie deeper in the cortex near its junction with the medulla. They have long, thin loops of Henle that penetrate into the outer and inner zones of the medulla and many that penetrate to the tips of the renal papillae (see Figure 1.4).

c. The medullary collecting ducts of all nephrons extend from the cortex-medulla junction through the outer and inner zones of the medulla to the tip of the papilla at the apex of the pyramids.

3. Vascular component (see Figures 1.4 and 1.5).
a. Each afferent arteriole divides into a tuft of capillaries called the glomerulus which is surrounded by Bowman's capsule.
b. Blood in the glomerulus is separated from fluid in Bowman's capsule only by its capillary membranes.
c. Permeability of the glomerular capillaries is about 100–500 times greater than the usual capillaries in other parts of the body. The glomerular capillaries are highly selective for the types of molecules that can pass through.
d. Glomerular capillary permeability and selectivity are related to the structure of the glomerular capillary membrane.

e. The membrane has three major layers (see Figure 1.5).
   (1) Endothelial layer lining glomerular capillaries is perforated by thousands of holes called fenestrae. Thus, glomerular capillaries are often called fenestrated capillaries. The large fenestrae allow filtration of water and small solutes with diameters up to about 100 nanometers.
   (2) Basement membrane layer, composed of collagen and proteoglycans, also has large spaces through which water and some solutes can pass.
   (3) Layer of epithelial cells (called podocytes) line outer surface of glomerulus and also serves as inner layer of Bowman's capsule. These cells have structures called foot processes that are not continuous, but have slit pores about 25–60 nanometers wide that allow water and some solutes to pass.
f. Reasons for selectivity of molecules that can filter through glomerular capillaries:
   (1) Size of pores. Solutes with molecular weights less than 5,000 daltons are easily filtered (e.g., water and ions). As the molecular weight of a solutes increases, there is less filtration, and solutes with

molecular weights greater than 69,000 daltons (diameters more than about 8 nanometers) filter very poorly or not at all.

(2) All three layers of the glomerular membrane have negative charges. Plasma proteins and other solutes with negative charges are therefore repelled by the negative charges and are not filtered by the membrane.

(3) Example. Albumin has a molecular diameter of about 6 nanometers. Therefore, based on size, it should filter through the glomerular membranes. Yet, almost no albumin is present in the glomerular filtrate because albumin has a strong negative electrical charge and the pores in the glomerular membrane have a strong negative electrical charge. Thus, electrostatic forces keep almost all the albumin from filtering across the glomerular membrane.

g. Glomerular capillaries are separated by mesangial cells, which provide support for the capillaries. Some mesangial cells also have phagocytic properties.

h. Glomerular capillaries reunite to form the efferent arteriole, which has two branches (see Figures 1.4 and 1.5).

(1) Peritubular capillaries.
(a) Surround the PT and DT, loops of Henle, and collecting tubules of cortical nephrons.
(b) Surround the PT, DT, cortical collecting tubules, and medullary collecting ducts of juxtamedullary nephrons.
(c) Drain into venules.

(2) Vasa recta capillaries are branches of peritubular capillaries, which wrap around and run parallel to long thin loops of Henle associated with juxtamedullary nephrons. Vasa recta and loops of Henle of juxtamedullary nephrons are located in renal medulla.

4. Tubular component.
a. Composed of Bowman's capsule, PT, loop of Henle, DT, cortical collecting tubule, and medullary collecting duct (see Figures 1.6 and 1.7).
b. Bowman's capsule is a concave sac that surrounds glomerular capillaries, creating Bowman's space. On one side Bowman's

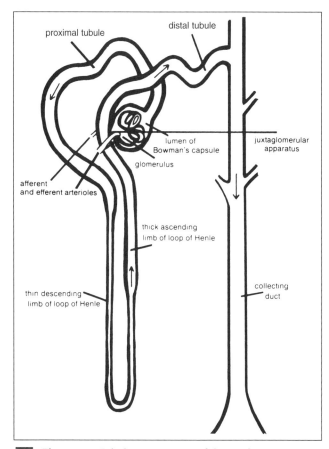

Figure 1.6. Tubular component of the nephron.

capsule shares cells with the glomerulus; on the other Bowman's space opens into the PT.

c. PT is composed of columnar epithelial cells with many mitochondria, which provide energy (adenosine triphosphate [ATP]) for active transport of solutes. Hundreds of microvilli (called brush borders) increase the surface area of the PT lumen about 20 times.

d. PT straightens and narrows to become the descending limb of the loop of Henle, which is composed of squamous epithelial cells with few organelles (e.g., mitochondria) and few microvilli. Because the walls of the descending segment are very thin, it is called the thin segment or concentrating segment of the loop of Henle.

e. The loop of Henle makes a sharp U turn and ascends through the cortex parallel with the descending limb. The early segment of the ascending limb is thin and is called the passive diluting segment. About halfway up the ascending limb, the diameter of the limb increases and the cells change to cuboidal epithelial, with more mitochondria and

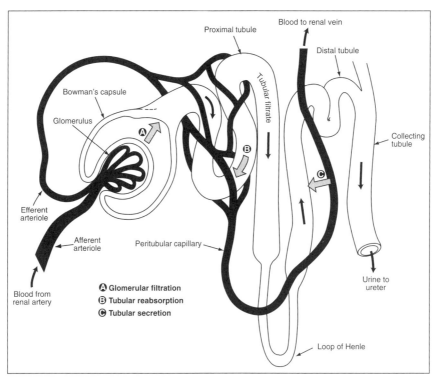

Figure 1.7. Summary of nephron structure and function. The plasma portion of blood flowing into the glomerular capillaries is filtered into Bowman's capsule (A). As the filtrate flows through the lumen of the tubule, some substances are reabsorbed from the filtrate into the peritubular capillaries (B), and other substances are secreted from the peritubular capillaries into the lumen of the tubule (C).

microvilli. This is called the thick ascending segment or active diluting segment of the loop of Henle.
(1) Cortical nephrons (80–85%) have short loops of Henle confined to the cortex and outer portion of the medulla.
(2) Juxtamedullary nephrons (15–20%) have long loops of Henle that descend deeply into the inner medulla before making a sharp U turn and ascending through the medulla back up to the cortex.
f. The loop of Henle empties into the DT. Several DTs join to form the cortical collecting tubule, which descends downward through the cortex into the medulla where it is then called first the outer and then the inner medullary collecting duct. The cortical collecting tubule and medullary collecting duct run parallel to the descending and ascending limbs of the loops of Henle. The early part of the DT functions almost identically to the thick ascending limb of the loop of Henle, and the late part of the DT

functions almost identically to the cortical collecting tubule.
g. Several collecting ducts join and open into the papilla of the pyramid (duct of Bellini) and then into a minor calyx of the ureter.

B. Interstitium.
1. Nephrons are separated by interstitial cells. More are located in the medulla than in the cortex.
2. Function of these cells is not well delineated. They probably are phagocytic and secrete hormones or hormone precursors.

C. Juxtaglomerular complex or apparatus (JGA).
1. Located at the junction where the DT of the nephron loops and passes through the angle between the afferent and efferent arterioles, and comes in contact with afferent and efferent arterioles of its own nephron unit (Figure 1.6).
2. Composed of:
a. Macula densa cells in wall of DT.
b. Juxtaglomerular cells in walls of afferent arteriole.

3. Functions are discussed in relation to tubuloglomerular feedback later in this chapter.

IV. Ureters.

A. Pair of retroperitoneal, mucosa-lined, fibromuscular tubes.

B. Transport urine from the renal pelvis to the urinary bladder.

C. Size: 30–33 cm long, 2–8 mm diameter, with narrowest diameter at the ureteropelvic junction and ureterovesical junction (bladder).

D. Oblique entrance into the bladder creates a mucosal fold. Pressure in the bladder creates a sphincter-like effect that prevents backflow of urine from the bladder into the ureters and renal pelvis.

V. Urinary bladder.

A. Pouch is composed of thick smooth muscle and is lined with epithelial cells.

B. Located in the pelvis anterior and inferior to the peritoneal cavity and posterior to the pubic bones.

C. Adult capacity: 300–500 mL.

D. Ureteral orifices enter and urethral orifice exits the bladder. These three orifices form a triangular area called the trigone.

VI. Urethra.

A. Tube that conveys urine from the bladder to the urinary meatus for excretion.

B. Internal urinary sphincter, formed by bladder smooth muscle, is located at junction of the urethra with the bladder.

C. External urinary sphincter is formed by skeletal muscle surrounding the urethra as the urethra passes through the pelvic floor.

D. Sphincters control movement of urine through urethra.

E. Male urethra is about 20 cm long. Much of it is external to the body. Meatus opens at the end of the penis.

F. Female urethra is about 3–5 cm long. It lies within the body. Meatus opens superior to the vaginal orifice.

Embryonic and Fetal Development

I. **Kidneys, adrenal glands, and gonads develop from mesodermal tissue.** Three successive types of kidneys that develop in the embryo: pronephros, mesonephros, and metanephros.

II. **Conception to 8 weeks.**

A. Pronephros develops during the 4th week, arises from urogenital ridge, then degenerates.

B. Mesonephros develops at the end of the 4th week, gives rise to ureteral bud, and then degenerates. The mesonephros functions through 8th week of development.

C. Ureteral bud gives rise to metanephros and metanephric blastema from which the kidney develops during the 5th week. Metanephros becomes functional at the end of the 8th week (beginning of fetal period). The paired metanephros form urine during fetal development; the urine is expelled through the urinary system into amniotic fluid.

III. **5th to 14th or 15th weeks.**

A. Ureter begins to form from a portion of ureteral bud.

B. Anterior bud dilates and gives rise to the renal pelvis, which grows and differentiates into calyces and collecting ducts.

C. Metanephric blastema differentiate into nephrons.

D. DT joins the end of the collecting ducts. Subsequently the loop of Henle, PT, Bowman's capsule, and glomerular capillaries form.

E. Kidneys originate in lower pelvic region. During first growth period, they rotate 90° medially and start ascent for adult position.

IV. **14th or 15th to 20th or 22nd weeks.**

A. Collecting system matures.

B. New nephrons develop.

V. **20th or 22nd to 32nd or 36th weeks.**

A. Collecting ducts grow toward renal capsules and gather nephrons.

B. Cortical nephrons originate.

VI. 32nd or 36th weeks kidneys are fully developed.

A. Nephrons lengthen and become tortuous.

B. Glomeruli enlarge.

C. Kidney surface becomes smooth during neonatal period.

D. Kidneys reach maturity by second year of life.

Physiology of the Kidney

I. Primary purposes of the kidney.

A. Regulate body fluid volume and osmolality.

B. Regulate electrolyte balance of body fluids.

C. Regulate acid-base balance of body fluids, in conjunction with body buffer systems and respiratory system.

D. Remove metabolic wastes from the body fluids, such as urea, creatinine, uric acid, beta-2 microglobulin, and many others.

E. Regulate blood pressure.

F. Regulate bone marrow production of red blood cells.

G. Synthesize vitamin D to its physiologic active form.

H. Perform gluconeogenesis (about 50% fasting state).

I. Synthesize hormones, such as prostaglandins, endothelin, and nitric oxide.

J. Excrete drugs and toxins from the body fluids.

II. Basic concepts (see Table 1.1 for summary).

A. Nephron regulation of blood and body fluid composition.
  1. The plasma portion of blood is filtered as it flows through the glomerulus. The filtrate enters Bowman's space and the lumen of the tubule.
  2. As the filtrate moves along and through the tubule, some substances, such as amino acids and glucose, are completely reabsorbed. Other substances, such as urea, creatinine, and excess water and electrolytes, are either not reabsorbed or only partially reabsorbed depending on the body's need for the substance.
  3. Other substances may be secreted into the tubule as the filtrate moves through the tubule.
  4. Substances that are not reabsorbed into the blood and those that are secreted into the tubule are then excreted in the urine.
  5. Thus substances in the glomerular filtrate needed by the body are returned to the blood whereas substances not needed are not returned and are lost in the urine.

B. Tubular reabsorption (see Figure 1.7).
  1. Water and solutes move from tubular lumen into the plasma of peritubular capillaries.
  2. 98–99% of glomerular filtrate is normally reabsorbed from the tubule.
  3. Tubular reabsorption involves both passive and active transport mechanisms.
    a. Passive transport requires no energy as it is based on concentration gradients. Urea, water, chloride, and some bicarbonate and phosphates are passively reabsorbed.
    b. Active transport requires energy (ATP) to move substances against an electrochemical gradient. Sodium, potassium, glucose, calcium, phosphate, and amino acids are actively reabsorbed.
  4. Most reabsorption (about 65%) occurs in the PT.
  5. Variable amounts of the remaining filtrate are reabsorbed in Henle's loop, DT, cortical collecting tubule, and medullary collecting duct, depending on the body's need to excrete or retain specific substances.

C. Tubular secretion (see Figure 1.7).
  1. Substance moves from peritubular capillary plasma into the tubular lumen.
  2. Substances secreted into the tubule include potassium, hydrogen, ammonia, uric acid, exogenous substances (e.g., drugs), and other wastes.

D. Tubular transport maximum (Tm).
  1. Definition: the point at which the tubular membrane transport proteins for a specific substance become saturated with it and cannot accept more.
  2. Renal tubules have a different Tm for different substances.
  3. Once the Tm is reached, a substance normally reabsorbed by a particular membrane transport protein is excreted in the urine, and a substance normally secreted by a particular membrane transport protein remains in the plasma. The most common example of a membrane transport protein that can become saturated and exceed its Tm is the one specific for glucose reabsorption (discussed later in this chapter).

Table 1.1

Summary of Physiologic Concepts Related to Renal Regulation of Water and Electrolyte Balance

GLOMERULAR FILTRATION RATE (GFR): volume of plasma filtered from the glomerular capillaries into Bowman's capsule each minute, expressed in mL/min. Average GFR for a young adult in 100–125 mL/min.

DIFFUSION: passive (does not require ATP) movement of particles from an area of higher to an area of lesser concentration of particles; diffusion ceases when equilibrium is reached.

ACTIVE TRANSPORT: movement of substances against an electrochemical or pressure gradient; requires energy from ATP.

OSMOSIS: movement of water across a semipermeable membrane from an area of lower concentration of solutes to an area of higher concentration of solutes. Osmosis ceases when concentration (osmolality) on the two sides of the semipermeable membrane equilibrates.

COLLOIDAL OSMOTIC (ONCOTIC) PRESSURE: the osmotic pressure related to proteins, especially albumin.

HYDROSTATIC PRESSURE: the pressure exerted by a fluid in a closed system.

OSMOLE (Osm): unit of osmotic pressure created by one mole of atoms or molecules in solution. Milliosmole (mOsm): one-thousandth of an osmole.

OSMOLALITY: concentration of a solution in terms of osmoles or milliosmoles per kilogram of water (osm/kg H_2O or mOsm/kg H_2O). In a solution, the fewer the number of particles in proportion to the volume of water, the less concentrated, or the lower the osmolality, of the solution.

OSMOLARITY: the concentration of solution in terms of osmoles or milliosmoles per liter of water (osm/L H_2O or mOsm/L H_2O).

HYPOSMOTIC: decreased osmolarity or osmolality of a solution.

HYPEROSMOTIC: increased osmolarity or osmolality of a solution.

ISO-OSMOTIC: solution with an osmolarity or osmolality equal to that with which it is compared.

TUBULAR REABSORPTION: process by which substances move from the tubular filtrate into the plasma of peritubular capillaries.

TUBULAR SECRETION: process by which substances move from the plasma of peritubular capillaries into the tubular filtrate.

TRANSPORT MAXIMUM (Tm): the point at which the tubular membrane transport proteins for a specific substance become saturated and cannot accept more. Reabsorption of a substance that has a Tm (e.g., glucose and amino acids) ceases when its Tm is exceeded, and the excess substance is excreted in the urine.

CLEARANCE (Cl): volume of plasma that is cleared of a specific solute by the kidneys per unit of time, expressed in mL/min. Renal clearance of a specific substance depends on several factors, including:

- if a substance is filtered at the glomerulus and is not reabsorbed or secreted in the tubule, then clearance of that substance equals the amount filtered.

- if a substance is filtered at the glomerulus and partially or completely reabsorbed from the tubule, then clearance of that substance equals the amount filtered minus the total amount reabsorbed.

- if a substance is filtered at the glomerulus and secreted into the tubule, then clearance of that substance equals the amount filtered plus the total amount secreted.

- if a substance is filtered at the glomerulus and both reabsorbed and secreted in the tubule, then clearance of that substance equals the amount filtered minus the total amount reabsorbed plus the total amount secreted. The amount cleared may be less than, equal to, or greater than the amount filtered, depending on the rates of filtration, reabsorption, and secretion.

E. Clearance (see Table 1.1).
   1. Definition: volume of plasma cleared of a specific solute by the kidneys per unit of time.
   2. Renal clearance depends on filtration of the substance by the glomerulus, reabsorption from the tubule, secretion into the tubule.

III. Glomerular filtration and its regulation.

A. Glomerular filtration begins as blood enters the glomerulus from the afferent arteriole under high pressure, called glomerular hydrostatic pressure (estimated about 60 mm Hg) (see Figures 1.7 and

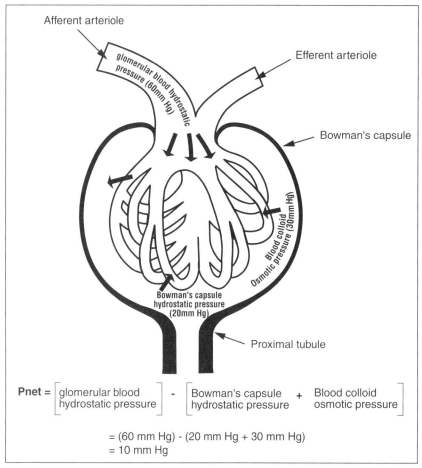

Pnet = $\left[\begin{array}{c}\text{glomerular blood}\\\text{hydrostatic pressure}\end{array}\right]$ - $\left[\begin{array}{c}\text{Bowman's capsule}\\\text{hydrostatic pressure}\end{array}\right.$ + $\left.\begin{array}{c}\text{Blood colloid}\\\text{osmotic pressure}\end{array}\right]$

= (60 mm Hg) - (20 mm Hg + 30 mm Hg)
= 10 mm Hg

Figure 1.8. Pressures involved in determining net filtration pressure.

1.8). *Note*: These pressures have never been measured in the human kidney. They have been measured in dogs and have been extrapolated to estimated human kidney pressures.

1. Hydrostatic pressure in glomerular capillary is opposed by glomerular capillary colloid osmotic pressure (also called oncotic pressure; it is caused by plasma proteins, especially albumin, which do not filter from the capillary into the tubule). This pressure is estimated as 30 mm Hg.

2. Hydrostatic pressure in glomerular capillary is also opposed by Bowman's capsule hydrostatic pressure, estimated as 20 mm Hg.

3. The colloid osmotic pressure in Bowman's capsule is normally 0 mm Hg because plasma proteins do not filter from the glomerular blood into Bowman's capsule. If plasma protein (e.g., albumin) does filter into Bowman's capsule, it creates a colloid osmotic pressure, which would enhance glomerular filtration because it would pull water from the glomerular capillaries into

Bowman's capsule. This occurs in disease states such as nephrotic syndrome.

4. Pressures that favor and oppose result in a net or effective filtration pressure of approximately 10 mm Hg (Figure 1.8). The following calculation illustrates the filtration pressure variables:

Glomerular capillary hydrostatic pressure **+60 mm Hg**
Pressures opposing glomerular hydrostatic pressure:
  Glomerular capillary colloid osmotic
    pressure   (30 mm Hg)
  Bowman's capsule hydrostatic
    pressure   (20 mm Hg)
  Total opposing pressures   **–50 mm Hg**
  Net or effective filtration pressure   **+10 mm Hg**

5. Effective glomerular filtration pressure forces fluid and some solutes of small molecular size through pores in the glomerular capillaries into Bowman's capsule.

6. Glomerular filtrate (also called tubular filtrate or simply filtrate) is similar to plasma except it lacks

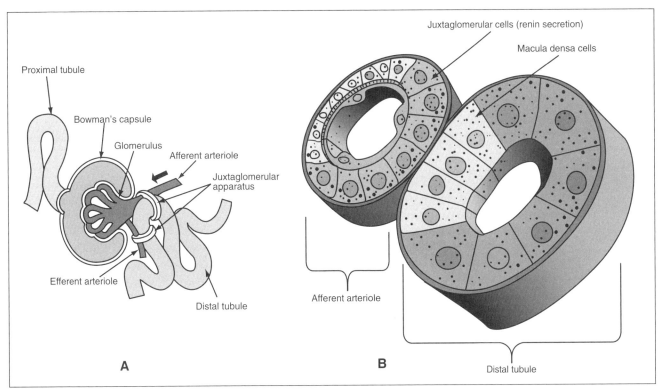

Figure 1.9. Juxtaglomerular apparatus (JGA).
A – arrangement of distal convoluted tubule and afferent and efferent arterioles and location of JGA.
B – cross section showing cells that compose the JGA.

proteins (or only in minute quantities) and blood cells. Proteins have a strong negative electrical charge which is repelled by the negative charge on the pores of the glomerular membranes. Red and white blood cells are too large to pass through the glomerular capillary pores.

7. Glomerular filtration rate (GFR), normally about 125 mL/min in young healthy adults, depends on three factors:
   a. Permeability and surface area of the glomerular capillary walls.
   b. Mean arterial blood pressure.
   c. Net filtration pressure.

B. Autoregulation of renal blood flow, glomerular blood flow, and glomerular filtration rate.
1. GFR normally remains constant despite wide variations in mean arterial blood pressure (MAP). For example, a change in MAP from about 70 mm Hg to 160 mm Hg has little effect on GFR. This ability of the kidneys to maintain a constant GFR is called autoregulation.
2. Mechanisms responsible for autoregulation.
   a. The process for autoregulation of glomerular blood flow is related to myogenic reflex of afferent arterioles and tubuloglomerular feedback.
   b. Myogenic reflex of afferent arterioles relates to baroreceptors in the walls of the arterioles. When the MAP increases, the baroreceptors sense the increased vessel stretch and cause afferent arteriole constriction. This constriction prevents major change in the glomerular capillary hydrostatic pressure. The opposite occurs when the MAP decreases; the afferent arteriole dilates and glomerular blood flow increases to preserve glomerular capillary hydrostatic pressure.
3. The two mechanisms involved in tubuloglomerular feedback are afferent arteriole vasodilator feedback and efferent arteriole vasoconstrictor feedback. The JGA controls most of the feedback mechanisms.
   a. The JGA consists of specialized cells located at the point at which the DT of each nephron loops and comes into contact with the angle of the afferent and efferent arterioles of that nephron (see Figure 1.9). The cells of the distal tubule located at this junction are called the macula densa, which respond to

changes in sodium and chloride concentration. The cells of the afferent arterioles at this point are called juxtaglomerular cells and secrete renin.

b. A decrease in glomerular filtrate decreases sodium and chloride concentration in the area of the macula densa. The macula densa, in turn, send a message by an unknown mechanism that causes afferent arteriole dilatation. As the afferent arteriole dilates, glomerular blood flow and capillary hydrostatic pressure increase, thus maintaining the glomerular capillary pressure and GFR. The opposite occurs if the GFR increases and there is an increased concentration of sodium and chloride at the macula densa. The macula densa stops (or does not) sending a message to dilate the afferent arteriole, resulting in a relative vasoconstriction.

c. The decrease in sodium and chloride at the macula densa also causes renin release from the juxtaglomerular cells.
   (1) Renin secretion by these cells also occurs in response to decreased blood flow and pressure in the afferent arteriole and in response to sympathetic nervous system (SNS) stimulation. SNS stimulation results in secretion of epinephrine and norepinephrine which excite alpha adrenergic receptors to constrict renal arterioles. Renin is secreted in response to decreased afferent arteriole pressure.
   (2) Epinephrine and norepinephrine also excite Beta-1 adrenergic receptors in the juxtaglomerular cells, which then secrete renin.

d. Through a series of several physiologic processes, renin is converted to angiotensin II, which causes efferent arteriole constriction (among other things). Efferent arteriole constriction impedes the flow of blood from the glomerular capillaries and helps maintain glomerular hydrostatic pressure and a normal GFR.

e. If the level of circulating angiotensin II is extremely high (as in hemodynamic instability), it also causes afferent arteriole constriction. The arteriole constriction would then decrease glomerular blood flow, hydrostatic pressure, and GFR and be detrimental to kidney function and can cause serious damage.

4. Regulation of renal blood flow is secondary to the regulation of glomerular blood flow. As blood flow to the glomerular capillaries increases or decreases, blood flow through the arteries and arterioles leading up to the glomerulus increases or decreases accordingly.

5. Other factors.
   a. Eicosanoid synthesis.
      (1) Eicosanoids are vasoactive substances and include prostaglandins, thromboxanes, and leukotrienes.
      (2) Produced in almost every body cell by the action of the enzyme phospholipase A2 on fatty acids from the phospholipid cell membrane (see Figure 1.10).
      (3) Arachidonic acid, which is synthesized from the fatty acids in the cell membrane, is acted on by one of two enzymes: cyclooxygenase or lipoxygenase. Prostaglandins and thromboxanes are synthesized in the cyclooxygenase pathway, and leukotrienes are synthesized in the lipoxygenase pathway.
      (4) In the kidney, eicosanoids are produced by the glomerular endothelium, nephrons, and interstitium.
      (5) Thromboxane and leukotrienes are vasoconstrictors. Their role in the kidney is unclear.
      (6) Some prostaglandins, such as PGE1, PGE2, and PGI2 (prostacyclin) are vasodilators. These substances are released in response to and counteract the effects of vasoconstrictors, such as norepinephrine, epinephrine, and angiotensin II. Prostaglandins are important in maintaining renal blood flow but have minimal systemic effect.
   b. Vasoactive peptides.
      (1) Vasoactive peptides endothelin, nitric oxide, and atrial natriuretic peptide (ANP).
      (2) Endothelin is synthesized in endothelial cells of kidneys, lungs, cerebellum, and some arteries in response to increased stretch of vessel walls, and is a potent vasoconstrictor. In the kidney, endothelin probably constricts both the afferent and efferent arterioles.
      (3) Nitric oxide is released from vascular smooth muscle in response to vaso-dilators, and is probably the mediator of the vasodilatation caused by these substances. In addition, nitric oxide may inhibit renin secretion.

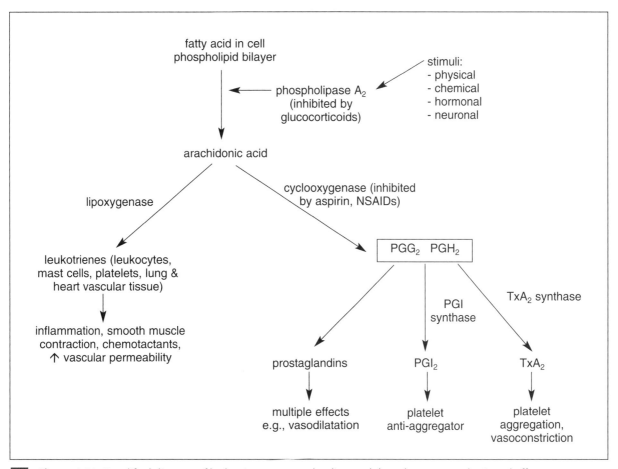

Figure 1.10. Simplified diagram of leukotrienes, prostaglandins, and thromboxanes synthesis and effects.

(4) ANP is secreted by cardiocytes in the atria and large veins in response to atrial distention and increased atrial pressure (as in increased volume states). ANP causes dilatation of the afferent arteriole and constriction of the efferent arteriole, thus enhancing GFR. ANP blocks ADH, angiotensin II, and aldosterone. The overall effects are diuresis (increases sodium and water excretion), natriuresis (decreases sodium reabsorption by the collecting ducts), decreased extracellular volume, vasorelaxation, and decreased blood pressure (see Figure 1.11).

6. In summary, by the process of autoregulation, renal blood flow, glomerular blood flow, and GFR are maintained within a narrow range despite wide fluctuations in MAP. However, once the MAP falls and is sustained below 70–80 mm Hg, the renal autoregulatory processes are no longer able to maintain adequate renal blood flow and GFR. As a result,

in states of prolonged hypotension and renal hypoperfusion, drastic changes occur in kidney function.

IV. Formation of urine (see Table 1.2 for summary).

A. Proximal tubule.
  1. Large amounts of the filtrate is reabsorbed through active and passive processes. About 65% of the glomerular filtrate is reabsorbed from the PT. Factors that favor reabsorption:
    a. The cells of the PT are large cuboidal epithelial cells with numerous mitochondria, which produce ATP to be used as the energy source for active transport.
    b. The luminal border (the cell membrane that faces the tubular lumen) consists of a very extensive brush border that increases the surface area of the luminal membrane about 20 times. The brush border membrane contains numerous protein transport molecules that enhance transport of solutes across the membrane.

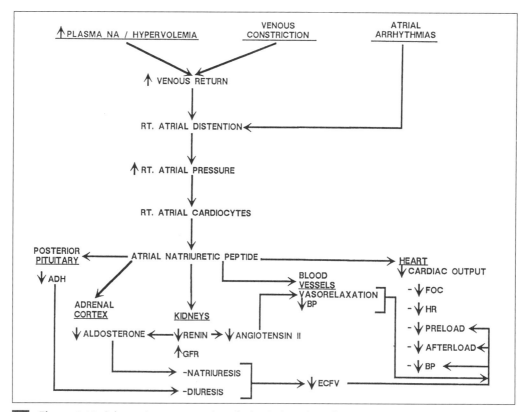

Figure 1.11. Schematic representation of stimulation of atrial natriuretic peptide (ANP) secretion and its physiologic effects. (GFR = glomerular filtration; ECFV = extracellular fluid volume; FOC = force of cardiac contraction; HR = heart rate; BP = blood pressure; ADH = antidiuretic hormone).

Source: Lancaster, L.E. (1991). Atrial natruretic peptide: Implications for nephrology nursing. *Dialysis and Transplantation, 20*(1), 17-19. Used with permission.

c. The basal border (the cell membrane facing the interstitium between the tubule and peritubular capillary) has an active sodium-potassium pump (requires ATP for operation).
   (1) For every three sodium ions that the sodium-potassium pump transports from the interior of the cell, two potassium ions are pumped into the interior of the cell.
   (2) Because more sodium ions are pumped out of the cell than potassium ions are pumped into the cell, an electrochemical gradient is created between the interior of the cell and the filtrate in the lumen of the tubule.
d. The pressure in the peritubular capillaries throughout the course of the nephron is less than the pressure inside the tubular lumen, which favors reabsorption of substances back into the capillaries.

2. Sodium regulation in PT (see Figure 1.12).
   a. Because of the active sodium-potassium pump on the basal membrane of tubular cells, the concentration of sodium inside the cells becomes less than the concentration of sodium in the tubular lumen. The sodium transport proteins on the luminal membrane of PT cells bind with sodium ions and then release them inside the cell, which provides for rapid reabsorption of sodium.
   b. After sodium moves to the interior of the cell, it is pumped across the basal membrane into the interstitium and then absorbed into the peritubular capillaries.
   c. 65% of the filtered sodium is reabsorbed from the PT.
3. Amino acid reabsorption in PT (see Figure 1.13).
   a. Amino acids are reabsorbed by cotransport with sodium ions.
      (1) On the luminal membrane, both a sodium ion and an amino acid bind with

---

Table 1.2

Summary of Major Functions of Nephron Components in Water and Electrolyte Regulation

GLOMERULUS
- filtration of plasma-like substance (filtrate) into Bowman's capsule.
- RBCs, WBCs, and plasma proteins normally not filtered.

PROXIMAL TUBULE (PT)
- 65% of sodium actively reabsorbed.
- obligatory passive reabsorption of water with sodium.
- 65% of potassium reabsorbed by cotransport with sodium.
- 25% magnesium actively reabsorbed.
- 65% calcium passively reabsorbed. Increases or decreases as water and sodium reabsorption change.
- most phosphate reabsorbed.
- acid-base balance begins: hydrogen ions secreted; bicarbonate reabsorbed; ammonia synthesized; hydrogen ions buffered with phosphates in filtrate.
- chloride ions reabsorbed along with cations.
- 100% amino acids reabsorbed by cotransport with sodium.
- 100% glucose reabsorbed by cotransport with sodium if Tm not exceeded.
- proteins reabsorbed by pinocytosis.
- some urea reabsorbed.
- exogenous substances (e.g., drugs) secreted.
- volume of filtrate decreased by 65% when it leaves PT, but it is iso-osmotic because equal amounts of water and solutes are reabsorbed.

LOOP OF HENLE
- countercurrent multiplying and exchange mechanism established in long, thin loops of Henle and vasa recta of juxtamedullary nephrons.
- about 25% of sodium, 65% of magnesium, 25% of calcium, and 27% of potassium are reabsorbed; chloride reabsorbed along with cations.

descending limb
- permeable to water; somewhat permeable to sodium, chloride, and urea.
- water moves by osmosis from tubular lumen into hyperosmotic interstitium.
- sodium, chloride, and urea move into tubular lumen from interstitium.
- because water leaves and solutes enter, the osmolality of the filtrate progressively increases.

thick ascending limb
- impermeable to water and urea.
- Na^+-K^+-$2Cl^-$ actively transported into interstitium, which makes the interstitium progressively hyperosmotic from cortex to deep inner medulla.
- because solutes are transported out and water is not, the osmolality of the filtrate progressively decreases and a hyposmotic filtrate leaves the ascending limb.
- the vasa recta act as countercurrent exchangers to maintain the hyperosmotic interstitium.

DISTAL TUBULE (DT)
- early DT functions same as thick ascending limb of loop of Henle; late DT functions same as cortical collecting tubule.

LATE DT, CORTICAL COLLECTING TUBULE, AND MEDULLARY COLLECTING DUCT
- hyposmotic filtrate empties from ascending limb of loop of Henle into collecting tubule.
- sodium is reabsorbed and potassium secreted in presence of aldosterone or vice versa if aldosterone is not present.
- calcium is reabsorbed if parathyroid hormone (PTH) or 1,25-DHCC is present; calcium is not reabsorbed and is lost in urine if PTH or 1,25-DHCC is not present. Calcitonin also decreases calcium reabsorption.
- varying amounts of magnesium reabsorbed or secreted.
- acid-base regulation continues by hydrogen ion secretion, bicarbonate reabsorption, ammonia synthesis, and hydrogen buffering with phosphates in the filtrate.
- ADH determines final urine osmolality.
- if ADH is not present, collecting tubule and medullary collecting duct are impermeable to water and a dilute urine (low osmolality) is excreted.
- if ADH is present, collecting tubule and medullary collecting duct are permeable to water; water is reabsorbed into the hyperosmotic interstitium and a concentrated urine (high osmolality) is excreted.
- when filtrate leaves medullary collecting duct, it is in final form of urine excreted from the body.

---

a transport protein that is specific for transporting this combination simultaneously.

(2) The transport protein then releases both the sodium ion and the amino acid to the interior of the cell.

(3) The amino acid is then transported by facilitated diffusion across the basal membrane into the interstitium and absorbed into peritubular capillaries.

b. 100% of filtered amino acids are normally reabsorbed.

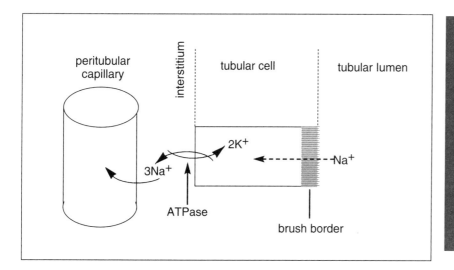

Figure 1.12. Diagram of reabsorption of sodium from the proximal tubular lumen into the plasma of peritubular capillaries. Note that the sodium-potassium pump on the basal membrane actively pumps 3 sodium ions out of the cell for every 2 potassium ions it pumps into the cell. This creates an electrochemical gradient between the filtrate in the tubular lumen and cytoplasm of the tubular cell. Thus, sodium moves into the tubular cell; it is then transported into the interstitium and reabsorbed into the plasma of peritubular capillaries.

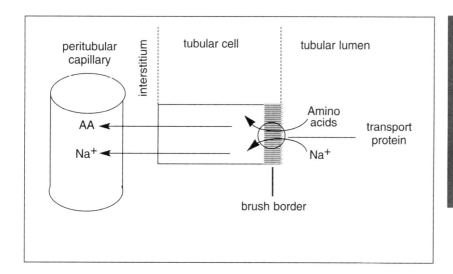

Figure 1.13. Diagram of cotransport of amino acids and sodium from the proximal tubule lumen into the plasma of peritubular capillaries. Both an amino acid and a sodium ion bind with a specific transport protein in the luminal membrane of the tubular cell. The amino acid and sodium are then released into the cytoplasm of the cell from where they are reabsorbed into the plasma of peritubular capillaries.

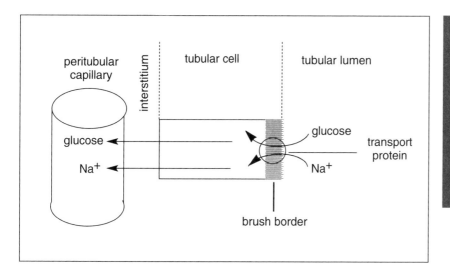

Figure 1.14. Diagram of cotransport of glucose and sodium from the proximal tubular lumen into the plasma of peritubular capillaries. Both a glucose molecule and a sodium ion bind with a specific transport protein in the luminal membrane of the tubular cell. The glucose and sodium are then released into the cytoplasm of the cell from where they are reabsorbed into the plasma of peritubular capillaries.

4. Glucose reabsorption in PT (see Figure 1.14).
   a. Glucose is reabsorbed by cotransport with sodium ions.
      (1) On the luminal membrane, both a glucose molecule and a sodium ion bind with transport proteins that are specific for transporting this combination simultaneously.
      (2) The transport proteins release the sodium ion and glucose molecule to the interior of the cell.
      (3) The glucose is then transported by facilitated diffusion across the basal membrane into the interstitium and absorbed into peritubular capillaries.
   b. 100% of filtered glucose is normally reabsorbed.
5. Tubular transport maximum for glucose and some other filtered substances.
   a. Substances that are reabsorbed by facilitated diffusion require a specific transport protein. When a transport protein becomes saturated with its specific substance, the remainder of that substance is excreted in the urine instead of being reabsorbed. The maximum rate at which a specific substance can be reabsorbed is called its transport maximum (Tm).
   b. Substances that have a Tm include glucose, amino acids, proteins, and phosphate. Sodium does not have a Tm. Its reabsorption depends on its high concentration gradient between the filtrate and the interior of tubular cells.
   c. Tm for a substance depends on the tubular load of that substance. Tubular load is the total amount of a substance that filters through the glomerulus into the tubular lumen each minute.
   d. For example, the normal blood glucose is about 100 mg/dL and the normal GFR is about 125 mL/min. Thus, the tubular load for glucose is normally about 125 mg/min. The Tm for glucose is about 320 mg/min and the threshold is about 220 mg/min. This means that as long as the tubular load of glucose is less than 220 mg/min (which corresponds with a blood glucose of about 180 mg/dL) all glucose is reabsorbed from the proximal tubule and none is excreted in the urine. At a tubular load of 220 mg/min the threshold for glucose reabsorption is exceeded and some glucose is excreted rather than being reabsorbed. At a tubular load of 320 mg/min (which corresponds with a

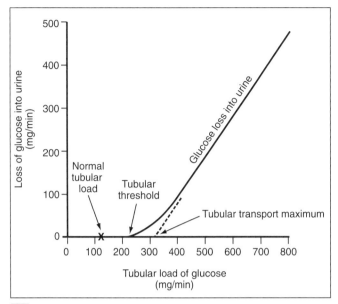

Figure 1.15. Relationship of tubular load of glucose to loss of glucose in the urine. If the tubular load of glucose is less than 220 mg/min, no glucose appears in the urine. At a tubular load of 220 mg/min (at a GFR of 125 mL/min, a tubular glucose load of 220 mg/min corresponds to a blood glucose of about 180 mg/dL) glucose begins to spill into the urine. When the tubular load exceeds 320 mg/min (blood glucose of about 260 mg/dL at a GFR of 125 mL/min) the tubular maximum for glucose reabsorption is reached and all the glucose above that amount is lost in the urine.

blood glucose of about 260 mg/dL) the Tm for glucose is exceeded and all glucose above this amount is excreted in the urine rather than being reabsorbed (see Figure 1.15).
6. Proteins are reabsorbed from the PT by pinocytosis. Once the proteins are inside the tubular cell they are broken down into their constituent amino acids, which are then reabsorbed into the interstitium and peritubular capillaries along with other amino acids. If the tubular load of proteins exceed the Tm, the excess amino acids are excreted.
7. Potassium regulation in PT. About 65% of potassium is reabsorbed from the PT by cotransport with sodium.
8. Magnesium regulation in PT. About 25% of magnesium is actively reabsorbed from the PT.
9. Calcium regulation in PT.
   a. About 65% of calcium is passively reabsorbed from the PT.
   b. Calcium reabsorption increases or decreases as water and sodium resorption increases or decreases.

10. Phosphate regulation in PT.
    a. Most phosphate is reabsorbed from the PT.
    b. If the tubular load of phosphate exceeds its Tm, the excess phosphate is excreted.
    c. Increased dietary intake of phosphate, parathyroid hormone, and the active form of vitamin D3 (1,25-dihydroxycholecalciferol [1,25-DHCC]) decrease phosphate reabsorption and vice versa.
11. Chloride ions (anions) are passively reabsorbed from the PT along with cations.
12. Metabolic end products.
    a. Small amounts of urea are reabsorbed from the PT.
    b. Filtered creatinine is secreted (about 10%) into the PT.
13. Kidney regulation of acid-base balance begins in the PT. This is discussed extensively later in this chapter.
14. Because of the osmotic gradient created by the reabsorption of solutes from the PT, about 65% of water is passively reabsorbed from the PT. This is called obligatory reabsorption of water. Because solutes and water are reabsorbed at the same rate from the PT, the osmolality of the filtrate does not change, and the filtrate that leaves the PT is iso-osmotic. The volume of the filtrate, however, has decreased by 65%.

B. Loop of Henle.
   1. The countercurrent multiplying and exchange mechanism is established between the long, thin loops of Henle and vasa recta of juxtamedullary nephrons. This mechanism is part of the process involved in regulating body water and is discussed in detail later in this chapter and diagrammed in Figure 1.16.
   2. About 25% of sodium, 65% of magnesium, 25% of calcium, and 27% of potassium are reabsorbed from the loop of Henle. Chloride is reabsorbed along with the cations.
   3. Descending limb of the loop of Henle.
      a. The epithelial cells of the descending limb of the loop of Henle are very thin and have few mitochondria and rudimentary brush borders.
      b. The descending limb is very permeable to water and somewhat permeable to urea, sodium and other ions. This limb is called the concentrating segment of the loop because water moves out and some solutes move in.
   4. Ascending limb of the loop of Henle.
      a. The early, thin segment of the ascending limb is much less permeable to water than the thin descending limb. This segment is called the passive diluting segment of the loop.
      b. The thick segment begins approximately half way up the ascending limb. The epithelial cells become thick and have many mitochondria, but only a rudimentary brush border.
         (1) This segment is called the active diluting segment and is impermeable to water, but the cells are adapted for active transport of sodium, chloride, and potassium ions from the tubular filtrate into the interstitium.
         (2) Solutes are reabsorbed in excess of water so hyposmotic filtrate leaves the ascending limb and empties into the DT. At this point the filtrate does have a high concentration of urea (see discussion of regulation of body water later in this chapter).

C. Distal tubule.
   1. The early part of the DT functions almost the same as the thick ascending segment of the loop of Henle.
   2. The late DT functions almost the same as the cortical collecting tubule.

D. Late DT and cortical collecting tubule.
   1. The late DT and cortical collecting tubule, formed by several DTs joining, is impermeable to urea.
   2. Sodium is reabsorbed from and potassium is secreted into the tubular lumen (or vice versa) depending on the level of potassium in the plasma and body fluids and the presence of aldosterone.
      a. When plasma potassium is greater than about 4.0 mEq/L, potassium diffuses from the interstitium into the tubular cell and increases the intracellular potassium.
      b. This creates a concentration gradient between the cell and the filtrate in the tubular lumen.
      c. As a result, potassium diffuses from the cell into the tubular lumen and is excreted in the urine.
      d. Aldosterone is secreted by the zona glomerulosa cells (outer layer) of the adrenal cortex. Stimuli for aldosterone secretion. (*Note*: The first two are particularly strong stimulants.)
         (1) Elevated potassium in plasma and interstitial fluids.
         (2) Angiotensin II.

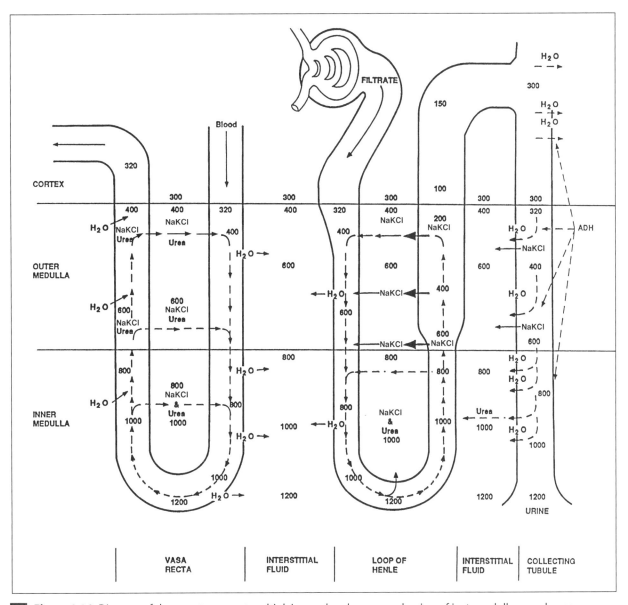

Figure 1.16. Diagram of the countercurrent multiplying and exchange mechanism of juxtamedullary nephrons.

(3) Decreased sodium in plasma and interstitial fluids.

(4) Adrenocorticotrophic hormone (ACTH).

e. Aldosterone attaches to receptors on the collecting tubule, which, in turn, activate transport proteins in the cell membrane that transport potassium from interstitium to tubular lumen and transport sodium from the tubular lumen to the interstitium. The potassium is excreted in the urine and the sodium is absorbed by peritubular capillaries.

f. If the plasma potassium is low or aldosterone is not present, sodium is not reabsorbed and postassium is not secreted.

g. Through the above processes, sodium and potassium levels in the body fluids are regulated within very narrow limits.

3. Calcium is reabsorbed in the late distal tubule if parathyroid hormone or 1,25-DHCC is present. Calcium is not reabsorbed (thus it is excreted in the urine) if parathyroid hormone or 1,25-DHCC is not present. Calcitonin also decreases calcium reabsorption.

4. The late DT and the cortical collecting duct are

permeable to water if antidiuretic hormone (ADH) is present. This is discussed in the following section of this chapter in relation to regulation of body water.
5. Regulation of acid-base balance continues in the late DT and cortical collecting duct (discussed later in this chapter).

E. Medullary collecting duct.
1. The medullary collecting duct is permeable to water and urea if ADH is present (see following discussion of regulation of body water).
2. The medullary collecting duct can secrete hydrogen ions into the tubular lumen, an important part of the kidney's regulation of acid-base balance.

Regulation of Body Water: Formation of a Dilute or a Concentrated Urine

I. Introduction.

A. Overview.
1. Of the 125 mL/min (180 L in 24 hours) filtered from the glomeruli into the tubules, approximately 98–99% of the filtrate is reabsorbed from the tubular lumen of the nephrons into the plasma of the peritubular capillaries and returned to the systemic circulation.
2. Thus, of the 180 L of glomerular filtrate each 24 hours, only about 1.5 to 2 L is excreted as urine. A smaller amount of concentrated urine is excreted in states of water deficit (increased extracellular osmolality) and a larger amount of more dilute urine is excreted in states of water excess (decreased extracellular osmolality).
3. Excretion of a dilute or concentrated urine facilitates return of the body's water volume and extracellular osmolality to normal.
4. The kidney's processes for regulating body water and extracellular osmolality primarily involve the descending and ascending limbs of the loop of Henle, DT, cortical collecting tubule, medullary collecting duct, and vasa recta of juxtamedullary nephrons.
5. Osmoreceptors in the hypothalamus and antidiuretic hormone (ADH), which is released from the posterior pituitary gland, operate along with the nephrons to regulate body water.

B. Changes in osmolality.
1. The glomerular filtrate is basically the same as plasma and has an osmolality about the same as plasma (290–300 mOsm/L) as it enters Bowman's capsule.
2. In the PT, about 65% of the glomerular filtrate is reabsorbed into peritubular capillaries (described earlier).
3. Due to reabsorption of proportional amounts of solutes and water in the PT, the filtrate leaving the PT and entering the descending limb of the loop of Henle remains at an osmolality of 290–300 mOsm/L.
4. In conditions of water deficit, the tubular filtrate can be maximally concentrated to about 1200 mOsm/L before the filtrate leaves the collecting duct as urine. Conversely, in states of water excess, the concentration of the tubular filtrate can be diluted to as low as 50 mOsm/L before it leaves the collecting duct as urine.

C. Regardless of whether a concentrated or a dilute urine is finally excreted, a hyperosmotic medullary interstitium is created by a complex process involving the countercurrent multiplying and exchange mechanism of the juxtamedullary nephrons and vasa recta.

II. Countercurrent multiplying and exchange mechanism.

A. The slow flow of blood in the vasa recta, slow flow of filtrate in the lumen of juxtamedullary nephrons, and the parallel arrangement of vasa recta, loops of Henle, cortical collecting tubule, and medullary collecting duct are essential for the formation of both a concentrated and a dilute urine. This arrangement allows for exchange of solutes and water between the lumen of the tubule, the renal interstitial fluid, and plasma of the vasa recta.

B. As Figure 1.16 shows, the osmolality of the renal interstitial fluid progressively increases from about 300 mOsm/L in the cortical-medullary junction to about 1200 mOsm/L in the deep inner medulla. Creation of this hyperosmotic interstitium is a prerequisite to the nephron's forming either a dilute or a concentrated urine.

C. Principal mechanisms responsible for creating the hyperosmolality of the medullary interstitium.
1. Tubular processes: the countercurrent multiplier.

a. The descending limb (concentrating segment) of the loop of Henle is permeable to water and somewhat permeable to solutes. Thus, as the filtrate flows down the descending limb water moves from the lumen into the interstitium and some sodium, chloride, and urea move from the interstitium into the lumen of the tubule. The water is removed from the interstitium by the capillary network so it does not dilute the interstitium. The result is a progressively concentrated (increase in osmolality) tubular filtrate as it moves down the descending limb into the medullary interstitium.

b. The thin ascending segment (passive diluting segment) of the loop of Henle is impermeable to water, but is permeable to solutes. Sodium and chloride move into the interstitium, and urea moves into the lumen of the tubule. The net movement of sodium and chloride out of the lumen exceeds the net movement of urea into the tubular lumen. As a result, the filtrate becomes progressively dilute (decreased osmolality) as it moves up the ascending limb. Because only passive transport is involved, the osmolality of the tubular fluid can decrease only to the osmolality of the surrounding interstitium, or about 800 mOsm/L, in this segment.

c. The thick ascending segment (active diluting segment) of the loop of Henle is impermeable to water, but actively transports sodium, potassium, and chloride ions from the lumen of the tubule into the interstitium. As a result, sodium, potassium, and chloride become concentrated in the interstitium, and the osmolality of the interstitium increases. Because solutes are actively pumped from the thick segment and because it is impermeable to water, the osmolality of the tubular filtrate progressively decreases (is more dilute) and is less than 100 mOsm/L by the time it reaches the late DT.

d. Small amounts of sodium ions are also actively transported from the collecting duct into the interstitium. This further increases the osmolality of the interstitium.

e. In the presence of high concentrations of ADH, urea diffuses from the medullary collecting duct into the interstitium. This also increases the osmolality of the interstitium.

f. The constant transport of sodium, potassium, and chloride from the thick ascending limb and continuous inflow of new sodium and chloride from the proximal tubule constitute the countercurrent multiplier mechanism.

g. The above mechanisms create an osmolality of about 1200 mOsm/L both at the sharp U turn of the loop of Henle and in the deep medullary interstitium.

2. Vasa recta processes: the countercurrent exchanger.

a. The arrangement of the vasa recta and the slow blood flow through the vasa recta prevent the removal of the solutes from the interstitium and maintain the interstitial hyperosmolality.

b. As Figure 1.16 shows, the descending and ascending limbs of the vasa recta are arranged parallel to each other. Thus, as blood flows down the descending limb it is concurrently flowing up the ascending limb. This arrangement allows the vasa recta to operate as countercurrent exchangers.

c. As blood flows down the descending limb of the vasa recta, sodium, potassium, and chloride ions and urea diffuse from the interstitium into the blood. At the same time, water diffuses from the blood into the hyperosmotic interstitium. Thus, because of influx of solutes and outflux of water, the osmolality of the blood in the vasa recta progressively increases from about 320 mOsm/L as it enters the vasa recta to about 1200 mOsm/L at the tip of the vasa recta, which is about the same as the osmolality of the interstitium at each point.

d. As blood flows up the ascending limb of the vasa recta, sodium, potassium, and chloride ions and urea diffuse out of the blood into the interstitium, and water diffuses back into the blood. Thus, when the blood in the ascending vasa recta leaves the renal medulla, its osmolality is almost the same as that of the blood that flowed into the descending limb of the vasa recta (i.e., about 320 mOsm/L).

e. As a result, the osmolality of the medullary interstitium has been maintained because only a slight amount of solutes was removed from the interstitium by the blood flow in the vasa recta.

D. Role of the osmoreceptor-antidiuretic hormone system.

1. ADH (also called vasopressin) controls the formation and excretion of either a dilute or a concentrated urine through its effect on the

cortical collecting tubule and medullary collecting duct.

    a. ADH is formed in neurons of the hypothalamus (specifically the supraoptic and paraventricular nuclei).

    b. After synthesis, ADH is packaged into vesicles, which are transported into synaptic bulbs at the tips of the neurons. The bulbs terminate in the posterior pituitary gland.

    c. Release of the contents of the vesicles in the synaptic bulbs results in release of ADH into the interstitium surrounding the posterior pituitary gland. The hormone then diffuses into the surrounding capillaries and is transported in the systemic circulation.

2. Other neurons, called osmoreceptors, are located in the hypothalamus near the supraoptic and paraventricular nuclei. These are extremely responsive to slight changes in extracellular osmolality.

    a. The osmoreceptors are stimulated by an increase in extracellular sodium (increased osmolality) and inhibited by a decrease in extracellular sodium (decreased osmolality). Extracellular sodium concentration can increase as either the result of increased sodium or decreased water. Conversely, extracellular sodium concentration can decrease as either the result of decreased sodium or increased water.

    b. The osmoreceptors signal the supraoptic and paraventricular nuclei to increase or decrease the secretion of ADH, depending on the extracellular osmolality.

3. Osmoreceptor-ADH-renal system integration.

    a. An increase in sodium (or a decrease in water) specifically, and other ions to some extent, increases the extracellular fluid osmolality.

    b. The increased extracellular fluid osmolality stimulates osmoreceptors.

    c. The stimulated osmoreceptors, in turn, stimulate the supraoptic and paraventricular nuclei.

    d. The supraoptic and paraventricular nuclei then cause release of ADH from the posterior pituitary gland.

    e. ADH causes increased permeability of the cortical collecting tubule and medullary collecting duct to water.

        (1) ADH binds with receptors on the basal membrane (interstitial side) of collecting tubule and duct cells.

        (2) ADH's binding with its receptors causes activation of the enzyme adenyl cyclase, which, in turn, causes the formation of cyclic adenosine monophosphate (CAMP) in the cell cytoplasm. CAMP acts as the second messenger to activate the enzyme protein kinase A.

        (3) Protein kinase A regulates the formation of water channels (called aquaporins) from the luminal membrane (the side of the tubular cell that faces the tubular lumen) to the basal membrane (the side of the membrane facing the interstitium).

        (4) Water is reabsorbed across the luminal membrane through these channels and exits the basal membrane into the interstitium from where it is reabsorbed into the vasa recta and returned to the systemic circulation. As the tubule becomes more permeable to water, urea is also reabsorbed into the interstitium, which enhances the interstitial hyperosmolality.

        (5) Although increased permeability of the tubules leads to increased reabsorption of water from the tubular lumen, most solutes are not reabsorbed and are excreted in the urine.

        (6) With reabsorption of water the extracellular osmolality is returned to normal.

        (7) Hypothalamic osmoreceptors sense the decrease toward normal in extracellular osmolality and cause decreased release of ADH.

        (8) In conditions of decreased extracellular sodium (or excess water), the osmoreceptors sense the low extracellular osmolality and cause decreased ADH release. With decreased circulating ADH, less water is reabsorbed from the renal tubules until the extracellular osmolality returns to normal.

III. Formation and excretion of urine.

A. Concentrated urine.

1. In conditions of body water deficit, a concentrated urine is excreted to correct the water deficit and extracellular hyperosmolality.

2. When the tubular filtrate enters the late distal tubule and cortical collecting tubule, it is hypotonic (about 100–150 mOsm/L) because more solutes than water have been reabsorbed from the ascending limb of the loop of Henle.

3. In the presence of high levels of circulating ADH, the cortical collecting tubule and medullary collecting duct become extremely

permeable to water. Thus water moves by osmosis from the lumen of the collecting tubule and duct into the hyperosmotic interstitium; that is, the fluid in the tubular lumen equilibrates with the fluid in the interstitium.

4. The water moves from the interstitium into the adjacent capillary network and then into the systemic circulation.

5. Solutes, however, are not reabsorbed along with the water.

6. The final outcome is concentration of the final urine to an osmolality as high as 1200 mOsm/L, which is comparable to the osmolality of the deep medullary interstitium.

7. Following reabsorption of water from the tubular lumen into plasma, the osmolality of the extracellular fluid returns to the normal level of about 290–300 mOsm/L.

B. Dilute urine.

1. In conditions of excess body water, a dilute urine is excreted to correct the water excess and extracellular hypo-osmolality.

2. Osmoreceptors in the hypothalamus detect the low extracellular osmolality and the release of ADH from the posterior hypothalamus decreases.

3. With decreased circulating ADH, the cortical collecting tubule and medullary collecting duct become relatively impermeable to water.

4. As a result, water cannot be reabsorbed from the tubular lumen into the interstitium and capillary network.

5. Without reabsorption of water, the osmolality of the tubular filtrate remains at or somewhat below the level it was when it entered the cortical collecting tubule from the ascending limb of the loop of Henle, that is, about 100–150 mOsm/L or less with maximal reabsorption of solutes.

6. A dilute urine is excreted until water excess is corrected and the extracellular osmolality returns to normal.

Regulation of Acid-Base Balance

I. Basic concepts.

A. Each day the body produces acids that must be neutralized to maintain a normal acid-base balance in the body.

1. Endogenous acid production in adults is about

1 mEq/kg/day, and about 2 or 3 times that amount in children.

2. States of high catabolism increase acid production.

3. Endogenous acids are produced in two forms by cellular metabolism: volatile acids and nonvolatile acids.

a. Metabolism of fats and carbohydrates yields 15,000 mmol of carbon dioxide (CO_2) daily. The CO_2 combines with water (H_2O) to form carbonic acid (H_2CO_3), which is a volatile acid because the CO_2 can be exhaled through the lungs.

b. A small percentage of endogenous acids is noncarbonic or nonvolatile. These acids cannot be exhaled through the lungs, e.g., sulfuric acid and phosphoric acid.

B. An acid is a molecule or ion that donates hydrogen ions (H^+) in a chemical reaction.

1. Acids that dissociate freely into H^+ and an anion are strong acids (e.g., hydrochloric acid (HCl) dissociates freely into H^+ and Cl^-).

2. Acids that dissociate minimally into H^+ and an anion are weak acids (e.g., carbonic acid (H_2CO_3) dissociates weakly into $H^+ + HCO_3$).

C. A base is a molecule or ion that combines with or accepts H^+ and removes them from solution.

1. Strong bases react powerfully with H^+; for example the hydroxide ion (OH-) reacts with H^+ to form H_2O.

2. Weak bases react weakly with H^+; for example, bicarbonate (HCO_3) reacts weakly with H^+ to form carbonic acid (H_2CO_3).

3. Proteins, such as hemoglobin and albumin, also serve as bases because some of their amino acids function as negative ions that bind with H^+. H^+ can also be released from the proteins, so they can also act as H^+ donors.

D. The hydrogen ion concentration of a solution is expressed as the pH value. Free hydrogen ions (i.e., those not bound to other ions or proteins) contribute to the hydrogen ion concentration of a solution; pH is the negative logarithm of the hydrogen concentration of a solution. The pH scale is on a continuum from 0 to 14.

1. A pH of 7 is neutral; that is, acid (H^+) and base (OH-) are equal.

2. A pH below 7 (0–6.99999) indicates a progressive increase in hydrogen ion concentration, and is acidic.

3. A pH above 7 (7.00001–14) indicates a

progressive decrease in hydrogen ion concentration, and is basic or alkaline.

E. The normal pH of arterial blood is 7.4 (range 7.35–7.45). The limits for life are about 6.9–7.8. A pH below 7.35 is called acidosis, and a pH above 7.45 is called alkalosis.
   1. An increase in HCO_3^- concentration or a decrease in CO_2 concentration causes a rise in pH (alkaline).
   2. An increase in CO_2 concentration or a decrease in HCO_3^- causes a decrease in pH (acid).
   3. To maintain an arterial blood pH of 7.4, 20 times more base than acid must be present. Although the acid or base level may change, the pH does not change as long as the 20:1 ratio of base to acid is maintained.
   4. The process by which the body maintains a normal pH by increasing acid to balance an increase in base or vice versa is called compensation. Examples of compensation:
      a. If a rise in HCO_3^- is offset by a proportional rise in CO_2, then the pH does not change.
      b. If a rise in CO_2 is offset by a proportional rise in HCO_3^-, then the pH does not change.
      c. If a decrease in HCO_3^- is offset by a proportional decrease in CO_2, then the pH does not change.
      d. If a decrease in CO_2 is offset by a proportional decrease in HCO_3^-, then the pH does not change.

F. Normal pH of body fluids is maintained by buffer systems of body fluids, the lungs, and the kidneys.
   1. Buffer systems in body fluids and cells operate within a fraction of a second to regulate pH.
   2. The respiratory system is stimulated in 1 to 12 minutes to make acute adjustments and in 1 to 2 days to make chronic adjustments.
   3. The kidneys respond within many hours to days and can continue to infinity to regulate pH.

G. Buffer systems.
   1. An acid-base buffer system is a solution that contains two or more chemicals that prevent major changes in H^+ concentration when an acid or a base is added to the solution.
   2. The bicarbonate-carbonic acid (a weak base and a weak acid) buffer system is the most important of the body buffers, although it is not the most powerful.
      a. The basis for the operation of this system relates to the following formula:

$$CO_2 + H_2O \overset{CA}{\underset{}{\rightleftarrows}} H_2CO_3 \rightleftarrows H^+ + HCO_3^-$$

      b. The reaction between CO_2 and H_2O to form H_2CO_3 is catalyzed by the enzyme carbonic anhydrase (CA), which increases the rate of the reaction about 5,000 times.
      c. H_2CO_3 dissociates into H^+ and HCO_3^-. The reaction is reversible and the breakdown of H_2CO_3 to CO_2 and H_2O is catalyzed by CA. The direction in which the reaction moves depends on the concentration of molecules on either side.
      d. CO_2 is regulated by the lungs and the HCO_3^- by the kidneys.
      e. If an acid (hydrogen ions) is added to a solution in which this buffer system is functional, the acid is buffered by the HCO_3^- ($H^+ + HCO_3^- \rightarrow H_2CO_3$). As a result, the strong acid is changed to a weak acid and the pH of the solution changes minimally. The H_2CO_3 in the presence of carbonic anhydrase breaks down into H_2O and CO_2 and the CO_2 exhaled through the lungs.
      f. If a base (hydroxide ions) is added to a solution in which this buffer is functional, the hydroxide ions combine with carbonic acid to form water and bicarbonate (OH- + $H_2CO_3 \rightarrow H_2O + HCO_3^-$). As a result, the strong base is changed to a weak base and the pH of the solution changes minimally. The HCO_3^- that is formed as an outcome is excreted by the kidneys.
      g. The pH of a solution in which the bicarbonate-carbonic acid buffer system is operational can be calculated using the Henderson-Hasselbalch Equation:

$$pH = 6.1 + \frac{\log HCO_3^-}{CO_2}$$

      To perform the calculation, the plasma concentration of HCO_3^- and dissolved CO_2 must be measured.
   3. Plasma proteins (e.g., albumin) and intracellular proteins (e.g., hemoglobin) are negatively charged and can donate or accept H^+. This provides a very plentiful, strong buffer system.
   4. Ions can diffuse across cell membranes to regulate the extracellular H^+ concentration.
      a. When the extracellular H^+ concentration is increased (acidosis), some of the H^+ diffuses to the interior of cells. To maintain electrochemical neutrality, a cation must

concomitantly diffuse out of the cell. Thus potassium ions (K^+), the most abundant intracellular cation, diffuses from inside the cell into the extracellular fluid.

b. When the extracellular H^+ concentration is decreased (alkalosis), H^+ diffuses from the interior of the cell into the extracellular fluid. To maintain electrochemical neutrality, K^+ diffuses from the extracellular fluid into the interior of the cell.

c. The relationship between pH and extracellular K^+ can be predicted by the following rule: For each change in pH of 0.1 from a normal of 7.40, the plasma K^+ changes in the opposite direction by 0.6 mEq/L from a normal of 4.0 mEq/L. (*Note*: Consider each pH change of 0.1 as 1 unit.) Examples:

(1) Arterial blood pH = 7.5 (0.1 or 1 unit higher than normal). Thus, plasma K^+ would be expected to be 4.0 mEq/L minus 0.6 mEq/L or 3.4 mEq/L.

(2) Arterial blood pH = 7.2 (0.2 or 2 units lower than normal). Thus, plasma K^+ would be expected to be 4.0 mEq/L plus 1.2 mEq/L or 5.2 mEq/L.

H. Respiratory regulation of acid-base balance.
  1. Respiratory system controls the CO_2 portion of the Henderson-Hasselbalch equation.
    a. An increase in CO_2 decreases pH toward acidity.
    b. A decrease in CO_2 increases pH toward alkalinity.
  2. When the level of CO_2 in arterial blood rises, CO_2 diffuses into cerebrospinal fluid (CSF) and combines with H_2O to form H_2CO_3, an acid, which lowers the CSF pH.
  3. Central chemoreceptors within the medulla are stimulated by the decreased pH of CSF. In addition, peripheral chemoreceptors in the carotid and aortic bodies are stimulated by the decreased pH of arterial blood. As a result, the medullary respiratory center is stimulated to increase the rate and depth of ventilation. Thus, CO_2 is exhaled through the lungs and the pH returns toward normal.
  4. The opposite of the above occurs with decreased CO_2 and increased pH of CSF and arterial blood.

I. Kidney regulation of acid-base balance.
  1. The kidneys regulate the HCO_3^- portion of the Henderson-Hasselbalch equation.

a. The kidney's mechanisms for regulating acid-base balance are HCO_3^- reabsorption and H^+ secretion, excretion of H^+ with urinary phosphates, and excretion of H^+ by synthesis of ammonia and excretion of ammonium chloride. The processes primarily occur in the PT, DT, and collecting duct.

b. An acid urine is formed if the pH of body fluids is in the acid range and the kidneys excrete more H^+ than HCO_3^-.

c. An alkaline urine is formed if the pH of body fluids is in the alkaline range and the kidneys excrete more HCO_3^- than H^+.

d. The kidneys can excrete a urine with a pH between 4.5 and 8.

  2. Reabsorption of filtered bicarbonate.
    a. Basic rule. For every H^+ secreted into the tubular lumen, a HCO_3^- and an Na^+ are reabsorbed into the plasma of peritubular capillaries.
    b. HCO_3^- cannot be reabsorbed from renal tubules directly because it is a large ion and has a negative electrical charge. Therefore HCO_3^- must be broken down and then regenerated to be reabsorbed. The following summarizes the processes involved (see Figure 1.17).
      (1) Na^+ and HCO_3^- are filtered from the glomerulus into filtrate of tubular lumen.
      (2) In PT and DT, Na^+ is reabsorbed and H^+ secreted into tubular filtrate.
      (3) H^+ reacts with HCO_3^- to form H_2CO_3.
      (4) Under influence of carbonic anhydrase (CA) that is present in the PT and DT cell membrane, H_2CO_3 breaks down into H_2O and CO_2.
      (5) H_2O is excreted in the urine and CO_2 diffuses into the cell.
      (6) In cell cytoplasm, CO_2 and H_2O in presence of carbonic anhydrase form H_2CO_3.
      (7) H_2CO_3 dissociates into H^+ and HCO_3^-.
      (8) HCO_3^- is reabsorbed into the plasma of peritubular capillaries.
      (9) H^+ is secreted into tubular lumen and Na^+ is reabsorbed from tubular lumen.
      (10) Although not the original HCO_3^- that was filtered into the tubular lumen, an equivalent amount is regenerated and reabsorbed by the above process.
      (11) The basic rule holds true: an H^+ is secreted and an HCO_3^- and Na^+ are reabsorbed.
  3. In the late DT and collecting tubule, specialized

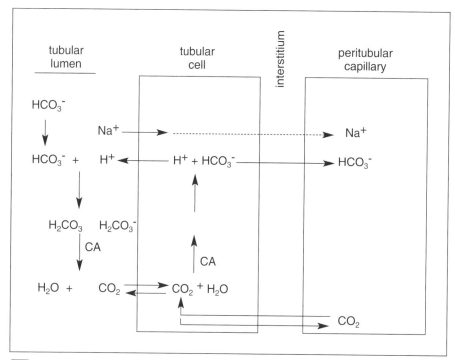

Figure 1.17. Diagram of tubular reabsorption of filtered bicarbonate.

cells, called intercalated cells, actively secrete hydrogen ions into the tubular lumen against a high concentration gradient. These cannot be transported as free H^+. Therefore, they first combine with buffers in the tubular filtrate and are excreted in the urine in this form. The two important buffers of the tubular filtrate are the phosphate buffer system and the ammonia buffer system. These processes allow for synthesis of new bicarbonate.

4. Transport of H^+ by phosphate buffers.
   a. The phosphate buffer system is composed of HPO_4^{--} (base phosphate) and $H_2PO_4^-$ (acid phosphate). HPO_4^{--} can accept H^+ and $H_2PO_4^-$ can donate H^+.
   b. Na_2PO_4 is filtered from the glomerulus into the tubular filtrate (see Figure 1.18).
   c. One of the Na^+ is reabsorbed and H^+ is secreted by countertransport.
   d. H^+ binds with HPO_4^{--} to form $H_2PO_4^-$.
   e. The other Na^+ binds with the $H_2PO_4^-$ to form NaH_2PO_4, which is excreted in the urine. (Note that this involves excretion of H^+.)
   f. In the renal cell, CO_2 binds with H_2O to form H_2CO_3, which dissociates to H^+ and HCO_3^-.
   g. The HCO_3^- is reabsorbed and H^+ is secreted into the tubular lumen.
   h. As an outcome, for each H^+ that binds with

HPO_4^{--}, a new HCO_3^- is formed and transported into the blood along with Na^+. The secretion and excretion of H^+ and the reabsorption of HCO_3^- contribute to acid-base regulation.

5. Transport of H^+ by the ammonia buffer system.
   a. Ammonia (NH_3) is synthesized in epithelial cells of almost all segments of the renal tubule. The NH_3 is synthesized primarily from the amino acid glutamine in the presence of the enzyme glutaminase, which is present in the tubular cell. The NH_3 is secreted into the tubular lumen (see Figure 1.19).
   b. In the filtrate of the tubular lumen, NH_3 binds with H^+ to form ammonium (NH_4^+), a cation.
   c. The NH_4^+ combines with Cl^- to form NH_4Cl, which is excreted in the urine. (Note that this involves excretion of H^+.)
   d. Ay the same time H^+ is secreted, Na^+ and a new HCO_3^- are reabsorbed.
   e. As an outcome, H^+ is secreted and excreted and new HCO_3^- is reabsorbed, which contributes to acid-base regulation.
   f. The synthesis of NH_3 increases in acidosis and decreases in alkalosis.

6. Summary of kidney's response to acidosis.
   a. HCO_3^- reabsorption increases.
   b. H^+ secretion increases so H^+ excretion increases.

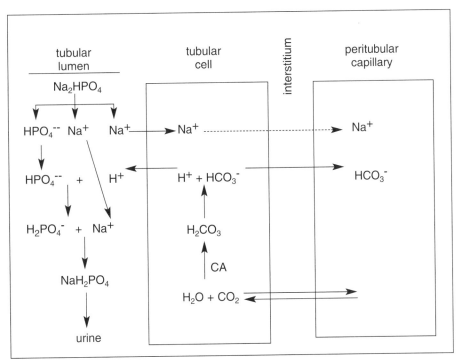

Figure 1.18. Diagram of excretion of hydrogen ions with phosphate buffers. Note that a hydrogen ion is secreted and excreted and a new bicarbonate ion is reabsorbed.

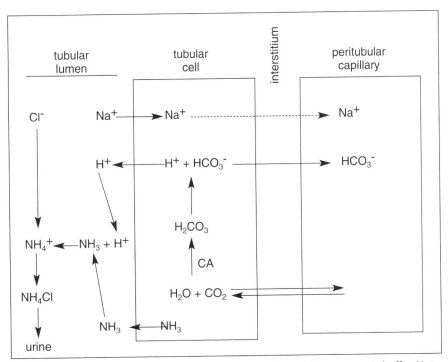

Figure 1.19. Diagram of excretion of hydrogen ions with an ammonia buffer. Note that a hydrogen ion is secreted and excreted and a new bicarbonate ion is reabsorbed.

  c. NaH_2PO_4 production increases.
  d. NH_3 synthesis and NH_4Cl excretion increase.
  e. Active secretion of H^+ by DT and collecting tubule increases.
  f. pH of urine decreases to as low as 4.5 as an acid urine is produced as excess H^+ are excreted and HCO_3^- is reabsorbed into body fluids.
 7. Summary of kidney's response to alkalosis.
  a. HCO_3^- reabsorption decreases, so HCO_3^- excretion increases.
  b. NH_3 synthesis decreases.
  c. Active secretion of H^+ by DT and collecting tubule decreases.
  d. pH of urine increases to as high as 8.0 as an alkaline urine is produced as excess HCO_3^- is excreted and H^+ is retained in the body fluids.

Other Functions of the Kidneys

I. **Vitamin D3 Synthesis to 1,25-DHCC.** See Section 2 for information in relation to bone problems and metastatic calcifications of kidney failure.

II. **Erythropoietin secretion.** See Section 2 for information regarding anemia and chronic kidney disease.

III. **Renin secretion.** See discussion earlier in this chapter regarding autoregulation of renal and glomerular blood flow. See Section 2 for discussion of hypertension and chronic kidney disease.

IV. **Eicosanoids, endothelin, and endothelium-derived relaxing factor.** See discussion earlier in this chapter regarding autoregulation of renal and glomerular blood flow.

Ureter and Bladder Function and Micturition

I. **Urine transport from the renal pelvis to the urinary bladder.**

A. Hydrostatic pressure in renal pelvis averages 0 mm Hg. Thus there is no pressure gradient to force urine to flow to the urinary bladder through the ureters.

B. Ureters have large amount of smooth muscle. Peristaltic contractions of the smooth muscle, which occur about every 2–3 minutes, progress from the renal pelvis to the urinary bladder. This forces urine to flow through the ureters at a velocity of about 3 cm/sec.

C. Parasympathetic stimulation increases and sympathetic stimulation decreases frequency of contractions.

II. Micturition.

A. When urine is not in the urinary bladder, the internal pressure is about 0 mm Hg. As urine collects in the bladder, there is a slow pressure increase until the volume reaches about 400–500 mL. Above this volume the pressure rises rapidly.

B. As the bladder fills, stretch receptors in the bladder wall are stimulated.

C. Afferent nerve signals are sent from bladder to sacral segments of spinal cord through pelvic nerves.

D. Reflex integration takes place in the spinal cord. Efferent nerve impulses are conducted from the spinal cord to the urinary bladder through parasympathetic portion of pelvic nerves. A conscious desire to urinate occurs when ascending tracts in spinal cord conduct nerve impulses to the brain.

E. Bladder muscles contract and internal and external urinary sphincters relax as result of efferent nerve impulses.

F. In normal adults and children over age 2 or 3, the reflex can be voluntarily inhibited or stimulated by higher brain centers.

G. During voluntary urination, the higher brain centers send impulses to the spinal cord to enhance the micturition reflex and inhibit contraction of external urinary sphincter.

Chapter 2

Pathophysiology

Purpose

The purposes of this chapter are to describe the etiology, pathology, and assessment data related to the causes of acute and chronic kidney failure, and other kidney disorders, and to briefly outline treatment of these disorders.

Objectives

Upon completion of this chapter, the learner will be able to:
1. Differentiate acute and chronic kidney failure.
2. Describe the etiology, pathophysiology, and assessment findings of prerenal, intrarenal, and postrenal acute failure.
3. Delineate patient care during the four stages of acute kidney injury.
4. Describe the characteristics of the stages of chronic kidney disease.
5. Explain the pathogenesis of diabetic nephropathy.
6. Explain how hypertension can affect kidney function.
7. Discuss the pathophysiology of the nephrotic syndrome.
8. Outline development and congenital disorders that affect kidney function.
9. Define the terminology related to glomerulopathies.
10. Review the incidence, clinical manifestations, and treatment of polycystic, medullary, and acquired cystic kidney diseases.
11. Compare the etiology and pathophysiology of renal tubular acidosis and Fanconi syndrome.
12. Summarize the types of kidney neoplasms, signs and symptoms, and management approaches.
13. Explain the causative agents, clinical manifestations, and treatment of pyelonephritis and renal tuberculosis.
14. Describe the pathogenesis and prognosis of acute poststreptococcal glomerulonephritis.
15. Discuss retroperitoneal fibrosis and its effect on kidney function.
16. Identify populations at risk, signs and symptoms, treatment, and complications of nephrolithiasis.
17. Explain the effects of hyperparathyroidism on the kidney.
18. Describe the hepatorenal syndrome.
19. Explain how gout can affect kidney function.
20. Outline the relationship between amyloidosis and kidney failure.
21. Distinguish between the immune mechanisms and the pathogenesis of kidney failure related to Goodpasture syndrome.
22. Describe the pathogenesis and treatment of kidney dysfunction related to systemic lupus erythematosus.
23. Relate the kidney effects and treatment of scleroderma.
24. Summarize the population affected, the kidney involvement, and management associated with Henoch-Schönlein syndrome.
25. Describe the effects of pregnancy on kidney function and potential problems that may occur.

Acute Kidney Injury

I. General concepts.

A. Definition.
1. Sudden, rapid deterioration of kidney function. Potentially reversible.
2. Frequently a complication of other potentially life-threatening illness or injury.
3. Diagnostic criteria includes:
   a. Serum creatinine increase > 0 .5 mg/dL or
   b. Serum creatinine increase from baseline > 25% or
   c. Creatinine clearance (calculated) decrease > 50%.
   d. Also consider:
      (1) Altered electrolytes.
      (2) Metabolic acidosis.
      (3) Cognitive, gastrointestinal, skin symptoms, or retained waste products.
      (4) Volume overload.
4. May be oliguric (< 500 mL/day [SI = 0.5 L/day]) or nonoliguric (> 800 mL/day [SI = 0.8 L/day]). *Note*: SI = International System of Units.
5. Azotemia (retention of nitrogenous substances in the blood) usually present.
6. Most frequent causes are hypoperfusion to the kidneys and nephrotoxins (see Table 1.3).
7. Signs and symptoms vary and can range from mild azotemia to uremia.
   a. Some patients experience similar problems (e.g., fluid and electrolyte imbalances) as patients with chronic kidney failure.
   b. Profound neurologic and musculoskeletal disorders usually not present.

B. Major treatment goals.
1. Supportive therapy to maintain homeostasis until the kidney lesion heals.
2. Prevent life-threatening complications such as infection, fluid/electrolyte imbalance, acid-base imbalance, and gastrointestinal bleeding.
3. Management varies based on the etiology and degree of kidney injury.
   a. Remove cause or contributing factors.
   b. Conservative interventions, such as rest, volume management, and mild dietary restrictions, are adequate for many patients.
   c. Aggressive interventions, such as dialysis and prolonged hospitalization, are necessary for some patients.

C. Mortality.
1. Approximately 40–60%. Generally due to primary illness, sepsis, and/or multiorgan failure rather than kidney failure.
2. Patients who survive usually have good return of kidney function.

II. Classifications.

A. Prerenal.
1. Etiology.
   a. Decreased blood flow to the kidneys, usually due to poor systemic perfusion.
   b. Hypovolemia related to hemorrhage, burns, shock, excessive diaphoresis, gastrointestinal or kidney losses, peritonitis, and malignancies.
   c. Diminished cardiac output related to congestive heart failure, myocardial infarction, cardiac tamponade, and cardiac dysrhythmias.
   d. Altered peripheral vascular resistance related to sepsis, antihypertensive medications, anaphylactic reactions, neurogenic shock, and drug overdose.
   e. Renal artery emboli, thrombi, stenosis, aneurysm, occlusion, and trauma.
   f. Hepatorenal syndrome (see discussion later in this chapter).
2. Pathophysiology.
   a. The kidneys adapt to hypoperfusion through autoregulation and release of renin.
   b. In autoregulation, the afferent arteriole dilates and efferent arteriole constricts to maintain glomerular filtration rate (GFR) and creatinine clearance.
   c. The release of renin activates the angiotensin-aldosterone system.
      (1) Results in peripheral vasoconstriction and increased sodium reabsorption (thus decreasing urinary sodium).
      (2) Increased plasma sodium causes the release of antidiuretic hormone, which enhances vasoconstriction and increases water reabsorption, resulting in decreased urinary output and increased blood volume.
      (3) With increased sodium and water reabsorption, urea reabsorption is increased and blood urea nitrogen (BUN) increases.
   d. The goal of the above mechanisms is to maintain systemic and kidney perfusion, and kidney function.
   e. If kidney hypoperfusion persists and exceeds

Table 1.3

Causes of Acute Kidney Injury

Prerenal Factors

Hypovolemia
Hemorrhage, burns, shock, excessive sweating, peritonitis, nephrotic syndrome, gastrointestinal losses, renal losses (e.g., diuretics, diabetes insipidus, malignancies)

Altered peripheral vascular resistance
Sepsis, antihypertensive medications, drug overdose, anaphylactic reactions, neurogenic shock
Nonsteroidal antiinflammatory drugs

Cardiac disorders
Congestive heart failure, myocardial infarction, cardiac tamponade, cardiac arrhythmias

Renal artery disorders
Emboli, thrombi, stenosis, aneurysm, occlusion, trauma

Hepatorenal syndrome

Nephrotoxins

Drugs
Anesthetics, antimicrobials, antiinflammatories, chemotherapeutic agents

Contrast media

Biologic substances
Toxins: tumor products
Heme pigments: hemoglobin, myoglobin

Environmental agents
Pesticides, fungicides
Organic solvents: carbon tetrachloride, diesel fuel, phenol

Heavy metals
Lead, mercury, gold, arsenic, bismuth, uranium, cadmium

Plant and animal substances
Mushrooms, snake venom

Intrarenal Factors

Nephrotoxic agents

Inflammatory processes
Bacterial, viral, toxemia of pregnancy

Immune processes
Autoimmunity, hypersensitivity, rejection

Trauma
Penetrating, nonpenetrating

Radiation nephritis

Obstruction
Neoplasm, stones, scar tissue

Intravascular hemolysis
Transfusion reaction, disseminated intravascular hemolysis

Systemic and vascular disorders
Renal vein thrombosis, malaria, nephrotic syndrome, Wilson disease, multiple myeloma, sickle-cell disease, malignant hypertension, diabetes mellitus, systemic lupus erythematosus

Pregnancy-related disorders

Postrenal Factors

Ureteral, bladder neck, or urethral obstruction
Calculi, neoplasms, sloughed papillary tissue, strictures, trauma, blood clots, congenital/developmental abnormalities, foreign object, surgical ligation

Prostatic hypertrophy

Retroperitoneal fibrosis

Abdominal and pelvic neoplasms

Pregnancy

Neurogenic bladder

Bladder rupture

Drugs
Antihistamines, ganglionic blocking agents, methysergide

---

the abilities of the kidney's adaptive mechanisms, acute kidney injury develops due to ischemia (see discussion later).
3. Assessment.
   a. History. Data indicates poor perfusion to the kidneys and/or poor systemic perfusion.
      (1) Surgery.
      (2) Persistent upper and lower GI losses (vomiting, diarrhea).
      (3) High fever.
      (4) Multiple tests that require NPO and/or bowel preparation.
      (5) Acute myocardial infarction.
      (6) Anaphylactic drug or transfusion reaction.
      (7) Cardiac arrest with successful resuscitation.
      (8) Low sodium diets with fluid restriction, diuretics, and antihypertensives.

(9) Exposure to consecutive days of hot, humid weather, with or without exercise and accompanied by poor fluid intake.
(10) Penetrating or nonpenetrating abdominal trauma.
4. Physical assessment.
    a. Findings vary depending on the etiology.
    b. Need to be correlated with laboratory and history findings.
    c. May include dry mucous membranes, poor skin turgor, reduced jugular venous pressure, hypotension, weight loss, decreased urine output (oliguria).
5. Laboratory findings.
    a. Increased BUN.
    b. Plasma creatinine may be normal.
    c. Ratio of BUN to plasma creatinine increases.
    d. Increased urine osmolality and specific gravity.
    e. Decreased urine sodium, fractional excretion of sodium, and urea.
    f. Urinary sediment usually normal.
6. Major treatment goal is to reestablish kidney perfusion.
    a. Administer fluids to increase circulatory blood volume (e.g., 500 mL [SI = 0.5 L]) over 30 minutes and repeat if no increase in urine volume). During the fluid bolus monitor cardiovascular response to the increased intravascular volume.
    b. Increase or support cardiac function (e.g., inotropes to increase ability to pump blood to the kidneys).

B. Intrarenal (parenchymal) azotemia.
1. Etiology.
    a. Results from injury to renal (parenchymal) tissue.
    b. Usually associated with intrarenal ischemia, toxins, or both.
    c. Often called acute tubular necrosis (ATN). ATN is the most common cause of intrarenal azotemia and acute kidney injury in general.
    d. Prolonged prerenal etiologies.
    e. Perfusion injury and/or prolonged ischemia in transplanted kidney.
    f. Nephrotoxic agents.
        (1) Drugs (e.g., antineoplastics, anesthetics, antimicrobics, antiinflammatory agents, and immunosuppressants).
        (2) X-ray contrast media (especially iodine-based dyes).
        (3) Biologic substances (e.g., toxins, tumor products, and heme pigments from hemoglobin or myoglobin).

(4) Environmental agents (e.g., pesticides and organic solvents).
(5) Heavy metals (e.g., lead, mercury, and gold).
(6) Plant and animal substances (e.g., mushrooms and snake venoms).
(7) Some herbal agents.
    g. Inflammatory processes related to bacteria, virus, and toxemia of pregnancy.
    h. Immune processes, such as autoimmunity, hypersensitivity, and tissue or organ transplant rejection.
    i. Trauma or radiation to the kidney.
    j. Obstruction (e.g., neoplasm, stones, and scar tissue).
    k. Intravascular hemolysis related to transfusion reaction and disseminated intravascular hemolysis.
    l. Systemic and vascular disorders.
        (1) Renal vein thrombosis.
        (2) Nephrotic syndrome.
        (3) Wilson disease.
        (4) Malaria.
        (5) Multiple myeloma.
        (6) Sickle cell disease.
        (7) Malignant hypertension.
        (8) Diabetes mellitus.
        (9) Systemic lupus erythematosus.
    m. Pregnancy related disorders (such as septic abortion, preeclampsia, abruptio placenta, intrauterine fetal death, and idiopathic postpartum kidney failure).
2. Pathophysiology.
    a. Figure 1.20 is a schematic representation of the pathophysiology of ischemic and toxic conditions that result in ATN.
    b. Ischemic acute tubular necrosis.
        (1) The ischemic event is prolonged hypoperfusion and ischemia of the kidneys with a sustained mean arterial pressure (MAP) of less than 75 mm Hg.
        (2) Renal autoregulation fails and the sympathetic nervous system (SNS) response, renin-angiotensin system, and (possibly) endothelin cause prolonged afferent arteriole constriction.
        (3) These mechanisms lead to decreased glomerular blood flow, glomerular hydrostatic pressure, and GFR.
        (4) The amount and degree of cellular damage depend on the length of the ischemic episode.
            (a) Ischemia of 25 minutes or less causes reversible mild injury.

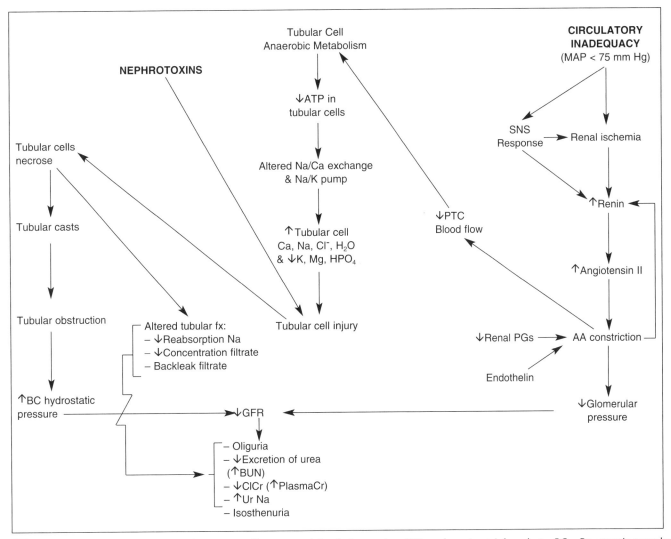

Figure 1.20. Pathophysiology of ATN. AA— afferent arteriole of glomerulus; ATP = adenosine triphosphate; BC – Bowman's capsule, BUN = blood urea nitrogen; Ca = calcium; Cl = clearance; Cl⁻ = chloride; Cr = creatinine; fx = function; GFR = glomerular filtration rate; H_2O = water; HPO_4 = phosphate; K = potassium; MAP = mean arterial pressure; Mg = magnesium; Na = sodium; PGs = prostaglandins; PTC = peritubular capillary; SNS = sympathetic nervous system; Ur = urine.

(b) Ischemia of 40–60 minutes causes more severe damage that may recover to some extent in 2–3 weeks.

(c) Ischemia lasting 60–90 minutes usually causes irreversible damage.

(5) Cellular damage often continues after MAP and renal perfusion are restored (ischemia reperfusion injury). Renal blood flow can be reduced by 50% after an episode of ischemia.

(6) Due to prolonged ischemia the kidneys are unable to synthesize vasodilating prostaglandins. Without them, the ischemic injury may be exacerbated/worsened.

(7) Sympathetic nervous system (SNS) stimulation and angiotensin II redistribute blood flow from the cortex to the medulla. This further decreases glomerular capillary flow and worsens tubular ischemia (because tubules are located primarily in the cortex).

(8) With ischemia, nutrients and oxygen for basic cellular metabolism and tubular transport systems are diminished.

(a) Production of adenosine triphosphate (ATP) by renal cell mitochondria decreases significantly.

(b) Without adequate oxygen and ATP, metabolism shifts from aerobic to anaerobic.

(c) A corresponding renal tissue extracellular and intracellular acidosis alters kidney function.

(9) Ischemia causes a decrease in renal cellular potassium, magnesium, and inorganic phosphates, and an increase in intracellular sodium, chloride, and calcium.

(a) Sodium/calcium exchange is abnormal due to low ATP, altered ca-ATPase, and increased cell sodium. As a result, there is an increase in cellular calcium, which increases cell injury.

(b) During reperfusion after a prolonged ischemic event to the kidneys, the formation of oxygen-free radicals further exacerbates cellular damage.

(10) The final outcome of prolonged tubular ischemia is swelling and necrosis of tubular cells, altering the function of the basement membrane.

(a) Tubular obstruction occurs due to sloughed necrotic cells and cast formation.

(b) Tubular obstruction increases tubular hydrostatic pressure and Bowman's capsule hydrostatic pressure.

(c) Increased hydrostatic pressure in Bowman's capsule opposes the glomerular hydrostatic pressure and decreases GFR.

(d) Injury to the basement membrane increases tubular permeability and allows tubular filtrate to leak back into the interstitium and peritubular capillaries, resulting in a further decrease in tubular filtrate.

(11) Ischemic ATN is usually associated with oliguria because of extensive nephron injury.

(12) Other clinical indications of ATN.

(a) Decreased urea excretion and elevated blood urea nitrogen (BUN).

(b) Decreased creatinine clearance and elevated plasma creatinine.

(c) Abnormal renal handling of sodium (usually sodium loss with urinary sodium equal to sodium filtered into the tubule from the glomerulus, fractional excretion of sodium > 1). *and*

(d) Inability to concentrate urine. Urinary osmolality approximates plasma osmolality or 300–320 mOsm/L (SI = 300–320 mOsm/L) (isosthenuria).

c. Toxic acute tubular necrosis.

(1) The toxic event may be the toxic products of organisms and/or nephrotoxic agents.

(2) Toxic ATN begins with injury to the tubular cells.

(3) Subsequent pathophysiology is similar to ischemic ATN. There is tubular cell necrosis, cast formation, tubular obstruction, and decreased GFR.

(a) The basement membrane is usually intact.

(b) Injured necrotic areas are more localized to proximal and distal tubules than with ischemic ATN.

(c) More likely to be nonoliguric (ischemic more likely to be oliguric).

(4) The injury can be less severe than with ischemic ATN, therefore healing more likely and more rapid than ischemic ATN.

(5) Kidneys are susceptible to toxic damage due to:

(a) Blood circulates through the kidneys approximately 14 times a minute. Therefore, the kidneys are repeatedly exposed to all substances in the blood.

(b) Kidneys are largely responsible for concentration and excretion of toxic substances and are therefore exposed to high concentrations of these substances.

(c) Renal tubule cells are highly susceptible to direct toxic effects of a large number of substances (e.g., drugs, heavy metals, organic solvents).

(d) In addition, the liver usually detoxifies substances, and, with liver disease, the kidney can be overloaded with underdetoxified substances.

3. Assessment.

a. History. Collect data that identify an event, series of events, agent, or agents that may have caused kidney injury.

(1) Exposure to nephrotoxins (see Table 1.3).

(2) Radiologic tests that require administration of a dye.

(3) Hypersensitivity reaction to a drug or dye.

(4) Recent infections, trauma, or sepsis.

(5) Antineoplastics with or without irradiation.

(6) Multiple myeloma or pregnancy.

(7) History of cardiac, renal, or liver disease.

Table 1.4

Typical Findings in Prerenal and Intrarenal Acute Kidney Injury

	Prerenal	Intrarenal
Volume	Oliguria	Oliguria or Nonoliguria
Urinary sediment	Normal (Hyaline and granular casts)	RBC casts Cellular debris
Specific gravity	High	Low
Osmolality (mOsm/Kg H_2O)	High	Low (isosthenuria)
Ratio Osm Urine to Osm Plasma	> 1.5	< 1.2
Urine Na (mEq/L)	Low (< 20)	Increased over prerenal (> 20)
Urine urea (g/24 hr)	Low (15)	Low (5)
Urine Creatinine (g/24 hr)	Normal (>1.0)	Low (< 1.0)
Ratio Urine Creatinine to Plasma Creatinine	> 15:1	< 10:1

Source: Lancaster, L.E. (1990). Renal response to shock. *Critical Care Nursing Clinics of North America, 2*(2), 221-223. Used with permission.

b. Physical assessment. No one specific finding pinpoints intrarenal azotemia. Correlate all findings with history and laboratory findings.
4. Differential diagnosis of prerenal azotemia and acute tubular necrosis.
   a. Differentiating prerenal problems and intrarenal ATN is a challenge. Prerenal problems often correspond with the onset phase of ATN. Because this is a reversible phase, it is essential for diagnosis and aggressive management to begin early in the course of prerenal problems. In addition, an acute obstruction should be ruled out (see *C. Postrenal azotemia*).
   b. Urinalysis, microscopic examination of the urine, and laboratory plasma values provide important data for differentiating prerenal azotemia from ATN. Table 1.4 summarizes typical urine and plasma findings in prerenal azotemia and ATN.
   c. Prerenal problems.
      (1) Urinary specific gravity and osmolality are high, and the urinary sodium and fractional excretion of sodium are low

because of decreased renal blood flow and decreased GFR (which the kidneys interpret as a state of dehydration).
      (2) As a response (under the influence of aldosterone and ADH), maximal sodium and water are reabsorbed from the distal tubule and collecting duct into the peritubular capillary plasma.
      (3) As a result, a small amount (oliguria) of very concentrated urine with high specific gravity and high osmolality is excreted.
      (4) Although maximal sodium is reabsorbed, the urine is concentrated due to urea or other solutes.
      (5) Urinary and plasma creatinine levels often show wide variation in prerenal problems.
   d. In contrast to prerenal problems, ATN is characterized by the kidney's inability to conserve sodium.
      (1) Clinically, this is seen as an increased urinary sodium (greater than 20 mEq/L [SI = 20 mmol/L]; FENa > 1).

(2) Serum sodium varies, depending on the state of hydration.

(3) Oliguria is usually associated with postischemic ATN. Nephrotoxic ATN is associated with either oliguria or nonoliguria (as explained above).

(4) The creatinine clearance is severely decreased, and the plasma creatinine rises at a rate of about 1 to 3 mg/dL/day (SI = 88–264 mmol/L/day) in ATN.

(5) The urine to plasma creatinine ratio is less than 10 to 1 in ATN.

(6) The BUN also rises. As a result, the BUN to creatinine ratio is normal.

e. Another distinguishing factor for prerenal problems and ATN is the response to therapy.

(1) In prerenal problems in which no actual nephron damage has occurred, the kidney's response to therapy aimed at correcting the underlying problem is often rapid with return to normal urine output and normal blood chemistries.

(2) In ATN, which indicates nephron damage, response to therapy of the underlying cause of the damage is minimal. ATN requires additional therapy aimed at correcting alterations related to inability of the kidneys to maintain their functions.

5. Major treatment goal is to remove the causative agent/event as soon as possible (such as discontinue administration of nephrotoxic drugs/agents).

C. Postrenal azotemia.

1. Etiology.

a. Results from interference with the flow of urine from the kidneys to the exterior of the body and is associated with obstruction or disruption of the urinary tract (see Table 1.3).

b. Ureteral, bladder neck, or urethral obstruction.

(1) Calculi, neoplasms, or sloughed papillary tissue.

(2) Strictures, trauma, or blood clots.

(3) Congenital/developmental abnormalities.

(4) Foreign objects or inadvertent surgical ligation.

c. Prostatic hypertrophy.

d. Retroperitoneal fibrosis.

e. Abdominal and pelvic neoplasms.

f. Pregnancy.

g. Neurogenic bladder.

h. Bladder rupture.

i. Drugs, such as antihistamines and ganglionic blocking agents.

2. Pathophysiology.

a. Bilateral obstruction results in anuria related to the impedance of urine flow past the obstruction.

b. Urine congestion increases backward/retrograde pressure through the collecting system and nephron and slows the tubular fluid flow and GFR.

(1) Increased reabsorption of sodium, water, and urea results in decreased urinary sodium, increased urine osmolality, and increased BUN.

(2) Decreased GFR results in a decreased creatinine clearance and increased plasma creatinine.

c. With prolonged postrenal obstruction, the collecting system dilates and compresses parenchymal tissue.

d. The nephrons are injured, resulting in dysfunction of the concentrating/diluting mechanism.

e. With a temporary postrenal obstruction, there is minimal dilation of the collecting system and loss of renal tissue.

(1) With complete obstruction abrupt anuria occurs and urine accumulates behind the obstruction.

(2) When the obstruction is relieved, the dammed up urine rushes out, and polyuria results.

3. Assessment.

a. Unilateral obstruction may result in few signs and symptoms.

b. History. Collect data that indicate obstruction or disruption of the urinary tract.

(1) History of change in urine volume.

(2) History of prostatic disease or abdominal neoplasms.

(3) History of urinary tract stones or nephralgia.

(4) Pregnancy.

(5) Recent abdominal surgery.

(6) Paralysis (e.g., quadriplegia).

c. Physical assessment.

(1) Findings vary with etiology and need to be correlated with laboratory and history findings (e.g., nephralgia associated with moving urinary tract stones or rapidly developing hydronephrosis. Bladder distention associated with prostate, bladder neck, and urethral disorders).

(2) Urine volume variable. May be oliguria

or polyuria or abrupt anuria. Asking about changes in urinary patterns is helpful in identifying urinary tract obstructions.
  d. Laboratory findings.
    (1) Urine osmolality variable. Increases or may be similar to plasma osmolality.
    (2) Urine specific gravity variable.
    (3) Urine sodium variable. Often similar to plasma sodium.
    (4) Urine urea decreases.
    (5) Urinary sediment usually normal (except if urinary tract infection is present).
    (6) BUN and plasma creatinine increase. Ratio normal to slightly increased.
  e. Radiologic findings.
    (1) Renal ultrasound often demonstrates obstruction and/or dilated collecting structures. Abdominal ultrasound may also be helpful.
    (2) Spiral CT and/or IVP is useful in locating an obstruction within the collecting/drainage structures (e.g., renal stones).
  4. Major treatment goals are to relieve the obstruction/disruption and reestablish urine flow.

III. Clinical course of acute kidney injury.

A. Initiating stage.
  1. Begins when kidney is injured and lasts from hours to days.
  2. Signs and symptoms of impaired kidney function present (e.g., decreased urine volume).
  3. Cause of acute kidney injury sought, and treatment plan to reverse initiated.
  4. Minimal effect on the endocrine functions of the kidneys.

B. Oliguric stage.
  1. Usually lasts from 5 to 15 days, but can persist for weeks.
  2. Healing begins.
    a. Tubular cells regenerate.
    b. Destroyed basement membrane replaced with fibrous scar tissue.
    c. Tubules clogged with inflammatory products.
  3. Functional changes include decreased glomerular filtration, decreased tubular transport of substances, decreased urine formation, and decreased renal clearance.
  4. When acute kidney injury persists for weeks or longer, the kidney's endocrine functions are altered (e.g., decreased secretion of erythropoietin).
  5. Approximately 50% of acute kidney injury

patients are nonoliguric and have less severe signs and symptoms than oliguric patients.
  6. Frequent causes of death are cardiac arrest due to hyperkalemia, gastrointestinal bleeding, and infection.
  7. Goal is to provide supportive and therapeutic care until kidney lesion heals. Day-to-day care is very important.
  8. Patient problems.
    a. Increased susceptibility to infection, especially urinary and respiratory, related to hospitalization and altered immune, nutritional, and biochemical status.
      (1) Implement preventive measures.
      (2) Avoid invasive procedures, especially urinary bladder catheters.
      (3) Strict aseptic techniques with all invasive procedures.
      (4) Maintain skin and mucous membrane integrity, nutrition, pulmonary hygiene, and exercise program.
      (5) Avoid contact with people who have infections (including a hospital roommate who has a urinary tract infection).
      (6) Instruct about increased susceptibility to infection, how to prevent, and signs and symptoms to report.
      (7) Assess for signs and symptoms of local or systemic infection.
      (8) Assess vital signs, lung sounds, and leukocyte count.
      (9) Assess changes in wounds, drainage, and body secretions. Culture immediately.
      (10) Assess chest x-ray.
      (11) Treat infections promptly to avoid septicemia.
      (12) Remove catheters, tubings, and invasive lines as soon as possible.
      (13) Use antibiotics/antiinfectives that are specific for the organism(s) cultured, but not nephrotoxic or excreted by the kidney.
    b. Fluid volume excess related to decreased excretion of water, excessive fluid intake, and sodium retention.
    c. Hyperkalemia related to decreased renal regulation and excretion of potassium, increased endogenous production of potassium, increased potassium intake, tissue breakdown, and metabolic acidosis.
    d. Hyperphosphatemia related to decreased renal excretion and regulation of phosphate, increased or continued intake of phosphate, and tissue breakdown (especially muscle).
    e. Metabolic acidosis related to decreased renal excretion of acid load and decreased

regeneration of bicarbonate, increased tissue catabolism, and endogenous production of acids.

f. Potential for gastrointestinal bleeding related to physiologic stress, retention of metabolic wastes and end products, altered capillary permeability, and platelet dysfunction.

g. Altered nutrition. Needs generally exceed intake, especially protein calories.

h. Potential for drug toxicity, adverse drug reactions, and nephrotoxicity related to inability of kidneys to excrete drugs and/or drug metabolites, continued administration of drugs excreted by the kidneys, and nephrotoxic drugs.

i. Anemia due to blood loss and decreased erythrocyte production.

j. Pericardial effusion/tamponade due to uremia.

k. Cardiac arrhythmias due to electrolyte imbalances.

l. Potential for skin breakdown related to bed rest, inadequate nutrition, fluid/electrolyte imbalances, metabolic products and toxins accumulation, edema, disrupted hemostasis and increased capillary fragility, repeated venipunctures, and other invasive procedures.

m. Disturbances in self-concept related to loss of bodily function, dependency, separation from family and friends, fatigue, cognitive dysfunction (e.g., memory), confusion, lack of knowledge, hopelessness, and lack of control.

n. Disturbances in sleep pattern related to biochemical disruption, anxiety, hospitalization, isolation from family/friends, fear regarding lack of recovery of kidney function, multiple tests, dietary and fluid restrictions.

o. Lack of knowledge related to kidney function, diagnostic tests, pathogenesis of acute kidney injury, effects of acute kidney injury on all body systems; course, management, prognosis, complications, and prevention of acute kidney injury.

C. Diuretic stage.
  1. Usually lasts from 1 to 2 weeks, but can persist for weeks.
  2. Self-limiting diuresis.
     a. Renal tubular patency is restored.
     b. Retained substances (e.g., urea and sodium) act as osmotic agents.
     c. Nephron's ability to concentrate urine not recovered.

3. With continued healing, the kidneys regain most lost functions (depends on degree of initial injury and of basement membrane loss), except concentrating ability.

4. Signs and symptoms of azotemia diminish toward the end of diuretic stage.

5. Oliguric patients have a greater diuresis than nonoliguric patients.

6. During diuresis, the patient is at risk for fluid volume deficit and reinjury to renal tissue due to hypotension and/or hypoperfusion.

7. Frequent causes of death are infection and gastrointestinal bleeding.

8. Goal of therapy is to provide supportive and therapeutic care until healing occurs.

9. Patient problems.
   a. Fluid volume deficit related to increased excretion of water, inadequate fluid intake/replacement, sodium loss, continued use of diuretics/dialysis, fluid loss through nonrenal sources.
      (1) Perform fluid assessment.
      (2) Daily weight, vital signs, intake and output. Correlate fluid intake/output record with weight.
      (3) Assess edema, skin turgor, mucous membranes.
      (4) Assess for dizziness, hypotension, orthostasis, hard stool.
      (5) Assess plasma sodium and osmolality, hematocrit, urine sodium, and urine osmolality.
      (6) Instruct patient how to participate in fluid assessment and to report signs and symptoms of fluid deficit.
      (7) Determine if fluid balanced, deficit, or overloaded.
      (8) Adjust fluid intake to approximate fluid loss plus 300–500 mL/day (SI = 0.3–0.5 L/day). Increase with fever or if losing fluids (e.g., wounds, GI tract).
      (9) Offer fluids throughout day.
      (10) Consult and coordinate fluid plan with dietitian.
      (11) Provide for excretory needs (e.g., commode, urinal, bedpan).
      (12) Avoid procedures that require NPO or bowel preparation until diuresis subsides and/or initiate intravenous therapy.
      (13) Develop fluid plan with patient.
      (14) Teach about kidney function and need for increased fluids.

b. Hypokalemia related to increased excretion of potassium, decreased potassium intake, metabolic alkalosis, continued administration of diuretics/resin exchangers, intravenous fluid without potassium, GI fluid losses.
    (1) Assess plasma potassium changes.
    (2) Assess for decreased neuromuscular irritability, constipation, weakness, diminished reflexes.
    (3) Monitor ECG and vital signs for signs and symptoms of hypokalemia.
    (4) Consult dietitian for adequate dietary intake of potassium.
    (5) Administer potassium parenterally if unable to ingest adequate dietary potassium.
    (6) Prevent metabolic alkalosis because of hydrogen-potassium cellular exchange.
    (7) Control GI losses.
    (8) Avoid drugs that cause potassium loss (e.g., diuretics).
    (9) Teach patient why at risk for hypokalemia and signs and symptoms to report.
c. Problems from the oliguric state often persist.
    (1) Increased susceptibility to infection.
    (2) Gastrointestinal bleeding.
    (3) Altered nutrition.
    (4) Skin breakdown.
    (5) Drug toxicity and nephrotoxicity.
    (6) Anemia.
    (7) Disturbances in sleep pattern.
d. Problems related to hyperphosphatemia and metabolic acidosis gradually resolve during the diuretic stage as kidney function improves and the kidneys are able to regulate and excrete hydrogen and phosphate, and reabsorb bicarbonate ions.

D. Recovery stage.
  1. Usually lasts several months to 1 year.
  2. Healing process completed.
    a. Contractile scar tissue replaces damaged basement membrane.
    b. Nephrons are maximally patent.
    c. Tubular cells regenerate.
    d. Some scar tissue probably remains in all kidneys affected by acute kidney injury, but the functional loss is not always clinically significant.
  3. Maximal kidney functions return (e.g., concentrating ability) and kidneys recover regulatory and excretory mechanisms.
  4. Urine osmolality increases, urine volume stabilizes; plasma substances normalize, body fluids balance, and uremia resolves.

5. No special form of treatment.
6. Major patient problem is lack of knowledge regarding the acute kidney injury episode, follow-up care, and prevention of another episode.
    a. Teach patient about the acute kidney injury episode.
    b. Interventions to prevent another episode (e.g., avoid Nephrotoxins, maintain fluid intake).
    c. Increased risk to develop acute kidney injury in future.

Chronic Kidney Disease and Failure

I. General concepts.

A. Definition and criteria.
  1. Kidney damage for > 3 months.
    a. Includes structural or functional abnormalities of the kidneys.
    b. With or without decreased GFR.
    c. Manifested by either pathologic abnormalities or markers of kidney damage (abnormal blood, urine, imaging tests).
  2. GFR < 60 mL/min/1.73 m² for > 3 months, with or without kidney damage.

B. Insidious, progressive, irreversible loss of kidney function.
  1. Frequent causes.
    a. Chronic systemic diseases that affect the kidneys (e.g., diabetes mellitus, hypertension).
    b. Chronic kidney diseases (e.g., polycystic kidney disease, immunologic disorders).
  2. Other causes increasing in frequency include herbal agents and nephrotoxins, such as immunosuppressants used for solid organ transplants.
  3. Signs and symptoms usually are mild at first, such as elevated plasma creatinine and BUN, but increase in number and severity until uremia occurs.
  4. Initial treatment goal is to preserve kidney function for as long as possible. Interventions vary with the etiology.
  5. As kidney function continues to decline, management focuses on controlling uremic symptoms, preventing complications, and preparing for kidney replacement therapy.
  6. Mortality rate is 100% if maintenance dialysis or kidney transplant is not implemented.

Table 1.5

Stages of Chronic Kidney Disease

Stage	GFR (mL/min/1.73 m²)	Effect on Homeostasis
1	> 90	Minimal. Excretory and secretory functions intact.
2	60–89	Excretory and secretory functions beginning to be affected.
3	30–59	Excretory, secretory functions failing. Ability to concentrate urine decreased. Complications present.
4	15–29	Excretory, secretory functions severely impaired.
5	< 15 or on dialysis	Excretory, secretory functions failed. Unable to maintain homeostasis without replacement therapy.

C. Stages of chronic kidney disease (see Table 1.5).
   1. Stage 1.
      a. GFR > 90 mL/min.
      b. Patient asymptomatic; normal BUN, creatinine.
      c. Excretory and regulatory functions intact.
      d. Homeostasis maintained.
      e. Goal of treatment is diagnosis and treatment of kidney dysfunction, slowing the progression of kidney disease, treatment of comorbid conditions (including cardiovascular risk assessment and reduction).
   2. Stage 2.
      a. GFR 60–89 mL/min.
      b. Decreased glomerular filtration rate, solute clearance, ability to concentrate urine, and hormone secretion.
      c. Signs and symptoms. Rising BUN and plasma creatinine, mild azotemia, polyuria, nocturia, and anemia.
      d. Signs and symptoms often become more severe if the kidneys are stressed, such as with fluid volume depletion or exposure to a nephrotoxic substance.
      e. Goal of therapy is to estimate progression of kidney dysfunction and continue interventions as in stage 1.
   3. Stage 3.
      a. GFR 30–59 mL/min.
      b. Excretory, regulatory, and hormonal functions more severely impaired.

      c. Goal of therapy is to evaluate and treat complications of failing kidney function.
   4. Stage 4.
      a. GFR 15–29 mL/min.
      b. Ability to maintain homeostasis severely impaired.
      c. Goal of therapy is to prepare for kidney replacement therapy.
   5. Stage 5.
      a. GFR < 15 mL/min, or on dialysis.
      b. Unable to maintain homeostasis (e.g., fluid, electrolyte, pH balance).
      c. Markedly elevated BUN and plasma creatinine, anemia, hyperphosphatemia, hypocalcemia, hyperkalemia, fluid overload, usually oliguria with urine osmolality similar to plasma osmolality.
      d. Uremic syndrome develops, and all body systems are affected.
      e. Replacement therapy needed to sustain homeostasis.
      f. Goal of therapy is to replace kidney function through technology and prevent/delay progression of complications.

II. Kidney diseases.

A. Developmental/congenital disorders.
   1. Approximately 10% of newborns have significant malformation of urinary tract.

2. Unilateral renal agenesis (absence of kidney) is compatible with life.
   a. Teach patient that he or she has one kidney.
   b. Should carry identification with that information.
   c. Avoid traumatizing the kidney.
   d. Inform health care providers of solitary kidney.
3. Bilateral renal agenesis is not compatible with life.
   a. Usually diagnosed within 48 hours of birth due to anuria.
   b. May be associated with infant's death within first week of life.
4. Bilateral aplastic kidneys (small, underdeveloped, and nonfunctional) are incompatible with life.
5. Bilateral renal hypoplasia.
   a. Kidneys fail to develop to normal size.
   b. Minimally functional and usually progress to CKD stage 5.
6. Bilateral renal dysplasia.
   a. Anatomically disorganized, malformed with aberrant substances present.
   b. Usually associated with CKD stage 5.
7. Unilateral renal aplasia, hypoplasia, or dysplasia is compatible with life. Teach patient similar precautions as for unilateral renal agenesis.
8. Ectopic or displaced kidneys.
   a. Usually structurally and functionally normal (see Figure 1.21).
   b. Because of abnormal placement and ureteral position (twisted, kinked, compressed), these kidneys are predisposed to infection and stone formation.
   c. Chronic urinary tract infection and calculi may lead to CKD stage 5.
   d. Patient teaching.
      (1) Location of ectopic kidney.
      (2) Predisposed to infection and stone formation.
      (3) Signs and symptoms of infection, stone formation to watch for and report.
      (4) Importance of seeking early health care to prevent CKD.
9. Fused kidneys.
   a. Horseshoe kidneys. Portion or portions of both kidneys grow together.
   b. Usually structurally and functionally normal, but predisposed to chronic infection, stone formation, and CKD for reasons similar to ectopic kidneys.
10. Ectopic, displaced, and fused kidneys frequently are diagnosed by x-ray for nonkidney problems and/or when patient presents with signs and symptoms of urinary tract infection.

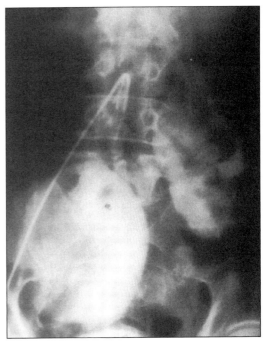

Figure 1.21. Pelvic kidneys. Both kidneys are ectopic and lower than the normal position. Possible cause for pelvic kidneys is inadequate ascension during fetal development. The right kidney is anterior to the vertebral column and the left kidney is lateral to the vertebral column. The white diagonal line is an angiogram catheter.

B. Cystic disorders.
   1. Polycystic kidney disease.
      a. Autosomal dominant.
         (1) PKD1 (most common) and PDK2 genotypes.
         (2) Accounts for < 5% of adult-onset CKD stage 5.
         (3) Onset usually 30–50 years of age, but as late as 70s or 80s.
         (4) Affects both genders equally.
         (5) Pathology.
            (a) Nephrons become cystic with outpouchings or distention of wall.
            (b) Functional tissue is lost (see Figure 1.22).
            (c) Kidneys become enlarged.
            (d) Progresses over continuous but variable time frame.
         (6) Signs and symptoms include hematuria, nephralgia, infection, hypertension, abdominal fullness, calculi, palpable abdominal fullness (from enlarged kidney), polyuria (from failure to concentrate urine), and proteinuria.

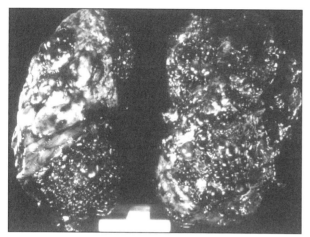

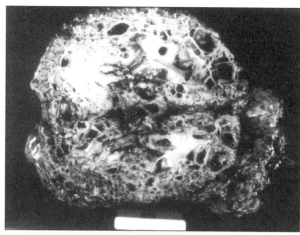

Figure 1.22. Polycystic kidneys.

A. Exterior view of two large cadaveric polycystic kidneys. The bubble-like structures are cysts. The ruler is 6 inches in length.

B. Interior view of a bisected large cadaveric kidney. Many cysts are present. The ruler is 6 inches in length.

(7) Not as anemic as other patients with CKD because polycystic kidneys still produce some erythropoietin.

(8) Treatment includes genetic counseling, prevention of infection, nephrectomy if intrarenal bleeding and infection are significant, and treatment for CKD.

(9) Individuals with PKD1 genotype progress to CKD stage 5 more rapidly than PKD2 genotypes.

b. Infant polycystic kidney disease. Rare autosomal recessive disorder that often results in death from kidney failure and liver fibrosis within the first year of life.

2. Medullary cystic disease.

a. Rare, progressive disorder that occurs sporadically or is autosomal dominant (adult) or recessive (child).

b. Onset usually 20–40 years of age, occasionally in older adults or infants.

c. Kidneys are small with medullary cysts and many functional inadequacies that lead to CKD.

d. Signs and symptoms include polyuria, severe anemia, and hyperchloremic metabolic acidosis.

e. Treatment includes genetic counseling and treatment of CKD.

3. Acquired cystic kidney disease (ACKD).

a. Occurs in patients with CKD without a previous history of kidney cysts.

b. Incidence is slightly higher in males and individuals of African descent.

(1) Incidence increases with increasing years on dialysis.

(2) May occur in transplanted kidneys with chronic rejection.

c. Pathogenesis of ACKD is unknown.

d. Signs and symptoms.

(1) Frequently absent. May have pain, hematuria, and fever.

(2) Noted on x-ray.

(3) Occasionally cysts rupture and bleeding occurs retroperitoneally.

e. Nephrectomy may be needed.

f. For unknown reasons, some people with ACKD develop renal cell carcinoma (see renal neoplasms).

C. Tubular disorders.

1. Renal tubular acidosis (RTA).

a. Genetically transmitted or acquired (e.g., from drugs – lithium carbonate).

b. Usually occurs with another renal tubular disorder and together these may cause CKD stage 4. RTA alone does not usually cause CKD stage 5.

c. Pathology.

(1) Proximal or distal renal tubule or both are affected.

(2) Results in a mild to moderate metabolic acidosis, hypokalemia or hyperkalemia, and fluid volume depletion.

(3) Proximal tubule has decreased ability to reabsorb bicarbonate. Therefore it is lost in the urine.

(4) Bicarbonate loss accompanied by sodium, potassium (to maintain electroneutrality), and water (to maintain osmotic pressure) excretion.

(5) Distal tubule has decreased ability to secrete hydrogen ions, which decreases the sodium-hydrogen exchange, further decreasing the sodium-potassium exchange and resulting in increased potassium and water excretion.

  d. Treatment goals are to maintain pH, electrolyte, and fluid balances.

2. Fanconi syndrome.
  a. Proximal tubular functions are impaired.
  b. Results in wasting of bicarbonate, glucose, amino acids, electrolytes, uric acid, and water.
  c. May be genetic or acquired and caused by multiple myeloma, nephrotic syndrome, tubulointerstitial disorders, and drugs.
  d. Progresses to CKD stage 5 if primary kidney disease.
  e. Treatment goals are to maintain pH, electrolyte, fluid and nutritional balances, and to treat CKD progression.

D. Renal neoplasms.
1. Benign renal neoplasms rare.
  a. Seldom cause CKD stage 5.
  b. Often removed due to pain, bleeding, and obstruction.
2. Malignant neoplasm.
  a. Incidence.
    (1) < 3% of all malignancies are primary cancer of the kidney.
    (2) Approximately 85% of primary renal neoplasms are malignant.
    (3) More common after 45 years of age.
    (4) Affects males twice more than females. 7th leading cause of cancer in males.
    (5) Metastasis to the kidney, usually from the lung, is more common than primary renal neoplasms.
  b. Two types of renal cancer.
    (1) Renal cell carcinoma.
    (2) Cancer of the renal pelvis.
  c. Risk factors.
    (1) Cigarette and pipe smoking.
    (2) Heavy use of phenacetin or acetaminophen-containing products.
    (3) Exposure to asbestos, chemicals.
    (4) Advanced kidney disease.
    (5) Positive family history.

  d. Tumor growth.
    (1) Renal cell carcinoma usually arises from tubular epithelium in the cortex, grows toward the medulla and out through the renal capsule into the perirenal fat.
    (2) Renal pelvis cancer arises from epithelial cells in the renal pelvis, grows down the ureter and into muscular layers.
    (3) Metastasis indicates a poor prognosis. Usually involves the lungs, lymph nodes, liver, bones, and contralateral kidney.
  e. Signs and symptoms.
    (1) Variable; depend upon size of tumor.
    (2) General signs and symptoms include weight loss, fatigue, and elevated erythrocyte sedimentation rate.
    (3) Specific signs and symptoms are hematuria (microscopic, macroscopic, and/or passing clots), palpable abdominal mass, and nephralgia.
  f. Tumor staging.
    (1) The cancer is staged to determine interventions and prognosis.
    (2) The TNM staging system describes the extent of the cancer at time of diagnosis by tumor (T) characteristics and growth, lymph node (N) involvement, and presence of distant metastasis (M).
    (3) Table 1.6 outlines the TNM stages for cancer of the kidney.
  g. Treatment.
    (1) Renal carcinoma is radioresistant. Therefore radiation is not effective.
    (2) Chemotherapy may be used.
    (3) Radical nephrectomy is usually indicated.
      (a) Prevent pulmonary complications (e.g., aggressive pulmonary toilet).
      (b) Assess for paralytic ileus and treat (e.g., ambulate).
      (c) Provide pain control (painful surgery because of location of surgery and trauma to muscles).
      (d) Emotional support to cope with cancer.
      (e) Stress it is safe to live with one kidney.
      (f) Educate to splint surgical site, avoid nephrotoxins, eat nutritional foods, and wear/carry medical alert with the information about solitary kidney.
      (g) Monitor/evaluate function of remaining kidney.
3. Wilms tumor.
  a. Most common tumor of urinary tract in children.

Table 1.6

TNM Staging System for Cancer of the Kidney

Primary Tumor (T)

TX	Primary tumor cannot be assessed.
T0	No evidence of primary tumor.
T1a	Tumor 4 cm or less in diameter; limited to the kidney.
T1b	Tumor 4–7 cm in diameter; limited to the kidney.
T2	Tumor more than 7 cm in diameter; limited to the kidney.
T3a	Tumor spread into the adrenal gland or perinephric fatty tissues but not beyond the fibrous Gerota's fascia.
T3b	Tumor spread into the renal vein(s) and/or vena cava within the abdomen.
T3c	Tumor reached the vena cava within the chest or invaded the wall of the vena cava.
T4	Tumor spread beyond Gerota's fascia.

Regional Lymph Nodes (N)

NX	Regional lymph nodes cannot be assessed.
N0	No regional lymph node metastasis.
N1	Metastasis to one regional lymph node.
N2	Metastasis to more than one regional lymph node.

Distant Metastasis (M)

MX	Presence of distant metastasis cannot be assessed.
M0	No distant metastasis.
M1	Distant metastasis; includes metastasis to nonregional lymph nodes and/or other organs.

Stage Grouping

Stage I T1a–T1b, N0, M0

Stage IIT2, N0, M0

Stage III T1a–T3b, N1, M0 or T3a–T3c, N0, M0

Stage IV T4, N0–N1, M0 or any T, any N, M1

Source: American Cancer Society, 2005.

b. Onset usually 3–5 years of age, occasionally in young adolescence.
c. Etiology unclear but hereditary and nonhereditary forms known. Associated with congenital anomalies of genitourinary system.
d. Signs and symptoms include abdominal mass, abdominal pain, hypertension (tumor secretes renin and causes renal ischemia), and hematuria.
e. Treatment includes radial nephrectomy,

irradiation, and chemotherapy. Long-term follow-up for metastasis.
f. Prognosis depends on child's age and stage and pathology of tumor.

E. Infectious diseases.
1. Pyelonephritis.
a. Inflammation of the kidney, including the renal pelvis.
b. Occurs primarily in females between the ages of 18 and 40 years. Rarely occurs in males.
c. Chronic pyelonephritis represents < 1% of the causes of CKD.
d. Usually caused by enterobacteriaceae (most common *E. coli*) that have ascended from the lower urinary tract into the kidneys.
e. Less commonly, pathogens can reach the kidneys via blood and cause pyelonephritis.
(1) Pathogens from the hematogenous route are different than the ones that ascend the urinary tract (e.g., unlikely enterbacteriaceae).
(2) The hematogenous uropathogens are *S. aureus, Salmonella, P. aeruginosa*, and *Candida* species.
f. Pathophysiology.
(1) Pathogens multiply and create a local and systemic inflammatory response, usually in the renal medulla.
(2) Medulla is susceptible to bacterial invasion because blood circulates more slowly in the medulla, which delays the arrival of leukocytes and thus bacterial phagocytosis.
(3) Kidney becomes edematous from interstitial inflammation, congested circulation, and tubular cell necrosis.
(4) Glomeruli are usually not affected.
(5) Inflammation can be spotty or diffuse. May be contained within the kidney or spread perirenally.
(6) Initial inflammatory phase lasts 1–3 weeks, then healing begins and is usually complete in 6–10 weeks.
(7) Increased susceptibility to pyelonephritis.
(a) Uroepithelial cells have a greater number of receptors for *E. coli* in some individuals.
(b) Kidney trauma, such as with renal transplantation and/or physical trauma.
(c) Urinary tract obstruction. Tissue pressure increased and decreases protective mechanisms.
(d) Ureteral reflux. Creates higher

pressure in calyces causing intrarenal reflux (movement of urine into papillae). Some papillae, because of their anatomic orientation and large ductal openings, are more susceptible to intrarenal reflux.

g. Signs and symptoms.
  (1) Depends on the severity of pyelonephritis. Range from mild to severe.
  (2) Fever, chills, sweats, headache, nausea, vomiting, fatigue.
  (3) Flank (especially at the costoveterbral angle), low back, or abdominal pain.
  (4) Urinalysis reveals leukocytosis, bacteriuria, pyuria, leukocyte casts, antibody-coated bacteria, and urine with nitrites and leukocyte esterase if gram-negative bacteria are present. With the first episode of pyelonephritis, antibody-coated bacteria may not appear for a week.
  (5) With greater severity, positive blood cultures are present and intrarenal and/or perirenal abscesses can develop.

h. Treatment goals.
  (1) Eradicate the pathogen.
  (2) Relieve symptoms.
  (3) Preserve kidney function.
  (4) Prevent septicemia.
  (5) Eliminate any pathogen reservoirs and prevent reoccurrence.

i. Treatment.
  (1) Antibiotic therapy specific to cultured organism; parenteral until clinical improvement (typically 72 hours), then 10 to 14 days of oral therapy.
  (2) Rest, high fluid intake, pain management, and patient education.
  (3) Assess kidney function because many antibiotics are potentially nephrotoxic. Vomiting and fever predispose the patient to fluid volume deficit and prerenal acute failure.

j. Recovery and prognosis.
  (1) If no clinical improvement within 72 hours, suspect an obstruction and/or abscess.
  (2) Prognosis is good. However, with repeated recurrences, scar tissue can replace healthy parenchyma and chronic kidney failure can occur.

k. Preventive measures.
  (1) Urinate when urge occurs, especially after intercourse.
  (2) Avoid intercourse until urinary tract infection (upper or lower) is resolved. May need to change contraception method (e.g., avoid spermicides).
  (3) Treat lower urinary tract infection promptly.
  (4) Avoid instrumentation and/or catheterization of urinary tract.

2. Renal tuberculosis (TB).
  a. Kidneys are the most frequent site for TB outside of the lungs.
  b. Results from hematogenous spread of *Mycobacterium tuberculosis* from the lungs to the kidneys.
    (1) Inflammation usually begins in the renal medulla near the papillae.
    (2) Causes necrosis. Cavities may form. May spread to the cortex and outside the kidney.
  c. Renal TB can develop before signs and symptoms of decreased function are present and result in irreversible kidney damaged. Early detection of renal TB is enhanced by examining urine for tubercle bacilli in all people with pulmonary TB.
  d. Signs and symptoms.
    (1) Dysuria, urinary frequency, flank, or abdominal pain.
    (2) Hematuria, pyuria, tubercle bacilli in urine.
    (3) Suspect with a sterile hematuria and/or pyuria.
    (4) Epididymitis in men.
  e. Kidney failure is rare with 2 months to 6 months of effective antituberculosis drug therapy.

F. Glomerulonephritis (GN).
  1. Introduction.
    a. Inflammatory process that primarily affects the glomerular capillaries.
    b. Third leading cause of CKD. Represents approximately 17% of patients with CKD.
    c. May be primary (occurs mainly in glomeruli), secondary (results from systemic disease that affects kidneys), or idiopathic (unknown or unclear etiology).
    d. Predominant pathology is immune mechanism.
      (1) Primary. Antigen-antibody complexes develop in the glomerular capillaries (e.g., Goodpasture syndrome). Antigen can be a substance found in the kidney (e.g., enzyme), kidney structure (e.g., the basement membrane), or a substance

Table 1.7

Terms Used to Describe Glomerular Diseases

Primary	Disease occurs mainly in the glomeruli and later may or may not involve extrarenal sites
Secondary	Glomerular disease occurs as a consequence of a systemic disease
Idiopathic	Cause is unknown
Acute	Pathologic changes occur over days or weeks
Chronic	Pathologic changes occur over months or years
Rapidly progressive	Constant loss of renal function with minimal recovery potential
Diffuse	Involves all glomeruli
Focal	Involves some glomeruli
Segmental	Involves portions of individual glomeruli
Membranous	Glomerular capillary wall thickens
Proliferative	Number of glomerular cells increases

that has circulated to the kidney (e.g., infectious product).

   (2) Secondary. Antigen-antibody complexes form in the circulation and are entrapped in the glomeruli (e.g., systemic lupus erythematosus).

   (3) Cell-mediated mechanisms include inflammation of inflammatory cells and proliferation of mesangial, epithelial, or endothelial cells.

   (4) Complement activation leads to additional inflammation and/or direct tissue injury.

e. Signs and symptoms.
   (1) Vary by etiology.
   (2) Most common are proteinuria, hematuria, red cell casts.
   (3) Edema and hypertension.

f. Classification systems for glomerulopathies.
   (1) Categorizing glomerular diseases is done by etiology, onset and duration, clinical signs and symptoms, morphologic findings, and pathophysiology.
   (2) Table 1.7 defines terms that describe glomerulopathies.

g. Treatment is based on the specific etiology (e.g., Steroids if lupus-related, controlling volume and hypertension if acute GN).

2. Goodpasture syndrome.
   a. Etiology.
      (1) Unclear, most likely autoimmune.
      (2) Incidence higher in males than females; increased between ages 18 and 35 years.
      (3) Antibodies form against the basement membrane of the glomerular and pulmonary alveolar capillaries resulting in an immune response.
      (4) Focal to diffuse proliferative glomerulonephritis develops rapidly.
      (5) Crescents and inflammatory substances, such as complement and antiglomerular basement membrane antibodies are present.
   b. Renal signs and symptoms.
      (1) Hematuria, proteinuria.
      (2) Casts and immunoglobulins in the urine.
      (3) Elevated plasma levels of antiglomerular basement membrane antibodies.
      (4) Eventually, azotemia, and kidney failure.
   c. Pulmonary involvement.
      (1) Necrosis of alveolar capillaries with pulmonary hemorrhage and poor gas exchange.
      (2) Signs and symptoms.
         (a) Cough, hemoptysis, dyspnea, rales.
         (b) Pallor, anemia, leukocytosis, schistocytes.

(c) Elevated levels of antiglomerular basement membrane antibodies in plasma and lung tissue.

d. Patients may present with either renal or pulmonary signs and symptoms or both.

e. Treatment.
   (1) Immunosuppressants, steroids, plasmapheresis.
   (2) Pulmonary support.
   (3) Supportive care and kidney replacement therapy.

3. Acute poststreptococcal glomerulonephritis (APSGN).
   a. APSGN is classified as a primary glomerular disease.
   b. Onset is 1-4 weeks after beta-hemolytic streptococcal infection of throat or skin.
      (1) Approximately 7–14 days after throat infection.
      (2) Approximately 14–28 days after skin infection.
   c. Occurs primarily during childhood and adolescence. Greater incidence in boys than girls.
   d. Pathogenesis signs and symptoms.
      (1) Antigen-antibody complexes are formed in the circulation and deposited in glomeruli, initiating an inflammatory response.
      (2) As glomeruli are damaged, function is compromised and signs and symptoms of kidney dysfunction appear.
      (3) Glomerular capillaries become more permeable.
      (4) Most patients have gross hematuria, mild proteinuria, and oliguria.
      (5) As glomerular filtration rate decreases, sodium and water are retained, leading to edema (especially periorbital in the morning), weight gain, and hypertension.
      (6) Cerebral and cardiopulmonary signs and symptoms of hypertension and fluid overload may be present including headache, decreased level of consciousness, convulsions, dyspnea, cough, pulmonary edema, and tachycardia.
      (7) Systemic signs and symptoms of infection may be present and include fever, nausea, vomiting, leukocytosis, and elevated antistreptolysin O titers.
      (8) In addition to the presence of blood and protein, the urine is rust colored, and contains red cell, leukocyte, tubular, and granular casts.
      (9) Anemia is secondary to fluid overload.
      (10) Plasma creatinine and BUN may be elevated.
   e. Treatment is nonspecific and primarily symptomatic.
      (1) Bed rest and/or activity as tolerated.
      (2) Diuretics, fluid restriction, and low sodium diet for hypertension and edema.
      (3) Immunosuppressants and/or steroids may be helpful to decrease the immune system response.
      (4) Antibiotics are not helpful.
      (5) Dietary consult for nutrition and low prealbumin/albumin.
      (6) Education about the disease process and treatment.
      (7) Consultation with a child life specialist for age-appropriate activities.
   f. Prognosis is favorable, especially for children and individuals without preexisting kidney disease.
      (1) Signs and symptoms usually resolve within a month.
      (2) Hematuria and proteinuria may require 6 months to a year to resolve.
      (3) Some adults develop chronic glomerulonephritis and CKD.

G. Nephrotic syndrome.
   1. Potential etiologies.
      a. Inflammatory process that damages glomerular basement membrane. Alters glomerular permeability.
      b. Result of degenerative, sclerotic process that alters glomerulus.
      c. Primary (idiopathic) or secondary (due to other systemic disease, e.g., diabetes mellitus).
   2. Clinical signs and symptoms.
      a. Proteinuria > 3.5 g/day (increased capillary permeability).
      b. Hypoalbuminemia (protein loss).
      c. Edema (renal sodium retention and loss of plasma oncotic pressure with hypoalbuminemia).
      d. Hyperlipidemia (increased hepatic production of lipids).
      e. Lipiduria.
      f. Hypercoagulability.
   3. Treatment.
      a. Treat underlying disease state and pathology.
      b. Slow the progression of CKD.
      c. Treat complications (e.g., relieve edema, decrease lipids).

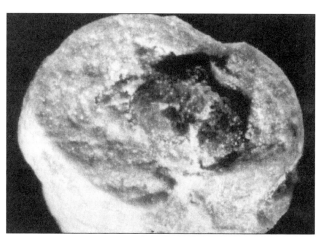

Figure 1.23. Renal calculus. Large kidney stone composed of calcium oxalate and uric acid core.

H. Obstructive disorders.
  1. Nephrolithiasis.
     a. Incidence.
        (1) Peaks between 20 and 50 years of age.
        (2) Higher in males than females.
        (3) More common in southeast, west, and midwest regions of the United States.
     b. Calculi vary in size and composition.
        (1) Most contain calcium.
        (2) Other substances include oxalate, phosphate, magnesium, struvite, uric acid, and cystine (see Figure 1.23).
     c. Etiology and pathogenesis of stone formation (calculogenesis) is unclear.
        (1) Most likely related to supersaturation of urine with a particular substance.
        (2) Compatible urinary pH for precipitation of that substance.
        (3) Presence or absence of inhibitors of crystal formation.
            (a) For example, with hypercalciuria, urine is supersaturated with calcium.
            (b) A nidus or cluster of calcium crystals forms, called nucleation.
            (c) The calcium crystalline mass enlarges, especially in an alkaline urine and in a higher degree of hypercalciuria.
            (d) The developing stone can adhere to any surface structure in the urinary tract, continue to enlarge, and remain in this location or move.
     d. Signs and symptoms.
        (1) Vary; range from none to many with stone movement.
        (2) Nephralgia, nausea, vomiting, hematuria, and weakness.

        (3) Urine and plasma may or may not have an elevated level of the stone forming substance.
     e. Treatment goals.
        (1) Prevent the recurrence of stones.
        (2) Decrease continued development of existing stones.
        (3) Decrease urinary concentration of stone forming substances.
        (4) General measures.
            (a) High fluid intake (3–4 L/day) is essential and must continue indefinitely.
            (b) Alterations in diet to avoid or decrease the stone-forming substance are controversial.
            (c) Some drugs help to reduce urinary excretion of stone-forming substances (thiazide diuretics and calcium, allopurinol and uric acid, penicillamine and cystine).
        (5) Sequelae to existing calculi are infection, bleeding, obstruction, recurrence, and CKD stage 5 (uncommon).
        (6) If stone does not pass spontaneously, invasive procedures to remove the stone may be needed (e.g., surgery, lithotriptic agent, nephroscope, or lithotripsy).
        (7) Approximately 40–85% recur. About one third of patients with recurrent stones will lose function of the affected kidney.
  2. Retroperitoneal fibrosis.
     a. Exact cause unknown but associated with administration of methysergide and systemic infections.
     b. Fibrotic tissue develops in the retroperitoneal abdominal cavity and grows around and compresses the ureters (see Figure 1.24).
     c. Postrenal obstruction occurs that can lead to failure if not diagnosed promptly.
     d. Signs and symptoms are similar to those of postrenal azotemia (see previous discussion).
     e. Treatment includes ureterolysis and administration of steroids.

III. Kidney problems due to systemic diseases.

A. Diabetic nephropathy.
  1. Introduction.
     a. Diabetes mellitus (DM) is a chronic disorder of carbohydrate metabolism resulting from inadequate production and/or inability to use endogenous insulin.
     b. DM is classified into type 1 (lack of insulin)

or type 2 (decreased production of insulin or inability of tissues to use endogenous insulin).
c. Long-term detrimental effects of DM include negative vascular effects throughout the body.
d. DM is a major cause of CKD. Approximately 40% of individuals with CKD stage 5 have diabetes mellitus (most have DM type 2).
e. Diabetic nephropathy refers to kidney disease associated with diabetes mellitus and occurs with both type 1 and type 2 DM.

2. Pathophysiology.
a. Affects and eventually destroys the ability of the afferent and efferent arterioles and glomerular capillaries to function.
b. Glomerular changes include basement membrane thickening, fusion of foot processes, glomerular enlargement, and diffuse sclerosis.
c. The glomerular capillaries lose their selective permeability, become increasingly permeable, causing proteinuria, and contribute to a decreased glomerular filtration rate (GFR).
d. The afferent and efferent arterioles have a decreased ability to respond to systemic blood pressure changes, also resulting in a decreased GFR.
e. Late in the disease, tubular atrophy and interstitial fibrosis occur.
f. Hyperglycemia is a major contributing factor to nephropathy.
g. Hypertension and elevated pressure within the glomeruli also contribute to diabetic nephropathy.

3. Signs and symptoms.
a. Microalbuminuria (30–300 mg/day [SI = 0.44–2.2 mmol/day]) is the hallmark sign of diabetic nephropathy.
b. Borderline hypertension is often present.
c. Progresses to proteinuria, hypoalbuminemia, hypertension, edema, azotemia (rising plasma creatinine and decreasing GFR).
d. By the time diabetic nephropathy has occurred retinopathy and neuropathy are also present.
e. The development of diabetic nephropathy is painless.

4. Progression of diabetic nephropathy.
a. At the onset of DM most people have increased GFR, slightly enlarged kidneys, and albuminuria that is reversible with control of blood glucose.
b. Within 5 years, glomerular changes are usually evident.
c. With progression (may occur after 10–25 years), overt proteinuria and hypertension are evident and are ominous signs.

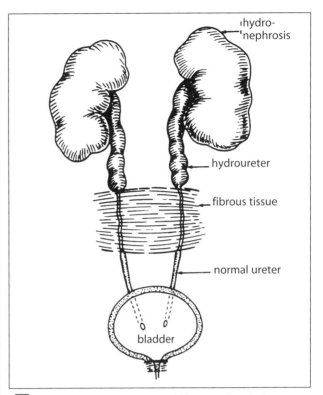

Figure 1.24. Retroperitoneal fibrosis. Fibrotic tissue develops in the retroperitoneal abdominal cavity and grows around and compresses the ureters. The compression creates a retrograde pressure up the urinary tract causing the ureters to enlarge (hydroureter) and the kidneys to enlarge (hydronephrosis).

Sourrce: Richard, C.J. (1986). *Comprehensive nephrology nursing.* Boston: Little, Brown. Used with permission.

d. CKD stage 5 develops within 7–10 years in 50% of these patients.

5. Preventive measures.
a. When the diagnosis of DM is confirmed, and yearly thereafter, patients should be tested for microalbuminuria.
(1) If microalbumin is present on dipstick/reagent strip, urine should be sent to the laboratory to quantify the amount of albumin/protein present.
(2) Research indicates that preventing and decreasing microalbuminuria slows the progression of diabetic nephropathy.
b. Preventive measures focus on preventing microalbuminuria and controlling blood glucose and hypertension.
(1) Angiotensin-converting enzyme (ACE) inhibitors are renoprotective independent of blood pressure lowering effects.

(2) Control blood pressure; < 130/80 mm Hg; < 125/75 if proteinuria present.

(3) Control blood glucose; fasting glucose < 120 mg/dL; hemoglobin A1c < 7%.

6. Patient education.
   a. Control of DM.
   b. Measures to prevent nephropathy.
   c. Importance of regular follow up of kidney function.
7. Treatment.
   a. Treatment goals are to minimize the complications of DM, including CKD.
   b. Patients with decreased kidney function are more susceptible to acute kidney injury from volume depletion (because of compromised autoregulation) and nephrotoxic substances (especially iodine-based dyes, nonsteroidal antiinflammatory drugs, antibiotics).
   c. As kidney failure progresses, the dosage of insulin needed to control blood glucose is reduced because of a decreased ability of the kidneys to metabolize insulin, increasing the half-life of insulin.
   d. Treatment options for CKD stage 5 include all kidney replacement therapies (hemodialysis, peritoneal dialysis, transplantation).
8. Mortality and morbidity of a person with CKD due to diabetic nephropathy is usually due to cardiovascular complications.

B. Hypertensive nephropathy.
   1. Introduction.
      a. Kidneys are major organs affected by hypertension.
      b. Nephrosclerosis refers to kidney disease associated with hypertension.
      c. Kidney damage develops slowly and is associated with chronic mild and moderate hypertension.
      d. 5% of patients with hypertension have kidney disease.
      e. Over 80% of patients with CKD stages 3–4 have hypertension.
      f. Over 90% of patient with CKD stage 5 have hypertension.
      g. Second most common cause (> 24%) of CKD stage 5.
   2. Pathophysiology.
      a. Renal arterial vessels become thickened and the lumens narrow.
      b. Results in decreased renal blood flow and autoregulation.
      c. Renal tubular changes correlate with the degree of reduction in renal blood flow.
      d. Arterioles and glomerular capillaries become thickened and necrotic. The tubules atrophy.
   3. Signs and symptoms.
      a. Consistently elevated blood pressure >140/90 mm Hg in general population; >130/80 in individuals with diabetes mellitus or chronic kidney disease.
      b. Headache (especially in the morning), blurred vision.
      c. Symptoms of congestive heart failure (e.g., edema, dyspnea).
   4. Treatment.
      a. Control blood pressure with goal of <125/75 mm Hg.
      b. Medications: antihypertensives, diuretics.
      c. Lifestyle modification: diet, exercise.
   5. Malignant hypertension.
      a. Associated with marked hypertension, headache, acute congestive heart failure, and blurred vision.
      b. Kidney failure may develop rapidly.
      c. Indicated by hematuria with red cell casts, proteinuria, and azotemia.
      d. Treatment is focused on immediate reduction of blood pressure to prevent permanent loss of kidney function and damage to other organs (e.g., brain, eyes).

C. Renovascular hypertension (RVH).
   1. Hypertension from renal artery stenosis.
      a. Results from overstimulation of the renin-angiotensin-aldosterone system.
      b. Accounts for approximately 5% of people with hypertension.
      c. Occurs more often before age 25 and after 60.
      d. May be the cause of new onset hypertension after kidney transplant.
      e. Usually treatable.
   2. Etiology.
      a. Renal artery and/or its branches become thickened, stiff, and narrow.
      b. Due to atheromatous plaques (atherosclerosis) or fibromuscular dysplasia (see Figure 1.25A).
      c. Fibromuscular dysplasia occurs more often in females, especially from 20 to 40 years of age.
      d. Less common causes include radiation fibrosis, thromboembolism, congenital anomaly, extrinsic compression, and Takayasu syndrome in people from South Asia.
   3. Pathophysiology.
      a. Decreased blood flow stimulates renin release.
      b. Renin converts angiotensinogen to angiotensin I.

c. Angiotensin-converting enzyme (ACE) converts angiotensin I to angiotensin II, causing vasoconstriction that leads to hypertension.
d. Angiotensin II also stimulates release of aldosterone.
   (1) Increases renal absorption of sodium.
   (2) Causes volume expansion and hypertension.
4. Signs and symptoms.
   a. Mild or severe hypertension.
   b. May be recent onset and difficult to control.
   c. Bruit auscultated in flank or abdomen.
   d. Elevated blood renin level from the renal vein of the affected kidney.
   e. Stenotic vessels on renal arteriogram or magnetic resonance angiogram.
   f. Positive response to ace inhibitors. ACE inhibitor test with or without renogram establishes RVH.
      (1) Baseline renin levels are established, ace inhibitor administered and renin levels measured at specified intervals. An increase in serum renin indicates renal artery stenosis.
      (2) With renogram, baseline glomerular filtration rate (GFR) is established by radionuclide clearance. ACE inhibitor administered and radionuclide clearance is again measured. With renal artery stenosis the clearance (and therefore GFR) decreases with the ACE inhibitor.
5. Treatment.
   a. Surgical repair/reconstruction of the stenotic vessels with a graft, renal arterial angioplasty, placement of stent in renal artery (see Figure 1.25 B-E).
   b. Antihypertensives and diuretics.
   c. Nephrectomy rarely indicated.

D. Systemic lupus erythematosus (SLE).
1. Incidence.
   a. Greater in females than males.
   b. Many organs and systems can be affected, especially musculoskeletal, skin, kidney, and cardiovascular.
   c. Onset usually between adolescence and fourth decade.
      (1) 80% of patients with SLE have some degree of kidney involvement.
      (2) 40% patients with SLE develop lupus nephritis.
      (3) Generally occurs within 5 years of onset of lupus.

(4) Represents about 2% patients with CKD stage 5.
d. May be due to an inherited trait involving chromosome 6 and represents a defect in genetic control of immune response.
e. Some drugs induce SLE-like syndrome. When drugs are discontinued, SLE-like signs and symptoms subside.
2. Pathophysiology.
   a. Most likely autoimmune.
   b. Chronic systemic inflammatory disorder of connective tissue, especially the arterial vasculature.
   c. Autoantibodies are formed against constituents of cells (e.g., DNA, RNA, cell membranes) and blood substances, such as coagulation factors.
   d. Antigen-antibody complexes form, lodge in blood vessels, and initiate an inflammatory response that injures the vasculature and surrounding tissue.
   e. Lupus nephritis.
      (1) Immune complexes are deposited in glomerular capillaries.
      (2) An inflammatory/immune response follows that injures the capillaries and adjacent structures.
3. Signs and symptoms.
   a. Vary depending upon degree of organ/system involvement.
   b. Many patients present with general signs and symptoms of inflammation, such as fatigue, fever, and weight loss, nondeforming arthritis, and a skin rash (characteristic "butterfly rash" occurs in about 30% of individuals).
   c. Elevated blood levels of antinuclear antibody (ANA) and/or anti-DNA antibody and serum complement changes.
   d. Lupus nephritis.
      (1) Urinalysis indicates proteinuria, hematuria, red cell casts.
      (2) Hypertension, edema, nephrotic syndrome.
4. World health Organization (WHO) classification system for the glomerular injury associated with lupus nephritis.
   a. Classification system is based on the findings of kidney biopsy (see Table 1.8).
   b. Use of the WHO classification system helps determine therapies and prognosis.
   c. Signs and symptoms do not always correlate with histologic findings (e.g., approximately 25% of the patients with class IV renal biopsy

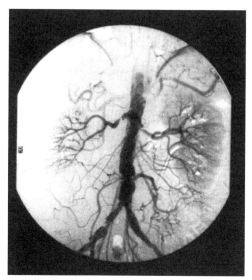

Figure 1.25 (A-E). Bilateral renal artery stenosis. Right femoral artery was used for access to the vascular system.

A
Abdominal aortogram and renal arteriogram. Bilaterally, renal arteries are narrowed near their exit from the aorta. The right kidney is small and the left kidney is normal size. The distal aorta and right common iliac artery have moderate to high-grade stenosis.

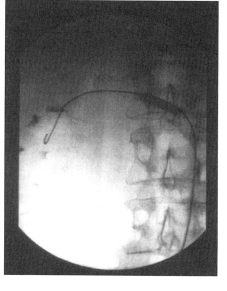

B
Right renal artery was catheterized and angioplasty attempted with balloon inflation.

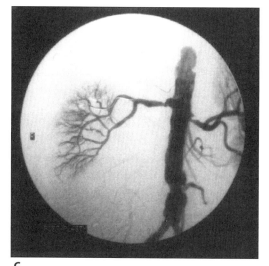

C
Renal artery stenosis remains after angioplasty.

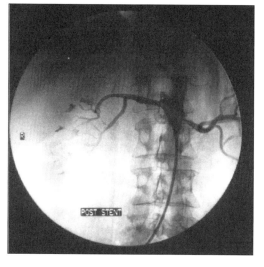

D
A stent was placed in the right renal artery and angiogram demonstrates adequate blood flow through the stent into the distal renal arteries.

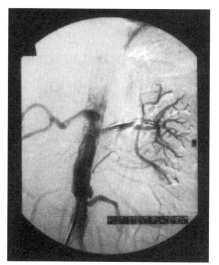

E
Left renal artery angioplasty was attempted, and the left renal artery stenosis remains. A stent was placed in the left renal artery and angiogram demonstrates normal blood flow through the stent into the distal left renal arteries.

Table 1.8

World Health Organization (WHO) Classification of Lupus Nephritis Lesions

Class		Description
I	Normal glomeruli	
II	Mesangial glomerulonephritis	Immune deposits found in mesangial regions only
III	Focal segmental glomerulonephritis	Mild or moderate mesangial alterations, Class II plus deposits of complement
IV	Diffuse proliferative glomerulonephritis	Injury more widespread and extensive than Class III
V	Diffuse membranous glomerulonephritis	All of the above classes plus granular deposits
VI	Advanced glomerulonephritis sclerosis	

findings have no clinical signs and symptoms of kidney involvement).

5. Prevention.
   a. For individuals with a diagnosis of SLE, assess the urine regularly, for hematuria, proteinuria, and casts (red and/or white cell).
   b. Monitor creatinine and BUN.
   c. Early detection and treatment of lupus nephritis is key to delaying progression of kidney involvement.
6. Treatment addresses systemic and kidney problems.
   a. Treatment of systemic problems addresses fatigue, sensitivity to sunlight, susceptibility to infection, decreased mobility.
   b. Patient teaching regarding the disease process, prognosis, treatment.
   c. Body image changes, altered emotional status, impaired coping mechanisms also need to be addressed.
   d. Pharmacologic agents include glucocorticoids, steroids (to a lesser degree), immunosuppressants, anticoagulants, cytotoxins, analgesics, and antimalarials for skin manifestations.
   e. Plasmapheresis may be helpful in some patients.
   f. Actions to preserve kidney function (e.g., control hypertension and avoid nephrotoxins). Early referral to a nephrologist is needed.
   g. Renal replacement therapy (dialysis, transplantation) if progresses to CKD stage 5.

E. Scleroderma or progressive systemic sclerosis.
   1. Systemic disease characterized by an accumulation of collagen in connective tissue and proliferative lesions in capillaries and small arteries.
      a. More common in females, especially 20–50 years of age.
      b. Increased risk in individuals of African ethnicity.
   2. Pathophysiology.
      a. Etiology unclear but related to autoimmune mechanisms and abnormal production of collagen.
      b. Vascular and collagen changes result in connective tissue thickening.
      c. Localized form of scleroderma mainly affects skin and viscera (gastrointestinal tract, lungs, heart, and musculoskeletal system).
         (1) Major cause of skin and viscera changes is ischemia.
         (2) Characteristic skin changes are Raynaud phenomenon and a feeling that the skin is turning to stone.
      d. Vascular changes lead to structural and functional organ changes, including the kidneys.
      e. Approximately 50% of patients with scleroderma develop renal ischemia and tubular changes.
         (1) About 15% of these patients develop a renal crisis, oliguric kidney failure that results from severe ischemia. Associated with malignant hypertension and very high renin blood levels (12 times normal).

      (2) Major preventive measure for a renal crisis is to control hypertension.

  3. Treatment.

    a. Goals.

      (1) Control collagen accumulation and vascular destruction.

      (2) Control hypertension.

      (3) Alleviate general signs and symptoms.

    b. Teach signs and symptoms, prevention, and interventions to alleviate Raynaud phenomenon.

    c. Maintain nutrition and physical mobility.

    d. Plasmapheresis may be helpful.

    e. If progresses to CKD stage 5, decreased clearances may occur with either type of dialysis because of widespread vascular abnormalities.

F. Amyloidosis.

  1. Systemic disease characterized by deposits of amyloid (beta-2 microglobulins), a fibrillar glycoprotein, in many organs including the kidneys.

  2. Pathophysiology.

    a. Etiology is idiopathic.

    b. Associated with multiple myeloma and any chronic inflammatory condition that continuously and intensely stimulates the immune system.

    c. May be primary or secondary.

      (1) Primary. Kidney disease results from amyloid fibrils produced by immunoglobulin light chains deposited in glomeruli, blood vessels, tubules.

      (2) Secondary. Amyloid fibrils produced by the liver as an acute phase reactant serum protein in response to a chronic inflammatory state deposited in glomeruli, blood vessels, tubules.

    d. Results in proteinuria and may progress to the nephrotic syndrome.

    e. With renal tubular involvement, renal tubular acidosis and nephrogenic diabetes insipidus (kidneys unable to respond to antidiuretic hormone) can occur.

    f. Onset of CKD stage 4 or 5 is approximately 1–4 years from the onset of proteinuria.

  3. Diagnosis.

    a. Positive Congo red test (dye is injected intravenously and binds to amyloid, producing a characteristic yellow-green fluorescence under the microscope).

    b. Proteinuria, hypoalbuminemia, peripheral edema.

    c. Signs, symptoms of decreasing kidney function.

  4. There is no specific treatment for primary amyloidosis. Treatment of secondary amyloidosis focuses on decreasing the underlying inflammatory process.

G. Gout.

  1. Metabolic disorder that results in hyperuricemia and inflammation of the joints.

  2. Kidney disease results from effect of hyperuricemia.

    a. All patients with gout do not develop kidney disease.

    b. Possible outcomes.

      (1) Massive precipitation of uric acid crystals within nephron leads to tubular obstruction and altered kidney function and potential kidney failure.

      (2) Formation of uric acid nephrolithiasis and subsequent potential for kidney failure.

  3. Treatment.

    a. Reduce hyperuricemia and prevent uric acid crystallization.

    b. High fluid intake, alkalinization of urine, administration of allopurinol.

H. HIV (human immunodeficiency virus) associated nephropathy (HIVAN).

  1. Introduction.

    a. Most common cause CKD in HIV-seropositive individuals.

    b. Highest incidence.

      (1) African Americans, 20–64 years old.

      (2) Associated with IV drug use.

      (3) More common in males.

    c. Progresses to CKD stage 5 within weeks to months without HIV treatment.

    d. Increases risk of overall mortality and after the initiation of dialyis (50% at 1 year).

  2. Pathophysiology.

    a. HIV genome present in kidney tissue.

    b. May or may not result in kidney disease (other immune mechanisms also needed).

    c. Tubular interstitium infiltrated with leukocytes.

    d. Thought to involve replication of virus within mesangial cells.

  3. Diagnosis.

    a. Present with nephritic syndrome symptoms: proteinuria, edema, hypoalbuminemia.

    b. Rapidly progressive loss of kidney function.

    c. Large, echogenic kidneys on ultrasound.

d. CD4 count < 200 mm^2; HIV viral load
   > 500 copies/mL.
4. Treatment.
   a. Angiotensin-converting enzyme inhibitors
      (decrease proteinuria, edema).
   b. Antiretroviral drugs (HAART: highly active
      antiretroviral therapy drug regimen).
   c. Steroids controversial. May slow progression
      to HIVAN.

I. Hepatorenal syndrome.
   1. Kidney failure that occurs in the presence of
      severe liver dysfunction.
      a. Characterized by systemic vasodilation and
         renal vasoconstriction that results in kidney
         hypoperfusion.
      b. May be related to humoral agents produced
         or inadequately deactivated by the poorly
         functioning liver.
      c. No structural kidney changes occur.
   2. Signs and symptoms.
      a. Oliguria.
      b. Increased BUN and creatinine (rarely
         > 5.0 mg/dL).
      c. Urine sediment is usually normal.
      d. Jaundice, hypoalbuminemia.
      e. Ascites, portal hypertension.
      f. Splenomegaly.
   3. Treatment.
      a. Maintain fluid balance (fluid depletion
         enhances the development of kidney failure).
      b. Avoid neomycin (potentially nephrotoxic).
      c. Prepare for liver transplant, if appropriate.
      d. Kidney function usually recovers with a
         functioning liver transplant.
   4. Prognosis is poor due to combined liver and
      kidney failure.

J. Henoch-Schönlein syndrome (HSS).
   1. Incidence.
      a. Affects children between the ages of 2 and 11
         years.
      b. Slightly higher incidence in boys than girls.
      c. Rarely occurs in adults (the adult form of
         HSS is Berger disease).
      d. Incidence of kidney involvement is variable
         (10–92% of patients have kidney
         involvement, most of which is mild).
   2. Pathophysiology.
      a. Etiology unclear, probably immune.
      b. Associated with streptococcal infections,
         varicella, mycoplasma pneumoniae, drugs,
         food, allergies, insect bites, vaccinations, and
         exposure to cold.

   c. An increased number of IgA complexes
      produce an immune-inflammatory response
      that injures the glomerular capillaries.
   d. Results in a generalized vasculitis that affects
      small blood vessels in the skin, joints, kidney,
      and GI tract.
   3. Signs and symptoms.
      a. General.
         (1) Elevated plasma IgA.
         (2) Presence of IgA immune complexes in
             blood vessels.
         (3) Asymmetric, nonpruritic, purpuric-
             petechial rash on extremities and
             buttocks.
         (4) Nondeforming arthralgia and arthritis,
             mostly of ankles and knees.
         (5) Abdominal pain, vomiting, GI bleeding.
      b. Kidney involvement.
         (1) Presence of IgA complexes and
             complement in glomerular capillaries
             on biopsy.
         (2) Hematuria, proteinuria.
         (3) Hypertension, azotemia, and nephrotic
             syndrome.
         (4) Skin and gastrointestinal signs and
             symptoms usually precede kidney
             manifestations.
   4. Treatment.
      a. Nonspecific and primarily symptomatic.
      b. Corticosteroids, nonsteroidal antiinflammatory
         agents, immunosuppressants, and
         anticoagulants may be used.
      c. Plasmapheresis.
      d. Renal replacement therapy as needed.

K. Primary hyperparathyroidism.
   1. Etiology. Hyperplasia and neoplasms of
      parathyroid glands, history of neck irradiation,
      and parathyroid hormone secreting tumors.
   2. Incidence greater in females. Age greater than
      40 years.
   3. Pathophysiology. Uncontrolled secretion of
      parathyroid hormone (PTH) results in elevated
      PTH blood levels despite hypercalcemia
      (normally acts as negative feedback control for
      the parathyroid gland to decrease PTH secretion).
   4. Kidney effects are the result of hypercalcemia.
      a. Hypercalciuria and nephrolithiasis (discussed
         earlier).
      b. Nephrocalcinosis (deposits of calcium
         phosphate in nephron).
      c. Nephrogenic diabetes insipidus (hypercalcemia
         interferes with action of ADH on the tubules).
      d. Additional effects from the elevated PTH are

hyperphosphaturia and hyperchloremic metabolic acidosis (bicarbonate reabsorption is decreased, hydrogen ions are not buffered, and chloride is reabsorbed).

5. Treatment.
   a. Usually includes partial parathyroidectomy, high fluid intake, and adequate ambulation.
   b. May include dietary calcium restriction, phosphate supplements, and estrogens.

IV. The kidney and pregnancy.

A. Normal changes in pregnancy.
   1. Kidneys and urinary tract structures undergo anatomic and physiologic changes during pregnancy.
   2. Changes begin to reverse during the first week postpartum and are completed by the 12th week postpartum.
   3. Changes.
      a. Kidneys enlarge approximately 1–2 cm due to increased intrarenal blood volume, dilation of the collecting system, and hypertrophy.
      b. Collecting system (calyces, renal pelvis, and ureters) dilates due to hormonal influences (termed physiologic hydronephrosis of pregnancy).
      c. Ureters dilate, become tortuous (hydroureter).
         (1) Causes decreased ureteral peristalsis.
         (2) Leads to increased urine stasis and susceptibility to pyelonephritis.
      d. Bladder is displaced anteriorly and superiorly. Capacity is increased.
      e. Renal blood flow (RBF).
         (1) Increases up to 50% above normal by second trimester and remains elevated throughout pregnancy.
         (2) Due to increased cardiac output, dilation of renal vessels.
         (3) Declines to normal just before delivery.
      f. Increased RBF increases glomerular filtration (GFR).
         (1) Begins to increase at 4 weeks gestation.
         (2) Peaks by 13 weeks and continues until delivery.
         (3) GFR varies with position. Lower in the supine than lateral recumbent.
      g. Increased GFR leads to increased solute clearances.
      h. Normal solute plasma values are lower in pregnant than nonpregnant woman.
         (1) Plasma creatinine is 0.46 mg ± 0.13 mg/dL (SI = 40.5 mmol ± 11.44 mmol/L) and BUN is 8.7 mg ± 1.5 mg/dL (SI = 3.13 mmol ± 0.54 mmol/L).
         (2) Creatinine greater than 0.9 mg/dL (SI = 80 mmol/L) and BUN greater than 14 mg/dL (SI = 50.4 mmol/L) generally indicates kidney dysfunction.
         (3) Serum uric acid values lower. Urine values higher.
         (4) Serum sodium is 5–10 mEq/L (SI = same) less; osmolality is approximately 10 mOsm/kg H_2O (SI = same) less.
      i. As a result of the increased GFR, the increased volume of glomerular filtrate exceeds tubular reabsorption capabilities.
         (1) Proteinuria 300–500 mg/day (SI = same).
         (2) Glycosuria, usually without hyperglycemia.
         (3) Aminoaciduria.
         (4) Increased nutrients in urine may enhance bacterial growth and subsequent urinary tract infection.
      j. Renal bicarbonate threshold decreases.
         (1) As a result, the plasma bicarbonate level is lower, approximately 10–20 mEq/L (SI = same).
         (2) Plasma pH decreases to 7.44 (SI = same).
         (3) Causes the urine to be alkaline in the early morning.
      k. Total body water increases by 6–8 liters, sodium reabsorption increases, and subsequent dependent edema may develop.
      l. Prostaglandins, renin, and angiotensinogen increase due to unclear mechanisms.
      m. The enlarging uterus may cause incomplete bladder emptying, vesicoureteral reflux, and ureteral obstruction, leading to an increased risk for pyelonephritis.

B. Pyelonephritis.
   1. Most common infectious complication in pregnancy.
      a. Overall incidence among pregnant women 1–2%.
      b. Often develops when asymptomatic bacteriuria is poorly or not treated.
         (1) 5% have asymptomatic bacteriuria.
         (2) 30% with asymptomatic bacteriuria will get pyelonephritis.
      c. *Escherichia coli* is the most common (80%) pathogen. Klebsiella, enterobacter, and proteus are less common.
      d. Prevention is accomplished through careful screening and treating all pregnant women with asymptomatic bacteriuria (>100,000 colonies/mL of urine without urinary tract symptoms).

2. Signs and symptoms.
   a. Fever, as high as 104°F (40°C), chills.
   b. Nausea, vomiting.
   c. Flank tenderness/pain, especially at costovertebral angle.
   d. Urinalysis indicates bacteria, white cell casts, red blood cells, leukocyte esterase, and nitrites.
   e. A small percentage of women may have positive blood cultures.
3. Treatment.
   a. Hospitalization for parenteral antibiotics.
   b. Moderate fluid intake.
   c. Follow-up care during the remainder of the pregnancy with possible prophylactic antibiotics to prevent recurrent infection.
4. Has been associated with premature labor and intrauterine fetal death.

C. Acute kidney failure.
1. Acute kidney failure occurs in 1 of every 2000–5000 pregnancies.
2. Frequency distribution is bimodal.
   a. First peak in early pregnancy. Associated with septic abortion and shock and fluid and electrolyte imbalances from hyperemesis.
   b. Second peak in final gestational month. Associated with preeclampsia, hemorrhagic complications, abruptio placenta.
   c. Associated with:
      (1) Urinary tract obstruction from stone and/or ureteral obstruction from the uterus.
      (2) Intravascular coagulation.
      (3) Prolonged intrauterine fetal death.
3. Treatment similar to nongravidas with acute kidney injury.
4. Dialysis may need to be implemented early to maintain a normal fetal environment because urea, creatinine, and other metabolic waste substances cross the placenta.

D. Pregnancy and chronic kidney disease.
1. Pregnancy does not generally affect early stages of kidney disease if hypertension is absent at conception (e.g., as in glomerulonephritis and renal tuberculosis).
2. In women with early stage CKD who become pregnant, acceleration in kidney dysfunction may occur. Reversal of decreased kidney function with termination of pregnancy cannot be assured/predicted.
3. When hypertension and kidney disease coexist, pregnancy is more likely to be associated with complications, such as severe hypertension and/or decline in kidney function.

a. Fetal surveillance is important (e.g., by ultrasound) because intrauterine retardation can occur.
b. Risk for small for gestational age and premature infant is greater than general population.
4. The ability to conceive decreases proportionally with the level of kidney impairment.
   a. With declining kidney function, plasma creatinine > 3 mg/dL (SI = 264 mmol/L) and BUN > 30 mg/dL (SI = 10.8 mmol/L) fertility decreases and normal gestation is unlikely.
   b. < 1% of women on dialysis conceive. 30% deliver a live infant.
   c. 20% of infants are premature and/or are small for gestational age.
   d. 10% of pregnancies that continue beyond the second trimester result in stillbirth.
5. Specific populations.
   a. Women with SLE.
      (1) Have variable courses during pregnancy.
      (2) Generally, the longer SLE has been in remission prior to pregnancy, the greater the possibility for a symptom-free gestation.
      (3) Serum complement should be monitored frequently to detect exacerbation and treatment initiated if serum levels decrease.
   b. Prognosis for successful pregnancy in women with periarteritis nodosa and scleroderma is generally poor because of the kidney involvement and hypertension.
6. After kidney transplant.
   a. Fertility usually returns 4–6 months after kidney transplantation.
   b. Women are encouraged to avoid conception for 1 to 2 years after transplant because of the increased incidence of graft rejection.
   c. Kidney function and fetal growth and development should be monitored carefully throughout the pregnancy.
   d. Immunosuppressive therapy increases the risk for maternal and fetal infections.

V. Acute and chronic kidney failure associated with nonkidney organ transplantation.

A. Incidence.
1. Acute and/or chronic kidney failure can follow solid organ (liver, heart, and lung) and bone marrow transplantation.
2. The incidence of some degree of kidney dysfunction/failure may be as high as 50%.

B. Contributing factors.
 1. Major cause of chronic kidney failure after transplantation is nephrotoxic immunosuppressant agents, especially cyclosporine a and tacrolimus that may contribute to the development of acute and/or chronic kidney failure.
 2. Pretransplant factors.
  a. High acuity of heart and liver failure patients pretransplant and the negative impact on kidney function.
  b. Hepatorenal syndrome with liver failure patients pretransplant and the challenge to accurately determine kidney function.
  c. CKD stage 1 or 2 before transplantation.
 3. Posttransplant factors.
  a. Prolonged intubation and ventilatory support.
  b. Development of hypertension.
  c. Development of proteinuria.
  d. Hyperlipidemia.
 4. Additional factors.
  a. Donor organ from an older person.
  b. Inherent perioperative risks.
  c. Kidney hypoperfusion during surgery.

C. Pathophysiology.
 1. Recipients of organ transplants receive immunosuppressants and other drugs to prevent graft rejection that are potentially nephrotoxic.
 2. Pathogenesis of acute and chronic kidney failure (CKF) are not fully understood.
 3. General concepts.
  a. Development of kidney failure is similar across patients although the specific organ or tissue transplanted is different.
  b. Acute kidney injury and CKD can occur independently of each other.
  c. All kidney structures are affected.
   (1) Glomeruli are ischemic and collapse.
   (2) Tubules atrophy.
   (3) Interstitial fibrosis occurs.
   (4) Afferent arteriole vasoconstriction and subsequent decreased glomerular filtration rate are common with acute and chronic kidney failure.
 4. Treatment.
  a. Similar to overall treatment of acute and/or chronic kidney failure.
  b. Tapering and eliminating nephrotoxic immunosuppressants may help.
  c. When CKD stage 5 occurs, all kidney replacement therapies may be instituted, including kidney transplant.

Chapter 3

Assessment of Kidney Structure and Function

Purpose

Standard 1 (Assessment) of the *The Nephrology Nursing Standards of Practice and Guidelines for Care* states: "The nephrology nurse collects comprehensive data pertinent to the patient's health or the situation." The purpose of this chapter is to provide a guide for history and physical assessment of patients with kidney disease and to provide an overview of methods used to assess kidney structure and function. The related nursing interventions are also summarized.

Objectives

Upon completion of this chapter, the learner will be able to:
1. Obtain a comprehensive health history on a patient experiencing kidney disease.
2. Perform a systematic physical examination on a patient experiencing kidney problems.
3. State typical history and physical assessment findings in patients with kidney disorders.
4. Explain the four physical examination techniques used to perform a kidney assessment.
5. Discuss limitations of the findings related to physical examination of the kidneys.
6. Describe nursing responsibilities for collection of urine specimens and distribution to the laboratory.
7. Relate abnormal urinalysis findings to underlying renal pathophysiology.
8. Compare plasma creatinine to blood urea nitrogen in terms of normal blood levels, significance to kidney assessment, and changes in kidney disease.
9. Explain the basis for using plasma electrolyte levels to assess kidney function.
10. Relate creatinine clearance to kidney function.
11. Discuss the nursing responsibilities related to performing a creatinine clearance test.
12. Identify the purpose and nursing responsibilities related to a renal scan and renogram.
13. Describe the indications, procedure, and patient care for renal arteriogram and venogram.
14. Differentiate kidney ultrasound, computerized axial tomography, and magnetic resonance imaging.
15. Outline patient teaching for a kidney ultrasound, computerized axial tomography, and magnetic resonance imaging.
16. Summarize the purpose, procedure, patient care, and potential complications of an intravenous pyelography.
17. Compare retrograde, antegrade, and intravenous pyelographies.
18. Discuss the potential for adverse reaction to radiopaque contrast media.
19. Explain the purpose, indications, contraindications, and potential complications associated with a kidney biopsy.
20. Describe the nursing care for a patient before, during, and after kidney biopsy.
21. Identify potential complications associated with a kidney biopsy.

I. History and physical assessment.

Format for the patient with kidney problems:
Table 1.9 provides a detailed outline for a history and physical assessment format for patients experiencing kidney problems. A basic understanding of interviewing and familiarity with physical assessment skills are prerequisites. See the reference list at the end of this section for readings that expand on the history and physical examination.

II. Physical assessment of the kidneys.

A. Patient preparation.
  1. Before beginning the physical assessment, tell the patient what will happen, address questions and concerns, provide privacy, and help the patient relax.
  2. The environment should be at a comfortable temperature with adequate lighting. The nurse needs to warm his or her hands and any equipment that will be used (such as a stethoscope).

B. Inspection.
  1. Patient is supine with examiner on right side.
  2. Inspect right and left upper quadrants at the midclavicular line, from a standing position and at eye level.
  3. Inspect for raised areas, masses, or unusual pulsations.
     a. Raised masses may be a large polycystic kidney or hypernephroma.
     b. Unusual pulsations may be an arterial aneurysm.
  4. Inspect lower quadrant at midline. A distended bladder may be visible midline across the lower quadrants.

C. Auscultation.
  1. Bell of the stethoscope is held lightly against the abdomen slightly to the right and left of the midline in both upper quadrants.
  2. With the patient in a supine position, listen for a renal or aortic bruit (a low pitched murmur), indicating renal arterial stenosis or aortic aneurysm.
  3. With the patient in a prone or sitting position, auscultate the entire costovertebral angle (area where the twelfth rib and vertebral column intersect) for bruits.

D. Palpation.
  1. Kidneys.
     a. The kidneys are located deep in the abdomen and are difficult to palpate.
     b. Moderate to deep palpation is required.
     c. Place one hand posteriorly under the flank and place the other hand anteriorly over the lower aspect of the upper quadrant on the same side of the body. Posteriorly elevate the kidney by pushing up, and ask the patient to breathe deeply. During exhalation, anteriorly palpate deeply for the kidney.
     d. Occasionally the lower pole of a normal sized right kidney is palpated as a solid, firm, but elastic mass that moves with inspiration. (Polycystic kidneys usually feel bumpy.)
     e. Enlarged kidneys may indicate hydronephrosis, neoplasms, or polycystic disease.
  2. Urinary bladder.
     a. Palpate bladder at midline 1 cm above symphysis pubis.
     b. A distended bladder feels smooth, round, and tense, and can extend above the umbilicus.
     c. The patient may feel pressure or the urge to void if the bladder is distended.

E. Percussion.
  1. Kidneys are difficult to percuss anteriorly because they are located deep and posterior in the abdominal cavity.
  2. Posteriorly percuss both sides of the costovertebral angle (CVA) for kidney tenderness or pain.
     a. Place the palm of one hand against the skin and gently strike the top of this hand with the ulnar surface of the other hand that has been made into a fist.
     b. CVA tenderness may indicate pyelonephritis, neoplasms, inflamed or bleeding cysts, calculi, or intermittent hydronephrosis.
  3. A distended bladder is dull to percussion above the symphysis pubis.

III. Kidney pain.

A. Assessment.
  1. Careful assessment of urinary tract pain aids in differential diagnosis of intrarenal, postrenal, and/or extrarenal disorders and provides information for the management of the pain.
  2. Assess the location, intensity, onset, pattern(s), and description/characterization of pain.
     a. Identify aggravating (what worsens) and alleviating (what improves) factors.
     b. Positional factors, change with body movement.

| Table 1.9 | Health History and Physical Assessment Guide for the Nephrology Patient |

Patient's Name: **Date:**

Nurse's Name:

I. COMPREHENSIVE HEALTH HISTORY

A. Identifying data
1. Age
2. Birth date
3. Sex
4. Race
5. Place of birth
6. Marital status
7. Occupation
8. Religious preference and spiritual practices and beliefs

B. Source of history (i.e., patient, relative, friend, medical record) and nurse's judgment about the validity of the information

C. Chief complaint(s): stated in the patient's own words, if possible.

D. History of the present illness: the patient's chronologic explanation of the health problems for which he/she is seeking care
The account should include:
1. Onset of the problem
2. The setting in which it developed
3. Its manifestations
4. Its treatments
5. Its impact on the patient's life
6. Its meaning to the patient
The symptoms of the problems should be described in terms of seven dimensions:
1. Body location
2. Quality
3. Quantity (severity)
4. Timing (i.e., onset, duration, and frequency)
5. Setting in which they occur
6. Factors that aggravate or relieve the symptoms
7. Associated manifestations

E. Past health history
1. General state of health
2. Childhood illnesses (i.e., measles, rubella, mumps, whooping cough, chicken pox, rheumatic fever, scarlet fever, polio, frequent "strep" throat)
3. Immunizations and dates (i.e., tetanus, pertussis, diphtheria, polio (Salk and/or Sabin), measles, rubella, mumps, hepatitis)
4. Adult illnesses: describe nature of each illness, date, treatment, and outcome in patient's own words if possible
5. Psychiatric illnesses: describe nature of each illness, date, treatment, and outcome in patient's own words, if possible
6. Operations: describe type of operation(s), date(s), and outcome(s), including organ/tissue transplants
7. Other hospitalizations: reason(s), date(s), and outcome(s)
8. Allergies: state substance(s) to which allergic; how each allergy manifests itself (signs and symptoms); prophylactic treatment, if any; date of past allergic response
9. Current medications: state all prescription, over-the-counter, home remedy nonprescription, and herbal drugs/teas, and dietary/nutritional supplements, vitamins, minerals, and flower essences that the patient uses. Give dosage, frequency, and length of time taking. Elicit patient's understanding of reason(s) for each, its desired effects, and its side effects.
10. Diet history
    a. ask for a 24-hour recall of all food and fluids consumed and dietary supplements, including amount of each and time of day
    b. ascertain any special dietary restrictions or requirements
    c. determine patient's understanding of reasons for dietary restrictions
    d. determine patient's ability to purchase and prepare necessary foods
11. Sleep patterns
    a. usual bedtime and time of awakening
    b. difficulty falling asleep or staying asleep and associated reasons; aids to sleep
    c. daytime naps: how many and how long for each
    d. any recent changes in any of the above
12. Habits
    a. describe exercise schedule
    b. coffee/tea: daily amount
    c. alcohol: type and usual daily consumption
    d. tobacco: type (cigarettes, cigars, pipe, chewing) and usual daily number
    e. recreational drugs: name drug and describe its use (Note: the patient may be reluctant to give this information about illegal drug use.)
13. Environmental hazards
    a. recent recipient of x-ray contrast media
    b. ingestion of lead
    c. exposure or ingestion of mercury
    d. prolonged use of NSAIDs
    e. prolonged sulfonamide use
    f. prolonged aminoglycoside use

Table 1.9 ———— **Health History and Physical Assessment Guide for the Nephrology Patient** (page 2 of 9)

g. "moonshine" ingestion
h. exposure to radiation
i. exposure to sprays, herbicides, pesticides, fumes (e.g., farmers, ranchers, loggers)
j. others
14. Ask patient to describe work and neighborhood where he/she live; look for evidence of new industrial park or nuclear waste site, fumes, air pollution, water pollution.

F. Family History
1. Give age and state of health or cause and age at death for each of the following family members:
   a. paternal and maternal grandparents
   b. parents
   c. siblings
   d. spouse
   e. children
2. Question about the occurrence of the following conditions in any family member:
   a. diabetes mellitus
   b. tuberculosis
   c. heart disease
   d. high blood pressure
   e. stroke
   f. kidney disease
   g. cancer
   h. arthritis
   i. anemia
   j. headaches
   k. mental illness
   l. symptoms similar to those the patient is experiencing

	Typical Findings in Patients with Kidney Failure
G. Psychosocial history. Have the patient describe in his/her own words: 1. His lifestyle, home situation, significant people in his life and any recent changes in each 2. A typical day and recent changes 3. The most important events in his life 4. Spiritual/cultural/religious beliefs that influence his health or therapeutic regimen 5. Educational background 6. Current occupation 7. Professional and personal goals 8. Financial status and effect of illness on it; ability to manage cost of illness 9. Travel in last year	changes in lifestyle because of illness often changes in occupation or unemployed because of illness major financial problems because of cost of kidney failure treatment

H. Review of systems (from the patient's *subjective* point of view)
Note: As abnormalities arise, ask what the person does to treat them.
1. General state of health
   a. usual weight
   b. recent decrease or increase in weight
   c. fever
   d. unusual weakness, fatigue, malaise
   e. pain
	losses in weight if anorexic or has nausea and vomiting
	gains in weight with fluid retention
	
	weakness, fatigue, malaise

2. Skin
   a. rashes
   b. bumps
   c. itching or dryness and how managed
   d. color changes
   e. changes in hair or nails
	dry, scaly skin
	severe itching
	
	grayish-bronze color with underlying pallor
	easy bruising, poor healing of cuts and scratches
	dry brittle hair
	brittle split nails

3. Head
   a. headache: location, frequency, and treatment
   b. head injuries
	frequent headaches

4. Eyes
   a. visual
   b. glasses or contact lenses: reason and length of time
   c. last eye examination
   d. pain
   f. excessive tearing
   g. double vision
   h. glaucoma
   i. cataracts
	decreased visual acuity
	redness
	pain
	double vision
	cataracts

5. Ears a. hearing acuity	

Table 1.9 _____Health History and Physical Assessment Guide for the Nephrology Patient (page 3 of 9)	**Typical Findings in Patients with Kidney Failure**
b. tinnitus	
c. vertigo	
d. earaches	
e. infection	
f. discharge	
6. Nose and sinuses	nose bleeds
a. frequent colds	
b. nasal stuffiness	
c. hay fever/allergies/sneezing	
d. nosebleeds	
e. sinus problems	
7. Mouth and throat	bleeding
a. condition of teeth and gums	ammonia or urine smell to breath
b. bleeding gums or mucous membranes	metallic taste in mouth
c. last dental examination	sore, cracked, bleeding tongue
d. history of cavities	and mucous membranes
e. sore, bleeding tongue	frequent "strep" throat may be
f. history of sore throat (especially "strep" throat)	precursor to some types of glomerulonephritis
g. hoarseness	
h. unusual taste in mouth	
i. unusual odor on breath	
8. Neck	
a. lumps	
b. "swollen glands"	
c. goiter	
d. pain	
9. Breasts	enlargement of breast tissue
a. lumps	(for men)
b. pain	
c. discharge from nipples	
d. self-examination knowledge and practice	
e. recent enlargement of breasts, especially for men	
10. Respiratory	tenacious sputum
a. cough	pneumonia
b. sputum (color, quantity, consistency)	
c. hemoptysis	
d. wheezing	
e. asthma	
f. bronchitis	
g. emphysema	
h. pneumonia	
i. tuberculosis	
j. pleurisy	
k. last tuberculin skin test and results	
l. last chest x-ray and results	
11. Cardiac	high blood pressure
a. heart trouble	dyspnea
b. high blood pressure	orthopnea
c. rheumatic fever	paroxysmal nocturnal dyspnea
d. heart murmurs	edema of feet and legs, and around eyes
e. dyspnea	palpitations
f. orthopnea	chest pain
g. paroxysmal nocturnal dyspnea	
h. edema	
i. chest pains	
j. palpitations	
k. last EKG or other cardiac evaluations and results	
12. Gastrointestinal	heartburn
a. dysphagia	anorexia
b. heartburn and treatment	nausea, especially in the early morning
c. change in appetite	
d. nausea	
e. vomiting (have patient describe emesis)	vomiting
f. indigestion	indigestion
g. frequency and description of bowel movements	constipation and/or diarrhea
h. change in bowel habits	blood in vomitus and/or stools
i. rectal bleeding	difficulty swallowing
j. constipation and treatment	
k. diarrhea and treatment	

Table 1.9 _____ **Health History and Physical Assessment Guide for the Nephrology Patient** (page 4 of 9)

	Typical Findings in Patients with Kidney Failure
l. abdominal pain m. food intolerances n. excessive flatus o. hemorrhoids p. jaundice q. liver or gall bladder problems r. hepatitis	

13. Urinary
  a. frequency of urination
  b. amount of each urination
  c. number of times gets up at night to urinate (nocturia)
  d. recent increase or decrease in amount of each urination
  e. pain during urination (dysuria)
  f. difficulty starting urinating (hesitancy)
  g. urgency
  h. dribbling at end of urination
  i. starting and stopping of stream during urination
  j. blood in urine (hematuria)
  k. color of urine
  l. burning during urination
  m. incontinence or enuresis
  n. history of urinary tract infections and treatment
  o. history of urinary tract stones and treatment
  p. operations, such as kidney donation, kidney transplant recipient, bladder surgery, or stents.
If patient on dialysis:
  a. date of initiation
  b. type of dialysis
  c. date of last dialysis
  d. where treated (home, in-center)
  e. complications
	polyuria in early kidney failure and in polycystic kidney disease
	nocturia in early kidney failure
	decreased amount of urine in late kidney failure
	blood in urine
	depending on cause of renal problem, patient may report history of:
	  dysuria
	  hesitancy
	  urgency
	  dribbling
	  burning during urination
	  incontinence or enuresis
	  history of frequent urinary tract infections
	  history of urinary tract stones

14. Genito-reproductive
  a. males
    (1) discharge from penis or sores on penis
    (2) history of sexually transmitted disease(s) and treatment
    (3) hernias
    (4) pain or masses in testicles
    (5) recent decrease in size of testicles
    (6) ability to achieve and maintain an erection
    (7) recent change in interest in sex
    (8) frequency of intercourse
    (9) contraceptive measures
  b. females
    (1) age at menarche
    (2) regularity, frequency, and duration of menstrual periods
    (3) amount of bleeding during menstrual periods
    (4) bleeding between periods or after intercourse
    (5) recent changes in frequency or duration of periods
    (6) frequency of intercourse; recent changes in interest in sex
    (7) ability to achieve orgasm
    (8) number of pregnancies; number of live births; number of spontaneous, therapeutic, or induced abortions
    (9) date of last menstrual period
    (10) dysmenorrhea
    (11) age of menopause
    (12) last Pap smear and results
    (13) contraceptive measures, use of hormones, creams
	problem achieving and/or maintaining erection
	
	decreased libido
	infertility
	
	failure to menarche (children)
	infertility
	amenorrhea or irregular menstrual periods
	decreased libido

15. Musculoskeletal
  a. joint pains or stiffness
  b. arthritis
  c. gout
  d. backache
  e. if any of above are present, describe location and symptoms (i.e., swelling, redness, pain, stiffness, weakness, limitation of motion or activity)
  f. muscle pains, cramps, or spasms
	joint pain
	gout
	arthritis
	stiff joints
	muscle pains
	leg cramps
	restlessness

16. Peripheral vascular a. pain on walking	

Table 1.9_____**Health History and Physical Assessment Guide for the Nephrology Patient** (page 5 of 9)

	Typical Findings in Patients with Kidney Failure
b. leg cramps c. varicose veins d. thrombophlebitis e. recent hair loss from extremities	leg cramps pain on walking

17. Neurologic
  a. fainting
  b. seizures
  c. localized weakness
  d. numbness
  e. tingling or burning sensations
  f. tremors
  g. paralysis
  h. memory loss
  i. alteration in state of mental acuity
	fainting
	seizures
	muscle weakness
	numbness, tingling, burning of soles of feet
	
	footdrop
	decreased interest in environment
	decreased ability to do abstract reasoning

18. Psychiatric
  a. unusual nervousness, anxiety
  b. mood changes
  c. depression
  d. loss of interest in usual recreation activities
  e. depression
	mood swings
	depression
	anger
	hostility

19. Endocrine
  a. thyroid problems
  b. heat or cold intolerance
  c. excessive sweating
  d. excessive thirst, hunger, or urination
  e. diabetes mellitus
  f. problems with conception
	heat and/or cold intolerance
	excessive thirst, hunger (diabetic nephropathy)
	infertility

20. Hematologic
  a. anemia
  b. easy bruising or bleeding
  c. history of blood transfusion: dates, reasons, and reactions
  d. fatigue, malaise
	anemia
	easy bruising and bleeding
	fatigue
	malaise

II. SYSTEMATIC PHYSICAL EXAMINATION (from the examiner's objective point of view) Note: As abnormalities arise, ask what the peron does to treat them.	

A. General survey
  1. Observe the patient's apparent state of health and signs of distress
  2. Height
  3. Weight
  4. Correlate height and weight to determine appropriateness for each patient.
  5. Observe posture, activity, gait, dress, grooming, personal hygiene, odors to breath or body, facial expressions, manner, affect, reaction to other people, state of awareness.
	low weight for height if patient anorexic
	high weight for height if patient has fluid overload
	appears chronically or acutely ill, often emaciated, apathetic, poorly groomed, low energy level, halitosis, body odor, uses defense mechanisms.

B. Vital signs
  1. Blood pressure: lying, sitting, and standing
  2. Oral or rectal temperature; observe for hypothermia or hyperthermia
  3. Count radial pulse rate
  4. Count respiratory rate
	usually hypertensive
	possible orthostatic hypotension
	hyperthermic (due to infection)
	abnormal pulse rate and rhythm

C. Skin
  1. Inspect color, evidence of bleeding, bruising, excoriation
  2. Palpate
    a. moisture: dryness, sweating, oiliness
    b. temperature (with backs of examiner's fingers)
    c. mobility and turgor: lift a fold of skin and note ease with which it moves (mobility) and speed with which it returns into place (turgor)
  3. Observe skin lesions and describe their anatomic locations, distribution, arrangement, type of lesion (macules, papules, vesticles, bulla, erosion, etc.), and color
  4. Inspect and palpate fingernails and toenails for color, shape, and lesions
  5. Inspect and palpate the head and body hair for quantity, distribution, and texture
	pale, grayish-bronze color
	ecchymoses
	purpura
	excoriated and reddened areas
	dry
	delayed wound healing
	poor turgor and mobility
	
	brittle, split nails
	red, brown, or white bands
	scant (do not confuse with normal male balding), dry, brittle hair

Table 1.9 ——————— **Health History and Physical Assessment Guide for the Nephrology Patient** (page 6 of 9)

	Typical Findings in Patients with Kidney Failure
D. Eyes 　1. Test visual acuity using a Snellen eye chart, or have the patient read small newspaper or magazine print up close and then large print several feet away 　2. Inspect eyebrows for quantity and distribution of hair and scaliness of skin 　3. Inspect eyelids for edema, color, lesions, adequacy with which the eyelids close to cover the corneas 　4. Inspect the conjunctivas and sclera for color, especially jaundice and pallor 　5. Using oblique lighting, inspect the cornea and lens of each eye for opacities 　6. Inspect the size, shape, and equality of the pupils 　7. Test direct and consensual pupillary reaction to light (CN III) 　8. Test the pupillary reaction to accommodation 　9. Assess the extraocular movements through the six cardinal fields of gaze (CN III, IV, VI) 　10. Using the ophthalmoscope, examine the fundus of each eye; note the outline and color of the optic disc; inspect for nicking of junctions of arterioles and veins	decreased visual acuity double vision dry, scaly skin under eyebrows edema of eyelids which may prevent their closing completely pale or red, inflamed conjunctiva yellow sclera opacities of cornea and lens nystagmus retinopathy outline of optic disc blurred hemorrhages nicking at arteriovenous crossings papilledema
E. Ears 　1. Inspect the auricles for deformities and lesions 　2. Using an otoscope, inspect the ear canal and drum; note discharge, redness, swelling of the drum 　3. Test auditory acuity by asking the patient to repeat numbers whispered by the examiner (CN VIII).	hard nodules or lumps in auricles decreased hearing acuity
F. Nose 　1. Inspect for deformity and inflammation 　2. Using a nasal speculum and light source, inspect the nasal mucosa for color, swelling, exudate, and bleeding	pale mucous membranes bleeding
G. Mouth and pharynx 　1. Inspect the lips for color, moisture, lumps, ulcerations, cracking, and bleeding 　2. Using a light source, inspect the buccal mucosa for color, pigmentation, ulcerations, nodules, and bleeding 　3. Inspect the gums and teeth for inflammation, swelling, retraction, bleeding, caries, and loose or missing teeth 　4. Inspect the tongue for color, ulcerations, bleeding 　5. Inspect under the surface of the tongue and floor of the mouth for redness, nodules, and ulcerations 　6. Note and describe the smell of the breath 　7. Using a tongue blade and light source, inspect the pharynx; describe color, exudate, edema, ulcerations, tonsillar enlargement	dry, cracked lips with bleeding pale, ulcerated, bleeding mucous membranes inflamed, bleeding gums dry, cracked, bleeding tongue smell of ammonia and urine to breath
H. Neck 　1. Palpate lymph nodes, using pads of index and middle fingers, and note enlargement 　2. Inspect and palpate trachea for deviation from midline 　3. Palpate the lobes of the thyroid; note size, shape, symmetry, tenderness, and nodules	
I. Thorax and lungs 　1. Inspect the posterior and anterior chest for rate, rhythm, and effort of breathing; deformities of the thorax; shape of chest; bulging interspaces during expiration 　2. Auscultate the anterior and posterior lung fields for normal vesicular breath sounds and adventitious sounds (crackles, rhonchi, rubs)	rapid, deep respirations in acidosis crackles pleural rubs
J. The heart 　1. Inspect and palpate each of the following areas for pulsations, lifts, heaves, and thrills 　　a. aortic area (2nd intercostal space, right sternal border) 　　b. pulmonic area (2nd intercostal space, left sternal border) 　　c. 3rd left intercostal space (Erb's point) 　　d. right ventricular area (lower half of sternum and parasternal area on the left) 　　e. apical (left ventricular) area (5th intercostal space, just medial to the left midclavicular line) 　　f. epigastric area (lower sternum and xiphoid process)	

Table 1.9 ————————**Health History and Physical Assessment Guide for the Nephrology Patient** (page 7 of 9)

	Typical Findings in Patients with Kidney Failure

2. Using the stethoscope, auscultate each of the following areas:
  a. aortic area (2nd intercostal space, right sternal border)
  b. pulmonic area (2nd intercostal space, left sternal border)
  c. Erb's point (3rd intercostal space, left sternal border)
  d. tricuspid area (5th intercostal space, left sternal border)
  e. mitral area (5th intercostal space, just medial to left midclavicular line)
  f. listen with bell and then diaphragm of stethoscope in each area
  g. assess the following
    (1) first heart sound for intensity and splitting
    (2) second heart sound for intensity and splitting
    (3) systolic and diastolic murmurs
    (4) pericardial friction rub
	murmurs
	pericardial friction rub

3. Assess the rate and rhythm of the radial and carotid pulses 4. Using a stethoscope and sphygmomanometer, measure the arterial blood pressure 5. With the patient's upper torso at a 15°–30° angle, assess the internal and external jugular veins for level of distension	irregular pulse rate hypertension paradoxical pulse (in pericardial effusion) distended jugular veins

K. Peripheral vascular system
1. Inspect arms, noting size and symmetry, color and texture of skin, nail beds, venous pattern, and edema
2. Inspect the legs, noting size and symmetry; color and texture of skin; nail beds; hair distribution on the lower legs, feet, and toes; rashes, scars, ulcers, venous enlargement, and edema.
3. Palpate each peripheral pulse:
  a. radial
  b. ulnar
  c. brachial
  d. femoral
  e. popliteal
  f. dorsalis pedis
  g. posterior tibial
4. Grade peripheral pulses based on a 4-point scale:
  0 – completely absent
  1 – barely palpable
  2 – expected, normal
  3 – full, increased
  4 – bounding
5. Perform an Allen test to assess patency of radial and ulnar arteries (especially important in patients who will have an artery in the forearm used for an AV shunt or fistula formation)
6. Assess external arteriovenous shunt or fistula or graft for patency and for adequate circulation to extremity distal to the shunt or fistula. Inspect exit site of external AV shunt for signs of inflammation. Inspect internal AV fistula or graft for scar tissue, redness, infection, presence of pulsation
	edema
	pale, cyanotic nail beds
	
	weak or absent peripheral pulses

L. Breasts and axillae 1. Inspect the female breasts for size and symmetry, masses, dimpling, flattening, color, edema, venous pattern, size and shape of nipples, direction in which nipples point, discharge from nipples 2. Palpate the female breasts for induration, tenderness, nodules 3. Inspect the male breasts for nodules, swelling, ulcerations 4. Palpate the male breasts for nodules, glandular enlargement (gynecomastia) 5. Inspect the axillae for rash and infection 6. Palpate auxiliary lymph nodes for enlargement and tenderness	gynecomastia
M. The abdomen 1. Inspect the skin for scars, striae, dilated veins, rashes, and lesions 2. Inspect the contour of the abdomen for masses, enlarged organs, peristalsis, pulsations 3. Using the diaphragm of the stethoscope, auscultate for bowel sounds 4. Auscultate for bruits over the aorta, iliac arteries, and femoral arteries 5. Lightly percuss in all four quadrants, checking for normal sound of tympany or dullness of ascitic fluid 6. Percuss the upper and lower liver borders, and measure the span at the right midclavicular line 7. Palpate in all four quadrants for masses and tenderness 8. Palpate the lower liver border for consistency, tenderness, enlargement 9. Palpate right and left kidneys, noting size, contour, and tenderness 10. Assess for kidney tenderness at left and right costovertebral angles	distended abdomen bruits ascites enlarged liver kidney tenderness

Table 1.9 ——————— **Health History and Physical Assessment Guide for the Nephrology Patient** (page 8 of 9)

	Typical Findings in Patients with Kidney Failure

N. Male Genitalia
   1. Assess sexual maturation
      a. size and shape of penis and testes
      b. color and texture of scrotal skin
      c. character and distribution of pubic hair
   2. Inspect foreskin, if present, for phimosis and paraphimosis
   3. Inspect the glans for ulcers, scars, nodules, and signs of inflammation
   4. Inspect the urethral meatus for size and discharge
   5. Palpate the penis, noting tenderness and induration
   6. Inspect the scrotum for lumps, swelling, excoriation, and signs of inflammation
   7. Palpate each testis and epididymis, noting size, consistency, nodules and swelling
   8. Inspect for scar of past kidney implant
	in pubescent boys, underdeveloped penis and testes and absence of public hair for age
	
	decreased size of testes

O. Female Genitalia
   1. Asses sexual maturation
      a. character and distribution of pubic hair
      b. breast development
   2. Inspect labia majora, labia minora, clitoris, urethral orifice, vaginal opening for inflammation, ulcerations, discharge, swelling or nodules
   3. Inspect for scar of past kidney transplant
	in pubescent girls, absence of pubic hair and decreased breast development for age

P. Musculoskeletal
   1. Assess each joint for
      a. limitation in range of motion
      b. swelling
      c. tenderness
      d. heat
      e. redness
      f. crepitation
      g. deformities
      h. symmetry
   2. For renal patients, especially important to assess the following joints:
      a. hands and wrists
      b. elbows
      c. shoulders
      d. ankles
      e. knees
      f. hips
      g. spine
	decreased range of motion of joints
	swelling
	tenderness
	skin warm to touch
	red skin over joints
	deformities

Q. Nervous system
   1. Cranial nerves assessment
      I. Olfactory: have patient identify familiar odors
      II. Optic: test visual acuity; using an ophthalmoscope, inspect the fundus
 	
      III. Oculomotor
      IV. Trochlear ⎰ Inspect shape and size of the pupils; test pupillary reaction to light; test extraocular movements
      VI. Abducens ⎱ through the six cardinal fields of gaze, noting loss of movement in any direction and nystagmus
 	
      V. Trigemial
         Motor: Assess strength of temporal and masseter muscles
         Sensory: Assess for pain and light touch on the forehead, cheek and chin, bilaterally
            Assess for corneal reflex
 	
      VII. Facial
         Motor: Inspect symmetry of face; assess ability to raise eyebrows, frown, show teeth, smile, puff out cheeks
      VIII. Acoustic: Assess hearing acuity
      IX. Glossopharyneal ⎰ Listen for hoarseness of the voice;
      X. Vagus ⎱ assess gag reflex
 	
      XI. Spinal Accessory: Assess strength of shoulder muscles (trapezil)
      XII. Hypoglossal: Assess ability of tongue to protrude in midline and to move side to side
 	
   2. Screening motor examination
      a. assess posture and balance during walking and standing
      b. perform a Romberg test
	decreased ability to identify odors
	
	nystagmus
	
	decreased sensation
	
	facial weakness
	
	decreased hearing acuity
	
	poor posture
	weakness of extremities

Table 1.9 _____ **Health History and Physical Assessment Guide for the Nephrology Patient** (page 9 of 9)

	Typical Findings in Patients with Kidney Failure

3. Screening sensory examination
   a. assess patient's ability (with his eyes closed) to identify points of sharp and light touch by the examiner
   b. stereognosis
	decreased sensation

4. Reflexes
   a. using a reflex hammer, assess each reflex:
     (1) biceps
     (2) triceps
     (3) brachioradialis
     (4) knee
     (5) ankle
     (6) plantar response (Assess plantar flexion or dorsiflexion of foot in response to stroking sole of foot.)
   b. grade each reflex on a 4-point scale:
     4+: very brisk; hyperactive
     3+: brisker than average
     2+: average; normal
     1+: somewhat decreased
     0 : no response
	decreased reflexes

R. Mental Status	

   c. Associated signs and symptoms that occur with the pain.
3. Clarify the location of the pain.
   a. Kidney pain or nephralgia is generally felt in the flank(s) and along the costovertebral angle in the back and is not altered by position changes.
   b. Ureteral pain is felt in the groin or genital area.
   c. Bladder pain is felt in the suprapubic to upper thigh area.
   d. Urinary tract pain is often perceived slightly below the ribs to the upper thighs and can be bilateral or unilateral.

B. Pain pathway.
1. Nociceptors (pain receptors) are located throughout the renal capsule and urinary collecting system (i.e., renal pelvis to external urethral sphincter).
2. Most of the kidney lacks nociceptors. Therefore extensive damage and complete loss of kidney function can occur without nephralgia.
3. Renal nociceptors transmit information to afferent (sensory) neurons that enter the dorsal spinal cord between T10 and T12.
4. Anterolateral spinal tracts transmit all pain information to the brain.

5. Testicular pain may accompany kidney pain because nerves from the renal plexus communicate with the spermatic plexus.

C. Nephralgia.
1. Kidney pain is classified primarily as nociceptive visceral pain, meaning it arises from an intact nervous system in the kidney. Neuropathic kidney pain occurs less frequently and generally indicates damage to the nervous system (e.g., loin pain–hematuria syndrome).
2. If the renal capsule is punctured, distended, or inflamed, nephralgia occurs.
   a. When the renal capsule is punctured (such as with a biopsy or trauma), dull deep pain or intense pressure is felt. True nephralgia is evident with a closed renal biopsy. Because cutaneous nociceptors are anesthetized, the needle passes through the skin painlessly. As the needle penetrates the renal capsule, deep nephralgia is felt because the capsule nociceptors are stimulated.
   b. Distention or inflammation of the renal capsule causes a dull, constant pain (as seen with neoplastic growths, bleeding from trauma, inflammation with edema formation, pyelonephritis, and inflamed or bleeding cysts).

3. Acute obstruction in the intrarenal collecting system can cause pain if the renal pelvis is distended. Slowly developing calculi in the renal pelvis, however, can be painless.
4. Ischemia caused by occlusion of renal blood vessels (e.g., from an embolus, arteriosclerotic disease, or tumor) results in constant dull or sharp pain.

D. Referred pain.
   1. Pain that originates in a viscera and is felt on the skin is referred pain.
   2. Renal (visceral) and cutaneous sensory/afferent neurons enter the spinal cord adjacent to each other.
   3. When renal sensory neurons are stimulated, concurrent stimulation of cutaneous neurons occurs and the nephralgia feels as though it originates in the skin.
   4. Renal pain is felt in dermatomes T10-L1.

E. Renal colic.
   1. Colic refers to spasm in a tubular or hollow organ accompanied by pain.
   2. Renal colic is often associated with movement of a stone down the ureter.
   3. Renal colic is an excruciating pain that increases in intensity, plateaus, and then decreases. The pain may radiate from the flank into the genital area (testicle or labia).
   4. Renal colic is treated with analgesia and fluid support.

IV. Urine collection for analysis.

A. Use clean catch or midstream method for bacterial and routine urine analysis.
   1. Cleanse external genitalia.
   2. Have patient urinate approximately 100 mL (if possible) to flush out urethral bacteria and leukocytes. Discard.
   3. Then collect urine in a sterile container.

B. Urine specimens also can be collected by bladder catheterization or suprapubic aspiration of the bladder.
   1. These are both invasive procedures that may lead to urinary tract infection. Therefore, these are done when no alternative noninvasive method is available.
   2. When a bladder catheter is in place, using aseptic technique, collect freshly excreted urine from the drainage system according to the manufacturer's instructions.

C. To ensure accurate analysis, deliver urine to the laboratory immediately. The specimen may be refrigerated up to 1 hour. Urine that remains at room temperature for 1 hour undergoes the following changes:
   1. Crystals form.
   2. Red blood cells hemolyze.
   3. Leukocytes lyse and release leukocyte esterase.
   4. Nitrites degrade.
   5. Tubercle bacilli die.
   6. Bacteria grow, consume glucose, and decompose urea to ammonia.
   7. Ammonia increases the urine pH.
   8. Many casts disintegrate in an alkaline environment.

IV. Macroscopic urinalysis (see Table 1.10).

A. Physical characteristics.
   1. Normal yellow color is due to the presence of urochrome and urobilin pigments.
   2. Concentration of urine affects color. Dilute urine is less colored and concentrated urine is more orange colored.
   3. Urine color may be changed by drug and dye excretion, pigments, type of foods eaten, and cellular substances (for example, leukocytes make urine white, bile pigments make urine yellow-brown or greenish, and beets make urine burgundy).
      a. Hematuria can be microscopic or macroscopic, resulting in a range of color from yellow to bright red. Hematuria can originate from anywhere along the urinary tract (see Sediment later in this chapter).
      b. Normal urine is clear. Cloudiness results from phosphates, urates, pH changes, bacteria, cells, crystals, or lipids.
      c. Normal urine foams slightly when shaken. Proteinuria causes increased foam and may indicate renal disease, such as the nephrotic syndrome (see Protein and Related Substances).
   4. Degradation of urea to ammonia causes the characteristic smell of urine. Bacteriuria can increase urea breakdown and cause urine to have a much stronger ammonia smell.
   5. Unusual urine odor may also result from ketonuria, phenylketonuria, alkaptonuria, hypermethioninemia, maple syrup urine disease, and the ingestion of certain foods such as asparagus.

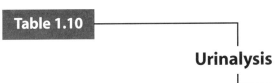

Table 1.10

Urinalysis

Macroscopic Analysis		
	Normal	**Alteration**
Color	Clear Pale yellow or amber	Cloudy with infection Lighter if dilute; darker if concentrated Changed by foods, cellular debris
Specific gravity	1.005–1.030	Increased with volume deficit Decreased with volume excess
Omsolality	100–1200 mOsm/kg	Increased with volume deficit Decreased with volume excess
pH	4.5–8	Increased with Fanconi Syndrome; renal tubular acidosis
Glucose	Negative	Diabetes mellitus
Ketones	Negative	Starvation, vomiting, ketoacidosis
Leukocyte esterase	Negative	Inflammation, infection
Nitrites	Negative	Infection
Red blood cells	Negative – few	Inflammation, trauma, calculi, neoplasm
Protein	Negative/trace or < 30 mg/day	Increase in glomerular disease, tubular disease

Microscopic Analysis/Sediment		
	Normal	**Alteration**
Crystals	Negative	Calculi – specific to type
Casts		
Hyaline	0–few	Stress, fever, volume deficit, renal parenchymal disease
Red cell	0	Glomerulonephritis
White cell	0	Inflammation, infection
Fatty	0	Nephrotic syndrome
Renal tubular epithelial	0	Interstitial nephritis, acute tubular necrosis, transplant rejection
Granular	0	Renal parenchymal disease
Waxy or broad	0	Advanced kidney disease

B. Volume.
   1. A minimal daily urinary volume of approximately 500 mL (SI = 0.5 L) is required to excrete wastes.
   2. The maximum diuretic volume is approximately 20 L (SI = 20 L).
   3. Urine is formed at about 1 mL/min (SI = .001 L/min).
   4. Clinically less than 30 mL/hour (SI = .03 L/hr) warrants investigation.
   5. Daily urine volume can vary and is influenced by multiple variables, such as fluid intake, hydration status, and adequacy of kidney function.

C. Specific gravity and osmolality. Urine specific gravity normally ranges from 1.005 to 1.030. Osmolality ranges from 100 to 1200 mOsm/kg H_2O.
   1. Specific gravity measures the density of a solution compared to the density of water, which is one (1.000). Specific gravity is altered by the presence of proteins, cells, casts, and other substances, whereas osmolality is not altered by these substances.
   2. Osmolality measures the number of solute particles per kilogram of water.
   3. Osmolality is the most accurate measurement of the kidney's ability to concentrate or dilute urine.
   4. The more concentrated the urine, the higher the osmolality (as with fluid volume depletion). The more dilute the urine, the lower the osmolality (as with fluid volume excess or diabetes insipidus).
   5. Blood and urine osmolality are measured simultaneously to determine if the kidneys are responding correctly to the body's fluid status. Blood osmolality is approximately 280–300 mOsm/kg H_2O (SI = 280–300 mOsm/kg H_2O). Healthy kidneys maintain a constant plasma osmolality by excreting urine with an increased osmolality when the plasma osmolality increases, or excreting urine with a low osmolality when the plasma osmolality decreases.

D. pH. Normal range of urine pH is 4.5 to 8 (SI = pH 4.5–8).
   1. pH is influenced by many extrarenal factors, such as drugs, electrolyte imbalances, and systemic pH changes.
   2. A change in urine pH seldom indicates kidney disease, except with renal tubular acidosis and

Fanconi syndrome (in these cases, the urine is alkaline).
   3. With pregnancy, urine pH is more alkaline, especially in the morning. This is normal and does not indicate kidney disease.

E. Glucose.
   1. Glycosuria with normally functioning kidneys is due to plasma glucose that exceeds the renal threshold for glucose reabsorption (e.g., diabetes mellitus, excessive carbohydrate intake, highly emotional states, pregnancy, and dysfunction of the pituitary gland). With pregnancy, glycosuria can occur without hyperglycemia.
   2. Glycosuria without hyperglycemia occurs with kidney impairment (e.g., Fanconi syndrome and with exposure to nephrotoxins).

F. Ketones.
   1. Ketones are an end product of fat metabolism.
   2. Ketonuria results from an increased catabolism of fatty acids due to starvation, vomiting, extreme temperature exposure, extreme overexertion/physical exercise, and alcoholic or diabetic ketoacidosis, and a large vitamin C intake.
   3. Ketonuria is a poor indicator of kidney disease.

G. Nitrites.
   1. Urine does not normally contain nitrites.
   2. In the bladder, many gram-negative and some gram-positive bacteria convert nitrates (substances related to protein metabolism) to nitrites.
   3. Bacterial conversion of nitrates to nitrites takes 4 hours or more. Therefore the best time to test is the first urine specimen of the morning.
   4. Presence of nitrites in urine is detected by a color change test and reported as positive or negative.
   5. A positive nitrites test indicates bacterial infection in the urinary tract (greater than 10,000 organisms per mL).
   6. Factors that interfere with accurate test results are high urine specific gravity, abundance of urinary ascorbic acid, low dietary intake of protein, urine pH less than 6, and prolonged storage of urine (nitrites will degrade).

H. Electrolytes.
   1. Many factors affect the quantity of electrolytes excreted in the urine. Their daily range is quite variable. It is beneficial to analyze urinary electrolyte composition from a 24-hour specimen and correlate the results with plasma electrolyte levels.

2. Certain electrolytes are altered with kidney disease (see Chapter 2) (e.g., sodium and potassium in acute kidney injury).
   a. Measuring urinary sodium assists in differentiating prerenal from intrarenal (also called acute tubular necrosis) acute kidney injury.
   b. In prerenal acute kidney injury, the kidneys are healthy although hypoperfused and respond by reabsorbing sodium and water. As a result, urine sodium is low.
   c. In intrarenal acute kidney injury, the kidneys are damaged and unable to fully reabsorb sodium. As a result, urine sodium is moderate to high.
3. Electrolyte and/or water wasting means that there is an increased urinary excretion of electrolytes or water because the kidneys have a diminished or no ability to regulate carefully the excretion of these substances.

I. Protein.
1. Normal urinary excretion of albumin is approximately 30 mg/day (SI = 0.73 μmol/day).
2. Microalbuminuria is defined as urine excretion of albumin between 30 and 150 mg/day (SI = 0.73–2.2 μmol/day).
   a. The presence of microalbuminuria helps to diagnose, plan, and evaluate treatment, and monitor disease progression of diabetic nephropathy.
   b. The reagent on most dipstick tests is sensitive to albumin with 99% sensitivity and specificity.
   c. Follow-up analysis of significant proteinuria should be done by sending a urine specimen to the laboratory.
   d. Table 1.11 describes how dipstick results correspond with laboratory values of proteinuria.
   e. With increasing amounts of protein in the urine, foaming occurs (like whisking an egg white).
3. Proteinuria greater than 150 mg/24 hr (SI = 2.2 μmol/24 hr) is significant and should be evaluated thoroughly. Proteinuria may indicate glomerular capillary disease, such as nephrotic syndrome or glomerulonephritis.
4. With pregnancy, proteinuria up to 300 mg/day (SI = 4.4 μmol/day) is considered within normal limits.
5. Proteinuria may be transient or persistent.
   a. Transient proteinuria reflects a temporary change in the glomerulus and is generally benign and self-limited. (e.g., congestive heart failure, exercise, fever).

Table 1.11

Proteinuria – Correlation of Dipstick and Amount of Protein

Dipstick Result	Amount of Protein
Trace	5–10 mg/dL
1+	30 mg/dL
2+	100 mg/dL
3+	300 mg/dL
4+	1000 mg/dL

   b. Persistent proteinuria reflects malfunction of the glomerulus or tubules and requires additional investigation.
6. Proteinuria can be estimated from a random spot urine.
   a. Collect a minimum of 10 mL and measure the protein and creatinine in the urine.
   b. Calculate the ratio of urinary protein in mg/urinary creatinine in mg. Normally the ratio in an adult is approximately 0.2 or 200 mg/day (SI = 2.92 μmol/day); in a child 0.5 or 500 mg/day (SI = 7.3 μmol/day).
   c. As proteinuria increases, the ratio increases (e.g., ratio of 3.5 = 3.5 gm/day [SI = 51.3 μmol/day] proteinuria).
   d. This method of estimating 24-hour proteinuria is useful when a 24-hour urine sample is difficult to obtain and/or when proteinuria has been established via a 24-hour collection and subsequent changes are monitored serially, such as with nephrotic syndrome.
7. Significant aminoaciduria occurs with elevated plasma amino acid levels (hepatic disorders), high protein intake, and renal tubular disorders (e.g., cystinuria and Hartnup disease).

J. Additional substances.
1. Uric acid.
   a. Daily urinary excretion is variable and influenced by diet and protein metabolism.
   b. Hyperuricosuria is associated with malignant neoplasms, antineoplastic agents, and gout. May result in calculi formation and renal impairment.
   c. Some hyperuricosuria is normal in pregnancy due to the increased glomerular filtration rate.

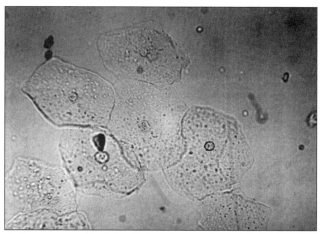

A. Squamous epithelial cells from lower urinary tract.

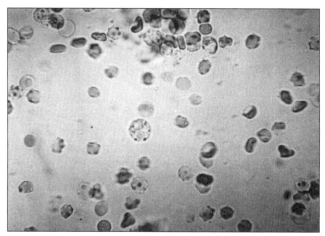

B. Numerous red blood cells and occasional white blood cells.

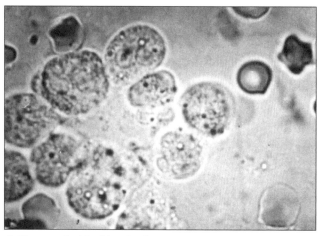

C. Clusters of white blood cells.

Figure 1.26. Urinary sediment.

2. Urea.
    a. Variable amount is excreted daily depending on diet, fluid balance, and kidney function.
    b. Altered urinary urea levels suggest kidney disease and need to be correlated with blood urea nitrogen levels. Urine urea levels usually decrease with kidney failure.
3. Myoglobin.
    a. Myoglobin is a protein found in muscle cells where it accepts oxygen from hemoglobin and stores oxygen for use by the mitochondria.
    b. Filtered by the nephron and excreted in the urine.
    c. Myoglobinuria occurs with excessive skeletal muscular trauma (called rhabdomyolysis) and does not necessarily indicate kidney disease.
    d. Excessive myoglobinemia may cause kidney impairment because one of myoglobin's metabolites is potentially nephrotoxic.

VI. Sediment.

A. Cells.
    1. Squamous epithelial cells represent normal desquamation from the lower urinary tract and a few are normal (see Figure 1.26A).
    2. Transitional cells, renal tubular cells, and oval fat bodies originate from the upper urinary tract with disorders such as acute tubular necrosis, acute glomerulonephritis, pyelonephritis, and nephrotic syndrome.
    3. Erythrocytes (red blood cells [RBCs]).
        a. A few RBCs are normally present in urine (see Figure 1.26B).
        b. An increased number indicates disruption of the genitourinary tract vasculature (e.g., inflammation, lesions, trauma, neoplasms, moving calculi, and cystic disease).
        c. Erythrocytes that originate from the kidney are usually broken and accompanied by red cell casts.
    4. Leukocytes, bacteria.
        a. A few leukocytes and bacteria normally are present in urine (see Figure 1.26C).
        b. An increased number of leukocytes, bacteria, or both nitrites and leukocyte esterase indicate inflammation in the urinary tract (e.g., pyelonephritis).
            (1) Leukocyte esterase is an enzyme found in azurophilic or primary neutrophil granules and released with inflammation.
                (a) Leukocyte esterase is reported as negative or positive and may be

quantified as trace, small (+), moderate (++), or large (+++).

(b) A false positive result may occur if urine has vaginal secretions or cells.

(c) An erroneous high positive result occurs when urine remains at room temperature because, over time, more leukocytes lyse and more leukocyte esterase is released.

(d) Substances that can affect test accuracy are the presence of ascorbic acid, glucose, albumin, cephalexin, tetracycline, cephalothin, and large quantities of oxalic acid in the urine.

(2) Casts usually accompany leukocytes and bacteria that originate in the kidney.

(3) Bacteria are surrounded by an antibody when they originate in the kidney. A full inflammatory reaction may take about a week, and that is when the antibody-coated bacteria will be visible in the urine. With repeated infections, the antibody-coated bacteria will appear more quickly.

(4) Persistent leukocyturia without bacteriuria may indicate the presence of fungi, yeast, or tubercule bacilli.

d. Eosinophils.

(1) Eosinophiluria indicates a hypersensitivity reaction intrarenally such as acute interstitial nephritis, or urinary tract infection and renal transplant rejection.

(2) Eosinophiluria is affirmed by Wright stain when urine pH is greater than 7 (SI = pH 7), or by Hansel stain when the urine pH is less than 7.

B. Crystals.

1. Crystalluria is an abnormal urinary finding and may or may not be related to kidney disease.

2. Crystal formation is pH dependent, occurs any place along the urinary tract, is enhanced by fluid volume depletion, and can result in calculi.

a. Crystals found in acid urine are uric acid, calcium oxalate, calcium sulfate, amorphous urate, cystine, leucine, and tyrosine (see Figure 1.27A).

b. Crystals found in alkaline urine are phosphates, calcium carbonate, and ammonium biuret (see Figure 1.27B).

c. Drugs and dyes can also crystallize.

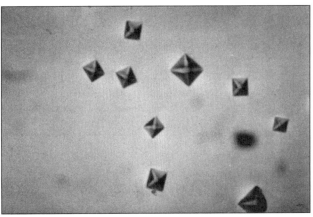

A. Calcium oxalate crystals.

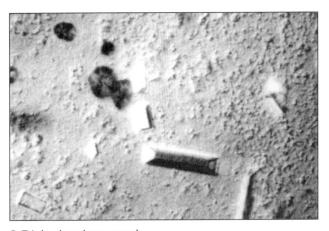

B. Triple phosphate crystals.

 Figure 1.27. Urinary crystals.

C. Casts.

1. Casts are formed or molded in the tubular lumen of the kidney and because of the molding process, are called casts (cylindruria).

2. Casts are composed of Tamm-Horsfall protein and other substances associated with inflammation (e.g., cellular debris, immunoglobulins, and pigments). Tamm-Horsfall protein is a mucoprotein that forms the base of casts, formed and secreted by cells of the ascending loop of Henle, distal tubule, and collecting duct.

3. Casts are important indicators of kidney disease and aid in identifying the type of disease.

a. Decreased tubular fluid flow or stasis, increased acidity, and increased solute concentration favor cast formation.

b. Casts generally form in the favorable environments of the distal tubule and collecting duct.

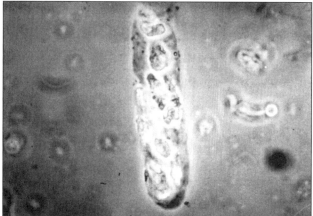

A. Tubular epithelial cell cast.

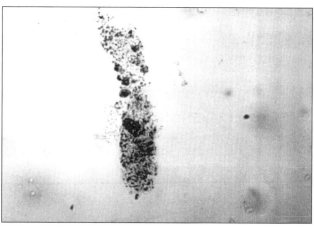

B. Coarse granular cast.

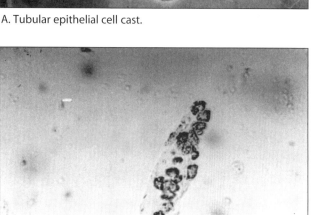

C. White blood cell cast.

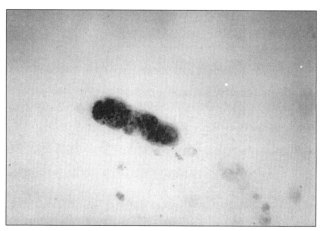

D. Red blood cell cast.

Figure 1.28. Urinary casts.

c. Casts can dissolve in alkaline urine.
d. Although casts vary in length, size, and width, they are cylindrical because the tubular lumen is cylindrical.
e. Casts are classified by their appearance and composition (see Figures 1.28A–D).

4. Types of casts.
a. Hyaline casts are acellular and a few in the urine are normal.
   (1) A transient increase in urinary hyaline casts can occur with stress, strenuous exercise, fever, and fluid loss.
   (2) A persistent increase may indicate renal parenchymal disease.
b. Red cell casts contain fragments of erythrocytes and are associated with glomerular disruption and bleeding (e.g., glomerulonephritis, Goodpasture syndrome, renal trauma, and lupus nephritis).
c. White cell casts contain leukocyte fragments and are associated with inflammation (e.g.,

pyelonephritis and interstitial nephritis).
d. Fatty casts contain lipoid material, are present with fatty degeneration of tubular epithelium, and are associated with nephrotic syndrome, diabetic glomerulosclerosis, and lupus erythematosus.
e. Renal tubular epithelial cell casts are composed of sloughed tubular epithelium and associated with acute tubular necrosis and transplant rejection.
f. Broad casts contain epithelium and are large because they form in the collecting duct.
g. Granular casts indicate kidney disease and represent final degeneration of cellular casts and/or aggregation of serum protein with Tamm-Horsfall protein.
   (1) Granular casts are described as fine or coarse. There is no clinical difference between them.
   (2) Pigmented granular casts contain portions of hemepigments, myoglobin,

hemoglobin, or a combination, and may be named for the pigment (e.g., hemoglobin cast).
  (3) Heavily pigmented granular casts may be called muddy brown casts and are one of the casts associated with acute tubular necrosis.
  h. Waxy casts are the final degeneration of granular casts.
  (1) Indicate advanced kidney disease, and are sometimes called kidney failure casts.
  (2) Associated with diabetic nephropathy, renal amyloidosis, and CKD Stage 5.

VII. Blood analysis.

A. Plasma creatinine.
  1. Normal 1 mg ± 0.3 mg/dL (SI = 88 mmol/dL) and pregnant woman 0.46 mg ± 0.3 mg/dL (SI = 37 mmol/dL).
  2. An end product of phosphocreatine, a high energy substance used to form ATP to be used as energy by muscles.
  3. Slightly higher in men than women because of larger muscle mass in men.
  4. Fluctuates minimally throughout the day and from day to day.
  5. Regulated and excreted by the kidneys.
  6. Rises with kidney failure, severe muscle breakdown, or both.
  7. An elevated creatinine is a good indicator of kidney function after it is established that no muscle breakdown exists.
  a. Plasma creatinine of 2 mg/dL (SI = 176 mmol) indicates an approximate 50% loss of kidney function. A plasma creatinine of 8–9 mg/dL (SI = 704–792 mmol/dL) indicates an approximate 90% loss of kidney function.
  b. The plasma creatinine rises when about 50% of kidney function is lost.
  8. As the ability of the kidneys to remove creatinine decreases, the plasma creatinine increases. As the plasma creatinine doubles, the creatinine clearance decreases by 50%.
  9. Because plasma creatinine varies from person to person related to muscle mass, it is important to obtain a baseline for each person and follow plasma creatinine levels over time.
  10. Plasma creatinine is less reliable as an indicator of kidney failure with malnourishment, liver failure, and heart failure. In these situations, creatinine clearance is more accurate.
  11. In pregnancy, plasma creatinine is lower because of increased clearance of creatinine. Therefore, a

slight rise in plasma creatinine (> 0.9 mg/dL [SI = 78 mmol/dL]) should be investigated.

B. Blood urea nitrogen (BUN).
  1. Normal 10–20 mg/dL (SI = 3.6–7.1 mmol/L); in pregnant woman 8.7 mg ± 1.5 mg/dL.
  2. An end product of endogenous or exogenous (dietary) protein metabolism.
  3. Influenced by fluid volume changes, dietary protein intake, and catabolism.
  4. 75% is excreted by the kidney and 25% by the bowel.
  5. BUN rises with kidney failure, increased protein breakdown (e.g., gastrointestinal bleeding and fever), and fluid volume depletion.
  a. With kidney failure, the kidney does not excrete urea and it is retained in the blood.
  b. With bleeding in the GI tract, the blood is digested (including plasma protein), and as with any protein, urea is an end product and absorbed into the blood.
  c. With fluid volume depletion, although the number of urea molecules stays constant, they appear increased in proportion to the low number of water molecules.
  6. Changes in BUN must be correlated with changes in plasma creatinine to assess kidney failure.
  7. In pregnancy, BUN is lower because of increased renal clearance. As with plasma creatinine, a slight rise should be investigated.
  8. BUN and plasma creatinine rise simultaneously in kidney failure.

C. Cystatin C.
  1. Cystatin C is a cysteine protease inhibitor produced by the body's cells at a constant rate.
  2. Filtered by the glomerulus and reabsorbed by the tubules.
  3. May be used as an alternative to serum creatinine or creatinine clearance for screening and monitoring.
  4. Elevated levels indicate decreased kidney function (decreased glomerular filtration rate).
  5. May be more useful in monitoring kidney function in critically ill patients and tends to rise more quickly than creatinine.
  6. May be useful in predicting higher risk of CKD among older adults without known kidney disease.
  7. Not affected by diet, inflammation, gender, age, or race.

D. Although many electrolytes, pH, and nonelectrolytes

are regulated and excreted by the kidney, numerous extrarenal factors influence their plasma levels and must be considered in assessing kidney function. For example, plasma potassium is regulated and excreted by the kidneys but is also influenced by insulin, aldosterone, cellular damage, and pH changes. After disorders of these extrarenal factors are excluded, a rise in plasma potassium along with a rise in creatinine and BUN is a good indicator of kidney failure.

E. Erythropoiesis is regulated by renal erythropoietin. With chronic kidney disease, anemia occurs, and the hematocrit, hemoglobin, and the erythrocyte count are decreased.

F. Substances that the kidney secretes can be measured, such as plasma renin.
  1. Renin is elevated in some forms of hypertension and renal artery stenosis.
  2. Renin is normally elevated in pregnancy.
  3. Plasma renin concentration is obtained with a blood sample drawn with the patient in an upright position (stimulates renin release).
  4. Concentration values.
    a. Normal sodium diet.
      (1) 2.9–24.0 ng/mL/hr ages 20–39.
      (2) 2.9–10.8 ng/mL/hr greater than 40 years old.
    b. Low sodium diet.
      (1) 0.1–4.3 ng/mL/hr ages 20-39.
      (2) 0.1–3.0 ng/mL/hr greater than 40 years old.

G. Plasma substances that are altered with specific kidney diseases can be measured (e.g., antibodies, complement, and autoantibodies).
  1. Antibodies are composed of globulin proteins and termed immunoglobulins (Ig).
    a. The classes of these antibodies and typical values are:
      (1) IgG   565-1765 mg/dL (SI = 5.65–17.65 g/L).
      (2) IgA   85–385 mg/dL (SI = 0.85–3.85 g/L).
      (3) IgM   55–375 mg/dL (SI = 0.55–3.75 g/L).
      (4) IgD   Minimal.
      (5) IgE   Minimal.
    b. A rise in IgG and IgM is associated with nephropathy, such as SLE or Sjögren's syndrome.
    c. IgA rises with Berger's disease (glomerular pathology) and pregnancy hypertension.
    d. IgE rises with allergic reactions.
  2. Normal complement values are:

    a. Total complement: 75–160 U/mL (SI = 75–160 U/L).
    b. C3 55–120 mg/dL (SI = 0.55–1.20 g/L).
    c. C4 20–50 mg/dL (SI = 0.20–0.50 g/L).
    d. Complement decreases with inflammatory kidney diseases.
  3. Autoantibodies are normally absent. Therefore their presence indicates pathology. Autoantibodies and kidney diseases associated with them include:
    a. Anti-DNA: systemic lupus erythematosus (SLE) and scleroderma.
    b. Antiglomerular basement membrane: Goodpasture syndrome.
    c. Antinuclear: SLE, scleroderma and Sjögren's syndrome.
    d. Anti-sm-B: SLE (sm = smooth muscle).
    e. Anti-ss-A and Anti-ss-C (ss = Sjögren's syndrome).

VIII. Creatinine clearance.

A. Creatinine clearance.
  1. The amount of blood cleared of creatinine in 1 minute by the glomerular capillaries.
  2. After creatinine is filtered through the glomerular capillaries, it passes through the nephron with minimal change and is excreted. Creatinine clearance is a measure of the glomerular filtration rate (GFR).
  3. Creatinine clearance is a good clinical indicator of kidney function. As kidney function decreases, creatinine clearance decreases.
  4. Normal creatinine clearance for a young adult is about 110 to 120 mL/min.

B. Procedure. Collect a 24-hour urine specimen and one blood specimen drawn at the midpoint of the urine collection.
  1. The volume of urine and quantity of creatinine in the blood and urine are measured.
  2. These values are inserted into formulas that calculate creatinine clearance.

C. Formulas for creatinine clearance.
  1. Basic formula:

$$\frac{\text{volume of urine (mL/min)} \times \text{urinary concentration of creatinine (mg/dL)}}{\text{plasma creatinine (mg/dL)}}$$

  2. Approximately 10% of urinary creatinine is secreted into the tubular lumen. Therefore, the above formula overestimates GFR by about 10%. Thus, a more accurate GFR is obtained by multiplying the results by 90% (.90).

3. Creatinine clearance can be estimated by the Cockcroft-Gault formula:

$$\frac{(140 - age) \times (adjusted\ body\ weight\ in\ kg)}{(72) \times (serum\ creatinine\ in\ mg/dL)}$$

  a. For females, the above result is multiplied by 85% (.85).
  b. This calculation does not require a 24-hour urine collection and is an estimate rather than direct measure of the creatinine clearance.

4. Another formula for creatinine clearance is the MDRD (Modification of Diet in Renal Disease) formula:

  a. $186 \times (plasma\ creatinine)^{-1.154} \times (age\ in\ years)^{-0.203}$
  b. For females, the above result is multiplied by 0.742.
  c. For African Americans, the above result is multiplied by 1.210.
  d. The MDRD formula is complex due to the negative log algebra functions. As a result, a calculator is needed to compute the creatine clearance.
  e. The MDRD formula is generally considered a more accurate estimate of creatinine clearance than the Cockcroft-Gault formula. However, many clinicians and reference books use the Cockcroft-Gault equation due to ease of calculation.

5. For children (1 week to 18 years), the Schwartz equation is often used:

  a. (length [cm] x k) / serum creatinine
  b. k = 0.45 for infants 1–52 weeks old.
  c. k = 0.55 for children 1 to 13 years old.
  d. k = 0.55 for adolescent females 13–18 years old.
  e. k = 0.7 for adolescent males 13–18 years old.

IX. Vascular studies.

A. Radionuclide tests.
  1. Renal scan.
    a. A radionuclide (low dose radioactive substance) is injected intravenously. The radioactive substance circulates through the kidneys and is excreted in the urine.
    b. Renal scans depict accumulation of the radionuclide by the kidneys and primarily provide information related to anatomy (for example, in renovascular disease hypoperfused areas visualize poorly).
  2. Renogram.
    a. Procedure is same as the renal scan.
    b. As the radionuclide circulates through the kidneys, scintillators count the agent's activity and curves are generated that describe blood

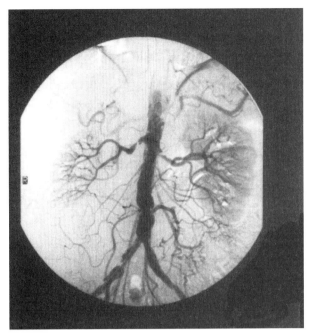

Figure 1.29. Abdominal aortogram and renal arteriogram. Bilaterally, renal arteries are narrowed near their exit from the aorta. The right kidney is small and the left kidney is normal size. The distal aorta and right common iliac artery have moderate to high-grade stenosis.

flow, glomerular filtration, and tubular secretion.
  3. Patient preparation for above tests.
    a. Explanation of the procedure, which is painless and noninvasive (except for the venipuncture).
    b. Required to sit or lie quietly during the test.
    c. No special posttest care.

B. Renal arteriogram.
  1. Outlines renal arterial vasculature and differentiates the type of renovascular disorder (for example, can identify high vascularity of a malignant neoplasm; differentiate between stenosed or misplaced vessels) (see Figure 1.29).
  2. Indications for an arteriogram include persistent hematuria, blunt trauma, hypertension, renal arterial disease, renal mass, and preparation for kidney surgery.
  3. Procedure.
    a. A radiopaque dye is injected intravenously (IV) or through a catheter.
    b. Numerous roentgenograms are taken.
    c. The IV catheter is removed and a pressure dressing applied to the catheter insertion site.

4. The iodine-based radiopaque dye is potentially nephrotoxic and allergenic.
   a. Should be used with caution, and in the lowest dose possible in patients with diabetes mellitus, diabetic nephropathy, preexisting kidney disease, vascular disease, multiple myeloma, older adults, and in the presence of fluid volume depletion.
   b. Individuals with an allergy to iodine or seafood may be unable to receive an iodine-based dye.
5. Patient care before the arteriogram.
   a. Description of the test.
   b. Assessment for allergy to the dye.
   c. Explanation that as dye is injected an unusual taste may be sensed in the mouth.
   d. Explanation of posttest care and vital signs monitoring.
6. Patient care after a renal arteriogram:
   a. Bed rest for 4–12 hours (variable; may be shorter or longer depending on the patient and length/difficulty of the procedure).
   b. Frequent assessment of vital signs and pedal pulses for peripheral circulation.
   c. Assessment for bleeding or hematoma formation at the catheter insertion site.
   d. Maintenance of the pressure dressing for 24 hours.
   e. Adequate hydration.
   f. Observation for nephrotoxic and/or allergic reactions to the dye.
7. Complications associated with a renal arteriogram include inflammation, hematoma, thrombus, embolus, arteriovenous fistula formation, atheroma dislodgement, acute decrease in kidney function (nephrotoxic reaction), and anaphylactic reaction to dye.

C. Renal venogram.
   1. Outlines the renal venous vessels.
   2. The procedure and patient care are same as for the renal arteriogram.

D. Magnetic resonance angiography (MRA).
   1. Arteries can be visualized with increasing accuracy.
   2. Can be an alternative to traditional renal angiography for people at risk for complications associated with contrast media.
   3. See MRI for additional discussion regarding patient care and procedure.

X. Roentgenograms.

A. Plain roentgenogram (x-ray) of the kidneys, ureters, and bladder (KUB).
   1. Visualizes the size, shape, position, and number of kidney, ureteral, and bladder structures.
   2. Identifies radiopaque objects, foreign bodies, calculi, neoplasms, or air.

B. Significance of findings.
   1. Size, shape.
      a. Large or irregular shaped kidneys may indicate hydronephrosis, cysts, neoplasms.
      b. Small kidneys may indicate chronic glomerulonephritis or nonfunctioning kidneys.
      c. The kidneys lengthen a few centimeters with pregnancy.
   2. Air around or inside the kidney may indicate severe infection.
   3. A nebulous or indistinct kidney border may indicate neoplasm or inflammation.

C. Patient teaching.
   1. A KUB is noninvasive, painless, requires no dyes, and can be done in an upright or lying position.
   2. No special patient preparation or posttest care is required.

XI. Ultrasound studies.

A. During renal ultrasound, inaudible nonharmful sound waves are reflected off the kidneys. Photographs are made that identify renal anatomy and true kidney depth.

B. Patient teaching.
   1. Procedure is noninvasive and painless.
   2. Requires that the patient remain in the prone or sitting position for about 30 minutes.
   3. No special care before or after the procedure is required.

C. Limitations.
   1. Ribs, adipose tissue, and gas in the bowel can interfere with sound wave reflections.
   2. Interpretation is difficult in obese individuals.
   3. Interpretation is difficult if the kidneys are high under the ribs and/or behind a gas filled gastrointestinal tract.

D. Significance of findings.
1. Outlines hydronephrosis.
2. Differentiates between a cyst that is fluid-filled versus a tumor that is solid.
3. During pregnancy, the kidneys will be larger.

XII. Computerized axial tomography (CAT/CT).

A. Numerous roentgenograms are taken, each about 10 degrees apart and transmitted into a computer that creates an image of the kidney and calculates its density.

B. Significance of findings.
1. CAT is more sensitive than ultrasound.
2. Detects and characterizes renal masses.
3. Visualizes renal vascular disorders, inferior vena cava tumors.
4. Identifies filling defects of the collecting system and regional lymph nodes.

C. CT can be performed with or without intravenous dye. The patient is observed for an allergic response to the dye during and after the test.

D. Patient teaching includes:
1. Test is painless.
2. A supine position for 10–15 minutes is required.
3. May have to hold breath for short periods of time during the test.
4. Machine makes some noise.
5. After the test no special care is required.

XIII. Magnetic resonance imaging (MRI).

A. MRI is a painless, noninvasive procedure that provides visual information about soft tissue.

B. The MRI scanner applies a strong magnetic field that causes protons to align themselves with the magnetic field. Emission of radiowaves causes the magnetic field to rotate or resonate.

C. The rotating fields generate electric signals that a computer analyzes and creates an image on a screen. Images are available in all planes.

D. Significance of findings.
1. Visualizes renal vessels, possible extension of neoplasm in the renal vein and/or inferior vena cava.
2. Visualizes retroperitoneal structures.
3. Identifies renal masses. MRI does not differentiate benign from malignant tumors.

E. Patient teaching includes:
1. Test is painless.
2. Need to lie still in a horizontal position on a table.
3. The table is moved into a tube-like structure that may create a feeling of claustrophobia ("open" MRI is also available that does not require a closed structure).
4. In general, metal objects must be removed before the test. Individuals with pacemakers and aneuryism clips should not undergo an MRI. Other indwelling metal is acceptable (e.g., braces, surgical clips and joint replacements after 6 weeks postoperatively).
5. Takes about 40–90 minutes.
6. The room may feel cool and it is warmer inside the magnet.
7. The magnet makes noise like a jack hammer so ear plugs or covering are worn.
8. Sedation is available based on the patient's need.
9. Individuals with CKD stage 4 and 5 should undergo MRI only if necessary. In about 2.5% of these individuals, an adverse reaction to gadolinium (the contrast agent used in MRI) may cause nephrogenic systemic fibrosis (NSF). NSF is characterized by thickening and hardening of the skin (most commonly in the extremities) that progresses to joint immobility and may present 2 weeks to 18 months after receiving gadolinium.

F. Posttest care is determined by the use or absence of sedation during the test.

XIV. Excretory urograms.

A. Intravenous pyelography (IVP).
1. Provides information about the size, shape, and position of the urinary tract structures, and renal excretory function (e.g., twisted ureters, misplaced kidneys, and obstructed calyces).
2. A radiopaque dye is injected intravenously, circulates through the kidneys, and is excreted in the urine. Roentgenograms are taken as the dye circulates through the urinary tract.
3. The iodine based dye used for the IVP is potentially nephrotoxic and allergenic.
   a. Should be used with caution, and in the lowest dose possible in patients with diabetes mellitus, diabetic nephropathy, preexisting kidney disease, vascular disease, multiple myeloma, older adults, and in the presence of fluid volume depletion.

b. Individuals with an allergy to iodine or seafood may be unable to receive an iodine-based dye.

4. Patient preparation for an IVP includes:
   a. Explanation of the procedure.
   b. A clear, empty gastrointestinal tract.
   c. Good hydration.
   d. Assessment of kidney function (creatinine clearance).
   e. Assessment of allergy to the dye, iodine, or seafood.

5. Posttest care includes:
   a. Maintaining good hydration.
   b. Watching for allergic reaction.
   c. Evaluating kidney function for nephrotoxicity to the dye.

B. Retrograde pyelogram.
   1. Provides anatomic information about the collecting system of the urinary tract (e.g., the position of a ureteral calculus).
   2. Procedure.
      a. Patient preparation is similar to an IVP.
      b. The procedure may be uncomfortable — pressure and an urge to void are felt.
      c. Bladder and ureteral catheterizations are performed.
      d. A radiopaque dye is injected through the catheters into the urinary tract and roentgenograms are taken.
         (1) As the catheters are removed, more dye is injected and x-ray is taken.
         (2) About 5 minutes after the catheters are removed, another x-ray is taken.
         (3) If a ureteral obstruction is identified, a stent may be left so urine can drain.
   3. Potential complications include:
      a. Urinary tract infection.
      b. Perforation of the bladder or ureter.
      c. Ureteral edema with possible obstruction.
      d. Hematuria.
      e. Discomfort from the dye (unusual taste).
   4. Postprocedure care includes:
      a. Assess for and treat complications.
      b. Assess for bleeding, infection, characteristics of the urine, ability to void and completely empty the bladder (using a bladder scanner may be helpful to determine bladder volume).
      c. Assess for pain and/or ureteral, bladder, or urethral spasms. Administer analgesics.
      d. Provide and encourage hydration.

C. Antegrade pyelogram (nephrostomogram).
   1. Provides anatomic visualization of the urinary collecting system.
      a. May include the renal pelvis.
      b. Will include the ureter.
      c. May include the bladder.
   2. Indicated with a ureteral, ureteropelvic, or ureterovesical obstruction when an intravenous or retrograde pyelography cannot be done.
   3. Procedure.
      a. Contrast material is injected into the renal pelvis via a percutaneous needle or a nephrostomy tube (if present), and x-rays are taken.
      b. Patient preparation and postcare are similar to a kidney biopsy (following section) and retrograde pyelogram (above).
         (1) Pain occurs with this procedure as with a kidney biopsy because a needle punctures the kidney.
         (2) No pain is felt if a nephrostomy tube is in place.
      c. Potential complications.
         (1) Allergic reaction to the dye.
         (2) Urinary tract bleeding.
         (3) Urinary tract infection.
      d. Generally, minimal concern about potential nephrotoxicity of the contrast material (unless it refluxes through the calyces and into the papillae).

XV. Kidney biopsy.

A. Purpose, indications, and contraindications.
   1. Determines the nature and extent of kidney disease for diagnosis, treatment, and prognosis.
   2. Indications.
      a. Unexplained acute kidney injury.
      b. Persistent proteinuria.
      c. Hematuria of renal origin.
      d. A kidney mass/suspected cancer.
      e. Glomerulopathies.
      f. Suspected kidney involvement in systemic disease.
      g. Transplant rejection.
   3. Contraindications.
      a. Hemorrhagic tendencies.
      b. Uncontrolled hypertension.
      c. Sepsis.
      d. Solitary kidney (relative contraindication).
      e. Small shrunken kidneys.
      f. Large polycystic kidneys.
      g. Hydronephrosis.
      h. Documented kidney neoplasm.
      i. Urinary tract infection.

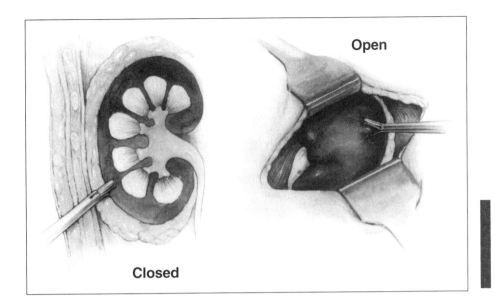

Open

Closed

Figure 1.30. Kidney biopsy. Technique for closed/ percutaneous and open kidney biopsy. The biopsy needle is enlarged for illustrative purposes.

j. Frequent coughing, sneezing (or both).
k. Uncooperative patient.

B. Procedure.
1. Invasive procedure requiring strict aseptic technique.
2. Small section of cortical tissue is obtained by a needle and examined histologically by light, immunofluorescence, and/or electron microscopy.
  a. Light microscopy magnifies tissue approximately 750 times and electron microscopy 54,999 times.
  b. Immunofluorescence is a staining technique used to study immunopathologic processes (e.g., identify complement and antibodies).
3. Kidney biopsy can be done by the open or closed/percutaneous method. The percutaneous method is done more frequently (see Figure 1.30).
4. Open method.
  a. Surgical procedure.
    (1) The kidney is exposed.
    (2) Biopsy needle is inserted into the kidney under direct visualization.
  b. Indicated when percutaneous biopsy is hazardous (e.g., with an obese or restless patient).
  c. Patient preparation is similar to any major abdominal operation and includes the preparation for a closed or percutaneous kidney biopsy (explained below).
  d. Advantages include direct visualization of kidney, better control of bleeding, and can be done with other abdominal surgeries.

e. Disadvantages include the risks of surgery (e.g., risk of anesthesia, an operation, lengthened recovery, and infection).
5. Closed or percutaneous method.
  a. Procedure.
    (1) Can be done at the bedside if patient is unable to go to medical imaging department.
    (2) Patient is prone with pillows under abdomen to elevate kidney.
    (3) Patient with transplanted kidney will be supine because of the position of the allograft in the iliac fossa.
    (4) Skin is cleansed and anesthetized.
    (5) Patient holds his or her breath and the biopsy needle is inserted with aid of ultrasound (needle moves slightly with breathing because the kidneys are in contact with the diaphragm).
    (6) Patient may complain of pain and/or intense pressure as the needle enters the innervated renal capsule.
    (7) Tissue samples are taken and prepared, needle removed, pressure dressing applied to puncture site.
    (8) Patient remains in position for 20–30 minutes.
    (9) An ultrasound may be completed after the biopsy to identify any immediate postprocedure bleeding.
  b. Patient preparation.
    (1) Explanation of the procedure and postprocedure care.
    (2) Signed informed consent.

(3) Pain will be felt when needle enters kidney (this is an example of visceral pain).

(4) Patient responsibilities (e.g., position and holding breath).

(5) Hematologic and kidney function assessment.

(6) Determination of kidney position and depth (usually by CT or ultrasound).

(7) Vital sign monitoring.

(8) Mild sedation.

(9) Urinate before procedure.

(10) NPO 8–12 hours before (variable).

6. Postprocedure care for percutaneous and open kidney biopsy.

   a. Monitor vital signs frequently for first 24–48 hours to detect intrarenal and/or extrarenal bleeding and infection.

   b. Assess for other signs and symptoms of bleeding including pallor, dizziness, lightheadedness, decrease in erythrocytes, hematocrit, and/or hemoglobin, backache and/or flank pain.

   c. Collect serial urine specimens to evaluate hematuria (redness should decrease with each sample).

   d. Maintain bed rest and pressure dressings to prevent bleeding.

   e. Assess puncture site for bleeding and/or signs and symptoms of inflammation.

   f. Assess pain with administration of analgesics (opioids often indicated. Cold therapy and therapeutic touch may also be beneficial).

   g. Educate and assist with splinting puncture site to decrease discomfort with coughing and deep breathing.

   h. Instruct patient to drink liberal amounts of fluids to maintain a dilute urine and prevent intrarenal clot formation.

   i. Give emotional and psychologic support.

   j. Limit strenuous activity, heavy lifting for 1–2 weeks.

7. Complications.

   a. Persistent hematuria.

   b. Infection.

   c. Perirenal and/or intrarenal arteriovenous fistula.

   d. Aneurysm.

   e. Laceration of organs and/or blood vessels adjacent to the biopsied kidney.

American Cancer Society. (2006). *How is kidney cancer (renal cell carcinoma) staged?* Retrieved August 3, 2006, from http://www.cancer.org.

Berne, R.M., Levy, M.N., Koeppen, B.M., & Stanton, B.A. (2005). *Principles of physiology* (5th ed.). Philadelphia: Elsevier.

Bickley, L.S., & Prabhu, F.R. (2004). *Bates' guide to physical examination and history taking* (8th ed.). Philadelphia: Lippincott Williams & Wilkins.

Brenner, B.M. (2003). *Brenner and Rector's the kidney* (7th ed.). Philadelphia: Saunders.

Burrows-Hudson, S., & Prowant, B. (Eds.). (2005). *Nephrology nursing standards of practice and guidelines for care* (2nd ed.). Pitman, NJ: American Nephrology Nurses' Association.

Chmielewski, C. , Molechek, M., Ludlow, M., Yucha, C., Gurthrie, D., Dungan, J., Candela, L., et al. (2006). Renal physiology. In A. Molzahn & E. Butera (Eds.), *Contemporary nephrology nursing: Principles and practice* (2nd ed., pp. 73-118). Pitman, NJ: American Nephrology Nurses' Association.

Copeland, S.D. (2006). Amyloidosis and its impact on patients with ESRD. *Nephrology Nursing Journal, 33,* 31-33.

Eaton, D.C., & Pooler, J. (2004). *Vander's renal physiology* (6th ed.). St. Louis: McGraw-Hill.

Foote, J., & Cohen, B. (1998). Medicinal herb use and the renal patient. *Journal of Renal Nutrition, 8*(1), 40-42.

Ganong, W.F. (2005). *Review of medical physiology* (22nd ed.). New York: McGraw Hill.

Gleeson, T., & Bulugahapitiya, S. (2004). Contrast-induced neph-ropathy. *American Journal of Roentgenology, 183,* 1673-1689.

Guyton, A.C., & Hall, J.E. (2006). *Textbook of medical physiology* (11th ed.). Philadelphia: Elsevier.

Headley, C.M., & Wall, B. (1999). Acquired cystic kidney disease in ESRD. *ANNA Journal, 26,* 381-389.

Hodge, P., & Ullrich, S. (1999). Does your assessment include alternative therapies? *RN, 62*(6), 47-49.

Hricik, D.E., Miller, R.T., & Sedor, J.R. (2003). *Nephrology secrets* (2nd ed.). Philadelphia: Hanley & Belfus.

Jacobs, D.S., DeMott, W.R., & Oxley, D.K. (Eds.). (2001). *Laboratory test handbook* (5th ed.). Hudson, OH: Lexi-Comp.

Kee, J.L. (2006). *Laboratory and diagnostic tests with nursing implications* (7th ed.). Upper Saddle River, NJ: Prentice Hall.

Lancaster, L.E. (1991). Atrial natriuretic peptide: Implications for nephrology nursing. *Dialysis & Transplantation, 20*(1), 17-19.

Liangos, O., Wald, R., O'Bell, J.W., Price, L., Pereira, B.J., & Jaber, B.L. (2006). Epidemiology and outcomes of acute renal failure in hospitalized patients: A national survey. *Clinical Journal of the American Society of Nephrology, 1,* 43-51.

Little, C. (2000). Renovascular hypertension. *AJN, 100*(2), 46-52.

Lochner, M.L., & Wolf, A. (2006). Human immunodeficiency virus-1 associated nephropathy (HIVAN): Epidemiology, pathogenesis, histology, diagnosis, and medical management. *Nephrology Nursing Journal, 33,* 259-267.

Mattson, D.L. (2003). Renal physiology. In H. Raff, *Physiology secrets* (2nd ed., pp. 123-158). Philadelphia: Belfus & Hanley.

Michota, F.A. (2001). *Diagnostic procedures handbook* (2nd ed.). Hudson, OH: Lexi-Comp.

Molzahn, A., & Butera, E. (Eds.). (2006). *Contemporary nephrology nursing: Principles and practice* (2nd ed). Pitman, NJ: American Nephrology Nurses' Association.

National Kidney Foundation (NFK). (2002). K/DOQI clinical practice guidelines for chronic kidney disease: Evaluation, classification, and stratification. *American Journal of Kidney Disease, 39*(Suppl. 2), S1-266.

Nelson, D.B. (2006). Minimal change glomerulopathy in pregnancy. *Nephrology Nursing Journal, 30,* 45-56, 122.

Olyaie, A.J., De Mattos, A.M., & Bennett, W. (1999). Immuno-suppressed-induced nephropathy: Pathophysiology, incidence, and management. *Drug safety, 21,* 471-488.

Otterness, S. (2006). Scleroderma: A case presentation. *Nephrology Nursing Journal, 33,* 39-41, 90.

Prahash, A., & Lynch, T. (2004). B-Type natriuretic peptide: A diagnostic, prognostic, and therapeutic tool in heart failure. *American Journal of Critical Care, 13,* 46-53.

Rabinovitch, A. (2001). *Urinalysis and collection, transportation, and preservation of urine specimens: Approved guideline* (2nd ed.). Wayne, PA: National Committee for Clinical Laboratory Standards.

Radke, K.J. (1994). The aging kidney: Structure, function, and nursing practice implications. *ANNA Journal, 21*(4), 181-190.

Rose, B.D., & Post, T. (2001). *Clinical physiology of acid-base and electrolyte disorders* (5th ed.). New York: McGraw-Hill.

Russell, T.A. (2006). Diabetic nephropathy in patients with type I diabetes mellitus. *Nephrology Nursing Journal, 33,* 15-30.

Schira, M., & Lough, M. (2006). Renal clinical assessment and diagnostic procedures. In L.D. Urden, K.M. Stacy, & M.E. Lough (Eds.), *Thelan's critical care nursing. Diagnosis and management* (5th ed., pp. 801-812). Philadelphia: Elsevier.

Schrier, R.W. (Ed.). (2001). *Diseases of the kidney and urinary tract* (6th ed.). Philadelphia: Lippincott Williams & Wilkins.

Seeley, R.R., Stephens, T.D., & Tate, P. (2006). *Anatomy & physiology* (7th ed.). New York: McGraw-Hill.

Seidel, H.M., Ball, J.W., Dains, J.E., & Benedict, G.W. (2003). *Mosby's guide to physical examination* (5th ed.). Philadelphia: Mosby.

Simerville, J.A., Maxted, W.C., & Pahira, J.J. (2005). Urinalysis: A comprehensive review. *American Family Physician, 71,* 1153-1162.

Smith, D.M., Fortune-Faulkner, E.M., & Spurbeck, B.L. (2000). Lupus nephritis: Pathophysiology, diagnosis, and collaborative management. *Nephrology Nursing Journal, 27,* 199-211.

Snyder, S., & Pendergraph, B. (2005). Detection and evaluation of chronic kidney disease. *American Family Physician, 72,* 1723-1732.

Turkoski, B.B., Lance, B.R., & Bonfiglio, M.F. (2005). *Drug information handbook for advanced practice nursing* (6th ed.). Hudson, OH: Lexi-Comp.

United States Renal Data System. (2005). *2005 annual data report.* Retrieved July 23, 2006, from http://www.usrds.org/2005

Vanherweghem, J.L. (2000). Nephropathy and herbal medicine. *Journal of Kidney Disease, 35,* 330-332.

Wilkinson, A.H., & Cohen, D. (1999). Renal failure in the recipients of nonrenal solid organ transplants. *Journal of the American Society of Nephrology, 10,* 1136-1144.

Section 2

Chronic Kidney Disease

Section Editor

Caroline S. Counts, MSN, RN, CNN

Authors

Gladys S. Benavente, MSN, ANP-C, CNN-NP

Caroline S. Counts, MSN, RN, CNN

Patricia Bargo McCarley, MSN, RN, NP, CNN

Nancy J. Pelfrey, MSN, RN, ACNP-C, CNN-NP

Suanne Petroff, APRN, BC, CNN

Lucy Stackiewicz, MSN, CNN, CRNP

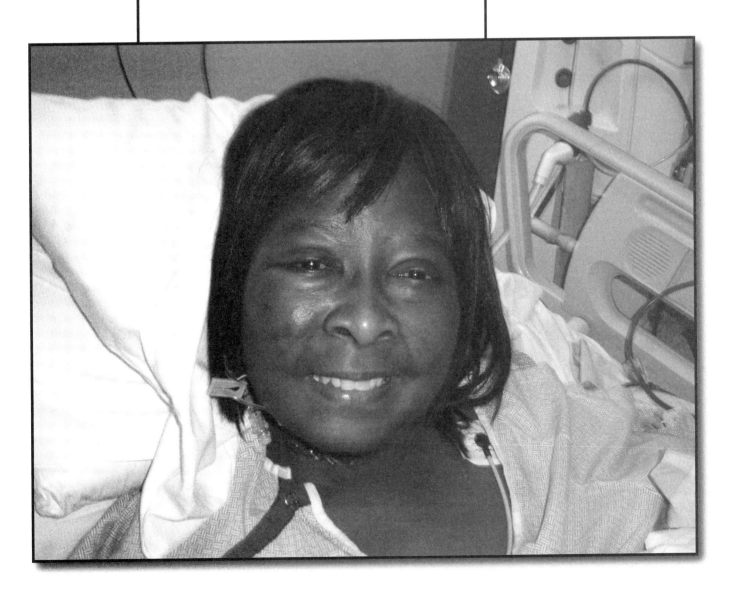

About the Authors

Caroline S. Counts, MSN, RN, CNN, Section Editor and Author, is Research Coordinator in the Division of Nephrology at the Medical University of South Carolina in Charleston, South Carolina.

Gladys S. Benavente, MSN, ANP-C, CNN-NP, is a Renal Nurse Practitioner & Primary Care Provider at Southern Arizona V.A. Healthcare Systems in Tucson, Arizona.

Patricia Bargo McCarley, MSN, RN, NP, CNN, is a Nurse Practitioner at Diablo Nephrology Medical Group in Walnut Creek, California.

Nancy J. Pelfrey, MSN, RN, ACNP-C, CNN-NP, is a Nurse Practitioner at DaVita, Inc., in Fairview, North Carolina.

Suanne Petroff, APRN, BC, CNN, is a Disease Management Consultant at CKD Consults in South Deerfield, Massachusetts.

Lucy Stackiewicz, MSN, CNN, CRNP, is a Nurse Practitioner in Nephrology and Transplant at University Physicians, Inc., University of Maryland Medical System in Baltimore, Maryland.

Section 2

Chronic Kidney Disease

Section

2

Chronic Kidney Disease

Purpose

Chronic kidney disease (CKD) has been declared a public health issue by the Centers for Disease Control and Prevention (Schoolwerth et al., 2006). It meets the four criteria to be designated as such. First, it places a burden on society that is getting larger despite existing control efforts. Second, the burden is distributed unfairly in that certain segments of the population are affected unequally. Third, there is evidence that preventive strategies could substantially lessen the burden of the condition. And, fourth, those preventive strategies are not yet in place. For many reasons, all nurses need to be prepared for the rise in the incidence and prevalence of CKD.

Objectives

Upon completion of this section, the learner will be able to:
1. Summarize the definition and stages of chronic kidney diseases.
2. Describe the pathophysiology of chronic kidney disease.
3. Recognize the comorbidities associated with CKD.
4. Relate the importance of early identification and treatment of chronic kidney disease and its comorbidities.
5. Discuss steps used to delay the progression of CKD.
6. Identify the complications of CKD.
7. List methods of empowering individuals with CKD to make changes needed to take control of their own health care.

Chapter 4

Introduction to Chronic Kidney Disease

I. Introduction.

A. Definitions.
1. Chronic kidney disease (CKD), as defined by the National Kidney Foundation's (NKF) Kidney Disease Outcomes Quality Initiative (KDOQI), includes the following criteria (see Table 2.1).
   a. Kidney damage for greater than or equal to 3 months with or without decreased glomerular filtration rate (GFR), *or*
   b. GFR < 60 mL/min/1.73 m² for greater than or equal to 3 months with or without kidney damage.
2. Kidney damage is defined as structural or functional abnormalities of the kidney. Initially there may be no drop in the GFR. Markers for kidney damage include:
   a. Abnormalities in the composition of the blood.
   b. Abnormalities in the composition of the urine.
   c. Abnormalities in imaging tests.
3. CKD is defined according to the stage of kidney damage or the level of kidney function (i.e., the GFR).

B. Quick statistics.
1. One in 9 American adults (age 20 and older) — an estimated 20 million people — have chronic kidney disease.
2. The number of people diagnosed with kidney disease has doubled each decade for the last 2 decades.
3. Each year, kidney disease kills more than 14 people out of every 100,000, making it America's ninth leading cause of death.
4. It is estimated that 800,000 patients in the United States have serum creatinine > 2 mg/dL and 6.2 million have serum creatinine > 1.5 mg/dL.
5. It is also estimated that by the year 2030, the annual number of people with new onset of end-stage renal disease (ESRD) will exceed 450,000. Those receiving dialysis or kidney transplant will exceed 2 million.

C. Risk factors for developing CKD.
1. Diabetes (DM) is the most common cause of CKD worldwide.
   a. For Americans born in 2000:
      (1) Males have a 33% lifetime risk of developing diabetes.
      (2) Females have a 39% lifetime risk.
      (3) Hispanic American males have a 45% lifetime risk.
      (4) Hispanic American females have a 53% lifetime risk.
   b. Obesity is an additional risk factor for diabetes.
   c. The recommended HbA1C (glycosylated hemoglobin) level for people without diabetes is between 4% and 6%; for persons with diabetes it is < 7%. Data from the National Health and Nutrition Examination Survey (NHANES) revealed that only 37% of participants diagnosed with diabetes achieved that goal. This lack of control leads to further damage.
2. Hypertension (HTN).
   a. More than 50,000,000 Americans have hypertension that requires treatment. The Seventh Report of the Joint National Commission on Prevention, Detection, Evaluation, and Treatment of High Blood Pressure (JNC 7) reported that only 59% receive treatment, and of those, only 34% achieved blood pressure control.

Table 2.1

Definition of Chronic Kidney Disease

Criteria

1. Kidney damage for 3 months, as defined by structural of functional abnormalities of the kidney, with or without decreased GFR (glomerular filtration rate), manifested by *either*:
   • Pathological abnormalities; or
   • Markers of kidney damage, including abnormalities in the composition of the blood or urine, or abnormalities in imaging tests
2. GFR < 60 mL/min/1.73 m² for ≥ 3 months, with or without kidney damage

Source: NFK KDOQI Guidelines, http://www.kidney.org/professionals/kdoqi/guidelines_ckd/p1_exec.htm.

b. Systolic blood pressure is particularly worrisome as it begins to rise at around 50 years of age and continues this upward progression. The diastolic pressure rises until 50 years of age and then levels off.

3. Other underlying diseases and conditions that are considered risk factors.
   a. Obesity.
   b. Dyslipidemia.
   c. Autoimmune disease.
   d. Urinary stones.
   e. Urinary tract infections.
   f. Lower urinary tract obstruction.
   g. Reduction in kidney mass.
   h. Recovery from acute kidney injury (AKI).
   i. Neoplasia.

4. Lifestyle factors.
   a. Tobacco.
   b. Inactivity.
   c. Low income.
   d. Education.
   e. Obesity.

5. Prenatal factors.
   a. Maternal diabetes mellitus.
   b. Low birth weight.
   c. Small for gestational age.

6. Exposure factors.
   a. Exposure to certain toxic drugs (e.g., cyclosporine, other immunosuppressive agents, corticosteroids, etc.).
   b. Exposure to certain chemical or environmental toxins (e.g., heavy metals, tobacco smoke, radiopaque dye, etc.).

7. Nonmodifiable factors.
   a. Family history.
   b. Age (over 60 years old; 50 years old has also been published).
   c. Race or ethnic background (African American, Hispanic, American Indian, Asian, Pacific Islander).

8. General recommendations.
   a. It is essential that persons with known risk factors have early and ongoing assessment for CKD.
   b. Patients remain asymptomatic until later stages and may not realize that they have CKD.
   c. Early detection and risk factor reduction can prevent or slow down the development of CKD.

D. Pathophysiology of CKD.
   1. The pathophysiologic changes within the kidney vary depending on the specific underlying etiology.

2. There are progressive mechanisms that occur following the long-term reduction of the mass of the kidney, regardless of the etiology. These include:
   a. Structural and functional hypertrophy of surviving nephrons.
   b. The hypertrophy is mediated by vasoactive molecules, cytokines, and growth factors.
   c. At first, the hypertrophy is due to adaptive hyperfiltration. Glomerular capillary pressure and flow increase.
   d. These changes eventually predispose the remaining viable nephrons to sclerosis.
   e. Increased intrarenal activity of the renin-angiotensin system appears to contribute to the hyperfiltration, the hypertrophy, and subsequent sclerosis.

3. Azotemia refers to the retention of nitrogenous waste products as CKD develops.

4. Uremia occurs in the last stage of kidney disease when complex, multiorgan systems become deranged, and clinical symptoms begin to manifest themselves. Uremia leads to disturbance in the function of all body systems. There are two sets of abnormalities that account for the uremic syndrome:
   a. The accumulation of products of protein metabolism.
   b. The loss of other kidney functions, e.g., resultant fluid and electrolyte imbalance and hormonal abnormalities.

5. See Figure 2.1 and Section 1 for further details regarding the pathophysiologic changes.

II. Stages of CKD.

A. The Kidney Disease Outcomes Quality Initiative (KDOQI) classification system of the stages of CKD is based on level of kidney function.
   1. It provides a common language for practitioners and patients in evaluation and treatment of patients with CKD.
   2. It promotes the conduct of clinical research.
   3. It allows for development of clinical action plans based on level of kidney function.

B. Glomerular filtration rate.
   1. The level of kidney function is based on calculation of the glomerular filtration rate (GFR).
   2. Serum creatinine alone is not an accurate index of kidney dysfunction.
      a. It is not an ideal filtration marker because it is secreted in the tubules.
      b. It is affected by age, gender, race, body mass,

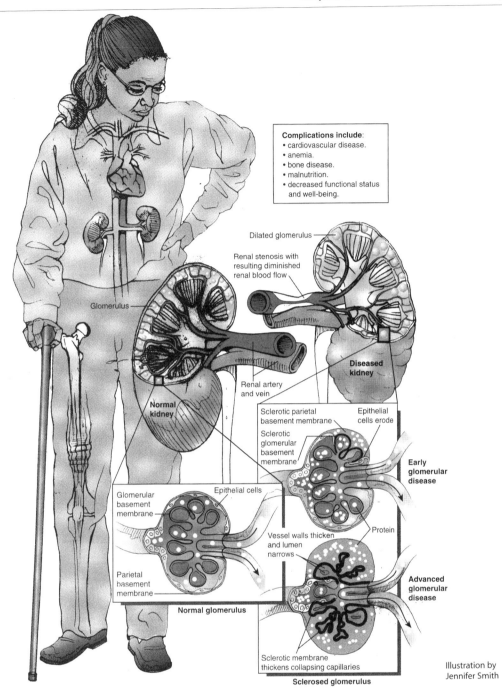

Complications include:
• cardiovascular disease.
• anemia.
• bone disease.
• malnutrition.
• decreased functional status and well-being.

Dilated glomerulus

Renal stenosis with resulting diminished renal blood flow

Glomerulus

Renal artery and vein

Diseased kidney

Normal kidney

Sclerotic parietal basement membrane

Epithelial cells erode

Sclerotic glomerular basement membrane

Early glomerular disease

Glomerular basement membrane

Epithelial cells

Protein

Vessel walls thicken and lumen narrows

Parietal basement membrane

Advanced glomerular disease

Normal glomerulus

Sclerotic membrane thickens collapsing capillaries

Illustration by Jennifer Smith

Sclerosed glomerulus

Figure 2.1. Pathophysiologic changes in chronic kidney disease. Chronic kidney disease may be a result of vascular injury, glomerulosclerosis, or tubulointerstitial injury. Decreased blood flow, inflammatory changes in the glomeruli, and thickening of the capillary walls lead to a loss of selective permeability and a reduced glomerular filtration rate. As the disease progresses, more nephrons are destroyed and kidney function continues to decline.

Source: Burrows-Hudson, S. (2005). Chronic kidney disease: An overview. *American Journal of Nursing, 105*(2), 40-49. Reprinted with permission.

muscle mass, body fat, metabolic state, pharmacologic agents, and lab analytical methods.
   c. It is, however, a factor used in the calculation of the eGFR.
3. GFR is the best measure of kidney function.
   a. It is the rate at which an ultrafiltrate of plasma is produced by the glomeruli per unit of time. Measured GFR is equal to the sum of its filtration rates in each functioning nephron.
   b. GFR provides a measure of the filtering capacity of the kidneys and an index of the functioning kidney mass.

c. It cannot be measured directly but can be assessed by measuring exogenous filtration markers.

d. In clinical practice, GFR is estimated by creatinine clearance, which is directly proportional to creatinine generation from muscle and inversely proportional to serum creatinine levels.

e. Inulin or iothalamate provides the most accurate measure of GFR, but the test is expensive and impractical for screening purposes.

f. Normal GFR based on inulin clearance and adjusted to standard body surface area of 173 m² is 127 mL/min for men and 118 mL/min for women (standard deviation is approximately 20 mL/min/1.73 m²).

g. GFR may vary in response to age, body mass, meals, exercise, posture, changes in blood pressure, level of protein in the diet and high salt intake, and laboratory measurement of creatinine.

h. GFR is affected by pregnancy, glucose control in diabetes, extracellular fluid volume, and antihypertensive medications.

i. GFR may be estimated by use of prediction equations. Two such equations are endorsed by the KDOQI guidelines: the Cockcroft-Gault formula and the Modification of Diet in Renal Disease (MDRD) study equation.

4. The Cockcroft-Gault formula is a prediction equation used to estimate the creatinine clearance (see www.medcalc.com/gfr.html).

$$CrCl \text{ (mL/min)} = \frac{(140 - age)\ (weight\ in\ kg)}{(serum\ Cr)(72) \times 0.85\ if\ female}$$

a. Accuracy of the formula in predicting creatinine clearance from 24-hour urine collections has been evaluated in many studies.

b. The formula takes into account age, weight, gender, and serum creatinine.

c. In a large study that evaluated the formula compared to the MDRD equation, the Crockcroft-Gault formula overestimated GFR by 23%.

5. The modification of diet in renal disease (MDRD) equation is a prediction equation used to estimate GFR.

$$GFR \text{ (mL/min/1.73 m}^2) = 186 \times (SCr)^{-1.154} \times (age)^{0.203}$$

$$(0.742\ if\ female)\ and \times (1.210\ if\ African\text{-}American)$$

a. The equation is based on GFR values measured by iothalamate clearance in 1628 adults and validated in 1775 adults.

b. It takes into account age, gender, and race

and serum creatinine.

c. The GFR is normalized for a standard body surface area of 1.73 m².

d. It has not been tested in children, the elderly > 75 years old, pregnancy, patients with serious comorbid conditions, or persons with extremes of body size, muscle mass, or nutritional status.

e. Performance of the equation in healthy individuals or patients with GFR > 90 mL/min/1.73 m² is unclear.

6. Sources of variability in GFR estimates by prediction equations exist.

a. Errors may occur in measurement of serum markers.

b. Variability exists in lab methods in measurement of serum creatinine.

c. Use of all prediction equations at the higher ranges of GFR (> 60 mL/min/1.73 m²) is less accurate and no longer recommended by the National Kidney Disease Education Program Laboratory Working Group.

C. Cystatin C is a low molecular weight protein produced by all human nucleated cells.

1. Cystatin C is a serum marker of kidney insufficiency.

2. It may improve detection of early CKD.

3. Preliminary studies suggest that it is a better indicator of CKD in children, transplant patients, and persons with cirrhosis. It appears to be more sensitive than serum creatinine (Lederer & Ouseph, 2007).

III. Proteinuria.

A. Definitions.

1. *Proteinuria* refers to the excretion of albumin and other proteins.

a. Persistent (>/= 3 months) increased protein excretion in the urine is an early marker of kidney damage.

b. Measurement of the level of albumin or protein in the urine helps to establish diagnosis, severity, and prognosis.

2. *Albuminuria* refers to increased excretion of albumin only and is the preferred measurement until the albumin in the urine is elevated > 500 mg/day. Then, due to cost, measuring protein in the urine is acceptable.

3. *Microalbuminuria* may be the first evidence of kidney damage and is the most common marker of kidney disease. It is albumin excretion above the normal range, but less than the test for total protein.

B. Type of protein to assess.
  1. Increased excretion of albumin is a more sensitive marker for CKD that is due to:
     a. Diabetes.
     b. Glomerular diseases.
     c. Hypertension.
  2. Increased excretion of low molecular weight globulins is a sensitive marker for CKD due to some types of tubulointerstitial disease.
  3. Testing and monitoring for albuminuria rather than total protein is recommended in kidney transplant recipients.
     a. Native kidneys may still be excreting small amounts of protein resulting in a positive test for albumin.
     b. Rejection or toxicity from immunosuppressive drugs are not characterized by proteinuria.
     c. Diabetic kidney disease may recur in the transplanted kidney.
     d. HTN after transplant can be associated with more rapid loss of kidney function.

C. Early identification and monitoring allows for treatment that can slow the course of CKD.
  1. Albumin or protein in the urine should be measured annually in patients with risk factors for CKD and routinely in patients being treated for CKD.
  2. Quantitative measurements should be used when monitoring patients with CKD.
  3. Albuminuria should be measured at diagnosis of type 2 diabetes.
  4. Albuminuria should be measured 1 year after diagnosis of type 1 diabetes.
  5. Patients with 2 or more positive quantitative tests spaced 1 to 2 weeks apart are considered to have persistent proteinuria. Further evaluation for and monitoring of CKD is recommended.

D. Specific tests.
  1. The 24-hour urine collection.
     a. 24-hour urine collection for albumin or protein is no longer considered as the preferred method for measuring albumin or protein levels in the urine.
     b. Significant collection errors can include improper timing, missed samples, and incomplete emptying of the bladder.
     c. A positive result for microalbuminuria is 30–300 mg/day.
     d. A positive result for albuminuria is > 300 mg/day.
  2. The spot urine sample (untimed).
     a. Since it is difficult to collect timed specimens, the measurement of the ratio of the concentration of albumin or protein to creatinine in a random, spot urine is now the preferred method for quantifying albumin or protein in the urine.
     b. First morning specimens are preferred, but random samples are acceptable.
     c. Excretion of creatinine is relatively constant throughout the day in an individual. The ratio of protein-to-creatinine in a spot urine sample reflects the excretion of protein.
     d. A positive result for microalbuminuria is > 17–250 mg/g in males and > 25–355 mg/g in females.
     e. A positive result for albuminuria is > 250 mg/g in males and > 355 mg/g in females.
  3. The urine dipstick.
     a. The colorimetric pH dye on the pad of the dipstick changes color when exposed to negatively charged serum proteins.
     b. Standard urine dipsticks detect total protein above concentration levels of 10–20 mg/dL.
     c. Standard urine dipsticks are not sensitive to microalbuminuria levels.
     d. An albumin-specific dipstick should be used when screening patients with CKD.
     e. A positive dipstick reading (1+ or greater) should be confirmed by a quantitative measurement within 3 months.
     f. False positive results can be caused by dehydration, hematuria, exercise, urinary tract infections, and extremely alkaline urine that will react with the dipstick's pad.
     g. False negative results can be caused by excessive hydration and urine proteins other than albumin.
     h. False negative results may inadvertently delay the initiation of treatment for CKD.
  4. Quantitative measurements are protein-to-creatinine ratios or albumin-to-creatinine ratios.

E. Limitations when assessing proteinuria.
  1. The potential for misclassification of an individual exists.
  2. Excretion of total protein or albumin in urine is highly variable. Influencing factors include:
     a. Activity.
     b. Urinary tract infections.
     c. Diet.
     d. Menstruation.
  3. Repeat studies should be considered when abnormal results are obtained.

F. Proteinuria is a key prognostic finding in CKD.

IV. Stages of CKD in the KDOQI Classification system are based on GFR and the presence of kidney damage regardless of the patient's diagnosis. The symptoms the patient experiences and the abnormal lab findings vary based on the level of kidney dysfunction. This categorization of the levels of kidney function does not negate the requirement for continuing to monitor the patient's level of kidney function. Table 2.2 summarizes the stages and prevalence of CKD in adults in the United States.

A. Stage 1 includes persons with normal or increased GFR with kidney damage.
   1. GFR ≥ 90 mL/min/1.73 m² is normal or even increased.
   2. Kidney damage is manifested by markers of kidney disease (e.g., proteinuria, abnormalities of the urinary sediment, or abnormalities in imaging test).
   3. No symptoms or lab abnormalities indicative of dysfunction in other organ systems are present.

B. Stage 2 includes persons with a mild decrease in GFR with kidney damage.
   1. GFR = 60–89 mL/min/1.73 m² demonstrates a mild decrease in kidney function.
   2. Kidney damage is manifested by markers of kidney disease.
   3. Patients are usually asymptomatic. Hypertension usually develops during this stage. Lab abnor-

malities indicative of dysfunction in other organ systems may or may not be present.
   4. Persons with a GFR = 60–89 mL/min/1.73 m² without kidney damage are classified as "mildly decreased GFR." Causes for the decrease may be attributed to:
      a. Age. This occurs frequently in older adults and is usually considered "normal for age." However, the risk for CKD exists.
      b. Vegetarian diets.
      c. Unilateral nephrectomy.
      d. Extracellular volume depletion.
      e. Systemic illnesses causing decreased kidney perfusion (e.g., heart failure, cirrhosis).

C. Stage 3 includes patients with moderate decrease in kidney function with or without kidney damage.
   1. GFR = 30–59 mL/min/1.73 m².
   2. Patients may or may not have manifestation of kidney damage.
   3. Patients may still be asymptomatic. Hypertension is almost always present. Patients begin to have lab abnormalities indicating dysfunction in other organ systems as manifested by development of anemia, hyperparathyroidism, and dyslipidemias.

D. Stage 4 includes patients with severe kidney disease.
   1. GFR = 15–29 mL/min/1.73 m².
   2. Patients typically have lab abnormalities in

Table 2.2

Stages and Prevalence of Chronic Kidney Disease in the Adult U.S. Population

Stage	Description	GFR mL/min/1.73 m²	Prevalence* N (1000s)
1	Kidney damage with normal or increased GFR	90 or greater	5900
2	Kidney damage with mild or decreased GFR	60–89	5300
3	Moderate decreased GFR	30–59	7600
4	Severe decreased GFR	15–29	400
5	Kidney failure	Less than 15 or dialysis	300

*Data for Stages 1-4 from NHANES III (1988-1994). Population 177 million adults age 20 years or older. Data for Stage 5 CKD from USRDS (1998) include approximately 230,000 patients treated by dialysis and assuming 70,000 additional patients not on dialysis. GFR estimated from serum creatinine using MDRD Study equation based on age, gender, race, and calibration for serum creatinine. For Stages 1 and 2, kidney damage estimated by spot albumin-to creatinine ratio greater than 17 mg/g in men or greater than 25 mg/g in women on two measurements.

Adapted from NKF. (2002). KDOQI clinical practice guidelines for chronic kidney disease: Evaluation, classification, and stratification. *American Journal of Kidney Diseases, 39* (Suppl. 1), S1-S266.

Table 2.3

Simplified Classification of Chronic Kidney Disease by Diagnoses

Disease	Major types (Examples)
Diabetic Kidney Disease	Type 1 and Type 2 diabetes

Nondiabetic Kidney Disease	Glomerular diseases
	   (autoimmune diseases, systemic infections, drugs,
	   neoplasia)
	Vascular diseases
	   (large vessel disease, hypertension, microangiopathy)
	Tubulointerstitial diseases
	   (urinary tract infection, stones, obstruction, drug toxicity)
	Cystic diseases
	   (polycystic diseases)

Diseases in the Transplant	Chronic rejection Drug toxicity (cyclosporin or tacrolimus) Recurrent diseases (FSGS) Transplant glomerulopathy

Adapted from NKF. (2002). KDOQI clinical practice guidelines for chronic kidney disease: Evaluation, classification, and stratification. *American Journal of Kidney Diseases, 39* (Suppl. 1), S1-S266.

several organ systems and usually begin to experience symptoms such as fatigue, anorexia, edema, apathy, impaired memory, and decreased cognitive function.

E. Stage 5 includes patients with kidney failure.
1. GFR < 15 mL/min/1.73 m^2.
2. Patients have lab abnormalities indicating dysfunction in many organ systems.
3. Symptoms vary from patient to patient and depend on the speed and severity of loss of kidney function.
4. Persons usually will start kidney replacement therapy (KRT) based on the severity of symptoms and uremic complications. Indications for initiation of KRT include:
    a. Uncontrolled hyperkalemia.
    b. Metabolic acidosis.
    c. Fluid overload.
    d. Gastrointestinal symptoms, such as nausea, vomiting, anorexia, gastrointestinal bleeding, diarrhea or constipation, malnutrition.
    e. Neurologic symptoms, which can be manifested as:
        (1) Encephalopathy (fatigue, impaired memory, inability to concentrate).
        (2) Peripheral neuropathy (burning sensation, pruritus, weakness).
        (3) Sleep disorders.
        (4) Autonomic dysfunction (blood pressure variability in response to postural changes).

V. Classification of CKD by diagnosis.

A. Although CKD can be classified by stages, the etiology should be included to assist with implementing evidence-based guidelines to slow progression and to prevent complications related to comorbid conditions.
1. Etiology is often determined by the inclusion of the most common causes of CKD by history (medical, CKD risk factors, etc.), and physical examination.
2. Inclusion of other diagnostic findings (e.g., imaging of the kidney, evaluation of urine sedimentation, kidney biopsy, etc.) is required when CKD interventions may require more invasive interventions to halt or reverse rapid decline in GFR.

B. Table 2.3 displays a simplified classification of CKD based on diagnoses.

Chapter 5

Comorbidities Associated with CKD

I. Diabetes mellitus (DM).

A. Diabetes mellitus is a metabolic disease.
  1. It is characterized by hyperglycemia resulting from defects in insulin secretion, insulin action, or both.
  2. It is associated with long-term damage and failure of various organs: eyes, heart, kidneys, nerves, and blood vessels.
  3. It is the most common cause of kidney disease.

B. Pathologic processes associated with the development of diabetes.
  1. Autoimmune destruction of the beta cells of the pancreas with subsequent insulin deficiency.
  2. Abnormalities that result in resistance to insulin action.

C. Long-term complications of DM.
  1. Retinopathy with potential loss of vision.
  2. Nephropathy leading to chronic kidney disease and need for KRT.
  3. Cardiovascular damage leading to myocardial infarction and/or stroke.
  4. Peripheral neuropathy with its risk of foot ulcers, amputations, and Charcot joints.
  5. Autonomic neuropathy leading to gastrointestinal, genitourinary, cardiovascular symptoms, and sexual dysfunction.
  6. Atherosclerotic, cardiovascular, peripheral, arterial, and cerebrovascular disease.
  7. Cardiovascular disease is the main cause of mortality in persons with diabetes.

D. Pathogenesis of hyperglycemia.
  1. The focus should be on effective treatment.
  2. Type 1 diabetes is an absence of insulin production and secretion and autoimmune destruction of the beta cells of the Islet of Langerhans in the pancreas.
    a. Accounts for 5–10% of persons with diabetes; results from a cellular-mediated destruction of the beta cells of the pancreas.
    b. Previously known by the terms *juvenile diabetes, insulin-dependent diabetes,* or *type I diabetes.*
    c. The rate of beta cell destruction is variable.
      (1) A rapid destruction rate takes place in some, mainly infants and children. Children and teens may present with ketoacidosis as the first manifestation of the disease.
      (2) A slower destruction rate occurs mainly in adults. Adults in particular, have moderate fasting hyperglycemia. However, this can rapidly change to ketoacidosis when compounded by stress or infection.
    d. Autoimmune disease is manifested by:
      (1) Low or undetectable levels of C-peptide. This commonly occurs in children and adolescents, but can occur later in life.
      (2) Ketoacidosis. The person will eventually become insulin dependent.
      (3) Little insulin secretion over time. This leads to the need for exogenous insulin.
  3. Type 2 diabetes is characterized by a relative deficiency of insulin production, decreased insulin action, and increased insulin resistance.
    a. 90–95% of persons with diabetes have type 2 diabetes.
    b. Previously termed type II diabetes, non-insulin-dependent diabetes, or adult-onset diabetes.
    c. Insulin resistance. Initially the person may have relative rather than absolute insulin deficiency, although this does not always occur.
    d. Does not need insulin to survive.

E. Diabetes and kidney disease.
  1. The risk of developing CKD increases with the length of time a person has diabetes.
    a. About one third of patients with diabetes eventually develop CKD.
    b. Diabetes is the single leading cause of kidney failure in the United States, accounting for 45% of people who start treatment for kidney failure each year.
    c. Persons with diabetes who are at higher risk for developing kidney diseases include:
      (1) Certain ethnic groups: African Americans, Native Americans, Hispanics,

Asians (Pacific Islanders). These groups are at increased risk because of type 2 diabetes (see Table 2.4).

   (2) Those with a previous past medical history of hypertension, poor glycemic control, dyslipidemia, and/or smoking increase their risk of developing CKD.

  2. Intense glycemic control (HbA1C < 7.0 and postprandial blood glucose < 180 mg/dL) can help control damage to the kidneys.

F. Several changes or imbalances account for the development of diabetic nephropathy.

  1. Hyperglycemic changes.
    a. Cause alterations in glomerular feedback.
    b. Forms advanced glycation end products, e.g., glycosylated proteins and polyols (alcohol sugars) that can accumulate in the glomeruli.

  2. Hormonal imbalances.
    a. Increases in both growth hormone and glucagons occur in patients with diabetes who are poorly controlled.
    b. Glucose elevations cause glomerular hyperfiltration.
    c. Changes in the levels of vasoactive hormones.
     (1) Angiotensin II, catecholamines, and prostaglandins, or changes in the responsiveness to these hormones.
     (2) These changes lead to hyperfiltration.

  3. Hemodynamic changes.
    a. Glomerular hypertension leads to hyperfiltration.
    b. Hyperfiltration leads to proteinuria and mesangial disposition of circulating proteins.
    c. Mesangial expansion and glomerulosclerosis lead to progressive loss of nephrons.

  4. A research study conducted by the National Institute of Diabetes and Digestive and Kidney Diseases (NIDDKD) found that periodontitis predicted the development of overt nephropathy and end-stage renal disease (ESRD) in individuals with type 2 diabetes. The effects of treating periodontal disease on reducing or delaying the risk of diabetic nephropathy remains to be seen.

G. Stages of CKD and changes seen in diabetic nephropathy.

  1. Stage 1.
    a. Hypertrophy.
    b. Hyperfiltration or GFR ≥ 90 mL/min.
    c. Microalbuminuria may be present.

  2. Stage 2.
    a. Basement membrane thickening.
    b. Enlargement of mesangium.
    c. GFR normal or decreased from stage 1.

Table 2.4

The Risk of Kidney Disease Is Not Equal

Relative risk compared to Caucasians:

African Americans	4.45 times
Native Americans	3.57 x
Hispanics	2.00 x
Asians	1.59 x

  3. Stage 3.
    a. Sclerosis or thickening of glomeruli.
    b. Microalbuminuria.
    c. GFR normal or slightly elevated.

  4. Stage 4.
    a. Decrease in the glomerular filtration surface.
    b. Impediment of the blood flow to the glomeruli.
    c. Proteinuria.
    d. The GFR is no longer elevated.
    e. Hypertension.
    f. Retinopathy.

  5. Stage 5.
    a. ESRD.
    b. Nodules of glomerular sclerotic lesions apparent.
    c. Severe hypertension that is difficult to control.
    d. Proteinuria.
    e. Hyperlipidemia.

H. Disease progression.
  1. Microalbuminuria is the first indication that kidney disease is present.
  2. Macroalbuminuria is an indication of overt diabetic nephropathy.
  3. As the amount of albumin in the urine increases, the filtering function, or GFR, of the kidney decreases.
  4. As kidney damage progresses, the blood pressure increases.
  5. In diabetes, a family history of HTN coupled with the presence of HTN, appears to increase the chances of developing kidney disease.

II. Hypertension (HTN).

A. Hypertension is the second leading risk factor in the development of kidney disease in people with and without diabetes.

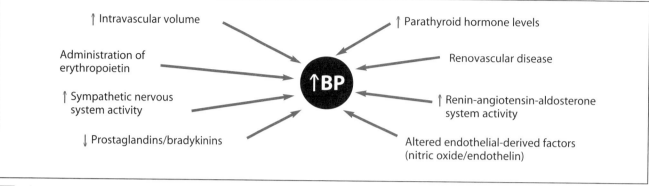

Figure 2.2. Overview of major factors that contribute to development or worsening of hypertension in patients with CKD. Elevated blood pressure also contributes to further structural injury to the kidney and progressive kidney disease (Kaplan, 2006).

Source: Burrows, L., & Muller, R. (2007). Chronic kidney disease and cardiovascular disease: Pathophysiologic links. *Nephrology Nursing Journal*, 34(1), 61.

1. See Figure 2.2 to examine an overview of factors that contribute to HTN in persons with CKD.
2. Uncontrolled HTN also accelerates the progression of kidney disease when kidney disease is already present.

B. Effects of kidney damage.
   1. As kidney disease progresses, physical changes in the kidney lead to increased blood pressure.
   2. Direct damage occurs to the small blood vessels in the nephron. The kidney loses its ability to autoregulate glomerular filtration flow and pressure.
   3. Early detection and treatment of even mild HTN is essential for everyone, especially people with diabetes.
   4. Despite the beneficial effect of lowering blood pressure, achieving target BP goals in diabetics and nondiabetics alike occurs at alarmingly low rates.

C. Goals of antihypertensive therapy in patients with CKD.
   1. Slow the rate of progression and reduce proteinuria.
   2. Prevent the progression of cardiovascular complications. Patients with CKD are at highest risk for the development of cardiovascular complications.
      a. If the BP is >115/75 there is an increased risk for cardiovascular mortality for every increase in 20 mm Hg systolic pressure and 10 mm Hg diastolic pressure.
      b. The goal for all people with CKD is a BP < 130/80. If proteinuria > 1 gram per gram of creatinine in 24 hours is present, the goal is lower.

D. The benefits of lowering blood pressure can be seen in Table 2.5.

III. Cardiovascular disease (CVD).

A. The kidney and the heart are closely integrated in a number of regulatory and hemodynamic functions.
   1. Studies have suggested that mild to moderate kidney dysfunction is associated with an increased rate of death from cardiovascular causes.
   2. There is also an association between the eGFR and the risk of death, cardiovascular events, and hospitalization.
   3. Cardiovascular mortality is 10 to 20 times greater in persons who are on dialysis.
   4. Figure 2.3 highlights a few of the postulated pathophysiologic links between CKD and increased CVD risks.

B. Reduced GFR is associated with increased CV morbidity and mortality.
   1. Reduced GFR may be associated with an increased level of nontraditional CVD risk factors.

Table 2.5

Benefits of Lowering Blood Pressure

Event	% Risk Reduction
Stroke	35-40
Myocardial Infarction	20-25
Heart Failure	50

Data from Chobanian et al. (2003).

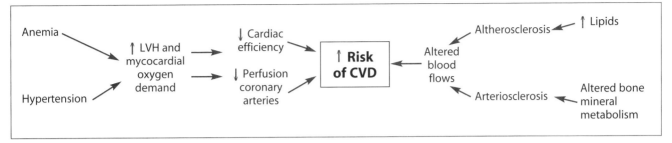

Figure 2.3. This figure highlights a few of the postulated pathophysiologic links between CKD and increased CVD risk.

Source: Burrows, L., & Muller, R. (2007). Chronic kidney disease and cardiovascular disease: Pathophysiologic links. *Nephrology Nursing Journal, 34*(1), 61.

2. Reduced GFR may be a marker of undiagnosed vascular disease, or alternatively, may be a marker for the severity of diagnosed vascular disease, especially in high-risk populations.
3. Reduced GFR may be a measure of residual confounding from traditional CVD risk factors. Patients with decreased GFR may have more severe HTN, dyslipidemia, and suffer worse vascular damage.
4. Those with reduced GFR may be less likely to receive those medications and therapies to reduce CVD risk factors such as angiotensin-converting enzyme (ACE) inhibitors, angiotensin-receptor blockers (ARBs), beta blockers, postmyocardial infarction, aspirin, and antiplatelet therapy.
5. Most important, reduced GFR itself may be a risk factor for progression of cardiac ventricular remodeling and cardiac dysfunction.
6. ACE inhibitors are not only effective antihypertensive medications, but in some studies they have also been shown to be effective in reducing the amount of left ventricular mass.

C. CKD and CVD risk factors (see Table 2.6).
   1. As in subjects with diabetes, persons without diabetes who have microalbuminuria or proteinuria have a higher prevalence of CVD risk factors as compared to those without microalbuminuria or proteinuria.
      a. Microalbuminuria and proteinuria are associated with a worse prognosis for both the progression of kidney disease and the development of CVD.
      b. Persistent microalbuminuria and proteinuria have important implications for the diagnosis of the type of kidney disease present.
   2. Traditional risk factors are based on the similarities of risk factors for both CKD and

Table 2.6

Cardiovascular Risk Factors in Adults with CKD

Traditional	CKD Related
Older age	Decreased GFR
White race	Proteinuria
Male gender	Peripheral renin-angiotensin-aldosterone activity
Hypertension	Anemia
Increased LDL cholesterol	Abnormal calcium and phosphorus
Decreased HDL cholesterol	Hypoalbuminemia
Diabetes mellitus	Hemodynamic overload
Tobacco use	Thrombogenic factors
Physical inactivity	Hyperhomocysteinemia
Obesity	Chronic inflammation
Physical inactivity	
Psychosocial stress	
Positive family history of CVD	
LVH	

Adapted from Mitsnefes, M.M. (2005). Cardiovascular disease in children with chronic kidney disease. *Advances in Chronic Kidney Disease, 12*(4), 397-405.

CVD. Those patients with CKD had greater rates of CVD than those without CKD.

3. Anemia is one example of a nontraditional risk factor for CVD in CKD.

   a. The role of anemia in CKD as a risk factor for CVD deserves careful attention because anemia is modifiable with erythropoietin therapy.

   b. Anemia has emerged as an important, independent risk factor for the development and progression of left ventricular hypertrophy (LVH), congestive heart failure (CHF), ischemic-heart disease, exacerbation of angina, and mortality in patients with CKD.

   c. Anemia is a precipitating factor for CHF.

   d. Anemia causes reductions in aerobic capacity, overall well-being, cognition.

D. Recommendations for practice.

1. All patients with CKD should be considered in the "highest risk" group for cardiovascular disease, irrespective of levels of traditional CVD risk factors.

2. All patients with CKD should undergo assessment of CVD risk factors, including "traditional" CVD risk factors used in the general population, and also "nontraditional" CKD-related risk factors.

3. Preventive strategies must take center stage.

4. Pharmacologic interventions may include the use of antilipemics and/or aspirin.

Chapter 6

Deterring Chronic Kidney Disease

I. Early identification.

A. The early identification of the underlying disease or condition causing kidney disease is important. Proper treatment could lead to delaying, preventing, or even reversing the progression of kidney disease.

1. A detailed history and physical identifying CKD risk factors, coupled with a detailed family history, can assist in the development of the clinical action plan.

2. Examples of potential beneficial actions.

   a. Removing toxic agents could improve outcomes; e.g., nonsteroidal anti-inflammatory drugs (NSAIDs), certain antibiotics, contrast dye, etc.

   b. Referring a patient to an urologist if an obstruction is present could potentially reverse damage.

   c. Evaluating renal artery stenosis can lead to early appropriate treatment.

B. Identification of the current stage of CKD can assist in identifying actions to slow the progression of the disease, as well as preventing complications that may occur, e.g., anemia and metabolic bone disease.

II. General recommendations for monitoring CKD.

A. Ongoing monitoring for the progression of proteinuria by routinely obtaining spot urine samples for protein/creatinine ratio.

B. Ongoing calculation of current eGFR (either through MDRD or Cockcroft-Gault calculation).

C. Ongoing blood pressure monitoring and assessment with accompanying medication management.

D. Ongoing monitoring and assessment of patient's medication regimen with dose adjustments made if necessary. Adjustments should be based on the level of kidney dysfunction as determined by the eGFR.

E. Monitoring for and attempting to prevent all other comorbid diseases.

F. Referring to a nephrologist for early diagnosis and comanagement of complications as they occur. It is recommended that this happen minimally when the eGFR is < 60mL/min.

G. Ongoing symptom assessment through the use of validated instruments.

1. Medical Outcomes Study 36-item short form

health survey (MOS SF-36). A sample form is available at www.sf-36.org/tools.
2. Kidney Disease Quality of Life tool (KDOQI).

III. Steps to delay the progression of CKD. Table 2.7 offers additional strategies to slow the progression of CKD and CVD.

A. Blood glucose control.
   1. The patient should follow the latest guidelines from the American Diabetes Association. The current Guidelines (2006) include:
      a. HbA1C < 7.0%.
      b. Preprandial blood glucose 90–130mg/dL.
      c. Postprandial blood glucose < 180mg/dL.
      d. HbA1C is the primary target for control. *Caution*: Tighter control can lead to an increase of hypoglycemic episodes.
   2. Yearly screening for microalbuminuria is recommended. Reduction of microalbuminuria may reflect:
      a. Control of the disease process.
      b. Success in controlling secondary factors, i.e., intraglomerular hypertension and hyperfiltration.
   3. Lifestyle changes should be instituted: following the recommended diet, ceasing smoking, losing weight if necessary, beginning an exercise program, e.g., brisk walking on a daily basis.
   4. ACE inhibitor and/or ARB therapy is recommended to decrease albuminuria.
   5. Maintaining blood sugar control reduces the risk of DM nephropathy. The patient should be monitoring blood glucose levels on a regular basis.
   6. Oral pharmacologic agents used to treat diabetes need to be reviewed whether the patient is on first or second generation sulfonyureas or metformin. Metformin should be discontinued when the eGFR is < 40 mL/minute/1.73m^2 due to risk of lactic acidosis.
   7. If the patient is on insulin, be aware that as GFR decreases, there is a potential for an increase in hypoglycemia. Therefore, there may be a need to decrease the insulin dose.
   8. Ensure the patient knows that diuretic use may cause fluctuations in blood glucose levels.

B. Blood pressure control.
   1. The goals of the KDOQI guidelines are to lower the blood pressure, slow the progression of kidney disease, and reduce the risk of CVD.
      a. BP < 130/80 for all persons with CKD.
      b. The goal is a lower blood pressure for those with proteinuria > 1 g/24 hr.
   2. JNC VII guidelines (see Table 2.8).
   3. In stages 1 through 3, a thiazide diuretic may be beneficial to help reach goal. In stages 4 and 5, a loop diuretic (e.g., furosemide) is more effective.
   4. Blood pressure control reduces cardiovascular risk and slows the progression of glomerulonephrosclerosis.
   5. The use of angiotensin-converting enzyme inhibitors (ACE-I) and/or angiotensin receptor blockers (ARBs) is highly recommended with the presence of albuminuria/proteinuria.
      a. ACE-I and ARBs have renoprotective, antihypertensive, and antiproteinuric effects in persons diagnosed with diabetes.
      b. These classes of drugs decreases intraglomerular pressure and improves glomerular barriers size selectivity.
      c. Some small studies have demonstrated that dual therapy with ACE-I and ARB may provide better long-term protection of the kidneys.
         (1) Initially, there may be a decrease in GFR, a mild increase in creatinine (< 20% of baseline), and a mild increase in the K+ level.
         (2) Blood levels should be monitored 1–2 weeks after initiating drug therapy.
         (3) Monitor for adverse reactions. Educate patients concerning the possibility of angioedema.
         (4) Caution should be used if the patient has a history of hyperkalemia. Patient education is needed regarding the control of dietary potassium. The potential need for the drug Kayexalate and the avoidance of other medications that can increase the potassium level. These drugs would include potassium supplements, NSAIDs, COX 2 inhibitors, and potassium sparing diuretics (see Sections 8 and 9).
         (5) ACE-I and ARBs may be contraindicated in acute kidney failure or if there is a history of renal artery stenosis.

C. Avoidance of nephrotoxic agents.
   1. Evaluate the current list of medications.
      a. Make required dose adjustments as the GFR decreases.
      b. This usually takes place when the GFR reaches < 50 mL/min.

Table 2.7

Strategies to Slow Progression of CKD and CVD

Risk Factor	Target/Treatment Recommendations	Nursing Considerations
Hypertension	• Target: less than 130/80 mmHg • ACE inhibitor/ARB preferred in patients with diabetes and patients with protein-to-creatinine ratio greater than 200 mg/g. • All antihypertensive agents effective in patients without diabetes and protein-to-creatinine ratio less than 200 mg/dL. Follow recommendations of JNC 7 for drug selection in other comorbidities. • Diuretics are ideal second drug (thiazides may not be effective at GFR less than 40 mL/min/1.73m^2). • Fluid restriction and sodium restriction critical.	• Initiate TLC (weight reduction, DASH diet, decreasing dietary sodium, increasing physical activity, alcohol moderation). • Side effects of ACE inhibitor or ARB include hyperkalemia and decreasing GFR (increasing SCr). • ACE inhibitors can cause angioedema and cough. • Monitor for hypotension with all agents. • Monitor for electrolyte abnormalities with diuretics.
Proteinuria	• Target: less than 500 mg – 1 g/24 hour • ACE inhibitor and ARB effective in reducing proteinuria. Combination may have increased effect.	• Monitor urine protein-to-creatinine ratio for improvements. • Side effects of ACE inhibitor/ARB listed above.
Hyperglycemia	• Targets: HbA1C less than 7.0% Preprandial glucose: 90–130 mg/dL Peak postprandial glucose less than 180 mg/dL	• Diabetes self-management education essential. • Monitor patients for side effects: hypoglycemia, weight gain, and edema. • Avoid Metformin due to development of lactic acidosis GFR less than 40 mL/min/1.73m^2.
Hyperlipidemia	• Targets: LDL less than 100 mg/dL Non-HDL less than 130 mg/dL Trig. less than 150 mg/dL HDL greater than 40 mg/dL (varies by gender) • TLC + statin recommended. • Fibrate and niacin as needed.	• Monitor patients for rhabdomyolysis and increased LFTs with statin. • Fibrates renally excreted; use lower doses.
Smoking	Target: cessation of smoking	• Counseling, nicotine replacement, bupropion are effective. • Address cessation at every encounter.
Nutrition	• Targets: HCO$_3$ greater than 22 mg/dL Albumin greater than 3.5 g/dL K$^+$ 3.5–5.5 mEq/L BMI 18.5–25.9	• Protein: 1.2–1.4 mg/kg/day 0.6–0.8 mg/kg/day (Stage 3/4) • Calorie: 35 kcal/kg/day < 60 years old 30–35 kcal/kg/day > 60 years old • Potassium: less than 2000 mg/day (based serum K$^+$ level) • Sodium: less than 2400 mg/day • Calcium: less than 2000 mg/day • Phosphorous: less than 1000 mg/day (Stage 3/4) • Fluid: 500 cc + 24-hr urine output/day • HCO$_3$ less than 22 mg/dL – alkali salts 0.5–1.0 meq/kg/day
Anemia	• Target: Hgb 11–12 mg/dL	• Anemia workup: Assess RBC indices, retic ct, iron profile, B$_{12}$ & folate levels • Initiate ESAs and target 11–12 mg/dL.
Bone metabolism	• Stage 3 Targets: Phos. 2.7–4.6 mg/dL iPTH 35-70 pg/mL – PTH Ca – normal for lab • Stage 4 Targets: Phos. 2.7–4.6 mg/dL iPTH 70 – 110 pg.mL Ca – normal for lab	• Stage 3 & 4 increased iPTH – Measure serum 25-hydroxyvitamin D < 30 ng/mL – ergocalciferolol (D2) > 30 ng/mL – active Vitamin D • Increased Phos. – low phos diet/binder • Increased Ca – dc Ca and Vitamin D

Abbreviations: TLC – therapeutic lifestyle changes; ACE – angiotensin converting enzyme; ARB – angiotensin receptor blocker; GFR – glomerularfiltration rate; Scr – serum creatinine; JNC VII – Joint National Committee on Treatment of Hypertension; LDL – low density lipoprotein; LFT – liver function test; Hgb – hemaglobin; RBC – red blood cell; Retic ct – reticulocyte count; BMI – body mass index; K$^+$ – potassium; HCO$_3$ – bicarbonate, BP – blood pressure; Phos – phosphorous; Ca – calcium; iPTH – intact parathyroid hormone
Sources: ADA, 2006; ATP III, 2001; Chobanian et al., 2003; National Kidney Foundation, 2002-2006.

Table 2.8

JNC VII Classification of Blood Pressure for Adults Aged 18 Years or Older

BP Classification	Systolic BP (mm Hg)		Diastolic BP (mm Hg)
Normal	< 120	and	< 80
Prehypertension	120–139	or	80–89
Stage 1 Hypertension	140–159	or	90–99
Stage 2 Hypertension	≥180	or	≥100

Source: Chobanian, A.V., Bakis, G.L., Black, H.R., Cushman, W.C., Green, L.A., Izzo, J.L., et al., & the National High Blood Pressure Education Programming Coordinating Committee. (2003). The seventh report of the Joint National Committee on Prevention, Detection, Evaluation, and Treatment of High Blood Pressure. *JAMA, 289*, 2560-2562

2. Discuss with the patient all current (and previous history) of self-administered medications such as over-the-counter (OTC) and herbal supplements.
   a. Avoid use of NSAIDs therapy. For example: ibuprofen, naproxen, COX 2 inhibitors, etc.
   b. Herbal supplements.
      (1) Aristolochic acid nephropathy can cause interstitial renal fibrosis.
      (2) Djenkol bean can lead to severe tubular necrosis.
      (3) Licorice, rhubarb, cascara sagrada can cause hypokalemia.
      (4) Noni juice can cause hyperkalemia.
      (5) A diuretic effect can be seen with dandelion, juniper berry, and goldenrod. A decrease in immunosuppression can occur with echinacea and St. John's wort.
   c. Incorporate into the patient's nursing care an open dialogue about alternative therapies. Patients are more willing to discuss their actions if they do not feel criticized. Stress the importance of drug interactions and encourage the patient to inform health care providers of any herbal supplements they may be taking.
3. Avoid contrast dye. If needed for diagnostics, hydration should be provided to reduce the risk of acute kidney failure.
   a. Radiocontrast nephropathy can be defined as an increase of 25% or more in the serum creatinine level.
   b. Contrast-induced nephropathy accounts for >10% of hospital acquired kidney failure and is a leading cause of acute kidney failure.
   c. Associated contributing factors include diabetes, high doses of the contrast, volume depletion, coadministration of nephrotoxic drugs, and preexisting CKD.
   d. A study by Merten et al. (2004) suggests that hydration with sodium bicarbonate before contrast exposure is more effective than hydration with sodium chloride in preventing contrast-induced nephropathy.
4. Antibiotics. Patients should be aware of medications that are prescribed for them in various health care arenas as the dose may need to be adjusted for a lower GFR. They should inform their primary care physician or nephrologist if they are already being followed for CKD.

D. Recommended lifestyle changes.
   1. Weight reduction if necessary.
   2. Exercise at least 30 minutes on daily basis.
   3. Low salt diet.
   4. Moderation of alcohol intake.
   5. Smoking cessation.

E. Self-care management activities should be promoted, including:
   1. Blood pressure monitoring.
   2. Taking medications as prescribed.
   3. Limiting salt intake by reading food labels and not adding salt to foods.
   4. Exercising.

F. Protein restriction.
   1. There is still controversy over restriction of protein to slow progression of CKD. The goal is to slow the progression while at the same time avoiding malnutrition (see Section 8).
   2. KDOQI recommendations for protein intake.

Table 2.9

Hypertension in Chronic Kidney Disease (CKD), Stages 1–4

Patient Outcomes
- The patient will achieve and maintain blood pressure (BP) within the targeted range.
- There will be a decrease in rate of progression of chronic kidney disease (CKD).
- The patient will demonstrate a reduction in modifiable risk factors for cardiovascular disease (CVD).
- The patient will demonstrate knowledge of hypertension and its relationship to CKD and CVD.

Nursing Care
Assessment
1. Measure BP at each health encounter.
   A. Measure BP at least two times and calculate the average of the readings
   B. Compare to the targeted goal of less than 130/80
2. Assess the patient's
   A. Weight
   B. Respiratory rate and quality
   C. Heart sounds
   D. Breath sounds
   E. Peripheral edema
   F. Neck vein distention, jugular venous pressure
   G. Adherence to recommended therapeutic lifestyle changes, dietary modifications and medication regimen
3. Assess the patient for personal and/or family history of hypertension.
4. Identify barriers to self-management.
5. Review home BP record.
6. Review lab tests for blood urea nitrogen (BUN), creatinine, and electrolytes.
7. Review results of electrocardiogram, chest x-rays, other diagnostic studies.
8. Assess the patient's understanding of
   A. Hypertension (HTN)
   B. Prescribed antihypertensive medications
   C. Prescribed dietary modifications
   D. Recommended therapeutic lifestyle changes
   E. Proper BP measurement technique
   F. Kidney function and its relationship to hypertension
   G. HTN and its relationship to CKD and CVD
   H. Causes, signs, and symptoms of cardiac alterations related to HTN
   I. Signs and symptoms of hypotension

Interventions
1. Collaborate with physician, primary care provider, and dietitian in planning appropriate BP goals and therapeutic regimen.
2. Administer antihypertensive medications as ordered.
3. Encourage adherence to prescribed medication regimen.
4. Encourage adherence to therapeutic lifestyle changes and dietary modifications.
5. Identify resources to assist patient to achieve goals of blood pressure control.
6. Initiate consultations/referrals, as appropriate (Dietician, Social Worker).

Patient Teaching
1. Teach the patient to measure and record his/her own BP, whenever possible.
2. Instruct the patient regarding
   A. HTN
   B. Prescribed antihypertensive medications
   C. Prescribed dietary modifications
   D. Recommended therapeutic lifestyle changes
   E. Proper BP measurement technique
   F. Kidney function and its relationship to hypertension
   G. HTN and its relationship to CKD and CVD
   H. Causes, signs, and symptoms of cardiac alterations related to HTN
   I. Signs and symptoms of hypotension

References
Chobanian, A.V., Bakis, G.L., Black, H.R., Cushman, W.C., Green, L.A., Izzo, J.L., et al., & the National High Blood Pressure Education Programming Coordinating Committee. (2003). The seventh report of the Joint National Committee on Prevention, Detection, Evaluation, and Treatment of High Blood Pressure. *Journal of the American Medical Association, 289,* 2560-2562.

National Kidney Foundation. (2004). KDOQI clinical practice guidelines on blood pressure management and use of antihypertensive agents in chronic kidney disease. *American Journal of Kidney Disease, 43,* S1-S268.

Adapted from Burrows-Hudson, S., & Prowant, B. (Eds.). (2005). *Nephrology nursing standards of practice and guidelines for care.* Pitman, NJ: American Nephrology Nurses' Association.

a. Dietary protein 0.75 g/kg/day in stages 1 through 3.
b. Dietary protein 0.6 g/kg/day in stages 4 and 5.
c. Individualized dietary counseling is recommended.
3. Uremia leads to decreased appetite, anorexia, a metallic taste, metabolic acidosis, and hyperphosphatemia. As the dietary plan is being developed, all of these issues need to be considered.
4. Early referral, by stage 3, to the nutritionist is recommended.

G. Smoking cessation.
1. Diabetic nephropathy occurs five times faster in CKD patients who smoke.
2. Smoking increases platelet aggregation, fibrinogen concentration, elevates the blood pressure, leads to hypoxia and vascular damage.
3. Smoking is a risk factor for cardiovascular mortality in patients with CKD.
4. Encourage smoking cessation at every visit.
   a. Help patients to self-identify their personal benefits of quitting such as financial gain, physical improvements, etc.
   b. Offer individual counseling, group or class support, community groups, nicotine patches, nicotine gum, and buproprion.
H. Table 2.9 demonstrates the incorporation of the ANNA *Nephrology Nursing Standards of Practice and Guidelines for Care* into a nursing care plan.

Chapter 7

Complications of Chronic Kidney Disease

I. Cardiovascular abnormalities.

A. Risk factors.
1. Patients with CKD are considered at highest risk for cardiovascular disease (CVD) and its associated mortality. The increased risk has been estimated to range from 10-fold to 200-fold.
2. The risk for CVD begins early in the course of CKD. By the time people reach ESRD, between 30% and 45% will have advanced cardiovascular complications.
3. Modifiable risk factor reduction should begin early to reduce morbidity and mortality.
4. Traditional risk factors.
   a. Older age.
   b. White race.
   c. Male gender.
   d. Hypertension.
   e. Left ventricular hypertrophy.
   f. Dyslipidemias, e.g., increased LDL cholesterol and decreased HDL cholesterol.
   g. Diabetes mellitus.
   h. Physical inactivity.
   i. Tobacco use.
   j. Obesity.
   k. Family history.
   l. Psychosocial stress.

5. Kidney-related risk factors.
   a. Decreased GFR.
   b. Anemia.
   c. Disturbances in mineral metabolism.
   d. Proteinuria.
   e. Peripheral renin-angiotensin-aldosterone activity.
   f. Extracellular fluid volume overload.
   g. Malnutrition.
   h. Inflammation.
   i. Elevated homocysteine.
   j. Elevated c-reactive protein.
   k. Thrombogenic factors.

B. Hypertension.
1. HTN is a complication of CKD and a major risk factor for accelerating the progression of CKD. Treatment of HTN is vital to slowing the downward spiral.
2. HTN can develop as a complication of CKD as early as stage 1.
3. Glomerular hypertension results in injury to kidney's endothelial, mesangial, and epithelial cells. The higher the pressure, the worse the resultant injury.
4. A primary cause of HTN is the diseased kidney's inability to handle salt and water resulting in volume expansion.

5. Other potential contributing factors.
   a. Sympathetic nervous system over activity with increased catecholamine production.
   b. Increased activity of the renin-angiotensin-aldosterone system.
      (1) High levels of angiotensin II yield increased levels of intracellular sodium and calcium leading to vasoconstriction.
      (2) Aldosterone excess can lead to vascular damage in the form of endothelial stiffness and fibrosis in both the heart and the kidney.
      (3) Primary vascular disease, e.g., renal artery stenosis, contributes to stimulation of the renin-angiotensin-aldosterone system.
   c. Administration of erythropoiesis stimulating agents (ESA).
   d. Increased levels of parathyroid hormone.
6. Benefits related to lowering the blood pressure.
   a. Risk of a stroke is decreased 35–40%.
   b. Risk of a myocardial infarction is decreased 20–25%.
   c. Risk of heart failure is decreased 50%.
   d. Table 2.10 displays the effects of lifestyle modifications on HTN.

C. Left ventricular hypertrophy (LVH).
   1. LVH refers to the adaptation of the myocardium to increased cardiac load. Contributing factors include:
      a. Volume overload, which is common in CKD.
      b. Pressure overload, which can be related to:
         (1) HTN, arteriosclerosis, aortic stenosis, or any combination of these factors.
         (2) Stiffness of the aorta, stiffness of the large central arteries, or peripheral vascular resistance increases the workload of the left ventricle.
         (3) The arterial stiffness generates an increase in the pulse wave velocity and

Table 2.10

Lifestyle Modifications to Manage Hypertension

Modification	Recommendation	Approximate Systolic BP Reduction Range
Weight reduction	Maintain normal body weight (BMI 18.5–24.9).	5–20 mm Hg/10 kg weight loss
Adopt DASH eating plan (CKD Stage 1–2 only)*	Consume a diet rich in fruits, vegetables, and low-fat dairy products with a reduced content of saturated and total fat.	8–14 mm Hg
Dietary sodium reduction	Reduce dietary sodium intake to no more than 100 mEq/L (2.4 g sodium or 6 g sodium chloride).	2–8 mm Hg
Physical activity	Engage in regular aerobic physical activity such as brisk walking (at least 30 minutes per day, most days of the week).	4–9 mm Hg
Moderation of alcohol consumption	Limit consumption to no more than 2 drinks per day (1 oz or 30 mL) ethanol in most men and no more than 1 drink per day in women and lighter-weight persons.	2–4 mm Hg

Abbreviations: BMI - body mass index calculated as weight in kilograms divided by the square of the height in meters; BP – blood pressure; DASH – Dietary Approaches to Stop Hypertension

Source: Chobanian et al. (2003).

* The KDOQI recommendations differ only in the area of diet. The DASH diet is recommended for patients with CKD in Stages 1 and 2. In Stages 3-5 however, modifications in the diet are necessary due to the possibility of hyperkalemia with a diet rich in fruit and vegetables and hyperphosphatemia with low fat dairy products. A dietary consult will be helpful in assisting the patients to meet the dietary recommendations and modifications required by CKD.

the subsequent early return of wave reflections. The resultant increase in pressure opposes LV ejection.
   (4) Aortic stenosis also creates an obstruction to LV ejection.
   c. A combination of volume overload and pressure overload.
2. LVH can be a normal adaptive process, e.g., pregnancy, high level exercise.
   a. The number of functional cardiac muscle units increases.
   b. Allows equal load distribution and maintenance of normal systolic function.
3. Sustained overload becomes maladaptive and leads to cardiomyopathy and heart failure.
4. Definitions.
   a. Concentric LVH: an increase in wall thickness but without a simultaneous increase in volume capacity.
      (1) Generally caused by pure BP overload.
      (2) Associated with increased systolic stress.
   b. Eccentric LVH: an increase in volume capacity of the chamber or chamber enlargement, but not relative wall thickness; associated with increased diastolic stress.
   c. Left ventricular mass.
      (1) Indexed for body size.
      (2) Reported as grams per metered square.
      (3) Increased in LVH no matter the type.
5. Diagnosis.
   a. Electrocardiogram.
   b. Echocardiography: the preferred method since it is more sensitive.
6. It has been estimated that 75% of adults and 69% of pediatric patients have LVH when dialysis is initiated.
7. Correction of anemia may lead to regression of left ventricular mass.
8. LVH and dilated cardiomyopathy are among the most ominous risk factors for excess cardiovascular morbidity and mortality in CKD and ESRD. Adverse effects of LVH include:
   a. Heart failure.
   b. Ventricular arrhythmias.
   c. Sudden cardiac death.
   d. Death following a myocardial infarction.
   e. Decreased left ventricular fraction.
   f. Cerebrovascular events.

D. Anemia.
1. Causes of anemia in CKD.
   a. Eythropoeitin (EPO) deficiency is main cause of anemia, but other causes should be ruled out.
   b. Shortened RBC life span.
   c. Blood loss due to platelet dysfunction.
   d. Low iron intake and absorption.
   e. Deficiency of folate or cobalamin (vitamin B12).
   f. Chronic disease factors inflammation.
   g. Hemolysis.
2. Erythropoietin is the endogenous hormone produced primarily by the kidney. Its functions include:
   a. Stimulation of the production of red blood cells (RBC).
   b. Stimulation of the division and differentiation of progenitor cells within the bone marrow.
   c. Bringing about the release of reticulocytes from the bone marrow into the bloodstream. There the reticulocytes mature into erythrocytes, i.e., mature red blood cells.
3. Erythrocytes carry oxygen to tissues and are scavengers of free radicals which leads to the reduction of oxidative stress.
4. Assessment of anemia in CKD.
   a. Normocytic (normal size red blood cell), normochromic (normal RBC color, indicating normal amount of Hgb) anemia most commonly found in CKD.
   b. Anemia can develop as early as CKD stage 2.
5. Anemia can contribute to the development of left ventricular hypertrophy (LVH), maladaptive cardiomyopathy, congestive heart failure, and ischemic heart disease.
6. Workup for anemia includes:
   a. Iron studies: iron (Fe), ferritin, transferrin, total iron binding capacity(TIBC), transferrin saturation (Tsat). To compute the Tsat: serum iron is divided by the TIBC X 100.
   b. Reticulocyte count (retic count).
   c. Complete blood count (CBC).
7. Symptoms can include pallor, fatigue, shortness of breath, decreased cognition, muscle weakness, decreased exercise tolerance, chest pain, tachycardia, and decreased quality of life.
8. Treatment of anemia in CKD.
   a. KDOQI guidelines. Treatment ranges includes:
      (1) Hgb 11.0–12.0 g/dL.
      (2) Ferritin level > 100 ng/mL in CKD stages 2–5; > 200 ng/mL in CKD stage 5 on hemodialysis.
      (3) Tranferrin saturation > 20%.
   b. Iron therapy.
      (1) Oral iron: at least 200 mg elemental iron a day.

(2) IV iron: various intravenous iron preparations are available. For example, iron sucrose, ferric gluconate. Iron dextran is rarely used because of the danger of anaphylactic reactions.

c. ESA therapy.
   (1) FDA Alert (11/16/06; 2/16/07; 3/9/07).
   (2) Correction of Hemoglobin and Outcomes in Renal Insufficiency (CHOIR) Study.
   (3) Demonstrated that serious and potentially life-threatening cardiovascular events occurred when the targeted Hgb was 13.5 g/dL as compared to a targeted Hgb of 11.3 g/dL.
   (4) Target Hgb should not exceed the dosing recommended 12 g/dL. A black box warning was issued.
   (5) In an August 30, 2007, press release from the National Kidney Foundation, the Kidney Disease Outcomes Quality Initiative (KDOQI) updated its 2006 Clinical Practice Guidelines on Anemia and CKD.
      (a) The selected target should generally be in the range of 11.0 to 12.0 g/dL.
      (b) They pointed out that because of natural fluctuations, actual Hb results will vary from targeted levels.
      (c) In patients with CKD receiving ESA therapy, whether they are on dialysis or not, the target Hb should not exceed 13.0 g/dL.
      (d) Additional research is needed.
d. The blood pressure should be monitored as it may tend to increase as the hemoglobin is corrected.

E. Dyslipidemia.
   1. Can occur early in CKD and can worsen as overall kidney function declines.
   2. Contributing factors to the occurrence of dyslipidemia.
      a. Type of underlying kidney disease.
      b. Level of kidney function.
      c. Presence of diabetes.
      d. Proteinuria.
      e. Use of certain medications, e.g., cyclosporine, corticosteroids.
   3. The lipid abnormalities in CKD consist of:
      a. Elevated total cholesterol.
      b. Elevated triglycerides.
      c. Elevated LDL cholesterol.
      d. Low HDL cholesterol.
   4. Because patients with CKD are in the highest

risk category for CVD, it is prudent to aggressively treat dyslipidemias. The NKF recommends that the goal for LDL be < 100 mg/dL for persons with CKD.
   5. Based on the Third Report of the Expert Panel on Detection, Evaluation, and Treatment of High Blood Cholesterol in Adults (Adult Treatment Panel or ATP III), a Quick Desk Reference was developed. It outlines cholesterol management in steps. The guidelines can be found at http://www.nhlbi.nih.gov/guidelines/cholesterol/dskref.htm

F. Vascular calcification.
   1. Vascular calcification is accelerated in CKD. Excess calcium is deposited into blood vessels, the myocardium, and cardiac valves.
   2. Calcium can be deposited in either the intimal or medial layers of arteries.
      a. Generally confined to the coronary, aortic, and iliofemoral vessels.
      b. Intimal calcification occurs within atherosclerotic plaques.
         (1) Narrows the arterial lumen.
         (2) Blood flow may be compromised leading to chronic ischemia and/or necrosis.
         (3) Acute ischemia can also result (e.g., when the plaques rupture and thrombosis occludes the vessel lumen as with acute coronary syndrome).
         (4) Atherosclerotic plaques develop more rapidly when uremia is present.
      c. Medial calcification is fundamentally different than intimal calcification.
         (1) Contributes to the stiffness of blood vessels and reduces vascular compliance.
         (2) Lesions cause the BP to worsen with the systolic pressure rising and the diastolic pressure remaining the same or going lower.
         (3) High systolic pressure increases the workload of the heart and therefore the amount of oxygen required by the myocardium.
         (4) Low diastolic pressure can result in decreased perfusion of the coronary arteries, thus predisposing the myocardium to ischemia.
         (5) The pulse pressure widens and pulse wave velocity increases, i.e., the stiffer the vessels, the faster the pulse wave travels along the vessel.
         (6) The faster traveling pulse wave gets reflected back to the central aorta during late systole or early diastole.

Table 2.11

Factors Associated with Development or Acceleration of Valvular Calcification in Patients on Dialysis

General Population	CKD-Related
Advancing age	Vascular calcification
Systemic hypertension	Hyperphosphatemia
Diabetes Mellitus	Hypercalcemia
Abnormal lipids	Elevated PTH levels
LVH	Elevated calcium and phosphorus product

Data from Cunningham, R., Corretti, M., & Henrich, W. (2006). *Valvular heart disease in patients with end-stage renal disease.* Retrieved October 23, 2006, from http://www.UpToDate.com

(7) This movement increases the cardiac afterload and contributes to LVH and compromising the perfusion of the coronary arteries.

(8) Arterial calcification has also been associated with MI, valvular heart disease, CHF, endocarditis, and death.

3. Vascular calcification is also associated with accelerated risk of stroke and amputation.

4. The prevalence of calcification of the aortic valve has been found to be 55%; for the mitral valve the rate is 59%. The tricuspid and pulmonic valves are rarely involved in relation to CKD. Factors associated with the development of valvular calcification can be seen in Table 2.11.

   a. CKD-related factors predisposing the patient to calcification of the valves include vascular calcification, hyperphosphatemia, hypercalcemia, elevated PTH, elevated calcium, and phosphorous product.

   b. Valvular calcification in CKD is linked to inflammation, carotid atherosclerosis, and arterial calcification.

G. Abnormal hemostasis.

1. Associated with prolonged bleeding time, decreased activity of platelet factor III, abnormal platelet aggregation and adhesiveness, and impaired prothrombin consumption.

2. Clinical manifestations include tendency for abnormal bleeding and bruising, bleeding from surgical wounds, GI bleeding, bleeding into the pericardial sac, or bleeding into the intracranial vault, i.e., sudural hematoma or intracerebral hemorrhage.

3. In spite of these bleeding tendencies, persons with CKD have a greater susceptibility to thromboembolic complications.

II. CKD – Mineral and bone disorder.

A. CKD-mineral and bone disorder is a broad clinical syndrome that can be manifested by any one or combination of the following:

1. Abnormalities of calcium, phosphorous, PTH, and vitamin D metabolism.

2. Abnormalities of bone turnover, mineralization, volume, linear growth, and strength.

3. Vascular and soft tissue calcification.

B. Potential abnormalities in bone.

1. High turnover bone disease, e.g., osteitis fibrosa related to elevated PTH levels.

2. Adynamic bone characterized by extremely low bone turnover.

3. Mineralization defects resulting in osteomalacia.

4. Mixed renal osteodystrophy.

5. The picture may be complicated by other systemic processes, e.g., accumulation of B-2 microglobulin, postmenopausal osteoporosis, steroid-induced osteoporosis.

C. Causes of alterations in calcium phosphorous balance (see Figure 2.4).

1. Alterations in calcium phosphorous balance can be seen at CKD stage 3, GFR < 60 mL/min.

2. Phosphorus retention suppresses vitamin D production by the kidney which leads to decrease in calcium absorption. The parathyroid gland senses a low calcium level. The gland hypertrophies as it attempts to compensate for the low calcium level.

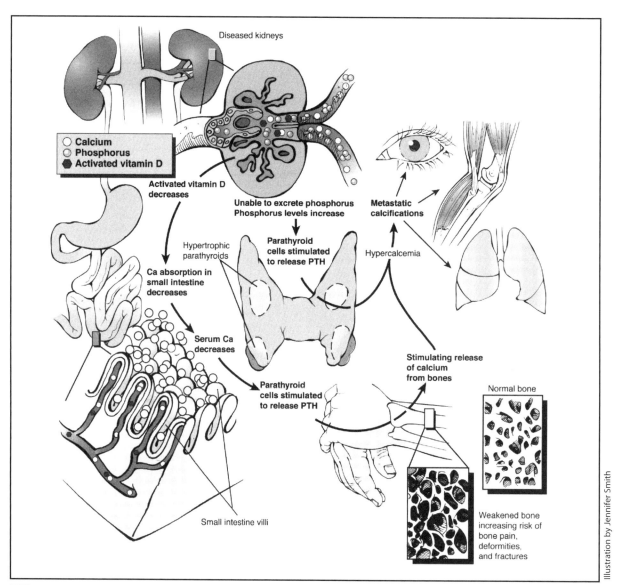

Figure 2.4. In diseased kidneys, there is a disruption of the normal feedback loop that controls serum calcium and phosphorus levels. Decreased production of activated vitamin D causes malabsorption of calcium form the intestine, stimulating the parathyroid glands to release parathyroid hormone (PTH). At the same time, the kidney's inability to excrete phosphorus stimulates the release of PTH. The PTH further stimulates the resorption of calcium and phosphorus from bone, resulting in hypercalcemia and metastatic calcifications.

Source: Legg, V. (2005). Complications of chronic kidney disease. *American Journal of Nursing, 105*(6), 40-49. Reprinted with permission.

D. High-turnover metabolic bone disease in CKD.
   1. Hyperplasia and resultant high levels of PTH are related to:
      a. Retention of phosphorous.
      b. Decreased levels of calcitriol.
      c. Changes within the parathyroid gland result in increased PTH secretion.
      d. Increased parathyroid growth.
      e. Skeletal resistance to the actions of PTH.
      f. Hypocalcemia.
      g. All of these abnormalities are related. One or more may dominate at any given time throughout the course of CKD.
   2. Potential roles of phosphorous retention.
      a. Phosphate retention, secondary to reductions in GFR, causes transient decreases in levels of ionized calcium which then triggers an increase in PTH secretion, thereby restoring a normal

state of calcium phosphate levels. Increased levels of PTH are then required to maintain homeostasis leading to hyperparathyroidism.
   b. Reductions in dietary phosphorous have been shown to prevent the development of hyperparathyroidism.
   c. It has been demonstrated that hypocalcemia is not an essential factor for the development of hyperparathyroidism.
   d. It has been demonstrated that production of calcitriol is regulated by phosphorous, e.g., phosphorous retention leads to decrease in the blood levels of calcitriol.
   e. It has been demonstrated in experimental animals that phosphate affects parathyroid function independently of calcium or calcitriol.
3. Potential roles of vitamin D 1-25 (calcitriol).
   a. The kidneys are the primary site for the production of calcitriol.
   b. In CKD, decreased production of calcitriol contributes to the development of secondary hyperparathyroidism.
   c. The increased level of PTH does not stimulate the kidneys to produce additional calcitriol.
   d. Other factors that can limit the actions of calcitriol include:
      (1) Decreases in the vitamin D receptors in target tissues.
      (2) Uremic toxins potentially interfering with the normal actions of vitamin D.
4. Potential roles of alterations in the parathyroid gland.
   a. Hypocalcemia is a powerful stimulus for PTH secretion and growth of the parathyroid gland.
      (1) Calcium-sensing receptors seem to mediate the effects of calcium.
      (2) In CKD there appears to be a decrease in calcium-sensing receptors that could lead to increased PTH secretion since the response of the parathyroid glands to stimulation by calcium may be diminished.
   b. Decreased levels of calcitriol may also play a role in the development of parathyroid abnormalities.
      (1) Calcitriol is a major regulator of PTH secretion and the vitamin D receptor is expressed in the parathyroid glands.
      (2) Calcitriol decreases PTH secretion by affecting the level of transcription of the PTH gene.
      (3) Calcitriol may also alter PTH secretion by increasing the parathyroid gland's vitamin D receptor, regulating parathyroid growth,

altering the expression of the calcium-sensing receptor, and possibly affecting the set point for calcium-regulated PTH secretion.
   c. Consequences of parathyroid growth in CKD.
      (1) Calcium-sensing receptors are decreased in the parathyroid gland.
      (2) Vitamin D receptors are decreased in the parathyroid gland.
5. Factors contributing to skeletal resistance to the action of PTH may include:
   a. Phosphorous retention.
   b. Decreased levels of calcitriol.
   c. Suppression of the PTH receptor.
   d. Potential actions of PTH fragments that can dull the calcemic effect of PTH.

E. Low-turnover metabolic bone disease.
   1. Characterized by an extremely slow rate of bone formation.
   2. Osteomalacia, defective bone mineralization, may also be present.
      a. Lesions are usually due to aluminum.
      b. Seen less commonly these days since aluminum binders are not routinely prescribed.
   3. Adynamic bone disease is characterized by reduced numbers of osteoblasts (bone forming cells) and osteoclasts (bone resorption cells) and low or absent bone formation.
      a. The pathogenesis of adynamic bone disease is unknown, but the number of cases is increasing.
      b. Susceptible populations include the elderly, women, persons with diabetes, and Caucasians.
      c. It is associated with a higher rate of fractures. Symptoms are usually absent until the disease is advanced.
   4. Factors contributing to low-turnover metabolic bone disease.
      a. Administration of high calcium loads. Potential sources take in:
         (1) Calcium-containing phosphate binders.
         (2) Use of dialysate fluid containing high levels of calcium.
      b. Administration of potent vitamin D sterols.
      c. Age.
         (1) Postmenopausal osteoporosis.
         (2) Osteopenia in association with systemic disease.
      d. Increases in circulating peptides that may decrease bone formation, e.g., N-terminal truncated PTH fragments.
      e. Undefined uremic toxins.

f. Acidosis.

g. Decreased expression of PTH receptors.

h. Alterations in concentrations of growth factors and cytokines that affect bone turnover.

i. Previous corticosteroid therapy, e.g., induced osteoporosis.

j. General malnutrition.

F. Signs and symptoms of metabolic bone disease.
  1. The patient is often asymptomatic. Symptoms appear only late in the development of metabolic bone disease.
  2. Nonspecific symptoms.
    a. Pain and stiffness in the joints.
    b. Spontaneous tendon rupture.
    c. Predisposition to fracture.
    d. Proximal muscle weakness.
  3. The control of metabolic bone disease, even in the absence of signs and symptoms, is important since metabolic bone disease also has consequences at extraskeletal sites.
  4. Extraskeletal involvement includes:
    a. Extraskeletal calcifications such as in the vasculature, the skin, and calciphylaxis. Calciphylaxis is a metastatic calcification of soft tissue and blood vessels that can lead to necrosis and extremity loss.
    b. Cardiovascular calcification.

G. Treatment of calcium phosphorous imbalance.
  1. NKF KDOQI guidelines.
    a. Phosphorus (PO_4) level at 2.7–4.6 mg/dL for CKD stage 3–4.
    b. Phosphorus (PO_4) level at 3.5–5.5 mg/dL for CKD stage 5.
    c. Intact PTH:
      (1) 35–70 pg/mL for CKD stage 3.
      (2) 70–110 pg/mL for CKD stage 4.
      (3) 150–300 pg/mL for CKD stage 5.
    d. Recommended frequency for lab draws.
      (1) CKD stage 3: PTH, Ca and PO_4 every 12 months.
      (2) CKD stage 4: PTH, Ca and PO_4 every 3 months.
      (3) CKD stage 5: PTH every 3 months; Ca and PO_4 every month.
  2. Diet should only have 800–1000 mg of phosphorus/day (see Section 8 for further details).
  3. Use of phosphate binders with meals (see Section 9 for further details).
    a. Calcium-based binders.
      (1) Calcium carbonate/acetate.
      (2) Can lead to hypercalcemia and soft tissue calcification.

(3) Should not be used if serum calcium level is elevated.

(4) Total elemental calcium intake should not exceed 2000 mg/day.

b. Non-calcium-based binders used in end-stage renal disease.
  (1) Sevelamer also assists in lipid control.
  (2) Lanthanum.

4. PTH reduction.
  a. If the PTH level is above the target range for the CKD stage, a serum 25-hydroxyvitamin D level should be obtained.
  b. If the result is < 30 ng/mL, it indicates the need to supplement the patient with vitamin D2-ergocalciferol 50,000 IU monthly for 6 months.
  c. Calcium and phosphorus levels should be monitored.
  d. When the intact PTH is >300 pg/mL, the use of a vitamin D analog is recommended, such as calcitriol, doxecalciferol.
  e. Cinacalcet acts on calcium receptors of the parathyroid gland. This drug can be used to decrease PTH synthesis in CKD stage 5 patients who are undergoing dialysis. Its use can lead to hypocalcemia.

III. Protein energy malnutrition (PEM).

A. Factors causing protein energy malnutrition in CKD.
  1. Low protein and caloric intake are important causes.
  2. The patient with CKD is at risk for lower levels of albumin and malnutrition. Both lead to poor outcomes for the patient.
  3. Uremic toxins that lead to decreased appetite and poor intake of dietary nutrients.
  4. The altered body's response to insulin that occurs in CKD.
  5. Accelerated protein catabolism.
  6. Chronic inflammation.
  7. Nausea.
  8. Proteinuria.

B. Assessment of protein energy malnutrition (see Section 8).

C. Treatment of protein energy malnutrition.
  1. Early referral to nutritionist at stage 3.
  2. There are concerns regarding the limitation of protein intake to delay the progression of CKD.

IV. Metabolic acidosis.

A. Mechanisms include:
  1. Accumulation of organic acids in plasma.
  2. Impairment of renal acidification mechanisms.
  3. Loss of nephron mass.

B. Metabolic acidosis usually occurs in the later stages of CKD.

C. Complications.
  1. Chronic bone loss.
  2. Muscle wasting.
  3. Anorexia and weight loss.
  4. Hypoalbuminemia.
  5. Acceleration of the loss of kidney function.
  6. Impaired cardiac function.
  7. Resistance to insulin.
  8. Abnormal growth hormone and thyroid hormone function.

D. Treatment of metabolic acidosis.
  1. The goal is to maintain the serum bicarbonate level at 22 mEq/L (mmol/L).
  2. Oral bicarbonate tablets ($NaHCO_3$): 0.5 meq/kg/day in divided doses. Side effects of sodium bicarbonate include fluid retention, edema, exacerbation of heart failure, elevated blood pressure.

V. Hyperkalemia.

A. Precipitating factors leading to hyperkalemia.
  1. Dietary indiscretions.
  2. Constipation.
  3. Protein catabolism.
  4. Hemolysis.
  5. Hemorrhage.
  6. Blood transfusion.
  7. Medications, such as ACE inhibitors, beta blockers, ARBs, potassium sparing diuretics, and nonsteroidal antiinflammatory drugs.
  8. Physiologic changes such as:
     a. Impaired tubular secretion of K+.
     b. Certain forms of renal tubular acidosis such as seen in persons with diabetes.
     c. Volume depletion leading to poor perfusion.
     d. Starvation.

B. Hyperkalemia is more prevalent at GFR < 15 mL/min.

C. Treatment.
  1. Dietary consult (see Section 8).
  2. Discontinue offending drugs, such as an ACE-I.
  3. In life-threatening situations, the patient may need medications to treat the hyperkalemia (see Table 2.12 and Section 9).
  4. Dialysis is indicated if the patient is not responding to medical treatment.
  5. Follow-up lab work should be done.

VI. Hypervolemia/volume overload.

A. Precipitating factors leading to hypervolemia/volume overload.
  1. Increase in serum sodium.
     a. The underlying disease process may disrupt glomerulotubular balance and promote sodium retention.
     b. Excessive sodium ingestion.
  2. Secondary to the increase in the extracellular fluid, the blood pressure increases. This in turn accelerates the progression of injury to the kidneys.
  3. As long as water intake does not exceed the capacity for free water clearance, balance will be maintained.

B. Assessment of hypervolemia/volume overload.
  1. Weight gain associated with volume expansion may be offset in patients with CKD if they are losing lean body mass.
  2. Blood pressure measurements; comparative weight; respiratory rate, quality, and breath sounds; heart rate and heart sounds; peripheral edema; neck vein distension.

C. Treatment of hypervolemia/volume overload.
  1. Restriction of salt intake (see Section 8).
  2. Use of diuretics: thiazides, loop diuretics (see Section 9).
  3. Monitor the patient for possible side effects of the medications: hypotension, dehydration, electrolyte imbalance.
  4. When extracellular fluid volume expansion does not respond to treatment, it may be time for the initiation of dialysis.

D. Patients with CKD also have an impaired mechanism for conserving sodium and water. When the patients have vomiting, diarrhea, sweating, or fever, they are more prone to volume depletion. This depletion can compromise kidney function with resulting signs and symptoms of uremia. Cautious volume repletion is necessary, usually with normal saline.

Table 2.12

Treatment of Hyperkalemia

Mechanism	Onset of Action
Antagonism of membrane actions • Calcium	Several minutes and then rapidly waves
Increased potassium entry into cells • Insulin and glucose • -2 adrenergic agonists • Sodium bicarbonate	Each of these modalities works within 30–60 minutes, lowers the serum potassium concentration by 0.5–1.5 mEq/L, and lasts for several hours
Potassium removal from the body • Diuretics • Cation exchange resin • Dialysis	Several hours but many patients with advance kidney failure show little response 2-3 hours Several hours

Source: Rose, B.D., & Rennke, H.G. (1994). *Renal pathophysiology – The essentials (p.183)*. Baltimore: Lippincott Williams & Wilkins. Reprinted with permission.

VII. Sexual function in CKD.

A. A variety of sexual problems affect both men and women with CKD.

B. Potential problems.
   1. Decreased libido.
   2. Erectile dysfunction.
   3. Dysmenorrhea.
   4. Infertility.

C. Contributing factors.
   1. The hormonal changes that occur.
   2. Vascular alterations.
   3. Neurologic alterations.
   4. Psychogenic factors.
   5. Certain medications.
      a. Antihypertensive medications, e.g., central acting agents such as clonidine, beta blockers, and alpha blockers. ACE inhibitors and ARBs have a lower incidence of impotence.
      b. Cimetidine.
      c. Tricyclic antidepressants.
      d. Phenothiazines.
      e. Metoclopramide.

D. Potential female sexual problems in CKD including those with stage 5 CKD.
   1. Premature menopause, averaging 4.5 years earlier than expected.
      a. Short-term effects include skin wrinkling, urinary incontinence, hypoactive sexual functioning, hot flashes, sleep disorders, and depression.
      b. Long-term effects include osteoporosis, disorders of cognitive functioning, and CVD.
   2. Most women report decreased libido consistent with sexual aversion disorder or hypoactive sexual desire disorder (HSDD), and inability to achieve an orgasm.
      a. HSDD is the persistent absence of sexual thoughts and/or desire for and receptivity to sexual activity that causes personal distress.
      b. Endocrine abnormalities leading to vaginal dryness and/or pain after intercourse also contribute to decreased sexual activity.
   3. Available treatment for women.
      a. Pharmacologic therapy with hormones.
      b. Correction of anemia.
      c. Adequate dialysis.
      d. Treatment of depression.
      e. Changes in lifestyle.
         (1) Smoking cessation.
         (2) Strength training and aerobic exercise may help depression as well as have a positive impact on body image and sexuality.
      f. Topical estrogen cream and vaginal lubricants.
   4. By the time stage 5 CKD is reached, women are

usually amenorrheic or have irregular menstrual cycles.
    a. Anovulatory cycles are not uncommon.
    b. Pregnancy is not likely to happen. However, women who do have menstrual cycles should be encouraged to use contraception.
    c. Because of poor pregnancy outcomes, restoring fertility is not an advisable therapeutic goal.
    d. Up to 65% of women on hemodialysis report problems with sexual functioning; 40% no longer engage in sexual intercourse.
5. Pregnancy in women with CKD.
    a. Information regarding outcomes is limited.
    b. When the serum creatinine is < 1.4 mg/dL, the pregnancy leads to a successful outcome and does not appear to affect the course of CKD.
    c. When the serum creatinine is > 2.0 mg/dL at the time of conception, one third of the women progress to stage 5 CKD over the first postpartum year.
    d. Fetal outcomes have been helped by improvements in prenatal care.
        (1) There is significant intrauterine growth restriction.
        (2) Prematurity occurs in 40% to 70% of the births.
        (3) Fetal survival is > 70% when the woman does not require dialysis.
        (4) Fetal survival is lower with uncontrolled HTN.
        (5) Proteinuria < 300 mg/day during pregnancy is associated with lower infant mortality.
        (6) Preeclampsia occurs in 30% of pregnancies in women with CKD.
    e. Women with CKD who become pregnant need to be followed closely by both a nephrologist and an obstetrician specializing in high risk pregnancies.
    f. Women with CKD stage 5 who become pregnant are faced with potential complications.
        (1) In the last 10 years, infant survival is reported to be 40% to 50%.
        (2) Over 80% of the infants are premature. The average gestational age is 32 weeks.
        (3) Early delivery is due to premature labor, premature rupture of the membranes, and/or cervical incompetence.
        (4) A much more intense dialysis regimen is required. The blood urea nitrogen should be maintained at less than or equal to 50 mg/dL and the rapidity of ultrafiltration should be reduced.
    g. A successful kidney transplant offers the best chance for pregnancy and a viable birth.
        (1) Many transplant centers encourage women to wait 18 to 24 months after transplant before conceiving.
        (2) Graft function should be stable and immunosuppressive drugs should be at baseline levels before conceiving.

E. Potential male sexual problems in CKD including those on dialysis.
1. Men with CKD have low levels of testosterone, both free and total.
    a. Contributes to decreased libido, erectile dysfunction (ED), decreased mature sperm cells, infertility, decreased muscle mass, osteopenia, osteoporosis, and anemia.
    b. ED may be as high as 70% to 80% in CKD with similar results in stage 5 CKD.
        (1) Risk factors for the development of ED include increasing age, diabetes, HTN, dyslipidemia, and smoking.
        (2) Psychological problems and anxiety also play major roles.
2. Hormonal changes exist in the early stages of CKD and progressively worsen as the disease worsens.
3. Evaluation and possible treatment of sexual dysfunction in men with CKD.
    a. Nocturnal penile tumescence testing is used to differentiate organic and psychological causes of impotence. Normal nocturnal erections during rapid eye movement sleep indicates the need for psychological testing and evaluation.
    b. Measurement of penile blood flow and blood pressure by Doppler may be helpful in determining a vascular etiology of ED.
    c. Impotence of neurologic origin is characterized by prolonged latency time of the bulbocavernous reflex or by the presence of a neurogenic bladder.
    d. Treatment includes:
        (1) Adequate nutritional intake.
        (2) ESA.
        (3) Adequate dialysis.
4. Successful kidney transplant can restore the hormonal balance.

Chapter 8

Empowerment Strategies and the Introduction to Kidney Replacement Therapies

I. The goals of treatment.

A. Preventing or slowing the progression of CKD.

B. Preventing, identifying and managing comorbidities and complications.

C. Controlling symptoms of CKD.

D. Minimizing the effects of CKD on lifestyles.

E. Preparing the patient for kidney replacement therapies when appropriate.

F. Managing other chronic conditions.

G. Empowering patients to actively participate and oversee their health care.

II. Basic strategies designed to empower the CKD patient.

A. The patient is the principal manager of CKD.
  1. Proficiency in specific skills and tasks is necessary to master this role.
  2. The role of the nurse in this process cannot be underestimated.

B. Definition of self-care/self-management.
  1. Engaging in activities that promote health and prevent illness and complications.
  2. Interacting with health care providers and adhering to recommended treatment.
  3. Monitoring physical and emotional status and being able to make decisions based on self-monitoring.
  4. Managing the effects of illness based on the individual's ability to function in important roles.

C. Collaborative management means that the medical providers and the patient are able to have shared goals, a working relationship, and a mutual understanding of their roles.
  1. Clinicians can and should encourage patients to be active participants in their own care.

2. Forming partnerships with the patient can be encouraged by:
  a. Ensuring the patient feels comfortable during visits.
  b. Avoiding rushed and insensitive interactions.
  c. Asking what the patient wants from an interaction; what are his/her current concerns, and what progress has been made to previously established goals.
  d. Encouraging the patient and family (as appropriate) to ask questions.
  e. Spending more time listening to the patient and less time offering advice.
  f. Showing concern for the patient first and the disease second.
  g. Keeping the patient informed of the findings of an assessment and progress toward goals.
3. Concordance is a healthy partnership between the patient and the clinician that implies a shared understanding or agreement on the nature of an illness and its treatment. It does not imply adherence.
  a. Concordance describes the outcome of the patient's and clinician's interaction.
  b. Adherence describes the patient's behavior.

D. Challenges associated with CKD education programs.
  1. Beliefs strongly influence self-management.
    a. Many patients with stage 1 or 2 CKD are asymptomatic.
    b. Encouraging these individuals to change their lifestyles can be difficult.
    c. Assessing the patient's perception is an important first step.
  2. Self-efficacy, that is, confidence in one's ability to perform a task, must be developed. Thomas-Hawkins and Zazworsky (2005) identified four essential ingredients to building self-efficacy.
    a. Performance mastery.
      (1) Helping patients to attain specific skills builds confidence.
      (2) Goals must be realistic.

(3) One task must be mastered before new responsibilities are introduced.

b. Modeling.
   (1) Teaching materials should be appropriate to the patient's age, ethnicity, and, when appropriate, the person's gender.
   (2) Support groups provide opportunities for modeling.

c. Interpretation of symptoms.
   (1) If done in a negative way, the patient can be left feeling vulnerable and may have difficulty coping.
   (2) The patient may try new self-management behaviors if given alternative explanations for symptoms' causes.

d. Verbal persuasion.
   (1) A credible source should provide the patient with a "you can do it" attitude.
   (2) Classes and support groups are two venues in which this can occur.

E. Transtheoretical model (TTM) of intentional change focuses on the decision making of the individual.
   1. Background.
      a. Developed by Prochaska, DiClemente, and colleagues. Based on over 15 years of research on a variety of problem behaviors.
      b. Behavioral change is a process rather than a discrete event. Relapse may occur. Individuals go through a series of changes on the road to adopting healthy behaviors and/or cessation of unhealthy behaviors.
   2. Five stages of change.
      a. Precontemplation: lack of awareness that a situation/problem can be improved by change in behavior.
         (1) The individual has no intention of changing in the near future, i.e., the next 6 months.
         (2) The patient is often characterized as resistant or unmotivated.
         (3) The person tends to avoid information, discussion, or thought about the situation or problem.
         (4) Traditional programs are often not designed for such individuals and their needs can go unmet.
      b. Contemplation: recognition of the problem.
         (1) Initial consideration is given to change in behavior.
         (2) Gathering information about potential solutions and actions begins.
         (3) Often seen as ambivalent to change or as a procrastinator.

(4) Like those in the precontemplation stage, these individuals are not ready for traditional action oriented programs.

c. Preparation: introspection about the decision.
   (1) Reaffirms the need and desire to change a behavior(s) usually within the next 30 days.
   (2) Completes the final pre-action steps.
   (3) A transition stage rather than a stable stage.

d. Action: implementation of the practices needed for successful behavior change (e.g., taking antihypertensive medication as prescribed).
   (1) Lifestyle modifications for fewer than 6 months.
   (2) Vigilance against relapse is critical.

e. Maintenance: consolidation of the behaviors initiated in the action stage.
   (1) Report the highest level of self-efficacy.
   (2) Less frequently tempted to relapse.

f. Termination: problem behaviors are no longer desirable.

F. Processes of change are covert and overt actions that individuals use to progress through the stages of change. The processes of change are important guides for intervention programs to assist the individual to move through these stages.
   1. Conscious raising: increasing the awareness about the causes, consequences, and cures for a particular problem; e.g., CKD. *Potential interventions*: feedback, education, confrontation, media campaigns.
   2. Dramatic relief: emotional arousal; produces increased emotional experiences followed by reduced affect if appropriate action can be taken. *Potential interventions*: role playing, grieving, personal testimonies, media campaigns.
   3. Environmental reevaluation: social reappraisal; assesses how the problem affects one's social environment. It can also include the awareness that one can serve as a role model in a positive or negative way. *Potential interventions*: empathy training, documentaries, and family interventions.
   4. Social liberation: environmental opportunities; requires an increase in social opportunities or alternatives especially for people who are relatively deprived or oppressed. *Potential interventions*: advocacy, empowerment procedures, appropriate policies.
   5. Self-reevaluation: self-reappraisal; assessment of

an individual's self-image with and without a particular unhealthy habit. *Potential interventions*: value clarification, appropriate role models, imagery techniques.

6. Stimulus control: re-engineering; removes cues for unhealthy habits and adds prompts for healthier alternatives. *Potential interventions*: avoidance, environmental re-engineering, self-help groups.

7. Helping relationships: supporting; combine caring, trust, openness, acceptance and support for healthy habits. *Potential interventions*: rapport building, therapeutic alliance, counselor calls, buddy system.

8. Counter conditioning: substituting; learning healthier behaviors that can substitute problem behaviors. *Potential interventions*: e.g., substitute hard candy for fluid to accommodate limitations in intake.

9. Reinforcement management: rewarding; self-changers rely more on rewards than on punishments. *Potential interventions*: contingency contracts, positive self-statements, group recognition.

10. Self-liberation: committing; the belief that one can change as well as the commitment and recommitment to act on that belief.

G. Enhancing change with motivational interviewing.
   1. Background. Motivational interviewing was developed by William Miller and Stephen Rollnick in the early 1990s. Its aim is to help someone make changes in behavior. Motivational interviewing can be integrated with other methods for facilitating change.
   2. Definition. A client-centered, directive method for enhancing intrinsic motivation to change by exploring and resolving ambivalence (Miller & Rollnick, 2002).
      a. It is person-centered and focuses on the concerns and perspectives of the individual. It relies heavily on the work of Carl Rogers.
      b. It intentionally seeks to resolve ambivalence, often in a particular direction of change. The interviewer selectively responds to speech in a way that resolves ambivalence and moves the person toward change.
      c. It is a method of communication rather than a set of techniques; a facilitative approach to communication that evokes natural change.
      d. Its focus is on eliciting the person's intrinsic motivation for change.
      e. It cannot be used to impose change that is inconsistent with the individual's own values and beliefs.

3. The goals of motivational interviewing.
   a. To create a safe and supportive rapport with a person and to facilitate thinking about one's own behavior(s).
   b. To help the individual explore that behavior(s).
   c. To make a cost-benefit analysis of the status quo.
   d. To decrease potential resistance to change.
   e. To clarify goals.
   f. To assist in developing realistic strategies for facilitating behavioral changes.
4. Addresses whether and/or how the individual might go about making changes.
5. Recognizes that if the idea of change was entirely positive then it would be easy.
6. Motivational interviewing techniques recognize both positive and negative aspects of change.
7. Situations to avoid during a motivational interview.
   a. The question/answer routine, which prevents elaboration and exploration.
   b. Confrontation/denial, which almost always demands the individual insist on the opposite perspective. Avoid arguments, struggles, or debates about what the person should do.
   c. The expert trap, which leads the individual into a passive role. The person will not work on his/her own to explore and resolve ambivalence.
   d. Labeling, e.g., troublemaker, which can provoke a lot of resistance. If a person asks about a labeling, reply that "a label is not of interest; what is of interest is the person's behavior and what it means to him/her."
   e. Blaming, which is not particularly relevant or important to the goals of the interview.
   f. Preaching, which no one likes. Avoid scolding, lecturing, or talking down to; give suggestions and feedback.

H. Impact of chronic illness on the family (see Section 4, Chapter 17).
   1. Stressors from role reversal.
   2. Increase in responsibility due to being caregiver.
   3. Conflict within family values, cultural needs.

I. Incorporating a plan of action (see Section 4, Chapter 18).
   1. The educational process should include the patient and family, joint discussion about goals from the medical perspective as well as from the individual's perspective.
   2. Patients need to be motivated and supported with self-empowerment skills.

3. Medical providers are guides. It is the patient who is making decisions about the choice of treatment.
4. Information should be provided in a variety of ways: verbally, written handouts, videos. If the patient is interested in computers and the Internet, refer to Web sites.
   a. Patients should be asked to identify their choice in education support.
   b. "How do you learn best? How do you like to learn?"

J. Examples of areas where self-care can be instituted.
   1. Interpreting and reporting symptoms.
      a. Patients should know that there may not be any symptoms in the early stages of CKD.
      b. In later stages patients should know that symptoms can include fatigue, malaise, sleep disturbance, nausea, vomiting, anorexia, changes in taste, weight loss, pruritus, skin rash, muscle cramping, edema, poor concentration, neuropathy, restless legs, and/or an increase in urination especially at night.
   2. Blood pressure monitoring: maintaining a log, understanding what the values mean, and how medications impact blood pressure control.
   3. Blood sugar control: monitoring blood sugar and being able to adjust insulin, apply readings to diet, or activity.
   4. Medications: understanding the purpose for each medication and relationship to kidney disease; e.g., the importance of phosphate binders in relation to the control of serum calcium and phosphorous levels and the prevention of possible complications.
   5. Lab values: what the numbers mean in relationship to illness; how the current lab values compare to the patient's trended lab results.
   6. Diet: why it may be modified, why fluids may need to be decreased, or the relationship between salt and high blood pressure.
   7. Exercise as tolerated.
   8. Nurses should routinely ask the patient about these topics and help them reshape their misperceptions and lead them to appropriate strategies that yield desired outcomes.

III. Preparation for kidney replacement therapy (KRT).

A. When and how KRT should be introduced to the patient and family/significant other(s).
   1. The risks and benefits of kidney replacement

therapy need to be discussed by CKD stage 4 or when the GFR is 25 mL/min or less. Ongoing education at different stages should be initiated.
   2. An objective and unbiased approach about all modalities should be used in presenting information.
   3. Referral to nurse educator for formal education on modality options should be done with reinforcement of information done by all health care providers.
   4. Education can be done in a group class for general information with a follow-up individual session where specific needs can be addressed.
   5. Group process can allay fears about illness and sharing of experience can also be a means of learning.
   6. A tour of the dialysis unit may assist patients in accepting treatment, especially if they are able to ask questions from one who is on dialysis.
   7. Written information should be provided for further reading or discussion with family.
   8. A multidisciplinary team approach should be used to reinforce all team members' specific roles.
   9. Decision making about choice is partially dependent upon how the individual is coping. Some individuals will be able to state what modality is of interest to them. Some individuals will not be able to or willing to make a choice if they are in denial or are overwhelmed. Some patients may verbalize that they feel fine and do not believe that their kidney disease will get worse. The earlier the education starts, the more time patients have to reevaluate modality choice, review information, and ask questions.

B. Selection of kidney replacement therapy (KRT).
   1. The risks, benefits, and complications of each modality should be thoroughly addressed so that the individual can make an informed consent.
   2. Palliative care (see Section 4, Chapter 22).
      a. Some individuals will be adamant about not choosing any replacement therapy and will want only comfort measures.
      b. Discuss advance directives, hospice care, and pain control.
      c. Assure the individual has a clear understanding of the process and outcomes of palliative care.
      d. Family members should also be involved in this discussion, so that everyone is aware of the patient's desires.

e. The individual should be assessed for depression to assure that the decision is made through the process of evaluating the risks and benefits of the choices available.
3. Home therapies (see Section 14).
4. Nocturnal hemodialysis (see Section 14). While this hemodialysis modality is usually performed at home, some in-center dialysis facilities offer this option.
5. Hemodialysis (see Sections 11 and 12).
   a. Referral for vascular access placement should be done when the GFR is < 25–30 mL/min if this modality is chosen.
   b. Vessel mapping and evaluation by the vascular surgeon and scheduling of surgery should be planned early to provide at least 3–4 months for healing and development of the fistula.
   c. Preservation of veins and protection of nondominant arm or arm identified for access should be stressed to the patient in the early stages of CKD.
   d. Instruct patient on hand exercises once surgery is done.
   e. Creation of access: an arteriovenous (AV) fistula is the preferred access. If the veins are too small, an AV graft would be next choice. Central lines should be used only as a last resort due to a high risk for infection. Central lines are associated with an increase in morbidity and mortality.
6. Peritoneal dialysis (see Section 13).
   a. Ensure that home environment will be adequate for home therapy e.g., is there enough storage space for supplies, a clean environment, etc.
   b. Referral to a interventional radiologist or nephrologist trained in the procedure for catheter placement is not required until the patient is approaching dialysis, GFR < 20 mL/min.
   c. Once placed the catheter will not be used until it is well healed to prevent leaks.
7. Transplant (see Section 10).
   a. With preemptive transplants the patient can be worked up when GFR is < 20mL/min.
   b. Stress that transplant is another treatment, not a cure.
   c. The importance of self-care with transplant and lifelong use of immunosuppressive agents needs to be addressed.
   d. Discussions should take place about risks, complications, medications and side effects, and long-term complications with transplant.

e. Organ donation and waiting list should also be discussed.

IV. Despite current recommendations, there are still barriers that impact CKD care. The Chronic Kidney Initiative was developed by multiple associations, and stakeholders to identify some of those barriers.

A. Barriers to early identification of CKD.
   1. There is an absence of coordinated care systems that insures that all CKD patients are identified and subsequently receive the care that is needed.
   2. Coordination between primary care providers and nephrologists is lacking.
   3. Primary care providers do not always refer the patient to the nephrologist until the patient has reached the last stage of CKD.
   4. A lack of public awareness and concern regarding risks associated with CKD exists.
   5. The GFR is not routinely reported by all laboratories.
   6. There is inadequate recognition of cardiovascular disease and its relation to a decreased GFR.
   7. Shortage of health care providers as well as time constraints.
   8. Unwillingness by some payers to reimburse for early CKD management and education is a problem.
   9. Payers need to recognize the value of early CKD management including education.

B. Barriers to referrals to the nephrology team.
   1. The number of nephrologists is decreasing. There will not be enough nephrologists to manage all of the CKD patients identified.
   2. Early referral (at least by eGFR < 60 mL/min) to a nephrologist is recommended to insure a clinical plan is put into place.
   3. Comanagement of CKD patients is going to be required. Early collaboration between the primary care provider and the nephrologist should occur.

C. Steps toward optimizing care of the CKD patient.
   1. It is important to enhance communication among providers.
   2. Centralized services would be beneficial to all.
   3. Efficient and effective systems of reimbursement need to be established.
   4. The enormity and diversity of the population at risk must be taken into account.
   5. Evaluation of the clinical effectiveness and cost-effectiveness of interventions currently working

should take place. Included should be disease management, the use of CKD clinics, nephrology multidisciplinary teams, etc.

6. Establishment of best practice guidelines in different settings through evidenced-based protocols and interventions is essential.

V. Outcome resources to evaluate target recommendations.

A. CMS – Centers for Medicare and Medicaid Services – www.cms.hhs.gov.
1. Pay for performance.
   a. Quality-based purchasing, also known as pay-for-performance, is the use of payment methods and other incentives to encourage quality improvement and patient focused, high value care.
   b. Many models, early stages of development, best method not yet determined.
   c. ESRD patients can compare dialysis facilities on several quality measures: anemia, hemodialysis, and patient survival (www.cms.gov/DialysisFacilitycompare).
2. Quality indicators – www.cms.hhs.gov/PQRI.
   a. 2008 Physician Quality Reporting Initiative (PQRI) establishes a financial incentive for eligible professionals to participate in a voluntary quality reporting program. Eligible professionals who successfully report a designated set of quality measures on claims for dates of service from July 1 to December 31, 2007, may earn a bonus payment, subject to a cap, of 1.5% of total allowed charges for covered Medicare physician fee schedule services; and
   b. PRQI measures include screening for microalbumin, use of ACEI or ARB in patients with CKD, CKD lab testing, CKD and BP management, and use of ESAs.

B. AV Fistula First – www.fistulafirst.org.
1. AV Fistula First is a coalition working to increase the use of AVFs by individuals who need hemodialysis and is led by renal, healthcare, trade organizations and government agencies.
2. A national initiative to increase the AVF use for all suitable hemodialysis patients.
3. Working together to meet KDOQI guidelines and the CMS stretch goal of increasing the percentage of hemodialysis patients using AVFs to 66% by 2009 nationwide.
4. Provides education to all renal health care providers and patients about AVFs.

C. ESRD networks – www.esrdnetworks.org.
1. The formation of ESRD Network Organizations was authorized in 1978 by Public Law 95-292 which amended Title XVIII of the Social Security Act by adding section 1881. CMS Today, 18 ESRD Network Organizations exist under contract to CMS and serve as liaisons between the federal government and the providers of ESRD services. The Network Organizations are defined geographically by the number and concentration of ESRD beneficiaries in each area. Some Networks represent one state, others multiple states.
2. The ESRD Network Organizations' responsibilities include the quality oversight of the care ESRD patients receive, the collection of data to administer the national Medicare ESRD program, and the provision of technical assistance to ESRD providers and patients in areas related to ESRD.

D. USRDS – United States Renal Data System – www.USRDS.org.
1. The United States Renal Data System (USRDS) is a national data system that collects, analyzes, and distributes information about end-stage renal disease (ESRD) in the United States. The USRDS is funded directly by the National Institute of Diabetes and Digestive and Kidney Diseases (NIDDK) in conjunction with the Centers for Medicare & Medicaid Services (CMS, formerly HCFA). USRDS staff collaborates with members of CMS, the United Network for Organ Sharing (UNOS), and the ESRD networks, sharing datasets and actively working to improve the accuracy of ESRD patient information.
2. CKD has received more attention as the precursor to ESRD since the 2002 publication of the National Kidney Foundation's KDOQI Clinical Practice Guidelines for Chronic Kidney: Evaluation, Classification, and Stratification.
3. USRDS uses diagnosis codes from hospital and outpatient encounters to determine the size of the CKD population.
4. In approximately two thirds of Medicare recipients > 65 years of age diagnosed with CKD, the CKD is accompanied by diabetes, CHF, or a combination of both diseases.
5. The USRDS offers educational materials (such as slides) about CKD that are available at their Web site.
6. Persons can request specific data from the USRDS.

7. The USRDS provides indicators and current data.

E. Healthy People 2010 – www.healthypeople.gov.
   1. Healthy People 2010 represents the third time the U.S. Department of Health and Human Services (HHS) has developed 10-year health objectives for the nation.
   2. Health Promotion and Disease Prevention Objectives for people with CKD.
      a. Reduce the rate of new cases of ESRD.
      b. Reduce deaths from cardiovascular disease in persons with CKD.
      c. Increase the proportion of treated CKD patients who receive counseling on nutrition, treatment choices, and cardiovascular care 12 months before the start of KRT.
      d. Increase the proportion of new hemodialysis patients who use AV fistulas as the primary mode of vascular access.
      e. Increase the proportion of dialysis patients registered on the waiting list for transplantation.
      f. Reduce kidney failure due to diabetes.
      g. Deter the progression of kidney disease in people with type 1 or type 2 diabetes with proteinuria, by increasing the proportions of this patient population that receive the recommended medical therapy.
      h. To review the status of these goals, visit www.usrds.org/2005.

F. KDIGO – Kidney Disease: Improving Global Outcomes – www.kdigo.org.
   1. KDIGO is a Belgian not-for-profit foundation with a 40-member international Board of Directors and managed by NKF. Its mission is to improve outcomes for kidney patients worldwide through coordination, development, and implementation of practice guidelines.
   2. Mission statement: to improve the care and outcomes of kidney disease patients worldwide through promoting coordination, collaboration and integration of initiatives to develop and implement clinical practice guidelines.
   3. Associated countries include Australia, Canada, Europe, the United States, and the United Kingdom.

G. The Joint Commission (on Accreditation of Health Care Organizations – JCAHO) – www.jointcommission.org.
   1. The Joint Commission's Certificate of Distinction for chronic kidney disease recognizes organizations that make exceptional efforts to foster better outcomes for CKD patients.
   2. Developed in 2005, it is based on the KDOQI Guidelines published by the National Kidney Foundation.

References

American Diabetes Association (ADA). (2004). Nephropathy in diabetes. Position statement. *Diabetes Care, 27*(Suppl. 1), 79-83.

American Diabetes Association (ADA). (2005). Diagnosis and classification of diabetes mellitus. *Diabetes Care, 28*(Suppl. 1), 37-42.

Anantharaman, P., & Schmidt, R.J. (2007). Sexual function in chronic kidney disease. *Advances in Chronic Kidney Disease, 14*(2), 119–125.

Burgess, E. (2004, March). The risk of CVD: How are patients with CKD affected? *Perspectives in Cardiology, 30-36.*

Burrows, L., & Muller, R. (2007). Chronic kidney disease and cardiovascular disease: Pathophysiologic links. *Nephrology Nursing Journal, 34*(1), 55-63.

Burrows-Hudson, S. (2005). Chronic kidney disease: An overview. *American Journal of Nursing, 105*(2), 40-50.

Burrows-Hudson, S., & Prowant, B. (2005). *Nephrology nursing standards of practice and guidelines for care.* Pitman, NJ: American Nephrology Nurses' Association.

Campoy, S., & Elwell, R. (2005). Pharmacology and CKD. *American Journal of Nursing, 105*(9), 60-72.

Cancer Prevention Research Center. (2007). *Detailed overview of the transtheoretical model.* Retrieved January 30, 2008, from http://www.uri.edu/research/cprc/TTM/detailedoverview.htm

Centers for Disease Control and Prevention (CDC). (2007). Prevalence of chronic kidney disease and associated risk factors – United States, 1999–2004. *MMWR Weekly, 56*(8), 161-165.

Chertow, G.M. (2004). Prevention of radiocontrast nephropathy back to basics. *Journal of the American Medical Association, 291*(19), 2376-2377.

Chobanian, A.V., Bakis, G.L., Black, H.R., Cushman, W.C., Green, L.A., Izzo, J.L., et al., & the National High Blood Pressure Education Programming Coordinating Committee. (2003). The seventh report of the Joint National Committee on Prevention, Detection, Evaluation, and Treatment of High Blood Pressure. *JAMA, 289*, 2560-2562.

Cimprich, B. (1992). A theoretical perspective on attention to patient education. *Advances in Nursing Science, 14*(3), 39-51.

Combest, W., Newton, M., Combest, A., & Kosier, J.H. (2005). Effects of herbal supplements on the kidney. *Urologic Nursing, 25*(5), 381-386.

Coyne, D.W., Cheng, S.C., & Delmez, J.A. (2007). Bone disease. In J.T. Daugirdas, P.G. Blake, & T.S. Ing (Eds.), *Handbook of dialysis* (4th ed.). Philadelphia: Wolters Kluwer/Lippincott Williams & Wilkins.

Cunningham, R., Corretti, M., & Henrich, W. (2006). *Valvular heart disease in patients with end-stage renal disease.* Retrieved October 23, 2006, from http://www.UpToDate.com

Curtin, R.B., & Mapes, D.L. (2001). Health care management strategies of long-term dialysis survivors. *Nephrology Nursing Journal, 28*(4), 385-394.

Deferrari, G., Ravera, M., Berruti, V., Leoncini, G., & Deferrari, L. (2004). Optimizing therapy in the diabetic patient with renal disease: Antihypertensive treatment. *Journal of the American Society of Nephrology, 15,* S6-S11.

Dinwiddie, L., Burrows-Hudson, S., & Peacock, E. (2006). Stage 4 chronic kidney disease: Preserving kidney function and preparing patients for stage 5 kidney disease. *American Journal of Nursing, 106*(9), 40-51.

Dombroski, J., Prentice, M., Walters, J., & Wells, E. (2004). *Diabetes and kidney disease: Independent study module.* Retrieved January 30, 2008, from http://www.diabetesin michigan.org/ISM/kidney.pdf

Food and Drug Administration (FDA). (2007). *Information for healthcare professionals erythropoiesis stimulating agents (ESA) [Aranesp (darbepoetin), Epogen (epoetin alfa), and Procrit (epoetin alfa)].* Retrieved August 2007, from http://www.fda.gov/cder/drug/InfoSheets/HCP/RHE_HCP.htm

Gnanasekaran, I., Kim, S., Dimitrov, V., & Soni, A. (2006, May). SHAPE UP – A management program for chronic kidney disease. *Dialysis and Transplantation,* 294-302.

Hsu, C., & Schieppati, A. (2006). Chronic kidney disease progression. *Nephrology Self-Assessment Program, 5*(3), 167-170.

Istre, S.M. (1989). The art and science of successful teaching (continuing education credit). *Diabetes Educator, 15*(1), 67-76.

Johnson, C., Levey, A.S., Coresh, J., Levin, A., Lau, J., & Eknoyan, G. (2004). Clinical guidelines for chronic kidney disease in adults: Part I. Definition, disease stages, evaluation, treatment, and risk factors. *American Family Physician, 70,* 869-876.

Johnson, R.J., & Fcchally, J. (2000). *Comprehensive clinical nephrology.* London: Mosby.

Kaplan, N.M. (2006). *Clinical hypertension* (9th ed.). Philadelphia: Lippincott Williams & Wilkins.

Laverman, G., Remuzzi, G., & Ruggeneti, P. (2004). ACE inhibition versus angiotensin receptor blockade: Which is better for renal and cardiovascular protection? *Journal of the American Society of Nephrology, 15,* S64-S70.

Lederer, E., & Ouseph, R. (2007). Core curriculum in nephrology. *American Journal of Kidney Diseases, 49*(1), 162-171.

Liddle, D.B. (2004). Assessment of musculoskeletal function. In S.C. Smeltzer & B. Bare (Eds.), *Brunner & Suddarth's textbook of medical surgical nursing* (10th ed.). Philadelphia: Lippincott Williams & Wilkins.

Lipetz, M.J., Bussigel, M.N., Bannerman, J., & Risley, B. (1990). What is wrong with patient education programs? *Nursing Outlook, 38*(4), 184-189.

Martin, K.J., & Gonzalez, E.A. (2007). Metabolic bone disease in chronic kidney disease. *Journal of the American Society of Nephrology, 18,* 875-885.

McCarley, P.B. (2006). Diagnosis, classification and management of chronic kidney disease. In A.E. Molzahn & E. Butera (Eds.), *Contemporary nephrology nursing: Principles and practice* (2nd ed.). Pitman, NJ: American Nephrology Nurses' Association.

McCarley, P.B., & Burrows-Hudson, S. (2006). Chronic kidney disease and cardiovascular disease – Using ANNA Standards and Practice Guidelines to improve care. Part 1: The epidemiology of chronic kidney disease: The risk factors and complications that contribute to cardiovascular disease. *Nephrology Nursing Journal, 33*(6), 666-674.

McCarley, P.B., & Salai, P.B. (2007). Chronic kidney disease and cardiovascular disease: A case presentation. *Nephrology Nursing Journal, 34*(2), 187-198.

McGraw-Hill. (n.d.). *AccessMedicine: Harrison's internal medicine part 11. Mechanisms of chronic renal failure.* Retrieved October 31, 2006, from http://www.acessmedicine.com

Merten, G.J., Burgess, W.P., Gray, L.V., Holleman, J.H., Roush, T.S., Kowalchuk, G.J., et al. (2004). Prevention of contrast-induced nephropathy with sodium bicarbonate a randomized controlled trial. *Journal of the American Medical Association, 291*(19), 2328-2334.

Miller, W.R., & Rollnick, S. (2002). *Motivational interviewing preparing people for change* (2nd ed). New York: Guilford Press.

Mitsnefes, M.M. (2005). Cardiovascular disease in children with chronic kidney disease. *Advances in Chronic Kidney Disease, 12*(4), 397-405.

National Kidney and Urologic Diseases Information Clearinghouse (NKUDIC). (2006). *Kidney disease of diabetes.* Retrieved January 24, 2008, from http://kidney.niddk.nih.gov/kudiseases/pubs/kdd/index.htm

National Kidney Foundation (NKF). (2001). Treatment of anemia of chronic renal failure update. *American Journal of Kidney Diseases, 37*(1).

National Kidney Foundation (NKF). (2002). KDOQI clinical practice guidelines for chronic kidney disease: Evaluation, classification and stratification. *American Journal of Kidney Diseases, 39*(Suppl. 1), S1-S266.

National Kidney Foundation (NKF). (2003a). KDOQI clinical practice guidelines for bone metabolism and disease in chronic kidney disease. *American Journal of Kidney Diseases, 42*(4)(Suppl. 3), S1-S201.

National Kidney Foundation (NKF). (2003b). Managing dyslipidemias in chronic kidney disease. *American Journal of Kidney Diseases, 41*(4).

National Kidney Foundation (NKF). (2004). Clinical practice guidelines on hypertension and antihypertensive agents in chronic kidney disease. *American Journal of Kidney Diseases, 43*(5).

National Kidney Foundation (NKF). (2007). *National Kidney Foundation releases anemia guideline update: New recommendations based on months of analysis of six new randomized trials.* Retrieved January 31, 2008, from http://www.kidney.org/news/newsroom/printnews.cfm?id=408

Nosadini, R., & Tonolo, G. (2004). Relationship between blood glucose control, pathogenesis and progression of diabetic nephropathy. *Journal of the American Society of Nephrology, 15*, S1-S5.

Padberg, R.M., & Padberg, L.F. (1990). Strengthening the effectiveness of patient education: Applying principles of adult education. *Oncology Nursing Forum, 17*(1), 65-69.

Parker, T., Blantz, R., Hostetter, T., Himmelfarb, J., Kliger, A., Lazarus, M., et al. (2004). The chronic kidney disease initiative. *Journal of the American Society of Nephrology, 15*, 708-716.

Pontremoli, R., Leoncini, G., Viazzi, F., Parodi, D., Ratto, E., Vettoretti, S., et al. (2004). Cardiovascular and renal risk assessment as a guide for treatment in primary hypertension. *Journal of the American Society of Nephrology, 15*, S34-S36.

Rose, B.D., & Rennke, H.G. (1994). *Renal pathophysiology – The essentials.* Baltimore: Lippincott Williams & Wilkins.

Rosenberg, M. (2003). Chronic kidney disease progression. *Nephrology Self-Assessment Program, 2*(3), 93.

Rosenberg, M., & Hsu, C. (2004). Chronic kidney and progression. *Nephrology Self-Assessment Program, 3*(6), 308.

Sarnak, M.J., Levey, A.S., Schoolwerth, A.C., Coresh, J., Culleton, B., Hamm, L.L., et al. (2003). Kidney disease as a risk factor for the development of cardiovascular disease. *Circulation, 108*(3), 14, 2114, 2154.

Schoolwerth, A.C., Engelgau, M.M., Hostetter, T.H., Rufo, K.H., Chianchiano, D., & McClellan, W.M., et al. (2006, April). Chronic kidney disease: A public health problem that needs a public health action plan. *Preventing Chronic Disease.* Retrieved January 31, 2008, from http://www.cdc.gov/pcd/issues/2006/apr/05_0105.htm

Shuitis, W.A., Weil, E.J., Looker, H.C., Curtis, J.M., Shlossman, M., Geneo, R.J., et al. (2007). Effects of periodontitis on overt nephropathy and end-stage renal disease in type 2 diabetes. *Diabetes Care, 30*, 306-311.

Singh, A.K., Szczech, L., Tang, K.L., Barnhart, H., Sapp, S., Wolfson, M., et al. (2006). Correction of anemia with epoetin alfa in chronic kidney disease. *The New England Journal of Medicine, 355*, 2085-2098.

Snively, C., & Gutierrez, C. (2004). Chronic kidney disease: Prevention and treatment of common complications. *American Family Physician, 70*, 1921-1928, 1929-1930.

Thomas-Hawkins, C., & Zazworsky, D. (2005). Self-management of chronic kidney disease: Patients shoulder the responsibility for day-to-day management of chronic illness. How can nurses support their autonomy? *American Journal of Nursing, 105*(10), 40-48.

Veteran Health Administration, Department of Defense. (2001). *VHA/DoD clinical practice guideline for the management of chronic kidney disease and pre-ESRD in the primary care setting.* Washington, DC: Author.

von Korff, M., Gruman, J., Schaefer, J., Curry, S.J., & Wagner, E.H. (1997). Collaborative management of chronic illness. *Annals of Internal Medicine, 127*, 1097-1102.

Watnick, S. (2007). Pregnancy and contraceptive counseling of women with chronic kidney disease and kidney transplants. *Advances in Chronic Kidney Disease, 14*(2), 126-131.

Wikipedia. (2007). *Transtheoretical model.* Retrieved January 24, 2008, from http://en.wikipedia.org/wiki/Transteoretical_Model

Section 3

Acute Care

Section Editors

Maureen Craig, MSN, RN, CNN, CCNS
Anne E. Harty, MS, APRN, FNP, CNN
Helen F. Williams, BSN, RN, CNN

Chapter Authors

Laurie Biel, BSN, RN, CNN
Jina L. Bogle, MSN, APRN, NP-C, CNN
Maureen Craig, MSN, RN, CNN, CCNS
Terrence L. Dalton, RN
Jaquelyn Davey-Tresemer, BSN, RN
Patricia L. Garrigan, BSN, RN
Maria Luongo, MSN, BA, RN
Regina M. Rohe, RN, HP(ASCP)
Sheila J. Smith, BSN, RN, HP(ASCP)
Helen F. Williams, BSN, RN, CNN
JoAnn Wilson, RN, HP(ASCP)

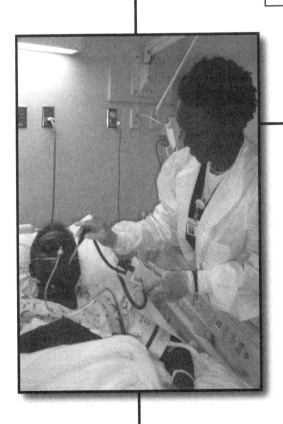

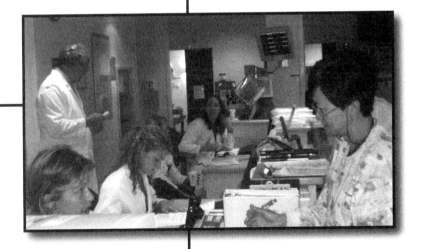

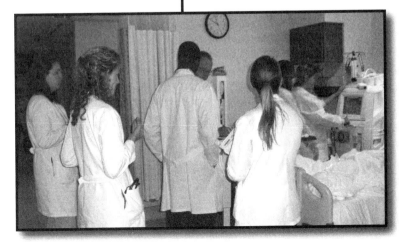

About the Authors

Maureen Craig, MSN, RN, CNN, CCNS, Section Co-Editor and Author, is a Clinical Nurse Specialist – Nephrology at the University of California Davis Medical Center in Sacramento, California.

Anne E. Harty, MS, APRN, FNP, CNN, Section Co-Editor, is a Nephrology Nurse Practitioner who has worked with hemodialysis patients. She developed and taught a CKD education class for patients and families facing ESRD.

Helen F. Williams, BSN, RN, CNN, Section Co-Editor and Author, is a Staff Nurse in Acute Dialysis at Western Nephrology in Denver, Colorado.

Laurie Biel, BSN, RN, CNN, is a Staff Nurse in the Peritoneal Dialysis Unit and Co-Coordinator in the Center for Renal Education at the Massachusetts General Hospital in Boston, Massachusetts.

Jina L. Bogle, MSN, APRN, NP-C, CNN, is a Nurse at DCI Acute Dialysis Services and at University of Nebraska Medical Center, Kidney and Pancreas Transplant Surgery, in Omaha, Nebraska.

Terrence L. Dalton, RN, is a Nurse Manager of Acute Dialysis Services at Dialysis Clinic, Inc., in Omaha, Nebraska.

Jaquelyn Davey-Tresemer, BSN, RN, is a Registered Nurse in the Trauma Intensive Care Unit at Creighton University Medical Center in Omaha, Nebraska.

Patricia L. Garrigan, BSN, RN, is an Acute Hemodialysis Registered Nurse at Dialysis Clinic Inc., in Omaha, Nebraska.

Maria Luongo, MSN, BA, RN, is CAPD Nurse Manager at Massachusetts General Hospital in Boston, Massachusetts.

Regina M. Rohe, RN, HP(ASCP), is Vice President of Operations at Apheresis Care Group, Inc., in San Francisco, California.

Sheila J. Smith, BSN, RN, HP(ASCP), is Director of Operations at Apheresis Care Group, Inc., in San Francisco, California.

JoAnn Wilson, RN, HP(ASCP), is an Apheresis Registered Nurse at Apheresis Care Group, Inc., in San Francisco, California.

Section 3

Acute Care

Acute Care

This section of the *Core Curriculum* is dedicated to recognizing the varied roles and specialized knowledge that encompass the practice of the nephrology nurse in the acute care setting. The acute care setting can present patients of any age group, from any background needing any variety of renal replacement or pheresis therapy and the accompanying education and placement assistance. The nephrology nurse practicing in acute care must integrate a basic understanding of all aspects of nephrology nursing, both acute and chronic, with the clinical skills to accurately assess and manage the ever-changing need of acutely ill patients. Acute care nephrology nurses cover call, frequently travel to many different facilities, and provide consistent staffing for a constantly changing workload. The acute care setting presents the extremes in diversity, demanding the nephrology nurse maintains flexibility while maximizing application of their critical thinking skills.

In the acute care setting, the nephrology nurse treats patients with acute kidney injury (AKI) as well as those with chronic kidney disease (CKD). Often the AKI patient may require only a few treatments. However, the acute care nephrology nurse also cares for trauma or septic patients who may require daily dialysis for weeks. This patient may progress from daily treatment with slow extended daily dialysis (SLEDD) in the intensive care unit (ICU) to every-other-day intermittent hemodialysis (IHD), then to "as needed" and, finally, to no treatments at all. During this progression, the treatment goals are adjusted to meet the patient's changing needs. The family's needs are assessed as well. Together, they are educated, supported, and encouraged by the acute nephrology nurse as they experience the transition of a return of renal function.

Continuous renal replacement therapy (CRRT) is initiated by the acute care nephrology nurse on the critically ill patient who will only survive for a few hours without the support that CRRT provides. This bridge of support may serve to give the family enough time to travel to the bedside for the death of their loved one. On the other hand, it may provide the patient's body enough time to heal and allow the patient to survive.

The acute nephrology nurse may initiate the first hemodialysis treatment on patients who have reached CKD stage 5. The nurse teaches the uncertain new patient about the experience of dialysis and prepares him for the busy, fast-paced world of the chronic dialysis unit setting. The acute nephrology nurse also cares for CKD patients who come into the acute care setting repeatedly with worsening illnesses. A rapport builds during these acute episodes among the acute nephrology nurse, the patient, and the family members. The strength of their relationship provides a safe and therapeutic environment for discussion of quality of life issues and the patient's desires regarding end-of-life care.

Plasmapheresis is provided by the acute nephrology nurse for a new mother with HELLP (hemolysis, elevated liver, low platelets) syndrome who is too ill to care for herself or her new baby. Support is also given to the new dad, recognizing his fears and uncertainties in dealing with a critically ill wife and a brand new infant. The acute nephrology nurse provides education and helps locate resources to address his needs, as he prays for the survival of his new family.

For acute dialysis nurses, the tasks are many. Skills are broad and yet meticulously detailed to relate to a variety of specific problems. Support and caring is provided for patients going through the stresses of acute illness, not only from a renal standpoint, but also from a nursing standpoint. Nephrology nurses in the acute care field have the assessment skills, the knowledge of kidney disease and its treatments, and the technical and mechanical skills they need. They also have the ability to improvise to make things come together so they can get the job done, whatever obstacles there may be. Plumbing and electrical issues, locating and moving equipment from one location to another, integrating and coordinating care when many essential things need to be done at the same time (intubation, x-ray, central line placement, stat EKG, blood cultures, blood gases, and dialysis at the bedside) are examples of the multitasking and problem solving that are frequently required of acute nephrology nurses.

The acute nephrology nurse is part of a multidisciplinary team. The nurse must recognize the role played by each member of the multidisciplinary team so that the variety of resources can be accessed, including the expertise offered by each member of the team in the plan of care for the patient. As nephrology nurses assist and teach their patients, they should work to complement the efforts of the multidisciplinary team. Acute nephrology nurses have to "fit in" while "standing out" in order to provide their unique and important service most effectively. They need to constantly teach while they are constantly learning.

The rewards of nephrology nursing in the acute setting are as varied as the types of care provided. The satisfaction of bringing a patient with a potassium of 9.6 back from their life-threatening cardiac arrthymias cannot be matched. The midnight trip to the hospital becomes worthwhile as the acute nephrology nurse watches the respirations of the patient in pulmonary edema ease as several liters of fluid are removed, allowing the patient to finally lie back on the pillow and get some sleep. Sitting at the bedside at the end of the patient's first hemodialysis treatment to hear the patient, with relief and gratitude in his/her eyes, say, "That wasn't as bad as I thought it would be," is a moment to be treasured. Seeing the young mother who survived HELLP syndrome walk in the door of the acute dialysis treatment room on the first birthday of her child to say "thank you" is a deep joy and satisfaction that cannot be explained. Reuniting a young family with their mother who was on the brink of death from a severe sepsis following multisystem organ failure makes the long hours put in to maintain the CRRT or SLEDD circuit all the more worthwhile.

These examples are but a few of the priceless experiences that are part of being an "acute nephrology nurse." This acute care section presents an exploration of the extensive and diverse knowledge base that supports people who work in the exciting and challenging field of acute nephrology nursing.

Chapter 9

Program Management in the Acute Care Setting

Purpose

The purpose of this chapter is to consider the variety of services, roles, and issues that are a part of providing nephrology nursing care in the acute care setting.

Objectives

Upon completion of this chapter, the learner will be able to:
1. Describe three settings and three services common to acute care nephrology.
2. Discuss the nephrology nurse's role in acute care program management.
3. Identify three challenges that the acute care nephrology nurse encounters.

I. Acute care nephrology services are provided in various types of facilities.

A. Facilities, locations, and treatment options.
1. Large teaching hospitals with multiple treatment sites on multiple campuses providing a full array of treatment options.
2. Large teaching hospitals with multiple intensive care units (ICU) on one campus providing a full array of treatment options.
3. Private hospitals with multiple ICUs on one campus providing a full array of treatment options.
4. Medium-sized hospitals with one or two ICUs and a dedicated dialysis treatment room (2–4 beds) providing hemodialysis, CRRT (continuous renal replacement therapy), and peritoneal dialysis (PD) coverage.
5. Small hospitals with a dedicated dialysis room (2 beds) providing hemodialysis treatments only.
6. Small hospitals with a dedicated dialysis storage area providing all hemodialysis treatments at the patient's bedside.
7. Acute care hospitals accepting patients on long-term ventilator management, complex wounds, and acute nursing needs with hemodialysis and peritoneal dialysis therapies.
8. Rehabilitation hospitals accepting patients with a need for chronic hemodialysis and/or peritoneal dialysis.
9. Multiple hospitals of various sizes contracting for a variety of levels of dialysis support with one provider.
10. Medium or larger hospitals using their own employees for dialysis services, floating them to other units in the hospital when census dictates.
11. Correctional institutions contracting for chronic hemodialysis services for their inmates onsite with an acute dialysis provider.

B. Departments within institutions where acute nephrology nursing services are provided.
1. Dialysis/pheresis treatment room.
2. Patient bedside.
3. ICU.
   a. Dialytic therapy right after surgery for fluid and electrolyte management.
   b. Maintenance dialytic therapy for the critically ill patient.
4. Emergency room (ER).
   a. Hemodialysis treatments for patients with hyperkalemia or fluid overload approaching intubation with no beds available in the ICU or telemetry unit.

b. Fistula needle removal from a patient who has arrived from outpatient dialysis with needles left in place to expedite rapid transfer to emergency care.
   c. Vascular access care for a patient with bleeding at the fistula needle site.
   d. Dialysis catheter care repairing disconnected or severed dialysis catheter ports or referring them to interventional radiology (IR).
   e. A peritoneal dialysis exchange performed to obtain a sample of effluent to send to the laboratory for rule out peritonitis.
   f. Assessing the PD catheter exit site and tunnel for signs and symptoms of infection.
5. The cardiac catheter lab.
   a. CRRT or intermittent hemodialysis (IHD) may be started or maintained on a patient sensitive to volume and electrolyte shifts during or shortly after a cardiac catheter procedure.
   b. Hemodialysis treatments during or immediately following contrast exposure to minimize contrast nephropathy on a patient with residual renal function.
6. The operating room (OR).
   a. During open hearts or other major vascular procedures, hemodialysis or CRRT may be started to assist with electrolyte and fluid management.
   b. During transplant surgery to maintain homeostasis.

II. The nephrology multidisciplinary team. Staff in the acute care setting can range from a small to a large team depending on the program needs. Positions may be filled by hospital employees, contracted dialysis employees, vendor-provided employees under contract, or a combination of these options.

A. Nephrologists/Nephrology Fellows/Advanced Practice Registered Nurses (APRN)/Clinical Nurse Specialists (CNS).

B. Nurse manager.

C. Administrative assistant.

D. Nephrology nurses.

E. Nephrology patient care technicians working under the direct supervision of the nephrology nurse.

F. Facility technician responsible for machine disinfection and culturing.

G. Biomed technician responsible for preventive maintenance and repairs.

H. Inventory technician responsible for ordering,

receiving, delivering to sites, and ensuring availability of supplies where and when needed.

I. Social worker.

J. Dietitian.

K. Home training nurse.

L. Transplant coordinators.

M. Case managers/discharge planners.

III. Nephrology nurse roles and responsibilities in the acute care setting.

A. Provide direct patient care using a variety of modalities of treatment.

B. Communicate with hospital care providers before, during, and after the dialysis treatment to ensure continuity of care.

C. Provide direct supervision of unlicensed dialysis personnel.

D. Provide dialysis coverage 24 hours a day, 7 days a week.

E. Educate hospital staff regarding care of the nephrology patient.

F. Educate hospital staff regarding treatment modalities used to treat acute kidney injury and CKD stage 5.

G. Coordinate schedule for dialytic procedures with hospital staff and departments.

H. Communicate patient care needs to physicians and other hospital care providers.

I. Educate patients and families regarding their diagnosis, the plan of care, and treatment options. (Refer to Appendix 3.1. Patient Education Pamphlet, at the end of Section 3).

J. Provide predialysis modality education for in-patients at CKD stage 4, approaching the need for dialysis treatments.

K. Use research to build evidence-based practice and to participate in personal education to improve the services provided.

L. Participate in Quality Assurance and Continuous Quality Improvement activities.

M. Participate in orientation and training of new employees, developing a mentoring relationship to strengthen our specialty.

N. Report equipment and supply issues to management to ensure a safe working environment.

O. Communicate with the patient's chronic dialysis unit providers prior to their discharge from acute care regarding the hospitalization, procedures performed, medication changes, vascular access issues, and other changes in the patient's condition as a result of their illness.

P. Serve as a positive representative of the nephrology service in every facility and unit with which they come in contact.

Q. Assist emergency room personnel in caring for patients with nephrology issues.

R. Coordinate with insurance providers for outpatient procedures such as therapeutic plasma exchange (TPE) or hemodialysis.

S. Coordinate uninsured or underinsured patient care when needed.

T. Help discharge planners and utilization review managers intervene with the Immigration and Naturalization Service (INS) or other governmental agencies (such as Centers for Medicare and Medicaid [CMS] or Social Security) as needed.

U. Coordinate insurance coverage and scheduling of treatments for acute kidney injury patients pending return of kidney function, as well as CKD stage 5 patients new to dialysis.

V. Provide weekly dialysis access catheter care, including site care, aspirating, flushing, and recapping the catheter, for patients discharged from the hospital but not being cared for in a chronic outpatient unit.

IV. Patients encountered in the acute care setting encompass a wide range of needs and interventions.

A. CKD stage 5 patients admitted for nonnephrology issue needing dialytic support during the acute care stay.

B. Newly diagnosed CKD stage 5 patients.
   1. Those patients living in areas where the chronic dialysis units are saturated and there is a waiting list for new patients.
   2. Patients who are without a funding source because they are undocumented or just uninsured may report to the ER or come to the hospital on a regularly scheduled basis for routine, urgent, or emergent dialysis care.

C. CKD stage 5 patients with urgent dialysis or vascular access needs.
   1. Outpatients who have had an access revision or

catheter placement and missed their outpatient appointment time can be dialyzed in the acute setting.

    a. In some states these treatments can be billed under a special Medicare billing code specific for this situation.

    b. Their treatment may be done by the acute nephrology nurse in the ER, in the dialysis unit, in an Infusion Center, or in an assigned patient room depending on the facility and the situation.

  2. Outpatients having dialytic needs for fluid overload or electrolyte disturbances not adequately managed by their regularly scheduled chronic dialysis unit treatments.

D. CKD stage 5 patients without chronic dialysis unit affiliation.

  1. Patients who have been dismissed from their chronic dialysis units because of nonadherence to the treatment plan. These patients will come to the ER for treatment until they can reestablish with a chronic dialysis unit.

  2. Patients who have been dismissed because of aggressive or violent behaviors against staff or patients at a chronic dialysis unit.

    a. These patients will come to the ER for treatment and will benefit from the help of the ESRD network to reestablish with a chronic dialysis center usually under a signed behavioral contract.

    b. These patients may not be able to reestablish with a chronic dialysis center.

E. Conservatively managed CKD stage 4–5 patients admitted for conservative management of uremic symptoms and palliative care.

F. AKI patients.

  1. Acutely ill patient with AKI still requiring hospitalization.

  2. Patients with acute kidney injury (AKI) stable enough to be managed as outpatient with ongoing dialytic support.

    a. These patients cannot find placement in a chronic outpatient unit because they have an "acute" process.

    b. They continue to require follow-up and intermittent hemodialysis and vascular access catheter care.

G. Patients needing therapeutic plasma exchange (TPE) treatments.

  1. Inpatients requiring ongoing TPE treatments for an acute illness.

  2. Outpatients with recurring admissions to receive TPE treatments on a regularly scheduled basis.

V. Approach to program management. In the acute care setting, program management will vary significantly from one location to another depending on the size of the program, the services provided, and the employment relationship between nephrology and other care providers.

A. Contracts.

  1. Establish contracted rates for all nephrology services.

    a. 1:1, 1:2, or 2:1 nephrology nursing care.

    b. Hemodialysis and SLEDD treatments in the ICU.

    c. CRRT treatment initiation and daily maintenance.

    d. Restarting a treatment after a clotted system.

    e. On-call treatments.

    f. Delayed and canceled treatments.

    g. Hourly rates for treatments over 5 hours.

    h. Nephrology nursing consultation.

    i. Peritoneal dialysis treatment initiation and daily maintenance.

    j. Educational classes provided for the hospital staff.

    k. Rates for storage space if not provided under the contract.

  2. Delineate responsibilities of nephrology and hospital staff.

    a. Transportation of patients.

    b. Administration of medications.

    c. Transporting blood samples to the lab.

    d. Picking up blood products from the blood bank.

    e. Submitting charge forms or entering charges in a computer for the services provided.

    f. Housekeeping duties.

    g. Plant operations and maintenance of water and electrical services.

  3. Specify communication channels between the hospital and nephrology staff, including the management level with an assigned liaison.

  4. Define expectation for reporting of quality monitoring, water system records, etc., including when reports are due and the person(s) to whom reports are submitted.

B. Staffing.

  1. Meet the credentialing requirements of the contracted hospital, which may include a payment of required fees for processing the

application for Allied Health Privileges.

2. Provide the level of professional personnel required by each contract.
3. Notify the hospital of changes in personnel.
4. Provide the dialysis staff with the necessary identification (ID) badge, parking permit, keys, and computer access appropriate for each facility contracted.
5. Provide education for nephrology staff to ensure quality patient care.
   a. Complete orientation at hire.
      (1) Plan for a minimum of 6–8 weeks orientation for nurses hired from an ICU or chronic dialysis unit.
      (2) Longer orientation may be needed for those with a general nursing background.
      (3) Appropriate orientation time varies with the individual.
      (4) Regular review and documentation of the orientees progress should occur by meeting with the nurse manager and preceptor on a regular basis, including documentation of the education plan moving forward.
   b. Provide and document training for any new procedure or new equipment prior to allowing staff to use or perform it.
   c. Provide learning opportunities to enhance professional development.
   d. Use annual performance reviews to determine individual educational needs and to develop a plan for obtaining or providing the appropriate training.
   e. Establish annual competency testing and a written plan to address any deficiencies discovered to ensure competent, safe, quality patient care.
      (1) Written exams.
      (2) Clinical simulations.
      (3) Case studies.
      (4) Observation of procedure performance.

C. Record keeping.
   1. Employee files.
      a. Application with education and job history.
      b. References and background check.
      c. Orientation completed.
         (1) Orientation checklist.
         (2) Skills checklist.
      d. Continuing education records.
         (1) Required CEU's.
         (2) Policy and procedure changes.
         (3) New equipment training.
      e. License records.

f. BCLS/ACLS (Basic Cardiac and Advanced Cardiac Life Support) training records.
      g. Certifications maintained.
      h. Performance appraisal and annual competency completed.
      i. Annual blood work and testing.
         (1) Hepatitis screening.
         (2) Rubella and rubeola immunity testing.
         (3) Tuberculin (TB) skin testing.
   2. Policy and procedure (P & P) manuals with copies at each contracted facility, with evidence of ongoing annual review and staff education regarding changes.
   3. Equipment and supply documentation.
      a. Hemodialysis, water treatment, and pheresis equipment use, repair, and preventive maintenance logbooks.
      b. Reports of equipment failure that result in patient injury or death and its subsequent investigation.
      c. Equipment recall notices.
      d. Electrical safety inspection reports of new equipment or equipment moved from one facility to another.
      e. Annual electrical safety inspection reports.
      f. Conductivity meter calibration log.
      g. Refrigerator temperature record log.
      h. Inventory audit and supply ordering records.
   4. Treatment records.
      a. Treatment log.
      b. Nursing treatment flowsheets.
      c. Results of documentation audits.
      d. Billing records.
   5. CQI/research records.
      a. Water quality testing.
         (1) Monthly water and dialysate cultures.
         (2) Monthly water LALs (Limulus amebocyte lysate).
         (3) Water analysis, annually or semiannually, depending on regional water quality.
      b. Infections, especially those related to vascular access.
      c. Research projects, including IRB (Investigational Review Board) applications and data collection materials.
   6. Inspection by any credentialing or accrediting body, i.e., State Department of Health, CMS, Occupational Safety and Health Administration (OSHA), Joint Commission on the Accreditation of Health Organizations (JCAHO).
      a. Inspection report.
      b. Facility response.
      c. Plan of action.
      d. Progress reports toward any deficiencies.

D. Communication.
1. Hospital or departmental liaison.
   a. Establish rapport.
   b. Anticipate problems before they escalate.
   c. Plan for solutions when things are not at crisis level.
   d. Coordinate scheduling of educational offerings for hospital staff regarding nephrology nursing and care of kidney patients.
   e. Discuss budgetary planning for new equipment or upgrading current equipment.
2. Hospital unit managers and charge nurses.
   a. Establish rapport.
   b. Use communication tools to ensure continuity of care.
3. Direct care providers and/or primary nurses.
   a. Discuss the schedule for dialysis treatment and any other procedures the patient may have planned for the same day.
   b. Receive report pretreatment.
   c. Obtain the patient's medical record along with the patient to ensure availability of medical information and records for the nephrology team during treatment.
   d. Complete medication and treatment charting in the medical record appropriate for each contracted facility.
   e. Inform primary nurse of significant changes in the patient's condition during dialysis treatment.
   f. Give report to primary nurse after the dialysis treatment, before the patient is transported back to their nursing unit.
4. Discharge planners, case managers, and social workers.
   a. Establish rapport.
   b. Identify ongoing patient needs for treatment as an outpatient.
      (1) Dialysis.
      (2) Transportation to and from treatment.
      (3) Vascular access follow-up.
      (4) Patient's mobility and ability to self-transfer.
      (5) Need for special dialysis chair or scale.
   c. Communicate changes in patient status to facilitate transfer or discharge of patient.
5. Dietitians and dietary department.
   a. Diet review.
   b. Set up renal diet based on patient's current nutritional needs.
   c. Request patient education on changes to diet as kidney function changes.
   d. Request meal trays are sent to the dialysis treatment room or kept for patient until after treatment.
   e. Record accurate intake and output (I & O) on the patient's record for his/her time in the dialysis unit.
6. Radiology and interventional radiology departments.
   a. Schedule procedures.
   b. Coordinate and prioritize procedures based on patient needs.
7. Surgery department to schedule and coordinate procedures.
8. Cardiac catheter lab to coordinate dialysis treatments after a procedure.
   a. Need for treatment based on amount of dye used in the procedure.
   b. Monitoring the groin line site.
   c. Monitoring changes in peripheral pulses.
   d. Maintaining bed rest and flat position as prescribed.
9. Hospital laboratory, blood gas laboratory, and blood bank.
   a. Ensure correct collection and handling of samples.
   b. Receive accurate results in a timely manner to allow changes to treatment plan.
10. Pharmacy.
    a. Coordinate obtaining medications needed during the dialysis treatment.
    b. Some dialysis units have Pyxis (or other automated medication dispensing systems) onsite.
    c. Some dialysis units keep narcotics on stock requiring counts and record keeping per pharmacy policy.
    d. Maintain a current supply of emergency drugs in the dialysis unit and replace when used or outdated.
    e. Coordinate maintaining a current stock of CRRT solutions and peritoneal dialysis solutions in Pharmacy to ensure they are available at all times so initiation of treatment will not be delayed.
    f. Facilitate updating the hospital formulary with new nephrology drugs.
11. Housekeeping department.
    a. Communicate special cleaning needs and protection of housekeeping staff due to potential contamination with blood or body fluids.
    b. Train personnel on safely moving dialysis equipment to facilitate adequate cleaning.
12. Central supply, materials management, supply distribution.

a. Work with each facility's procedures to record and monitor PAR levels, order stock (routine or special order), and rotate stock on shelves.

b. Negotiate lowest prices for dialysis-related supplies in conjunction with dialysis vendors. Include contracted facilities in those rates if possible.

13. Architectural services or space planners.

a. Consult for new space or remodeling of existing hospitals to incorporate adequate space for dialysis services.

b. Plan for correct square footage per station requirements to accommodate the dialysis equipment in addition to the patient's bed and equipment (approximately 100–120 square feet per station).

c. Water requirements.

(1) Selection of appropriate water treatment system based on water quality testing and use of a central or portable system.

(a) Reverse osmosis (RO).

(b) Deionization (DI) as backup or polisher.

(c) Carbon filtration.

(d) Softener.

(2) Adequate water pressure in pounds per square inch (PSI) to meet equipment requirements.

(3) Blending valves.

(4) Back-flow preventor.

(5) Drains at correct height with capacity for adequate volume.

(6) Dedicated water hook-up in ICUs and designated units and patient rooms.

d. Electrical requirements.

(1) Dedicated 20-amp circuit for each dialysis machine station or the amperage required by the brand of equipment being used.

(2) Adequate number of regular outlets at each station to accommodate the patient's bed, several IV pumps, and other equipment.

e. Adequate and secure square footage for storage of equipment when not in use as well as the large volume of supplies required.

f. Location in the facility with preference to proximity to the ICU, telemetry floor, kidney floor, or the cardiac floor to enhance support for an emergency in the dialysis unit.

g. Request a dedicated dialysis treatment room as opposed to doing treatments at bedside to increase efficiency of staffing in the dialysis unit.

14. Plant operations/facility management/maintenance.

a. Maintain water resources and quality for central or portable reverse osmosis (RO) water treatment system.

b. Maintain electrical resources for equipment needs.

15. Information technology and telecommunication departments.

a. Development of electronic medical record templates for dialysis procedures.

b. Maintain access to electronic records while maintaining patient privacy with user access codes and passwords.

c. Maintain electronic backup of all electronic records.

d. Supply and maintain adequate equipment for communication (faxes, copiers, computers, phones, pagers, Vocera).

e. Supply and maintain electronic entry access cards.

f. Communicate nephrology staff on-call schedule to telecommunications center or answering service.

VI. Challenging issues facing practitioners in the acute care setting.

A. Communication with chronic outpatient dialysis clinics.

1. Share information regarding patient's hospitalization including any surgical procedures, changes in vascular access, and/or adjustment of dry weight to enhance continuity of care.

2. Notify outpatient unit of doses of antibiotics and/or iron therapy given, the number of doses needed, and the schedule for continuing administration.

3. Notify outpatient units when patients present to the hospital with a vascular access infection or sepsis related to the access.

4. Ensure that patients have a functional vascular access prior to discharge to prevent frequent readmissions.

5. Share information to facilitate completion of the CMS 2728 form by the chronic unit and coordinate placement of new chronic dialysis patients in the outpatient setting.

a. Electrocardiogram.

b. Chest x-ray.

c. Blood chemistry prior to first dialysis treatment.

d. Complete blood count prior to first dialysis treatment.

e. Lipid panel.
f. TB skin test if done.
g. Hepatitis panel.
6. Provide predialysis modality training to hospitalized patients.
7. Communicate the next scheduled outpatient treatment day and time to the patient in cooperation with the unit to avoid missed treatments immediately after discharge.
8. Dialyze the patient on the day of discharge when needed to get him/her back on or keep him/her on the regular outpatient schedule.

B. Staffing issues.
1. Orienting to multiple therapies with different machines.
2. Maintaining competency in low volume, high complexity treatments.
3. Variability of caseloads and work hours.
4. RN supervision of unlicensed personnel.
5. Distance between facilities.
6. Orientation to multiple facilities with varying expectations and different standard procedures.
7. Limited recruitment options due to high skill level required.
8. Financial issues.
    a. Pay per hour or per case.
    b. Overtime pay.
    c. Bonus payment systems.
        (1) Shift differential.
        (2) On-call treatments.
        (3) On-call available time.
        (4) Charge nurse.
        (5) Preceptor.
    d. Working the day after being on call and working through the night.
    e. Benefits.
9. Safety in the workplace.
    a. Working conditions.
    b. Violent and/or hostile patients.
    c. Coming and going from facilities unescorted after dark.

C. Equipment.
1. Getting repairs done in a timely manner.
2. Moving machines between facilities.
3. Performing routine disinfection and preventive maintenance on equipment in remote or low use locations.
4. Not enough machines or support equipment at every facility.
5. Multiple machines down at one time for cultures and LALs, causing a longer work day for staff.

D. Contracted employees.
1. Credentialing process.
    a. Length of time to complete process.
    b. Amount of documentation required.
2. Relationships with facility staff.
    a. Communication.
    b. Coordination of care.
    c. Support services.
    d. Different practice approaches in multiple facilities.
    e. Power struggle regarding space, involvement in patient care decisions, and nursing care issues.

E. Relationships with physicians.
1. Conflicts with scheduling treatments for multiple physician groups.
    a. Establishing policy regarding prioritization.
    b. Avoiding late day add-ons for nonemergent care.
2. Negotiating physician cooperation to establish consistent policies and procedures in all facilities.
3. Interactions that are aggressive and/or disrespectful.
4. Disagreement among physician specialists regarding plan of care.
5. Participation in coordination of care with hospital units or outpatient clinics and acute nephrology staff.
6. Nonemergent treatments done by on call staff for physician convenience.

F. Interactions with patients.
1. Angry, hostile, and violent patients.
    a. Psychiatric diagnoses vs. recreational drug abuse vs. response to life's issues.
    b. Set parameters for accepted behavior and when treatment will be discontinued due to violation of those parameters.
    c. Hospital or family to provide a "sitter" at the bedside during treatment.
    d. Physician to manage chemical or physical restraint choices.
    e. Security officer onsite when needed.
2. Cultural and religious diversity.
    a. Need for staff to be educated about respecting diversity.
    b. Language barriers.
        (1) Hospital-based translator.
        (2) Computer or telephone translator availability.
        (3) www.Babelfish.com.
        (4) Provide written educational materials in patient's language.

(5) Provide consent for treatment(s) in patient's language.

(6) Blood products – acceptable or not?

(7) Native healers and traditional ceremonies.

(8) Evaluating quality of life in consideration of end-of-life care and the influence of cultural and religious leaders.

3. Nonadherence to schedule and fluid management in chronic treatment setting, leading to frequent emergency treatments in the acute setting.

4. Financial issues.
   a. Underinsured.
   b. Uninsured.
   c. Disposition during the 90-day waiting period for Medicare coverage at outpatient clinic.

5. Legal complexities.
   a. Undocumented residents.
   b. No Durable Power of Attorney for Health Care (DPAHC) or Conservator.

G. Interactions with patient's family.
   1. Family willingness to adhere to patient's decision.
   2. Overwhelming family involvement at the bedside.
      a. Boisterous or argumentative.
      b. Disruptive to patient or roommate.
      c. Attention seeking for their own issues over the patient's needs.
   3. No family available to make decisions.
   4. Family members contesting plan of care.
   5. Who makes decisions in the absence of a DPAHC?
   6. Evaluation of patient's quality of life.
   7. Participation in planning end-of-life care.

H. Ethical dilemmas.
   1. Definitions to consider.
      a. Respect for autonomy: the right of people to make choices.
      b. Beneficence: the obligation to help people in need.
      c. Nonmalificence: the duty to do no harm.
      d. Justice: treating everyone fairly.
      e. Distributive justice: all must receive a reasonable level of medical care.
   2. Examples of patient and staff concerns and issues.
      a. Initiating kidney replacement therapy on a Do Not Resuscitate (DNR) patient.
      b. Treatment of undocumented residents knowing they will not be able to get adequate follow-up care in this country.
      c. Patients who have been discharged from the outpatient clinic due to violent and aggressive behavior now come to the acute care setting regularly. What do the acute care providers do to address the behavior issues when there is no alternative for the patient to receive treatment?
      d. Patients who have verbalized clearly their end-of-life care to the acute care staff. Family arrive and demand the staff "do everything to save" their loved one.
   3. Factors to consider.
      a. Patient Self Determination Act (PSDA)(see Table 3.1).
         (1) Shared decision making includes physician, nurses, patient, and family in health care decisions.
         (2) Informed consent or refusal of treatment based on understanding of the personal decision.
      b. Emergency Medical Treatment & Labor Act (EMTALA) (see Table 3.2).
         (1) Obligation to treat everyone.
         (2) Staff must take precautions to minimize their personal risk.

Table 3.1

Patient Self–Determination Act (PSDA)

On November 5, 1990, Congress passed this measure as an amendment to the Omnibus Budget Reconciliation Act of 1990. It became effective on December 1, 1991. The Patient Self-Determination Act (PSDA) requires many Medicare and Medicaid providers (hospitals, nursing homes, hospice programs, home health agencies, and HMOs) to give adult individuals, at the time of inpatient admission or enrollment, certain information about their rights under laws governing advance directives, including: (1) the right to participate in and direct their own health care decisions; (2) the right to accept or refuse medical or surgical treatment; (3) the right to prepare an advance directive; (4) information on the provider's policies that govern the utilization of these rights. The act also prohibits institutions from discriminating against a patient who does not have an advance directive. The PSDA further requires institutions to document patient information and provide ongoing community education on advance directives.

Source: Ascension Health. (2005). Retrieved June 27, 2006, from www.ascension health.org/ethics/public/issues/patient_self.asp. Used with permission.

Emergency Medical Treatment and Labor Act

In 1986, Section 1867 of the Social Security Act imposed specific obligations on Medicare participating hospitals that offered emergency services to provide a medical screening examination (MSE) when a request is made for examination or treatment for an emergency medical condition (EMC), including active labor, regardless of an individual's ability to pay. Hospitals were then required to provide stabilizing treatment for patients with EMCs. If a hospital is unable to stabilize a patient within its capability, or if the patient requests, an appropriate transfer should be implemented (Center for Medicare & Medicaid Services, 2006).

Source: Centers for Medicare and Medicaid Services. (2006). *Medicare coverage for ESRD patients, section 1881* (42 U.S.C. 1395rr). Retrieved April 6, 2006, at www.ssa.gov/OP_Home/ssact/title18/1881.htm. Used with permission.

4. Resources available in the acute care setting.
   a. Ethics committee.
   b. Palliative care team.
   c. Pastoral care.
   d. Patient representative.
   e. End stage renal disease (ESRD) Networks.
   f. Kidney End-of-Life Coalition at www.kidneyeol.com
   g. ANNA's Ethics Committee.
   h. Hospital liaison.
   i. Case managers and/or social workers.

Chapter 10

Acute Kidney Injury (AKI) and Acute Renal Failure (ARF)

Purpose

The purposes of this chapter are to describe acute kidney injury, the etiology, pathology, assessment, and nursing care specific to this group of patients.

Objectives

Upon completion of this chapter, the learner will be able to:
1. Describe the debate surrounding the definition of acute kidney injury.
2. Describe the at-risk and special populations and their nursing care needs.
3. Describe the etiology, pathophysiology, assessment findings, presentation, and care management of patients with prerenal, intrarenal, and postrenal acute kidney injury.

I. Definitions and descriptions of acute kidney injury and acute renal failure.

A. Traditional definitions.
   1. Sudden, rapid deterioration of kidney function.
   2. Potentially reversible.
   3. Associated with:
      a. Oliguria: < 500 mL/day (International System [SI] = 0.5 L/day), or

   b. Nonoliguria: > 800 mL/day (SI = 0.8 L/day).
   c. Oliguria indicates a more severe insult to the kidney compared to nonoliguria.
4. Usually associated with azotemia (retention of nitrogenous substances in the blood) although the actual levels of accumulation (indicated by serum creatinine levels) necessary to be considered acute kidney injury are still under extensive debate.

5. Some patients experience similar problems with fluid and electrolyte imbalances as chronic kidney patients, but not usually the profound neurologic and musculoskeletal disorders that develop over time.

B. Patients at risk for acute kidney injury.
1. The elderly.
2. Postsurgical patients, especially cardiovascular.
3. Patients who develop sepsis.
4. Patients who experience major trauma that results in significant blood loss and muscle damage.
5. Patients with multiple organ dysfunction syndrome (MODS), also called multisystem organ failure (MSOF).
6. People with compromised underlying kidney disease who develop a serious illness or suffer an exposure to a nephrotoxic agent.
   a. "Acute on chronic."
   b. Important to preserve blood vessels for future vascular access placement.
   c. Avoid placement of PICC (peripherally inserted central catheter) lines if possible to preserve vessels.
   d. Exercise extra vigilance in monitoring to prevent and/or intervene quickly at first sign of AKI.

C. Incidence data.
1. The development of AKI increases the mortality associated with any primary disease.
2. AKI develops in 5% of all hospitalized patients.
3. Approximately 20–60% of hospitalized patients who develop AKI require dialysis treatment.
4. Of patients developing AKI, 50–60% will regain most, if not all, of their kidney function.
5. Depending on the severity of the kidney injury, mortality averages 50–80%.
6. Infection accounts for 75% of deaths in patients with AKI.
7. Cardiorespiratory complications are the second most common cause of death.
8. Incidence and prevalence of AKI are significantly increased in the elderly.
9. AKI occurs in 1 of every 2000–5000 pregnancies.
10. A conservative estimate of the incidence of AKI following nonrenal organ transplantation is 50%. Probably most transplant recipients have some degree of AKI.
11. Following cardiac transplant, early AKI (in the immediate postoperative period of 0–30 days) incidence is approximately 50%; late AKI (occurring after 30 days) has an incidence of 1–2%.

D. Search for consensus in AKI research.
1. Numerous studies have looked at treatment modalities, outcomes, prevention, and management of ARF/AKI over the past 5 decades.
2. Since the studies have used different criteria for defining what acute renal failure/acute kidney injury is, the results have limited generalizability to other locations and patient populations.
3. The PICARD (Program to Improve Care in Acute Renal Disease) experience, a large multicenter international study, confirmed the wide variation in definition on ARF/AKI, and the practice patterns for management of care and choice of renal replacement therapy (RRT).
4. Scoring systems available in the acute setting to predict patient outcomes.
   a. APACHE II.
      (1) Acute Physiology and Chronic Health Evaluation II Score.
      (2) Designed to measure the severity of disease for patients (aged 16 or more) admitted to ICUs.
      (3) A point score is calculated during the first 24 hours from 12 routine physiologic measurements, information about previous health status, and information obtained at admission.
      (4) The calculated score is used to establish a predicted death rate.
      (5) There are differing opinions about whether this tool is effective in patients with acute renal failure/acute kidney injury.
   b. SOFA score.
      (1) Sequential Organ Failure Assessment score.
      (2) A score is assigned to each of six organ systems (respiratory, cardiovascular, hepatic, coagulation, renal, and neurologic) with a grade range from 0 to 4.
      (3) Calculated on admission and then daily or every 48 hours to evaluate changes.
      (4) The initial, highest, and mean SOFA scores are evaluated to predict mortality rate.
      (5) Has been used successfully to evaluate and predict mortality in acute renal failure/acute kidney injury patients in the ICU.
   c. ATN-ISS.
      (1) Acute Tubular Necrosis Individual Severity score.
      (2) Produces a percent likelihood of mortality on the basis of several physiologic and laboratory parameters.

(3) Limited to patients with acute tubercular necrosis (ATN); does not address other forms of ARF/AKI.

d. SHARF scores.
  (1) Stuivenberg Hospital Acute Renal Failure scores.
  (2) Factors included in the formula: age, serum albumin, and partial thromboplastin time (PTT) lab values are entered. Respiratory support (vent) and heart failure are given a numeric value as absent (0) or present (1).
  (3) Measurements calculated at both Time 0 (T0) and Time 48 hours (T48) were found to improve the predictive value of the model.

e. RIFLE (see Table 3.3).
  (1) Risk of kidney failure, injury to the kidney, failure of kidney function, loss of kidney function, and end-stage renal failure.
  (2) Product of the Acute Dialysis Quality Initiative group (ADQI).
  (3) Patients classified based on estimated glomerular filtration rate (GFR) ranges and/or urine output in mL/kg/hour.
  (4) May prove helpful in deciding timing of initiation of RRT as well as offering a prediction of prognosis for consideration in allocation of financial and personnel resources.

II. Prevention of further acute kidney injury/acute renal failure.

A. Maintaining hydration.
  1. May require placement of pulmonary artery catheter to measure filling pressures, cardiac output, and systemic vascular resistance to determine patient volume.
  2. Preoperatively.
    a. Prevent kidney hypoperfusion and ischemia.
    b. Prophylactic dopamine should not be used specifically for prevention of AKI/ARF since studies have not supported any protective effect on kidney outcome or mortality.
  3. In patients receiving nephrotoxic drugs.
    a. Adjust the initial drug dose based on the patient's GFR.
    b. Monitor serum levels and adjust doses accordingly.
    c. Avoid daily dosing in the presence of elevated creatinine level.
  4. Prior to radiographic studies:
    a. Pathology may involve kidney vasoconstriction.
    b. Hydration with saline has shown improved kidney outcomes.
    c. Mannitol and furosemide infusions increase urinary output, but do not reduce the risk of worsening kidney function.
    d. Acetylcysteine (Mucomyst) administration orally the day before and the day of administration of contrast.

Table 3.3

RIFLE classification

GFR Criteria		Urine Output Criteria
Risk	Serum creatinine increased 1.5 times	< 0.5 mL/kg^{-1} h^{-1} for 6 h
Injury	Serum creatinine increased 2 times	< 0.5 mL/kg^{-1} h^{-1} for 12 h
Failure	Serum creatinine increased 3 times or creatinine – 355 µmol/L when there was an acute rise of > 44 µmol/L	< 0–3 mL/kg^{-1} h^{-1} for 24 h or anuria for 12 h
Loss	Persistent acute renal failure; complete loss of kidney function for longer than 4 weeks	
End-stage renal disease	End-stage renal disease for longer than 3 months	

Source: Bellomo, R., Ronco, C., Kellum, J.A., Mehta, R.L., Palevshy, P., & the ADQI Workgroup. (2004). Acute renal failure – Definition, outcome measures, animal models, fluid therapy and information technology needs: The second international consensus conference of the Acute Dialysis Quality Initiative (ADQI) group. *Critical Care, 8*(4), R204-R212. Used with permission.

(1) Is an inexpensive alternative treatment.
(2) May have some benefit in protecting kidney function.
(3) Has antioxidant and vasodilatory properties.
(4) May minimize vasoconstriction and oxygen-free radical generation from radiocontrast materials.
5. Normal saline administration.
   a. Aggressive in patients with rhabdomyolysis to maintain urine output of 200–300 mL/hr.
   b. For patients with other risk factors, administration of saline to achieve a rate of urine output of 150–200 mL/hr is adequate.
6. Furosemide (Lasix) use should be limited to times when diuresis is needed. Using as a prophylactic approach to prevent AKI/ARF may actually worsen kidney outcomes.

B. Maintaining kidney perfusion.
   1. Vasoactive agents.
      a. Low-dose dopamine is no longer shown to improve, and may actually decrease return of kidney function. It can also contribute to adverse complications, such as cardiac arrhythmias, myocardial infarction (MI), and gastrointestinal (GI) ischemia.
      b. Calcium channel blockers may be effective in reducing the incidence and severity of AKI/ARF following cadaveric kidney transplantation.
      c. Atrial natriuretic peptide (ANP) has been shown to increase (GFR), reverse kidney vasoconstriction, and block sodium reabsorption in animal studies. Its effectiveness in the setting of AKI/ARF in humans is still being evaluated.
   2. Volume expanders. The comparable effectiveness of crystalloids vs. colloids continues to be debated.
      a. Crystalloids: 0.9% saline (normal), 0.45% saline (half normal), dextrose 5% in water (D5W), and lactated Ringer's solution (LR).
      b. Colloids: albumin, dextran, and hetastarch.

C. Minimizing exposure to nephrotoxins.
   1. Antibiotics.
      a. Aminoglycosides are well-recognized nephrotoxins.
      b. Kidney hypoperfusion or kidney ischemia predisposes this nephrotoxicity.
   2. Radiocontrast materials.
   3. Nonsteroidal antiinflammatory drugs (NSAIDs).

D. Infection control.
   1. Skin care.
   2. Respiratory care.
   3. Management of indwelling lines and exit site care.
   4. Removal of indwelling urinary catheters as soon as possible.

E. Nutritional support to maintain the building blocks for cellular reproduction and to mitigate the response to the stress and insult of acute illness.

F. Continual assessment and monitoring of kidney function to facilitate early interventions.

G. When to initiate dialysis in patients with AKI.
   1. Ideally, to minimize morbidity, treatment should be initiated prior to the onset of complications due to kidney failure.
   2. Indications include one or more of the following:
      a. Refractory fluid overload.
      b. Hyperkalemia (serum potassium concentration > 6.5 mEq/L) or rapidly rising potassium levels.
      c. Metabolic acidosis (pH < 7.1).
      d. Azotemia with BUN > 80–100 mg/dL (29–30 mmol/L).
      e. Signs of uremia.
         (1) Pericarditis.
         (2) Bleeding disorders from uremia platelet dysfunction.
         (3) Neuropathy or an otherwise unexplainable decline in mental status.
            (a) Asterixis.
            (b) Tremor.
            (c) Seizures.
      f. Severe dysnatremias with serum sodium levels < 120 mEq/L or > 155 mEq/L.
      g. Hyperthermia.
      h. Overdose with a dialyzable drug or toxin.
   3. Less common indications.
      a. Drug intoxication requiring hemoperfusion.
      b. Hypothermia.
      c. Hyperurcemia.
      d. Hypercalcemia.
      e. Metabolic alkalosis requiring a special dialysis solution.

III. Acute kidney injury and acute renal failure.

A. Prerenal acute renal failure.
1. Incidence: approximtely 35% of cases of ARF depending on the definition of ARF used (see Figure 3.1).
2. Etiology.
   a. Decreased blood flow to the kidneys.
      (1) Intraoperative.
      (2) Blood vessel obstruction.
   b. Decreased intravascular volume (hypovolemia).

(1) Sepsis and systemic inflammatory response syndrome (SIRS).
(2) Hemorrhage.
(3) Dehydration.
(4) Overdiuresis.
(5) Vomiting.
(6) Diarrhea.
(7) Peritonitis.
(8) Integumentary loss from burns.
   c. Decreased effective circulating volume to the kidneys related to decreased cardiac output or altered peripheral vascular resistance.

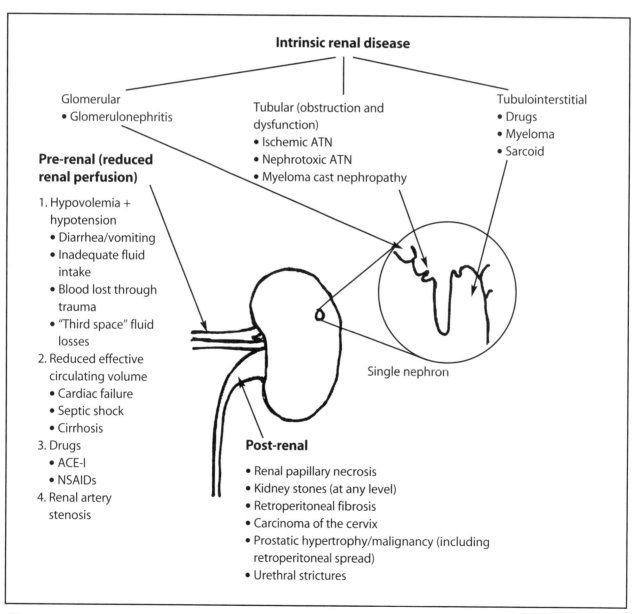

Figure 3.1. Etiology of acute renal failure.

Source: Fry, A.C., & Farrington, K. (2006). Management of acute renal failure. *Postgraduate Medicine Journal, 82*, 106-116. Used with permission.

(1) Congestive heart failure.
(2) Myocardial infarction.
(3) Cardiac tamponade.
(4) Cardiac dysrhythmias.
(5) Cirrhosis or hepatorenal syndrome.
(6) Nephrotic syndrome.
(7) Cardiogenic shock.
(8) Vasodilatation.
(9) Anaphylactic reactions.
(10) Neurogenic shock.
(11) Systemic septic shock.
(12) Drug overdose.
d. Impaired kidney blood flow because of exogenous agents.
(1) Angiotensin-converting enzyme inhibitors (ACE).
(2) NSAIDs.
e. Impaired kidney blood flow because of kidney artery disorders.
(1) Emboli.
(2) Thrombi.
(3) Stenosis.
(4) Aneurysm.
(5) Occlusion.
(6) Trauma.
3. Pathophysiology.
a. The parenchyma is initially undamaged.
b. Kidneys respond as if volume depletion has occurred, using adaptive mechanisms of autoregulation and release of renin.
(1) Autoregulation: afferent arteriole dilation and efferent arteriole constriction in an attempt to increase kidney blood flow and maintain normal GFR.
(2) Release of renin.
(a) Renin activates the angiotensin-aldosterone system, which results in peripheral vasoconstriction and increased sodium reabsorption, decreasing urinary sodium.
(b) Increased plasma sodium causes the release of antidiuretic hormone (ADH) that enhances vasoconstriction and increases water reabsorption, thus decreasing urinary output and increasing circulating blood volume.
(c) With increased sodium and water reabsorption, urea reabsorption increases. Therefore, blood urea nitrogen (BUN) increases.
(d) These mechanisms attempt to maintain systemic and kidney perfusion to protect kidney function.
c. If kidney hypoperfusion persists and exceeds

the capabilities of the kidney's adaptive mechanisms, AKI/ARF develops from ischemia.
d. In congestive heart failure (CHF), decreased kidney blood flow can be caused by overdiuresis or by hypervolemia that causes elevated filling pressures in the left ventricle and leads to decreased cardiac output.
e. ACE inhibitors and angiotensin receptor blocking (ARB) agents reduce angiotensin II production or block its action on kidney tissue. Angiotensin II constricts the efferent arteriole. Blocking the effect of angiotensin II on kidney tissue reduces the pressure on the glomerulus by allowing the efferent arteriole to dilate. This effect is desired in many patients and reduces proteinuria. However, patients with kidney artery stenosis should avoid ACE I's and ARB agents as kidney failure can result when the efferent arteriole dilation drops the pressure in the glomerulus and decreases the GFR.
f. NSAIDs block prostaglandin production, allowing constriction of the afferent arteriole, decreasing kidney perfusion, and potentially lowering GFR.
4. Assessment.
a. History: collect data that could indicate poor kidney perfusion and/or poor systemic perfusion.
(1) Surgery.
(2) Fever.
(3) Multiple tests that require no oral intake (NPO) and/or bowel preparation.
(4) Acute myocardial infarction.
(5) Anaphylactic drug or transfusion reaction.
(6) Cardiac arrest with successful resuscitation.
(7) Low sodium diets with fluid restriction, diuretics, and antihypertensives.
(8) Exposure to consecutive days of hot, humid weather, with or without exercise.
(9) Penetrating or nonpenetrating abdominal trauma.
b. Physical assessment: findings related to fluid volume depletion vary depending on the etiology and need to be correlated with laboratory and history findings.
(1) Dry mucous membranes.
(2) Poor skin turgor.
(3) Reduced jugular venous pressure.
(4) Hypotension.
(5) Weight loss.

Table 3.4

Blood and Urine Studies to Distinguish Prerenal from Intrinsic Acute Renal Failure

Type of renal failure	BUN-to-creatinine ratio	Urine osmolality	Fractional excretion of sodium*
Prerenal acute renal failure	> 20:1	> 500 mOsm	< 1%
Intrinsic acute renal failure	< 20:1	250 to 300 mOsm	> 3%

BUN = blood urea nitrogen (mg per dL).
* The fractional excretion of sodium is calculated using the following formula:
100 x (urine sodium/serum sodium) / (urine creatinine/serum creatinine).

Source: Agrawal, M., & Swartz, R. (2000). Acute renal failure. *American Family Physician, 61*, 2077-2088. Used with permission.

c. Laboratory findings (see Table 3.4).
(1) Decreased urine output (oliguria).
(2) Increased urine osmolality and specific gravity.
(3) Decreased urine sodium and urea.
(4) Increased blood urea nitrogen (BUN), plasma creatinine usually normal. Therefore, the ratio of BUN to plasma creatinine increases.
(5) Urinary sediment usually normal.
(6) Fractional excretion of sodium is less than 1% in most patients. *Calculation*: 100 x (urine sodium/serum sodium) / (urine creatinine/serum creatinine)
5. Goal of treatment: early restoration of kidney perfusion to shorten the ischemic time and prevent parenchymal injury.
6. Treatment.
a. Treat the underlying disorder.
b. Administer fluids to increase circulatory blood volume: 500 mL (SI = 0.5 L) over 30 minutes and repeat if no increase in urine volume.
c. Achieve and maintain euvolemia.
d. Eliminate causative agents.
7. Nursing care interventions by hospital staff.
a. When administering fluid bolus/es, monitor for cardiovascular response to the increased intravascular volume, expecting an increase in blood pressure (BP) and central venous pressure (CVP).
b. Measure and document accurate intake and output (I & O).
c. Exercise infection control measures.

d. Review medications for nephrotoxins.
e. Monitor volume status, including I & O, body weight, BP, heart rate, jugular venous distention (JVD), and edema (periorbital, sacral, pretibial, and peripheral).
8. Nursing care interventions by dialysis staff.
a. In most cases the acute dialysis staff will not be involved with this patient's care because early intervention on the part of nephrology staff will resolve the problems before kidney replacement therapy is needed.
b. If the conditions are not resolved in a timely manner, the patient will progress to intrarenal kidney damage, for which nursing care will be addressed in that section.

B. Intrarenal acute renal failure.
1. Incidence.
a. Approximately 50% of cases of AKI/ARF.
b. Patients at risk include the elderly, those with diabetes, congestive heart failure (CHF), or chronic renal insufficiency (CRI).
2. Etiology: usually caused by intrarenal ischemia or toxins or both.
a. Tubular disease: acute tubular necrosis (ATN) (see Figure 3.2).
(1) Ischemia.
(a) Failure to reverse hypovolemia due to prolonged prerenal azotemia.
(b) Perfusion injury and/or prolonged ischemia in transplanted kidney.
(2) Nephrotoxic agents.
(a) Drugs: antineoplastics, anesthetics, antimicrobials, antiinflammatory agents, and immunosuppressants.

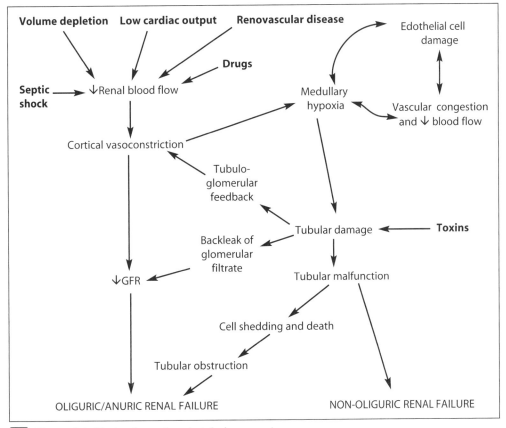

Figure 3.2. Mechanisms of acute tubular necrosis.

Source: Fry, A.C., & Farrington, K. (2006). Management of acute renal failure. *Postgraduate Medicine Journal, 82,* 106-116. Used with permission.

(b) Radiocontrast agents.
(c) Poisons.
  [1] Environmental agents: pesticides and organic solvents.
  [2] Heavy metals: lead, mercury, and gold.
  [3] Plant and animal substances: mushrooms and snake venom.
  [4] Some herbal agents.
(d) Blockage of tubules.
  [1] Pigments: myoglobin in rhabdomyolysis, hemoglobin with hemolysis.
  [2] Tumor products in myeloma.
b. Interstitial disease: acute interstitial nephritis (AIN).
  (1) Patients frequently present with fever, rash, and eosinophilia.
  (2) Allergic reaction to drugs.
    (a) Antibiotics: cephalosporins, penicillins, sulfonamides.
    (b) NSAIDs.
    (c) Diuretics.

(d) Allopurinol (Zyloprim).
(3) Some herbal agents: mutong and fangchi contain aristolochic acid, which causes focal interstitial nephritis.
(4) Autoimmune disease.
  (a) Systemic lupus erythematosis (SLE).
  (b) Mixed connective tissue disease.
(5) Pyelonephritis.
(6) Infiltrative disease.
  (a) Lymphoma.
  (b) Leukemia.
c. Glomerular disease.
  (1) Characterized by hypertension, proteinuria, and hematuria.
  (2) Rapidly progressive glomerulonephritis.
    (a) Systemic lupus erythematosis.
    (b) Small vessel vasculitis.
      [1] Wegener's granulomatosis.
      [2] Polyarteritis nodosa.
    (c) Henoch-Schonlein purpura (immunoglobulin A nephropathy).
    (d) Goodpasture syndrome.

(3) Acute proliferative glomerulonephritis.
  (a) Endocarditis.
  (b) Poststreptococcal infection.
  (c) Postpneumococcal infection.
d. Vascular disease.
  (1) Present with microangiopathic hemolysis and acute renal failure.
  (2) Microvascular disease.
    (a) Thrombotic thrombocytopenia purpura (TTP).
    (b) Hemolytic uremic syndrome (HUS).
    (c) HELLP syndrome (hemolysis, elevated liver enzymes, and low platelets).
    (d) Atheroembolic disease (cholesterol-plaque microembolism).
  (3) Macrovascular disease.
    (a) Renal artery occlusion.
    (b) Severe abdominal aortic disease (aneurysm).
    (c) Renal vein thrombosis.
e. Systemic and vascular disorders.
  (1) Wilson disease.
  (2) Malaria.
  (3) Multiple myeloma.
  (4) Sickle cell disease.
  (5) Malignant hypertension.
  (6) Diabetes mellitus.
  (7) Systemic lupus erythematosis.
  (8) Pregnancy related disorders.
    (a) Septic abortion.
    (b) Pre-eclampsia.
    (c) Abruptio placenta.
    (d) Intrauterine fetal death.
    (e) Idiopathic postpartum kidney failure.
3. Pathophysiology.
  a. Ischemic intrarenal acute renal failure (ischemic ATN).
    (1) The ischemic event refers to prolonged hypoperfusion and ischemia of the kidneys with a sustained mean arterial pressure (MAP) of less than 75 mm Hg.
    (2) Kidney autoregulation fails and the sympathetic nervous system (SNS) response, renin-angiotensin system, and possibly endothelin cause severe afferent arteriole constriction.
    (3) These mechanisms cause decreased glomerular blood flow, glomerular hydrostatic pressure, and GFR.
    (4) The amount and degree of renal cellular damage depends on the length of the ischemic episode.
      (a) Ischemia of 25 minutes or less causes reversible mild injury.
      (b) Ischemia of 40–60 minutes causes more severe damage that may recover to some extent in 2–3 weeks.
      (c) Ischemia lasting 60–90 minutes usually causes irreversible damage.
      (d) Cellular damage often continues after MAP and kidney perfusion are restored.
      (e) Renal blood flow can be reduced by 50% after an episode of ischemia; this is termed *no reflow phenomenon*.
      (f) The kidneys are unable to synthesize vasodilating prostaglandins without which the ischemic injury may be exacerbated.
    (5) Sympathetic nervous system (SNS) stimulation and angiotensin II redistribute blood flow from the cortex to the medulla. This further decreases glomerular capillary flow and worsens tubular ischemia because these structures are located primarily in the cortex.
    (6) With kidney ischemia, the nutrients and oxygen for basic cellular metabolism and tubular transport systems within the kidney are diminished.
      (a) Production of adenosine triphosphate (ATP) by kidney cell mitochondria decreases significantly.
      (b) Without adequate oxygen and ATP, kidney cell metabolism shifts from aerobic to anaerobic. There is a corresponding kidney tissue extracellular and intracellular acidosis that alters kidney function.
    (7) Ischemia causes a decrease in kidney cellular potassium, magnesium, and inorganic phosphates, and an increase in intracellular sodium, chloride, and calcium.
      (a) Sodium (Na)/calcium (Ca) exchange is abnormal owing to low ATP, altered Ca-ATPase, and increased cellular sodium. As a result, there is an increase in cellular calcium, which increases cell injury.
      (b) During reperfusion after a prolonged kidney ischemic event, the formation of oxygen-free radicals further exacerbates cellular damage.
    (8) As the final outcome of prolonged tubular ischemia, tubular cells swell and become necrotic, altering the function of the basement membrane.

(a) Tubular obstruction occurs from sloughed necrotic cells and cast formation.

(b) The tubular obstruction increases tubular hydrostatic pressure and Bowman's capsule hydrostatic pressure, which opposes the glomerular hydro-static pressure and decreases GFR.

(c) Injury to the basement membrane increases tubular permeability and allows tubular filtrate to leak back into the interstitium and peritubular capillaries, further decreasing tubular filtrate.

(9) Ischemic ATN is usually associated with oliguria because of extensive nephron injury (see Table 3.5). Other clinical indications include:

(a) Decreased urea excretion and elevated BUN.

(b) Decreased creatinine clearance and elevated plasma creatinine (Cr).

(c) Abnormal kidney handling of sodium. Usually there is sodium loss with urinary sodium equal to sodium filtered into the tubule from the glomerulus.

(d) Inability to concentrate urine. Urinary osmolality approximates plasma osmolality or 300–320 mOsm/L (SI = 300–320 mOsm/L) a condition called isosthenuria.

b. Toxic intrarenal acute renal failure (toxic ATN).

(1) The toxic event refers to toxic products of organisms and/or nephrotoxic agents, which begin by causing injury to the tubular cells.

(2) There is tubular cell necrosis, cast formation, tubular obstruction, and altered GFR.

(a) The basement membrane is usually intact and the injured necrotic areas are more localized than with ischemic ATN.

(b) Nonoliguria occurs more often with toxic ATN than with ischemic ATN.

(3) The injury with toxic ATN can be less than with ischemic ATN. Therefore the healing process can be more rapid with toxic ATN.

Table 3.5

Typical Findings in Prerenal and Intrarenal Acute Renal Failure

	Prerenal	Intrarenal Renal
Volume	Oliguria	Oliguria or nonoliguria
Urinary sediment	Normal (hyaline and granular casts)	RBC casts Cellular debris
Specific gravity	High	Low
Osmolality (mOsm/Kg H_2O)	High	Low (Isosthenuria)
Ratio Osm Urine to Osm Plasma	> 1.5	< 1.2
Urine Na (mEq/L)	Low (< 20)	Increased over prerenal (> 20)
Urine urea (g/24 hrs)	Low (15)	Low (5)
Urine creatinine (g/24 hrs)	Normal (> 1.0)	Low (< 1.0)
Ratio urine creatinine to plasma creatinine	> 15:1	< 10:1

Source: Lancaster, L.E. (1990). Renal response to shock. *Critical Care Nursing Clinics of North America, 2*(2), 221-223. Used with permission.

(4) Reasons the kidney is so susceptible to toxic damage.
   (a) Blood circulates through the kidney approximately 14 times a minute. Therefore, the kidney is repeatedly exposed to all components in the blood.
   (b) The kidney is the major excretory organ for toxic substances, and as these substances await transport, they are held within kidney cells where they can disrupt cellular function.
   (c) The liver usually detoxifies substances, and, with liver disease, the kidney can be overloaded with underdetoxified substances.
   (d) The kidney transforms many substances. Some of these new metabolites can be toxic to the kidney.
   (e) The countercurrent mechanism (the method in which the sodium pump concentrates urine as it travels through the hair pin turns made by the loop of Henle, folding back on itself, creating a higher osmotic gradient between the descending and ascending flows) concentrates bodily substances as well as other substances. This increased concentration can result in toxicity to the kidney.

4. Assessment.
   a. History. Collect data that identify an event, series of events, agent, or agents that have caused kidney injury, especially those related to ischemia or toxins.
      (1) Exposure to nephrotoxins.
      (2) Radiologic tests that require administration of a dye.
      (3) Hypersensitivity reaction to a drug or dye.
      (4) Recent infections.
      (5) Sepsis.
      (6) Recent trauma.
      (7) Antineoplastics with or without irradiation.
      (8) Multiple myeloma.
      (9) Pregnancy.
      (10) History of cardiac, kidney, or liver disease.
   b. Physical assessment. No one specific finding pinpoints intrarenal azotemia. Correlate all findings with history and laboratory findings.
   c. Laboratory findings and other considerations for differentiating prerenal azotemia from ATN.

(1) Because prerenal problems often correspond with the onset phase of ATN and because prerenal is a reversible phase, it is essential for diagnosis and aggressive management to begin early in the course of prerenal problems.
(2) Urinalysis, microscopic examination of the urine, and laboratory plasma values provide important data for differentiating prerenal azotemia from intrinsic.
(3) In prerenal problems, the urinary specific gravity and osmolality are high and the urinary sodium is low because of decreased kidney blood flow and decreased GFR, which the kidneys interpret as a state of dehydration. As a response, under the influence of aldosterone and ADH, maximal sodium and water are reabsorbed from the distal tubule and collecting duct into the peritubular capillary plasma. Thus, a small amount (oliguria) of very concentrated urine with high specific gravity and high osmolality is excreted.
   (a) Although maximal sodium is reabsorbed, the urine is concentrated due to urea or other solutes.
   (b) Urinary and plasma creatinine levels often show wide variation in the prerenal period.
(4) In contrast to prerenal problems, ATN is characterized by parenchymal damage that causes impaired sodium reabsorption.
   (a) This results in an increase in urinary sodium, greater than 20 mEq/L (SI = 20 mmol/L). The serum sodium varies, depending on the state of hydration.
   (b) The fractional excretion of sodium is > 3% and urine osmolality between 250 and 300 mOsm.
   (c) Oliguria is usually associated with postischemic ATN, whereas nephrotoxic ATN can be associated with either oliguria or nonoliguria, as explained above.
   (d) The creatinine clearance is severely decreased and the plasma creatinine rises at a rate of about 1–3 mg/dL/day (SI = 88–264 mmol/L/day) in ATN.
   (e) The urine to plasma creatinine ratio

is less than 10 to 1 in ATN compared to more than 15 to 1 in prerenal.

(5) Another distinguishing factor between prerenal and ATN is the response to therapy.

(a) In prerenal illness in which no actual nephron damage has occurred, the kidney's response to therapy aimed at correcting the underlying problem is often rapid with return to normal urine output and normal blood chemistries.

(b) In ATN, which indicates nephron damage, response to therapy aimed at the underlying cause of the damage is minimal. ATN requires additional interventions aimed at correcting the abnormalities resulting from the inability of the kidneys to maintain their functions.

5. Goals of treatment.
   a. Correct the primary disorder.
   b. Correct fluid and electrolyte disorders.
   c. Prevent infection.
   d. Maintain optimal nutrition.
   e. Treat systemic effects of uremia.
   f. Provide education and support to patient and family.

6. Treatment.
   a. Must be tailored to address the specific presentation of the AKI/ARF.
   b. Pharmacologic interventions, clinical interventions, medical and nursing treatments, and laboratory monitoring all play a role in sustaining the patient through this acute illness.

7. Nursing care interventions by hospital staff.
   a. Monitor closely volume status including I & O, body weight, BP, heart rate, jugular venous distention (JVD), and edema (periorbital, sacral, pretibial, peripheral).
   b. Concentrate IV infusions.
   c. Utilize medication protocols, such as Lasix.
   d. Monitor changes in mental status that can indicate an electrolyte imbalance or hypoxemia.
   e. Monitor lab values for electrolyte imbalances.
   f. Increase awareness of nephrotoxic agents, such as contrast media and antibiotics.
   g. Provide skin care for rash, ischemia ("purple toes"), and tissue integrity.
   h. Monitor dialysis access site for infection.

8. Nursing care interventions by dialysis staff.
   a. Educate patient and family.
   b. Educate hospital staff.

c. Comprehensive nursing assessment, including lab values, changes in weight and fluid status, mental status changes, cardiac and respiratory condition, prior to initiating kidney replacement therapy.

d. Report assessment findings and collaborate with nephrologist to tailor the treatment plan for optimal patient treatment outcomes.

e. Collaborate with hospital staff caring for patient.

(1) Receive report prior to initiating RRT and incorporate information into assessment and treatment plan.

(2) Review medications for nephrotoxins, dialyzability, and impact on hemodynamics.

(3) During treatment, advise hospital staff of changes in condition and interventions used to respond to changes.

(4) Participate in infection control procedures.

(5) Perform dialysis access catheter care, inform hospital staff of assessment, and document condition of site.

(6) Assist with skin care and turning when appropriate.

(7) Following treatment, report to hospital staff regarding patient's response to treatment, amount of fluid removed, post-treatment vital signs, medications given, blood products administered, access status, and plan for next treatment if known.

f. Avoid hypotension during dialysis treatments.

g. Document patient education provided.

h. Evaluate dialysis treatment outcome and communicate need to modify next treatment to supervisor and/or nephrologist as appropriate.

C. Postrenal acute renal failure.
   1. Incidence: 5–10 % of cases of AKI/ARF.
   2. Etiology.
      a. Interference with flow of urine from the kidneys to the exterior of the body.
      b. Most often due to obstruction of the lower urinary tract.
      c. Obstruction.
         (1) Ureteral, bladder neck, or urethral obstruction.
            (a) Calculi, neoplasms, or sloughed papillary tissue.
            (b) Strictures, trauma, or blood clots.

(c) Congenital/developmental abnormalities.

(d) Foreign objects or inadvertent surgical ligation.

(2) Benign prostatic hypertrophy or prostatic cancer.

(3) Cervical cancer.

(4) Retroperitoneal fibrosis.

(5) Intratubular obstruction (crystals or myeloma light chains).

(6) Pelvic mass or invasive pelvic malignancy.

(7) Intraluminal bladder mass.

(8) Neurogenic bladder.

(9) Pregnancy.

(10) Drugs, such as antihistamines and ganglionic blocking agents.

3. Pathophysiology.

a. Obstruction of urine outflow may lead to a sudden decrease in urine output.

b. Obstruction in the urinary tract causes an increase in pressure near the obstruction due to the continued production of urine by glomcrular filtration.

c. The increased pressure from the obstruction is transmitted retrograde through the collecting system to the nephron.

d. When the pressure in the tubule exceeds the pressure in the glomerulus, glomerular filtration is stopped.

(1) Increased reabsorption of sodium, water, and urea results in decreased urinary sodium, increased urine osmolality, and increased BUN.

(2) Decreased GFR results in a decreased creatinine clearance and increased plasma creatinine.

e. Prolonged obstruction can result in:

(1) Dilation of the collecting system and compression of parenchymal tissue.

(2) Increased tubular hydrostatic pressure.

(3) Kidney interstitial edema.

(4) Reduced kidney blood flow.

(5) Secondary tubular damage.

f. Temporary obstruction results in little dilation of the collecting system and little or no loss of kidney tissue.

g. The obstruction can be total or partial with resulting symptoms depending on the amount of change in GFR.

4. Assessment.

a. History. Collect data that indicate obstruction or disruption of the urinary tract.

(1) History of change in urine volume and/or urinating pattern.

(2) History of prostatic disease or abdominal neoplasms.

(3) History of urinary tract stones or nephralgia.

(4) Pregnancy.

(5) Recent abdominal surgery.

(6) Paralysis (quadriplegia).

b. Physical assessment. Findings vary with etiology and need to be correlated with laboratory and history findings.

c. Laboratory findings.

(1) Urine volume variable: may be oliguria or polyuria or abrupt anuria.

(2) Urine osmolality variable: increases or may be similar to plasma osmolality.

(3) Urine specific gravity: variable.

(4) Urine sodium variable: decreases (often similar to plasma sodium).

(5) Urine urea decreases.

(6) BUN and plasma creatinine increase: ratio normal to slightly increased.

(7) Urinary sediment usually normal, unless urinary tract infection is present.

d. Diagnostic studies that may be used:

(1) X-ray of kidneys, ureters, and bladder (KUB) to determine size, shape, and placement of kidneys.

(2) Intravenous pyelogram (IVP) to detect location and/or type of obstruction.

(3) Radionuclide studies to screen for tumors, cysts, and blood flow.

(4) Ultrasound, computed tomography (CT), or magnetic resonance imaging (MRI) to screen for hydronephrosis and location of obstruction.

5. Goals of treatment.

a. Relieve the obstruction as soon as possible. The potential for recovery of kidney function is often inversely related to the duration of the obstruction.

b. Ongoing prevention and detection of urosepsis.

6. Treatment.

a. Bladder catheterization can be both diagnostic and therapeutic in bladder or urethral obstruction.

b. Other treatments may include percutaneous nephrostomy, lithotripsy, ureteral stenting, and urethral stenting.

7. Nursing care interventions by hospital staff.

a. Stoma and skin care.

b. Nephrostomy and urostomy care and dressing changes.

c. Appliances.

d. Identify early stent tissue overgrowth.

8. Nursing care interventions by dialysis staff.
   a. Resource and support for hospital staff.
   b. Provide kidney replacement therapy options for potential acute complications.

IV. Complications of acute kidney injury/acute renal failure. Not all AKI patients experience all of these complications, but they can occur in some natural sequence.

A. The diagnosis of AKI/ARF.
   1. Signs and symptoms of kidney impairment are present, such as decreased urine volume.
   2. Treatment goals are to determine the cause of the AKI/ARF and establish a treatment plan based on the etiology.
   3. Nursing care interventions are supportive and responsive to signs and symptoms.

B. Oliguria or nonoliguria.
   1. If it occurs, it usually lasts from 5 to 15 days, but can persist for weeks.
   2. Approximately 50% AKI/ARF patients are nonoliguric, which may indicate a less severe insult to the kidney than patients who are oliguric.
   3. Kidney pathology.
      a. Kidney healing occurs.
         (1) Tubular cells regenerate.
         (2) Destroyed basement membrane is replaced with fibrous scar tissue.
         (3) Tubules are clogged with inflammatory products.
      b. Functional changes.
         (1) Decreased glomerular filtration.
         (2) Decreased tubular transport of substances.
         (3) Decreased urine formation.
         (4) Decreased kidney clearance.
      c. When ARF persists for weeks or longer, kidney endocrine functions are altered, including decreased secretion of erythropoietin.
   4. Frequent causes of death are cardiac arrest due to hyperkalemia, gastrointestinal bleeding, and infection.
   5. Treatment goals are to keep the patient alive until the kidney damage heals.
   6. Signs, symptoms, and related nursing (hospital and nephrology) care interventions.
      a. Increased susceptibility to infection (especially urinary and respiratory) related to altered immune, nutritional, and biochemical status, and hospitalization.
         (1) Implement infection preventive measures.

            (a) Avoid invasive procedures, especially urinary bladder catheters.
            (b) Use aseptic technique for all invasive procedures and dressing changes.
            (c) Wash hands before and after contact with patient.
            (d) Turn, cough, and deep breathe; provide incentive spirometry equipment for regular use.
            (e) Frequent position changes and skin care to prevent skin breakdown.
            (f) Remove catheters, tubings, and lines as soon as possible.
         (2) Instruct patient on increased susceptibility to infection.
            (a) Signs and symptoms to report.
            (b) Avoid contact with people who have infections.
            (c) Importance of hand washing.
            (d) Encourage level of activity tolerated to facilitate deep respirations.
         (3) Assess for changes in infection status.
            (a) Assess vital signs for elevated temperature, increased respiratory rate, increased heart rate, and/or decreased BP.
            (b) Monitor lung sounds and productivity of cough.
            (c) Monitor lab values: white blood cell count (WBCs), blood culture results.
            (d) Review reports of chest x-rays.
            (e) Observe dialysis access catheter exit sites for infection and remove sutures from new tunneled catheter exit sites two weeks after placement.
            (f) Perform dressing changes per protocol using aseptic technique.
      b. Fluid volume excess related to decreased kidney excretion of water, inappropriate fluid intake, and/or sodium retention.
         (1) Instruct patient and family on appropriate fluid intake and dietary restrictions.
         (2) Monitor intake and output (I & O) accurately.
         (3) Weigh patient daily using correctly calibrated scale.
         (4) Observe for BP changes, orthostatic hypotension, and increased heart rate.
         (5) Observe for JVD or, when available, elevated CVP.
         (6) Observe for edema (periorbital, sacral, pretibial, peripheral).
         (7) Observe skin turgor.

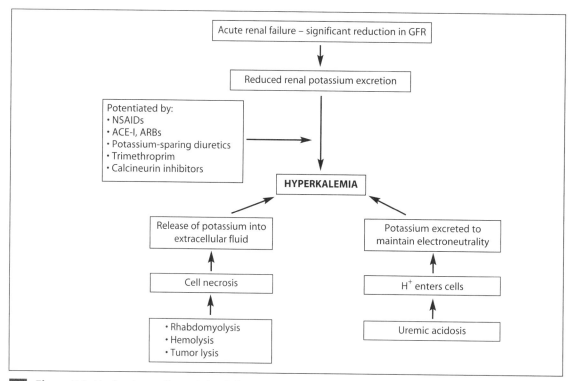

Figure 3.3. Mechanisms of hyperkalemia in acute renal failure.
Source: Fry, A.C., & Farrington, K. (2006). Management of acute renal failure. *Postgraduate Medicine Journal, 82,* 106-116. Used with permission.

(8) Check lab values of brain natriuretic peptide (BNP) and for hyponatremia.

c. Hyperkalemia related to decreased kidney regulation and excretion of potassium, increased endogenous production of potassium, increased potassium intake, tissue breakdown, and/or metabolic acidosis (see Figure 3.3).

(1) Instruct patient and family on dietary potassium and its affect on the heart.

(2) Monitor electrocardiogram (EKG) for signs of hyperkalemia.
   (a) Tall, peaked T waves.
   (b) Prolonged PR interval.
   (c) ST depression.
   (d) Widened QRS.
   (e) Loss of P wave.

(3) Monitor for signs and symptoms of hyperkalemia.
   (a) Irritability.
   (b) Anxiety.
   (c) Abdominal cramping.
   (d) Diarrhea.
   (e) Weakness, especially of lower extremities.
   (f) Paresthesias.

(4) Administer blood products during hemodialysis treatments if possible to remove extra potassium resulting from cell breakdown in handling and administration.

(5) Monitor signs of tissue breakdown and/or GI bleeding and report to nephrologist or appropriate medical doctor (MD).

(6) Administer emergency medications as needed while waiting for initiation of hemodialysis: insulin and glucose, calcium, and/or resin exchange products (Kayexalate).

(7) Use apple or cranberry juice to treat hypoglycemia instead of the traditional orange juice to prevent hyperkalemia.

d. Hyperphosphatemia related to decreased kidney excretion and regulation of phosphate, increased or continued intake of phosphate, and tissue breakdown, especially muscle tissue.

(1) Monitor for signs and symptoms of hyperphosphatemia (most of the symptoms are related to the development of hypocalcemia).
   (a) Anorexia.
   (b) Nausea.
   (c) Vomiting.

(d) Muscle weakness.
(e) Hyperreflexia.
(f) Tetany.
(g) Tachycardia.
(2) Instruct patient and family on dietary phosphorus and its relationship to calcium in maintaining good balance.
(3) Administer phosphate binders with meals to increase effectiveness.

e. Metabolic acidosis related to decreased kidney excretion of acid load, decreased regeneration of bicarbonate, increased tissue catabolism, and endogenous production of acids.
(1) Administer sodium bicarbonate and/or other medications for electrolyte repletion as needed.
(2) Coordinate schedule of RRT to correct electrolyte imbalances.

f. Potential for GI bleeding related to stress, retention of metabolic wastes and end products, altered capillary permeability, and platelet dysfunction.
(1) Instruct patient and family to report any signs of GI bleeding.
(2) Monitor lab values for changes in Hct and Hgb.
(3) Monitor vital signs to detect volume loss.
(4) Guaiac test nasogastric (NG) drainage, emesis, and stool for occult blood.
(5) Administer erythropoietin (EPO) during hemodialysis treatments and/or as ordered, subcutaneously (SC) or intravenously (IV).

g. Alteration in nutrition.
(1) Review diet prescription for appropriateness.
(2) Address uremia caused anorexia, nausea, and vomiting.
(3) Provide antiemetic medications prior to mealtime as needed.
(4) Encourage dietary selection of foods that are appealing to patient.
(5) If meals are missed due to tests or treatments, arrange for snacks between meals.
(6) Avoid scheduling other activities (exercise, dressing changes, etc.) at mealtimes.
(7) Dietary supplements, tube feedings, and/or total parenteral nutrition (TPN) may be necessary to meet caloric and protein needs while this catabolic state persists.

(a) Mild degree of catabolism.
[1] Urea nitrogen appearance (UNA) level < 5 g/24 hours. UNA is measured as the amount of urea excreted in urine plus the net amount accumulated in body water (Maroni formula).
[2] Adequate nutritional support can usually be achieved with oral intake alone.
[3] Caloric needs: 30–35 cal/kg edema-free body weight.
[4] Protein needs: 0.6–0.8 mg/kg provided as both essential and nonessential amino acids.
[5] Fluid and electrolyte restrictions usually not indicated.

(b) Moderate degree of catabolism.
[1] Urea nitrogen appearance level 5–10 mg/24 hours.
[2] Nutritional support is by tube feeding or TPN.
[3] Caloric needs: 30–35 cal/kg edema-free body weight.
[4] Protein needs: 1.0–1.2 g/kg provided as both essential and nonessential amino acids.
[5] Fluid requirements adjusted for intake and output and dialysis losses.
[6] Electrolytes usually limited unless lab results indicate otherwise.

(c) Severe degree of catabolism.
[1] Urea nitrogen appearance level greater than 10 g/24 hours.
[2] Nutritional support most often TPN as GI dysfunction occurs frequently in this setting.
[3] During the first 24–48 hours after injury, nutrition support should be withheld. Infusion of large quantities of amino acids or glucose during this time can increase oxygen demand and further aggravate tubular damage.
[4] Caloric needs: 35–45 cal/kg edema-free body weight.
[5] Protein needs: 1.5–2.0 g/kg provided as essential and nonessential amino acids.
[6] Fluid requirements adjusted for intake and output and dialysis losses.
[7] Electrolytes are usually limited

unless laboratory results indicate otherwise.

[8] Hyperkalemia and hyperphosphatemia can be significant secondary to catabolism of lean body mass as well as secondary to impaired excretion and should be monitored closely.

(8) Maintain normoglycemic state using frequent bedside glucose monitoring and insulin IV drip or sliding scale injections.

h. Potential for drug toxicity and nephrotoxicity related to inability of kidney to excrete all drugs, continued administration of drugs excreted by the kidney, and nephrotoxic drugs.

(1) Adjust doses of medications by clinical pharmacist based on patient's residual kidney function as well as the type of dialytic therapy and membrane characteristics being used.

(2) Review medications for kidney toxicity prior to administration.

(3) Review serum drug levels (digoxin, antibiotics) prior to administering the next dose to be sure they are not in a toxic range.

(4) Monitor pain medications to avoid oversedation due to decreased metabolism and/or excretion.

(5) Do not administer medications prior to the hemodialysis treatment that will be removed by the dialytic process.

(6) Hold medications that will lower the patient's blood pressure prior to their scheduled hemodialysis treatment.

(7) Do not withhold pain medications from patients on dialysis because they may be partially removed by the treatment. Arrange for an extra dose if necessary to respond effectively to the patient's pain level.

(8) Hospital staff and nephrology nurses will collaborate to provide appropriate medication administration during the dialysis treatment.

i. Potential for skin breakdown related to bed rest, fluid/electrolyte imbalances, metabolic products and toxin accumulation, edema, disrupted hemostasis and increased capillary fragility, repeated venipunctures, and other invasive procedures.

(1) Maintain skin cleanliness and dry bedding at all times.

(2) Treat skin breakdown with appropriate protective agents; consult wound care nurse if needed.

(3) Turn patient and provide skin care regularly.

(4) Position patient off bony prominences.

(5) Consider the possibility of allergy to soaps and request extra-rinse, nonallergenic linens if needed.

(6) Use linen and pads appropriate for the specific therapeutic bed, when one is in use.

(7) Consider the fragility of the patient's skin when selecting the kind of tape to use on a wound or exit site dressing.

j. Disturbances in self-concept related to loss of bodily function, dependency, separation from family and friends, fatigue, inability to meet personal and professional responsibilities, confusion, lack of knowledge, hopelessness, and loss of control.

(1) Provide support to patient and family as they transition through the various stages of their acute illness experience.

(2) Provide education at the bedside and use printed materials to increase level of understanding and to provide an element of hope.

(3) Use the expertise of the nephrology nurse at the bedside to educate hospital staff, patients, and family members about the AKI/ARF process.

(4) Allow the patient to make as many decisions about their care as possible to return some element of control to them while they are in a world where many things are beyond their control.

(5) Allow frequent rest periods with opportunities for naps.

(6) Encourage family involvement in care and decision making when possible.

(7) Provide regular reorientation to place and time.

k. Disturbances in sleep pattern related to biochemical disruption, anxiety, hospitalization, isolation from family/friends, fear regarding lack of recovery of kidney function, multiple tests, dietary and fluid restrictions.

(1) Encourage a realization of time of day by using "dark hours" for sleep during the night shift.

(2) Administer sleeping medications when needed to facilitate a good night's sleep.

    (3) Minimize interruptions of patient's sleep when only related to staff convenience for performing procedures.

    (4) Encourage family and friends presence at the bedside within the hospital's visitation policies.

    (5) Develop a professional relationship of listening and supporting to help alleviate the patient's anxiety, fear, and uncertainty.

l. Lack of knowledge related to kidney function, diagnostic tests, pathogenesis of AKI/ARF, effects of AKI/ARF on all body system; course, management, prognosis, complications, and prevention of AKI/ARF.

    (1) Explain all tests, procedures, and interventions prior to performing them.

    (2) Consult nephrologist and nephrology nurses for intervention and education related to return of kidney function.

    (3) Review lab tests and other measures of potential return of function with the patient and family so they know what to be aware of and to know the level of progress.

C. Diuresis.

1. If it occurs, it usually lasts from 1 to 2 weeks, but can persist for weeks.

2. Oliguric patients have a greater diuresis than nonoliguric patients.

3. Self-limiting diuresis occurs because:
   a. Kidney tubular patency is restored.
   b. Retained substances (e.g., urea and sodium) act as osmotic agents.
   c. Nephron's ability to concentrate urine is not recovered.

4. With continued kidney healing, the kidney regains most of its lost function except its concentrating ability. The amount regained is dependent on the degree of initial injury and of permanent basement membrane loss.

5. Frequent causes of death are infection and gastrointestinal bleeding.

6. Treatment goals are to keep the patient alive until the kidney lesion heals.

7. Signs, symptoms, and related nursing (hospital and nephrology) care interventions.
   a. Signs and symptoms of azotemia gradually diminish.
   b. Fluid volume deficit related to increased kidney excretion of water, inadequate fluid intake, sodium loss, continued use of diuretics/dialysis, fluid loss through nonrenal sources.

    (1) Perform fluid status assessment: edema, JVD, hypotension (including orthostatic), heart rate, lung sounds, skin turgor, mucous membranes, constipation and/or hard stool, and weight changes.

    (2) Weigh patient daily on a correctly calibrated scale.

    (3) Record accurate I & O.

    (4) Correlate the physical assessment with the weight and I & O to determine fluid status: balanced, deficit, or overload.

    (5) Educate the patient and family about the kidney's response to the diuresis, including the need for increased fluid intake.

    (6) Develop fluid plan for the day with the patient and coordinate with dietitian.

    (7) Adjust fluid intake to approximate fluid losses to protect the returning kidney function, increasing or decreasing as the kidney responds.

    (8) Provide for excretory needs, keeping commode, urinal, or bedpan within easy access of the patient.

    (9) Avoid procedures that require the patient to have nothing by mouth (NPO) or to have a bowel preparation until diuresis subsides or initiate intravenous therapy to maintain fluid balance.

c. Hypokalemia related to increased excretion of potassium, decreased potassium intake, metabolic alkalosis, continued administration of diuretics/resins exchangers, intravenous fluid with out potassium, and GI fluid losses.

    (1) Educate the patient and family regarding the risk of hypokalemia and the signs and symptoms they should report.

    (2) Review lab values for serum potassium levels.

    (3) Assess for decreased neuromuscular irritability, constipation, weakness, and/or diminished reflexes; severe hypokalemia can lead to ineffective breathing due to weakness or paralysis of respiratory muscles.

    (4) Monitor EKG for signs of hypokalemia.
      (a) ST segment depression.
      (b) Flattened T wave.
      (c) Presence of U wave.
      (d) Ventricular arrhythmias.

    (5) Consult dietitian for adequate dietary intake of potassium.

    (6) Administer potassium parenterally if unable to ingest adequate dietary potassium.

(7) Prevent metabolic alkalosis because of hydrogen-potassium cellular exchange.

(8) Control GI losses.

(9) Avoid medications that cause potassium loss (e.g., diuretics).

8. The following problems, described in the oliguria/nonoliguria section, persist and require continued nursing monitoring and interventions.

   a. Increased susceptibility to infection.

   b. Gastrointestinal bleeding.

   c. Alteration in nutrition.

   d. Skin breakdown.

   e. Drug toxicity and nephrotoxicity.

   f. Disturbances in sleep patterns.

9. The problems of hyperphosphatemia and metabolic acidosis gradually resolve during diuresis as kidney function improves and the kidneys are once more able to regulate and excrete hydrogen and phosphate and to reabsorb bicarbonate ions.

D. Recovery of kidney function.

1. If it occurs, the process usually lasts several months to 1 year.

2. Healing process completed.

   a. Contractile scar tissue replaces damaged basement membrane.

   b. Nephrons are maximally patent and tubular cells regenerated.

   c. Probably some scar tissue remains in all AKI/ARF kidneys, but the functional loss is not always clinically significant.

   d. Maximal kidney functions return (e.g., concentrating ability) and kidneys respond to body's needs through regulatory and excretory mechanisms.

   e. Urine osmolality increases, urine volume stabilizes, plasma substances normalize, body fluids balance, and uremia resolves.

3. No special form of treatment is required other than general healthy living.

4. Major patient issues requiring nursing (hospital and nephrology) care and intervention.

   a. Lack of knowledge regarding the AKI/ARF episode, including follow-up care and prevention of another episode.

   b. Educate the patient and family about the ARF episode and interventions to prevent another episode.

     (1) Avoid nephrotoxins.

     (2) Drink plenty of water.

V. Manifestations of frequently occurring acute kidney injury processes.

A. Acute tubular necrosis (ATN).

1. The most common cause of intrinsic AKI/ARF, responsible for 38–76% of cases.

2. Can be the result of septic, toxic, or ischemic insults.

3. Mortality rate in patients requiring dialysis is between 50 and 80%.

4. Presentation and assessment.

   a. Lab values show increased urine sodium concentration and fractional excretion of sodium.

   b. ATN is a part of a catabolic illness, making nutritional support critical, including administration of essential amino acids. Use of enteral feedings rather than parenteral is recommended when possible.

5. Nursing interventions and collaborative treatments.

   a. Continuous or intermittent forms of RRT may be used.

   b. The avoidance of hypotension is key with either modality.

B. Rhabdomyolysis is necrosis of skeletal muscle (see Table 3.6).

1. It is the cause of 7–10% of AKI/ARF.

2. It can occur from direct traumatic injury or nontraumatic (compression or exertional) injury.

3. The most common causes are alcohol abuse, muscle overexertion, muscle compression, and the use of certain medications or illicit drugs.

   a. When injured, muscle cells release myoglobin, which enters the circulation (see Figure 3.4).

     (1) Myoglobin is normally filtered by the glomerulus, but when excessive amounts damage the kidney tubule cells glomerular filtration is overwhelmed.

     (2) The myoglobin also precipitates and forms casts, which can obstruct flow through the tubules. AKI/ARF can occur.

   b. CPK (creatine phosphokinase) is also released from damaged muscle.

     (1) The level of CPK can indicate the likelihood of complications.

     (2) AKI/ARF usually occurs with creatine kinase "MM" isoenzyme (CK-MM) levels of more than 15,000, but treatment may be initiated at a lower level.

Table 3.6

Clinical Features of Rhabdomyolysis

Local features	Systemic features
Muscle pain	Tea-colored urine
Tenderness	Fever
Swelling	Malaise
Bruising	Nausea
Weakness	Emesis
	Confusion
	Agitation
	Delirium
	Anuria

Source: Sauret, J.M., & Marinides, G. (2002). Rhabdomyolysis. *American Family Physician, 65*, 5, 907-912. Used with permission.

c. Large amounts of fluid can accumulate in the necrotic muscle tissues, leading to hypovolemia, which is one of the causes of AKI/ARF in these patients.
d. Compartment syndrome can occur requiring fasciotomy to prevent secondary tissue necrosis.
e. Disseminated intravascular coagulation (DIC) and multiorgan dysfunction syndrome (MODS) can also occur.
f. Hyperkalemia, hyperphosphatemia, and lactic acidosis are other electrolyte disturbances likely to occur.
g. Changes in the urine are also evident (see Table 3.7).

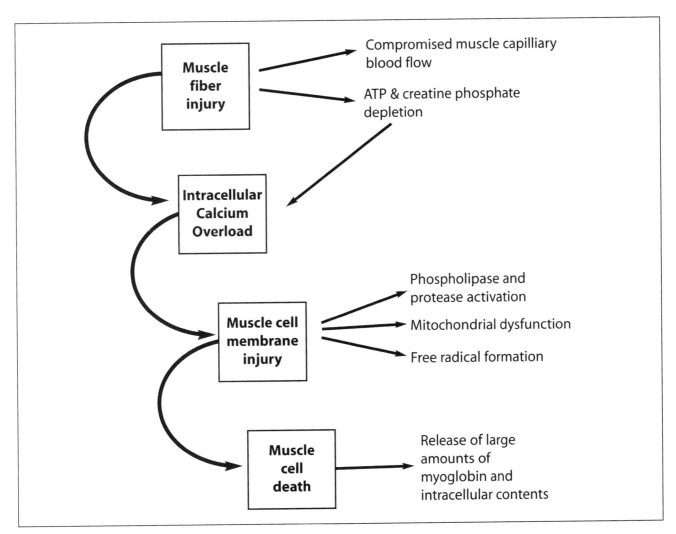

Figure 3.4. Pathogenesis of exertional rhabdomyolysis.

Source: Russell, T.A. (2005). Acute renal failure related to rhabdomyolysis: Pathophysiology, diagnosis, and collaborative management. *Nephrology Nursing Journal, 32*, 409-417. Used with permission.

Table 3.7

Urinalysis Findings in Rhabdomyolysis

Color	Dark (cola-colored)
pH	Acidic

Blood
  Benzidine reagent
  Microscopy
	3+ to 4+
	Less than 5 RBCs per high power field

Sediment	Pigmented brown granular casts Renal tubular epithelial cells
Urinary sodium concentration	> 20 mEq/L
FE$_{NA}$	> 1%

FE$_{NA}$ = fractional excretion of sodium

Source: Russell, T.A. (2005). Acute renal failure related to rhabdomyolysis: pathophysiology, diagnosis, and collaborative management. *Nephrology Nursing Journal, 32,* 409-417. Used with permission.

4. Nursing interventions and collaborative treatments.
   a. Treatment includes aggressive attempts to maintain high urine volume with IV infusions at 200–300 mL/hr.
   b. Continuous or intermittent forms of renal replacement therapy (RRT) may be used depending on the severity of the necrosis and catabolism, electrolyte imbalances, and hemodynamics.

C. Acute interstitial nephritis (AIN).
   1. Causes approximately 10–15% of ARF.
   2. For many years, AIN was known as the complication of streptococcal infections.
   3. With increased development and use of antibiotics, AIN became the complication of antibiotics and other drugs.
   4. It is an immune-mediated cause of AKI/ARF that is identified on kidney biopsy as inflammatory cell infiltrates in the interstitium of the kidney.
   5. Most frequently caused by drug hypersensitivity reactions that create an allergic reaction within the interstitium, but the tubules can also be involved.
   6. NSAIDs and antibiotics are the most frequent source of the reaction. Other medications that have been found to induce AIN include

analgesics, and diuretics.
   7. The elderly are the age group most at risk of experiencing this complication due to their increased use of prescription drugs and the reduced ability of their kidneys to clear drugs.
   8. Presentation and assessment.
      a. Classic symptoms on presentation are fever, rash, and eosinophilia.
      b. Other symptoms can include oliguria, arthalgia, and loin pain.
   9. Nursing interventions and collaborative treatments.
      a. The treatment of choice is removal of the causative agent.
      b. Renal replacement therapy support is frequently needed.
      c. Corticosteroids are often used in treatment based on the assumption of an immune system response in this disease process.
      d. Current studies are bringing the effectiveness of this use of steroids under scrutiny.

D. Goodpasture syndrome.
   1. It is characterized by pulmonary hemorrhage and crescentic glomerulonephritis.
   2. It is a disease of serum antibodies attacking the glomerular and alveolar basement membranes (see Figure 3.5).
   3. Presentation and assessment.
      a. Initially the patient may exhibit flu-like symptoms with malaise and a rapid onset of microscopic hematuria and proteinuria.
      b. 50%–75% of patients exhibit pulmonary symptoms, such as cough, mild shortness of breath, and hemoptysis.
      c. The pulmonary symptoms may have occurred days, weeks, or months before the kidney symptoms present.
   4. Nursing interventions and collaborative treatments.
      a. Pulmonary hemorrhage can be severe and lead to iron deficiency anemia and a significant increase in mortality.
      b. Airway management and pulmonary failure with increasing oxygen needs must be closely monitored.
      c. Therapeutic plasma exchange (TPE) is performed to decrease the circulating antibodies.
      d. To prevent exacerbation of pulmonary hemorrhage, fresh frozen plasma is used as the replacement fluid for TPE to replace the clotting factors lost by the removal of the patient's plasma.
      e. Immunosuppression is used to prevent further

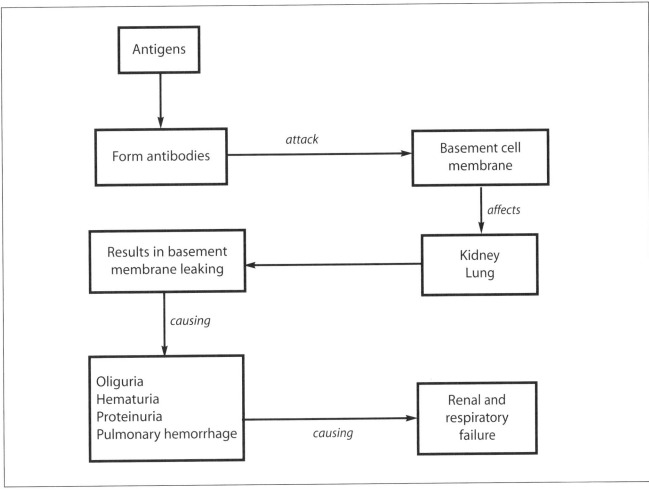

Figure 3.5. Type II hypersensitivity in Goodpasture syndrome.

Source: Bergs, L. (2005). Goodpasture syndrome. *Critical Care Nurse, 25*, 50-58. Used with permission.

antibody formation. Acute renal failure may develop, requiring RRT treatments.
f. Heparin should be avoided on RRT.

E. Sepsis and SIRS (systemic inflammatory response syndrome).
1. The septic response can be triggered by both infectious and noninfectious events (see Table 3.8).
2. Infectious causes are bacteria and fungi. Noninfectious causes include pancreatitis, burns, and trauma. SIRS is the term used to refer to noninfectious causes.
3. Presentation and assessment.
a. The pathophysiology of sepsis is, at least in part, an inappropriate and overwhelming inflammatory response: increased production of proinflammatory cytokines and decreased production of cytokines that normally inhibit inflammation.
b. The clotting cascade is activated and fibrinolysis is inhibited, frequently leading to development of DIC.
c. Peripheral vasodilation occurs resulting in decreased systemic vascular resistance (SVR). At the same time, catecholemines and angiotensin II are elevated, as evidenced by resistance of the vascular smooth muscles to constrict, leading to poor response to vasopressors.
d. Early in sepsis, cardiac output (CO) is increased and is able to maintain blood pressure in spite of the reduced afterload that results from the vasodilation.
e. As sepsis progresses, myocardial function becomes impaired and CO decreases.

Table 3.8

Definition of Terms for the Septic State

Bacteremia or fungemia	Blood cultures positive for bacteria or fungi

SIRS[a]	A syndrome characterized by at leat two of the following:
	   Hyperthermia or hypothermia (oral temp > 38°C or < 36°C)
	   Hyperventilation (respiratory rate > 20 breaths/min)
	   Tachycardia (> 90 beats/min)
	   Leukocytosis (>12,000/μL) or leukopenia (< 4000/μl)

Sepsis[a]	SIRS of suspected or proven microbial origin
Severe sepsis[a]	Sepsis with organ dyfunction or lactic acidosis
Septic shock[a]	Sepsis with systolic blood pressure < 90 mm Hg or 40 mm Hg below patient's baseline that is unresponsive to fluid resuscition
MODS[a]	Dysfunction of more than one organ (e.g., lungs, kidney, heart, liver, CNS)

[a] Terms suggested by the American College of Chest Physicians in 1992.

Source: Abernathy, V.E., & Lieberthal, W. (2002). Acute renal failure in the critically ill patient. *Critical Care Clinics, 18,* 203-222. Used with permission from Elsevier.

f. Intravascular fluid loss occurs because of capillary leak syndrome and third spacing.
g. There is decreased preload due to vasodilation and loss of intravascular volume due to increased vascular permeability. The combination of all these factors leads to hypotension.
h. Sepsis and SIRS are often associated with MODS.
i. The cause of ATN in sepsis is renal hypoperfusion and ischemic injury to proximal tubule cells (see Figure 3.6).
4. Nursing interventions and collaborative treatments.
    a. Recombinant human activated protein C (Xigris) is a natural anticoagulant and an antiinflammatory agent that has proved effective in the treatment of sepsis.
        (1) Effect appears to be a feedback mechanism between the coagulation system and the inflammatory cascade.
        (2) Inhibition of thrombin generation by activated protein C decreases inflammation by inhibiting platelet activation, neutrophil recruitment, and mast-cell degranulation.
        (3) A major risk of using activated protein C is hemorrhage. It should not be used with a platelet count less than 30,000 per cubic millimeter (mm).

        (4) No anticoagulation should be used in extracorporeal systems for hemodialysis, SLEDD, or CRRT while a patient is being given activated protein C.
    b. Intensive insulin therapy to keep blood glucose level between 80 and 110 has resulted in lower morbidity and mortality rates in critically ill patients with sepsis.
        (1) The protective mechanism of insulin is unknown.
        (2) Correcting hyperglycemia may improve the bacterial phagocytic action of neutrophils that is impaired in sepsis.
    c. Volume resuscitation to optimize preload, afterload and contractility of the heart in patients with severe sepsis has improved the likelihood of survival.
        (1) Use of crystalloid, vasoactive agents, and transfusions of red blood cells to increase oxygen delivery have all been found to have positive influence.
        (2) Monitors for adequacy of oxygen delivery includes normalizing values of mixed venous oxygen saturation, lactate concentration, base deficit, and pH.
    d. RRT support is provided as needed.

F. TTP-HUS (thrombotic thrombocytopenia purpura-hemolytic uremic syndrome).
    1. This is a disorder in which microthrombi

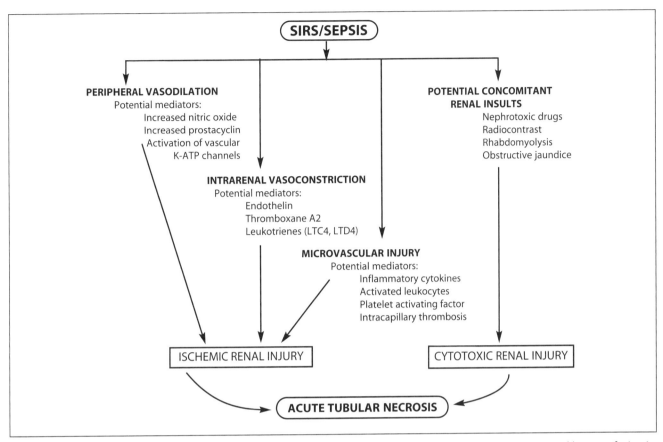

Figure 3.6. Mechanisms of ATN in sepsis. ATN associated with sepsis is largely caused by ischemic injury. Renal hypoperfusion is the combined result of peripheral vasodilation, intrarenal vasocontriction, and microvascular injury to the renal vasculature. These events commonly cause renal ischemia in sepsis even in the absence of hypotension. When septic shock develops, the incidence of ATN markedly increases. Because patients with sepsis often are subject to nephrotoxic events, cytotoxic injury to tubular cells often compounds the ischemic damage associated with sepis. LTC4 = leukotriene: C4: LTD4 = leukotriene: D4: K-ATP = ATP-sensitive potassium channels.

Source: Abernathy, V.E., & Lieberthal, W. (2002). Acute renal failure in the critically ill patient. *Critical Care Clinics, 18,* 203-222. Used with permission.

occlude the terminal ends of arterioles and capillaries.
2. It leads to ischemia in various organs, including the kidneys.
3. Presentation and assessment.
   a. Classic symptoms of TTP-HUS include microangiopathic hemolytic anemia, thrombocytopenia, fever, neurologic changes, and kidney failure (see Table 3.9).
   b. The occluding lesions in the terminal arterioles and capillaries consist of platelet aggregation and von Willebrand Factor (vWF) of unusually large molecular weight.
   c. Metalloproteinase is an enzyme that normally breaks up large clumps of vWF, which seems to be decreased or ineffective in patients with TTP-HUS.

d. Thrombocytopenia with counts dropping below 10,000/mm³ is classic.
   e. LDH (lactic dehydrogenase) is the primary indicator of intravascular red cell destruction (hemolysis).
   f. TTP and HUS are often difficult to differentiate.
      (1) In general, patients who develop kidney failure are described as having HUS. Compared to TTP patients, they may have less severe thrombocytopenia, less elevation in LDH, and fewer schistocytes on smear. Kidney failure develops due to infarction and kidney cortical necrosis, leading to occlusion of tubular lumina with the debris of the necrosis, fibrin, and hemolyzed red blood cells (RBCs).

Table 3.9

Diagnostic Criteria for TTP – HUS to Initiate Therapeutic Plasmapheresis Exchange

Classic pentad of symptoms TTP-HUS	Current dyad of symptoms TTP-HUS (in the absence of another apparent cause)
Microangiopthic anemia (MAHA) Thrombocytopenia purpura Neurologic disease Renal disease Fever	Microangiopathic anemia (MAHA) Thrombocytopenia purpura

Adapted from George, J.N., Gilcher, R.O., Smith, J.W., Chandler, L., Duvall, D., & Ellis, C. (1998). Thrombotic thrombocytopenic purpura-hemolytic uremic syndrome: Diagnosis and management. *Journal of Clinical Apheresis, 13,* 120-125. Printed in Myers, L. (2002). Thrombotic thrombocytopenia purpura-hemolytic uremic syndrome: Pathophysiology and management. *Nephrology Nursing Journal, 29,* 171-182. Used with permission.

(2) TTP patients may arrive more acutely ill than HUS patients, with signs of systemic platelet aggregation causing ischemia involving the central nervous system and/or the GI system. They will also have extreme thrombocytopenia, significantly elevated LDH, and more schistocytes on smear in comparison to HUS patients.

(3) When the diagnosis of TTP or HUS is unclear, TPE may be used initially.

g. There are several variations of TTP and HUS.

(1) Acute idiopathic TTP.

(a) Single episode occurs without a known cause in late adolescence and middle life with no recurrence.

(b) Intermittent recurs intermittently up to 8 years after the initial illness.

(2) Chronic relapsing TTP: rare, congenital condition of infancy or early childhood with frequent episodes of hemolysis that respond to infusions of FFP to replace the metalloproteinase.

(3) Chronic unremitting TTP: adult patients with persistent elevations of LDH, elevated reticulocytes, and thrombocytopenia despite treatment.

(4) Acquired HUS: occurs after GI infection with *E. coli* or other gram-negative organisms.

(5) Childhood HUS: most occur before age 6 months and present with bloody diarrhea; usually self-limiting with intravenous (IV) fluids and supportive care.

(6) Familial HUS: rare condition with defect of Factor H gene with high mortality rate, recurrence rate, and development of chronic kidney failure.

4. Nursing interventions and collaborative treatments for TTP.

a. Treatment of choice is therapeutic plasma exchange (TPE).

b. Increasing platelet count and decreasing LDH are markers of successful treatment.

G. HELLP.

1. A potentially fatal syndrome for the mother related to a progression of severe preeclampsia.

2. Can also decrease perfusion of the placenta and threaten the fetus with a potential for hypoxia, malnutrition, small size for gestational age, acidosis, mental disabilities, or death.

3. Presentation and assessment.

a. In HELLP.

(1) Hemolysis is a microangiopathic hemolytic anemia.

(2) Elevated liver enzymes are related to obstruction of hepatic blood flow by fibrin deposits.

(3) Thrombocytopenia (low platelets) is a result of increased consumption and/or increased destruction of platelets (see Figure 3.7).

b. This syndrome can begin in the third trimester of pregnancy or as late as 7 days after delivery.

c. HELLP can be ranked into three classes.

(1) Class 1 = Platelet count < 50,000/mm³.

(2) Class 2 = Platelet count 50,000 to < 100.000/mm³.

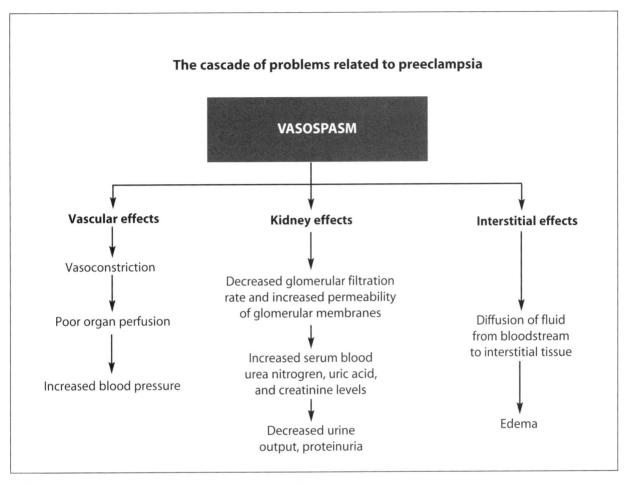

Figure 3.7. The cascade of problems related to preeclampsia.

Source: Pillitteri, A. (Ed.) (2002). *Maternal & Child Health Nursing* (4th ed.). Lippincott, Williams & Wilkins. Used with permission.

(3) Class 3 = Platelet count 100,000 to 150,000/mm³.
d. Lab values.
  (1) Tend to worsen following delivery and then start to normalize after 3 or 4 days.
  (2) Monitor LDH and platelet count to determine changes in disease process.
4. Nursing interventions and collaborative treatments.
  a. In Class 1, expediting delivery of the fetus (within 48 hours) is the treatment of choice.
  b. In Class 2 and 3, more conservative management can be considered based on gestational age along with close monitoring of the condition of the mother and the fetus.
  c. TPE has been effective in treating HELLP patients with severe lab values, such as platelet count less than 30,000/mm³ and persistent elevation of LDH.

d. TTP-HUS can occur in complicated pregnancies causing AKI/ARF requiring treatment with both TPE and hemodialysis to support full recovery.

H. Patients with drug intoxication.
  1. Aspirin (ASA) intoxication.
    a. Most common cause of death is acute noncardiogenic pulmonary edema.
    b. One of our oldest medications and is widely used.
    c. Rapidly metabolized when ingested into salicylic acid.
    d. Other sources of salicylate products.
      (1) Wart remover compounds.
      (2) Methylsalicylates are commonly used in creams and liniments for musculoskeletal pain.
        (a) Oil of wintergreen (if ingested).
        (b) Some herbal remedies.

e. Presentation and assessment.
 (1) Manifestations.
  (a) Nausea and vomiting.
  (b) Tinnitus and vertigo.
  (c) Diarrhea.
  (d) Respiratory alkalosis or mixed respiratory alkalosis-metabolic acidosis.
  (e) Hyperthermia or normothermia.
  (f) Hypovolemia.
  (g) Hypotension.
  (h) Tachycardia.
  (i) Agitation.
  (j) Altered mental status.
  (k) Cerebral edema.
  (l) General distress.
 (2) Serum salicylate level greater than 40 mg/dL indicates toxicity.

f. Nursing interventions and collaborative treatment.
 (1) Monitor for bleeding and use no heparin during hemodialysis.
 (2) Draw serial serum salicylate levels peripherally rather than from a dialysis access catheter to avoid recirculation that could alter serum drug levels.
 (3) Consult with nephrologist to discontinue bicarbonate IV solution prior to initiating HD treatment to prevent over compensating for metabolic acidosis.
 (4) Dialysis is the treatment indicated for the patient with acute pulmonary edema even with an ASA level not at a toxic level.
 (5) Laboratory toxicity reference ranges are different among commercial laboratories.
 (6) Volume resuscitation and glucose supplementation may be needed in severe intoxication, which can impact the hemodialysis treatment (see Table 3.10).

2. Ethylene glycol.
 a. An ingredient of automotive antifreeze, windshield wiper fluid and solvents, which may produce lethal serum levels with only a 100 mL ingestion.
 b. Toxicology and nephrology physicians collaborate to determine the most efficient course of treatment.
 c. Presentation and assessment.
  (1) Serum ethylene glycol level exceeding 50 mg/dL indicates toxicity.
  (2) Manifestations.
   (a) Confusion.
   (b) Drunkenness.
   (c) Convulsions.
   (d) Tachypnea.
   (e) Pulmonary edema.
   (f) Severe high anion gap with metabolic acidosis.
   (g) Coma.
   (h) Myocarditis.
   (i) Increased plasma osmolar gap.
  (3) AKI/ARF occurs due to urine oxalate precipitation that delays excretion of toxic metabolites.
 d. Nursing interventions and collaborative treatment.
  (1) Hemodialysis is required to remove the toxic metabolites using a large surface area dialyzer (> 1.5 m^2), a blood flow rate of 300 mL/min or greater, and a bicarbonate dialysate bath.
  (2) Fomepizole IV rapidly and competitively inhibits alcohol dehydrogenase, more potently than alcohol. It is the antidote of choice for ethylene glycol and methanol intoxication.
   (a) To compensate for fomepizole elimination during dialysis, clarify fomepizole dosing with nephrologist.
   (b) The frequency of dosing should be increased to every 4 hours during HD.
   (c) Administer an additional dose at the beginning of dialysis if greater than 6 hours since the last dose.
   (d) During HD, administer fomepizole after blood pump in the infusion port of the venous chamber if no other central line or IV catheter is available.
  (3) Treat metabolic acidosis with sodium bicarbonate infusion. Clarify with nephrologists if this infusion should be discontinued once HD is initiated.
  (4) If fomepizole is not available, ethanol should be used as an antidote to decrease the toxic effects of the poisoning. Once HD has been initiated, administer the ethanol infusion after blood pump in the infusion port of the venous chamber if no other central line or IV catheter is available.
  (5) Serial serum ethylene glycol levels should be monitored.
   (a) HD should be continued until levels are less than 20 mg/dL.
   (b) Rebound can be expected within 12 hours.
   (c) Repeat HD treatment may be necessary.

Table 3.10

Overview of Aspirin Intoxication

Clinical and laboratory features
- Common: tachypnea, tinnitus, nausea, vomiting, acid-base abnormalities
- Severe cases: hyperthermia, altered mental status, pulmonary edema

Diagnostic evaluation
- Salicylate level, arterial blood gas, basic metabolic panel (Chem-7), chest radiograph
- Repeat salicyclate level every 2 hours until level declining
- Repeat blood gas every 2 hours until acid-base status stable or improving

Treatment
- Avoid intubation if possible
- Administer supplemental oxygen as needed
- Volume resuscitate unless cerebral or pulmonary edema is present
- Administer multiple doses of activated charcoal (first dose: 1 g/kg up to 50 grams PO)
- Administer supplemental glucose in patients with altered mental status, even if serum glucose concentration is normal
- Alkalinize with sodium bicarbonate
  - Bolus therapy: $NaHCO_3$, 2–3 mEq/kg IV push (adults)
  - Maintenance therapy: 132 mEq $NaHCO_3$ in 1 L of D5W, run at 250 cc/h (adults) or 50–100 meq $NaHCO_3$ in 1 L D5W, run at 1.5 to 2 times maintenance (children)
  - DO NOT USE ACETAZOLAMIDE TO ALKALINIZE THE URINE
- Alert nephrology team early in the patient's clinical course; consider hemodialysis for:
  - Profoundly altered mental status
  - Pulmonary or cerebral edema
  - Renal insufficiency that interferes with salicylate excretion
  - Fluid overload that prevents the administration of sodium bicarbonate
  - A plasma salicylate concentration >100 mg/dL (7.2 mmo1/L)
  - Clinical deterioration despite aggressive and appropriate supportive care

Source: Traub, S.J. (2007). ASA intoxication overview. In B.D. Rose (Ed.), *UpToDate*. Waltham, MA. Copyright 2007 UpToDate, Inc. For more information visit http://www.uptodate.com. Used with permission.

(6) Monitor metabolic acidosis with arterial blood gases (ABGs). Continue HD until it is corrected.
(7) If the lab is unable to perform timely ethylene glycol levels, HD treatment should continue for no less than 8 hours, depending on the serum level at initiation.
(8) Systemic heparin anticoagulation during HD to prevent clotting the system is acceptable.
  (a) These patients usually have normal hemoglobin and hematocrit levels.
  (b) Reconsider if the patient has underlying chronic kidney injury or disease.
(9) Forced diuresis with fluids and mannitol may preserve kidney function during ethylene glycol intoxication by preventing oxalate formation. However, if the patient develops pulmonary edema during HD.
  (a) Mannitol may need to be discontinued due to its osmotic pull.
  (b) Ultrafiltration rate should be clarified with the nephrologist.
3. Methanol.
  a. A component of solvents, varnish, de-icing solutions, and other solutions containing wood alcohols to include "moonshine."
  b. Mortality rate is 80% or greater in patients who present with seizures, coma or pH < 7.0. Without these symptoms, the mortality rate is less than 6%.

c. Presentation and assessment.
  (1) Serum methanol level greater than 50 mg/dL indicates toxicity.
  (2) Methanol poisoning presents similarly to ethylene glycol poisoning.
    (a) Early presentation is confusion.
    (b) Metabolic acidosis begins 12–36 hours after ingestion.
    (c) Retinal involvement also occurs in 12–36 hours.
  (3) Manifestations include:
    (a) Weakness.
    (b) Nausea.
    (c) Headache.
    (d) Decreased vision.
    (e) High risk of permanent blindness.
  (4) Nursing interventions and collaborative treatments are similar to ethylene glycol intoxication. See Section 3, Chapter 10, V.H.2.d.
4. Lithium carbonate.
  a. Mortality rate is approximately 25% with an acute overdose.
  b. In patients intoxicated during maintenance therapy, 10% suffer permanent neurologic damage and the mortality rate is 9%.
  c. Presentation and assessment.
    (1) Serum lithium greater than 4.0 mEq/L indicate toxicity, regardless of the clinical status of the patient, and treatment with HD is indicated.
    (2) Manifestations.
      (a) Common characteristics.
        [1] Neuromuscular irritability.
        [2] Nausea.
        [3] Diarrhea.
      (b) Other possible symptoms.
        [1] Muscle weakness.
        [2] Increased deep tendon reflexes.
        [3] Somnolence.
        [4] T-wave flattening.
        [5] Coma eventually leading to death.
  d. Nursing interventions and collaborative treatment.
    (1) Primary medical management includes discontinuing diuretics and initiating 0.45% normal saline IV for rehydration.
    (2) The initial HD treatment should last 6–8 hours, until the serum level is 0.6 mEq/L or lower.
    (3) Hemodialysis is very effective at clearing lithium. However, levels may rebound within 12 hours of treatment.
    (4) Consecutive HD should be performed

until lithium levels stay at or below 1.0 mEq/L for 6–8 hours after treatment.
    (5) Continuous renal replacement therapy (CRRT) may be an effective modality choice to minimize rebound.

VI. Special patient populations and ARF.

A. Pregnancy.
  1. AKI/ARF occurs in 1 of every 2000–5000 pregnancies.
  2. Presentation and assessment.
    a. Frequency distribution is bimodal.
      (1) First peak in early pregnancy: associated with septic abortion and shock or fluid and electrolyte imbalances from hyperemsis.
      (2) Second peak in final gestational month: associated with preeclampsia, hemorrhagic complications, and abruptio placentae.
    b. AKI/ARF also associated with prolonged intrauterine fetal death, disseminated intravascular coagulation (DIC), urinary tract obstruction from stones, and/or ureteral obstruction from size and position of the uterus.
  3. Nursing interventions and collaborative treatment.
    a. Treatment similar to nongravidas with ARF.
      (1) Since urea, creatinine, and other substances cross the placenta, dialysis may need to be implemented early and performed more frequently to maintain a normal fetal environment.
      (2) Dialysate may need to be adjusted to lower levels of bicarbonate and higher levels of magnesium.
    b. Intradialytic monitoring to prevent hypotension and hypertension.
    c. Collaborate with obstetric (OB) nurses for fetal monitoring during hemodialysis treatments.

B. Gerontologic patients.
  1. Older adults experience an increased incidence of AKI/ARF; prevalence is increased threefold.
  2. Factors influencing the occurrence of AKI/ARF in the elderly.
    a. Increased systemic diseases.
    b. Structural changes in the aging kidneys.
    c. Functional changes in the aging kidneys.
  3. Presentation and assessment.
    a. Similar to younger patients, but more likely

to be superimposed on underlying kidney insufficiency.

b. Presence of other comorbidities may interfere with expedient diagnosis in the elderly.

c. Interpretation of diagnostic data may vary in the elderly (see Table 3.11).

d. Up to 90% mortality in the elderly in AKI/ARF occurring in an ICU and/or associated with sepsis.

e. Iatrogenic factors also put the elderly patient at risk for AKI/ARF.

 (1) Aggressive treatment of congestive heart failure with diuretics, leading to volume contraction and decreased kidney perfusion.

 (2) Salt restriction and diuretics for treatment of hypertension.

 (3) Medication management.

  (a) NSAIDs.

  (b) ACE inhibitors.

  (c) Combinations of medications (e.g., NSAIDs, ACEI, diuretics).

4. Causes of acute prerenal failure in the elderly.

 a. External losses of fluids with inadequate fluid replacement (dehydration).

  (1) Decreased concentrating ability of the

Table 3.11

Diagnostic Parameters in the Elderly

Test	Rationale	Adult	Elderly	Implications
Renal Ultrasound	Renal weight decreases 20–40% between the ages of 30 and 90	Renal Length – 9 cm Abnormal – Less than 9 cm or a difference of 1.5 cm	Decrease in renal length by 2 cm	Decrease in size of kidneys in elderly does not necessarily imply chronicity as it would in the adult
Serum Creatinine	Decreased muscle mass and diminished production of endogenous creatinine	Age 40–60 M 1.1–1.5 mg/dl F 1.0–.97 mg/dl	Age 60–99 M 1.5–1.20 mg/dl F 0.99–0.91 mg/dl	Serum creatinine can not be used as a marker for kidney function in the elderly
Creatinine Clearance	Age-related reduction in renal plasma flow and glomerular filtration rate	140 mL/min/1.73 m^2	97 mL/min/1.73 m^2	Cockcroft and Gault formula should be used to determine Cr clearance (kidney function) in the elderly
Urine Osmolarity	Tubular function decreases causing less effective concentration of urine	1,109 mOsm/kg	882 mOsm/kg	Measurement of urine osmolality is of limited value in differentiating prerenal azotemia from acute tubular necrosis in the elderly
Fractional Excretion of Sodium (FENa$^+$)	Decreased capacity to reabsorb sodium by the ascending loop of Henle	Prerenal < 1% Intrinsic > 1%	Not reliable values	Cannot be used to differentiate between prerenal azotemia and acute tubular necrosis in the elderly

References: Davison, A. (1998). Renal disease in the elderly. *Nephron, 80,* 6-19; Pascual, J., Fernando, F., & Ortuno, J. (1995). The elderly patient with acute renal failure. *Journal of the American Society of Nephrology, 6*(2), 144-149.

kidney.
  (2) Inability of kidney to retain sodium.
  (3) Impairment of thirst regulation.
  b. Internal redistribution of volume from intravascular to interstitial space.
    (1) Sepsis.
      (a) Decreased urine output may precede temperature spike by hours.
      (b) Absence of temperature spike is not unusual in the elderly.
    (2) Hypoproteinemia.
      (a) Nephrotic syndrome.
      (b) Cirrhosis/hepatorenal failure.
      (c) Malnutrition.
      (d) Tissue injury, e.g., burns, pancreatitis.
    (3) Decreased cardiac output.
      (a) Myocardial dysfunction.
      (b) Pericardial disease.
    (4) Drug induced nephropathy, by altering intrarenal hemodynamics.
      (a) ACE inhibitors.
        [1] Mechanism: fall in blood pressure and efferent glomerular arteriolar tone that decreases transglomerular hydraulic pressure and thereby glomerular filtration rate (GFR).
        [2] Used to treat hypertension, congestive heart failure, and secondary prevention of myocardial infarction.
        [3] Risk factors.
          [a] The presence of bilateral renovascular disease.
          [b] Arterial stenosis in a solitary kidney.
          [c] Volume depletion.
          [d] Concomitant treatment with diuretics.
          [e] Low salt diet.
          [f] Cardiac failure.
          [g] Combined treatment with NSAIDs.
          [h] Presence of diabetes mellitus.
        [4] Withdrawal of drug and volume repletion, if indicated, will result in kidney recovery.
      (b) NSAIDs.
        [1] Incidence of NSAID-induced uremia in patients with baseline kidney insufficiency may be as high as 30%.
        [2] Mechanism A.
          [a] NSAIDs inhibit

cyclooxygenase-mediated arachidonic acid metabolites.
          [b] They, in turn, inhibit production of prostaglandins, leaving the vasoconstrictive hormones (norepinephrine and angiotensin II) unopposed.
          [c] Decrease in circulating volume may result in severe kidney vasoconstriction and a rapid decrease in renal blood flow and GFR.
        [3] Mechanism B.
          [a] Immunologically mediated nephrotic syndrome.
          [b] Release of lymphokines and eosinophil chemotactic factors cause a diffuse infiltration of the kidney interstitium by mononuclear inflammatory cells and eosinophils.
          [c] Leads to tubulitis.
        [4] Risk factors.
          [a] Heart failure.
          [b] Cirrhosis.
          [c] Nephrotic syndrome.
          [d] Volume depletion.
          [e] Combined treatment with ACE inhibitors.
        [5] Withdrawal of medication usually results in recovery of kidney function.
      (c) Calcineurin inhibitors: cyclosporine and tacrolimas.
        [1] Mechanism: vasoconstriction of the afferent kidney arterioles caused by excessive endothelin-1 production.
        [2] Kidney function improves or recovers completely after reducing the dosage or discontinuing the drug.
5. Causes of acute renal parenchymal (intrarenal) failure in the elderly.
  a. Acute tubular necrosis (ATN).
    (1) Drug-induced nephrotoxicity occurrence is increased in the elderly.
    (2) Elderly patients have a longer recovery period.
    (3) Recovery may be compromised by the presence of comorbidities.
  b. Tubulointerstitial nephritis.
    (1) May be idiopathic or related to infection or a drug.

(2) Increased incidence over age 60.

(3) Discontinuation of medication will frequently result in return of kidney function.

c. Acute glomerulonephritis (GN).

(1) Responsible for 19% of AKI/ARF in the elderly.

(2) Rapidly progressive glomerular nephritis (RPGN) is most common type in the elderly.

(3) Treatable glomerular and tubulointerstitial diseases are common in the elderly, underscoring the importance of early diagnosis.

(4) Kidney biopsy, the gold standard for establishing diagnosis of these diseases, is well tolerated by older adults.

d. Atheroembolic kidney disease.

(1) This age group makes up approximately 36% of reported cases.

(2) Strong association between atrial fibrillation and atheroembolic kidney disease has been made.

e. Cholesterol embolization.

(1) The elderly make up 63% of the reported cases.

(2) Prognosis is dependent on the extent of organ(s) involvement. Kidney function may recover even if a course of kidney replacement therapy is required during the acute stage.

6. Acute obstructive uropathy (postrenal acute kidney failure) in the elderly.

a. Responsible for 10–15% of the cases of AKI/ARF in the elderly.

b. Prostatic disease is the most common cause of obstructive uropathy in males.

c. In females, bladder involvement and tumors of the pelvic organs are primarily responsible for obstruction.

d. 4.5% of the elderly population with obstructive uropathy did not demonstrate upper tract dilation with ultrasound or CT scan.

(1) This may be caused by a tumor encapsulating the kidneys and ureters.

(2) Also may be present in patients with retroperitoneal fibrosa.

e. Treatment will focus on relieving obstruction and supportive RRT until kidney function returns.

7. Nursing care and collaborative interventions.

a. Elderly patient generally become symptomatic at lower levels of BUN and serum creatinine than younger patients.

b. Symptoms the elderly patient may present.

(1) Exacerbation of previously well-controlled heart failure.

(2) Unexplained changes in mental status.

(3) Changes in behavior.

(4) Personality changes.

(5) Change in sense of well-being.

c. Indications for treatment.

(1) Pulmonary edema.

(2) Hyperkalemia.

(3) Severe acidemia.

(4) Catabolic state.

d. Modalities for treatment of elderly include intermittent hemodialysis, daily hemodialysis, SLEDD, and continuous renal replacement therapy.

e. Continuous cyclic peritoneal dialysis (CCPD) works well with elderly patients who cannot tolerate hemodialysis, e.g., heart failure.

f. Choice of treatment modality will depend on the clinical presentation of the patient as well as the patient's hemodynamic status.

g. Osmolality and fluid shifts associated with intermittent hemodialysis are not well tolerated by elderly patients because of their altered compensatory mechanisms associated with the aging process.

Chapter 11

Hemodialysis in the Acute Care Setting

Purpose
The purpose of this section is to describe the care of patients undergoing hemodialysis in the acute care setting.

Objectives
Upon completion of this chapter, the learner will be able to:
1. Develop a nursing care plan for hemodialysis patients in the acute care setting.
2. Discuss pharmaceutical and dialytic interventions for treatment of intradialytic hypotension and other complications experienced by patients in the acute care setting.
3. Describe tools available to the nurse in the acute setting to evaluate the care needs and patient responses to therapies used.

I. Patients with hemodialysis (HD) needs in the acute care setting.

A. Patients with acute kidney injury (AKI) with solute or fluid imbalance.

B. Patients with AKI superimposed on chronic kidney disease (CKD) ("acute on chronic") with solute or fluid imbalance.

C. Patients with CKD stage 5/end-stage renal disease (ESRD) in the acute care setting.
   1. Patients with a dialysis access-related event.
   2. Patients with a medical or surgical complication.
   3. Patients needing physical or mental rehabilitation.

D. Patients with CKD stages 3 and 4. The frequency and severity of AKI episodes is an indication of a patient's progression to CKD stage 5/ESRD.

II. Prehemodialysis patient assessment.

A. The purpose of an acute patient nephrology nursing assessment is to obtain baseline information relative to the patient's physical and/or mental status to determine appropriate interventions to achieve an adequate and safe dialysis treatment.

B. An assessment of the patient must be done prior to initiation of every dialysis treatment and documented on the treatment record (refer to Appendix 3.2: Acute Hemodialysis Flowsheet, at the end of Section 3).

C. Medicare guidelines and nursing scope of practice regulations designate a registered nurse as the appropriate professional to:
   1. Complete the pre-, intra-, and post-hemodialysis treatment assessment.
   2. Collaboratively formulate a treatment plan.
   3. Delegate care that does not require nursing judgment and ongoing nursing assessment to trained and supervised unlicensed personnel when appropriate.
   4. Perform and oversee treatment interventions.
   5. Evaluate the patient's response to treatment.

D. Patient history.
   1. Do not resuscitate (DNR) and advance directive status.
   2. Isolation precautions.

a. Reason for isolation.

b. Organisms cultured and when. Resistant organisms such as methicillin-resistant *Staphylococcus aureus* (MRSA) and vancomycin-resistant enterococcus (VRE) may require additional precautions.

c. Type of isolation and necessary precautions.

   (1) Standard precautions/universal precautions apply to all patients.

   (2) Airborne precautions are used to prevent transmission of the smallest airborne microorganisms. These pathogens can remain suspended in air for long periods of time and travel long distances. Transmission mechanism is inhalation. Patients are placed in negative pressure rooms.

   (3) Droplet precautions are used to distinguish the largest airborne organisms generated during coughing, sneezing, singing, talking, suctioning, and bronchoscopy. It is used for droplets that are propelled a short distance (usually 3 feet or less) in the air and are deposited on a host or in the environment. The transmission method is touch. Patients do not need to be placed in a negative pressure room.

   (4) Contact precautions are used for patients known or suspected to be infected or colonized with epidemiologically important microorganisms that can be transmitted by direct contact with the patient (direct transmission) or the patient's environment (indirect transmission). Resistant organism precautions are implemented for infections/colonizations caused by microorganisms resistant to several antimicrobial agents.

   (5) Strict isolation is used to control an outbreak occurrence or conditions requiring both airborne and contact precautions. It is a category of precautions that can be used to call attention to an epidemiologically important organism.

   (6) Neutropenic precautions are used when caring for patients with a compromised immune system.

3. Reason for admission.

a. Identifies the specific event or events that brought the patient to the acute care setting.

b. May be an exacerbation of a chronic condition or a new acute illness.

4. Current problem list.

a. Current medical diagnosis. Examples of expected diagnosis of patients requiring renal replacement therapy include the following:

   (1) CKD stages 1-5.

   (2) AKI.

   (3) Diabetes.

   (4) Hypertension.

   (5) Dyslipidemia.

   (6) Anemia.

   (7) Congestive heart failure.

   (8) Diastolic dysfunction.

   (9) Atrial fibrillation.

   (10) Atherosclerosis.

   (11) Systemic lupus erythematosis.

   (12) Cirrhosis.

   (13) Calcific uremic arteriolopathy also known as calciphylaxsis.

   (14) Infection.

     (a) Dialysis access-related.

     (b) Diabetic ulcer-related.

b. Recent surgical interventions.

   (1) Type and date of surgery. Examples of expected surgical procedures occurring on patients with concurrent renal replacement therapy needs would include the following:

     (a) Coronary artery bypass graft.

     (b) Heart valve replacement.

     (c) Kidney or other solid organ transplant.

     (d) Dialysis vascular access creation.

     (e) Ultrasound guided or open kidney biopsy.

     (f) Amputation.

   (2) Intraoperative or postoperative events.

     (a) Length of surgery.

     (b) Hypotension.

     (c) Blood loss.

     (d) Relative kidney hypoperfusion, e.g., cross-clamp time.

   (3) Wound healing considerations.

     (a) Minimize systemic anticoagulation.

     (b) Minimize edema.

     (c) Minimize uremic environment.

     (d) Optimize nitrogen balance with good nutrition and adequate dialysis.

   (4) Ventilation.

     (a) Cough and deep breathe.

     (b) Mobilization at least every 2 hours even while on renal replacement therapy.

     (c) Optimize fluid balance for good pulmonary function.

   (5) Pain control.

c. Recent diagnostic procedures.

(1) Chest x-ray.
 (a) Presence of pulmonary edema, effusion, and/or congestion.
 (b) Verify line placement.
(2) Computed tomography (CT), interventional radiology (IR), or magnetic resonance imaging (MRI) scan.
 (a) Placement of tunneled dialysis catheter.
 (b) Dialysis vascular access study.
 (c) Coronary angiogram.
 (d) Other diagnostic studies.
  [1] Rule out or define a tumor.
  [2] Define blood vessels anatomically or functionally.
  [3] Observe and define other systemic functions.
 (e) Exposure to contrast agents (see Section 3, Chapter 10, AKI).
 (f) FDA warns that gadolinium (MRI contrast agent) exposure is contraindicated in patients with reduced kidney function such as CKD stage 5/ESRD, due to risk of nephrogenic systemic fibrosis (NSF) also known as nephrogenic fibrosing dermopathy (NFD).
(3) Echocardiogram.
 (a) Heart size.
 (b) Ventricular function.
 (c) Vegetation on heart valves.
(4) Ultrasound.
 (a) Rule out hydronephrosis.
 (b) Vein mapping in preparation for dialysis access placement.
 (c) Guidance for kidney biopsy.
(5) Colonoscopy to look for gastrointestinal bleeding.
5. Medications.
 a. Allergies.
 b. Dose adjustment. Patients with compromised kidney clearance may need to have their medication doses adjusted. Some medications have a narrow therapeutic window and are subject to over or under dosing.
 c. Those medications that have significant clearance during hemodialysis may need dosing after hemodialysis or supplemental dosing to adjust for this clearance.
 d. Clearance of medications with dialysis increases for medications with a small molecular size, small volume of distribution, higher water solubility, and low protein binding.
 e. If protein binding exceeds 90%, the

medication will be minimally cleared with dialysis and does not need supplemental dosing.
 f. Examples.
  (1) Analgesics.
   (a) Narcotic analgesics produce sedation that may be more profound in patients with renal insufficiency. The smallest effective dose should be used.
   (b) Meperidine, and morphine to a lesser degree, has metabolites that may accumulate and decrease the seizure threshold in patients with reduced kidney function.
  (2) Anticoagulants.
   (a) Patients may be on more than one form of anticoagulant, such as heparin and warfarin, affecting different points in the clotting cascade.
   (b) Heparin dosing during hemodialysis may need to be adjusted if patient is on maintenance anticoagulant therapy.
  (3) Antihypertensives.
   (a) Medication administration of antihypertensive medications should be correlated to minimize hypotensive complications during hemodialysis.
   (b) For once or twice a day medications, they should administered right after dialysis and/or 12 hours later.
  (4) Vasopressors (see Table 3.12).
   (a) Type.
   (b) Dose and recent titrations.
   (c) Patient's previous response to ultrafiltration.
  (5) Cardiovascular.
   (a) Digoxin is initiated at a reduced dose and maintained at a reduced dose, e.g., 0.125 mg every 2–3 days.
   (b) Diuretics.
    [1] Diuretics lose effectiveness on patients with reduced kidney function and larger doses may be necessary to achieve the desired effect.
    [2] Larger doses are associated with more adverse events, e.g., ototoxicity.

Table 3.12

Pressors and Their Actions

Pressors	Heart Rate (Chronotropic)	Contractility (Inotropic)	Vasoconstriction
Dopamine	+ +	+ +	+ +
Vasopressin	0	+/-	+ + +
Neosynephrine	0	0	+ + +
Levophed (Norepi)	+ +	+ +	+ + +
Dobutamine	+	+ + +	- (Dilates)
Epinephrine	+ + +	+ + +	+ +

Source: Dr. David Gillum, Western Nephrology Acute Dialysis Medical Director, Denver, Colorado (2005). Used with permission.

[3] Potassium-sparing diuretics are not typically used in patients with a GFR < 30 mL/min because of the risk for hyperkalemia.

(6) Antimicrobial agents. Dose adjustments to antibiotics are common in patients who are dependent on renal replacement therapy.
  (a) Therapeutic drug monitoring may be required to achieve the desired drug level for the patient.
  (b) If significant clearance is expected with intermittent hemodialysis, administer the antimicrobial agent after dialysis or provide a supplemental dose.

(7) Sedatives or hypnotics:
  (a) Patients with reduced kidney function taking a sedative or hypnotic experience excessive sedation as the most common adverse effect.
  (b) The etiology of somnolence or encephalopathy (e.g., uremic symptoms or oversedation) may be difficult to differentiate.

(8) Neuromuscular blocking agents (NMBA). Extreme caution should be taken in assessing mental status and respiratory effort on a patient dependent on renal replacement therapy after NMBA administration.
  (a) Curarization effect may last for > 24 hours after dosing with some NMBA.

  (b) Pancuronium should be avoided in patients dependent on renal replacement therapy because of the potential for a prolonged recurarization effect.

(9) Hypoglycemic agents.
  (a) Oral hypoglycemic agents may result in prolonged hypoglycemia in patients with reduced kidney function.
  (b) Renal metabolism of insulin decreases with declining GFR.

(10) Antidepressants or selective serotonin-reuptake inhibitors (SSRIs). Side effects may include tremors and changes to gastrointestinal motility, sleep patterns, appetite, and sexual response.

(11) Eyrthropoietic-stimulating agents and iron.
  (a) Maintain outpatient dosing to avoid need for transfusion.
  (b) Dose adjustment may be indicated for inflammatory block related to acute illness.

(12) Immunosuppressants.
  (a) Maintain transplanted organ.
  (b) Suppress autoimmune disease activity.

E. Physical assessment.
  1. General assessment.
    a. Perform the physical assessment, documenting findings on the hemodialysis treatment record, and compare them to previous treatments to determine any changes in patient's clinical status that may require attention.

b. Assess patient for changes in energy and overall well-being.
2. Vital signs.
   a. Blood pressure (BP).
      (1) Noninvasive blood pressure (NIBP).
         (a) Place the BP cuff about 1 inch above the antecubital space of the upper arm.
         (b) BP readings taken on the wrist, ankle or thigh may provide falsely elevated BP measurements.
         (c) Use a cuff that reaches 1.5 times around the arm.
            [1] Using a cuff that is too small will provide a falsely high reading.
            [2] Conversely, using a cuff that is to large will provide a falsely low reading.
      (2) Arterial BP (ABP).
         (a) The arterial catheter is inserted into the radial, brachial, or femoral artery and connected to a continuous flush transducer system leveled to the right atrium and zeroed to atmosphere. The transducer is connected via pressure tubing to a pressurized flush system.
         (b) Provides continuous blood pressure monitoring and calculated mean arterial pressure (MAP) reading:
            MAP = (2 x diastolic BP + systolic BP)/3
         (c) Can be used for blood gas analysis or other laboratory test blood specimen sampling. Verify that the pressure line is anticoagulant-free if test results will be impacted by the presence of an anticoagulant.
         (d) Obtain NIBP readings for comparison to the ABP for accuracy at least once per shift.
         (e) Flush and observe the A-line waveform to evaluate accuracy of reading.
      (3) Obtain both sitting and standing BPs as patient condition permits to observe for orthostatic changes.
         (a) For the immobile patient, simulate sitting and standing by taking the BP with the head of the bed (HOB) down and then with the HOB elevated at an 80–90 degree angle.
         (b) Make certain repositioning patient does not compromise the patient's condition.
            [1] Keep the patient's head of bed at ≥ 30 degrees for patients with elevated intracranial pressure (ICP) to minimize intracranial pressure.
            [2] Patients who are ventilator dependent or receiving a tube feeding are at risk for aspiration of secretions or feeding and should not be left flat.
         (c) Orthostatic changes are defined as a systolic BP decrease > 20 mm Hg, a diastolic decrease > 10 mm Hg, or a pulse increase > 20 beats per minute between position changes.
         (d) Orthostatic changes in BP and or pulse readings taken within 2 minutes of the position change may reflect hypotension and/or vascular disease, which could be volume and/or medication related.
      (4) Elevated diastolic pressures along with other clinical manifestations may indicate right heart failure.
      (5) Auscultating the patient's blood pressure may be difficult when a patient is hypotensive, experiencing atrial fibrillation, or has vascular anomalies such as multiple vascular surgeries. Palpable BPs may be necessary with those patients to estimate systolic pressure.
         (a) To palpate the blood pressure, place a cuff on the upper arm.
         (b) Palpate the brachial pulse or the radial pulse.
         (c) Inflate the cuff until the pulse is no longer felt.
         (d) Slowly deflate the cuff, noting the point at which the pulse is felt again, this is the systolic pressure.
         (e) Example: If patient's blood pressure was palpated at 90 mm Hg, document "90/P."
         (f) If the patient's arm is too swollen or BP is so low that a pulse cannot be palpated, a Doppler may be used to obtain systolic BP readings and documented as "90/P obtained from Doppler."
   b. Temperature.
      (1) Uremic patients often manifest a body temperature < 37° C. Setting the dialysis solution temperature higher than the patient's temperature will cause vasodilation and increase the incidence of hypotension.

(2) Elevated temperature may indicate infection, malignancies, or other illness. The patient should be assessed to find the potential cause of the temperature elevation.

(3) Elevated temperature will cause an increase in insensible fluid loss.

3. Fluid balance.
   a. Intake and output (I/O).
      (1) Intake.
         (a) IV infusions.
         (b) Oral (PO) intake.
         (c) Gastric tube feeds.
      (2) Output.
         (a) Urine.
         (b) Ultrafiltrate removed.
         (c) Stool.
         (d) Drains, e.g., chest tube, nasogastric suction, and wounds.
         (e) Insensible losses related to burns, wounds, ventilation, or temperature elevation.
   b. Weight.
      (1) Patients on renal replacement therapy should be weighed at the same time daily to increase the likelihood of meaningful data.
      (2) Weights performed using a bed scale should standardize the linen and bed position.
      (3) Compare daily weight to "dry" weight in the outpatient setting or to the hospital admission weight, for an additional assessment of volume status.
   c. Edema.
      (1) Assess dependent areas for edema as fluid may shift to this position.
         (a) Sacral for supine patients.
         (b) Legs, feet, scrotum for sitting or ambulatory patients.
         (c) Facial or periorbital in the prone or reclined patient. Facial and upper extremity edema may also indicate blockage of venous return from occluded subclavian and jugular veins.
      (2) Pitting edema is the presence of fluid in tissue that mobilizes with pressure and does not rapidly refill after applied pressure is released.
      (3) Brawny edema presents with dark colored skin that appears distended but is resistant to pressure. The skin is so tight due to the excess fluid that the fluid cannot be displaced.

Table 3.13

Severity of Edema Classification Grading

Grading Level	Amount of Edema
0	No pitting
1+	Trace
2+	Mild
3+	Moderate
4+	Severe

Source: Springhouse Corporation. (1997). *Fluid & electrolytes made incredibly easy (p. 71)*. Philadelphia: Lippincott Williams & Wilkins. Used with permission.

      (4) Edema may be classified by grading 1-4. (see Table 3.13).
      (5) Anasarca is generalized edema.
      (6) Severe edema with venous status may result in skin ulceration and weeping.
   d. Ascites.
      (1) Fluid third-spaced in the peritoneal cavity.
      (2) Related to increased portal vein pressure, inflammation, and/or malignancy.
      (3) Ascitic fluid has relatively high protein content and resulting high oncotic pressure, making it difficult to mobilize into the vasculature for removal with ultrafiltration.
   e. Neck vein distention.
      (1) Have patient sit up to a 45-degree angle.
      (2) Have patient turn head to one side.
      (3) Locate external jugular vein and check for pulsation.
      (4) If vein pulsation ascends higher than 5 centimeters above the manubrium, positive neck vein distention is noted.
      (5) May indicate right heart failure.
   f. Skin turgor. Skin tenting indicates intravascular volume depletion.
   g. Mucous membranes. Dry mucous membranes indicate volume deficit.
   h. Evaluate results of hemodynamic monitoring devices.
   i. Review serum sodium levels for indications of hemoconcentration or hemodilution.

4. Dialysis access (see Section 12, Vascular Access, for further detail on assessment).
   a. Bruit.
   b. Thrill.
   c. Catheter exit site and dressing.
5. Skin. Assess for changes in integrity or suppleness. Patients on renal replacement therapy are at increased risk for calcific uremic arteriolopathy also known as calciphylaxis.
6. Cardiovascular.
   a. Heart rate.
      (1) Patients with a rate < 50 or > 120 beats/minute should be placed on a cardiac monitor during dialysis, especially if newly onset.
      (2) Rapid heart rate may be a result of anemia, hypotension, hypovolemia, or atrial fibrillation.
      (3) Auscultated heart rate < 50 beats/min may indicate digitalis toxicity requiring an adjustment in dialysate potassium and other medications.
   b. Heart rhythm. Arrhythmias (see Figure 3.8) may be due to:
      (1) Electrolyte and pH changes.
      (2) Heart failure.
      (3) Severe anemia.
      (4) Underlying ischemic and/or hypertensive cardiovascular disease.
      (5) Pericarditis.
      (6) Conduction system calcification.
   c. Heart sounds.
      (1) Friction rub indicates the development of pericarditis or may indicate recent myocardial infarction.
      (2) Gallop may indicate myocardial infarction, valvular disease, ventricular hypertrophy, hypertension, cardiomyopathy, volume overload, or ischemia.
      (3) Muffled or distant heart sounds may indicate fluid volume excess. Report to the nephrologist if this is a new onset.
      (4) Murmurs can be the result of increase in rate and velocity of blood flow, abnormal flow across stenosed or incompetent valves, or abnormal passages between chambers.
      (5) Muffled or diminished heart sounds during inspiration, may indicate pericardial effusion or cardiac tamponade.
         (a) Checking for a paradoxical pulse is indicated with these signs.

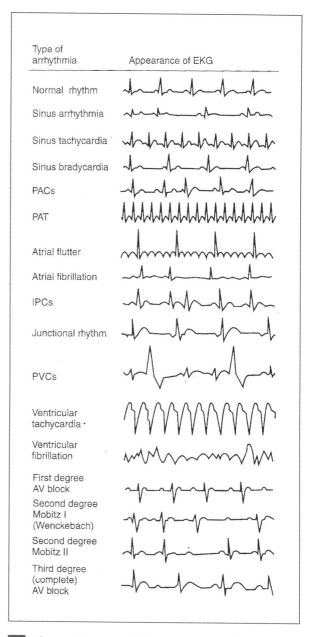

Figure 3.8. Normal EKG and types of arrhythmias.

Source: Monahan, L. (2002). *A practical guide to health assessment.* Philadelphia: W.B. Saunders Company. Used with permission.

         (b) Paradoxical pulse of 10 mm Hg or more is considered a hallmark of cardiac compression, pericardial effusion and/or cardiac tamponade (see Table 3.14).
   d. Noninvasive hemodynamic monitoring: bioimpedance or impedance cardiography (ICG).
      (1) Provides hemodynamic monitoring by electrodes that are placed on the neck and lower thorax (see Figure 3.9).

Table 3.14

Measuring Paradoxical Pulse

1. After placing BP cuff on patient, inflate it above the known systolic BP. Instruct patient to breathe normally.

2. While slowly deflating the cuff, auscultate BP.

3. Listen for the Korotkoff's sounds, which will occur during expiration with cardiac tamponade.

4. Note the manometer reading when the first sound occurs, and continue to deflate the cuff slowly until Korotkoff 's sounds are audible throughout inspiration and expiration.

5. Record the differences in millimeters of mercury between the first and second sounds. This is the pulsus paradoxus.

Source: Lokhandwala, K.A. (2002). Clinical signs in medicine: Pulsus paradoxus. *Clinical Signs, 48*(1), 46-49. Used with permission.

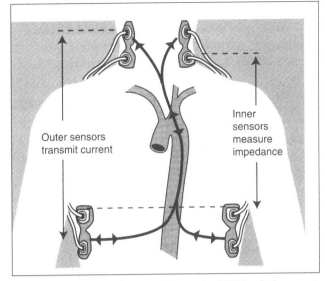

Figure 3.9. Impedance cardiography (ICG) lead placement.

Source: Hodges, R.K., Garrett, K.M., Chernecky, C., & Schumacher, L. (2005). *Real world nursing survival guide: Hemodynamic monitoring*, p. 145. St. Louis: Elsevier Saunders. Used with permission.

(2) Waveforms are reflective of the volume and velocity of aortic blood flow rather than blood pressure.

(3) Parameters measured are stroke volume (SV), cardiac output (CO), indices of myocardial contractility, and afterload.

e. Pulmonary artery (PA)/Swan-Ganz catheter (see Figure 3.10).

(1) Multi-lumen catheter with an inflatable balloon at the tip.

(2) Provides hemodynamic monitoring.

(3) Provides information about the left and right heart, differentiation of pressures, structures, and function.

(4) The ports include proximal port for measuring central venous pressure (CVP)/pulmonary artery pressure (PAP); cardiac output port/thermistor connector; PA distal infusion port, and balloon inflation port.

(5) It is inserted at the bedside through central venous approach in the external jugular or subclavian vein into the right side of the heart and into the pulmonary artery (see Figure 3.11).

(6) The PA catheter measures pressures within the right and left sides of the heart through a transducer creating a waveform on the monitor screen (see Figure 3.12).

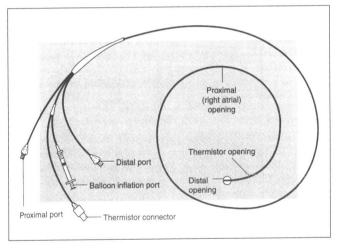

Figure 3.10. Swan-Ganz catheter ports.

Source: Hodges, R.K., Garrett, K.M., Chernecky, C., & Schumacher, L. (2005). *Real world nursing survival guide: Hemodynamic monitoring*, p. 39. St. Louis: Elsevier Saunders. Used with permission.

(7) Catheter provides an accurate picture of the patient's fluid volume status through measurements of PAP, including pulmonary artery systolic (PAS) and pulmonary artery diastolic (PAD) (see Figure 3.13), pulmonary artery wedge pressure (PAWP), CO (see Figure 3.14), and CVP (see Table 3.15). They provide information about how the left side of the heart is functioning, including its pumping ability, filling pressures, and

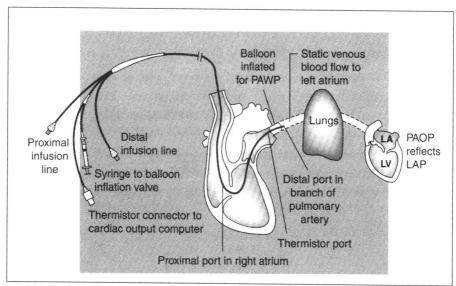

Figure 3.11. Advancement of the Swan-Ganz catheter into the heart.

Source: Hodges, R.K., Garrett, K.M., Chernecky, C., & Schumacher, L. (2005). *Real world nursing survival guide: Hemodynamic monitoring*, p. 115. St. Louis: Elsevier Saunders. Used with permission.

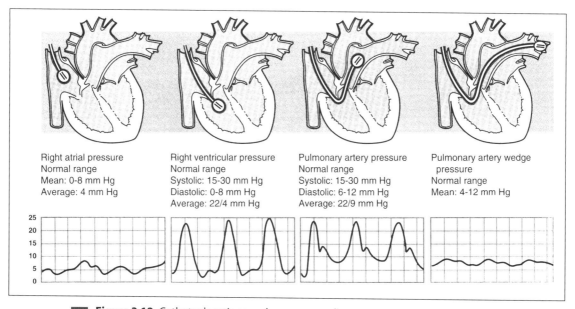

Figure 3.12. Catheter locations and pressure readings.

Source: Hodges, R.K., Garrett, K.M., Chernecky, C., & Schumacher, L. (2005). *Real world nursing survival guide: Hemodynamic monitoring*, p. 31. St. Louis: Elsevier Saunders. Used with permission.

vascular volume (see Table 3.16 and Table 3.17).

  f. Central venous pressure (CVP) monitoring.
    (1) Can be measured from a triple lumen catheter or through a Swan-Ganz catheter (see Figure 3.11).
    (2) Catheters are usually placed in the internal jugular vein (IJ) or subclavian vein.
    (3) Measures the pressure of the blood in the central venous circulation.

    (4) Useful indication of the patient's fluid status.
  7. Pulmonary.
    a. Oxygenation (see Table 3.18).
      (1) Assess oxygenation by checking oxygenation saturation using spot or continuous pulse oximeter.
      (2) Assess FiO$_2$ (fraction of inspired oxygen).
      (3) Review patient's arterial blood gas trend and current values.
      (4) Review chest x-ray.

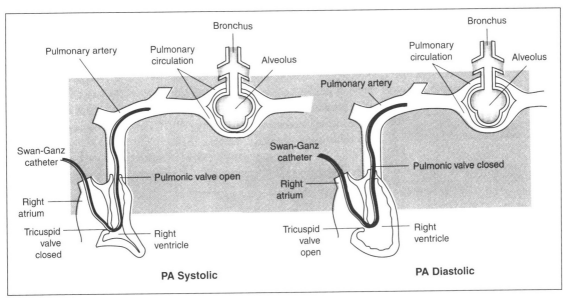

Figure 3.13. PA systolic and PA diastolic pressure readings.

Source: Hodges, R.K., Garrett, K.M., Chernecky, C., & Schumacher, L. (2005). *Real world nursing survival guide: Hemodynamic monitoring*, p. 107. St. Louis: Elsevier Saunders. Used with permission

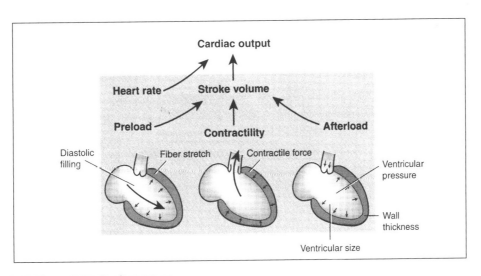

Figure 3.14. Cardiac output.

Source: Hodges, R.K., Garrett, K.M., Chernecky, C., & Schumacher, L. (2005). *Real world nursing survival guide: Hemodynamic monitoring*, p. 22. St. Louis: Elsevier Saunders. Used with permission

(5) Assess patient for signs and symptoms of cyanosis.
   (a) Central cyanosis is a blue coloration of the mucous membranes, ears, lips, and nose.
   (b) Peripheral cyanosis is a blue coloration to the upper and lower extremities.
b. Respiratory rate, rhythm, and pattern.
  (1) Respiratory distress/failure can develop from any condition that increases the work of breathing and/or decreases the respiratory drive (see Table 3.19).
  (2) Respiratory distress may respond to ultrafiltration with dialysis depending on the etiology.
  (3) When the lungs cannot adequately maintain tissue oxygenation or eliminate carbon dioxide, acute respiratory arrest and cardiac arrest can result.

Table 3.15

Hemodynamic Monitoring Definitions

Measurement		Definition	Normal Range
	Preload	Amount of blood filling the ventricle at the end of diastole.	
	Afterload	Amount of resistance against which the ventricle pumps.	
MAP	Mean arterial pressure	The average pressure in the peripheral arterial system during systole and diastole.	80–100 mm Hg
PAP	Pulmonary artery pressure	Measurement of right side of heart pressures.	average: 22/9
PAS	Pulmonary artery systolic	Pressure needed to open the pulmonic valve and send blood to the pulmonary circulation.	15–30 mm Hg
PAD	Pulmonary artery diastolic	Amount of resistance in the lungs between heartbeats.	6–12 mm Hg
CVP/RAP	Central venous pressure/Right atrial pressure	Measurement of pressure from the right atrium. CVP taken from superior or inferior vena cava; RAP from the right atrium.	2–8 mm Hg
PAWP PAOP PCWP	Pulmonary artery wedge Pulmonary artery occlusion Pulmonary capillary wedge	An indirect measurement of pulmonary venous pressure. Also reflects left atrial pressure and left ventricular end diastolic pressure. Measurement of preload.	6–12 mm Hg
CO	Cardiac output	Amount of blood ejected from the heart in one minute. Determined by heart rate and stroke volume.	4–8 L/min
CI	Cardiac index	Cardiac output that is corrected for body size (body surface area).	2.5–4 L/min
SV	Stroke volume	Volume of blood ejected from the left ventricle during systole. Affected by preload, afterload, and contractility.	60–130 mL
EF	Ejection fraction	The percentage of the total volume in the left ventricle that is ejected during systole. Used as a major indicator of LV function.	60%–75%
SVR	Systemic vascular resistance	The resistance to blood flow within the peripheral blood vessels (arterioles) in the systemic circulation. LV afterload.	800–1200 dynes/sec/cm^{-5}
PVR	Pulmonary vascular resistance	The resistance to blood flow within the pulmonary blood vessels (arterioles) in the pulmonary circulation. RV afterload.	< 250 dynes/sec/cm^{-5}
SaO$_2$	Arterial oxygen saturation	Relationship between the partial pressure of oxygen (PaO$_2$) and how well saturated with O$_2$ the hemoglobin is in the arterial system.	95%–100%
SVO$_2$	Mixed venous oxygen saturation	The amount of O$_2$ in Hgb in venous blood that has returned to the RV and the PA. Helps determine balance between oxygen supply and demand in the body.	60%–80%

Adapted from Hodges, R.K., Garrett, K.M., Chernecky, C., & Schumacher, L. (2005). *Real world nursing survival guide: Hemodynamic monitoring*. St. Louis: Elsevier Saunders. Used with permission.

Table 3.16

Typical Hemodynamic Profiles in Various Acute Conditions

Condition	HR	MAP	CO/CI	CVP/RAP	PAP/PAWP	Notes
Left ventricular failure	↑	↓	↓	↑	↑	
Pulmonary edema (cardiogenic)	↑	N,↓	↓	↑	↑PAWP > 25 mm Hg	
Massive pulmonary embolism	↑	↓,V	↓	↑	↑PAD > PAWP by > 5 mm Hg	↑ PVR
Acute ventricular septal defect	↑	↓	↓	↑	↑giant "v" wave on PAWP trace	O₂ step up noted in SvO₂
Acute mitral valve regurgitation	↑	↓	↓	↑	↑giant "v" wave on PAWP trace	No O₂ step up noted in SvO₂
Cardiac tamponade	↑	↓	↓	↑	↑CVP, PAD & PAW equalized	↓ RVEDVI
Right ventricular failure	↑,V	↓,V	↓	↑	PAP ↑ PAWP N, ↓	↑ RVEDVI
Hypovolemic shock	↑	↓	↓	↓	↓	↑O₂ extraction ↑SVR
Cardiogenic shock	↑	↓	↓	↑	↑	↑O₂ extraction ↑SVR
Septic shock	↑	↓	↑,↓	↓,↑	↓,↑	SVR changes, ↓O₂ extraction ↓ SVR

Key: ↑ = increased, ↓ = decreased, N = normal, V = varies

(4) If respiratory rate is elevated > 30 breaths per minute and the oxygen saturation is < 90%, the patient is in severe distress and immediate intervention is necessary.
(5) Note labored respirations and use of accessory muscles.
(6) Check equal expansion of the chest bilaterally.
c. Breath sounds.
   (1) Wheezes (sibilant): high-pitched musical sounds heard during exhalation.
      (a) May be caused by passage of air through a narrowed airway.
      (b) Consider asthma and bronchitis.
   (2) Rhonchi (gurgles/sonorous wheeze): deep-rumbling sounds heard during exhalation.
      (a) May be caused by passage of air through narrowed airway.
      (b) Consider asthma and bronchitis.
   (3) Rales (crackles): sounds like the crinkling of cellophane.
      (a) Caused by air passing through small airways in the presence of fluid, mucus, or pus.
      (b) Consider pulmonary edema.

Table 3.17 — Selected Drugs, Dosages, and Responses

Drug	Actions	Dose Range	HR	MAP	CO	PAWP (preload)	SVR (afterload)	PVR	Notes
Amrinone (Inocor)	Phosphodiecrease inhibitor with strong vasodilation properties	IV loading dose: 0.75 mg/kg over 3-5 min followed by a continuous infusion of 5-10 mcg/kg/min. The bolus may be repeated in 30 minutes if required. The total daily dose should not exceed 10 mcg/kg.	O/↑	O/↑	↓	↓	↓	↓	ACLS Guideline state requires hemodynamic monitoring.
Atropine Sulfate	Antiarrythmic which directly blocks vagal effects on SA node	0.5 to 1 mg IV push. Repeat every 3-5 minutes. Maximum dose 0.03 to 0.04 mg/kg.	↑	↑	↑	O	O	O	
Digoxin	Cardiatonic glycoside. Increases inaccophism by promoting extracellular calcium to move to intercellular cytoplasm. Inhibits adenosine triphospharase. Decrease conductivity through AV mode.	Loading dose 0.5 to 1 mg IV or in divided doses PO over 14 hours. Maintenance dose 0.125 to 0.5 mg IV or PO daily 0.25 mg.	O/↓	O/↑	↑	O/↓	O	O	
Dobutamine	Directly stimulates beta 1 receptors. Moderate stimulation of beta 2 receptors. Minimal stimulation of alpha receptors.	5-15 mcg/kg/min	O/↑	↑	↑	↓	↓	↓	Potential for arrythmias and ↑ O_2 consumption
Dopamine	Dopaminergic effects: Renal, mesenteric vasodilation. Beta effects: Increased inotrophism. Alpha effects: Vasoconstriction	0.5-3 mcg/kg/min 5.0-10 mcg/kg/min > 10.0 mcg/kg/min	↑	↑	↑	↓	↑	O	Potential for arrythmias, ↑ O_2 consumption, peripheral ischemia
Epinephrine	Low doses = Beta effect High doses = Alpha effect	0.005 – 0.02 mcg/kg/min 1 mg or > IV push; 1-4 mcg/min infusion	↑	↑	↑	↑	↑	↑	Potential for arrythmias and ↑ O_2 consumption, peripheral ischemia
Esmolol	Beta blocker	Loading dose 0.5 mg/kg over 1 minute followed by infusion titrate to desired effect range 50-300 mcg/kg/min	↓	↓	O/↓	O/↑	↓	↓	
Neo-synephrine (Phenylephrine)	Alpha stimulator	0.10- 0.18 mg/min until BP stable, then 0.04 0.06 mg/min	↓	↑	↓	↑	↑	↑	peripheral ischemia
Nitroglycerin	Vasodilator with stronger effects on peripheral venous bed and coronary arteries than peripheral arterial bed	Start infusion @ 10 mcg/min and increase in increments of 10 mcg/min as needed to achieve desired effect	O	↓	O/↑	↓	↓	↓	HA & hypotension
Norepinephrine (Levophed)	Low doses = Beta stimulation High doses = Alpha stimulation	Start at 0.05 – 0.01 mcg/kg/min and titrate up to 2.0 – 4.0 mcg/kg/min	↑	↓	↓	↓	↑	↓	peripheral ischemia
Morphine	Dilate pulmonary vascular system						↓		
Lasix	Diuresis					↓			

Alpha 1 receptors, vasoconstrict arterioles and coronary arteries
Beta 1 receptors, increase contractility, of Myocardial cells and increase conductivity to SA /AV Nodes
Beta 2 receptors, vasodilation of coronary arterioles and bronchodilation of bronchioles
Dopamine 1 and Dopamine 2 receptors vasoconstrict and vasodilate

Key ↓ = decrease ↑ = increase O = unknown

Source: Lichtenthal, P.R. (1998). *Quick guide to cardiopulmonary care.* Irvine, CA: Edwards Lifesciences. Used with permission.

Table 3.18

Oxygen Guideline for Estimating FiO$_2$ (varies with rate and depth of ventilation)

Method of Delivery	Oxygen Flow Rate	Estimated FIO$_2$ (fractionated inhaled oxygenation)
Nasal cannula • Oxygen delivery is extremely variable depending on tidal volume and ventilator pattern	1 liter/minute 2 liters/minute 3 liters/minute 4 liters/minute 5 liters/minute	24% 28% 32% 36% 40%
Simple mask • Need minimal flow of 5 LPM to flush out CO$_2$ • Oxygen delivery varies with changes in tidal volume, ventilator pattern, inspiratory flow rate, and whether the mask is loose or tight fitting	5–10 liters/minute	35% to 50%
Partial nonrebreathing mask • Mask with reservoir bag, still considered a low flow oxygen delivery system • Reservoir bag must not collapse during inspiration and must remain at least one third to one half full on inspiration	6–10 liters/minutes	40% to 70%
Nonrebreathing mask • Is similar to the partial rebreathing mask except it has a one way valve between the bag and the mask to prevent exhaled air from returning to the bag • Ideal method of delivering high O$_2$ concentration for short-term purposes	Minimum of 10 liters/minutes	60% to 80%

Source: Kallstrom, T.J. (2002). American Association of Respiratory Care clinical practice guideline: Oxygen therapy for adults in the acute care facility 2002 revision & update. *Respiratory Care, 47*(6), 717-720. Used with permission.

(4) Pleural friction rub: a dry, crackling, grating, low-pitched sound heard during inspiration or exhalation.
  (a) Caused by inflamed pleural surfaces rubbing against one another.
  (b) May indicate pleurisy.
(5) Absent or diminished sounds.
  (a) Indicates presence of fluid or pus in the lung fields, muscular weakness, or splinting from pain.
  (b) If unilateral, consider mucus plug, or hemo/pneumothorax that is spontaneous or related to central line placement.
(6) Mediastinal crepitus.

  (a) Indicates air in the pericardium, mediastinum or both.
  (b) Often associated with pericardial friction rub.
8. Gastrointestinal.
  a. Bowel sounds.
  b. Include stool in output.
  c. Hold anticoagulation for suspected GI bleed.
9. Genitourinary.
  a. Primary etiology of AKI or CKD.
  b. Avoid nephrotoxins (see Section 3, Chapter 10, *AKI*).
10. Endocrine: presence of diabetes and stability of serum glucose.

Table 3.19

Etiology of Respiratory Distress and Failure

Pulmonary	Extrapulmonary
Acute respiratory distress syndrome (ARDS)	Acidosis
Airway obstruction	Anesthesia
Aspiration	Brain or spinal cord injury
Asthma	Cardiopulmonary bypass
Bronchitis	Disseminated intravascular coagulation (DIC)
Chronic obstructive pulmonary disease (COPD)	Drug overdose
Cystic fibrosis (CF)	Multiple sclerosis
Inhalation injury	Muscular dystrophy
Pneumonia	Myasthenia gravis
Pneumo/hemothorax	Neuromuscular blocking agents
Pulmonary emboli	Sepsis
Pulmonary edema	Severe obesity
Oxygen toxicity	Sleep apnea
Lung cancer	Shock
Radiation	Systemic inflammatory response syndrome (SIRS)
Surgical resection	Transfustion related acute lung injury (TRALI)

Courtesy of Maureen Craig, University of California Davis Medical Center, Sacramento, CA. Used with permission.

11. Neurologic.
    a. Level of consciousness/mental status.
        (1) Altered concentration.
        (2) Change in alertness.
        (3) Change in orientation to person, place, or time.
    b. Identify risk factors for dialysis disequilibrium syndrome (DDS).
    c. Brain injury.
        (1) Intracranial pressure (ICP) monitoring.
        (2) ICP can be monitored from a burr hole through the skull via a small catheter inserted into the white matter.
            (a) Licox monitor can also provide a reading of brain tissue oxygenation and brain temperature in addition to the ICP reading.
            (b) Ventriculostomy catheter can drain the excess spinal fluid in addition to providing an ICP reading. Consider effects of fluid removal on ICP and brain oxygenation results.
        (3) When dialyzing a patient with ICP monitoring, anticoagulation should not be used and precautions should be taken to prevent further brain swelling or DDS.

F. Laboratory assessment.
    1. Blood chemistry (see section G: Dialysis solution, for further discussion of electrolytes present in dialysis solution and their physiologic importance).
        a. Sodium. Normal serum sodium is 136–146 mEq/L. Low serum sodium may indicate excess fluid. Elevated serum sodium may correlate with hypertension.
        b. Potassium. Normal serum potassium is 3.5–5 mEq/L. Elevated serum potassium may be related to diet, medications, blood transfusions, or under-dialysis.
        c. Normal CO_2 is 24–32 mEq/L and reflects acid/base balance. This should be evaluated along with an arterial blood gas (ABG) to determine respiratory or metabolic acid base disturbances.
        d. Blood urea nitrogen (BUN).
            (1) The BUN is elevated in patients with renal replacement therapy needs.
            (2) A low predialysis serum level may indicate malnutrition.
            (3) BUN will increase with a GI bleed or steroid administration.
            (4) BUN is used to assess treatment

adequacy using either the urea reduction ratio (URR) or the Kt/V$_{urea}$.

(5) Solutes that are easily cleared from the plasma water during a hemodialysis treatment may rebound after the treatment ends. Urea is often the marker used to assess this rebound effect.

d. Creatinine.

(1) Creatinine is used to determine creatinine clearance and estimate the patient's GFR when the patient's kidney function is stable.

(2) Creatinine levels are impacted by dialysis treatments and changing kidney function, so assessing trends in creatinine levels in light of these events is more meaningful than a single creatinine level.

e. Glucose. Normal range is 65–100 mg/dL.

(1) Glucose levels may be altered in diabetic patients.

(2) Hypoglycemic episodes during dialysis treatment are typically prevented by the presence of dextrose (200 mg/dL) in the dialysate.

f. Albumin. Normal range is 4–5.2 g/dL. Low albumin levels are associated with inflammation and/or inadequate dietary protein intake and are associated with increased morbidity and mortality in chronic hemodialysis patients.

g. Calcium. Normal range is 8.4–10 mg/dL.

(1) Phosphorus binders may be a significant source of calcium intake.

(2) Patients with excess calcium may be at increased risk for vascular calcifications and associated coronary events.

(3) Calcium functions on a reciprocal basis with phosphorus.

(4) Patients dependent on hemodialysis may experience calcium reabsorption from bone related to a state of chronic metabolic acidosis and experience loss of bone density.

h. Phosphorus levels. Normal range is 2.6–4.2 mg/L.

(1) Phosphorus dietary intake is typically limited to 600–1200 mg/day.

(2) Phosphorus binders are often prescribed to facilitate phosphorus excretion through the GI tract.

(3) For the patient with significant phosphorus clearance in daily dialysis, the dietary phosphorus may need to be liberalized and additional phosphorus

may be required by infusion or in the dialysis solution.

i. Calcium phosphorus product (mg/dL) = calcium x phosphorus:

(1) The calcium/phosphorus product should be < 55mg/dL.

(2) A higher product can lead to the deposition of calcium phosphate crystals in the body, e.g., heart valves, lungs, joints, soft tissue, and skin.

j. Magnesium levels. Normal range is 1.8–2.3 mg/dL. Patients dependent on hemodialysis should avoid magnesium containing laxatives or antacids.

k. Cholesterol. Normal is < 200 mg/dL. Elevated cholesterol may increase a patient's risk for coronary events.

l. Transaminase. Elevated transaminase levels may indicate liver malfunction or possible hepatitis.

m. Ferritin. Normal range is 9–200 ng/mL.

(1) Ferritin reflects the patient's iron stores.

(2) Low levels reflect iron deficiency.

(3) Elevated levels result from frequent blood transfusions.

n. Iron. Normal range is 40-175 μ/dL.

o. Iron-binding capacity. Normal is 225–410 μ/dL.

p. Iron saturation (%). Calculation: Iron/iron binding capacity. If iron saturation is < 20%, the patient is iron deficient and may benefit from iron repletion.

2. Hematology.

a. White blood cell (WBC) count. Normal 4,500–10,000/mm^3. Suspect infection if WBC count is elevated.

b. Hemoglobin (Hgb) and hematocrit (Hct) related to anemia:

(1) If the Hgb is < 8.0–9.0 g/dL, the patient may need a type & cross match for transfusion of packed red blood cells (PRBC) during dialysis.

(2) It is beneficial to administer the PRBC during HD to remove the excess volume and potassium.

(3) Potassium content in PRBCs increases as the unit of blood approaches its expiration date due to cell death.

(4) Platelet count is related to clotting ability. Decrease in platelet count > 50% from baseline (prior to heparin exposure) may indicate heparin-induced thrombocytopenia. Low platelet counts represent an increase risk for bleeding.

3. Coagulation.
   a. Protime (PT), partial thromboplastin time (PTT), and international normalized ratio (INR) are used to evaluate coagulation.
   b. D-dimer is used to evaluate for disseminated intravascular coagulation (DIC) or deep vein thrombosis (DVT).
   c. Heparin-induced thrombocytopenia (HIT) antibody is used to assess for safe heparin exposure.
   d. Need for transfusion of blood products to treat bleeding disorders.
      (1) Fresh-frozen plasma (FFP) can be administered during HD allowing for removal of fluid volume.
      (2) Platelets may be administered during or after HD, as specified by nephrologist, since some platelets may be captured in the dialyzer if given during HD. Anticoagulation needs to be adjusted as platelet counts change.
      (3) If ordered to be given during HD, administer platelets using an infusion pump via venous chamber the last 30 minutes of treatment.
      (4) An intravenous (IV)infusion pump that is administering an infusion into the venous chamber may need its pressure parameters adjusted to administer the infusion against a positive pressure in the venous chamber. The positive pressure present in the venous chamber is typically higher than that in a vein. The infusion pump may interpret this higher positive pressure inaccurately as a down stream occlusion.
4. Other laboratory data for analysis, such as drug levels.
   a. Digoxin to adjust potassium in bath.
   b. Therapeutic antibiotic levels.
   c. Beta-type natriuretic peptide (BNP) levels during congestive heart failure episodes.

III. The hemodialysis treatment plan.

A. In the acute setting, the dialysis prescription will vary according to the patient's clinical presentation and lab results.
   1. The role of the acute dialysis nurse is unique and requires experience and critical thinking skills.
   2. This role is autonomous and often there is only intermittent onsite contact with the nephrologist.

3. The treatment plan is determined by an accurate patient assessment, application of treatment protocols and collaboration with the nephrologist.
4. Refer to Appendix 3.3: Acute Hemodialysis Order Form.

B. Dialysis adequacy.
   1. The effectiveness of the dialysis treatment is dependent on the session length, the blood flow rate, and the dialysis solution flow rate.
   2. In the acute setting, dialysis adequacy is complicated by the following:
      a. Increased use of venous catheters for dialysis access that may deliver a substantially lower blood flow rate.
      b. Increased recirculation in venous catheters, especially those placed in the femoral vein.
      c. Decreased treatment time due to intradialytic patient complications.
      d. Increased sequestration of urea in muscles due to use of vasopressors resulting in decreased blood flow to muscles and skin.
      e. Interruptions to the prescribed dialysis treatment plan.
         (1) The patient's primary reason for hospitalization with its subsequent procedures, therapies, surgeries, and tests may take precedence over a single planned hemodialysis treatment.
         (2) It is the duty of the nephrologist and the acute care nephrology team to assess the patient's renal replacement therapy needs and to make every effort to provide adequate dialysis, which is often more dialysis than is required in the out patient setting.

C. Dialysis disequilibrium syndrome (DDS).
   1. Etiology. DDS is a set of neurologic and systemic symptoms related to an acute increase in brain water content.
      a. DDS is most likely to occur when a patient is first dialyzed or when the dialysis treatment aggressively lowers solutes in the patient's plasma.
      b. Occurs when BUN values are very high > 175 mg/dL.
      c. When plasma solute levels are rapidly lowered during a dialysis treatment, the solute concentration in brain cells and cerebral spinal fluid is much higher than that of plasma due to the difference in

Table 3.20

Osmolar Molecule Table

Urea	Na+	Glucose
Depending on the body weight of the patient, only a 30% reduction in plasma urea nitrogen is desired on the initial treatment. Low blood flow rates (BFR) 150–250 mL/min or a BFR that is about three times the body weight in kg is recommended and gradually increased with consecutive treatment. Shortened length of treatment (2 hours) is recommended (and gradually increased with consecutive treatment).	A dialysate sodium level of at least 140 mEq per L helps maintain serum osmolality during hemodialysis. Use of sodium gradient dialysis with dialysate sodium level > 145 mEq/L reduces incidence of DDS. In patients who are already hypernatremic it is safer to set the dialysate sodium level to a value close to the patients plasma sodium level, not lower. In these cases, sodium modeling may not be appropriate.	A dialysate solution that contains at least 200 mg/dL of dextrose should be used.

Courtesy of DCI Acute Program, Omaha, Nebraska. Used with permission.

permeability of the blood-brain barrier. Water shifts from plasma into the brain tissue causing cerebral edema.

   d. Acute changes in pH of the cerebral spinal fluid during hemodialysis are caused by a more rapid diffusion of carbon dioxide than bicarbonate across the blood/brain barrier.

   e. Patients who are very young, elderly, small body size or who have primary CNS disease (seizure disorders, stroke, brain aneurysms) are more susceptible to DDS.

   f. Chronic patients who are under-dialyzed are also susceptible.

2. Review predialysis labs and patient history to identify those at risk for DSS.

3. Support the osmolality of the blood during dialysis.
   a. Urea, sodium, and glucose are all important osmolar molecules.
   b. Each represents an important role (see Table 3.20).

4. Consider prophylactic use of anticonvulsants in patients predisposed to seizures until uremia is controlled.

5. Signs and symptoms (see Table 3.21).
   a. Headache.
   b. Nausea and vomiting.
   c. Restlessness.
   d. Hypertension.
   e. Increased pulse pressure.
   f. Decreased sensorium.
   g. Convulsions.
   h. Coma.

Table 3.21

DDS Signs and Symptoms

Mild To Early Disequilibrium
Nausea/vomiting
Blurred vision
Restlessness
Headache
Hypertension
Increased pulse pressure
Muscle cramps
Dizziness not related to BP
Asterixsis

Severe Disequilibrium
Confusion
Disorientation
Muscle twitching/tremors
Seizures
Arrhythmias
Coma (improved within 24 hours)
Death

Courtesy of DCI Acute Program, Omaha, Nebraska. Used with permission.

6. Prevention (see Table 3.22).
   a. Short inefficient dialysis treatments with slow solute removal.
      (1) Small dialyzer.
      (2) Slow dialysate flow rate.
      (3) Slow blood flow rate.

b. Administration of a suitable osmotic agent, such as mannitol, to counteract the rapid fall in plasma osmolality.

7. When DDS occurs, the hemodialysis treatment may need to be terminated, or at the very least slowed.

8. After the initial dialysis session, the patient should be re-evaluated.
   a. Is usually dialyzed again the following day.
   b. Gradually increase the length of treatment and the BFR over a series of treatments.
   c. Dialysate flow rates are slowly raised toward a goal of 500–800 mL/min.

9. If a longer dialysis session is required for purposes of fluid removal, isolated ultrafiltration (UF or PUF) can be performed in which dialysate flow bypasses the dialyzer resulting in a decreased effect on osmolality during isolated UF.

D. Depending on the clinical presentation, those patients not at risk for DDS are generally dialyzed three times per week for 3–4 hours at maximum BFR attainable.
   1. Extremely ill or hypercatabolic patients may benefit from more frequent or daily dialysis sessions.
   2. The length of a single dialysis session rarely exceeds 6 hours unless the purpose of the treatment is acute overdose.

E. Determining dialysate flow rates (DFR).
   1. Generally, for acute hemodialysis, the DFR is 500–600 mL/min.
   2. The rate may be higher for the hypercatabolic patient if DDS is not a risk.
   3. DFR is most efficiently set at twice the BFR.
   4. With the advent of newer dialysis machines, technology provides the capability of very rapid DFR.

F. Dialyzer.
   1. Biocompatible synthetic membranes obtain the best patient outcomes in the acute setting.
   2. The AN69 membrane (co-polymer of polyacrylonitrile and sodium methallyl sulfonate) has caused an increased risk of anaphylactic reactions in patients taking angiotensin converting enzyme (ACE) inhibitors and should be avoided in this group.
   3. To maintain economics in the acute setting, consider using one type of primary dialyzer and have a small supply of another dialyzer with a different membrane material available in case of

a dialyzer membrane reaction.
   4. Prepare the dialyzer for use by first rinsing with 1 liter of normal saline (following manufacturer's recommendations if more stringent) to remove residual sterilant and other manufacturing materials.
   5. Dialyzer membrane reaction.
      a. Signs and symptoms.
         (1) Dyspnea.
         (2) Feeling of warmth at the exit site or throughout the body.
         (3) Sense of impending doom.
         (4) Chest pain.
         (5) Back pain.
         (6) Anaphylaxis.
         (7) Cardiac arrest.
         (8) Death.
      b. Treatment.
         (1) Stop dialysis treatment without returning the patient's blood.
         (2) Provide patient oxygen by nasal cannula.
         (3) Monitor patient's vital signs.
         (4) Treat anaphylaxis with IV antihistamines (diphenhydramine), steroids, and epinephrine until patient stabilizes.
   6. Refer to Section 11 on various dialyzer filters and membrane types, sizes and specific attributes.

G. Dialysis solution.
   1. Dialysis solution composition should be tailored according to the patient's clinical presentation and laboratory values.
   2. The "standard" composition prescribed for chronic dialysis patients may not be appropriate in an acute care setting while the patient is experiencing an acute illness.
   3. Plasma bicarbonate levels are normally 24 mEq/liter.
      a. In the absence of renal function, patients may present with metabolic acidosis as the generated acids are not excreted.
      b. These acids may be buffered by bicarbonate and the patient will then have a lower bicarbonate level.
      c. Bicarbonate is delivered during a dialysis treatment when the dialysis solution bicarbonate concentration, e.g., 35 mEq/L, is higher than the plasma bicarbonate concentration, e.g., 20 mEq/L.
      d. Patient's plasma bicarbonate levels typically rise during a dialysis treatment to 26 or even 28 mEq/L.

Table 3.22

Sample DDS Prevention Protocol

Treatment Day 1

1. The prescribed BFR for the 1st treatment is calculated by taking the patient's approximate dry weight multiplied by 3 = _____ mL/min.
   Examples:
   50 kg patient x 3 = 150 mL/min BFR
   70 kg patient x 3 = 210 mL/min BFR
   90 kg patient x 3 = 270 mL/min BFR, not to exceed 300 mL/min

2. Treatment time: 2 hours

3. DFR = 500 mL/min

4. Heparin free until BUN < 100 mg/dL
   Tight low total heparin if BUN ≤ 100 mg/dL

5. HyperOsmolar agents to prevent DDS
   a. 25% mannitol, 6.5 to 12.5 g mannitol administered IVP hourly, do not administer last 30 minutes of treatment. Mannitol will be used on all patients with preexisting seizure conditions, patients exhibiting mild or moderate to severe CNS symptoms from dialysis disequilibrium.
   b. Exponential sodium modeling of 150

6. Weight loss according to fluid assessment

Treatment Day 2

1. If BUN > 100 mg/dL predialysis, use the same protocol as treatment #1 except increase treatment time to 2.5 hours.

2. If BUN < 100 mg/dL increase BFR by 50 mL/min from last treatment.

3. DFR = 500 mL/min

4. Heparin free until BUN < 100 mg/dL
   Tight low total heparin if BUN ≤ 100 mg/dL

5. HyperOsmolar agents to prevent DDS
   a. 25% Mannitol, 6.5 to 12.5 g mannitol administered IVP hourly, do not administer last 30 minutes of treatment. Mannitol will be used on all patients with preexisting seizure conditions, patients exhibiting mild or moderate to severe CNS symptoms from dialysis disequilibrium.
   b. Exponential sodium modeling of 150

6. F160 NR dialyzer or equivalent _____.

7. Weight loss according to fluid assessment.

Treatment Day 3

1. 3-hour treatment

2. DFR = 500 mL/min

3. Maximum BFR as tolerates

4. Tight low total heparin

5. Sodium modeling as indicated

6. F160 NR dialyzer or equivalent _____.

7. Weight loss according to fluid assessment.
   If BUN is still > 100 mg/dL on day 3, access is functioning adequately and/or patient is in a catabolic state, call nephrologist for treatment order clarification. If access is a potential problem associated with clearance, notify nephrologist.

Adapted from Creighton Nephrology, Creighton University, Omaha, Nebraska. Used with permission.

e. The dialysis solution bicarbonate concentration should be selected to achieve the desired changes in the patient's plasma bicarbonate level.

4. Dialysis solution sodium.

a. The normal range for serum sodium is 135–145 mEq/L.

b. Sodium and water are closely related in the body. The normal range of serum sodium reflects the relationship between sodium and volume status.

c. To learn the definitions and signs and symptoms of hyponatremia and hypernatremia clinical presentations, see the following tables:

Table 3.23: Hyponatremia and Hypovolemic/Hyponatremia

Table 3.24: Hypervolemic/Hyponatremia

Table 3.25: Isovolemic/Hyponatremia

Table 3.26: Hypernatremia

Table 3.27: Hypervolemic/Hypernatremia

Table 3.28: Hypovolemic/Hypernatremia

d. Sodium correction with hemodialysis.

(1) The goal is to achieve euvolemic status and normal body sodium at the end of the dialysis treatment (postdialysis serum sodium level of 140 mEq/L).

(2) This can be achieved by using osmotic agents, ultrafiltration, and a dialysis solution with the desired sodium content.

(3) Review serum sodium levels predialysis.

(4) Attempt to determine if patient is volume overloaded or depleted.

(a) Assess the patient's fluid balance to determine if sodium imbalance is due to hemodilution or hemoconcentration.

(b) If predialysis serum sodium levels are < 130 mEq/L and the hyponatremia is of long duration, it may be dangerous to achieve normonatremia quickly.

Table 3.23

Hyponatremia and Hypovolemic/Hyponatremia

Electrolyte Imbalance	Cause	Signs and Symptoms
Hyponatremia Serum sodium level < 135 mEq. Critically low levels may be < 125 mEq.	1) Sodium deficiency in relation to body water; body fluids are diluted and cells swell from decreased extracellular fluid osmolality.	1) Signs and symptoms vary depending on how quickly the sodium level drops. If the level drops quickly, the patient will be more symptomatic.

Hypovolemic/hyponatremia	1) Is defined as deficits of both total body water and sodium, but sodium loss is greater than water loss (true hyponatremia).
	a) Renal Causes
	   i) Osmotic diuresis
	   ii) Salt-losing nephrites
	   iii) Adrenal insufficiency
	   iv) Diuretic use (primarily thiazides)
	b) Nonrenal causes
	   i) Vomiting
	   ii) Diuresis
	   iii) GI fistulas
	   iv) Gastric suctioning
	   v) Excessive sweating
	   vi) Cystic fibrosis
	   vii) Burns
	   viii) Wound drainage
		1) Signs and symptoms include:
		a) Apprehension
		b) Dizziness
		c) Postural hypotension
		d) Cold, clammy skin
		e) Decreased skin turgor
		f) Tachycardia
		g) Oliguria
		h) Decreased CVP, PAP, PAW
		i) Elevated HCT

Courtesy of DCI Acute Program, Omaha, Nebraska. Used with permission.

Table 3.24

Hypervolemic/Hyponatremia

Electrolyte Imbalance	Cause	Signs and Symptoms
Hypervolemic/Hyponatremia	1) Both water and sodium levels increase in the extracellular area, but the water gain is more impressive. Serum sodium levels are diluted. a) Heart failure b) Liver failure c) Nephrotic syndrome d) Excessive administration of hypotonic IV fluids e) Hypoaldosteronism f) Severe hyperglycemia in diabetic dialysis patients. For every increase of 100 mg/dL in serum glucose, there is a corresponding initial decrease of 1.3meg/L in the serum sodium concentration due to osmotic shift of water from the intercellular to the extracellular compartment. Because osmotic diuresis does not occur, the excess plasma water is not excreted. Insulin administration reverses the water shift and corrects the hyponatremia.	1) Signs and symptoms include: b) Disorientation c) Muscle twitching d) Nausea/vomiting e) Abdominal cramps f) Headache g) Seizures h) Edema i) Hypertension j) Weight gain k) Rapid bounding pulse l) CVP and PAP elevated

Courtesy of DCI Acute Program, Omaha, Nebraska. Used with permission.

Table 3.25

Isovolemic/Hyponatremia

Electrolyte Imbalance	Cause	Signs and Symptoms

Isovolemic/Hyponatremia	1) Extracellular fluid is equal to intracellular fluid volume.
	a) Glucocorticoid deficiency (inadequate fluid filtration by the kidneys)
	b) Hypothyroidism (limited water excretion)
	c) Renal failure
	d) Syndrome of inappropriate antidiuretic hormone (SIADH) secretion
	  i) Concerns especially of duodenum, pancreas and oat cell carcinoma of the lung
	  ii) CNS disorders, trauma, tumors and stroke
	  iii) Pulmonary disorder, tumors, asthma and COPD
	  iv) Medications, oral antidiabetic drugs, chemotherapeutic drugs, psychoactive drugs, diuretics, synthetic hormones, and barbituates
		1) No physical signs and symptoms of volume excess.

Courtesy of DCI Acute Program, Omaha, Nebraska. Used with permission.

Table 3.26

Hypernatremia

Electrolyte Imbalance	Cause	Signs & Symptoms
Hypernatremia Serum sodium level > 145 mEq/L	An excess of sodium relative to body water occurs when there is an increase in sodium or loss of free water. Can occur with decreased, normal, or increased body water.	Body fluids become hypertonic; more concentrated fluid moves by osmosis from inside the cell to outside the cell to balance the concentration in the two compartments. As fluid leaves them, the cells become dehydrated, especially those of the CNS. Patients may show signs of fluid overload from increased extracellular fluid volume in the blood vessels. Symptoms are more severe if high sodium level develops rapidly instead of overtime. Neurologic symptoms Include: 1) Restlessness/agitation 2) Weakness 3) Lethargy 4) Stupor 5) Confusion 6) Seizures/coma 7) Neuromuscular irritability (twitching) 8) Low grade fever/flushed skin

Courtesy of DCI Acute Program, Omaha, Nebraska. Used with permission.

Table 3.27

Hypervolemic/Hypernatremia

Electrolyte Imbalance	Cause	Signs and Symptoms

Hypervolemic/Hypernatremia	1) Excessive sodium gain
	2) Food and medication (kayexalate)
	3) Excessive IV administration of sodium solutions (sodium bicarbonate, hypertonic saline solutions)
	4) Excessive adrenocortical hormones
	   a) Cushing's syndrome
	   b) Hyperaldosteronism
		1) Signs and symptoms include:
		   a) Increased BP
		   b) Bounding pulse
		   c) Dyspnea

Courtesy of DCI Acute Program, Omaha, Nebraska. Used with permission.

[1] Rapid correction, by more than 8–12 mEq/L per day, may cause osmotic demyelination syndrome (ODS), characterized clinically by an acute progressive dysarthria, dysphagia, weakness progressing to quadriplegia, and alterations of consciousness.

[2] It may be beneficial to correct hypokalemia prior to correction of the serum sodium to further reduce the incidence of ODS.

[3] The dialysate solution sodium level should be set no higher than 15–20 mEq/L above the plasma level.

Table 3.28

Hypovolemic/Hypernatremia

Electrolyte Imbalance	Cause	Signs and Symptoms
Hypovolemic/Hypernatremia	1) Loss of a small amount of sodium and a large amount of water, with a greater emphasis on loss of body water. a) Impaired thirst regulation (hypothalamic disorders) b) People who can't drink voluntarily (infants, confused elderly, immobile or unconscious patients) c) Fever, heat stroke d) Pulmonary infections/hyperventilation e) Excessive burns f) Diarrhea/GI losses g) Hyperglycemia/osmotic diuresis	1) Signs and symptoms include: a) Dry mucous membranes b) Oliguria c) Orthostatic hypotension

Courtesy of DCI Acute Program, Omaha, Nebraska. Used with permission.

[4] Patients at greatest risk of the syndrome include those with chronic alcoholism, malnutrition, prolonged diuretic use, liver failure, extensive burns, or a history of an organ transplant.

(c) If predialysis serum sodium levels are > 145 mEq/L, it is dangerous to attempt to correct hypernatremia by dialyzing against a low-sodium dialysis solution.

[1] May cause cerebral edema, hypotension, and muscle cramping.

[2] In this case, the dialysate sodium level should be set close (within 5 mEq/L) to that of the pre-treatment plasma level.

5. Dialysis solution potassium.
   a. Potassium is the major cation (positive charge) in the intracellular fluid and plays a critical role in many metabolic cell functions. Normal range for a serum potassium is 3.5–5 mEq/L.
      (1) Only 2% of the body's potassium is found in the extracellular fluid.
      (2) 98% is in the intracelluluar fluid.
      (3) Small, untreated alterations in serum potassium levels can seriously affect neuromuscular and cardiac functioning.
   b. Normal renal function is needed to maintain the potassium balance.
      (1) 80% of the daily excretion of potassium is done by the kidneys.
      (2) 20% is lost via the bowel and sweat glands.
   c. The sodium/potassium pump is an active transport mechanism that moves ions across the cell membrane against a concentration gradient. The pump moves sodium from the cell into the extracellular fluid and maintains high intracellular potassium levels by pumping potassium into the cell.
   d. Magnesium helps sodium and potassium ions across the cell membrane, affecting sodium and potassium levels both inside and outside the cell.
   e. A change in pH may affect serum potassium levels because hydrogen ions move into the cells and push potassium into the extracellular fluid.
      (1) Acidosis and/or hyperglycemia can cause hyperkalemia as potassium moves out of the cell to maintain balance.
      (2) Alkalosis and/or insulin can lower serum potassium levels as potassium moves into the cell to maintain balance.
      (3) To learn the potential causes and signs and symptoms of hypokalemia and hyperkalemia (see Tables 3.29 and 3.30).
   f. Potassium imbalance is corrected with HD to achieve a serum potassium level within safe range of 3.5 mEq/L to 5.0 mEq/L.
      (1) Hypokalemia.

Table 3.29

Hyperkalemia Imbalances

Electrolyte	Cause	Signs and Symptoms

Hyperkalemia Serum potassium level rises above 5.5 mEq/L	1) Pseudohyperkalemia
	   a) Hemolysis
	   b) Improper phlebotomy techniques
	     i) Prolonged tight tourniquet prior to lab draw
	     ii) Fist clenching and unclenching prior to drawing specimen may increasing serum K$^+$ levels by as much as 2.5 mEq/L
	     iii) Use of small gauge needle or finger sticks to obtain blood sample
	   c) Thrombocytosis (chemotherapy)
	   d) Leukocytosis (chemotherapy)
	2) Decreased renal excretion – acute or chronic oliguric renal failure
	   a) Decreased renal perfusion (CHF, sepsis)
	   b) Adrenal insufficiency (hypoaldosteronism/Addison's)
	   c) HIV
	   d) Drugs: ACE inhibitor/angiotension receptor blockers, heparin, cyclosporine and K$^+$ sparing diuretics
	3) Transcellular shift (intracellular to extracellular)
	   a) Metabolic acidosis (moves K$^+$ out of the cells as hydrogen ions shift into the cell). For each 0.1 decrease in pH typically there is an increase in K$^+$ of 0.5–0.8 mEq/L.
	   b) Drugs: beta blockers, angiotension receptor blockers, succinylcholine, digitalis (in large doses poisons the NA^{++}/K$^+$ ATPase pump resulting in K$^+$ release from the cells)
	   c) Tissue destruction: rhabdomyolysis, crush injuries, lungs, severe infections
	   d) Tumor lysis, hemolysis
	   e) Cardiac surgery
	   f) Diabetes – insulin deficiency (elevated blood sugar causes K$^+$ to rise)
	4) Factors due to increased intake
	   a) PRBC transfusions close to expiration date
	   b) Oral supplement, salt substitutes, IV potassium, tube feedings
	   c) GI bleeding related to gut reabsorption of hemolyzed RBCs
		1) Muscle weakness is usually the first sign, spreads from the legs to the trunk eventually involving the respiratory muscles. Paralysis seen with serum K$^+$ > 8.0, patients often report falling due to leg weakness
		2) Smooth muscle hyperactivity causing nausea, cramps, and diarrhea
		3) Paresthesias of face, tongue, feet, and hands (stimulation of pain receptors)
		4) EKG changes occur in the following progression as K$^+$ rises (see Figure 3.15, EKG changes with hypo/hyperkalemia)
		   a) Tall, peaked t-wave
		   b) Prolonged P-R internal (greater than 2.0 sec.)
		   c) Loss of P wave
		   d) Slight widening of QRS complex
		   e) Very wide QRS complex
		   f) Bradycardia
		   g) Sine wave pattern (QRS complex merges with T-wave)
		   h) Ventricular fibrillation or standstill

Courtesy of DCI Acute Program, Omaha, Nebraska. Used with permission.

(a) Review serum potassium levels predialysis to determine the correction needed.

(b) Assess patient for clinical evidence of hypokalemia.

(2) Hyperkalemia. Review serum potassium levels predialysis to determine the severity of the hyperkalemia and how much correction is needed.

(a) Make sure the results are current and accurate.

(b) A hemolyzed lab sample will cause a false high serum potassium level.

(c) Mild hyperkalemia:

   [1] Patients with some renal function may be treated with a loop diuretic to increase potassium removal by the kidneys or to resolve any acidosis present.

Table 3.30

Hypokalemia Imbalances

Electrolyte	Cause	Signs & Symptoms

Hypokalemia Serum potassium level < 3.5 mEq/L	1) Gastrointestinal losses
	  a) Diarrhea
	  b) Prolonged gastric suctioning/vomiting
	  c) Secretory tumors (villous adenoma)
	  d) Intestinal drainage (fistulas, surgical drains)
	  e) Recent ileostomy
	2) Renal losses: not uncommon in patients with nonoliguric acute renal failure
	  a) Drugs: duretics, high dose corticosteroids, insulin, high dose penicillins, drugs causing hypomagnesemia (amphotericin B, aminoglycosides, cisplatin), beta agonists (including pressors and broncho dilators such as albuteral), insulin overdose
	  b) Magnesuim depletion (magnesuim is needed for sodium and potassium ions to cross the cell membrane)
	    i) See drugs causing hypomagnesemia
	    ii) Hyperalimentation (causes hypomagnesemia due to shifting of magnesium into cells during anabolism)
	  c) Renal tubular acidosis
	  d) Cushing's syndrome
	  e) Increased GFR (osmotic diuresis with hyperglycemia, newly functioning transplanted kidney)
	3) Severe diaphoresis
	4) Poor dietary intake (anorexia, alcoholism, debilitation)
	5) Transcellular shift (extracellular to intracellular)
	  a) Alkalosis (potassium moves into the cell as hydrogen ions move out)
	  b) Elevated beta-adrenergic activity related to stress, coronary ischemia, or delerium tremens
	  c) Drugs (Beta agonists and insulin overdose)
	  d) Hypothermia
	  e) Hyperalimentation
		Hypokalemia: symptoms are rare if serum K^+ is > 3.0 mEq/L
		1) Skeletal muscle weakness, especially in the legs
		2) Paresthesia, leg cramps, restless legs and decreased or absent deep tendon reflexes
		3) Ascending paralysis with respiratory compromise
		4) Rarely, prolonged hypokalemia can cause rhabdomyolysis, a condition where there is breakdown of muscle fibers leading to myoglobin in the urine, eventually leading to hyperkalemia
		5) Anorexia, nausea and vomiting, decreased bowel sounds, constipation, ileus
		6) Cardiac problems
		  a) Weak, irregular pulse
		  b) Orthostatic hypotension
		  c) EKG changes
		    i) Flattened T wave
		    ii) Depressed ST segment
		    iii) Enlarging U wave superimposed on T wave to give appearance of prolonged Q-T
		    iv) Increased potential for bradycardic response to digitalis glycoside toxicity, as potassium is needed to balance the level of digoxin in the blood and cells
		    v) Cardiac arrest
		    vi) Frequent PVCs unresponsive to lidocaine
		    vii) Tachyarrhythmias if patient is volume depleted
		  d) Worsens the effects of digoxin toxicity, as potassium is needed to balance the level of digoxin in the blood

Courtesy of DCI Acute Program, Omaha, Nebraska. Used with permission.

[2] Educate patient and restrict PO and IV potassium intake.

[3] Screen medications and nutritional supplements for potassium.

[4] Treat underlying disorders leading to the high potassium: hyperglycemia, hypomagnesemia and acidosis.

(d) Moderate to severe symptomatic hyperkalemia usually requires HD. While arrangements for HD are being made, the patient may need to be treated medically.

[1] Assess cardiac rhythm changes associated with potassium (see Figure 3.15).

[2] Kayexalate 30 grams in 50 mL of

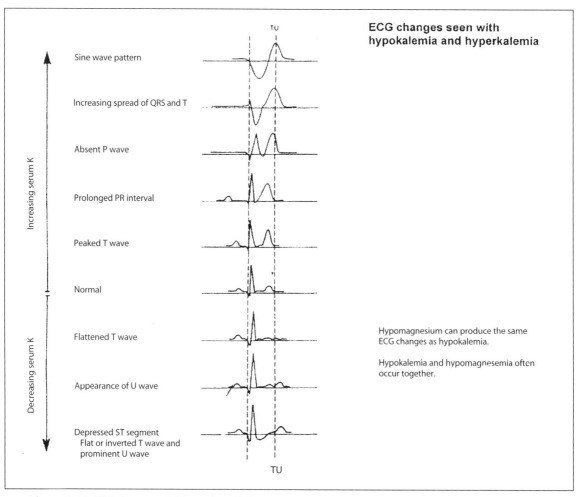

ECG changes seen with hypokalemia and hyperkalemia

Increasing serum K →

- Sine wave pattern
- Increasing spread of QRS and T
- Absent P wave
- Prolonged PR interval
- Peaked T wave
- Normal

Decreasing serum K →

- Flattened T wave
- Appearance of U wave
- Depressed ST segment
  Flat or inverted T wave and
  prominent U wave

Hypomagnesium can produce the same ECG changes as hypokalemia.

Hypokalemia and hypomagnesemia often occur together.

Figure 3.15. EKG changes with hypo/hyperkalemia.

Courtesy of DCI Acute Program, Omaha, Nebraska. Used with permission.

sorbitol by mouth or 50 grams of Kayexalate without sorbitol if given as a retention enema, as sorbitol can cause intestinal necrosis if given as an enema.
  [a] Onset 1–2 hours with duration of action 4–6 hours.
  [b] As the medication coats the intestines, sodium moves across the bowel wall into the blood and potassium moves out of the blood into the intestines.
  [c] Loose stools remove potassium from the body.
  [d] Watch for development of congestive heart failure due to sodium retention.

[3] 10% calcium gluconate (10 mL IV over 3 min). This is not a treatment for hyperkalemia; it is only used to protect the myocardium from the effects of hyperkalemia.
  [a] Onset is 1–3 minutes and the effects last 1–3 hours.
  [b] AVOID in suspected digitalis toxicity since calcium and digitalis have similar effects on the heart and can result in undesired bradycardia, even to the point of cardiac arrest.
[4] Sodium bicarbonate 50 mEq IV over 5 min: Effects last 1–3 hours.
  [a] Decreases serum potassium level by temporarily shifting

potassium into the cells in a patient with acidosis.

[b] This is a hypertonic solution and may exacerbate fluid overload and hypernatremia.

[c] Bicarbonate is a temporary alkalizing agent. Bicarbonate will, however, increase acidosis at the cellular level.

[d] Bicarbonate administration is no longer indicated once dialysis is initiated as hemo-dialysis provides bicarbonate to the patient via diffusion from the dialysate to the blood.

[5] Regular insulin 10 units and D50W in 50 mL IV, if glucose level is < 250 mg/dL.

[a] Onset 30 minutes with duration of 4–6 hours.

[b] This option moves potassium intracellular but does not reduce total body potassium.

[6] Beta 2 adrenergic agonist-nebulized albuterol 10 mg.

[a] Onset in 30 minutes with a duration of 24 hours.

[b] This option moves potassium intracellular but does not reduce total body potassium.

g. Dialysis solution potassium may affect the stability of a HD treatment.

(1) Obtain the most recent serum potassium level.

(2) Use a serum potassium level drawn just prior to dialysis if changes are suspected.

(3) Dialysis solution potassium concentrations are prescribed to correct potassium imbalance at a safe rate while avoiding patient complications of hyper or hypokalemia.

(4) For patients having the serum potassium level drawn by the dialysis nurse, consider initiating treatment with a 2 K$^+$ bath and adjust the bath if required when the serum level is available.

(5) Increased ectopy during a treatment may be resolved by increasing the potassium in the bath.

h. When determining the potassium dialysate bath to be used during acute HD, consider the following options: two potassium dialysate protocols are provided (see Table 3.31 and Table 3.32).

6. Dialysis solution calcium.

a. Calcium is a positively charged cation found in both the extracellular fluid and the intracellular fluid.

(1) The normal range for the total serum calcium is 8.4–10.0 mg/dL.

(2) About 99% of all calcium is concentrated in the skeletal system. Calcium, along with phosphorus, is responsible for bone and teeth formation.

(3) Only 1% of all calcium is found in the serum and soft tissue.

(4) Nearly half of all serum calcium is bound to albumin. Changes in serum albumin correlate with changes in serum calcium (see Figure 3.16).

(a) Evaluate the patient's albumin and calcium level together.

(b) Calculate a corrected calcium:

Corrected calcium (mg/dL) = measured total calcium (mg/dL) + 0.8(4 – serum albumin [g/dL]), where 4.0 represents the average albumin level.

(c) Example:

Serum calcium of 9 (mg/dL), albumin of 3 (g/dL)

(d) 9(mg/dL)+ 0.8(4- 3[g/dL]) = 9.8 (mg/dL) corrected calcium level

(5) Ionized or free calcium is the active form of calcium. Several systemic functions are dependent on ionized calcium levels:

Table 3.31

Potassium Dialysate Protocol – Option A

Standard Dialysate Bath Adjustments	
Serum potassium	Dialysate potassium
> 5.0 mEq/L	2.0 mEq/L
4.0–5.0 mEq/L	3.0 mEq/L
3.5–3.9 mEq/L	3.5 mEq/L
< 3.5 mEq/L	4.0 mEq/L
Notify nephrologist of serum K+ < 3.5 mEq/L	
Consider higher than usual bath for patients at high risk for arrhythmias: cardiomyopathy, s/p CABG, cardiac catheterization, or other cardiac compromise.	

Source: Western Nephrology Acute Dialysis, Denver, Colorado. Courtesy of Dr. David Gillum, Medical Director. Used with permission.

Table 3.32

Potassium Dialysate Protocol – Option B

Potassium dialysate bath considerations play an important role in achieving the goal of safe and effective hemodialysis treatment stability for the acutely ill renal patient.

1. The K^+ bath should be collaboratively verified with the orders of the nephrologist on the following patients:
   a. Renal impaired patients receiving digitalis medications, which are exhibiting signs and symptoms of digitalis toxicity.
   b. ESRD patients ordered to receive blood transfusions.
   c. ESRD patients ordered to receive isolative UF on a routine dialysis day.
   d. Renal impaired patients presenting with hyperglycemia and hyperkalemia.
   e. Renal impaired patients recently experiencing a cardiac condition or cardiac surgery.

2. If serum K^+ is < 4.0 mEq/L, use 4K^+ mEq/L dialysate bath.

3. If serum K^+ is 4.1 to 4.5 mEq/L, use 3K^+ mEq/L dialysate bath.

4. If serum K^+ is 4.6 to 5.5 mEq/L, use 2K^+ mEq/L dialysate bath.

5. If serum K^+ is 5.6 to 6.5 mEq/L, use 1K^+ mEq/L dialysate bath.

6. If serum K^+ is > 6.5 mEq/L, obtain direct K^+ bath orders from nephrologist.
   a. In patients exhibiting cardiac arrhythmias, draw a serum K+ level at baseline and hourly. Monitor patient closely for arrhythmias, refer to Table 3.15: EKG changes related to high or low potassium.
   b. A 0 K^+ bath is always contraindicated. The steep gradient between the serum potassium and the dialysis solution potassium may result in additional arrhythmias.
   c. Reducing the gradient between the serum potassium and the dialysis solution potassium will reduce this risk of arrhythmia, e.g., for a serum potassium of 10 mEq/L select a dialysis potassium of 2 mEq/L. The dialysis treatment may need to be lengthened to achieve the desired removal of potassium from the patient.
   d. The potassium content in the dialysis solution may also be stair-stepped down each hour to achieve the final desired serum potassium for the patient.

7. The potassium (K^+) dialysate protocol Option B listed, is a guideline only and does not replace communication with the ordering nephrologists, critical nursing assessment and evaluation of the acute and chronic renal failure patient.

Source: Creighton Nephrology, Creighton University, Omaha, Nebraska. Used with permission.

(a) Cell membrane permeability and nerve impulse transmission.
(b) Contraction of skeletal, smooth, and cardiac muscle.
(c) Blood clot formation.
b. Calcium is absorbed in the small intestine and excreted in the urine and feces. Several factors influence calcium levels in the body:
(1) Serum pH has an inverse relationship with the ionized calcium level.
(a) If the serum pH rises (the blood becomes alkaline) more calcium binds with protein and the ionized calcium level drops.
(b) The patient with alkalosis is usually hypocalcemic, and the patient with acidosis is usually hypercalcemic.
(2) For the definition, etiology, signs, and symptoms of hypocalcemia and hypercalcemia, see Table 3.33 and Table 3.34.
(3) Assess the patient for clinical evidence of hypocalcemia if total calcium level is < 8.7 mg/dL or ionized calcium is < 1.1 mMol/L.

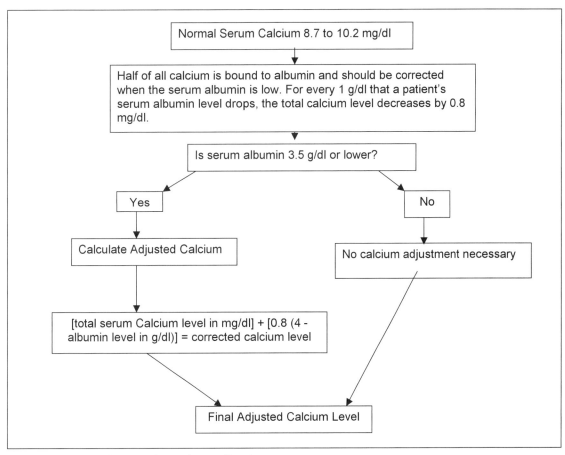

Figure 3.16. Calcium's relationship to albumin.

Courtesy of DCI Acute Program, Omaha, Nebraska. Algorithm compiled from: Springhouse Corporation. (1997). *Fluid and electrolytes made incredibly easy* (p. 135). Philadelphia: Lippincott, Williams & Wilkins. Used with permission.

c. Calcium is present in dialysis solution to prevent precipitous loss of calcium during treatment and resulting hypocalcemia.
  (1) KDOQI guidelines recommend that in patients receiving calcium-based phosphate binders, the dialysate calcium concentration should be targeted to physiologic levels of 2.5 mEq/L. In patients not receiving calcium-containing phosphate binders, the dialysate calcium should be targeted to 2.5–3.0 mEq/L based on serum calcium levels and the need for therapy with active vitamin D sterols.
  (2) The dialysis solution calcium directly effects the serum ionized calcium during a hemodialysis treatment.
    (a) A dialysis solution calcium of 2.5 mEq/L is equivalent to a 1.25 mMol/L.
    (b) The normal range for serum ionized calcium is 1.2-1.4 mMol/L.
  (3) Some authorities do not support using a dialysate solution containing 2.5 mEq/L of calcium in the critically ill patient.
    (a) For an adjusted serum calcium > 10.2 mg/dL use a dialysis solution with 2.5 mEq/L of calcium.
    (b) For an adjusted serum calcium < 10.2 mg/dL use a dialysis solution with 3–3.5 mEq/L of calcium.
    (c) Patients receiving large volumes of blood products may use a dialysis solution calcium of 3.0–3.5 mEq/L to counteract the effect of the citrate anticoagulant present in most blood products.
      [1] Citrate binds to available calcium and is metabolized by the liver to bicarbonate.

Table 3.33	Hypocalcemic Imbalances	
Electrolyte	**Cause**	**Signs & Symptoms**

Hypocalcemia Serum calcium levels drop below 8.7 mg/dL	1) Decreased intake or absorption
	  a) Insufficient dietary intake
	  b) Protein malnutrition (decreased albumin)
	  c) Alcoholism
	  d) Hypoparathyroidism/parathyroidectomy
	  e) Radical neck surgery
	  f) Hypomagnesemia (PTH is magnesium dependent)
	  g) Acute & chronic renal failure (the kidney is unable to activate vitamin D)
	  h) Liver disease
	  i) Steroids/Cushings
	  j) Sepsis
	  k) Anticonvulsants (phenobarb and dilantin interfere with calcium absorption)
	2) Increased excretion
	  a) Diuretics
	  b) Chronic diarrhea
	  c) High phosphorus levels
	  d) Diuretic phase of acute renal failure
	  e) Pancreatic insufficiency/acute pancreatitis cause malabsorption of calcium
	  f) Burns (distressed tissues trap calcium ions from extracellular fluid)
	3) Increased calcium binding
	  a) Citrate containing blood products
	  b) Alkalosis (causes increased protein bonding)
	  c) Drugs
	    i) Anticonvulsants (phenytoin & Phenobarbital)
	    ii) Calcitonin
	    iii) Drugs that lower serum magnesium levels (cisplatin & gentamycin)
	    iv) Edetate disodium (disodium EDTA)
	    v) Loop diuretics
	    vi) Mithramycin
		1) Neurologic
		  a) Anxiety
		  b) Confusion
		  c) Irritability
		  d) Seizures (usually generalized)
		2) Neuromuscular
		  a) Paresthesia of the toes, fingers or face (especially around the mouth)
		  b) Twitching/tremors
		  c) Muscle cramps (laryngeal & abdominal muscles are particularly prone to spasm)
		  d) Tetany (positive Trousseau or Chvostek's signs)
		  e) Hyperactive deep tendon reflexes
		3) Cardiac response
		  a) Diminished response to digoxin
		  b) Decreased cardiac output
		  c) Prolonged ST segment
		  d) Lengthened QT interval (risk for ventricular tachycardia)
		  e) Hypotension

Courtesy of DCI Acute Program, Omaha, Nebraska. Used with permission.

[2] Once the citrate has been metabolized, the calcium is then released back into the serum.
  d. Alternate methods to correct serum calcium.
    (1) For hypocalcemia administer 1 gram of calcium gluconate IV push over 10 minutes.
    (2) Calcium gluconate is preferable to calcium chloride as calcium chloride must always be infused into a central line as it may cause sloughing and necrosis of tissue if a peripheral IV site infiltrates.
    (3) Gram for gram, calcium chloride contains three times the available calcium as calcium gluconate; if given too rapidly calcium chloride may cause bradycardia and even cardiac arrest.
    (4) Correction of hypomagnesia (< 1.5 mEq/L), hyperphosphotemia (> 4.5 mg/dL), and alkalosis is imperative for IV calcium to be effective (see Figure 3.17).
    (5) If a patient is receiving IV calcium, watch for arrhythmias, especially if the patient is also taking digoxin.
      (a) Calcium and digoxin have similar effects on the heart.
      (b) Place patient on cardiac monitor and evaluate for changes in rate and rhythm.

| | Table 3.34 Hypercalcemic Imbalances | | | |

Table 3.34

Hypercalcemic Imbalances

Electrolyte	Cause	Signs & Symptoms

Hypercalcemia Adjusted serum calcium levels above 10.2 mg/dL	1) Increased calcium intake
	  a) Excessive intake of supplement or calcium antacids
	2) Increased absorption
	  a) Low phosphorus levels
	  b) Vitamin A & D overdose/toxicity
	3) Increased mobilization of calcium from bone
	  a) Hyperparathyroidism
	  b) Malignancy (especially breast, lung, lymphoma, multiple myeloma) causes bone destruction
	  c) Multiple fractures
	  d) Prolonged immobilization
	4) Decreased calcium excretion
	  a) Lithium & thiazide diuretics
	  b) Renal tubular acidosis
	5) Acidosis (increases calcium ionization)
	6) Children have higher serum calcium levels than adults and may be markedly increased during bone growth (especially adolescence)
		Caused by the effects of excess calcium in the cells, which causes a decrease in cell membrane excitability.
		1) Effects on skeletal muscle
		  a) Muscle weakness – flaccidity
		  b) Hyporeflexia
		  c) Decreased muscle tone
		2) Effects on heart muscle
		  a) Bradycardia/cardiac arrest
		  b) Shortened QT interval
		  c) Shortened ST segment
		  d) Increased PR interval
		  e) Evidence of digoxin toxicity
		  f) Hypertension
		3) Effects on nervous system
		  a) Confusion
		  b) Personality changes/psychosis
		  c) Lethargy/coma
		4) Decrease in GI motility causing: anorexia, nausea, vomiting, decreased bowel sounds, constipation, paralytic ileus
		5) Bone pain due to pathologic fractures
		6) Flank pain due to development of kidney stones

Courtesy of DCI Acute Program, Omaha, Nebraska. Used with permission.

H. Ultrafiltration.
 1. Ultrafiltration is the removal of water from the plasma through the semipermeable membrane of the dialyzer by hydrostatic pressure or osmotic force.
 2. Fluid assessment and calculations.
  a. Use the information obtained during the pre-dialysis patient assessment to anticipate the patient's volume status and available fluid for ultrafiltration (see section I.E.3. in this chapter).
   (1) Calculate the fluid balance since the last hemodialysis treatment or hospital admission for patient new to hemodialysis, using I/O and weight measurements.
    (a) For established ambulatory or wheelchair bound patients, the ultrafiltration goal can be calculated by the difference in weight since the last HD treatment.

    (b) Fluid removal based on weight gain should include correlation with intake and output measurements since different scales can produce different results and may not be accurate.
   (2) Assess patient's intravascular fluid status using BP, CVP, PAWP, hematocrit, and serum sodium levels. Excess fluid in this space responds well to ultrafiltration.
   (3) Assess the patient for edema, ascites, changes to skin turgor, and mucous membranes. Excess fluid in the form of edema and ascites is more resistant to removal with ultrafiltration than excess fluid in the intravascular space.
  b. Calculate anticipated intake during the hemodialysis treatment.
   (1) Saline for prime and rinseback.
   (2) Saline flushes.
   (3) Volume from anticoagulant, e.g., citrate and calcium.

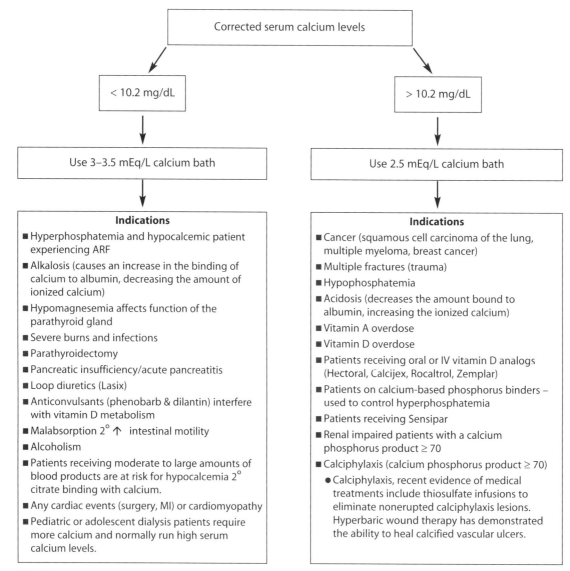

Figure 3.17. Selecting calcium concentration in dialysis solution based on serum calcium.

Adapted from Creighton Nephrology, Creighton University, Omaha, Nebraska. Algorithm compiled using references from Santos, P.W., Hartle, J.E., II, & Quarles, L.P. (2006) & Daugirdas, J.T., Blake, P.G., & Ing, T.S. (2001). Used with permission.

(4) Volume from blood products administration.

(5) Other PO or IV intake.

3. Review the prescribed ultrafiltration goal with the nephrologist as needed. Discrepancies may exist between the UF goal prescribed earlier and the current patient assessment of fluid excess.

4. Interventions that may assist with ultrafiltration.

a. Third spacing, poor cardiac function, and/or intravascular hypovolemia, may necessitate the use of osmotic agents to facilitate shifting the fluid back into the intravascular compartment for removal with dialysis.

b. Anticipate the need for osmotic agents and collaborate with the nephrologist to select and make these agents available (see Table 3.35).

c. Blood products act like osmotic agents to pull fluid into the vascular space.

d. Lower the dialysate temperature (35–36° C) to improve vascular tone.

e. UF profiling. A continuously decreasing linear pattern of UF is well tolerated and is associated with fewer hypotensive episodes.

f. Conductivity profiling, also known as sodium modeling:

Medication	Administration	Special Considerations
25 % albumin	50 mL administered IV via the arterial chamber, The mechanism of action causes approximately 175 mL of additional fluid shift into circulation within 15 minutes. Administer up to 2 times during HD session, 30 minutes apart, not in last hour of treatment.	Is expensive and sometimes in shortage in certain geographic areas. Is an effective osmotic agent. Is not an effective agent for fluid shifting when the serum albumin level is normal.
25% mannitol (12.5 g)	10–20 mL IVP into venous dialysis tubing. Mechanism of action, promotes osmotic fluid shift. Administer up to 3 times during HD session, 30 minutes apart, not in last hour of treatment.	
50% dextrose	10–25 mL IV via venous chamber port over 3–5 minutes. The mechanism of action is an immediate increase in plasma osmolarity contributing to a fluid shift. Administer up to 3 times during HD session, 30 minutes apart, not in last hour of treatment.	For use in the nondiabetic patient.

Adapted from DCI Acute Program, Omaha, Nebraska. Used with permission.

(1) Use cautiously to avoid leaving the patient with an elevated serum sodium that will drive rapid fluid gain post hemodialysis.

(2) Most effective when used in conjunction with UF profiling.

g. Sequential (isolated) ultrafiltration.

h. Online blood volume monitoring (BVM). BVM devices measure blood plasma refill via a relative hematocrit.

i. Position patient with feet elevated, lower head of bed as needed.

(1) Make certain positioning patient does not compromise the patient's condition.

(2) Keep the patient's head of bed at ≥ 30 degrees for patients with elevated intracranial pressure (ICP)to minimize intracranial pressure.

(3) Patients who are ventilator dependent or receiving a tube feeding are at risk for aspiration of secretions or feeding and should not be left flat.

j. Ted hose or sequential lower leg compression device.

I. Anticoagulation.

1. Use the information obtained during the predialysis patient assessment to determine the patient bleeding risk and response to anticoagulation. Bleeding risk may be elevated by any of the following:

a. BUN > 100 mg/dL may cause uremic platelet dysfunction.

b. Low platelet count.

c. Impaired liver function.

d. Medications such as NSAIDs, coumadin, activase, SQ heparin, and Plavix.

e. Chemotherapeutic agents causing thrombocytopenia.

f. Antibiotics affecting platelet function (cephalosporins, erythromycin, amphotericin B, Xigris, and most aminoglycosides).

2. Patients with minimal bleeding risk.

a. These patients may receive "tight" or "low" total heparinization to minimize patient bleeding risk.

b. The goal is to prolong the patient's clotting time to avoid thrombus formation in the extracorporeal circuit.

c. Anticoagulation is achieved with an initial heparin bolus followed by a constant infusion of heparin at a prescribed rate during the hemodialysis treatment.

d. The nephrologist may adjust the heparin dose based on the patient's and/or extra corporeal circuit's response in previous hemodialysis treatments.

e. PTTs may be used to titrate intradialytic heparin administration.

f. Goal PTT may be 45–65 seconds.

g. Heparin dosing in this low range is more accurately monitored and titrated by PTT measurements rather than ACT (activated clotting time) measurements. High dose heparin, as is used in extracorporeal membrane oxygenation (ECMO), is best monitored using ACTs in the range of 180–220 seconds.

h. Heparin adjustment in the acute care setting is under the direction of a registered nurse in collabration with the nephrologist and established protocols.

i. Patient response to heparin varies. Heparin half-life is patient dependent and ranges from 30 minutes to 2 hours. Rebound anticoagulation may occur posttreatment.

3. Patients with high bleeding risk.

a. Patients who are actively bleeding, who are at high risk of bleeding, or in whom the use of heparin is contraindicated should have hemodialysis without heparin.

b. Indications for heparin-free dialysis include:
(1) Pericardial effusion/pericarditis.
(2) Recent surgery with bleeding complications or risk (especially vascular, cardiac, eye, renal transplant, and brain).
(3) Known coagulopathy/thrombocytopenia.
(4) Heparin allergy (HIT).
(5) Active bleeding.
(6) Severe uremia (especially during the first three dialysis treatments).
(7) Patients receiving dialysis immediately before or after an operation or interventional procedure, e.g., kidney biopsy, cardiac cath.
(8) Patients at risk for GI bleed (esophageal varices, ulcer disease).
(9) Recent stroke, trauma, or burn.

c. Heparin-free dialysis may include the following techniques.
(1) Heparin rinse of the extracorporeal circuit with heparinized saline (3000 units/L) during the priming procedure, followed by a normal saline flush prior to initiating dialysis so the heparin in the circuit is not given to the patient. CAUTION: NOT APPROPRIATE FOR PATIENTS WITH HIT.
(2) The blood flow is set as high as tolerated during dialysis (at least 250 mL/min). CAUTION: NOT APPROPRIATE FOR PATIENTS AT RISK FOR DDS.
(3) A 25–200 mL rapid saline rinse of the dialyzer is performed every 30–60 minutes throughout the dialysis treatment. The rinsing allows inspection of the extracorporeal circuit and may assist in avoiding circuit clotting. The ultrafiltration calculations are adjusted to remove the fluid given as flushes.

d. Alternative anticoagulation options.
(1) Regional citrate anticoagulation using anticoagulant citrate dextrose formula A (ACD-A) or 4% trisodium citrate.
(2) Hemodialysis using dialysate containing citric acid.
(3) Other systemic anticoagulants, such as lepirudin, may also be used.

IV. Intradialytic assessment and interventions.

A. The goal of intradialytic patient care is to assess, apply interventions, and to evaluate the patient's response to the interventions, providing a safe, effective, and comfortable hemodialysis treatment.

B. Both the hemodialysis system and the water treatment system must be monitored throughout the hemodialysis treatment and findings documented.

C. Patient assessment and documentation of findings.

1. The intradialytic assessment will include the hemodialysis system BFR, arterial pressure (AP), venous pressure (VP), transmembrane pressure (TMP), and ultrafiltration rate (UFR), the patient's vital signs, pain level, I/O, vascular access, anticoagulation received, lab results, and any patient complaints or changes in patient behavior.

2. The patient on intermittent hemodialysis must be monitored continuously by the patient care provider. The patient's vascular access must be visible throughout the entire treatment. Changes in the patient's condition or vascular access can happen quickly and it is critical that the patient care provider be present to quickly resolve any treatment complication, e.g., hypotension, catheter disconnection, or needle dislodgement.

3. Documentation should occur every 15 minutes in critical care settings and in patients receiving HD for the first time.

4. Documentation may occur every 30 minutes in general acute care settings.
5. During unstable patient situations, documentation occurs as often as interventions are occurring and patient responses are being evaluated.

D. Patient parameters.
1. Vital signs.
    a. Blood pressure and pulse are indicative of the patient's tolerance to fluid removal. Hypotension and increased pulse rate often signal intravascular hypovolemia.
    b. Assess both the apical and radial heart rate for signs of atrial fibrillation or other arrthymias intermittently and when hypotension occurs.
    c. Respirations.
        (1) Increased respirations initially can indicate decreasing blood pressure or acidosis.
        (2) Decreased respirations can indicate severe hypotension or alkalosis.
    d. Temperature as warranted by changes in patient condition, e.g., shaking chills, or during the administration of blood products.
2. Fluid removal and blood pressure monitoring.
    a. Most patients that require renal replacement therapy have some UF needs.
    b. The total volume ultrafiltrated as well as rapid removal of fluid volume (high ultrafiltration rate) contribute to hypotension.
        (1) Hypotension is the most common complication during HD occurring in up to as many as 30% of treatments.
        (2) Defined as:
            (a) Systolic blood pressure (SBP) < 100 mm Hg.
            (b) Diastolic blood pressure (DBP) < 40 mm Hg.
            (c) Drop in SBP > 40 mm Hg.
            (d) Mean arterial pressure (MAP) < 65.
        (3) Hypotension is related to intravascular volume, cardiac output, and systemic vascular resistance.
        (4) 20–25% decrease in cardiac output = decrease of > 20 mm Hg in SBP or DBP upon standing.
    c. Contributing factors to intradialytic hypotension.
        (1) Solute gradient changes.
        (2) Eating a large meal immediately before or during treatment, has been known to

cause severe hypotension as well as nausea and vomiting.
        (a) Every effort should be made to assist the patient to maintain nutritional intake in the hospital setting to promote healing.
        (b) One option is to order the patient's meal to be delivered early so they can eat 1 hour prior to the planned treatment.
        (c) A nutritional supplement can be prescribed and offered in small amounts to the patient during treatment to maintain caloric intake and avoid hypotension.
        (d) The bedside nurse should be instructed to hold the patient's tray until the patient's hemodialysis treatment is complete, even when the patient is receiving the hemodialysis in the dialysis treatment room.
        (3) Decreased compensatory mechanisms.
        (4) Oxygen saturation level.
            (a) Decrease in saturation can be induced by ultrafiltration depleting the intravascular blood volume.
            (b) During HD the PO_2 may drop 5–30 mm Hg, creating a problem in patients with severe preexisting pulmonary or cardiac disease, especially in the elderly.
        (5) Autonomic dysfunction.
        (6) Medications, e.g., antihypertensive medications.
        (7) Laboratory values, e.g., low blood glucose, hypocalcemia, or low hematocrit.
    d. Prevention of hypotension and promotion of safe ultrafiltration with plasma refill occurs by following the interventions that may assist with UF (see III.H.4 in this chapter).
    e. Treating intradialytic hypotension. Each step should be taken and blood pressure reassessed until hypotension resolves.
        (1) Stop ultrafiltration.
        (2) Recline the patient if this position is not contraindicated.
        (3) Bolus with normal saline (volume dependent on the patient size and condition) and/or titrate vasopressors if available.
        (4) Additionally, apply the interventions that may assist with UF as indicated (see III.H.4 in this chapter).

3. Vascular access monitoring.
    a. Monitor the hemodialysis system AP and VP.
    b. Directly observe the catheter, fistula, or graft. Observe and verify the security of needle placement and/or bloodline connections.
    c. The patient's vascular access must be visible throughout the entire treatment.
4. Response to treatment. The patient should be encouraged to report complaints of dizziness, cramping, and restlessness as these symptoms may indicate hypotension or volume depletion.
5. Observe and document the patient's level of consciousness.

E. Equipment parameters.
    1. Integrity of the extracorporeal circuit:
        a. Verify that all lines are open and that connections are intact, and secure every 30 minutes.
        b. Keep connections visible at all times.
    2. Observe color of blood in dialyzer and bloodlines.
        a. Dark color can precede filter clotting.
        b. Cherry-pop appearance indicates hemolysis.
    3. Monitor pressure readings.
        a. Venous pressure (VP) measures the resistance encountered when blood is being returned to the patient through the venous access.
            (1) Should not exceed 250 mm Hg.
            (2) High VP pressure may indicate clotting in venous chamber, bloodline, or venous needle.
            (3) Low VP may indicate clotted dialyzer or venous access disconnection.
        b. Arterial pressure (AP) measures the negative pressure applied by the blood pump between the needle site and the blood pump.
            (1) Should not exceed 250 mm Hg.
            (2) Low AP indicates hypotension, excessive suction on wall of access or a clotted arterial needle or access port.
            (3) Sudden drop in AP may indicate needle migration or infiltration.
            (4) High AP may indicate clotting of dialyzer or system.
        c. Transmembrane pressure (TMP) is a calculated pressure derived from the venous pressure minus the dialysate pressure in mm Hg.
            (1) The TMP is influenced by the porosity of the dialyzer membrane.
            (2) High-flux dialyzers will have a lower TMP.
            (3) TMP rises slowly throughout a

hemodialysis treatment in response to ultrafiltration with resultant increased blood viscosity.
            (4) TMP must be monitored to detect rapid large shifts in pressure, which may indicate excess ultrafiltration, a dialysate leak, or system clotting.
    4. Anticoagulant delivery and effectiveness.
        a. The anticoagulant pump should be observed to make certain the anticoagulant is being infused as prescribed.
        b. Monitor patient and system response to anticoagulant by direct observation or blood specimen testing.
        c. Discontinue anticoagulant as indicated in treatment order, typically 30-60 minutes prior to treatment termination for patients who need to achieve hemostasis after needle removal from their graft or fistula.
        d. For patient bleeding, discontinue anticoagulation and consult the nephrologist for additional laboratory and/or medication orders.
    5. Blood and dialysate flow rates ensure that prescribed rates are being delivered to achieve desired patient solute clearance. Dialysis time may need to be increased if the prescribed rates are not achievable.
    6. Ultrafiltration rate (UFR) should be set and adjusted based on patient response to treatment.
    7. Conductivity. Dialysate conductivity monitoring ensures the delivery of a dialysis solution with an electrolyte concentration that will not harm red blood cells by causing hemolysis or crenation.

F. Intradialytic patient education.
    1. An acute nephrology nurse should assess the patient receiving hemodialysis for knowledge deficits, readiness to learn, and preferred method of learning.
    2. Patient education should meet the identified knowledge deficits using a method that meets the patient needs, e.g., audio, visual, or kinesthetic.
    3. The 1:1 bedside education helps to allay concerns about the dialysis process and offers an opportunity to educate and answer questions related to kidney health, whether the patient is experiencing AKI or CKD. Refer to Appendix 3.1: Patient Education Brochure, at the end of this section.
    4. Education should be provided for the CKD

patient approaching stage 5. This education should include exposure to all treatment options that are available to the patient, e.g., in-center hemodialysis, home hemodialysis, continuous ambulatory peritoneal dialysis, automated peritoneal dialysis, living donor kidney transplant, deceased donor kidney transplant, and conservative care. Refer to Section 4.
5. Vascular access.
   a. Educate the patient about the care and maintenance of their existing access.
   b. Educate the patient about vascular access options and the steps the patient will take to achieve a successful fistula or graft if needed.
   c. Educate the patient about care of a catheter vascular access. Refer to Appendix 3.4: Catheter Instructions for the Patient and Appendix 3.5: Patient Catheter Release Form at the end of this section.
6. Most importantly, education of the patient with CKD and/or family should include the information that renal replacement therapy may be integrated into a person's life, helping him/her feel better so he/she can fully live the life they have.

V. Posthemodialysis assessment and evaluation.

A. The purpose of the posthemodialysis assessment and evaluation is to evaluate the patient, their response to treatment, changes in their overall condition, and the achievement of treatment goals.
   1. Any unexpected changes in patient condition or failure to achieve the expected treatment goals should be reported to the charge nurse and/or nephrologist. Changes to the patient's care should be anticipated.
   2. The posthemodialysis patient assessment should be performed as indicated below and verbally reported to the receiving bedside nurse. The report should include the following:
      a. Blood glucose monitoring and laboratory tests drawn, pre-, intra-, or postdialysis.
      b. Amount and type of anticoagulation administered.
      c. All medications administered (oral, intravenous, and parenteral).
      d. Amount and type of blood products administered.
      e. Pre and post vital signs.
      f. Net fluid balance.
      g. Condition of vascular access.
         (1) Fistula or graft: patent with bruit and thrill and type of dressing.

      (2) Catheter: exit site condition and dressing change.
      h. Response or complications experienced throughout treatment.
      i. Clarify any orders to be carried out after dialysis to avoid an assumption that they may have already been completed, such as administration of antibiotics.
   3. If the hemodialysis treatment occurred in a dialysis treatment room, the pateint's condition and mode of departure should be documented on the hemodialysis treatment record as well.

B. The patient and extracorporeal circuit are evaluated after the treatment is discontinued and the assessment documented on the hemodialysis treatment flowsheet.
   1. Vital signs.
      a. BP: lying, sitting or standing, as patient condition permits. Consider a sitting and standing BP prior to removing needles so that additional saline may be infused if hypotensive.
      b. Standing BP is taken to assess for orthostatic hypotension; if patient is unable to stand, consider elevating the head of the bed to 80–90 degrees.
      c. Assess the pulse rate and rhythm by apical auscultation and radial pulse comparison.
         (1) Increased rate may indicate fluid volume depletion or atrial fibrillation in response to volume depletion.
         (2) A change in heart rate to > 120 or < 50 beats/min should be reported to the nephrologist.
      d. Temperature.
         (1) Compare to predialysis temperature.
         (2) Elevation may indicate access infection or infection related to other illness manifestations.
      e. Respiration.
         (1) Rate and quality: labored or rapid.
         (2) Auscultate breath sounds.
         (3) Oxygen saturation rate.
   2. Weight.
      a. Compare to predialysis weight to determine amount of fluid removed during dialysis.
      b. Compare to dry weight to determine if fluid removal achieved euvolemia.
   3. Vascular access (whether newly placed or established) condition.
      a. Estimate blood loss, length of time bleeding, type of dressing applied, and patency of access at time the patient is returned to the care of the bedside nurse.

b. Observe vascular access for signs and symptoms of infection, e.g, redness, warmth, swelling, and drainage. Obtain culture as needed.
4. Sense of well-being.
   a. Record the patient's response to treatment, e.g. "tolerated treatment without complications."
   b. Level of consciousness (LOC).
      (1) Note changes in patient's LOC prior to return to general care.
      (2) Include description such as alert, oriented, disoriented, agitated, confused, obtunded, unconscious, combative, depressed, etc.
5. Dialyzer and extracorporeal circuit condition.
   a. Residual blood loss.
      (1) Estimate and document after the rinseback of blood from the dialyzer.
         (a) Small = 25% clotted/streaked fibers noted.
         (b) Moderate = 25-50% clotted/streaked fibers noted.
         (c) Large = 50–100% clotted/streaked fibers noted.
      (2) Estimate the amount of surfaced area clotted in the chambers, correlating the total amount of anticoagulant administered during treatment.
   b. A large amount of clotting and streaking would be an indicator of inadequate anticoagulation and adjustments should be anticipated on subsequent hemodialysis treatments.

C. Obtain postdialysis laboratory tests.
   1. BUN for Kt/V$_{urea}$ or URR, blood cultures, serum drug levels.
   2. Ensure that blood chemistries are drawn no sooner than 1–2 hours after treatment, to allow the patient's body to re-equilibrate serum electrolyte levels and avoid treating an electrolyte level in the midst of equilibration, e.g., giving IV potassium for a low serum potassium level.

D. Provide patient education.
   1. The approximate date of next dialysis treatment.
   2. Access care.
   3. Diet.
   4. Fluid restrictions.
   5. Medications.
   6. Instruction and reinforcement in any areas needed.
   7. For the ARF patient undergoing hemodialysis for the first time, use ARF patient educational material. Refer to Appendix 3.1: Patient Education Brochure, at the end of this section. to provide patient and family education relative to ARF and the hemodialysis treatment.

Chapter 12

Peritoneal Dialysis in the Acute Care Setting

Purpose

The purpose of this chapter is to describe the care of patients undergoing peritoneal dialysis (PD) in the acute care setting

Objectives

Upon completion of this chapter, the learner will be able to:
1. Describe the nephrology nurse role in coordinating and facilitating the care of the PD patient in the acute care setting.
2. Outline the steps to initiate and manage the admission and discharge of the PD patient in the acute care setting.
3. Discuss assessment of potential PD patient complications in the acute care setting.

I. **Nursing management of the PD patient in the acute care setting.**

A. The PD patient on the medical/surgical unit may be admitted for:
1. PD catheter insertion or catheter-related complications.
2. Infectious or noninfectious dialysis complications.
3. Transferred from a critical care setting.
4. Admitted for elective, nonemergent reasons.
   a. Elective and nonemergent surgery.
   b. Elective diagnostic procedures.
      (1) Invasive cardiac studies.
      (2) Complicated endoscopy and/or colonoscopy.
      (3) Arthroscopy.
   c. Medical indications.
      (1) Cardiac ischemia.
      (2) Pulmonary problems.
         (a) Pneumonia.
         (b) Asthma.
         (c) Chronic obstructive pulmonary disease (COPD).
         (d) Evaluation of sleep apnea.
         (e) Gastroparesis.
      (3) Gastrointestinal issues.
         (a) Hiatal hernia.
         (b) Severe reflux disease.
         (c) Gastrointestinal bleeding.
         (d) Pancreatitis.
      (4) Metabolic and endocrine disorders.
      (5) Orthopedic procedures.
      (6) Diabetes and complications.
      (7) Neurologic disorders.
      (8) Peripheral vascular disease.
      (9) Localized and systemic infections.
      (10) Psychiatric disorders.

B. Preparations for an elective admission.
1. The home training or acute care PD nurse may be active in the coordination of the patient's admission.
2. Preparation will vary with each institution and may include the following:
   a. Determine if the hospital unit can safely perform PD therapy.
   b. Establish a channel of communication between the hospital unit and the outpatient PD nurses.
   c. Identify the hospital PD resource for the staff nurse on the unit.
   d. Provide inservice educational programs for the hospital staff.
   e. Provide written educational information and tools for the hospital staff.
   f. Provide the patient's chronic kidney disease (CKD) and dialysis history following Health

Insurance Portability and Accountability Act (HIPAA) guidelines.

g. Share information concerning the patient's learning style and coping mechanisms.

h. Identify and/or provide PD tubings, transfer sets, and other necessary PD equipment.

i. Identify the PD nurse as both a patient and a PD advocate.

j. Provide liaison service for hospital staff and the PD health care team.

C. Specific issues that may need to be addressed during the PD patient's hospitalization (see Figure 3.18).

1. Staff may lack experience with PD and need frequent coaching.

2. Staff may need review of policies and procedures.

3. PD orders/prescription may need clarification.

4. Ordering adequate supplies.

5. Protocols for adjustment of intraperitoneal PD solution volume for invasive procedures.

   a. A patient who is having a cardiac catheterization, for example, may need a temporary reduction in fill volume during the procedure to provide patient comfort and to diminish the possibility of respiratory embarrassment.

   b. These adjustments will vary according to physician's preference and experience.

6. Changes to the patient's PD exchange routine to accommodate delays due to invasive procedures and/or surgery.

7. Reminders about the need for thorough hand washing, wearing of face masks, and the use of universal precautions.

8. Securing of catheter at all times during invasive procedures, surgery, and transfers from bed to stretchers or wheelchairs.

9. Accurate and consistent documentation of the patient's PD therapy.

10. Preparation of a discharge plan.

D. Preparation for PD patient discharge.

1. The discharge planning process should be started early in the patient's hospitalization to facilitate a timely and smooth transition.

2. All the members of the patient's health care team may be involved, but the coordination is usually shared among case managers, the primary/bedside nurse, the home PD nurse, the nephrologist, and the social worker.

3. The discharge plan should include:

   a. Team discussion about safe discharge plan.

   b. Active patient and family involvement in the discharge plan.

   c. Identification of the PD unit that will resume patient follow-up.

4. Adequate supplies must be ordered and delivered to the patient's home prior to discharge.

5. Schedule a follow-up appointment with the nephrologist and the PD unit.

6. If the patient is unable to resume self-care responsibility at discharge:

   a. Discuss options with case manager, social worker, primary nurse, nephrologists, and PD nurse.

   b. Determine whether patient qualifies for either short- or long-term rehabilitation care.

   c. Evaluate rehabilitation center for PD experience and safety.

   d. Provide inservice instruction and written references to rehabilitation staff if needed.

   e. Identify PD resource individuals among the rehabilitation staff.

   f. Use the above-mentioned criteria in evaluation for long-term care facility placement.

7. Document all plans in the patient's hospital record.

8. Send discharge summaries to all involved PD unit and health care team members.

II. Nursing management of the PD treatment in the acute care setting.

A. The PD experience of the acute care nursing staff will vary.

1. Identification of resources for the staff nurse is crucial in providing safe PD therapy.

2. Communication and collaboration of all involved health care providers is vital to achieve appropriate clinical outcomes for the PD patient.

3. The acute care PD nephrology nurse may need to be facilitator, educator, and coordinator of this process.

4. Clarify who will perform the PD procedures.

   a. A designated in-hospital nephrology PD nurse team.

   b. An acute care hemodialysis nurse.

   c. An acute care dialysis technician with nurse supervision.

   d. The critical care nurse.

   e. An expert medical/surgical floor nurse.

   f. A per diem or contracted nurse from a nursing agency or vendor.

Daily Bedside Inservice Checklist for CAPD Patient Care

1. Review the patient's prescription
   a. Number of exchanges per day
   b. Volume of exchanges
   c. Dextrose and Calcium concentrations
   d. Effect of dextrose on fluid removal
   e. Medications to be added
   f. Where to get supplies needed for treatment
   g. Mask everyone, close the door, and wash your hands

2. Review the steps in performing a CAPD exchange - Tri-fold reference sheet
   a. Connect and drain
      - Assess effleuent for color, clarity, fibrin
      - Length of drain time
      - Difficulty or pain with draining
   b. Fill
      - Length of time to fill
      - Difficulty or pain with filling
   c. Disconnect and cap off the catheter
      - Weighing the effluent
      - Disposing of the effluent

3. Exit site and tunnel assessment
   a. Exit site care
   b. Tunnel palpation
   c. Securing the catheter

4. Documentation on the CAPD Treatment Record
   a. Exchange Record - out and in
   b. Patient Volume Net
   c. Effluent Characteristics
   d. Exit Site and Tunnel
   e. Observation of patient exchanges
   f. Labs
   g. Vital signs
   h. Patient assessments

5. When to call the nephrologist:
   a. If the effluent becomes cloudy or has fibrin in it.
   b. If the lab values are out of the normal range for a dialysis patient.
   c. If the catheter exit site or tunnel appear inflamed, sore, or draining.
   d. If the patient's fluid status is changing and the prescription for ulltrafiltration needs to be adjusted.

Hospital Staff

Western Acute Dialysis Staff

Date   Time

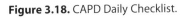

Figure 3.18. CAPD Daily Checklist.

Source: Western Nephrology Acute Dialysis, Denver, Colorado. Used with permission.

5. For general inforation regarding PD therapy, please refer to the following:
   a. Section 13, Chapter 61: Peritoneal Dialysis Access.
   b. Section 13, Chapter 62: Peritoneal Dialysis Therapy.
   c. Section 13, Chapter 63: Complications of Peritoneal Dialysis.

B. Initiating PD in the acute care setting.
   1. Educate the patient and family about PD care in the acute care setting.
   2. Evaluate the patient's need for a private room to limit exposure to possible infections.
   3. Identify nursing staff's ability to safely perform PD.
   4. Identify nursing staff's resources.
      a. Expert PD nurses in the institution.
      b. Outpatient home training PD nurses.
      c. Acute care hemodialysis nurses who may cover inpatient PD patients.
      d. Nephrology clinical nurse specialists (CNS) or nurse practitioners (NP).
   5. Inform the necessary health care team members of PD patient admission.
      a. PD resource nurses, inpatient and outpatient.
      b. Nurse manager or charge nurse on patient's unit to evaluate staff's ability to:
         (1) Safely perform PD.
         (2) Provide appropriate staffing.
         (3) Assess PD patient acuity.
      c. CNS or NP to provide additional education and support.
      d. Nephrologist.
   6. For the established PD patient in the acute care setting, contact the home PD nurse and consult with the patient, family member(s), or significant other to obtain:
      a. Current dialysis prescription.
      b. Membrane transport characteristics.
      c. Most recent Kt/V$_{urea}$ results.
      d. Medication list.
      e. Infection history.
      f. Allergies.
      g. Other pertinent health care information.
   7. Obtain and review pertinent hospital policies and procedures.
   8. Obtain PD prescription orders.
   9. Identify and obtain necessary PD equipment.
   10. Order adequate supplies to prevent delays in providing dialysis.
   11. Clarify how nursing management of PD will be communicated and documented, which is especially important when there are multiple

nurses involved in providing PD therapy (see Figures 3.18, 3.19, 3.20, and Table 3.36).

C. Performing PD as renal replacement therapy specific to the acute care setting.
   1. The nephrologist, renal fellow or attending physician should be notified of the following changes in condition:
      a. Severe abdominal pain or distention.
      b. Poor infusion or drainage.
      c. Leakage of dialysate from the exit site.
      d. Suspected exit site or tunnel infection.
      e. Cloudy effluent.
      f. Grossly bloody effluent.
      g. Diminished ultrafiltration.
      h. Hyperglycemia.
      i. Rapid shifts in serum electrolytes.
      j. Increased respiratory distress.
      k. Unusual changes in abdominal girth.
      l. Suspected migration of catheter tip away from the left lower quadrant of the abdomen.
      m. Unintentional tubing disconnections.
   2. Inspection of effluent (drained dialysate).
      a. Color.
         (1) Colorless.
         (2) Light to dark yellow.
         (3) Pink, in female patient, may indicate menstruation.
         (4) Red indicates bleeding.
         (5) Tea colored may indicate old bleeding or certain medications.
      b. Clarity.
         (1) Clear.
         (2) Cloudy is a sign of peritonitis. Send effluent for cell count, gram stain, and culture and sensitivity.
      c. Presence or absence of fibrin.
      d. Report unexpected changes to nephrologist.
   3. Monitoring the patient's weight. Daily weight is part of the global assessment of fluid balance.
      a. Obtain baseline weight prior to initiation of PD therapy.
      b. Weight should be obtained daily, consistently either with or without fluid dwelling.
      c. Patient should use same scale and wear similar clothing.
      d. Daily weight and fill volume needs to be documented in progress notes, PD flow sheets, or other sites according to institution's policy.
   4. Maintaining accurate documentation of intake and output. Document on unit specific PD treatment flow sheet (see Figures 3.19 and 3.20).
      a. Frequency of exchanges, fill volume, and dextrose %.

b. How much dialysate was infused.

c. How much dialysate was drained.

d. Subtract amount of infused dialysate from the drained dialysate to determine if the patient has a net negative or positive ultrafiltration.

e. Calculate intake.
(1) Oral intake.
(2) Intravenous infusions.
(3) Tube feedings.
(4) PD net negative ultrafiltration, i.e., retained dialysate.

f. Calculate output.
(1) Urine production.
(2) Nasogastric tube drainage.
(3) PD net positive ultrafiltration.
(4) If catheter site is leaking, weigh saturated dressings for accurate accounting of dialysate.

5. Facilitating infusion and draining of solution in the acute care setting.
a. Secure catheter carefully to prevent kinking or occlusion.
b. Use gravity.
(1) Lower patient or raise dialysis solution to increase rate of infusion.
(2) Raise patient or lower drain bag to increase rate of drainage.
c. Patient may need to be turned from side to side to facilitate draining.
d. If possible, elevate the patient's head and upper torso during infusion and draining of dialysis solution.
(1) To prevent respiratory compromise when infusing dialysate.
(2) To maximize use of gravity when draining dialysate.
e. The patient may need to be carefully positioned with respect to other monitoring devices and/or ventilator connections.

6. If ultrafiltration is diminished, consider the following:
a. Rule out problems related to catheter issues.
(1) Obstruction from fibrin.
(2) Kink in tubing or catheter.
(3) Patient position.
(4) Failure to open appropriate clamps on tubing set.
(5) Failure to open frangible(s) in-line on tubing set.
b. Assess abdominal wall for catheter exit site leak or subcutaneous leaking.
c. Assess for dehydration.
d. Assess for constipation.

e. Assess for unusual insensible loss of fluid.
f. Consult with nephrologists.

7. Infections.
a. Refer to Section 13 for peritoneal dialysis access catheter related infections.
b. Refer to Section 13 for complications of peritoneal dialysis.
c. Refer to Section 13, Table 13.24: Evidence-Based Practice Guidelines for PD Associated Peritonitis.
d. Assess for signs and symptoms of infection.
(1) Assess patient for:
(a) Abdominal pain or tenderness.
(b) Constipation/diarrhea.
(c) Nausea/vomiting.
(d) Elevated temperature.
(e) Blood leukocytosis, i.e, elevated white blood cell count.
(2) Assess exit site and tunnel for:
(a) Erythema.
(b) Pain or tenderness.
(c) Inflammation.
(d) Exudate at exit site.
(e) Purulent drainage (may be gently expressed from tunnel).
(f) Elevated skin temperature over tunnel.
(g) Fluid or fluctuance over the catheter tunnel.
(h) Dialysate leak.
(i) Edema over the catheter tunnel.
(3) Assess PD effluent for:
(a) Elevated white blood cell count, i.e., > 100/mL.
(b) Cloudiness.
(c) Blood.
(d) Fibrin.
e. Document and report any of the above changes to the nephrologist (see Figures 3.19 and 3.20).
(1) Send effluent sample for cell count, gram stain, and culture and sensitivity, including fungal culture, as ordered.
(2) Send swab of drainage for culture and sensitivity as ordered.
(3) Anticipate initiating antibiotics.
(4) Communicate change in plan of care to hospital nurse assigned to patient.

8. Patient and nursing safety issues:
a. Careful, thorough hand washing is mandated to protect both patient and caregiver from transmission of infection.
b. A mask must be worn by patient, if possible. All caregivers and/or family members present

Acute Peritoneal Dialysis Flow Sheet

Patient Name John Doe   Medical Record # 000-00-00
Nephrologist   Dr. G.F. Rate

Date	Time	Ex.#	Previous Fill Vol. (PFV)	% Dex.	Medication Added	Drain Vol. (DV)	Description Of effluent	(PFV)-(DV)= Ex. Balance	24hr.bal.	Daily Wt.
12-5-06	2 AM	1	2000 ml	1.5 %	none	2100 ml	Clear, no fibrin	2000-2100=-100	-100	169 lbs.
12-5-06	6 AM	2	2000 ml	2.5 %	none	2500 ml	Clear (+) fibrin	2000-2500=-500	-600	
12-5-06	10AM	3	2000 ml	1.5%	Heparin 2000u	2700 ml	Clear, no fibrin	2000-2700=-700	-1300	
"	2 PM	4	2000 ml	2.5 %	Heparin 2000u	2200 ml	Clear, no fibrin	2000-2200=-200	-1500	
"	6 PM	5	2000 ml	2.5 %	Heparin 2000u	2700 ml	Clear, no fibrin	2000-2700=-700	-2200	
"	10PM	6	2500 ml	2.5 %	Heparin 2000u	2700 ml	Clear, no fibrin	2500-2700=-200	-2900	
12-6-06	2 AM	7	2500 ml	2.5 %	Heparin 2000u	2800 ml	Clear, no fibrin	2500-2800=-300	-300	
12-6-06	6 AM	8	2500 ml	2.5%	Heparin 2000u					166 lbs.

Figure 3.19. Acute Care PD Flow Sheet.

Courtesy of Maria Luongo. Used with permission.

must mask when doing PD exchanges or procedures.

c. Nurses/caregivers must use universal precautions when performing PD therapy.

d. Effluent must be disposed of as a hazardous waste. Receptacles and procedures will vary with each institution.

D. Components of PD prescription and orders (see Figures 3.21, 3.22, 3.23, and 3.24).
1. Fill volume: Average fill is 2 to 2.5 liters.
   a. 500 to 1000 mL for initial exchanges on patients with new catheters.
   b. 2000 mL to 2500 mL for maintenance therapy.
   c. 3500 mL or greater only for unusual situations, since larger fill volumes may contribute to respiratory difficulty.
2. Frequency of exchanges will depend on:
   a. Current patient fluid balance.
   b. Need for emergent fluid removal.
   c. Need for emergent correction of electrolyte imbalance.
   d. Hemodynamic instability.
   e. Membrane transport characteristics.
   f. Metabolic stability or instability.
   g. Manual PD: 4 to 12 exchanges per 24 hours.
   h. APD: 4 to 12 exchanges per 24 hours.
   i. In unusual circumstances, exchanges may be done every 60 to 90 minutes, but this increases the risk of developing dialysis disequilibrium syndrome in patients with advanced uremia.
3. PD solutions.
   a. 1.5% dextrose.
   b. 2.5% dextrose.
   c. 4.25% dextrose.
   d. Either low calcium (2.5 mEq/L) or regular calcium (3.0 mEq/L) formulation.
   e. Extraneal® (Baxter, Deerfield, Illinois): icodextrin 7.5%.
      (1) Nonglucose polymer.
      (2) Used for selected patients for fluid removal.
      (3) Used for only one exchange every 24 hours.
      (4) Used as a long dwell exchange (10–12 hours).
         (a) With manual PD, is typically done as overnight dwell.
         (b) With APD, is typically done as the long daytime dwell.
      (5) Can interfere with select glucose monitoring devices. The Federal Drug Administration (FDA) warning indicates, "Blood glucose measurement in patients receiving Extraneal must be done with a glucose-specific method (monitor and test strips) to avoid interference by maltose, released from Extraneal®.

Western Acute Dialysis Peritoneal Dialysis Record

Date: _____   Date PD Initiated: _____   Hosp Day# _____

Hospital: _____   Patient Name: _____

Primary Diagnosis: _____ Set up:_____ Nurse visit:_____ On call:_____

Pager:_____

Out Patient Unit/Contact: _____ Phone: _____   Supplies: Adequate _____

Order placed _____

Physician CAPD Orders:

Number of exchanges _____

Volume: 2500ml or _____ ml

Dianeal: 2.5mEq Ca or _____mEq Ca

   : Add K+ _____mEq/L

Dry Weight _____

1. 6am _____%
2. 10 am _____%
3. 2 pm _____%
4. 6 pm _____%
5. 10 pm _____%

1. 8am _____%
2. 1 pm _____%
3. 6 pm _____%
4. 10 pm_____%

CAPD EXCHANGE RECORDS:

Date	BP	Exch No	Time	OUT ml's drained	Drain Time	Dextrose Solution % Selected	IN Meds added	ml's infused	Patient Volume Net	Staff Signature

Daily Total Net

Labs:

	Prev	Today
Na		
K+		
Cl		
CO2		
BUN		
Cr		
Gluc		
Ca		
Alb		
Phos		
WBC		
Hgb		
Hct		
Plt		

Cell Count:

Gram Stain:

Culture Results:

Assessment:

	Prev	Today
BP		
HR		
Temp		
Weight		
02		
Lungs		
Edema		
Muscle Cramping		

EXIT SITE:		**TUNNEL:**
Skin Color		Red
Clean		
Crusted		Warmth
Tender		
Drainage		Tender
Cleaned with		
Ointment applied		
Dressing		

Comments:

Effluent Characteristics:

Time	Color	Clarity	Fibrin

Mental Status	
Mobility	
Dexterity	
Appetite	
N/V	
Pain	
Observed Technique	
Mask	
Washed Hands	

Figure 3.20. CAPD Treatment Record.

Courtesy of Helen Williams, Western Nephrology Acute Dialysis, Denver, Colorado. Used with permission.

Peritoneal Dialysis Orders for the Hospitalized Patient   Date_____

Patient Name:_____   Diagnosis:_____

Nephrologist: _____   PD RN Resource phone # _____

CAPD orders:

Dialysate Solution   Low Ca+ 2.5 mEq/1L solution ____
1.5%_____   Reg. Ca+ 3.5 mEq/L solution   ____
2.5% ____
4.25% _____
or alternate_____% and _____ %

Fill volume (FV) per exchange   _____mL

Frequency of exchange: Every _____hrs. or _____ times per day

Assess drained effluent past each exchange. Report cloudy or bloody drainage.

Dialysate specimens to lab:
(Baseline upon admission and prn cloudy fluid)

Hematology – Cell count ____and differential__ _

Microbiology – Gm Stain_____and C & S_____

Medications Added to Dialysate Bag: **Allergies:** _____

Heparin _____units per solution bag prn fibrin

Antibiotic:_____Start Date_____ Frequency_____
Antibiotic:_____Start Date_____ Frequency_____

Potassium Chloride (KCl) _____ mEq per bag

Other medications: _____ _____

Exit Site Care:

Keep catheter secured to abdomen with tape.

Change tape and dressing daily and more frequently if needed.

Wash exit site daily with soap and water.

Apply: Bactroban ointment_____ Gentamycin ointment_____

Report signs and symptoms of infection of exit site to nephrologist.

Send swab for: Gm stain_____ C & S _____

Diet: High protein and low concentrated sweets

Figure 3.21. Peritoneal dialysis orders.
Courtesy of Maria Luongo. Used with permission.

CONTINUOUS AMBULATORY PERITONEAL DIALYSIS (CAPD) STANDING ORDERS

1. CAPD #_____ Exchanges/day of 2500 ml or _____ ml Dianeal with 2.5 mEq or _____mEq C

    Exchanges:
    1. 6 am _____%
    2. 10 am_____%
    3. 2 pm_____%
    4. 6 pm_____%
    5. 10 pm_____%

    1. 8 am _____%
    2. 1 pm_____%
    3. 6 pm_____%
    4. 10 pm_____%

2. Reassess weight gain or loss with Nephrologist and adjust % of dextrose prn.

3. Measure drain volume and record on flow sheet for each exchange every day.

4. Check peritoneal dialysis drainage bag with each exchange for fibrin, blood, or cloudiness. If present, notify nephrologist.

5. If peritonitis is present, the initial antibiotic regimen is as follows:
    __a. Vancomycin _____ mg per bag one 6 hour dwell (15-30 mg/kg I.P. with maximum dose of 2000 mg). Note: This is a one-time dose order.
    __b. Ciprofloxacin 500 mg p.o. bid or equivalent available on Formulary.
    __c. Once the organism is identified, narrow the antibiotic spectrum to cover the specific organism.

6. If fibrin is present, add Heparin_____ units per bag (recommended range of 500-1000 units Heparin/Liter of dialysate solution) after checking with nephrologist.

7. Pharmacy only to add any medication to dialysis bag.

8. Daily weight and record on graphic and CAPD flow sheet. (Weight should be done at the same time each day with abdomen full.)

9. If patient has had no bowel movement for 2 days, contact Nephrologist for prn laxative/stool softener order.

10. Diet: 1.3-1.5 g protein/kg/day, no added salt, no potassium restriction.

11. Daily exit site care should be done by cleansing with liquid soap via pump dispenser. Follow by applying Gentamicin 1% cream to site daily and covering with non-occlusive dressing If new (fresh post-op) exit site, use sterile technique to change dressing once a week or if dressing is soiled (bloody). Continue for first 3 weeks post-op.

12. Call Western Acute Dialysis team for nursing issues:
    M-F from 0600-1600 at 303-595-2660 and after hours 303-231-6552

    MD Signature_____ Date_____

Figure 3.22. CAPD orders.

Courtesy of Helen Williams, Western Nephrology Acute Dialysis, Denver, Colorado. Used with permission.

UNIVERSITY OF CALIFORNIA, DAVIS
MEDICAL CENTER
SACRAMENTO, CALIFORNIA

PHYSICIAN'S ORDERS

CONTINUOUS CYCLING PERITONEAL DIALYSIS

Directions: Check (√) and complete those orders to be carried out on this patient.

Date: _____ For Date: _____

Time: _____ For Time: _____

1. √ Fax orders to Tower Four x43505 and call x43333

2. ☐ Daily Weight in Kg

3. ☐ Daily exit site care with 3% saline followed by mupirocin 2% ointment at time of disconnection

4. ☐ Number of 5 liter dialysate bags____ 1.5% dextrose ____ 2.5% ____ 4.25%
   (Only one fill volume will be used from a loading dose bag)
   ☐ Delflex dialysate concentrations (mEq/L)
   | Ca^{++} 2.5 | Na^+ 132 | **Lactate** 40 |
   | K^+ 0 | Mg^{++} 0.5 | **Chloride** 95 |

5. ☐ Fills _____ (6-7) (includes last fill)   Total daily Fill volume_____ liters

6. ☐ CCPD volume _____ (2 - 3) liters (single fill volume)

7. ☐ Last Fill volume _____(2 - 3) liters (zero if patient to be left dry)

8. ☐ Fill Time 15 minutes

9. ☐ Dwell Time _____(1-3) hours (shorter dwell times increases ultrafiltration)

10. ☐ Drain Time 30 minutes

11. ☐ Manual drain of last fill volume at _____(4-6) hours post CCPD last fill

Laboratory:

12. ☐ Dialysate effluent cell count (send 5 ml sample of first drain in lavender top tube)

13. ☐ Dialysate effluent gram stain, culture and sensitivity (send 100 ml sample of first drain)

14. ☐ Catheter exit site culture and sensitivity (swab exit site with culturette swabstick)

15. ☐ _____(antibiotic) serum level (draw if suspected bacteremia)

Medications: Complete the antibiotic order from for any antibiotics ordered below.

16. ☐ Heparin _____(1000) units / liter Intra peritoneal

17. ☐ Deliver Antibiotics as follows:
    During first Fill cycle Loading bag is open and all Maintenance bags are clamped.
    After first Fill cycle, clamp Loading bag, and unclamp all Maintenance bags.

18. ☐ Loading Bag (LB):   Antibiotic:_____ _____ mg / liter Intraperitoneal
    ____% dextrose   Antibiotic:_____ _____ mg / liter Intraperitoneal

19. ☐ Maintenance Bags (MB): Antibiotic:_____ _____ mg / liter Intraperitoneal
                              Antibiotic:_____ _____ mg / liter Intraperitoneal

Dosing guide in mg/L: Gentamicin LB 60 (max LB volume = 2L) MB 4, Cefazolin LB 500 MB 125, Vancomycin LB 1000 MB 25, Ceftazidime LB 500 MB 125

Nephrologist (signature/print name): _____   P.I.:   Pager:

Nephrology Nurse(signature/print name): _____   Date/Time:

AR4098 (9/07)   **CONTINUOUS CYCLING PERITONEAL DIALYSIS ORDERS**   MR#07/00566

Figure 3.23. CCPD orders.

Courtesy of Maureen Craig, University of California, Davis Medical Center, Sacramento, California. Used with permission.

UNIVERSITY OF CALIFORNIA, DAVIS
MEDICAL CENTER
SACRAMENTO, CALIFORNIA

PHYSICIAN'S ORDERS

CONTINUOUS CYCLING PERITONEAL DIALYSIS "SUSPECT PERITONITIS"

Directions: Check (√) and complete those orders to be carried out on this patient.

Date:	For Date:
Time:	For Time:

1. √ Fax orders to Tower Four x43505 and call x43333

2. ☐ Daily exit site care with 3% saline followed by mupirocin 2% ointment at time of disconnection

3. ☐ Number of 5 liter dialysate bags _____ 1.5% dextrose
☐ Delflex dialysate concentrations (mEq/L)
Ca++ 2.5   Na+ 132   **Lactate** 40
K+ 0   Mg++ 0.5   **Chloride** 95

4. ☐ Fills _____ (3) (includes last fill)   Total daily Fill volume_____ liters

5. ☐ CCPD volume _____ (1- 2) liters (single fill volume)

6. ☐ Last Fill volume _____(1 - 2) liters (membrane is typically more permeable during peritonitis)

7. ☐ Fill Time   15 minutes

8. ☐ Dwell Time   5 minutes

9. ☐ Drain Time   20 minutes

10. ☐ Routine CCPD orders should begin within 4 hours

Laboratory:

11. ☐ Dialysate effluent cell count (send 5 ml sample of first drain in lavender top tube)

12. ☐ Dialysate effluent gram stain, culture and sensitivity (send 100 ml sample of first drain)

13. ☐ Catheter exit site culture and sensitivity (swab exit site with culturette swabstick)

Catheter Inflow / Outflow Treatment:

14. ☐ _____ (50) units of Heparin in 50 ml normal saline in syringe for flushing.

15. ☐ Vigorously flush PD catheter with ordered flush solution. Flush in and out to reestablish flow.

16. ☐ If poor flow, abdominal X-ray 2 views to check Peritoneal Dialysis catheter placement.

17. ☐ If poor flow fill PD catheter with Alteplase 5mg/5ml (use volume to fill catheter) Dwell for 2 hours and aspirate Alteplase. Repeat heparinized saline flush above.

18. ☐ If flow is not reestablished call Nephrologist.

19. ☐ Lactulose 30ml by mouth, twice a day, until stooling occurs.

Nephrologist (signature/print name):   P.I.:   Pager:

Nephrology Nurse (signature/print name):   Date/Time:

AR5937 (9/07)   **CCPD "SUSPECT PERITONITIS" DIALYSIS ORDERS**   MR 08/05993

Figure 3.24. CCPD suspect peritonitis orders.

Courtesy of Maureen Craig, University of California, Davis Medical Center, Sacramento, California. Used with permission.

Glucose dehydrogenase pyrroloquin-olinequinone (GDH PQQ) or glucose-dye-oxidoreductase based methods must not be used. If GDH-PQQ or glucose-dye-oxidoreductase based methods are used, using Extraneal may cause a falsely high glucose reading. Additionally, falsely elevated blood glucose measurements due to maltose interference may mask true hypoglycemia and allow it to go untreated. The maltose released from Extraneal may be present in the patient's blood for up to 72 hours after exposure to Extraneal." Check manufacturer's warnings and recommendations.
4. Medication additives to the PD solution.
   a. Refer to Section 13, Chapter 62: *Peritoneal Dialysis Therapy*.
   b. Meticulous sterile technique must be used to prevent bacterial or fungal contamination of the solution bag.
      (1) Anyone instilling medications into PD solution must be specifically trained to do so.
      (2) Alternatively, the pharmacy may instill medications into PD solution using a laminar airflow hood.
   c. Vials without preservative must not be reused.
   d. After medication is added, the solution bag must be labeled with name and dose of medication, time and date of addition, and initials of person who added them.
   e. Medication additives must be documented on the PD solution bag, PD flow sheet, and the medication record.
   f. Mix dialysis solution bag well by inverting bag several times after addition of medication(s).
   g. Heparin.
      (1) Used to treat formation of fibrin in the effluent and to prevent fibrin accumulation in the catheter.
      (2) Typical dose is 500 to 1000 units per liter of solution.
      (3) For patients with heparin-induced thrombocytopenia (HIT), consult with the nephrologist for anticoagulation alternatives.
   h. Antibiotics.
      (1) Refer to Section 13, Chapter 63: *Peritoneal Dialysis Complications*.
      (2) Obtain all specimens (culture and/or cell count of drainage or effluent) prior to addition of antibiotics to the dialysate.

      (3) Clarify route of administration.
         (a) Oral (PO).
         (b) Intraperitoneal (IP).
         (c) Intravenous (IV).
      (4) Clarify dosage and frequency of administration.
      (5) If antibiotic is administered IP, clarify length of dwell time of that solution bag to facilitate absorption of antibiotic.
   i. Potassium.
      (1) If patient is unable to take oral potassium or if vascular access prohibits IV administration, it can be added to dialysis solution bags.
      (2) Clarify dose and frequency of administration.
      (3) Obtain order for monitoring serum potassium levels.
      (4) Infuse slowly as potassium can be irritating to the peritoneum.
   j. Insulin.
      (1) Refer to Section 13, Chapter 62: *Peritoneal Dialysis Therapy*.
      (2) Insulin may be added to dialysis solution bags.
      (3) Insulin should be added immediately before infusion.
      (4) Insulin binds to the plastic bag and tubings, and only a fraction is absorbed, so dosage will be larger than the patient would be taking as a subcutaneous injection.
      (5) Frequent monitoring of blood glucose is imperative.
      (6) The needles on conventional insulin syringes may be too short to consistently and completely penetrate the medication port of the dialysis solution bags.
         (a) 1 mL syringe with a larger needle may only be used if the insulin is manufactured as 100 units per mL.
         (b) When adding insulin to PD solution, use extreme caution. Double check dosage with a second RN.
5. Specimens.
   a. Send dialysate effluent sample when ordered.
      (1) For suspected peritonitis.
         (a) Cell count.
         (b) Gram stain.
         (c) Culture and sensitivity.
         (d) Fungal culture.
      (2) For suspected exit site or tunnel infection.
         (a) Culture and sensitivity.
         (b) Gram stain of exudate or drainage.

b. Follow the institution's clinical laboratory procedures for appropriate containers and documentation.

E. Documentation of PD therapy in the acute setting (see Figures 3.19 and 3.20 and Table 3.36).
1. Documentation of PD therapy may be required on each nursing shift or daily.
2. The requirements should be part of the policy and procedures established by the hospital and/or the patient care unit in collaboration with the nephrology nursing team.
3. Documentation may be accomplished by the use of a daily treatment flow sheet, nursing Kardex tool, progress notes, or a combination of methods.
4. May be written, electronic, or a combination.
5. Components that should be included:
   a. Patient assessment.
      (1) Vital signs.
      (2) Lung sounds and oxygenation status.
      (3) Presence of:
         (a) Nausea/vomiting.
         (b) Constipation/diarrhea.
         (c) Abdominal pain/tenderness.
         (d) Edema.
   b. PD effluent.
      (1) Color.
      (2) Clarity.
      (3) Presence or absence of fibrin.
      (4) Ease of infusion and drainage.
   c. Dialysate and fluid balance.
      (1) Schedule of exchanges.
      (2) Fill and drain volume of each exchange.
      (3) Dextrose percentage used for each exchange.
      (4) Medications added to dialysate solution bags.
      (5) Number of exchanges prescribed and completed.
      (6) Intake and output of all fluids.
      (7) Calculation of ultrafiltration and net fluid balances.
      (8) Exchange dwell time.
   d. Patient's disposition during exchanges.
      (1) Positioning that facilitates infusion and/or drainage.
      (2) Comfort with PD exchanges.
      (3) Pain with infusion and/or drainage.
      (4) Presence of rectal pain, shoulder pain, and/or abdominal pain.
      (5) Unusual abdominal distention.
   e. Exit site and tunnel condition and care.
      (1) Appearance of exit site and tunnel.
         (2) Presence or absence of:
            (a) Exudate/drainage.
            (b) Pain/tenderness.
            (c) Leakage of dialysate.
         (3) Exit site care with hypertonic saline or other agent.
         (4) How catheter is secured.
         (5) Dressing condition or dressing change performed.
   f. Infection.
      (1) If the patient has peritonitis demonstrated by cloudy effluent, document:
         (a) Color and clarity of effluent.
         (b) Presence or absence of fibrin.
         (c) Acquisition of laboratory specimens.
         (d) Administration of prescribed antibiotic therapy.
      (2) If patient has an exit site or tunnel infection, document:
         (a) Antibiotic therapy.
         (b) Changes in local care.
         (c) Presence of absence of exudate.
         (d) Erythema.
         (e) Pain.
         (f) Tenderness.
         (g) Edema.

F. Supplies needed at the bedside in the acute care setting.
1. PD solutions with prescribed additives.
2. Dialysis tubings, transfer sets, cycler supplies if doing APD.
3. Masks.
4. Clamps for tubing.
5. Springscale.
6. IV pole.
7. Dry heat source.
8. Povidone iodine for medication port prep.
9. Unsterile gloves for universal precautions.
10. Specimen containers.
11. Dressing supplies.
12. PD treatment flow sheets or required forms for documentation in that institution.

III. Nursing management of the patient with urgent/emergent needs for PD.

A. Indications.
1. Urgent/emergent need for renal replacement therapy with limited or absent vascular access or the need to avoid a vascular access complication, e.g., hemorrhage, thrombosis, or infection.

Table 3.36

Nursing Documentation for Hospitalized PD Patient

Education
Who was involved – Patient/Family
Topic discussed
Assessment of understanding
Plan for further education

Procedure: Acute PD catheter placement at bedside
Pain assessment, intervention and evaluation of effectiveness
Catheter function (drain and fill), need for heparin
Exit site dressing
Drainage:
Frequency of changes
Color of drainage
Check drainage for glucose
Secured:
Immobilization

Fluid balance
Schedule of exchanges: e.g., every 2 hours, every 4 hours
Fill volume of each exchange
Dextrose percentage used for each exchange
Medications added to dialysate solution bags
Number of exchanges completed
Amount of effluent drained (Ultrafiltration)
Intake and output of all fluids

Patient's disposition during exchanges
Positioning that facilitates infusion or drain
Comfort with exchange sensations
Presence of pain with infusion or draining of solutions
Presence of rectal pain, shoulder pain, abdominal pain
Unusual abdominal distention

PD effluent (drainage)
Color (clear, yellow)
Presence of fibrin
Clarity (clear, bloody, cloudy, tea colored)
Ease of infusion and drainage

Exit site
Color of site
Presence of exudate
Presence of pain
Leakage of dialysate at exit site
How catheter is secured

Infection

Peritonitis
Cloudy fluid
Abdominal pain
Nausea, vomiting, and/or diarrhea
Antibiotic therapy – medication, dose, route, and frequency
Color and clarity of solution
Collect PD fluid for cultures and sensitivity prior to 1st dose of antibiotics
Organism causing the infection if known

Exit site infection
Presence of:
Exudate
Erythema
Pain or tenderness
Any change or leaking at site
Pending cultures and antibiotics ordered

Assessment of the serum laboratory levels of the 3 H's associated with PD patients

1 Hyperglycemia
% dextrose of PD solution
Increase requirement of oral diabetes medication or insulin

2 Hypokalemia
Potassium loss into drained effluent can significantly decrease serum potassium levels
Monitor serum potassium
Individualized nutrition consult

3 Hypoalbuminia
Protein loss with PD can be as high as 10–20 g/day and twice as much with peritonitis
Does patient have nutritional support
Consult dietitian

Courtesy of Maria Luongo. Used with permission.

2. Treatment of hypothermia.
3. Treatment of hemorrhagic pancreatitis.
4. Treatment of toxic and/or metabolic abnormalities.

B. Contraindications for use of PD.
1. Traumatic injury to the abdomen, either surgical or accidental.

2. Traumatic injury to the diaphragm and pulmonary cavity.
3. Acute diverticulitis with or without peritonitis.
4. Suspected bowel perforation or traumatic puncture.
5. Recent abdominal surgeries.
6. Severe gastrointestinal reflux disease.
7. Recent cardiothoracic surgery.

8. Life-threatening electrolyte and/or metabolic imbalance.
9. Recent fungal peritonitis.
10. Documented inadequate peritoneal clearances.
11. Lack of experienced nurses who can safely manage PD.

C. Initiating emergency PD with a temporary PD catheter.
   1. Rarely if ever performed, only consider in the absence of better alternative such as acute hemodialysis.
   2. Educate the patient and family about PD management.
      a. Catheter insertion procedure.
      b. PD as renal replacement therapy.
      c. PD exchange routine.
      d. Prevention of infection.
      e. Use of masks and hand washing.
      f. Provide time for questions.

D. Peritoneal dialysis catheter placement.
   1. Refer to Section 13: Peritoneal Dialysis Therapy for information on acute catheters and their insertion, surgical complications, and exit site infection.
   2. Care of the patient with a temporary PD catheter.
      a. Temporary catheter is inserted, ideally, in the interventional radiology (IR) suite or the operating room (OR) where visualization will minimize the risk of complications, e.g., bowel or other organ perforation, or trauma. Bedside or blind placement should only be performed in the absence of a better alternative.
      b. Staff nurse or nephrology nurse may need to assist with bedside PD catheter placement.
         (1) Obtain and organize catheter insertion equipment.
         (2) Set up sterile field for physician and assistants.
         (3) Position patient and complete skin preparation.
         (4) Assist with first exchange of dialysate while positioning catheter and/or after catheter placement.
         (5) Dress and secure catheter.
         (6) Initiate PD exchanges as ordered.
      c. Temporary catheters are often rigid and need to be carefully secured to the abdominal wall.
      d. The less rigid temporary catheter may or may not be sutured to the abdominal wall.
      e. The right angle component of the catheter

requires a multilayered dressing to support and immobilize the catheter.
      f. Temporary catheters are intended for short-term use (48 to 72 hours).
      g. Lack of subcutaneous tunnel can result in leaking of dialysate, leading to the development of exit site infection or peritonitis.
      h. Dressing changes must be done promptly when wet or bloody and performed per hospital policy and procedure.
      i. Observe and document characteristics of effluent.
         (1) May be bloody due to the trauma of catheter insertion or possible perforation of the abdominal viscera.
         (2) May be cloudy due to infection or bowel perforation.
      j. Assessment of pain.
         (1) A newly inserted temporary or chronic catheter may create pain perceived as cramping during infusion or draining.
         (2) Slowing the rate of infusion or drainage may diminish the cramping sensation.
         (3) Dialysis solution that is either too hot or too cold may cause cramping and pain.
         (4) Warm solution according to established policy.
         (5) Patient may experience incisional or exit site pain with newly placed PD catheter.
            (a) Obtain appropriate pain medication orders.
            (b) The conscious patient should rate pain using the institution's pain scale assessment tool.
            (c) The unconscious patient should be assessed for pain according to their physical responses.
               [1] Unusual movement or restlessness.
               [2] Facial grimacing.
               [3] Changes in vital signs.
                  [a] Increased pulse rate.
                  [b] Increased respiratory rate.
               [4] Agitation.
   3. Complication of PD associated with emergent temporary catheter placement.
      a. Refer to Section 13: Complications of Peritoneal Dialysis.
      b. Additional issues that may specifically occur with temporary catheters include:
         (1) Referred pain to shoulders, primarily related to free air in the abdomen.
         (2) Accidental disconnection of temporary catheter and/or tubing.

(3) Migration of catheter tip with difficulty filling or draining.

(4) Bowel or other organ perforation or trauma.

4. Chronic catheter placement and associated management of care.

 a. A chronic catheter can be inserted for emergent PD.

 b. The procedure is usually done in the operating room (OR) by surgical dissection or by laparoscopy.

 c. Refer to Section 13, Chapter 61: *Peritoneal Dialysis Access.*

 d. Refer to Section 13, Chapter 63: *Peritoneal Dialysis Complications.*

5. Development of disequilibrium syndrome.

 a. Usually associated with hemodialysis, but can also be seen in patients with a serum urea nitrogen ≥ 100 mg/dL receiving frequent PD exchanges with a 4.25% dextrose dialysis solution.

 b. Etiology. Different theories include the following:

(1) Plasma solute level is rapidly lowered during dialysis.

(2) Cerebral edema occurs due to a lag in osmolar shift between blood and brain.

(3) An acute increase in cerebral water content.

 c. Manifestations.

(1) Nausea.

(2) Vomiting.

(3) Headache.

(4) Restlessness.

(5) Seizures.

(6) Obtundation.

(7) Coma.

 d. Prevention of disequilibrium syndrome.

(1) Reduce elevated serum urea slowly with less frequent PD exchanges.

(2) More likely to occur in patients with advanced uremia.

Chapter 13

Slow Extended Daily Dialysis (SLEDD) and Continuous Renal Replacement Therapies (CRRT)

Purpose

The purposes of this chapter are to define various forms of SLEDD and CRRT for patients with kidney injury or disease in the intensive care unit (ICU) setting, to provide examples of SLEDD/CRRT equipment and coordinating documentation, to provide an outline for developing a new SLEDD/CRRT program in various ICU environments and to define the nursing care necessary to assure safe, effective therapy for the patients receiving SLEDD/CRRT.

Objectives

Upon completion of this chapter, the learner will be able to:
1. Define the various forms of SLEDD/CRRT.
2. Explain the theory supporting the clinical application of SLEDD/CRRT.
3. Describe the various anticoagulation options, and parameters to monitor for a SLEDD/CRRT treatment.
4. Define nephrology and ICU nursing responsibilities for collaborative patient management to provide safe, effective SLEDD/CRRT treatments.
5. Identify the role of administrators, nephrologists, intensivists, nephrology nurses, ICU nurses, pharmacists, nurse managers, and pediatric health care providers, in the development of a SLEDD/CRRT program.

I. History.

A. 1967 – Pioneer work of Henderson and colleagues with hemodiafiltration using hemodialyzers.

B. 1974 – Silverstein uses a technique to perform ultrafiltration isolated from hemodialysis by modification of a standard hemodialysis circuit and the addition of a hemofilter.

C. 1975 – Henderson proposes a hemofiltration technique by collecting an ultrafiltrate of plasma and then reconstituting the blood volume with a fluid composition similar to normal plasma.

D. 1977 – Kramer and colleagues in West Germany first use continuous arteriovenous hemofiltration (CAVH) to treat fluid overload.

E. 1979-82 – Efforts focus on creating a method to perform ambulatory hemofiltration such as "the machineless kidney" or "wearable glomerulus" for chronic renal failure.

F. 1979-82 – Paganini (MD) and Whitman (RN) use slow continuous ultrafiltration (SCUF) and CAVH at Cleveland Clinic.

G. 1982 – Food and Drug Administration (FDA) approves use of hemofilters for the management of acute renal failure.

H. 1983 – Geronimus and colleagues start investigating clinical applications of continuous arteriovenous hemodialysis (CAVHD) and continuous arteriovenous hemodiafiltration (CAVHDF).

I. 1982-84 – Kaplan and colleagues extend work with

CAVH using suction assistance to enhance ultrafiltration.

J. 1987 – Pump-assisted CRRT introduced.

K. 1988 – Regional citrate anticoagulation used as an alternative to heparin in CRRT.

L. 1989-91 – Dirkes, Price, and Whitman make contributions to the CRRT literature helping improve and standardize nursing practice.

M. 1990 – CRRT considered state of the art therapy for treatment of acute renal failure.

N. 1992 – Continuous venovenous hemofiltration (CVVH), continuous venovenous hemodialysis (CVVHD), and continuous venovenous hemodiafiltration (CVVHDF) are widely accepted in clinical practice.

O. 1993 – Standards of Clinical Practice for CRRT published by ANNA and endorsed by American Association of Critical Care Nurses (AACN).

P. 1995 – Mehta (MD), assisted by Martin (RN), chairs the First International Conference on CRRT.

Q. 1998 – Depner (MD) and Craig (RN) introduce SLEDD at UC Davis Medical Center, Golper (MD) at University of Arkansas, and Amerling (MD) at Beth Israel in New York City as alternative to CRRT in the ICU environment.

R. 1999 – Venovenous continuous therapies nearly replace arteriovenous continuous therapies.

S. 2000 – CRRT equipment integrates blood pump and fluid balance systems.

II. Definitions.

A. CRRT.
1. SCUF is the continuous removal of fluid from the blood in response to hydrostatic pressure as it passes across a semipermeable membrane. SCUF is used for fluid management.
   a. The ultrafiltrate has solute concentrations matching plasma water for those solutes that are cleared by the semipermeable membrane.
   b. Solute clearance is minimal and convective in nature. SCUF can be performed with either an arteriovenous or venovenous circuit.
   c. SCUF can be done independently or in

combination with another extracorporeal circuit such as extracorporeal membrane oxygenation (ECMO), i.e., the hemofilter or hemodialyzer can be added to the ECMO circuit. The removed fluid is measured to maintain accurate intakes and outputs (I/O).
2. CAVH, CAVHD, and CAVHDF all use the arteriovenous extracorporeal circuit.
   a. Blood is driven from an artery through a filter and back to a vein usually by the patient's own pump, i.e., the heart. Therefore, these therapies depend upon the patient's mean arterial pressure (MAP) to establish and maintain blood flow in the extracorporeal circuit. In addition, blood flow through the extracorporeal circuit is dependent on the patient's hematocrit (HCT). The higher the HCT, the slower the blood flow rate (BFR), secondary to the increased viscosity of the blood (see Figure 3.25).
   b. Experience has demonstrated that for many ICU patients with kidney injury/disease, the MAP is inadequate (≤ 60 mm Hg) or so variable that it is difficult to maintain the

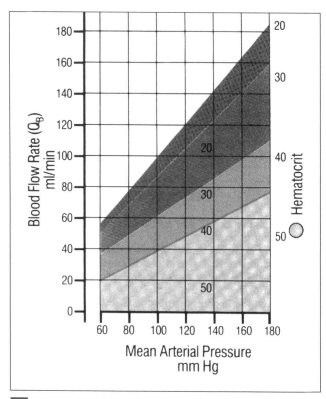

Figure 3.25. Blood flow rate related to mean arterial pressure and hematocrit.

Courtesy of Amicon, Inc.

blood flow in an arteriovenous extracorporeal circuit. A blood pump can be added to the arteriovenous circuit to maintain the desired blood flow.

c. The potential complications that can result from using an arterial access leave these therapies largely of historical interest in contrast to today's venovenous therapies.

d. The simplicity of the arteriovenous circuit makes it the choice for some ICUs, but considerations need to be taken for thermoregulation, hemoconcentration in the filter, and high doses of anticoagulants (see Figure 3.26).

e. CAVH, CAVHD, and CAVHDF may be performed on the arteriovenous circuit used in ECMO. A hemofilter or hemodialyzer may be added to the ECMO circuit. Intravenous (IV) fluid may be given through another access to provide volume replacement and/or dialysis solution may be pumped through the ultrafiltrate-dialysate compartment of the hemofilter or hemodialyzer depending on the solute clearance and/or fluid removal desired.

3. CVVH is the process where blood is driven from a vein through a filter and back to the patient's vein by a blood pump.

a. The ultrafiltrate produced during transit through the semipermeable membrane is largely replaced with IV fluids also referred to as replacement fluids.

b. Clearance is largely convective (see Figure 3.27).

4. CVVHD is also called continuous hemodialysis (CHD).

a. This is the process where blood is driven by a pump through a hemodialyzer with blood access originating and terminating in a vein.

b. Dialysis solution is pumped through the ultrafiltrate-dialysate compartment of the hemodialyzer counter-current to the blood flow.

c. Clearance is largely diffusive (see Figure 3.28).

5. CVVHDF is the modification of the CVVHD circuit by the addition of replacement solution to the blood either before or after the hemodialyzer. Clearance is both convective and diffusive (see Figure 3.29).

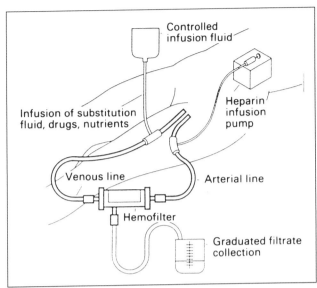

Figure 3.26. CAVH circuit: CAVH using a femoral cannulation.

Reprinted with permission from Millipore Corporation.

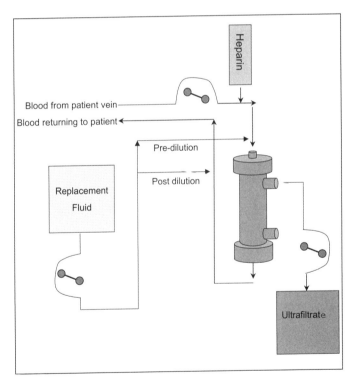

Figure 3.27. CVVH circuit: CVVH circuit with heparin anticoagulation.

Courtesy of Maureen Craig, UC Davis Medical Center, Sacramento, CA.

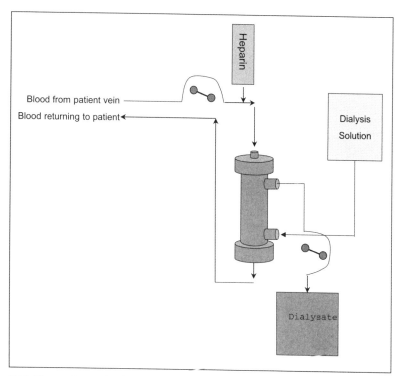

Figure 3.28. CVVHD circuit: CVVHD circuit with heparin anticoagulation.

Courtesy of Maureen Craig, UC Davis Medical Center, Sacramento, CA. Used with permission.

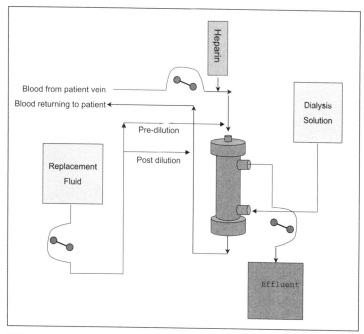

Figure 3.29. CVVHDF Circuit: CVVHDF circuit with heparin anticoagulation.

Courtesy of Maureen Craig, UC Davis Medical Center, Sacramento, CA. Used with permission.

B. SLEDD is a modification of traditional intermittent hemodialysis (IHD) to match the needs of the ICU patient with kidney injury or disease.
   1. University of California Davis Medical Center.
      a. SLEDD treatments are 8 hours in length performed 6 or 7 days per week.
      b. Blood flow rates are 100–200 mL/minute (min).
      c. Dialysis solutions flow rates are 100–300 mL/min.
      d. Net ultrafiltration rate (UFR) is ≤1000 mL/hour, based on the patient's need.
   2. University of Arkansas for Medical Sciences.
      a. SLEDD treatments are 6–12 hours in length and performed 5 days or nights per week.
      b. Blood flow rates are 200–250 mL/min.
      c. Dialysis solutions flow rates are 100–300 mL/min.
   3. Beth Israel Hospital, New York City.
      a. SLEDD treatments are 6–12 hours in length, performed 4–7 days per week.
      b. Blood flow rates are 200–350 mL/min.
      c. The dialysis solution flow rate is 300 mL/min.
      d. Net UFR is ≤ 500 mL/hour based on the patient's need.
   4. Commonalities among SLEDD programs.
      a. All forms of SLEDD result in modification of IHD by extending the time, while decreasing the rate at which both solute clearance and ultrafiltration (UF) occur.
      b. The composition of the dialyzing solution is similar to that used in continuous hemodialysis: sodium 138–145 mEq/L, potassium 3–4 mEq/L, bicarbonate 30–35 mEq/L (25–30 mEq/L when using regional citrate anticoagulation), calcium 2.5 mEq/L (0 mEq/L when using regional citrate anticoagulation), and phosphorus 0–3.5 mEq/L.
      c. All adult SLEDD treatments are performed using high-flux dialyzers

to maximize clearances. Clearance is largely diffusive.

d. These treatment modifications result in larger net solute clearances and fluid removal if desired. SLEDD allows the time to achieve a euvolemic state and remove the fluid intake the patient received during the previous 24-hour period.

e. Daily dialysis offers excellent solute and volume control with fewer episodes of hypotension in comparison to IHD.

f. Considering the improved patient management SLEDD/CRRT should be considered for every ICU patient with kidney injury and/or disease that requires renal replacement therapy.

III. Indications for SLEDD/CRRT in the ICU.

A. Fluid removal. SLEDD/CRRT can provide effective fluid removal and achieve fluid balance in an ICU patient who is receiving IV intake > urine output, and is relatively hemodynamically unstable.

B. Solute removal. SLEDD/CRRT provides excellent solute control in the catabolic ICU patient even while the patient is receiving hyperalimentation and having little or no residual renal function.

C. Examples of patients that may benefit from SLEDD/CRRT to assist in achieving volume and/or solute balance.
1. Patients with chronic kidney disease (CKD) stage 5 when they have other acute medical complications requiring an ICU stay.
2. Patients with acute kidney injury (AKI) who are catabolic and/or volume overloaded such that they will benefit from daily clearance of uremic toxins, management of fluid and electrolytes, and interventions to maintain acid-base balance.
   a. Acute tubular necrosis secondary to ischemic injury to the kidney. Following are examples of conditions that may lead to this injury.
      (1) Congestive heart failure.
      (2) Gastrointestinal bleed.
      (3) A recent myocardial infarction with or without cardiogenic shock.
      (4) Status postsurgery with intraoperative or postoperative hypotension.
      (5) Hepatic dysfunction.
      (6) Burn wounds.
      (7) Rhabdomyolysis.

      (8) Sepsis or systemic inflammatory response syndrome (SIRS).
      (9) Multisystem organ failure (MSOF).
   b. Nephrotoxin exposure.
      (1) Antineoplastic agents.
      (2) Antimicrobial agents.
      (3) Radiocontrast agents.
      (4) Poisons, such as ethylene glycol.
3. Patients with acute rejection following kidney or other solid organ transplant.
4. Patients with cardiac dysfunction who are resistant to diuretics or oliguric despite inotropic support, e.g., dopamine infusion, and have poor compensation to rapid UF.
5. Patients with anuria or oliguria who require large quantities of IV fluids including medications, hyperalimentation, and/or blood products.
6. Neonates with inborn errors of metabolism such as hyperammonemia.
7. Patients with hemolytic uremia syndrome (HUS) after *Escherichia coli* exposure.
8. Patients with tumor lysis syndrome (TLS) after receiving antineoplastic agents.

IV. Therapeutic effects of SLEDD/CRRT.

A. Initiate treatment early.
1. SLEDD/CRRT should be initiated when the patient's heart and kidneys are unable to remove the fluid or keep the patient in fluid balance or when the kidneys are unable to keep up with the solute load, e.g., the patient's blood urea nitrogen (BUN) and creatinine are rising each day.
2. Postponing SLEDD/CRRT treatment initiation in these circumstances increases the likelihood that the patient will experience hypotension and/or multisystem organ failure (MSOF) and will struggle to survive the fluid and/or solute imbalances that ensue.

B. Fluid removal/balance: SLEDD/CRRT can achieve a net ultrafiltration rate (UFR) of 0–1000 mL/hr. Alternatively, a patient can be kept in a positive fluid balance if insensible fluid losses are large as in a burn patient.
1. Rapid UF that occurs with IHD may be poorly tolerated in an ICU patient, resulting in hypotension and/or the inability to remove fluid. Hypotensive episodes have been linked to delayed renal recovery. SLEDD/CRRT can help the patient achieve the desired UF and/or fluid removal to match fluid intake by decreasing the

rate of UF while removing the fluid over a longer period of time. This results in a larger total fluid removal and/or better fluid control over the entire 24-hour period, with overall improved hemodynamic stability, when compared to IHD.

2. When removing fluid, the filtration fraction can estimate the amount of hemoconcentration within the circuit and should be ideally kept below 10% to minimize filter clotting. However a treatment with a filtration fraction up to 20% can be successful with effective anticoagulation.

3. The filtration fraction (FF) is the fraction of plasma water removed by ultrafiltration. This value can be calculated.

$$FF~(\%) = \frac{UFR~(mL/hr)}{BFR~(mL/min)} \times \frac{100}{60~(min/hr)} \times \frac{100}{(100-Hct)}$$

C. Solute clearance: SLEDD/CRRT can gently and effectively clear solutes and/or toxins from the plasma and balance electrolytes, minimizing the risk of changes to intracranial pressure. Decreased rebound of solutes occurs after treatment termination following SLEDD/CRRT when compared to IHD.

1. Convection.
   a. Convection is the process of transporting solutes across the semipermeable membrane together with fluid, which occurs in response to a transmembrane pressure (TMP)

gradient. Small solutes freely pass across the semipermeable membrane into the ultrafiltrate in a concentration matching the concentration of that solute in the plasma (see Figure 3.30).

   b. Increased solute size (5000–50,000 daltons) may decrease convective solute removal depending on the permeability (porosity) of the membrane. In general, however, larger molecules move across the same membrane better by convection than by diffusion.

   c. Convective clearance (CC) can be calculated.

$$CC~(mL/min) = \frac{UFR~(mL/hr)}{60~min/hr} \times \frac{ultrafiltrate~concentration}{plasma~concentration}$$

2. Diffusion.
   a. Diffusion is the process of transporting solutes across a semipermeable membrane from an area of higher solute concentration to an area of lower solute concentration (see Figure 3.31).

   b. Diffusion occurs in response to the concentration gradient. The greater the difference between the two sides of the membrane, the more solute moves across the membrane.

   c. Dialysis solution flow is counter-current to blood flow to maximize the diffusive gradient across the entire hemodialyzer.

   d. Diffusive clearance (DC) is more dependent on molecular size than convective clearance

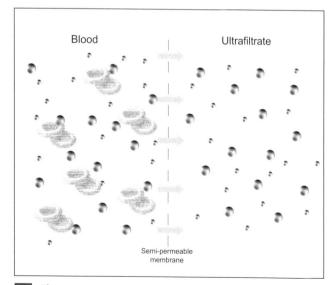

Figure 3.30. Convection: Solutes are transported across the semipermeable membrane together with fluid, which occurs in response to a transmembrane pressure gradient.

Courtesy of Maureen Craig, UC Davis Medical Center, Sacramento, CA.

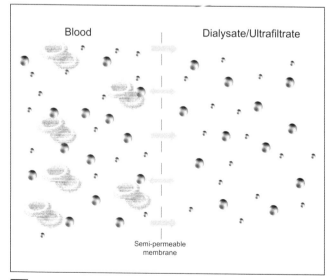

Figure 3.31. Diffusion: Solutes are transported across a semipermeable membrane from an area of higher solute concentration to an area of lower solute concentration.

Courtesy of Maureen Craig, UC Davis Medical Center, Sacramento, CA.

and works well for smaller size molecules (less than 200 daltons).

e. DC can be calculated using the dialysis flow rate (DFR).

$$DC\ (mL/min) = DFR\ (mL/min) \times \frac{dialysate\ concentration}{plasma\ concentration}$$

D. Medication clearance is dependent on several factors. There may be notable variations in drug removal and dosing that should be considered on an individual basis.

1. Patients may have residual kidney function resulting in some medication clearance into the urine.
2. A pathway other than the kidney, such as the liver or lung, may clear medications.
3. Medications may be cleared through a hemodialyzer or hemofilter.
   a. Clearance of any medication is impacted by the sieving coefficient (SC) of that substance as it passes across the membrane, and is different for different hemofilters or hemodialyzers.
      (1) The sieving coefficient is the fraction of a substance that will pass through a semipermeable membrane in relation to the concentration of the substance in the patient's plasma (see Table 3.37).
      (2) SC can be calculated.

$$SC = \frac{ultrafiltrate\ concentration}{plasma\ concentration}$$

   b. Several references predict medication clearance during dialytic therapies. Textbooks, pamphlets, drug information handouts, and charts have all been created to provide the clearance information for a particular medicine during a particular dialytic therapy. The practitioner implementing SLEDD/CRRT should exercise caution when referencing these medication clearance resources due to the many variations between forms of dialysis or filtration and within a specific form of dialysis or filtration.
   c. The more protein bound a medication is, the lower the clearance of that substance during SLEDD/CRRT. Albumin's molecular weight is 66,000 daltons, so solutes bound to it will be minimally cleared.
   d. Due to the longer duration of SLEDD/CRRT, even those medications that are highly protein bound may be more readily removed than anticipated with IHD.

Table 3.37

Comparison of Serum and Ultrafiltrate Chemistries with Sieving Coefficients

Substance	Serum	Ultrafiltrate	Seiving Coefficient
Sodium	140 mEq/L	140 mEq/L	1.00
Potassium	3.9 mEq/L	3.9 mEq/L	1.00
Chloride	105 mEq/L	111 mEq/L	.94
Bicarbonate	26 mEq/L	28 mEq/L	1.07
Urea	81 mg/dL	80 mg/dL	.99
Creatinine	4.0 mg/dL	3.8 mg/dL	.95
Calcium	8.3 mEq/L	5.2 mEq/L	.62
Phosphate	4.0 mEq/L	3.9 mEq/L	.98
Albumin	3.6 g/dL	0 g/dL	0
Total protein	4.6 g/dL	.1 g/dL	.02
Uric acid	8.4 mg/dL	7.7 mg/dL	.92
Total bilirubin	1.9 mg/dL	.1 mg/dL	.05
Direct bilirubin	.6 mg/dL	0 mg/dL	0
Alkaline phosphatase	65 IU/L	10 IU/L	.15
SGPT	31 IU/l	3 IU/L	.10
SGOT	29 IU/L	3 IU/L	.10
LDH	311 IU/L	7 IU/L	.02
CPK	55 IU/Ll	29 IU/L	.53
Cholesterol	89 mg/dL	8 mg/dL	.09
Glucose	89 mg/dL	108 mg/dL	1.21

   f. Medication clearance can occur via convection, diffusion, and adsorption. Clearance can be increased or decreased by changes in the BFR, DFR, replacement fluid rate (RFR), UFR, size or type of dialyzer/hemofilter, or available surface area

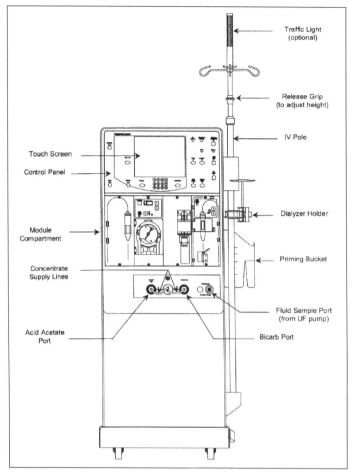

Figure 3.32. Fresenius 2008K Hemodialysis, SLEDD, and CRRT System.

Source: Fresenius, USA. (2002a). *2008K hemodialysis machine operator's manual* (p. 18). Walnut Creek, CA. Reprinted with permission from Fresenius.

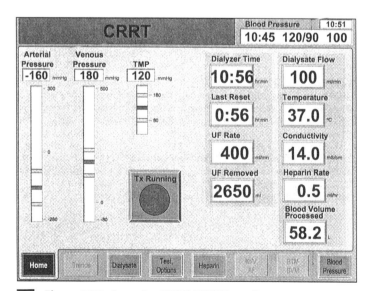

Figure 3.33. Fresenius 2008K CRRT Home Screen.

Source: Fresenius, USA. (2002a). *2008K hemodialysis machine operator's manual* (p. 172). Walnut Creek, CA. Reprinted with permission from Fresenius.

of the membrane. Membrane surface area decreases with clotting, and/or time on treatment.

4. Dose adjustment of medications.
   a. Medications such as vasopressors or sedatives may be titrated based on the effect on the patient.
   b. Medications such as heparin or citrate may be titrated based on patient laboratory parameters.
   c. Medications such as immunosuppressant medications or antibiotics may require monitoring of therapeutic serum levels. Achieving the desired level of a medication in the blood in a consistent fashion is challenging and the assistance of the pharmacist should not be undervalued.

V. Equipment and system components for SLEDD/CRRT.

A. Fresenius 2008K® (Fresenius Medical Care, Bad Homburg, Germany). The 2008K with the CRRT option can be used for IHD, SLEDD or CRRT (see Figure 3.32).
   1. System components: The Fresenius 2008K incorporates complex electronic and computerized technology with integrated fluid management systems and all the features of modern dialysis equipment. The machine can be divided into three main parts. The monitor with the CRRT screen, the extracorporeal blood circuit, and the dialysis solution circuit.
      a. CRRT home screen (see Figure 3.33).
         (1) Arterial pressure (AP): a visual display of the pressure in the arterial drip chamber in mm Hg. A transducer protector is fastened over the pressure port to guard against contamination of the transducer.
         (2) Venous pressure (VP): a visual display of the pressure in the venous drip chamber in mm Hg. The venous pressure limit cannot be set lower than + 9 mm Hg. A transducer protector is fastened over the pressure port to guard against contamination of the transducer.
         (3) TMP: equal to the venous pressure minus the dialysate pressure in

mm Hg. The TMP gradually increases when blood viscosity increases, and the alarm window for this pressure automatically adapts for this.

(4) Dialyzer time: a timer displays elapsed time, in hours/minutes, that the dialyzer has been used for the current treatment. The timer starts when the treatment button is pressed and resets to zero when the dialysate lines are placed back in the machine housing.

(5) Last reset: displays the amount of time, in hours/minutes, since the UF Removed button was cleared to zero. Automatically resets when UF Removed is set to 0.00 mL.

(6) UF rate: displays the current rate of ultrafiltration in mL/hour. UF rate flashes when the UF pump is turned off and there is no ultrafiltration.

(7) UF removed: displays the volume of fluid removed from the patient through UF. This value should be reset to zero at the end of each nursing shift and documented as an output.

(8) Dialysate flow: displays the current dialysate flow in mL/min.

(9) Temperature: displays the current temperature of the dialysate. The dialysate temperature can be adjusted here as well. The heated dialysate will minimize the heat loss from the patient's blood and keep the patient normothermic.

(10) Conductivity: displays the current conductivity of the dialysate. If the conductivity varies outside of the alarm limits, both visual and audible alarms will occur, and the dialysis solution flow will go into bypass.

(11) Heparin rate: displays the rate, in mL/hour, at which the syringe pump is infusing heparin into the blood. The rate can be adjusted from this screen.

(12) Blood volume processed: displays, in liters, the amount of blood that has passed through the dialyzer.

b. Extracorporeal blood circuit. The blood is continuously circulated from the patient through the filter or dialyzer where fluid and toxins are removed before being returned to the patient. The circuit is monitored for transmembrane pressure, venous and arterial pressures, for the presence of air in the blood, and for the presence of blood in the circuit.

(1) Heparin can be administered by a heparin syringe pump into the extracorporeal blood circuit evenly throughout the treatment.

(2) Blood Volume Monitor™: detects the change in blood volume relative to the initial blood volume at the start of the treatment. The graphic display is only available in the dialysis mode.

c. Dialysis solution circuit.

(1) The dialysis solution concentrates are mixed with reverse osmosis water that is further purified, heated, and degassed prior to delivery to the dialyzer. Balancing chambers ensure that the incoming flow of dialysate is volumetrically equal to the outgoing flow in order to accurately control UF.

(2) The dialysis solution is delivered at 100, 200, or 300 mL/min (6 to 18 liters/hour). This dialysis solution flow provides sufficient clearance to allow the flexibility of scheduling daily treatments from 4 to 24 hours a day.

(3) The dialysis solution is prepared from acid and bicarbonate concentrates. One 10-liter container of each concentrate will provide 12–14 hours of treatment with 12 liters/hour of dialysis solution flow.

2. Therapy considerations.

a. Online dialysis solution production allows the clinician to customize the electrolyte composition at the bedside at any time rather than wait for the pharmacy to prepare a new custom dialysis solution.

b. The dialysis solution is always bicarbonate buffered. The bicarbonate level can be adjusted from 20–40 mEq/L as desired.

c. When selecting dialysis solution flow rates of 100–300 mL/min on the Fresenius 2008K it will take longer for the equipment to adjust to changes in temperature or conductivity in comparison to dialysis solution flow rates > 300 mL/min.

d. At DFR of 100 mL/min with a high-flux filter, there may be more TMP alarms. To resolve the TMP alarms, you can increase the DFR, change the filter to a filter of a lower flux, or add in normal saline replacement fluid at 100 mL/hr and ultrafilter that fluid off again.

e. When preparing online dialysis solution, an ultrapure dialysis solution filter will prevent passage of endotoxins from dialysis solutions to the blood stream.

f. The dialysis solution temperature can be adjusted to meet the patient's needs. A dialysis solution temperature of 35°C has been shown to reduce the incidence of hypotension.

g. UF profiles are only available in the dialysis mode and can be used for a SLEDD treatment. UF profile 2 provides a linear decreasing UFR and has been shown to reduce the incidence of hypotension.

h. Fresenius recommends equipment disinfection and a new CRRT setup every 48 hours.

i. Pediatric tubing and filters are available to establish total circuit volumes as low as 48 mL.

3. Configuration of SLEDD/CRRT system.

a. SLEDD/CRRT with heparin anticoagulation. Heparin may be administered in the syringe pump or alternatively heparin may be diluted (5000, 10,000 or 20,000 units) in a liter of normal saline and infused into the heparin line on the extracorporeal blood circuit using a standard IV pump.

b. SLEDD/CRRT with regional citrate anticoagulation. When using citrate anticoagulation, it is essential that, whenever the blood pump stops, the IV infusion pump administering the citrate must also be stopped to prevent backflow, which would result in direct administration of citrate to the patient.

(1) Best option: Ideally the patient should have a dialysis catheter, a separate central line for calcium, and an additional line such as an arterial line, for blood draws (see Figure 3.34).

(2) Alternate option: The patient with limited vascular access, e.g., neonate, pediatric or vascular-compromised patient, may present with only a dialysis catheter. Although more challenging, this patient can still receive regional citrate anticoagulation. Several considerations should be taken to maximize the effective delivery of SLEDD/CRRT with regional citrate anticoagulation.

(a) A well placed catheter with a good blood flow.

[1] A poorly placed catheter with low blood flow will increase calcium

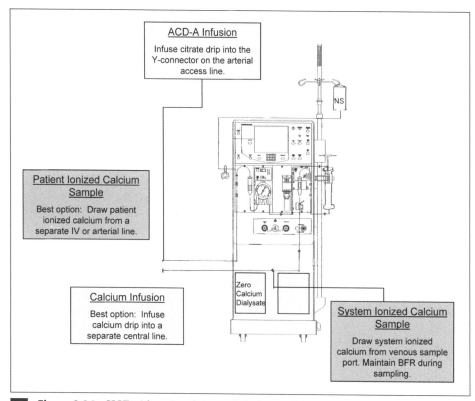

ACD-A Infusion
Infuse citrate drip into the Y-connector on the arterial access line.

NS

Patient Ionized Calcium Sample
Best option: Draw patient ionized calcium from a separate IV or arterial line.

Calcium Infusion
Best option: Infuse calcium drip into a separate central line.

Zero Calcium Dialysate

System Ionized Calcium Sample
Draw system ionized calcium from venous sample port. Maintain BFR during sampling.

Figure 3.34. CRRT with regional citrate: infusions and laboratory sampling.

Courtesy of Fresenius and Maureen Craig, UC Davis Medical Center, Sacramento, California.

recirculation resulting in the need to increase the citrate infusion, leading to the need for increasing the calcium infusion to reverse the citrate effect.

[2] This vicious cycle makes it impossible to deliver a safe and effective SLEDD/CRRT treatment.

(b) The calcium may be infused using a Y-connector on the venous return line or 3rd limb of the dialysis catheter if present. There will be some recirculation of calcium infused at this point.

(c) The patient ionized calcium sample, drawn from a stopcock on the arterial limb of the dialysis catheter, may be lower than the peripherally drawn sample due to the proximity of the citrate (ACD-A) fusion to the sampling port (see Figure 3.35). Draw the patient ionized calcium sample using the following steps to maximize an accurate result.

[1] Draw system-ionized calcium sample before patient ionized calcium sample maintaining the BFR.

[2] Stop citrate infusion.

[3] Reduce or maintain the BFR at ≤ 50 mL/min.

[4] Clamp venous port (and 3rd port if present) of central catheter to prevent recirculation.

[5] Await increased VP alarm (allows time for patient's blood to enter arterial line).

[6] Scrub the stopcock hub with alcohol, turn the stopcock off to the system, draw 1 mL blood to waste and then draw patient ionized calcium sample from the stopcock of the arterial port of the central catheter.

[7] Flush stopcock with 1 mL of normal saline to clear stopcock. Return system to standard position.

[8] Turn stopcock off to syringe, unclamp all catheter ports.

[9] Resume BFR and citrate infusion.

[10] Send samples to stat laboratory (see Figure 3.35).

4. Coordinating documentation: Designed for use on the Fresenius 2008K.

a. Order sets.
   (1) SLEDD/CRRT orders with regional citrate anticoagulation (see Figure 3.36).
   (2) SLEDD with heparin anticoagulation: These orders are similar to standard IHD orders but the time of the treatment is lengthened and the blood and dialysate flow rates have been slowed (see definitions above).
   (3) CRRT orders with heparin or no anticoagulation (see Figure 3.37).
   (4) Pediatric CRRT orders with regional citrate anticoagulation (see Figure 3.38).
   (5) Pediatric CRRT orders with heparin or no anticoagulation (see Figure 3.39).

b. Bedside inservice checklists.
   (1) SLEDD bedside inservice checklist (see Figure 3.40).
   (2) CRRT with regional citrate bedside inservice checklist (see Figure 3.41).

c. Nursing documentation.
   (1) Nephrology nursing flowsheet: An IHD flowsheet will work with minor additions (see Figure 3.42).
   (2) ICU nursing flowsheet: The ICU nurse should use the existing ICU flowsheet adding in documentation lines for patient and system pressure readings, intake lines for the replacement fluids and anticoagulation, and output lines for the volume of ultrafiltrate removed.

B. Prisma® system (Gambro, Stockholm, Sweden) http://www.usa-gambro.com and Prismaflex® system (Gambro, Stockholm, Sweden) are fully integrated systems for automated CRRT and continuous fluid management (see Figure 3.43).

1. System components. The Prisma system control unit has three functional parts.
   a. The communication unit is where the operator receives information and communicates with the system.
      (1) Has a display of information and machine status lights.
      (2) A touchscreen with softkeys is used to navigate through the screens and to change parameters.
      (3) Service screens provide guidance for calibration and testing procedures for technicians and users.
   b. The flow control unit manages and controls the different flow pumps and pressures. Alarms are built into the system to alert the user of any abnormal pressure within the system.

(1) Pumps include blood pump, dialysate pump, replacement pump, and effluent pump.

   (a) Blood pump moves blood through the system at the prescribed rate for all modalities available with this machine, including SCUF, CVVH, CVVHD, and CVVHDF.

   (b) Dialysate pump is used when performing CVVHD and CVVHDF to pump dialysate through the hemofilter using a countercurrent flow path to the blood flow direction.

   (c) Replacement pump is used when performing CVVH and CVVHDF to pump replacement solution, mixing with the blood as it enters (prefilter) or as it leaves (postfilter) the filter.

   (d) Effluent pump is the master pump controlling fluid removal by automatically removing the dialysate and replacement solution volumes being administered in addition to the desired net loss of fluid from the patient programmed into the system on an hourly basis.

(2) A syringe pump is available for administering anticoagulant and offers bolus and/or continuous infusion options.

(3) Pressure pods monitor and display access line pressure, filter pressure, return line pressure, and effluent line pressure.

   (a) The pressure pods are built into the circuit.

   (b) They fit into a pressure sensor housing on the flow control unit.

   (c) They provide noninvasive pressure measurements, without an air-blood interface, to continuously monitor system pressures.

(4) Safety monitoring includes a blood leak

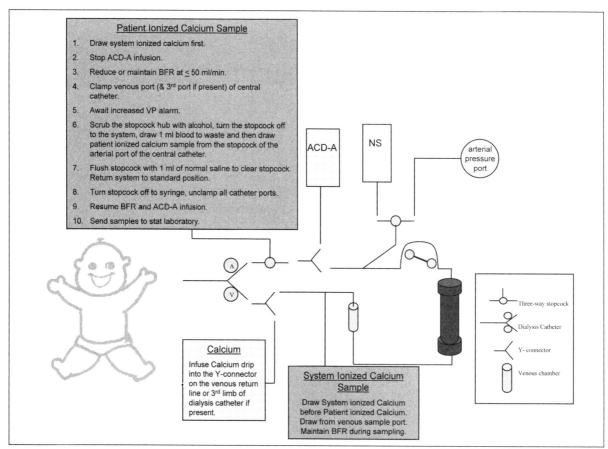

Figure 3.35. CRRT with regional citrate: line set up, infusions and laboratory sampling for a pediatric patient with only a dialysis catheter

Courtesy of Maureen Craig, UC Davis Medical Center, Sacramento, CA. Used with permission.

UNIVERSITY OF CALIFORNIA, DAVIS
MEDICAL CENTER
SACRAMENTO, CALIFORNIA

PHYSICIAN'S ORDERS

SLOW EXTENDED DAILY DIALYSIS (SLEDD) OR CONTINUOUS HEMODIALYSIS (CHD) ORDERS
WITH REGIONAL CITRATE ANTICOAGULATION

Date:	For Date:
Time:	

Directions: Check (√) and complete those orders to be implemented (order renewal daily before noon).

For assistance, Monday – Friday 0700-1930 call x48730, other hours call operator for on-call nurse.

1. ☐ Priority: ☐ 1   ☐ 2   Dialysis type: ☐ SLEDD _____ (8) hours ☐ CHD (24 hours/day)

2. ☐ Monitor EKG (required)

3. ☐ Weigh daily at 0500 (CHD)

4. ☐ Ultrafiltration volume: _____liters (SLEDD)   Ultrafiltration Rate = Total patient input +/-_____ ml/hour(CHD)
   ☐ (Optional) Ultrafiltration Profile (linear-continuously-decreasing) (SLEDD) ⊾

5. ☐ Dialyzer: _____

6. ☐ Blood Flow Rate _____ (100-200) mL/min.   Vascular Access: _____

7. ☐ Dialysate Flow Rate_____ (SLEDD 300 or CHD 200)ml/min.
   ☐ Dialysis solution temperature_____ (35-36)°C
   ☐ Dialysate: K+_____(0-4) mEq/L   Na+_____ (135) mEq/L   Phos_____(0-3) mg/dL
                 Ca++_____(0) mEq/L   HCO3_____(25-30) mEq/L

8. ☐ Support systolic blood pressure less than _____ mm Hg with 0.9% NaCl or _____PRN. (SLEDD)

9. ☐ Call Nephrology if fluid bolus greater than 250mL/shift is given for BP support or if MAP falls below 60mmHg. (CHD)

10. ☐ (Optional) Replacement Fluid: Normal Saline(NS)_____(1000-2000)mL/hour

11. ☐ (Optional) Replace patient Output (urine, stool, drains) mL for mL with normal saline.

Medications

12. ☐ Anticoagulant Citrate Dextrose (ACD-A) through dialyzer inflow (arterial) line _____ (150-250) mL/hour

13. ☐ Adjust ACD-A to maintain ionized calcium in the **extracorporeal outflow (venous)** blood at 0.35-0.50 mMol/L.

If **extracorporeal outflow** ionized calcium is:	Adjust ACD-A:
Less than 0.35	decrease by 25 mL/hour
0.35-0.50	no change
Greater than 0.50	increase by 25 mL/hour

14. ☐ Calcium gluconate 40mg/mL (20grams in 500 mL NS) at _____(60-180) mL/hour in a patient IV line or in venous return line.

15. ☐ Adjust calcium gluconate to maintain **Patient** ionized calcium of 1.11 – 1.31 mMol/L

If **Patient** ionized calcium is:	Adjust calcium gluconate:
Less than 1.01	increase by 20 mL/hour, see order #19, and call Nephrologist
1.01-1.10	increase by 20 mL/hour
1.11-1.31	no change
Greater than 1.31	decrease by 20 mL/hour

16. ☐ Give calcium gluconate 1g in 50mL NS over 15mins for symptoms of hypocalcemia or for patient ionized calcium below 1.01 mMol/L.

Laboratory:

17. ☐ Draw pre treatment patient ionized calcium.
   ☐ Draw ionized calciums from both system and patient 60 minutes after start and 60 minutes after prescribed BFR, DFR, ACD-A, or calcium gluconate infusion rate change, then every 2-3 hours for SLEDD or every 4-6 hours for CHD when rates are stable.
   ☐ Draw ionized calciums if patient is symptomatic of hypo or hyper-calcemia.
   ☐ Draw patient ionized calcium 20 minutes after discontinuing treatment.

18. ☐ CMP, ☐ CBC, ☐ Pre BUN, ☐ Post BUN, ☐ Hepatitis B surface Antigen, ☐ Hepatitis C Antibody

Treatment Termination:

19. ☐ Return blood with a _____(250)mL normal saline flush.
   ☐ Do not return blood.

20.   Pulsatile flush to each limb of catheter with 10 mL (adult) or 5 mL (pediatric) normal saline. Fill Arterial and Venous lumen of dialysis catheter (volume printed on catheter A_____mL, V_____mL) with:
   ☐ Heparin 5000 units/mL (adult standard).
   ☐ Heparin 1000 units/mL (pediatric standard).
   ☐ ACD-A from pharmacy.

Nephrologist (Signature/Print Name):	P.I.:	Pager:
Nephrology Nurse (Signature/Print Name):	Date/Time:	
ICU Nurse (Signature/Print Name):	Date/Time:	

AC6504 (9/07)   **SLEDD OR CHD WITH REGIONAL CITRATE ANTICOAGULATION**   MR#10/071142

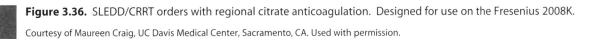

Figure 3.36. SLEDD/CRRT orders with regional citrate anticoagulation. Designed for use on the Fresenius 2008K.

Courtesy of Maureen Craig, UC Davis Medical Center, Sacramento, CA. Used with permission.

UNIVERSITY OF CALIFORNIA, DAVIS
MEDICAL CENTER
SACRAMENTO, CALIFORNIA

PHYSICIAN'S ORDERS

CONTINUOUS RENAL REPLACEMENT THERPY ORDERS
WITH HEPARIN ANTICOAGULATION

Directions: Check (√) and complete orders to be implemented (order renewal daily before noon).	
For assistance, Monday – Friday 0700-1930 call x48730, other hours call operator for on-call nurse.	
Date:	For, Date:
Time:	
1.	☐ Weigh daily at 0500
2.	☐ Blood Flow Rate (BFR) _____ (100-200) mL/minute.
3.	☐ Hemofilter _____
4.	☐ Ultrafiltration Rate = Total patient input +/-_____mL/hour
5.	☐ Dialysate Flow Rate_____ (100-300) mL/minute. ☐ Dialysis solution temperature_____ (35-36)°C
6.	☐ Dialysate: K⁺_____(3-4) mEq/L Na⁺ _____ (140) mEq/L Phos_____(2-3) mg/dL Ca⁺⁺_____(2.5) mEq/L HCO₃_____(30) mEq/L
7.	☐ Call Nephrology if fluid bolus greater than 250mL/shift is ordered for blood pressure support or if MAP is less than 60mmHg.
8.	☐ (Optional) Replacement Fluid: Normal Saline (NS)_____(1000-2000mL/hour)
9.	☐ (Optional) Replace patient Output (urine, stool, drains) mL for mL with Replacement Fluid.
Medications	
10.	☐ Prime hemofilter with 5000 units heparin in normal saline.
11.	☐ Heparin bolus: _____units (10-30 units/kg) IV. ☐ Based on goal APTT (see below), repeat bolus _____units (5-15 units/kg) IV to maximum of 80 units/kg heparin.
12.	☐ Heparin infusion: Initial rate_____units/hour (10-25 units/kg/hour)IV . Concentration: 1000 units/mL
13.	☐ Maintain goal APTT (see below) by repeat bolus and /or infusion adjustment per primary MD.
Laboratory:	
14.	☐ Goal APTT: _____-_____ (45-65) seconds. ☐ Check APTT BID, After each heparin bolus, Four hours after all heparin dosing changes, and Immediately after blood product administration.
15.	☐ Pre treatment draw: APTT, INR, CBC, CMP, Magnesium, and ionized Calcium.
16.	☐ Draw: CBC, BMP, Magnesium, Phosphorus, and Calcium every 12 hours x 2 then daily.
Treatment Termination:	
17.	☐ Return blood with a _____ml normal saline flush. ☐ Do not return blood.
18.	Pulsatile flush to each limb of catheter with 10 mL (adult) or 5 mL (pediatric) normal saline. Fill Arterial and Venous lumen of dialysis catheter (volume printed on catheter A_____mL, V_____mL) with: ☐ Heparin 5000 units/mL (adult standard). ☐ Heparin 1000 units/mL (pediatric standard). ☐ ACD-A from pharmacy.
Nephrologist (Signature/Print Name):	P.I.: Pager:
Nephrology Nurse (Signature/Print Name):	Date/Time:
ICU Nurse (Signature/Print Name):	Date/Time:

AM2555 (9/07)   **CRRT ORDERS WITH HEPARIN ANTICOAGULATION**   MR# 10/96/371

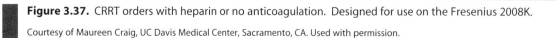

Figure 3.37. CRRT orders with heparin or no anticoagulation. Designed for use on the Fresenius 2008K.

Courtesy of Maureen Craig, UC Davis Medical Center, Sacramento, CA. Used with permission.

UNIVERSITY OF CALIFORNIA, DAVIS
MEDICAL CENTER
SACRAMENTO, CALIFORNIA

PHYSICIAN'S ORDERS

PEDIATRIC CONTINUOUS RENAL REPLACEMENT THERAPY (CRRT) ORDERS
WITH REGIONAL CITRATE ANTICOAGULATION

Directions: Check the appropriate boxes and complete those orders to be implemented (order renewal daily before noon).

For assistance, Monday-Friday 8-5 call x48730, other hours call operator for on-call Nephrology Nurse.

Date:	For Date:
Time:	

Fluid/ Solute Balance:

1. ☐ Daily Weights (kg).   Admission Weight (kg):
2. ☐ Dialyzer _____ (See Pediatric Specification Sheet).
3. ☐ Blood Tubing: ☐ Neonate, ☐ Husky, ☐ Pediatric, ☐ Adult **(See Pediatric Specification Sheet to set Pump Segment Diameter)**.
4. ☐ Prime circuit with: ☐ Saline, ☐ 5% Albumin, ☐ PRBC & normal saline for a HCT of_____ % (Sign Pediatric Specification Sheet).
5. ☐ Blood Flow Rate (BFR) _____ (20-200) ml/min (5-10 ml/kg/min) (consider reducing to decrease clearance).
6. ☐ Pediatric UFR = _____ ml/hr (0.5-1 ml/kg/hr) + Total Intake rate – patient's previous hour Output.
7. ☐ Dialysate Flow Rate (DFR) _____ (100) ml/min at _____ (36°-38°) C.
   ☐ (Optional) Dialysate Flow Co-current to Blood Flow (consider when needing to decrease clearance).
8. ☐ Dialysate: K^+ _____ (3-4) mEq/L Na^+ _____ (135) mEq/L PO_4^{-3} _____ (2.5) mg/dL
            Ca^{+2} ___0___ (0)mEq/L HCO_3^- _____ (25-30) mEq/L Mg^{+2} _____ (2 - 2.5) mEq/L
                                                                           (1 mEq/L Mg^{+2} = 1.2 mg/dL Mg)
9. ☐ (Optional) Replacement Fluid: Infuse normal saline at _____ (10% of BFR) ml/hour.
10. ☐ Call Nephrology if fluid bolus greater than 60ml/Kg/shift is ordered for BP support.

Medications:

11. ☐ Anticoagulant Citrate Dextrose (ACD-A) _____ ml/hour (BFR x 2, in ml/hour, i.e., BFR of 150 ml/min, ACD-A 300 ml/hr) Rx.
12. ☐ Adjust ACD-A to maintain the System (venous port) ionized Calcium 0.25-0.35 mMol/L.

For System (venous port) ionized Calcium (mMol/L)	Patient less than 5Kg Adjust ACD-A infusion	Patient 5-20 Kg Adjust ACD-A infusion	Patient more than 20 Kg Adjust ACD-A infusion
Less than 0.25	Decrease by 2.5 ml/hour	Decrease by 5 ml/hour	Decrease by 10 ml/hour
0.25-0.35	**No Change**	**No Change**	**No Change**
0.36-0.45	Increase by 2.5 ml/hour	Increase by 5 ml/hour	Increase by 10 ml/hour
Greater than 0.45	Increase by 5 ml/hour	Increase by 10 ml/hour	Increase by 20 ml/hour
Notify Nephrologist ASAP if ACD-A infusion is greater than 300 ml/hour			

13. ☐ Calcium Chloride (8 g/L 0.9% saline) _____ ml/hour (2/3 of BFR in ml/hour, i.e., BFR of 150 ml/min, CaCl 100 ml/hour) Rx.
14. ☐ Adjust Calcium Chloride to maintain the Patient (arterial) ionized Calcium 1.2 – 1.4 mMol/L

For Patient Ionized Calcium (mMol/L)	Patient less than 5Kg Adjust Calcium infusion	Patient 5-20 Kg Adjust Calcuium infusion	Patient greater than 20 Kg Adjust Calcium infusion
Less than 0.9	**Notify PICU MD. Increase calcium infusion by 10%. Hold ACD-A for 1 hour, and then restart at 30% of previous ACD-A rate.**		
0.90-1.00	Increase by 5 ml/hour	Increase by 10 ml/hour	Increase by 20 ml/hour
1.01-1.19	Increase by 2.5 ml/hour	Increase by 5 ml/hour	Increase by 10 ml/hour
1.20-1.40	**No Change**	**No Change**	**No Change**
1.41-1.60	Decrease by 2.5 ml/hour	Decrease by 5 ml/hour	Decrease by 10 ml/hour
Greater than 1.60	**Notify PICU MD**	**Notify PICU MD**	**Notify PICU MD**
Notify Nephrologist ASAP if Calcium infusion is greater than 200 ml/hour			

Laboratory:

15. ☐ Pretreatment draw: Patient ionized Calcium, CBC, BMP, Calcium, Magnesium, Phosphorus, and Albumin.
16. ☐ Every six hours x 2, then every 12 hours draw: CBC, BMP, Calcium, Magnesium, Phosphorus, and _____.
17. ☐ 30 minutes after treatment initiation or blood product administration draw Patient and System ionized Calcium.
18. ☐ 30-60 minutes after a change in BFR, DFR, ACD-A or Calcium infusion rate draw Patient and System ionized Calcium.
19. ☐ Every four hours draw Patient and System ionized Calcium.
20. ☐ For patient symptoms of hypocalcemia or hypercalcemia draw Patient ionized Calcium and System ionized Calcium.

Treatment Termination:

21. ☐ Return blood with a _____ ml normal saline flush (see Pediatric Specification Sheet for standard volume = circuit volume).
   ☐ (Optional) Do not return blood.
22.   Pulsatile flush to each limb of catheter with 5 ml normal saline. Fill Arterial and Venous lumen of dialysis catheter (volume printed on catheter A_____mL, V_____mL) with:
   ☐ Heparin 1000 units/ml (standard).
   ☐ ACD-A from pharmacy.
   ☐ _____
23. ☐ 20 minutes after treatment termination draw Patient ionized Calcium, notify PICU MD if not in range of 1.20-1.40mMol/L.
24. ☐ Notify Nephrologist of treatment termination.

Nephrologist signature / print name:	P.I.:	Pager:
Nephrology Nurse signature / print name:	Date/Time:	
ICU Nurse signature / print name:	Date / Time:	

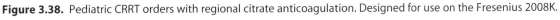

Figure 3.38. Pediatric CRRT orders with regional citrate anticoagulation. Designed for use on the Fresenius 2008K.

Courtesy of Maureen Craig, UC Davis Medical Center, Sacramento, CA. Used with permission.

UNIVERSITY OF CALIFORNIA, DAVIS
MEDICAL CENTER
SACRAMENTO, CALIFORNIA

PHYSICIAN'S ORDERS

PEDIATRIC CONTINUOUS RENAL REPLACEMENT THERAPY (CRRT) ORDERS
WITH HEPARIN OR NO ANTICOAGULATION

Date:	For Date:
Time:	

Directions: Check the appropriate boxes and complete those orders to be implemented (order renewal daily before noon).
For assistance, Monday-Friday 8-5 call x48730, other hours call operator for on-call Nephrology Nurse.

Fluid/Solute Balance:

1. ☐ Daily Weights (kg). _____   Admission Weight (kg): _____

2. ☐ Dialyzer _____ (See Pediatric Specification Sheet).

3. ☐ Blood Tubing: ☐ Neonate, ☐ Husky, ☐ Pediatric, ☐ Adult **(See Pediatric Specification Sheet to set Pump Segment Diameter).**

4. ☐ Prime circuit with: ☐ Saline, ☐ 5% Albumin, ☐ PRBC & normal saline for a HCT of _____% (See Pediatric Specification Sheet).

5. ☐ Blood Flow Rate (BFR) _____ (50-200) ml/min (consider 5-10 ml/kg/min).

6. ☐ Pediatric UFR = _____ ml/hr (0.5-1ml/kg/hr) + Total Intake rate – patient's previous hour Output.

7. ☐ Dialysate Flow Rate (DFR) _____ (100) ml/min at _____ (36°-38°) C.
    ☐ (Optional) Dialysate Flow Co-current to Blood Flow (consider when needing to decrease clearance).

8. ☐ Dialysate: K^+ _____ (3-4) mEq/L Na^+ _____ (135-140) mEq/L PO_4^{-3} _____ (2.5) mg/dL
    Ca^{+2} _____ (2.5)mEq/L HCO_3^- _____ (30) mEq/L Mg^{+2} _____ (2 - 2.5) mEq/L
    (1 mEq/L Mg^{+2} = 1.2 mg/dL Mg)

9. ☐ (Optional) Replacement Fluid: Infuse normal saline at _____ (10% of BFR) ml/hr.

10. ☐ Call Nephrology if fluid bolus greater than 60ml/Kg/shift is ordered for BP support.

Medications:

11. ☐ No Anticoagulation

12. ☐ Flush circuit with _____ (25-100) ml normal saline every 15-30 minutes.

13. ☐ Heparin bolus _____ units IV (25-50 units/kg/dose) and rebolus _____ units IV (10 units/kg) to achieve range.

14. ☐ Heparin (100 units/ml) infusion _____ units/hr IV (10-20 units/kg/hr).

15. ☐ Adjust Heparin infusion to achieve a PTT in the range of 45-65.

PTT	Bolus (units/kg)	Hold (minutes)	Rate Change (units/kg/hr)
Less than 34	25	0	Increase by 2
35-44	0	0	Increase by 1
45-65	**0**	**0**	**No Change**
66-75	0	0	Decrease by 1
76-100	0	30	Decrease by 2
Greater than100	0	60 Notify PICU MD	Decrease by 2

Laboratory:

16. ☐ Pretreatment draw: BMP, Calcium, Magnesium, Phosphorus, Albumin, CBC, INR, PTT, Fibrinogen, FDP, and D-dimer.

17. ☐ Every 12 hours draw: BMP, Calcium, Magnesium, Phosphorus, CBC, PTT, and _____.

18. ☐ Check PTT 5 minutes after a heparin bolus, 4 hours after an heparin infusion change, and after blood product administration.

19. ☐ Call PICU attending for a decrease in platelet count ≥ 50% from baseline at start of CRRT therapy.

Treatment Termination:

20. ☐ Return blood with a _____ml normal saline flush (see Pediatric Specification Sheet for standard volume = circuit volume).
    ☐ (Optional) Do not return blood.

21.   Pulsatile flush to each limb of catheter with 5 ml normal saline. Fill Arterial and Venous lumen of dialysis catheter (volume printed on catheter A_____mL, V_____mL) with:
    ☐ Heparin 1000 units/ml (standard).
    ☐ ACD-A from Rx.
    ☐ _____

22. ☐ Notify Nephrologist of treatment termination.

Nephrologist signature / print name:	P.I.:	Pager:
Nephrology Nurse signature / print name:	Date/Time:	
ICU Nurse signature / print name:	Date / Time:	

A5805-1 (9/07)   **PEDIATRIC CRRT ORDERS WITH HEPARIN OR NO ANTICOAGULATION**   MR#020/05964

Figure 3.39. Pediatric CRRT orders with heparin or no anticoagulation. Designed for use on the Fresenius 2008K.

Courtesy of Maureen Craig, UC Davis Medical Center, Sacramento, CA. Used with permission.

Slow Extended Daily Dialysis (SLEDD) Bedside Inservice Checklist
(Given at the beginning of each treatment, when a patient is on SLEDD)

Date/Time:

The ICU RN should verbalize:	Neph RN	ICU RN
Reason for treatment, how SLEDD works - fluid/solute balance, medication adjustments		
Where the blood, fluid, and dialysate pathways are		
How to respond to patient hypotension - Stop UF, titrate vasopressors, give ordered fluids		
How to interpret Ionized Calcium and adjust ACD-A and calcium gluconate IV rate when on ACD-A anticoagulation. Follow ordered titration of drips.		
How to assess hypocalcemia (Chvostek's sign) and associated changes in treatment (increase IV calcium gluconate per orders) when on regional citrate anticoagulation		
When and how to contact the Nephrology Nurse		
How and why to trouble shoot equipment alarms (if not resolved, call Nephrology Nurse)		
Alarm Action - Slow response to alarms may lead to the blood circuit clotting	**Neph RN**	**ICU RN**
AP/VP check lines for kinks, when open press Areset@, change transducer if wet, notify Nephrology Nurse if unable to achieve BFR		
Other contact Nephrology Nurse		
The ICU RN should demonstrate:	**Neph RN**	**ICU RN**
How to assist in drawing and processing Ionized Calcium labs when on ACD-A anticoagulation		
How to assess for system clotting and procedure to return patient=s blood with a saline flush		

Inservice Provided by:_____   Inservice Received by:_____
                                    Nephrology RN   ICU RN

Figure 3.40. SLEDD bedside inservice checklist. Designed for use with the Fresenius 2008K.

Courtesy of Maureen Craig, UC Davis Medical Center, Sacramento, CA. Used with permission.

detector, an air bubble detector, and a return line clamp.

c. The fluid control unit manages fluids through coordination of information between its scales and the pumps in the flow control unit.

(1) The three scales independently monitor the weight of the fluid bags and notify the practitioner when it is time to change bags.

(2) The three scales continuously and precisely weigh the fluid removed, the replacement fluid returned to the patient, and the dialysis solution used and alert the user when there is a discrepancy with the weight change it is expecting. FDA public heath notification (original publication August 23, 2005, updated February 27, 2006) states, "Caregivers must pay particular attention to the 'Incorrect Weight Change Detected' alarms. These alarms are designed to alert the user of a potential fluid imbalance that has occurred during the course of CRRT. If treatment is continued without resolving the cause of these alarms, excessive fluid may be removed from the patient, and this can result in serious injury or death."

(3) The scales and the corresponding parts of the tubing sets are color-coded for easy identification.

CRRT with Regional Citrate Bedside Inservice Checklist
(Given at the beginning of each shift when a patient is on CRRT)

Date:

The ICU RN should verbalize:	Neph RN	ICU RN
Reason for treatment, how CRRT works - fluid/solute balance, nutrition and medication changes		
Where the blood, fluid, and dialysate pathways are. Adult prime volume is ≈ 250 ml saline. See Pediatric Hemodialysis Specification Sheet for prime volume and pump segment diameter. Set CRRT machine to match		
How the R.O. works - purifies water		
How to respond to patient hypotension		
When and how to terminate CRRT and care for the catheter and access site (see CRRT Termination diagram)		
How to interpret patient and system ionized Calciums and adjust ACD-A and Calcium IV rates (see Regional Citrate diagram). When stopping ACD-A or Calcium drips, a new order set must be written.		
How to assess symptoms of hypocalcemia (seizures, Chvostek's sign, hypotention, prolonged Q-T interval) and hypercalcemia (lethargy, H/A, N/V) and associated changes in treatment		
When and how to contact the Nephrologist (clotted system or prescription changes) or Nephrology Nurse (equipment and documentation)		
How and why to trouble shoot equipment alarms (if not resolved or concerns exist, call Nephrology Nurse)		

Fresenius Alarm	Action - Slow response to alarms may lead to the blood circuit clotting	Neph RN	ICU RN
AP/VP	check lines for kinks, change transducer if wet, notify Neph MD if unable to achieve BFR		
Low TMP	increase rate and compensate with maintenance fluids, change transducer if wet		
Conductivity	Check wand connections, if concentrate jugs are empty, call Nephrology Nurse for refill. Concentrate jugs should be filled and tightly capped every 12-14 hours.		
Blood pump	check blood pump door is latched		
Air detector	raise venous chamber level with ^ arrow to 1cm of top, check lines below venous chamber are free of air, reset, replace transducer protector prn, check all blood line connections are tight		
No Water	check water tap is on (no hot water), hose connections are tight, RO plugged in and on, water pre filter "IN" pressure is at 20 PSI or more		
Blood leak	Hemastick dialysate, if + stop treatment without blood return, if - reset alarm		
Power failure	plug machine into red plate, turn machine on, select CRRT mode, confirm dialysate screen, select "Home" screen, touch "Tx Paused" button to turn it to "Tx Running" and confirm		
RO TDS	set TDS (Total Dissolved Solids) limit to 10 mg/L		

The ICU RN should demonstrate:	Neph RN	ICU RN
How to verify dialysate. How to verify and adjust ACD-A and Calcium solutions and rates. Zero Calcium dialyzing fluid must be used in tandem with ACD-A and IV Calcium solutions.		
How to draw/process patient and system ionized Calcium labs PRN (see Regional Citrate diagram).		
How to determine and set UF Rate (calculate Calcium and ACD-A fluid input into UF Rate). Nephrology Nurse will set up the Calcium and the ACD-A IV's on an IV pump on top of the Fresenius 2008K.		
How to reset "UF Removed" every hour for Pediatric treatments and every shift for Adult treatments.		
When and how to adjust BFR e.g. lab draws, frequent negative AP alarms (BFR should be > 20 ml/min) (If unable to achieve the prescribed BFR, notify the Nephrologist).		
How to assess clotting in the system		
How and when to adjust arterial and venous chamber levels		
How to complete ICU documentation (BFR, ACD-A, and Calcium rate, I/O's and system pressures). For Pediatric treatments refer to the "EMR Documentation Sheet."		

Inservice Provided by: _____   Inservice Received by: _____
Signature/Print Name   Signature/Print Name

Craig, 1/30/2008

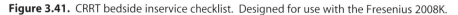

Figure 3.41. CRRT bedside inservice checklist. Designed for use with the Fresenius 2008K.

Courtesy of Maureen Craig, UC Davis Medical Center, Sacramento, CA. Used with permission.

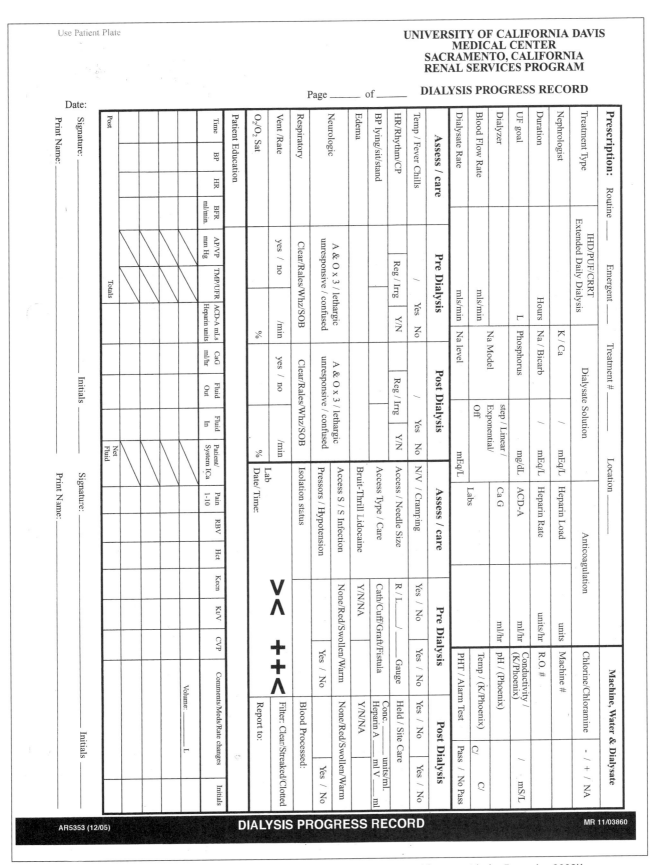

Figure 3.42. Nephrology nursing flowsheet for IHD, SLEDD, or CRRT. Designed for use with the Fresenius 2008K.

Courtesy of Maureen Craig, UC Davis Medical Center, Sacramento, CA. Used with permission.

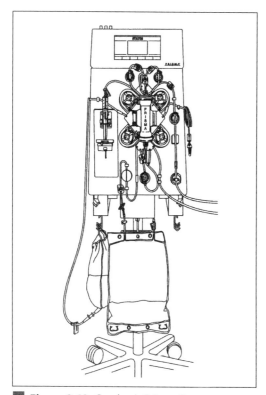

Figure 3.43. Gambro's Prisma System.

Source: Gambro: Prisma M60 instructions for use. Reprinted with permission from Gambro.

2. Therapy considerations.
   a. Software calculates the UFR needed to achieve the patient fluid removal rate (PFR) set by the practitioner.
   b. Software, pumps, and scales manage the fluid balance under the control of the ICU nurse at the bedside.
   c. Software records and displays all Prisma related I/O volumes. Patient I/O volumes are monitored by the bedside nurse to allow for hourly adjustments of machine settings to maximize the accuracy and effectiveness of the therapy.
   d. An ultrasonic air detector is built into the return bloodline.
   e. The alarm system lists alarms in order of importance and offers on-screen instructions for appropriate interventions. A log of the last 100 events is recorded and stored in the system memory for review.
   f. Anticoagulation can be achieved using heparin for systemic anticoagulation or citrate and calcium for regional anticoagulation.
      (1) Heparin can be administered on the Prisma by syringe pump or through a central line using an IV pump.
      (2) When using heparin, some users deliver an hourly flush of the system with 25–200 mL of normal saline to observe the patency of the system. The saline can be connected to a Y port or stopcock on the access line.
      (3) When using citrate and calcium for anticoagulation, the citrate is administered through a Y port or stopcock on the access line. The calcium is administered through a central line or through the third port on the dialysis catheter, if that type of catheter is being used.
      (4) When using citrate anticoagulation, it is essential that, whenever the blood pump stops, the IV infusion pump administering the citrate must also be stopped to prevent backflow, which would result in direct administration of citrate to the patient.
      (5) When treating patients for whom anticoagulation is not feasible, 25–200 mL normal saline flushes should be performed. The frequency can be adjusted based on the condition of the hemofilter.
      (6) Saline flushes, heparin, citrate, calcium, and all other patient intake must be included in the patient's I/O calculations. These intakes are not administered by the Prisma system and, therefore, need to be included in the PFR set by the practitioner.
   g. Flow rates available on the Prisma system include:
      (1) Blood flow can be set between 10 and 180 mL/min.
      (2) PFR can be set at 0 or from 10 to 1000 mL/hr in CVVH, CVVHD, and CVVHDF modes and at 10 to 2000 mL/hr in SCUF mode.
      (3) Dialysate flow can be set at 0 or from 50 to 2500 mL/hr in CVVHD and CVVHDF modes.
      (4) Replacement solution may be set to infuse at 0 or from 100 to 4500 mL/hr in the CVVH mode. Replacement solution may be set to infuse at 0 or from 100 to 2000 mL/hr in CVVHDF mode.
   h. There is no blood warmer built into the Prisma, so the patient's temperature should be monitored closely.
      (1) The Prismatherm II® (Gambro,

Stockholm, Sweden) is a blood warmer available that attaches to the return line to warm the blood as it returns to the patient.

(2) The Prismaflo® (Gambro, Stockholm, Sweden) is a blood or dialysate warmer that uses a thermal sleeve to warm the blood or dialysate within the line.

(3) A Bair Hugger® (Arizant Healthcare, Eden Prairie, Minnesota) or some variety of blanket warmer is an alternative method of warming the patient, should the blood warmer not be available.

3. Prismaflex® (Gambro, Stockholm, Sweden) is an updated version of the Prisma machine released by Gambro in 2005.

a. The system includes a 12-inch touch screen with improved color and graphics.

b. The step-by-step instructions on screen have been expanded and now include an illustration with color codes to match the hemofilter set.

c. An ultrasonic air detector is built into the return line.

d. Multiple external connections will allow connection to an ICU central monitoring system.

e. The four scales system has been ergonomically redesigned for ease of handling with improved alarm sensitivity to decrease the number of nuisance alarms from sudden bag movement.

f. A temporary disconnection procedure, allows recirculation to accommodate up to 2 hours off the treatment to move the patient.

g. An additional fifth "pre-blood pump," allows infusion of anticoagulant or solutions for the purpose of hemodilution.

h. The option of delivering infusions prefilter or postfilter by use of integral pinch valves, including changing from one to the other during a treatment using the same set is another upgrade on this system. The pinch valve system also allows for simultaneous predilution and postdilution.

i. Prismaflex disposable sets continue to be fully preconnected and color-coded and are available in 4 models with a range of filter surface area from 0.6 m² to 1.4 m². All sets are validated for 72 hours of use.

j. The flow rates available with the Prismaflex system are.
(1) Blood flow: 10 to 450 mL/min. in increments of 10 mL/min.

(2) Replacement solution: 0 to 8,000 mL/hr in increments of 50 mL/hr.

(3) Dialysate: 0 to 8,000 mL/hr in increments of 50 mL/hr.

(4) Pre-blood pump solution/anticoagulant: 0 to 8,000 mL/hr in increments of 10 mL/hr.

(5) PFR: 0 to 2,000 mL/hr.

(6) Effluent removal: 0 to 10,000 mL/hr.

4. Coordinating documentation: designed for use on the Prisma or Prismaflex.

a. Ordersets.
(1) CRRT orders with regional citrate anticoagulation (see Figure 3.44).

(2) CRRT orders with heparin or citrate anticoagulation (see Figure 3.45).

(3) Pediatric CRRT orders with regional citrate anticoagulation (see Figure 3.46).

b. Bedside inservice checklist (see Figure 3.47).

c. Nursing documents.
(1) Nephrology nursing flowsheet with regional citrate or heparin anticoagulation (see Figure 3.48).

(2) ICU Kardex for CRRT with regional citrate (see Figure 3.49).

(3) ICU nursing flowsheet with regional citrate or heparin anticoagulation (see Figure 3.50).

C. Other CRRT equipment.

1. NxStage System One® (NxStage Medical, Inc., Lawrence, Massachusetts). Product and supplies information available from NxStage at http://www.nxstage.com/acute_renal_care.

2. Accura™ (Baxter, Deerfield, Illinois). Product and supplies information available from Baxter at www.baxter.com/products/renal/crrt/sub/accura.html.

3. Diapact CRRT® (B. Braun Melsungen AG, Melsungen, Germany): Product and supplies information available from Braun at www.bbraunusa.com/products/diapact.html.

D. Other system components.

1. Vascular access.

a. CAVH, CAVHD, and CAVHDF require cannulation of both an artery and a vein for extracorporeal blood flow.

(1) Single-lumen dialysis catheters, (8 FR x 15 cm) may be placed in a femoral artery and femoral vein (preferred), or subclavian vein for the arteriovenous circuit.

(2) Femoral artery to a Cordis® catheter (Cordis Corporation, Miami Lakes,

---

ACUTE HEMODIALYSIS SERVICES
CITRATE CRRT ORDERS

Addressograph

Allergies:

Page 1 of 2

1. ☐ Consent for CRRT by Dr. _____.   ☐ Consent for vascular access by Dr. _____.
2. **Therapy type:**
   ☐ SCUF (ultrafiltration only)   ☐ CVVHD (using dialysate)
   ☐ CVVH (using replacement solution)   ☐ CVVHDF (using dialysate and replacement solution)
3. Blood Flow Rate: 100 ml/min
4. Hemofilter: M100 (AN69)
5. **Fluid Balance:**
   ☐ Start-up CRRT Weight: _____   ☐ Desired Net Negative Ultrafiltration _____ ml/hr
   ☐ Daily Weight & Hourly I & O   ☐ Desired Net Positive Fluid Gain _____ ml/hr
   ☐ Zero Balance Ultrafiltration   ☐ 24-hour Fluid Balance Goal _____ liters
       ☐ Other _____
6. **Lock Hemodialysis Catheter when not in use with:**
   ☐ Heparin 5000 units/ml: Red lumen __ ml Blue lumen _____ ml
   ☐ Heparin 1000 units/ml: Red lumen __ ml Blue lumen _____ ml
   ☐ Heparin 100 units/ml: 3rd Infusion lumen _____ ml
   ☐ For catheter thrombosis instill Alteplase Cathflo® 2 mg/2 ml: Red lumen _____ ml
       Blue lumen _____ ml   Infusion lumen _____ ml PRN for patency/thrombosis
7. ☐ For Heparin Induced Thrombocytopenia patients, lock catheter with Anticoagulant Citrate
       Dextrose Formula A 2% / 5 ml syringe, PRN for patency: Red lumen _____ ml Blue lumen _____ ml
       Infusion lumen _____ ml
8. ☐ Change circuit every 72 hr. If system fails between 2200 & 0600, restart: ☐ in AM   ☐ ASAP
9. **IV Replacement/Substitution Fluid:**
   ☐ A. 1 liter of 0.45% Sodium Chloride (1/2 strength Normal Saline) with 75 mEq Sodium Bicarbonate at _____ ml/hr
   ☐ B. 1 liter of 0.9% Sodium Chloride (Normal saline) at _____ ml/hr
   ☐ C. 1 liter of 0.45% Sodium Chloride (1/2 strength Normal Saline) at _____ ml/hr
   ☐ D. Other: _____ ml/hr
10. **Dialysate:**
    ☐ A. Dialysate flow rate _____ ml/hr (0-2500 liter/hr)
    ☐ B. Normocarb® base solution (total volume 3246.5 ml) (Normocarb 240 ml, Sterile Water 3 L, Dextrose 50% 6.5 ml)
        Total Anions 141.5 mEq/L   Total Cations 141.5 mEq/L

Components	Sterile Water	Na+	Mg	Cl	HCO$_3$	Ca^{2+}	KCl	Dextrose
Concentration mEq/L	3 Liters	140	1.5	106.5	35.0	0	0	0.1%

POTASSIUM MUST BE ADDED TO ALL ORDERS!
    ☐ C. To customize dialysate, check desired additives to 3246 ml base solution (Pharmacy to add/mix).
       ☐ Potassium Chloride 3.2 mEq (provides 1 mEq KCl/liter)
       ☐ Potassium Chloride 6.5 mEq (provides 2 mEq KCl/liter)
       ☐ Potassium Chloride 9.7 mEq (provides 3 mEq KCl/liter)
       ☐ Potassium Chloride 13 mEq (provides 4 mEq KCl/liter)
       ☐ Potassium Chloride 16.2 mEq (provides 5 mEq KCl/liter)
    ☐ D. Other _____
11. **Circuit Management:**
    ☐ Stop Citrate and Calcium infusions if:
        - Filter clots / termination of therapy
        - Machine alarms that stop blood pump
        - Stop for 1 minute only during NS flush or when returning blood
    ☐ Hang 1000 ml 0.9% Sodium Chloride to flush circuit (pharmacy to provide). Flush circuit with 100 ml 0.9% Sodium Chloride PRN to check circuit patency, add flush volume to patient fluid removal and follow instructions per circuit management.

Acute Unit\CRRT Forms\Citrate CRRT Orders 6-07

Figure 3.44 – page 1 of 2. CRRT orders with regional citrate. Designed for use on the Prisma.

Courtesy of Jina Bogle, DCI Acute Program, Omaha, Nebraska. Used with permission.

Addressograph

ACUTE HEMODIALYSIS SERVICES
CITRATE CRRT ORDERS

Allergies:

Page 2 of 2

12.　**Anticoagulation:**
　　☐ CRRT Regional Citrate Anticoagulation infusion
　　　　1.　☐ 1 liter Anticoagulant Citrate Dextrose Solution Formula A ACD(A) Citrate Solution 2% IV rate 150 ml/hr via CRRT access bloodline
　　　　2.　☐ 1 liter D5W + 6 grams Calcium Chloride IV rate 60 ml/hr via central line.
　　　　3.

Citrate Titration Table	
Post-Filter ionized Calcium (mmol/L)	Citrate Infusion Adjustment
Less than 0.25	↓ Rate by 10 ml/hr
0.25 – 0.35 (optimal range)	NO ADJUSTMENT
0.36 – 0.45	↑ Rate by 10 ml/hr
Greater than 0.45	↑ Rate by 20 ml/hr

Safety Parameters – Notify Nephrologist if the following occur:
　　　　1.　Citrate Rate greater than 200 ml/hr
　　　　2.　Systemic ionized Calcium less than 0.75 mmol/liter
　　　　3.　Serum Na^+ greater than 150 mEq/liter consider changing replacement solution to 0.45% Sodium Chloride.
　　　　4.　If the patient is hypotensive consider holding the citrate protocol for ½ hour until BP stable
　　　　4.

Calcium Titration Scale	
Systemic (Patient) ionized Calcium (mmol/L)	Calcium Infusion Adjustment
Greater than 1.3	↓ Rate by 10 ml/hr
1.1 – 1.3 (optimal range)	NO ADJUSTMENT
0.9 – 1.0	↑ Rate by 10 ml/hr
Less than 0.9	↑ Rate by 20 ml/hr

　　　　5.　➢ Serum Bicarb greater than 26 mEq/liter – Call Nephrologist to adjust replacement rate. If no replacement solution ordered, add NS as a replacement solution rate @ 200-400 ml/hr and decrease the dialysate rate by this amount. This will remove the excess bicarb in the ultrafiltered fluid and replace it with Normal Saline And reduce the Bicarbonate from the dialysate **OR**
　　　　　➢ Alternatively the amount of replacement can be calculated as follows:
　　　　　= bicarb current – desired bicarb) x 0.3 x patient weight (kg)
　　　　　　Time between the bicarb samples (hours) x current bicarb
　　　　　i.e. (26-24) x 0.3 x 78　=　0.30 liter/hr　=　300 ml/hr replacement solution rate
　　　　　　　6 x 26

13.　**Labs 1 hour after initiation and every 6 hours thereafter while on CRRT:**
　　☐ Post filter (Prisma) ionized Ca^{2+} (draw from blue sample port)
　　☐ Systemic ionized Ca^{2+} (draw from patient [true] arterial line or peripherally)
　　☐ For lab draws via central line, stop Citrate/Calcium Chloride infusions x 1 minute, waste 10 ml prior to draw
　　Labs 1 hour after initiation and every 12 hours thereafter while on CRRT:
　　☐ CBC
　　☐ Renal Function Panel: Alb, Ca^{2+}, CO_2, Cl^-, Creatinine, BUN, Glucose, Phosphorus, K^+, NA^+
　　☐ Mg^{2+}
　　☐ ABG
　　Miscellaneous Labs:
　　☐ Hepatic Function Panel (Alb, Total Bilirubin, Direct Bilirubin, Alk Phos, Total Protein, AST, ALT) at initiation of therapy
　　☐ Lactic acid at initiation of therapy
　　☐ If Platelet trend decreases at day 4 of therapy, draw Heparin Induced Antibody
　　☐ Other _____

Date/Time: _____　　Nephrologist: _____　　Noted by: _____
For initial notification call DCI-Acute (402) 449-5355 or (after-hours) Answering Service (402) 231-1032.

Acute Unit\CRRT Forms\Citrate CRRT Orders 6-07

Figure 3.44 – page 2 of 2. CRRT orders with regional citrate. Designed for use on the Prisma.

Courtesy of Jina Bogle, DCI Acute Program, Omaha, Nebraska. Used with permission.

STAT: Place an "X" in the box if STAT.   Please rule off unused lines after order sent to Pharmacy.

DATE / TIME	ORDERS	DATE	PROGRESS NOTES
	Rev: 01/06 PPO.430		
	Page 1 of 2		
	CONTINUOUS RENAL REPLACEMENT THERAPY (CRRT)		
	Date: _____ Procedure: ☐ SCUF ☐ CVVHD		
	☐ CVVH ☐ CVVHDF		
	Filter: ☐ M100		
	BFR: ☐ 150mL per min. OR _____mL per min		
	☐ Daily Wts.		
	Desired net fluid loss _____mL per hour		
	Replacement Solution		
	☐ Pre-Filter		
	Rate: ☐ 1200mL per hour OR _____mL per hour		
	Type A: ☐ 1L 0.9NaCl + 5mL 10% CaCl2		
	Type B: ☐ 1L 0.45NaCl + 75mL 8.4% NaHCO₃		
	Type C: ☐ PrismaSate® 5L (KO/Ca3.5)		
	add KCL _____ mEq/L and Glucose _____. mg/dL		
	Type D: ☐ Other_____		
	Mode: ☐ Simultaneous ("Y" connector)		
	(May use with type A / B)		
	☐ Sequential (alternate every L)		
	Dialysate Solution		
	Rate: ☐ 1200mL per hour OR _____mL per hour		
	Type A: ☐ PrismaSate® Formula (Bicarb with KO/Ca3.5)		
	Sodium 140 mEq per L		
	Calcium 3.5 mEq per L		
	Magnesium 1 mEq per L		
	Potassium 0 or _____ mEq per L		
	Chloride 109.5 mEq per L		
	Lactate 3 mEq per L		
	Bicarbonate 32 mEq per L		
	Glucose 0 or _____ mg per dL		
	(suggest 1gm per L=100 mg per dL, 2gm per L=200 mg per dL)		
	Type B: ☐ No Lactate Formula (made in pharmacy)		
	Na (variable) _____ mEq per L (suggest 140 mEq per L)		
	Bicarb (variable) _____mEq per L (suggest 35 mEq per L)		
	Cl (variable) _____mEq per L (CL = Na – Bicarb)		
	K (variable) _____ mEq per L		
	Magnesium sulfate 2 mEq per L		
	Dextrose (variable) _____ mg per dL		
	(suggest 1gm per L=100 mg per dL, 2gm per L=200 mg per dL)		
	Zero Calcium		
	Type C: ☐ Formula for use with Citrate ONLY		
	Na 117 mEq per L		
	K (variable) _____ mEq per L		
	Magnesium sulfate 1.5 mEq per L		
	Cl (variable) _____mEq per L (CL = Na + K)		
	Dextrose (variable) _____ mg per dL		
	(suggest 1gm per L=100mg per dL, 2 gm per L=200mg per dLI)		
	Zero Calcium		

DRUG ORDERS: UNLESS INITIALED PBO (PRESCRIBED BRAND ONLY) ANOTHER BRAND OF A GENERICALLY EQUIVALENT PRODUCT IDENTICAL IN CONTENT OF ACTIVE INGREDIENT(S) MAY BE ADMINISTERED

PHYSICIAN'S ORDERS AND PROGRESS NOTES INSTRUCTIONS

1. Attach patient's label or complete required information before placing in chart.
2. Rule off unused lines.
3. If STAT order, please rule off unused lines after order sent to Pharmacy.

PATIENT LABEL

Patient Name:

DOB:

Date of Procedure:

Diagnosis:

Patient Room#/Unit _____

Figure 3.45 – page 1 of 2. CRRT orders with heparin or regional citrate anticoagulation. Designed for use on the Prisma.

Courtesy of Helen Williams, Western Nephrology Acute Dialysis, Denver, Colorado. Used with permission.

STAT: Place an "X" in the box if STAT.   Please rule off unused lines after order sent to Pharmacy.

DATE / TIME	ORDERS	DATE	PROGRESS NOTES

ORDERS

Rev: 01/06   PPO.430
                                                                              Page 2 of 2

CONTINUOUS RENAL REPLACEMENT THERAPY (CRRT)

Anticoagulation   Current Weight _____ kg

1.   Select dose (check one box only)
☐ Heparin: Bolus 5,000 units then start 10 units/kg/hour infusion
☐ Tight Heparin: Bolus 1,000 units then start 5 units/kg/hour infusion

2.   Select method of administration (check one box only)
☐ Heparin via syringe on Prisma pump. Pharmacy to prepare 500
    units/mL, 20mL syringe.
    Use for heparin doses of 250 units/hour or greater
☐ Heparin drip via pump (25,000 units/500 mL D5W bag)
    Use for heparin doses less than 250 units/hour
    Select heparin protocol to use: (See other orders)
        ☐ Neuro Protocol (goal aPTT 51-70)
        ☐ Cardiac Protocol (goal aPTT 70-90)
☐ No Heparin: Flush with 0.9% NS 100 mL every hour

☐ Citrate Regional Anticoagulation
    Initiate 4% sodium citrate solution at 180 mL/hour pre-hemofilter using
    a pump. (Infusion will be connected to access port and be directed
    toward filter.)
***Citrate infusion should not exceed 210 mL/hr unless ordered by MD.
    Pharmacy will prepare a solution of Calcium Chloride 8.2 gm/L (82 mL
    of 10% calcium chloride in 0.9% NS 1L). Initiate Calcium Chloride
    infusion at 60 mL/hr via a central venous catheter.
    **CAUTION: Both IV pumps-Citrate/Calcium Chloride must be
    stopped when Prisma pump is stopped.**
☐ Do not use algorithm. Adjust per specific MD orders only.
☐ Use algorithm in table at right to adjust citrate infusion using post-filter
    ionized calcium.
CAUTION: Infuse to Prisma circuit ONLY. NOT for IV infusion.

Labs
☐ Chem. Panel, Phos, Mg Baseline and every _____ hours.
    (labs can only be drawn pre replacement fluid or arterial line)
☐ PT, aPTT Baseline and every _____ hours.
☐ CBC Baseline and every _____ hours.
☐ Lactate Baseline and every _____ hours.
☐ Post filter ICa every 6 hours X 24 hours, then per MD order with use of
    Citrate ONLY
☐ **Serum ICa every 6 hours x 24 hours, then per MD order.**

Filter to be replaced every 72 hours or earlier if indicated.

_____
Physician Signature   Date/Time

_____
Nurse Signature   Date/Time

PROGRESS NOTES

Citrate Anticoagulation for Continuous Renal Replacement Therapy
(CRRT)

Purpose
To provide an alternative to heparin-based anticoagulation for patients
requiring CRRT who are also at risk for serious hemorrhage or in whom
heparin is otherwise contraindicated (e.g. HIT). Such conditions include, but
are not limited to (HIT), post-surgical bleeding and traumatic bleeding.

Policy
1.   Citrate anticoagulation requires a physician order.
2.   Citrate should not be employed for CVVH, but is reserved for methods
     in which there is dialysate flow (i.e. CVVHD or CVVHDF). This is to
     ensure adequate removal of the citrate complex.
3.   An adequate supply of 4% sodium citrate will be dispensed by the
     hospital pharmacy in a pre-mixed 250 mL bag.
4.   Initiate citrate solution at 180 mL per hour pre-hemofilter, or other rate
     ordered by physician. (Infusion will be connected to access port and
     be directed toward filter.)
     **CAUTION: FOR INFUSION TO PRISMA CIRCUIT ONLY. IV
     pump must be stopped when PRISMA pump is stopped.**
5.   Pharmacy will prepare a solution of 8.2 gm per L Ca++ (82 mL of 10%
     CaCl$_2$ inj., U.S.P.) in 1000 mL 0.9% saline. Initiate CaCl$_2$ infusion at
     60 mL per hour via central venous catheter.
     **CAUTION: IV pump must be stopped when PRISMA pump is
     stopped.**
6.   In the event of premature clotting of the hemofilter, checking the post-
     filter ionized calcium (ICa) level will permit adjustment of the citrate
     infusion. Ideally, the post-filter ionized calcium (ICa) should be
     maintained between 0.25-0.35 mmol per L to reduce the risk of
     clotting.
7.   Measurement of post-filter ionized calcium and adjustment of the
     citrate infusion will be done by physician order. In general, the citrate
     infusion should not exceed 210 mL / hour *unless* ordered by a
     physician.
8.   Adjust citrate infusion by following algorithm:

Post-filter ionized Ca++		Change in 4% Sodium Citrate Infusion rate
mg/dL	mmol/L	
>2.00	>0.50	↑ rate by 30mL per hour
1.60-1.99	0.40-0.50	↑ rate by 20 mL per hour
1.41-1.59	0.36-0.39	↑ rate by 10 mL per hour
1.00-1.40	0.25-0.35	No change
<1.00	<0.25	↓ rate by 10 mL per hour

     *4% Sodium Citrate – Do not exceed 210 mL per hour unless ordered
     by physician.
     *Ideally, the post filter ionized calcium should be maintained between
     0.25-0.35 mmol per L to reduce risk of clotting.
9.   Potential complications of citrate anticoagulation include metabolic
     alkalosis, hypernatremia, hyper- or hypocalcemia, and bleeding.

DRUG ORDERS: UNLESS INITIALED PBO (PRESCRIBED BRAND ONLY) ANOTHER BRAND OF A GENERICALLY EQUIVALENT PRODUCT IDENTICAL IN CONTENT OF ACTIVE
INGREDIENT(S) MAY BE ADMINISTERED

PHYSICIAN'S ORDERS AND PROGRESS NOTES INSTRUCTIONS
1.   Attach patient's label or complete required information before placing in chart.
2.   Rule off unused lines.
3.   If STAT order, please rule off unused lines after order sent to Pharmacy.

PATIENT LABEL

Patient Name:

DOB:

Date of Procedure:

Diagnosis:

Patient Room#/Unit _____

Figure 3.45 – page 2 of 2. CRRT orders with heparin or regional citrate anticoagulation. Designed for use on the Prisma.

Courtesy of Helen Williams, Western Nephrology Acute Dialysis, Denver, Colorado. Used with permission.

RENAL DIALYSIS: Continuous Renal Replacement Therapy (CRRT) - Acute

Orders need renewal in 3 days. For 24-hour assistance Monday-Friday 8-5 call x 6-0851, other hours call operator x 4-2099 to page the on-call dialysis nurse.

ACCESS:

☐ Catheter site:_____ size:____F____cm
    ☐ triple lumen ☐ dual lumen ☐ single lumen ☐ uncuffed ☐ cuffed
    packing volume: arterial port ____mL; venous port ____mL; pigtail (triple lumen only) ____mL

CIRCUIT SET-UP AND PRIMING (* Dialysis nurse responsibility):

1.* Please ☐ initiate or ☐ restart CRRT using ☐ PRISMA® machine ☐ PRISMAFLEX® machine. Extracorporeal blood volume is ____mL, which equals ____% of patient's blood volume.

2.* Set PRISMA /PRISMAFLEX® to CVVHDF mode.

3.* Discard prime: ☐ Yes ☐ No
If prime not discarded, use one of the following:
☐ 5% Albumin
☐ 5% Albumin mixed with PRBC to final Hct 40%
☐ 50 ml PRBC, 50 mL (50 mEq) 8.4% NaHCO₃ and 4 mL (400 mg) 10% calcium gluconate. PRBC and NaHCO₃ mixed via blood transfusion y-set during manual CRRT prime. Calcium gluconate should be infused separately into venous limb of CRRT circuit during initiation.
☐ 0.9% Saline with 50 mL 8.4% NaHCO₃ and ____mL 10% calcium gluconate (50 mg/kg, maximum 2 g). NaHCO₃ should be infused into CRRT circuit over 2 minutes during initiation. Calcium gluconate should be infused separately into venous limb of CRRT circuit during initiation.

4.* Warm blood in CRRT circuit with blood warmer (35-36° C) as needed.

CRRT MACHINE SETTINGS

5. Set Blood Pump flow rate (Qb) at ____ mL/min
(2-8 mL/kg/min; minimum 20 mL/min; maximum 400 mL/min/1.73m²)

6. ☐ No Replacement Fluid ☐ Begin Replacement Fluid (☐ Pre ☐ Post) with _____ at rate ____ mL/hr
(*For PRISMAFLEX®, always use post-replacement fluid of 50 mL/hr minimum*).

7. Set Patient Removal flow rate (UFR=ultrafiltration rate) at ____ mL/hr
Keep total UFR rate <10% of Blood Pump flow rate.

Remember to account for ACD-A rate and CaCl₂ infusion rate in Patient Removal rate if given by separate IV pump.

8. Increase UFR mL for mL during administration of the following blood products:
☐ PRBC   ☐ FFP   ☐ Albumin   ☐ Platelets

9. Call Renal Service to adjust UFR, if patient has other new peripheral or central IV fluids added or an increase or decrease in existing IV fluid rates of more than 10 mL/hr.

Figure 3.46 – page 1 of 2. Pediatric CRRT orders with regional citrate anticoagulation. Designed for use on the Prisma or Prismaflex.

Courtesy of Helen Currier, Texas Children's Hospital, Houston, Texas. Used with permission.

Florida), that is, the introducer for a pulmonary artery catheter, e.g., Swan-Ganz, will support the extracorporeal flow, if the MAP is maintained continuously at greater than 70 mm Hg.
(3) The ECMO circuit can have a hemofilter or hemodialyzer added to it to provide SCUF, CAVH, CAVHD, or CAVHDF.
b. For SLEDD, CVVH, CVVHD, or CVVHDF, a standard dual or triple lumen hemodialysis

catheter is placed in an internal jugular, femoral, or subclavian vein.
(1) Internal jugular and subclavian catheters must have placement confirmed by x-ray.
(2) Femoral catheters require assessing the limb for signs of compromised blood flow each shift. The leg with the catheter in the femoral vein should remain relatively still which can be challenging for pediatric patients.

DIALYSIS FLUID (DIALYSATE)
10.   Normocarb® 240 mL in 3 L of sterile water (final volume 3.24 L)
          Other additives:
          • Potassium chloride _____ mEq/L (max conc: 4 mEq/L)
          • Potassium phosphate _____ mmol/L (2-3 mmol phos/L) (Each mmol Kphos =1.4 mmol K and 2 mmol phos)
          • Dextrose   □ None   □ 6 mL $D_{50}W$ (~90 mg/dl)   □ 12 mL $D_{50}W$ (~ 180mg/dl)
          • Other: _____

11.   Set Initial Dialysate flow rate (Qd) at _____mL/hr (2000 mL/$1.73M^2$/hr)

CITRATE REGIONAL ANTICOAGULATION
Baseline Monitoring
12.   Prior to initial set-up, check Chem-7, ionized calcium, total calcium, phosphorus, magnesium, total serum protein, glucose, CBC with diff & platelets, serum HbSAg and HbSAb if not already done.

Initial Citrate anticoagulation
13.   Order from pharmacy: □ ACD-A 1000 ml   □ 8000 mg calcium chloride in 1000 ml NS
14.   Start IV ACD-A at _____ mL/hr (rate=1.5min/hr X Qb) into arterial limb of CRRT circuit
15.   Infuse IV calcium chloride 8000 mg/L NS in □ central line other than CRRT circuit or □ pigtail of triple lumen access or □ venous limb of catheter via stopcock. Run at _____ mL/hr (rate = 0.4 min/hr X Qb)

Citrate anticoagulation monitoring and adjustments
Optimal range: CRRT circuit ionized calcium (0.2-0.4 mmol/L); patient ionized calcium (1.1-1.3 mmol/L)
16.   Check the CRRT circuit ionized calcium (draw from venous port) and patient's ionized calcium and total calcium (draw from site other than CRRT circuit) 10 minutes after initiation of therapy, then again 2 hours after initiation of therapy and every 6 hours thereafter (10 AM, 2PM, 10 PM, 2 AM).

17.   Re-check CRRT circuit ionized calcium and patient's ionized calcium 1 hour after any change in anticoagulation orders.

PROBLEMS/TROUBLE SHOOTING
18.   Notify Renal Service for
          • Patient ionized calcium less than 1.0 mmol/L or greater than 1.5 mmol/L
          • Circuit ionized calcium less than 0.2 mmol/L or greater than 0.4 mmol/L
          • Patient's total calcium less than _____ or greater than _____
          • Hourly UFR greater or less than_____ mL for 2 hours (+/- 30 mL per hour from prescribed UFR)
          • Access pressure less than   _____ (Default @ -250 mmHg)
          • Filter pressure greater than   _____ (Default @ 300 mmHg)
          • Return pressure greater than   _____ (Default @ 350 mmHg)
          • Patient BP less than _____/_____ or greater than _____/_____

19.   Notify the Renal Dialysis Nurse if the CRRT circuit clots.

Noted by:_____ RN (Renal Dialysis nurse) Noted by:_____ RN (ICU nurse)

_____ MD   Pager #_____

Format update November18, 2005

Figure 3.46 – page 2 of 2. Pediatric CRRT orders with regional citrate anticoagulation. Designed for use on the Prisma or Prismaflex.

Courtesy of Helen Currier, Texas Children's Hospital, Houston, Texas. Used with permission.

c. For neonates, the umbilical artery or umbilical vein is an alternative choice for vascular access.
d. For pediatric patients, smaller indwelling catheters are available, such as, 4 or 5 fr single lumen, 7, 8, 9, or 11.5 fr double lumen, but the same arterial and/or venous sites should be used.
    (1) Cuffed catheters with softer material and better memory (resumes manufactured shape and preserves intra-lumenal space even after kinking) can be inserted and left untunneled for use during SLEDD/CRRT, resulting in more dependable blood flow rates over time.
    (2) Adequate blood flow rates in the pediatric catheters can be challenging to achieve. Catheters must be carefully

Date:_____ Patient Name:_____

List Modality on screen:_____ and modality prescribed for pt._____

Solute transport mechanism: Diffusion_____ Convection_____

Setting Flow Rates & Patient Removal rate:_____

Type of Dialysate:

PrismaSate:	**Type B:**	**Type C Citrate:**
Frangible broken	Calcium infusion Y / N	No Calcium in Dialysate or Replacement
Expiration Date & Time	Bicarb Sources	Low Na Dialysate
		Bicarb Sources

Dual Check of Solutions Documented on MAR: Y / N

Impact of Solutions on pt:

K_____   Ca_____   ICa_____   Post Filter ICa_____

pH_____   CO2_____   PO4_____   Mg_____

Table of Critical Lab Values & when to call the Nephrologist @ bedside: Y / N

Where & How to draw Post Filter Ionized Ca:_____No other labs drawn from system._____

How to hang 2 1L bags of replacement solution & use of blue line clamps when Δ bags:_____

What to do if you run out of replacement or dialysate solutions:_____
Anticoagulaton:
Systemic Anticoagulation: Heparin_____ Xigris_____ NS Flush_____

Regional Anticoagulation Citrate & How it works:_____ & Why we need Calcium:_____

I&O Sheet reviewed:

Citrate & Calcium included:_____   Finding Actual Fluid Removed on Tx History Screen:_____

Calculations reviewed:_____

Incorrect Weight Change Alarm and Alarm screen reviewed:_____

Effluent Bags: Date & Time: Y / N Δ q24hrs   Keep connections clean and capped_____

Catheter Issues: Are lines reversed Y / N Type of catheter: Temporary   Tunneled

How to reposition temporary catheters:_____   Site care of HD Catheters:_____

Machine & Emergency Procedures:
Emergency Rinseback:_____ NS for blood return with free flow IV tubing:_____

Blue line Clamps in room (2):_____ Diaphragm reposition procedure card on machine: Y / N

Prisma Status Lights Illuminated: Red_____   Yellow_____ Green_____

How to contact MD & Dialysis staff:_____   Gambro Help line # posted on machine:_____

_____   _____
Western Dialysis Staff Signature   Hospital Staff Signature

Figure 3.47. CRRT bedside inservice checklist. Designed for use with the Prisma.

Courtesy of Helen Williams, Western Nephrology Acute Dialysis, Denver, Colorado. Used with permission.

PROCEDURE: ☐ SCUF   ☐ CVVHD
            ☐ CVVH   ☐ CVVHDF

Western Acute Dialysis

CRRT Record

Primary Dx _____

Date: Date CRRT Initiated

PHYSICIAN CRRT ORDER   **ACCESS**

Hospital:

Filter ☐ M100

Patient Name: _____

	Prev	Time	Time
BP			
MAP			
HR			
TEMP			
WT			
Hgb/HcT	/	/	/
PLT			
PTT			
PT/INR	/	/	/
Na			
K			
Cl			
CO2			
BUN			
CR			
Glucose			
Mg			
Ionized Ca			
Serum Ca			
Lactate			

Blood Flow Rate _____   Type _____
Dialysate Flow Rate _____   Redness _____
Replacement Flow Rate _____   Edema _____
Heparin Bolus _____   Bruising _____
Continuous _____   Drainage _____
Citrate _____   Insertion Date _____
Calcium Chloride _____   Insert by _____
Net Fluid Removal _____   Dressing Changed: _____
Dialysate Solution _____   Date Setup due
Replacement Solution _____   to be Changed _____

MACHINE CHECKLIST

	Previous	Time	Time
Dr. Ordered Net Loss			
Access			
Filter			
Effluent			
Return			
Blood Flow Rate			
Dialysate Flow Rate			
Replacement Flow Rate			
Heparin			
Citrate			
Calcium			
Machine #			
Lot #			

Date Time Nursing Notes
_____

Setup _____   Technical Assist _____   Nursing Visit _____

Staff Signature _____   Physician Signature _____

Western Acute Dialysis CRRT Record   PATIENT LABEL

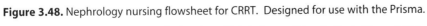

Figure 3.48. Nephrology nursing flowsheet for CRRT. Designed for use with the Prisma.

Courtesy of Helen Williams, Western Nephrology Acute Dialysis, Denver, Colorado. Used with permission.

ADDRESSOGRAPH

Citrate Kardex for CRRT

Diagnosis: _____   Allergies: _____
Recent Surgery: _____
CRRT Start Date: _____
Therapy Mode: _____   **CODE STATUS:** _____

CIRCUIT MANAGEMENT

Stop Citrate and Calcium drips if:
- **- filter clots / termination of therapy**
- **- machine alarms that stop the blood pump**
- **- during NS flush or returning blood for any reason**

Therapy Prescription:
Net Fluid Removal: _____
Replacement Solution: _____
_____
_____

Replacement Flowrate: _____ ml/hr
Dialysate Solution: _____
_____
_____
Dialysate Flow: _____ ml/hr
Blood Flow Rate: _____ ml/min
Lab draws from Circuit:
- During SCUF or CVVDH, draw labs from <u>any</u> red port.
- During CVVH or CVVHDF, draw labs from access red port.
- When anticoagulating, draw coags from blue port.
- When not anticoagulating, draw coags from access port.

Ca^{++} Labs 1° before initiation & q6hr thereafter:
- Prisma Post-Filter ionized Ca^{++} (blue sample port)
- Systemic ionized Ca^{++} (pt. (true) art. line or peripherally)
- Labs draws via central line, stop citrate/CaCl infusion x1min, waste 10ml prior to draw
- **ALL IONIZED Ca^{++} to RUN STAT IN LAB—results obtained within 15 min.**
- CBC
- CMP, Phos, Mg
- Miscellaneous: (check)
  - ☐ Liver panel @ initiation of Tx
  - ☐ Lactic acid @ initiation of Tx
  - ☐ ABG in AM
  - ☐ Heparin Induced Antibody PRN

Anticoagulation:
- ☐ 1L ACD(A) Citrate 2% rate @ _____ ml/hr via CRRT access blood line
- ☐ 1L D5W + 6 grams CaCl IV rate @ _____ ml/hr via central line

Citrate Titration Table

Prisma Post-Filter ionized Ca^{++} (mmol/L)	Citrate Infusion Adjustment
< 0.25	↓ Rate by 10 ml/hr
0.25 – 0.35 (optimal range)	NO ADJUSTMENT
0.36 – 0.45	↑ Rate by 10 ml/hr
> 0.45	↑ Rate by 20 ml/hr

Safety Parameters – **Notify Nephrologist** if the following occur:
1. Citrate Rate > 200 ml/hr
2. Replacement Rate > 1000 ml/hr
3. Systemic ionized Ca^{++} < 0.75 mmol/l (compare to total Ca^{++}). Consider holding citrate for 3 hours and resuming infusion at 150 ml/hr.
4. Serum Na+ > 150 mEq/L consider changing replacement solution to 0.45% NaCl.
5. Serum Bicarb is > 26 mEq/L

Calcium Titration Table

Systemic (Patient) ionized Ca^{++} (mmol/L)	Calcium Infusion Adjustment
> 1.3	↓ Rate by 10 ml/hr
1.1 – 1.3 (optimal range)	NO ADJUSTMENT
0.9 – 1.0	↑ Rate by 10 ml/hr
< 0.9	↑ Rate by 20 ml/hr

Vascular Access:
CXR Verified   Y or N
Access Physician: _____
Date: _____
Type: _____
Location: _____
Prep: _____
Dressing: _____

Dialysis Catheter Loads:
☐ Heparin 5,000 units/ml   ☐ Heparin 1,000 units/ml   ☐ 0.9% NS
☐ Citrate 2% ACA-A Sol.   ☐ Cathflo 2 mg/ml
Arterial/Red or Proximal Port _____ Volume ml
Blue/Venous or Distal Port _____ Volume ml

☐ Heparin 100 units/ml   ☐ 0.9% NS   ☐ Citrate 2% ACA-A Sol.
☐ Cathflo 2 mg/ml
INF/infusions/3rd Port _____ Volume ml

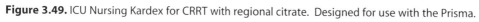

Figure 3.49. ICU Nursing Kardex for CRRT with regional citrate. Designed for use with the Prisma.

Courtesy of Jina Bogle, DCI Acute Program, Omaha, Nebraska. Used with permission.

Time	1900	2000	2100	2200	Total	2300	2400	0100	0200	Total	0300	0400	0500	0600		

24 Hour Flow Sheet for CRRT

Previous Wt. _____ Current Wt. _____ Today's Date _____ 12 HR 24 HR

A. Intake
 IV's (CITRATE AND CALCIUM MUST BE INCLUDED)
 Saline Flush
 Extended Bolus Amt.
 Other — Total Intake (A)
 Total intake
B. Output
 Urine
 Other
 Gastric — Total Output (B)
 Total Output
C. Intake minus output
D. Dr. ordered fluid removal
E. Line C + D = E (Removal goal)
F. Adjust from previous hour (difference from machine)
 If too much removed, subtract from goal
 If too little removed, add to goal
G. Machine set to remove this hour
H. Actual fluid removed (from machine)
Difference between (G-H)   4 hr   4 hr   4 hr
I. Net Fluid Removal (H-C)
J. Flow Rates
 Blood
 Dialysate
 Replacement
K. Pressures
 Access
 Filter
 Effluent
 Return
 TMPa
 △ P Filter
L. Anticoagulant
 Heparin continuous
 Heparin bolus
 Citrate infusion rate
 CaCl₂ infusion rate

Figure 3.50. ICU nursing flowsheet for CRRT. Designed for use with the Prisma.

Courtesy of Western Nephrology Acute Dialysis, Denver, Colorado. Used with permission.

placed to achieve desired blood flow so as not to limit the effectiveness of the treatment. Access difficulties should be corrected immediately.
(3) Blood flow rates should be ≥ 50 mL/min for systemic heparinization and ≥ 20 mL/min when using regional citrate anticoagulation to minimize patient and system complications such as clotting from an elevated filtration fraction.
e. Good blood flow in a hemodialysis catheter is critical to a successful SLEDD/CRRT treatment.
(1) Blood flow in the catheter can be compromised because of poor location in the blood vessel or because of a kink in the catheter or bloodline.

(2) Frequent (more than three per hour) equipment alarms related to poor blood flow in the catheter results in blood stasis in the hemofilter or hemodialyzer, setting the environment up for a clotted SLEDD/CRRT system.
(3) If good blood flow cannot be maintained consistently, the catheter must be replaced to accomplish an effective SLEDD/CRRT treatment.
f. Recirculation. Blood that has just left the venous or return line is drawn back in for another pass through the filter instead of returning to the patient's systemic circulation.
(1) Some recirculation occurs with any hemodialysis catheter.

(2) When recirculation is ≥ 15%, the SLEDD/CRRT treatment effectiveness begins to be compromised.

(3) Recirculation should be checked when:

(a) The patient does not achieve the expected change in solutes related to the SLEDD/CRRT treatment.

(b) The hemofilter or hemodialyzer clots easily (hemoconcentration of recirculated blood).

(4) Recirculation can be calculated using any freely diffusible small molecule such as BUN.

$$\text{Recirculation (\%)} = 100 \times \frac{(BUN_{peripheral} - BUN_{arterial})}{(BUN_{peripheral} - BUN_{venous})}$$

(5) If excessive recirculation is occurring, the catheter should be changed over a guide wire or placed in a new location depending on the reason for the increased recirculation.

g. Site care. The exit site and dressing should be kept clean, dry, and intact to minimize the chance of microorganisms entering the patient via this route.

(1) A sterile dressing change should be performed every other day for a standard occlusive gauze dressing and once every 7 days when using a chlorhexidine gluconate (CHG) sponge disc with a transparent semipermeable membrane occlusive dressing.

(2) The old dressing should be removed taking care not to tug at the exit site.

(3) The exit site should then be cleansed with alcohol or CHG.

(4) The catheter should be anchored with Steri-Strips and then covered with an occlusive dressing that can later be removed without tugging on the catheter exit site. (For more details, refer to Section 12: Vascular Access.)

h. The hemodialysis catheter should be accessed using aseptic technique to minimize the chance of microorganisms entering the patient via the lumen of the catheter. (For more details, refer to Section 12: Vascular Access.)

i. Infection. The patient with a hemodialysis catheter should be monitored for signs and symptoms of local and/or systemic infection.

j. Patients who have a fistula or synthetic graft must be constantly observed during treatment to decrease the risk of inadvertent needle dislodgement with potential patient exsanguination, or needle migration with hematoma formation. Arteriovenous

fistulas/grafts should be protected during the ICU stay, but should not be used for SLEDD/CRRT where the access is left unobserved for any substantial length of time.

2. Hemofilters, hemodialyzers, and blood tubing.

a. Membranes. Hollow fiber hemofilters and hemodialyzers are available in many different membranes including polysulfone, polyamide, polycarbonate, polyacrylonitrile (PAN), polymethylmethacrylate (PMMA), and polyaryl ether sulfone (PAES) and polyvinylpyrrolidonee (PVP), or a blending of these membranes.

(1) Nearly any hemofilter or hemodialyzer with a biocompatible membrane can be used.

(2) Synthetic membranes have increased biocompatibility and minimize patient complement activation. These membranes may decrease infection, morbidity, and mortality rates associated with AKI.

(3) Low-flux dialyzers and filters clear solutes ≤ 5000 daltons, while high-flux dialyzers and filters clear solutes ≤ 50,000 daltons. The size of the solute that needs to be cleared may impact the dialyzer or filter choice.

(4) Choosing a high-flux dialyzer assists in maximizing clearance. Hemofilters have essentially the same coefficient membrane properties as high-flux dialyzers, which explain their ability to achieve significant ultrafiltration and clearance.

(5) Some hemofilters are designed specifically for SLEDD/CRRT like the AV 400S, AV600S.

b. Volumes. Hemofilters and hemodialyzers range in volume from about 20 mL to 120 mL. Blood tubing ranges in volume from 20 mL to 140 mL.

(1) When providing SLEDD/CRRT to smaller patients, volume may be a concern.

(2) The smaller tubing sets sacrifice volume by reducing the lumen of the tubing and/or eliminating the arterial chamber. When no arterial chamber is present, AP monitoring should be accomplished by using two 24" pressure-tubing lines. The first one is filled with normal saline and attached to a 3-way stopcock on the saline line of the extracorporeal blood circuit. The second pressure tubing line is filled with air and connects the first pressure tubing line to a transducer

protector and then to the AP port on the Fresenius 2008K® hemodialysis system (see Figure 3.35).

  (3) Dialyzer and tubing combinations can be selected based on patient weight (see Figure 3.51).

c. Prisma® and Prismaflex® sets combine the hemofilter and blood tubing and are offered in a variety of sizes and filter types.

  (1) The AN69 membrane is available in the M60 and M100 sets for the Prisma® and Prismaflex®.

  (2) The PAES membrane is available for high volume therapies in the HF1000 on the Prisma® and in the HF1000 and HF1400 on the Prismaflex®.

  (3) The Prisma® M100 set has an extracorporeal volume of 110 mL ± 10 mL. Additionally there is the smaller M60 set, which can be used in patients ≤10 kg.

  (4) The blood tubing comes in a color-coded preconnected set, which can be directly mounted on the Prisma or Prismaflex, with automatic loading and priming capabilities.

  (5) The set has pressure pods built into the circuit that fit into a pressure sensor housing on the flow control unit.

  (6) The set includes the disposable pre-connected hemofilter and blood circuit, a prime collection bag, and an effluent bag.

d. Prime.

  (1) The SLEDD/CRRT circuit is usually flushed and primed with 1–2 liters of normal saline.

  (2) Sometimes 5000 units of heparin are added to the final liter of saline.

  (3) Flushing and priming the circuit removes the air, flushes out packing material, and may coat the membrane with heparin, if used.

e. Pediatric blood prime: When using a circuit volume that is ≥ 15% of the patient circulating blood volume, a blood prime should be considered.

  (1) For infants (0–12 months) circulating blood volume is about 80mL/kg, for a child (1–12 years) about 75 mL/kg, and for an adolescent (13–19 years) about 70 mL/kg.

  (2) The circuit is first flushed and primed with saline.

  (3) The volume of saline required for dilution of the mini (≤ 30 mL) packed red blood cells (PRBC) is calculated to achieve a HCT that matches the infants.

$$V_{saline} = \frac{V_{PRBC}\,(HCT_{PRBC} - HCT_{infant})}{HCT_{infant}}$$

  (4) Connect both the mini PRBC and a 50 mL bag of normal saline to a volutrol. Fill the volutrol with the entire volume of the mini PRBC and the calculated volume of saline (V_{saline}) in the volutrol. Gently agitate the PRBC and saline mix.

  (5) The mix is then primed into the SLEDD/CRRT circuit at a BFR of 20 mL/min.

  (6) Prior to starting the treatment, the circuit should be recirculated with a calcium containing dialysis solution for several minutes to remove some of the citrate that is present in PRBC. Infusing the fully citrated blood product directly into the patient can result in a rapid drop in patient ionized calcium.

  (7) Then the dialysis solution concentrate is changed to the ordered solution and a standard connection to the patient is performed.

  (8) The BFR is started at 10 mL/min and slowly increased to the prescribed BFR.

  (9) Typically when a blood prime is used for initiating the SLEDD/CRRT circuit, the blood is not returned upon discontinuation of the treatment.

3. Replacement solutions.

a. Normal saline. During SLEDD or CVVHDF normal saline, by itself or mixed with selected electrolytes, can be used as the replacement fluid. The dialysis solution is then used to keep the patient's electrolytes in the desired range, providing the DFR is ≥ 100 mL/min.

b. Custom pharmacy prepared replacement solutions.

  (1) Custom pharmacy prepared solutions are cost, time, and labor intensive for the pharmacy and have the inherent risk of being prepared with an unintended electrolyte composition.

  (2) At lower flow rates (1800 mL/hr or less) replacement solutions may be composed to correct electrolyte imbalances such as lowering the potassium content for a high serum potassium.

  (3) The more rapid the replacement solution flow, the more critical the electrolyte composition becomes as the patient's serum chemistry will more quickly begin to match the electrolyte composition of

Pediatric Hemodialysis Specification Sheet

-Volutrol on all IV's
-Crying may increase patient blood pressure even though patient is volume depleted

Dialyzer	Prime (ml)	Surface Area (m^2)
F3	28	0.4
F4	42	0.7
F5	63	1.0
F6	82	1.3
Polyflux 140 (high-flux)	94	1.4
F8	110	1.8

Blood Tubing	Prime (ml)	Pump Segment Diameter Set blood pump to coincide
Neonate (no arterial chamber)*	19 ml	2.6 mm
Husky Neonate (no arterial chamber)*	44 ml	4.8 mm
Pediatric	73 ml	6.35 mm
Adult	140 ml	8.0 mm

* When no arterial chamber is present, Arterial Pressure (AP) monitoring should be accomplished by using two 24" pressure-tubing lines. The first one is filled with normal saline and attached to a 3-way stopcock on the saline line of the blood tubing. The second pressure tubing line is filled with air and connects the first pressure tubing line to a transducer protector and then to the Arterial Pressure port on the Fresenius 2008K Hemodialysis System.

Suggested combinations based on Patient weight	Dialyzer	Tubing
Less than 13 kg	100 HG / F3	Neonate/Husky neonate
13kg-20 kg	F4 / F5	Husky neonate
20-40 kg	F6/Polyflux 140	Husky/Pediatric
Greater than 40 kg	F8/Polyflux 140	Pediatric/Adult

Blood Prime: Consider if the combined dialyzer / blood tubing volume is greater than **15%-20%** of the patient's total blood volume (TBV), i.e., patients less than 3 kg.

Estimate TBV using patient's weight.
Infant (0-1 year)   TBV = Weight x 80 ml/kg,
Child (1-12 years)   TBV = Weight x 75 ml/kg,
Adolescent (greater than 12 years)   TBV = Weight x 70 ml/kg.

Complete the Physician's Blood Order Form: 1. Select one Mini-Neonate type unit for anticipated blood loss. **2.**Select irradiated and CMV negative blood for infants less than 6mos. **3.**Indicate if patient is a transplant candidate and request *"Limited Donor Protocol"* blood in comments section for pediatric patients.

1. Fax both sides of this order form to Blood Bank at 734-8636
2. Prime the blood tubing circuit with normal saline.
3. Calculate $V_{saline} = \dfrac{V_{PRBC}\,(HCT_{PRBC} - HCT_{Infant})}{HCT_{Infant}} = \underline{\hspace{2cm}}$ **ml saline**
   Where V_{PRBC} is volume printed on PRBC unit and HCT_{PRBC} = 74%.
4. Obtain "Leukoreduced" labeled "Limited Donor Protocol" Mini-PRBC from blood bank.
5. Mix Mini-PRBC with V_{saline} using a 150 ml volutrol.
6. Prime the blood tubing at BFR of 20ml/min from the volutrol of PRBC and saline mix.
7. Recirculate the blood primed circuit for two minutes with a dialysis bath that contains 2.5 mEq/L Calcium.
8. Change dialysate bath to ordered solution and perform standard connection to the patient.

Nephrologist Signature / Print Name:	Date/Time:
Nephrology Nurse Signature / Print Name:	Date/Time:

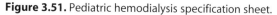

Figure 3.51. Pediatric hemodialysis specification sheet.

Courtesy of Lavjay Butani, Pediatric Nephrology, UC Davis Medical Center, Sacramento, California. Used with permission.

the replacement solution. Sodium, potassium, bicarbonate, chloride, magnesium, and phosphorus electrolyte content all need to be considered.

(4) Some electrolytes such as calcium and bicarbonate will precipitate at certain concentrations, so care needs to be taken when customizing a solution with a hospital pharmacy.

(5) The pharmacy can custom mix a solution to include 0.45% NaCl with 35 mEq NaCl, 35 mEq $NaHCO_3$, 3 mEq KCl, and 1.5 mEq $MgSO_4$. In a separate line infuse $CaCl_2$ 40 mEq in 125 mL D5W at 1% of the replacement fluid rate. This results in a replacement fluid that mimics the normal plasma water with the exception of phosphorus.

(6) Alternatively, the pharmacy can provide a combination of replacement solutions to be administered simultaneously when rates are greater than 1200 mL/hr or alternating between the two solutions using a Y-connector on the replacement infusion line for lower rates. Two solutions commonly used are:
   (a) 1 L 0.9 NaCl + 5 mL 10% $CaCl_2$
   (b) 1 L 0.45 NaCl + 75 mL 8.4% $NaHCO_3$

(7) Another custom formulation includes citrate in the replacement solution.
   (a) This solution provides adequate regional anticoagulation with a dilute concentration of citrate administered at a high rate with the prefilter tubing set.
   (b) Calcium is then infused through a separate central line.
   (c) When administering citrate in this fashion, a customized dialysate solution is also required. Since the citrate provides a bicarbonate source, the bicarbonate level in the dialysate must be decreased.
   (d) The benefit of this process is putting the citrate under the control of the Prisma® system so infusion will stop automatically when the blood pump has stopped.

c. Commercially available solutions.
   (1) Prismasol™ (Gambro, Stockholm, Sweden) is a commercially available sterile electrolyte replacement solution available in several different formulations to meet the needs of patients with a variety of electrolyte replacement needs on either heparin or citrate anticoagulation (see Table 3.38).
   (2) Normocarb HF™ (Dialysis Solutions INC., Richmond Hill, Ontario, Canada) is a commercially available sterile electrolyte concentrate. This 240 mL concentrate is available as NC 25 HF or NC 35 HF and must be diluted into 3 L of sterile water for injection to make 3.24 L of infusate solution. Normocarb HF™ is dextrose, calcium, and potassium-free (see Table 3.38 for the final electrolyte composition).

d. Replacement fluid can be put into the SLEDD/CRRT circuit either prefilter/predilution or postfilter/postdilution. Many arguments have been made supporting one over the other, but advocates of both still stand by the option they prefer.
   (1) Today's SLEDD/CRRT systems accommodate either option.
   (2) Adding replacement fluid into a SLEDD/CRRT circuit increases the volume of ultrafiltrate and thereby increases convective clearance.

4. Dialysis solutions.
   a. PrismaSate® (Gambro, Stockholm, Sweden).
      (1) PrismaSate® is available in a number of optional combinations of electrolytes and is bicarbonate buffered.
      (2) The 5-liter bag has two compartments: one for the electrolyte solution, the other for the buffer. The electrolyte solution must be mixed with the buffer prior to its use as a dialysis solution. This two-compartment system keeps the product stable for a reasonable shelf life, while providing bicarbonate as a buffer at the bedside.
      (3) When the bag is ready to be used, the frangible that is between the two compartments must be broken to allow the two solutions to mix.
      (4) Once the PrismaSate solution is mixed, it must be used within 24 hours.
   b. Normocarb HF™ can be diluted and used as a dialysis solution or as an electrolyte solution for infusion (see above for description).
   c. Pureflow™ (NxStage Medical, Inc., Lawrence, Massachusetts) and Accusol™ (Baxter, Deerfield, Illinois) are also commercially available dialysis solutions for CRRT equipment, and are bicarbonate buffered.

Table 3.38

Electrolyte Composition of Commercially Available Replacement Fluids

Replacement Solution	Normocarb 25 HF	Normocarb 35 HF	PrismaSol BK 0/3.5	PrimsaSol BGK 2/0	PrismaSol BGK 2/3.5	PrimaSol BGK 4/2.5	PrimaSol BGK 0/2.5
Sodium (mEq/L)	140	140	140	140	140	140	140
Potassium (mEq/L)	0	0	0	2	2	4	0
Chloride (mEq/L)	116.5	106.5	109.5	108	111.5	113	109
Bicarbonate (mEq/L)	25	35	32	32	32	32	32
Lactate (mEq/L)	0	0	3	3	3	3	3
Calcium (mEq/L)	0	0	3.5	0	3.5	2.5	2.5
Magnesium (mEq/L)	1.5	1.5	1	1	1	1.5	1.5
Phosphorus (mg/dL)	0	0	0	0	0	0	0
Dextrose (mg/dL)	0	0	0	100	100	100	100

Courtesy of Maureen Craig, UC Davis Medical Center, Sacramento, California. Used with permission.

d. Peritoneal dialysis solutions were used prior to the CRRT dialysis solutions becoming commercially available.
   (1) The disadvantages of peritoneal dialysis solution are the heavy concentrations of dextrose and lactate.
   (2) Peritoneal dialysis solution may not be well tolerated by some patients who either develop glucose intolerance or lactic acidosis secondary to their catabolic state and/or hepatic dysfunction.
   (3) Peritoneal dialysis solution should not be used on a CRRT treatment as it is an off-label use and complications may occur.
e. Custom pharmacy dialysis solutions:
   (1) The advantage of custom-made pharmacy solution is that solutions can be formulated with sodium, potassium, bicarbonate, calcium, and glucose concentrations that are prescribed to effectively meet the patient's specific metabolic needs.
   (2) The disadvantages are the considerable cost, time, and labor that these solutions may add to the procedure, and the inherent risk of being prepared with an unintended electrolyte composition.
f. Dialysis solution can also be prepared from

dialysate acid and bicarbonate concentrates and mixed with reverse osmosis water. This is the option used on the Fresenius 2008K® machine, the same as in IHD. This method produces a dialysis solution flow rate of 100-300 mL/min.
g. Phosphorus. During SLEDD/CRRT with higher clearance rates, phosphorus may need to be replaced to minimize removal of phosphorus from the patient.
   (1) When using the Prisma or any CRRT system, phosphorus can be replaced intravenously or added to the dialysis or replacement solutions.
   (2) When using the Fresenius type 34:1 proportioning dialysis solution delivery system, some units report adding 45 mL of oral Fleet, Phospha-soda, solution (CB Fleet Company, Lynchburg, Virginia) to the 9.45 L of dialysate bicarbonate concentrate solution to raise the phosphorus in the dialysis solution to 2.5 mg/dL (low physiologic). This will typically eliminate the need for further phosphorus replacement.
   (3) Proportionally more can be added to achieve a higher dialysis solution phosphorus if this is desired.
h. For patients less than 10 kg, the dialysis

solution may need to be warmed to 38° C to maintain the patient's temperature in the normal range. Alternatively, for dialysis solution flow rates of 100 mL/min, the heat loss to the environment can be reduced by insulating the dialysis tubing lines with foam insulation.

5. Anticoagulation.
   a. Regional citrate, heparin, and saline flushes were compared during CAVH treatments and noted that the extracorporeal system lasted longest with the regional citrate method followed by the heparin. Since the time of this study, variations to the delivery of CRRT treatments and the associated anticoagulation have occurred. These changes can result in the CRRT system lasting even longer than demonstrated in this article. Each form of anticoagulation has challenges and benefits that must be considered before applying them to the patient on a SLEDD/CRRT treatment.
   b. Regional citrate anticoagulation.
      (1) Anticoagulates the SLEDD/CRRT system and not the patient.
      (2) Citrate ideally should be infused as soon as the blood enters the SLEDD/CRRT circuit. When this set up is used, it is essential that whenever the blood pump stops, the IV infusion pump administering the citrate must also be stopped to prevent backflow, which would result in direct administration of citrate to the patient.
      (3) Citrate binds with calcium in the blood, interrupting the clotting cascade.
      (4) The calcium/citrate complexes are then removed by diffusing into the dialysate.
      (5) The effects of any complexes that are not removed are reversed in the patient by infusion of IV calcium either as calcium gluconate or calcium chloride in a central line.
      (6) This infusion also replaces the calcium lost from the patient in this process to prevent systemic hypocalcemia.
      (7) Citrate must not be infused directly into the right atrium, as this is associated with increased risk of cardiac arrhythmias.
      (8) Regional citrate anticoagulation is performed with a zero calcium dialysate on SLEDD, CVVHD, or CVVHDF.
         (a) The dialysate may need to be adjusted by reducing the sodium and bicarbonate content as citrate is delivered as sodium citrate and citrate is metabolized in the liver to bicarbonate.
         (b) The patient should periodically be monitored for hypernatremia and metabolic alkalosis.
      (9) BFR, DFR, IV citrate, and IV calcium must be initiated and terminated together to avoid undesired changes in the patient's serum chemistry.
      (10) Citrate is commercially available as anticoagulant citrate dextrose solution formula A (ACD-A) in 500 mL or 1000 mL bags. ACD-A is approximately a 3% citrate solution containing both sodium citrate and citric acid.
         (a) The ACD-A solution is infused at approximately 2–2.5% of the BFR, with a DFR of 100–200 mL/min.
         (b) The ACD-A solution rate must be adjusted when the BFR or DFR changes.
      (11) Citrate is also available in a 4% tri-sodium citrate solution from Baxter.
      (12) The system ionized calcium, measured postfilter, should be targeted to 0.25–0.5 mmol/L (1–2 mg/dL). The patient's ionized calcium should remain near normal.
         (a) The lower the system ionized calcium is targeted, the more calcium is required to normalize the patient's ionized calcium.
         (b) If both the citrate and calcium rates are being titrated in the same direction the provider should accept a higher ionized calcium in the system.
      (13) Alternatively a citrate solution can be custom made by the pharmacy, but this increases the time it takes to get the product, the expense, and the chance the product will not be made as intended.
      (14) During regional citrate anticoagulation, the patient and system-ionized calcium must be closely monitored and carefully differentiated. The citrate and calcium solutions are then titrated to achieve and maintain the desired ionized calcium range. Ionized calciums are monitored every 30 to 60 minutes after a change in BFR, DFR, ACD-A, or calcium infusion rate until the patient and system ionized calcium are in the prescribed range. Monitoring continues every 2–6 hours and whenever there is a concern that the patient is hypocalcemic.

(15) The nurse caring for the patient receiving regional citrate anticoagulation must monitor the patient for signs and symptoms of hypocalcaemia. Hypocalcemia symptoms include circumoral tingling, muscle cramps, tetany, seizures, positive Chvostek's or Trousseau's sign, prolonged QT interval, decreased heart rate, cardiac arrhythmias, and hypotension related to vasodilatation.

(16) Most blood gas or STAT labs will provide an ionized calcium result in 15–30 minutes. The quick ionized calcium results aid in titrating the citrate and calcium solutions into the safe and effective range.

(17) The patient on regional citrate anticoagulation can become alkalemic as citrate from the citrate/calcium complexes returned to the patient metabolizes to bicarbonate. The dialysis solution bicarbonate should be lowered to physiologic concentrations and the flow rate increased to correct this state.

c. Heparin.
(1) Heparin is a standard anticoagulant for SLEDD/CRRT. When using heparin as an anticoagulant, it is critical to heparinize the patient with a bolus (10–30 units/kg) five minutes prior to connection to the SLEDD/CRRT system.

(2) The patient's partial thromboplastin time (PTT) will rise during those 5 minutes minimizing clotting on the first few passes of blood through the circuit.

(3) PTT should be drawn immediately upon starting SLEDD/CRRT to determine if the patient is in the desired range (45–65 seconds or based on unit protocol).
   (a) PTT is the preferred form of monitoring heparin anticoagulation, as activated clotting time (ACT) monitoring is not reliable in this lower target range of heparin therapy. Point of care testing will result in the fastest results, but if those are unavailable, send the sample to the laboratory.
   (b) Smaller repeat boluses may be necessary to bring the PTT values into range.
   (c) A heparin infusion (10–25 units/kg/hr) should be given to maintain the patient in the desired PTT range.
   (d) The PTT should be rechecked after each bolus, 4 hours after any heparin dosing change, and immediately after blood product administration.

(4) Heparin is highly protein bound therefore it is not readily removed during SLEDD/CRRT.

(5) A heparin syringe pump typically delivers small amounts of very concentrated heparin (1:1000) Alternatively, heparin can be diluted and infused in a separate line to improve consistent delivery of the desired dose. Examples include 5,000, 10,000, or 20,000 units of heparin in 1000 mL normal saline.

(6) Patients with heparin-induced thrombocytopenia (HIT) cannot be exposed to heparin because of the danger of white clot syndrome which results in a drop in the patient's platelet count and potentially lethal clots. Alternative forms of anticoagulation must be sought for these patients.

d. Citrasate™ (Advanced Renal Technologies, Seattle, Washington). Citrasate is a citric acid containing dialysis solution concentrate that may be used for SLEDD treatments. Citrasate is more effective than normal saline flushes as an anticoagulant and does not adversely affect patient serum calcium levels.

e. Saline flushes.
(1) SLEDD/CRRT can be managed with 25–200 mL normal saline flush every 30 minutes to 1 hour, especially in patients who may be auto-anticoagulated with low platelet counts.

(2) The flush volume needs to be calculated into the volume to be removed from the patient.

(3) Adding a predilution solution and/or increasing the BFR may decrease the need for anticoagulation as well, but flushing accomplishes a better anticoagulation result than predilution of the same volume of saline.

(4) Regional citrate anticoagulation is the most effective at preserving filter life, followed by heparin and then normal saline flushes.

f. Other anticoagulants.
(1) Alternative anticoagulating agents are available like warfarin, argatroban, bivaliruden, r-Hirudin, lepirudin, and fondaparinux.

(2) These forms of anticoagulation are not likely to be used to manage SLEDD/ CRRT. However a patient receiving one of these less common anticoagulants could require SLEDD/CRRT. When this occurs, the anticoagulation for SLEDD/ CRRT needs to be adjusted to accommodate any additive influences from the other anticoagulants.

6. Supply basket.
   a. A supply basket should be left at bedside for the nurse to use.
   b. This should contain items that may be needed during the SLEDD/CRRT but are not on the ICU supply cart or must be close at hand.
   c. The supply basket can contain a separate container identified for system discontinuation to assist the nurse in having all the items needed for the end of the treatment in one place.
   d. The system support kit may include an extra cartridge or hemofilter/ hemodialyzer and blood line tubing, IV tubing, extra normal saline, Y-connectors, 3 mL, 10 mL, and 20 mL syringes, arterial blood gas (ABG) syringes, needle-less needles, standard needles, alcohol, betadine, and CHG pads, plastic hemostats, extra tape, 2x2 gauze sponges, transparent dressings, biodisc, hemasticks, recirculation tubes, eye protection wear, and transducer protectors.
   e. The discontinuation kit may include: normal saline, IV tubing, female-female IV adaptor, sterile drape, sterile gloves, alcohol pads, catheter caps, 3 mL and 10 mL syringes, and a catheter lock solution.

VI. Nursing care interventions for SLEDD/CRRT.

A. Standards of nursing care.
   1. SLEDD standards.
      a. SLEDD treatments are currently delivered by a number of medical centers across the United States and around the world. These treatments are similar in their delivery of solute clearance and ultrafiltration as outlined earlier. However, the nursing care interventions for SLEDD treatments are still being standardized.
         (1) The description of the nursing care for SLEDD in the following section focuses on the practice standards of a university medical center with a 10-year experience with SLEDD.

(2) As SLEDD therapy evolves further, additional acceptable variations will undoubtedly be expressed in the literature.
   2. CRRT guidelines.
      a. CRRT has existed in various forms for nearly 40 years. In 1993, the American Nephrology Nurses' Association (ANNA) established and published Nephrology Nursing Guidelines for Care: CRRT.
         (1) These guidelines are endorsed by American Association of Critical Care Nurses (AACN) and have recently been updated.
         (2) These guidelines are a reference for all nephrology and ICU nurses looking for guidance in providing care for patients on CRRT.

B. Nephrology and ICU collaboration. Nursing care for the patient on a SLEDD/CRRT is delivered differently in different settings.
   1. Nursing care for patients on SLEDD treatments requires the collaboration of the nephrology and ICU nurses.
      a. The nephrology nurse provides more of the care and documentation.
      b. The nephrology nurse provides a bedside inservice and physically is away from the bedside of the ICU patient between the 30–60 minute checks.
      c. The ICU nurse responds to the patient's needs as indicated in the bedside inservice and has the nephrology nurse available by pager for phone or bedside response within five minutes (see Figure 3.40).
      d. By design, SLEDD is intended to deliver a dose of therapy very similar to CRRT but to have the advantage of providing a period of time in which the patient is off treatment so that other interventions can occur.
      e. The treatment, as stated earlier, is a modification of IHD by extending the time and slowing the maximum rate that solute clearance and UF occur. This makes the SLEDD treatment reasonably familiar to most nephrology nurses because of its similarity to IHD.
      f. Ongoing communication between the nephrology and ICU nurses is a critical element to an effective and safe SLEDD treatment.
   2. Nursing care provided to the patient on CRRT may be predominately nephrology or ICU driven.
      a. Collaboration between the nephrology and

ICU disciplines leads to the best opportunities, care, and outcome for the patient.

b. For those facilities that do not have nephrology nursing backup, the ICU nurses deliver the CRRT treatment. Ideally these nurses are trained and supported by a clinical nurse specialist (CNS) or advanced practice nurse (APN) with a strong nephrology background.

c. The nephrologists, intensivists, nephrology nurses, and ICU nurses must all work together to meet the needs of the patient on CRRT.

d. The input from a pharmacist and nutritionist should not be undervalued in optimizing the delivery of care to the patient on CRRT (see Figure 3.52).

C. Education.
1. SLEDD training. A successful SLEDD program also must have an ongoing educational component to maintain competency of all the nurses providing the treatment.
   a. The acute care nephrology nurse will be able to learn this treatment option and provide this therapy with either a 1–2-hour SLEDD class or the eight-hour CRRT class (if the same equipment is used) followed by a mentored SLEDD treatment due to its similarity with the IHD treatments they do every day.
   b. The ICU nurse will be able to care for a patient on SLEDD with a SLEDD bedside inservice (Figure 3.40).
2. CRRT training: A successful CRRT program must have an ongoing educational component to establish and maintain competency of all the nurses providing the treatment. CRRT should only be performed by an ICU and nephrology nurse who have taken and passed the eight-hour CRRT class.
   a. When a CRRT treatment is ordered, the CRRT treatment is initiated by the nephrology nurse, and a bedside inservice is provided to the ICU nurse (Figure 3.41) emphasizing most common alarm conditions and providing a refresher of the content of the class the ICU nurse has taken earlier.
   b. ICU and nephrology nurses who have had the 8-hour CRRT class, but not yet cared directly for a patient on the therapy, should be mentored by an experienced nurse providing backup for their first patient care assignment.

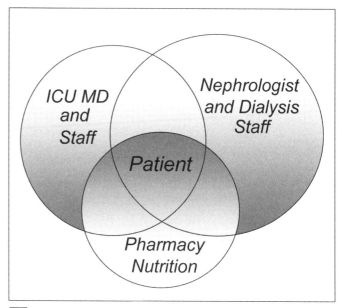

Figure 3.52. Models of collaboration for CRRT

Courtesy of Maureen Craig, UC Davis Medical Center, Sacramento, California.

3. SLEDD theory. The SLEDD class/inservice should include theoretical content that includes the definition of SLEDD and how it accomplishes solute clearance and ultrafiltration for the ICU patient. For the nephrology nurse, emphasis should focus on both the similarities and differences between SLEDD and IHD.
4. CRRT theory. A CRRT class should have theoretical content that covers the definitions of CRRT and related concepts, indications for CRRT, and benefits and challenges of CRRT.
5. SLEDD equipment. Typically the equipment used to perform SLEDD is the same equipment the nephrology nurse uses to perform IHD so the SLEDD class/inservice should emphasize the importance of not exceeding the prescribed maximum BFR, DFR, and UFR.
   a. Slowing the dialysis therapy, as is done during SLEDD, minimizes hemodynamic instability and reduces alarm conditions allowing the nephrology nurse to walk away from the bedside after inservicing the ICU nurse.
   b. The ICU nurse must understand the SLEDD treatment and the equipment used to adequately:
      (1) Respond to the patient's hypotension, arterial, and venous pressure alarms.
      (2) Titrate anticoagulation.
      (3) Assess system clotting.

(4) Return the patient's blood using normal saline.

c. The ICU nurse's response to other less common alarms or concerns should be to page the nephrology nurse and troubleshoot the situation together (Figure 3.41).

6. CRRT equipment. The CRRT equipment to be used should be reviewed and demonstrated in the 8-hour CRRT class along with related system components such as vascular access, hemofilters, or hemodialyzers, replacement solutions, dialysis solutions, and anticoagulation.

   a. The equipment review should emphasize the most frequently asked questions and most common alarm conditions, so the learner is not overwhelmed with memorizing detail that they may never need, while forgetting the critical points.

   b. References and personnel resources should be identified for more uncommon alarm conditions or concerns and a standard approach sought.

   c. Each class participant should have hands-on time with a system setup as close to a patient scenario as possible (use a catheter in a fluid bag for a patient to establish +/- pressures). This helps develop some familiarity with interacting with the CRRT equipment and serves to decrease anxiety as understanding occurs.

   d. The equipment time should include a review of the bedside inservice checklist (Figure 3.41) with an opportunity for the learner to initiate and resolve alarm conditions.

7. SLEDD documentation. The nephrology nurse provides most of the documentation for the patient on SLEDD.

   a. The documentation is very similar to that associated with an IHD treatment and should occur every 30–60 minutes with both patient and system assessments.

   b. The nephrology nurse is best trained on the few changes to documentation during the mentored SLEDD treatment.

   c. The ICU staff will document that the SLEDD treatment was initiated/terminated and the volume changes that occurred during the treatment, similar to the way they might document following an IHD treatment.

   d. Additionally, during treatment the ICU nurse may document alarm conditions and the action taken.

8. CRRT documentation. Documentation for the patient on CRRT must be taught to both the

nephrology and the ICU nurse.

   a. Documentation examples and scenarios improve effective and accurate documentation. Ideally, two shifts of a patient scenario should be documented during the eight-hour CRRT class to show how I/O are totaled and documented at change of shift.

   b. Elements of adjusting the UFR or PFR in response to changes in patient I/O or condition should be emphasized.

   c. Examples of resolving patient/system condition changes, such as hypotension and equipment alarms, should be included.

   d. Documentation should be developed emphasizing the principle of simplicity.

      (1) When introducing new documentation there is a tendency to "double document" to "just make sure."

      (2) Each entry and calculation is a chance for an error because humans are performing this task.

      (3) Increasing the number of entries or calculations increases the likelihood of errors.

      (4) A simple method of documentation that minimizes calculations is best, and likely to be implemented by more staff successfully.

      (5) The area of documentation of fluid balance and I/O during CRRT is especially challenging for the beginner.

         (a) The best way to keep the patient safe is to keep the nurse's eyes on the patient and the patient's parameters as the patient responds to treatment.

         (b) This does not happen when the nurse is spending > 50% of nursing care time documenting.

         (c) Correlating the documentation to the order in which tasks are performed and to the principles taught in the training program will faciliate learning, accuracy, and efficiency.

      (6) The documentation the ICU nurse is to complete should be blended with the existing ICU documentation if possible, e.g., pressures with pressures, labs with labs, intake with intake, and output with output. This can be done by revising the ICU flowsheet or the electronic medical record (EMR).

9. SLEDD bedside inservice. SLEDD treatments must also include a bedside inservice.

   a. The entire treatment can occur during one

ICU nursing shift, so frequently the bedside inservice is only provided at the beginning of the SLEDD treatment.

b. The SLEDD bedside inservice should include the reason for treatment, how to respond to and care for the patient, and the SLEDD system.

c. Emphasis should be placed on how to respond to the essential elements of a SLEDD treatment.
  (1) Hypotension.
  (2) Arterial or venous pressure alarms.
  (3) Titratation of anticoagulation.
  (4) Assess system clotting.
  (5) How to return the patient's blood using normal saline.
  (6) When and how to contact the nephrology nurse.

10. CRRT bedside inservice: The importance of the bedside inservice for CRRT cannot be overemphasized.

a. Several months may have passed since the ICU nurse has taken the CRRT class or since he/she has managed a CRRT treatment.

b. The bedside inservice is provided just-in-time (JIT) and includes:
  (1) A refresher of all the major points of the CRRT class.
  (2) Reason for treatment.
  (3) How treatment is to be accomplished.
  (4) How to respond to and care for the patient and CRRT system in a particular time frame.
  (5) How to document the care provided.
  (6) When and how to contact the nephrology nurse.

c. A bedside inservice checklist is a critical tool for both the nephrology and ICU nurse to make certain the inservice is as comprehensive as the ICU nurse desires.

d. The bedside inservice is best provided by the nephrology nurse who will be covering the CRRT call over the next shift.

e. The inservice can last up to 1 hour depending on the educational needs of the ICU nurse.

f. The bedside inservice must be repeated by the nephrology nurse near the beginning of each shift and can be coordinated with the time the nephrology nurse comes to do a patient/system assessment and to refill solutions and supplies needed for the CRRT treatment.

11. Competency.

a. If a nurse's exposure to the SLEDD/CRRT equipment and therapy is less than once every 6 months, add a competency program with equipment demonstration lab to be reviewed every 6 months.

b. A competency assessment should contain an examination and a demonstration checklist on equipment and documentation similar to the SLEDD/CRRT bedside inservice.

c. Maintaining the nephrology and ICU nurse competency without performing treatments is challenging, time consuming, and costly.

d. Every effort should be made when planning a SLEDD/CRRT program that once the initial training has occurred, treatments should be routinely ordered and supported by all the nephrology and ICU physicians, nurses, and administration. (See VII: Program selection and development for SLEDD/CRRT in various ICU environments.)

e. Initially, challenging experiences should be buffered by the fact that repetition smoothes and improves the road of experience. Do not stall a new program with the "paralysis of analysis."

12. Keep It Super Simple (KISS) principle: The reality of patient care is it is frequently fraught with complexities. Some of them are innate and others self-imposed, based on the knowledge of the importance of patient care outcomes.

a. SLEDD/CRRT are no exception and although they are relatively complex, the KISS principle is a great reminder to not make it more complex than it must be.

b. Developing a SLEDD/CRRT workgroup with the KISS principle focus can move a program forward, by addressing concerns, solving problems, and creating innovative solutions all in the spirit of simplicity like that intended by the original guru of CRRT, Peter Kramer.

D. Treatment overview.

1. SLEDD.

a. When a SLEDD treatment is ordered by the nephrologist, a nephrology nurse will set up the SLEDD system, assess the patient, initiate therapy, and document this care.

b. The nephrology nurse will then provide the SLEDD bedside inservice to the ICU nurse.

c. The nephrology nurse will return every 30–60 minutes to assess the patient and system and document the progress of the SLEDD treatment.

d. The nephrology nurse is available by pager for an immediate telephone response and/or a 5-minute bedside response time.

e. The nephrology nurse terminates the SLEDD treatment and completes his/her documentation.

f. Last, the nephrology nurse reports the final patient assessment and UF volume to the ICU nurse.

2. CRRT.

a. When a CRRT treatment is ordered by a nephrology physician, a nephrology nurse will set up the CRRT system and initiate therapy in collaboration with the ICU nurse.

b. The nephrology and ICU charge nurses should both be made aware of the pending treatment as soon as possible to take into consideration the staffing that the CRRT treatment may require.

c. Some facilities practice a 1:1 nurse to patient ratio when a patient is on CRRT.

(1) This planned 1:1 ratio is preferred especially in new and growing programs where the group's expertise is still emerging and several nurses may be involved to assist with the treatment or to learn from the more experienced nurses caring for the patient.

(2) As the group's expertise grows and the CRRT program becomes simpler and more systematic, the ICU charge nurse will make staffing assignments based on the overall level of care the patient will require and the application of CRRT to the patient's treatment plan will be one of, but not the only consideration.

d. The nephrology nurse is responsible for providing a bedside inservice and some system monitoring at the beginning of every shift or treatment.

e. The nephrology nurse will change the CRRT circuit as needed and is always available by phone to assist with system troubleshooting.

f. The ICU nurse is responsible for ongoing patient monitoring, CRRT system maintenance, treatment termination if emergently indicated and documentation of all assessments and care provided.

E. Initiation of SLEDD/CRRT treatment.

1. Nephrology nurse.

a. Notify ICU nurse of treatment orders and time treatment to be initiated; indicate supplies, medications, and equipment needed; verify consent is on chart.

b. Set up SLEDD/CRRT equipment, complete equipment calibration and safety checks, test

system alarms. All equipment related to the treatment should be kept on one stand or machine if possible. This setup prevents inadvertently leaving an IV infusion, e.g., calcium or heparin, related to SLEDD/CRRT behind upon treatment termination.

c. Prime blood pathway with normal saline or if indicated heparinized saline (5,000 units/L). Make certain to flush heparin from system with saline after recirculation time.

d. Prime, label, and connect calcium, citrate, and/or heparin IV lines to SLEDD/CRRT circuit or patient as ordered.

e. Ensure a supply of replacement solutions, dialysis solutions, calcium, citrate, and/or heparin is available to last until the next scheduled check (30–60 minutes SLEDD or 12–14 hours CRRT).

f. Assess patient, catheter and system; review medications; document assessment and care on nephrology nursing progress record.

g. Cleanse both dialysis ports of catheter. Using a syringe, aspirate two times the catheter fill volume of blood from each lumen of the dialysis ports of the catheter. Administer heparin load followed by saline flush as ordered. Wait 5 minutes.

h. Attach and secure the ends of the extracorporeal blood circuit to the patient's dialysis catheter. Initiate treatment per physician order.

i. Review care of patient on SLEDD/CRRT and documentation with ICU nurse using the bedside inservice checklist as a guide.

j. Monitor patient for a minimum of 15 minutes before leaving bedside.

k. Document treatment initiation and patient care on nephrology nursing progress record.

2. ICU nurse.

a. Draw baseline labs. Alternatively, the nephrology nurse can draw these labs from the dialysis catheter at the start of CRRT if no tests are ordered that will be impacted by the anticoagulant fill in the catheter such as PTT.

b. Verify that a dialysis catheter has been inserted in the patient and placement verified by x-ray for subclavian or internal jugular placement. For a femoral line placement, check the cannulated limb for circulation, including pedal pulses.

c. Assess and document treatment initiation, patient's fluid and electrolyte balance, vital signs (VS), weight, BP, edema, lab values, lung and heart sounds and overall condition.

d. Keep a 500 mL normal saline flush bag with gravity tubing for emergency termination at the bedside.

e. Receive inservice from nephrology nurse.

F. Maintenance of SLEDD treatment.
1. Nephrology nurse.
a. Every 30–60 minutes assess patient, catheter, and system.
b. Maintain MAP > 60 mm Hg.
c. Document assessment and care on nephrology nursing progress record.
d. Provide and document patient and family education and support.
2. ICU nurse.
a. Monitor patient, catheter, and SLEDD system.
b. Document any system alarms and the resolution of those alarm conditions.
c. Perform routine ICU patient assessment and document on ICU nursing flowsheet.
d. Provide and document patient and family education and support.

G. Maintenance of CRRT treatment.
1. Nephrology nurse.
a. Near the beginning of every ICU nursing shift (every 12 hours) and as needed (PRN), the nephrology nurse should do a bedside patient and system check followed by an inservice for the bedside nurse. In some facilities this timing is not possible, and a remote inservice between the ICU nurse and the nephrology nurse on-call occurs. The nephrology nurse must make this check at least once per day, and ideally once per shift to improve the consistency of delivery of CRRT to the patient.
(1) Assess patient, catheter, and system; review medications; document assessment and care on nephrology nursing progress record using a new note each day.
(2) Note CRRT order changes. Refill supply basket, dialysate, replacement fluid, saline and heparin as needed.
(3) Verify calcium, citrate, or heparin pumps are operating as expected.
(4) Verify the air detector line is engaged, if appropriate for the equipment you are using.
(5) Review care of patient on CRRT and flowsheet documentation with the ICU nurse.

(6) Provide and document patient and family education and support.
b. Every 2–3 days.
(1) Change CRRT filter and blood tubing.
(2) Clean and disinfect the CRRT machine prior to reinitiation of treatment (per manufacturer recommendations).
c. Every 2 days to 1 week.
(1) Change dialysis catheter dressing every 7 days if using a chlorhexidine gluconate (CHG) sponge disc with antimicrobial activity and a transparent semipermeable membrane (TSM) occlusive dressing.
(2) Other dialysis catheter dressings should be changed every other day.
2. ICU nurse.
a. Every 1–2 hours and PRN:
(1) Assess patient, catheter, and system. Monitor system for any changes or alarm conditions. Maintain MAP $\geq$ 60 mm Hg.
(2) Document VS, BFR, I/O, equipment alarms, resolution of alarms, equipment pressures and rates.
(3) Assess patient and laboratory findings, e.g., hypocalcemia. Titrate and document calcium and citrate or heparin infusions.
(4) Prisma.
(a) Clear all IV fluid pumps every hour.
(b) Determine and document patient's hourly I/O.
(c) Calculate hourly fluid removal goal, and set that target on the appropriate screen.
b. Every shift and PRN.
(1) Clear all pumps.
(2) Determine and document patient I/O for shift.
(3) Review and note changes of CRRT orders as applicable.
(4) Assess and document patient's fluid balance and overall condition. Consider weight, pulmonary artery wedge pressure (PAWP), VS, edema, laboratory values, heart and lung sounds.
c. PRN.
(1) To prevent system clotting or patient bleeding, titrate anticoagulants based on patient and system laboratory findings.
(2) Change catheter dressing if dressing is not clean, dry, and intact.
(3) Provide and document patient and family education and support, e.g., SLEDD/CRRT acts as a filter to clean the patient's blood, removing fluid and waste.

H. Termination of SLEDD treatment.
1. Nephrology nurse.
   a. Return blood to patient with normal saline flush.
   b. For regional citrate anticoagulation, stop citrate and calcium infusions simultaneously.
   c. Check patient ionized calcium value 20–30 minutes after SLEDD termination.
   d. Provide catheter care with normal saline flush and anticoagulant fill. Label dressing with date, initials, solution, solution concentration and volume used for catheter fill, e.g., heparin 5000 units/mL, arterial 1.8 mL, venous 1.9 mL or 3% citrate, arterial 1.8 mL, venous 1.9 mL.
   e. Change catheter dressing if dressing is not clean, dry, and intact. Document condition of exit site on treatment record.
   f. Remove and dispose of tubing using standard precautions. Disinfect equipment and return to appropriate storage area.
   g. Assess patient and document care provided and termination of treatment.
2. ICU nurse should assess and document patient condition, fluid removed, and termination of treatment.

I. Termination of CRRT treatment.
1. ICU nurse.
   a. Pediatric patients: consult with physician before returning blood. Blood return is usually contraindicated if blood prime was used.
   b. In adult patients return blood to patient with normal saline flush (see Figure 3.53).
   c. For regional citrate anticoagulation, stop citrate and calcium infusions simultaneously.
   d. Check a patient ionized calcium value 20–30 minutes after CRRT termination.
   e. Provide catheter care with normal saline flush and anticoagulant fill. Label dressing with date, initials, solution, solution concentration and volume used for catheter fill, e.g., heparin 5000 units/mL, arterial 1.8 mL, venous 1.9 mL or 3% citrate, arterial 1.8 mL, venous 1.9 mL.
   f. Document time and reason for termination of treatment.
2. Nephrology nurse.
   a. Assess patient condition and document on nephrology nursing note.
   b. Remove and dispose of tubing using standard precautions. Disinfect equipment and return to appropriate storage area.

   c. Document time and reason for termination of treatment.

J. Troubleshooting during SLEDD/CRRT treatments.
1. Nephrology nurse. Provide ICU nurse with support throughout each shift.
2. ICU nurse.
   a. Hypotension.
      (1) For MAP < 60 mm Hg, stop UF and administer a fluid bolus (not to be removed) as ordered by the intensivist or nephrologist.
      (2) For SLEDD, call the nephrology nurse to assess and determine changes to the UFR. Consider UF profiling to prevent hypotension. Patients using a linear decreasing UFR show a reduced incidence of hypotension.
      (3) For CRRT, call the nephrologist for changes to UFR.
      (4) Setting the dialysis solution temperature to 35–36° C may increase vasoconstriction and minimize hypotension.
      (5) Assess volume status changes and evaluate the need for initiating or titrating vasopressors to maintain BP and MAP within established range.
   b. Hemofilter clotting.
      (1) For rising TMP or VP, clotting should be suspected. Reducing the time that the blood flow is stopped due to alarm conditions decreases the risk for clotting.
      (2) For SLEDD, call the nephrology nurse to assess and potentially terminate treatment.
      (3) For CRRT, notify the nephrologist and follow procedure for end of treatment as outlined above.
   c. Hypothermia.
      (1) During CRRT with unwarmed dialysis or replacement solutions the patient temperature may fall to < 35° C.
      (2) Warm patient by warming dialysis or replacement solutions or by warming the blood or patient directly until patient is at desired temperature.
   d. Hyperthermia. The patient may be unable to elevate body temperature during exposure to large volumes of dialysis or replacement solutions at ≤ 37° C, clouding the use of temperature as an indicator of infectious processes.

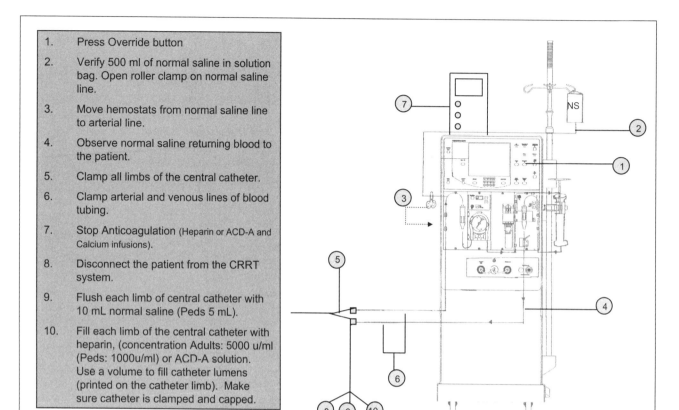

1. Press Override button
2. Verify 500 ml of normal saline in solution bag. Open roller clamp on normal saline line.
3. Move hemostats from normal saline line to arterial line.
4. Observe normal saline returning blood to the patient.
5. Clamp all limbs of the central catheter.
6. Clamp arterial and venous lines of blood tubing.
7. Stop Anticoagulation (Heparin or ACD-A and Calcium infusions).
8. Disconnect the patient from the CRRT system.
9. Flush each limb of central catheter with 10 mL normal saline (Peds 5 mL).
10. Fill each limb of the central catheter with heparin, (concentration Adults: 5000 u/ml (Peds: 1000u/ml) or ACD-A solution. Use a volume to fill catheter lumens (printed on the catheter limb). Make sure catheter is clamped and capped.

Figure 3.53. Treatment termination. Designed for use with the Fresenius 2008K.

Courtesy of Maureen Craig, UC Davis Medical Center, Sacramento, California. Used with permission.

e. Patient bleeding.
 (1) Stop heparin infusion.
 (2) Notify physician for signs and symptoms of bleeding or for a hematocrit decrease ≥ 5%.
 (3) Contact nephrologist to determine need for changes to anticoagulation orders.
f. Cardiopulmonary resuscitation (CPR). Initiate CPR and follow Advanced Cardiac Life Support (ACLS) guidelines. Return blood to patient if possible, stop treatment, clamp lines and call nephrology nurse and nephrologist for assistance.
g. Equipment alarms.
 (1) Refer to bedside inservice for most common alarm conditions.
 (2) Contact the nephrology nurse for less common alarm conditions.
 (3) Consult the operator's manual and/or contact the manufacturer's clinical

resources for unusual or irresolvable alarm conditions.
h. Serum electrolyte and solute imbalance.
 (1) Review the dialysis and/or the replacement solutions being used.
 (2) When necessary adapt solutions so patient can achieve desired serum electrolytes.
i. Procedure or test out of the ICU.
 (1) Schedule procedure during a time patient is off SLEDD treatment or the CRRT system is scheduled for a change.
 (2) Alternatively, interrupt treatment as indicated and resume SLEDD/CRRT treatment when patient is available and as ordered by the nephrologist.
j. Procedure in the ICU. If a procedure may cause patient agitation or disruption of dialysis circuit, contact nephrology nurse for additional monitoring of dialysis system during the procedure.

K. Nutrition for patient on SLEDD/CRRT.
1. Inadequate nutrition increases morbidity and mortality.
2. SLEDD/CRRT enables full fluid volume and solute control even with hyperalimentation or tube feedings.
3. Minimize negative nitrogen balance in ICU patients.
4. Decrease the time the patient goes without feeding during the ICU stay.

VII. Program selection and development for SLEDD/CRRT in various ICU environments.

A. Program interest and viability. Determine the hospital's need for and ability to support a SLEDD/CRRT program.

B. Patient population.
1. The ICU must have a minimum number of patients with AKI requiring dialytic therapy.
2. The number of patient cases required to build a SLEDD/CRRT program is based on the number of nurses that need to gain and maintain expertise on the therapy.
3. The more centralized these patient cases are (one ICU versus multiple ICUs), the fewer bedside nurses need to be trained to provide the care of the patient on SLEDD/CRRT and the more likely the bedside nurse can maintain the expertise with minimal assistance from other experts such as nephrology nurses, because of more frequent exposure.
4. To maintain nursing expertise, the potential AKI cases in the ICU requiring renal replacement therapy should be greater than 12 cases per year with a minimum of 5 to 7 days of SLEDD/CRRT therapy prescribed.
5. The scenario of having a few AKI cases spread over many ICUs perhaps even in different hospitals increases the benefit of using the model of training the nephrology nurses as experts to support the ICU nurses with bedside inservices at the beginning of every ICU nursing shift. This minimizes the training effort while maximizing the benefit of having information at the time of implementation.
6. The pediatric patient population has great variability in patient size and treatment orders with more stringent monitoring requirements of hourly and cumulative fluid balance. An integrated fluid management system is essential to accurate fluid handling.
7. Burn patients may have large volumes of

insensible fluid losses, requiring low to no ultrafiltration rates. Burn patients may have large dressing changes occurring over long time periods and possibly in a water tank. Consider SLEDD for more patient free time for these other essential interventions.
8. Choose a therapy that will effectively accomplish the goal of fluid removal and/or solute clearance for the identified patient population.
9. Choose a therapy that is relatively simple to learn for the health care providers that will be involved in its implementation.

C. Financial viability.
1. Expenses.
   a. Equipment and supplies.
      (1) Some equipment and supplies are relatively inexpensive.
      (2) However, the cost of training to safely use that system can overwhelm that cost savings.
      (3) Equipment should be chosen that will safely deliver the desired therapy with minimal training effort.
   b. Training.
      (1) The largest SLEDD/CRRT program expense will be the cost of training staff to establish and maintain competency.
      (2) A simpler SLEDD/CRRT program will result in fewer training requirements and fewer dollars spent meeting those requirements.
      (3) Smaller hospitals may contract services from providers that own the equipment, generally service the equipment, and oversee the education of dialysis and ICU staff.
      (4) In the larger hospital setting, consider working collaboratively with the ICU's CNS/APN, nurse manager and/or renal coordinator to establish an education program of the dialysis and critical care staff.
2. Revenues.
   a. Reimbursement for anticipated number of treatments.
   b. Therapy is likely to be ordered and implemented more frequently if it is simple and similar to what care providers already know.
3. The daily cost of providing SLEDD has been demonstrated to be considerably less than the cost of providing CRRT. This difference in cost

is dependent on several factors, e.g., staffing, equipment, and supplies.

D. Program coordinator.
1. CNS/APN or other resource nurse preferably with experience in both the nephrology and ICU environment.
2. The program can be led by either a nephrology or ICU discipline, but a collaborative practice should be sought as the program is implemented.
3. Develop expertise in the therapy of choice based on facility's needs and resources.
   a. Attend conferences, review the literature, and visit other working programs.
   b. The program must be designed to complement the existing patient population and the nursing, medical, and administrative resources.
4. Evaluate and purchase equipment to best perform the therapy chosen.
5. Develop documentation to support the delivery of SLEDD/CRRT in the current facility.
6. Establish and implement the training program as outlined in the Education section above.
7. Chair the SLEDD/CRRT workgroup.

F. SLEDD/CRRT Workgroup.
1. Determine the role each stakeholder will play.
2. Hospital and/or dialysis unit (for contracted dialysis services) administration.
   a. Focus on financial viability, program liability, ability and expense to train and maintain nursing resources.
   b. Determine who owns and maintains the SLEDD/CRRT equipment.
3. Intensivists: Identify ICU patients with potential renal replacement needs and consult nephrology.
4. Nephrologists.
   a. Develop SLEDD/CRRT order sets.
   b. Assess ICU patients requiring dialytic therapy for SLEDD/CRRT before considering IHD.
   c. Provide daily SLEDD/CRRT orders reflecting patient assessment and response to treatment.
5. Nephrology nurses.
   a. Develop outcome and patient care standards for patients on SLEDD/CRRT.
   b. Provide training for nephrology and ICU nurses on caring for patients on SLEDD/CRRT.
   c. Provide ICU nurse bedside inservice and treatment support during SLEDD/CRRT as outlined in the patient care standards.
6. ICU nurses.
   a. Train on providing SLEDD/CRRT as outlined in the patient care standard.
   b. Provide the SLEDD/CRRT treatment to the ICU patient with renal replacement therapy needs.
7. Nursing unit managers: Orchestrate getting adequate numbers of staff trained and then maintain unit competency.
8. Pharmacists.
   a. Provide customized or stock anticoagulant, replacement, and/or dialysis solutions, and information to support the use of each of these solutions in SLEDD/CRRT.
   b. Perform therapeutic drug monitoring of patient serum levels as indicated on patients receiving SLEDD/CRRT.
9. Pediatric ICU health care providers. Customize the existing adult SLEDD/CRRT program to meet pediatric needs or develop a new SLEDD/CRRT program based on the existing pediatric patient population using the literature and other pediatric centers offering SLEDD/CRRT as resources.

F. Initiate first SLEDD/CRRT treatment within 1–2 months of training the nursing staff.

G. Patient selection.
1. The first few patients chosen for SLEDD/CRRT may be those whose outcome is guarded at best.
2. The goal should be to apply the SLEDD/CRRT treatments to all patients in the intended population as soon as possible so care providers do not associate SLEDD/CRRT with only poor outcomes.

H. Follow the first several SLEDD/CRRT cases with a debriefing/evaluation session chaired by the program coordinator and attended by all interested parties in the SLEDD/CRRT workgroup. Continue to gather and evaluate ideas that evolve to improve the SLEDD/CRRT program. Make program changes judiciously and disseminate them to all involved parties.

Chapter 14

Therapeutic Plasma Exchange

Purpose

The purpose of this chapter is to present the history of apheresis, facilitate cognitive understanding of the concepts, principles, and clinical application of therapeutic plasma exchange (TPE), and to assist nephrology nurses in providing care for patients receiving TPE treatment.

Objectives

Upon completion of this chapter, the learner will be able to:
1. Define the terms and the history of apheresis.
2. Discuss the variety of treatment procedures and equipment alternatives available for TPE.
3. Describe the anticoagulation and medical support for the patient needed while providing TPE therapy.

I. Definition of terms.

A. Apheresis: derived from a Greek word meaning to remove or to separate a part from its whole. It has become synonymous with hemapheresis as an umbrella term encompassing all blood separation procedures.

B. Plasmapheresis: a separation of plasma from whole blood. Plasma exchange (PE) and TPE are terms used interchangeably to describe the separation of plasma along with the infusion of an equal amount of either plasma or another replacement fluid.

C. Leukapheresis: separation and removal of white cells (leukocytes).

D. Thrombocytapheresis or plateletpheresis: separation and removal of platelets.

E. Erythrocytapheresis: separation and removal of red blood cells.

F. Cytapheresis: separation and removal of a particular cellular component.

G. Cascade or secondary filtration: separated plasma is passed through a plasma filter that is specific for removal of a certain plasma element. The cascade, or second column, adsorbs the specific element, and the plasma is then returned to the patient.

II. History of apheresis.

A. 400 BC – Bloodletting, leeches, and manual phlebotomy all thought to be useful in removing toxins and treating diseases.

B. 1877 – Manual continuous flow centrifugation instrument is designed by a Swiss physician, Carl Gustav Patrik DeLaval, and used throughout Europe for cream separation.

C. 1881 – DeLaval device patented for use in the United States.

D. 1914 – Plasma exchange procedure done on uremic dogs which consisted of phlebotomy, separation by centrifuge and the removal of plasma cells while returning RBCs and saline through a separate intravenous (IV) line.

E. 1940s – Dr. Edwin Cohn adapts a cream separator to separate plasma from whole blood for use in injured soldiers during WWII.

F. 1950s – Dr. Cohn, while at the Harvard Medical School, invents the "Cohn Fractionator" which was successful in separating blood into all of its components.

G. 1952 – Human plasma is made commercially available.

H. 1959 – Plastic containers are introduced increasing storage time and cutting down on cost of producing and distributing plasma.

I. 1960s – Engineers and physicians at the National Cancer Institute and International Business Machines design an automatic continuous flow blood cell separator called "model 2990." This machine does not have a completely disposable unit and the separation bowl must be washed and sanitized by hand.

J. 1970s – Celltifuge® (Aminco Corporation, Silver Spring, Maryland) markets a completely disposable continuous flow blood cell separator that is adapted for use in TPE treatments.

K. 1982 – Century TPE System® (Gambro BCT, Lakewood, Colorado) introduces the first plasma membrane exchange system.

L. 1987 – COBE Spectra® (Gambro BCT, Lakewood, Colorado) introduces a continuous-flow centrifugation device used for plasma exchange, cytapheresis, and other clinical applications.

M. 1987 – Prosorba Protein A column® (Fresenius Hemocare Bad Homburg, Germany) is approved by the Food and Drug Administration (FDA) for idiopathic thrombocytopenia purpura (ITP) and later approved for refractory rheumatoid arthritis (RA).

N. 1994 – AS 104® (Fresenius Hemocare Bad Homburg, Germany) is FDA approved as another continuous flow centrifugation device.

O. 1996 – Liposorber® system (Kaneka, Osaka, Japan) introduces a plasma column for reducing low density lipids (LDL) in patients with familial hypercholesterolemia.

P. 1997 – Heparin-induced Extracorporeal Lipoprotein Precipitation (HELP®) system (B. Braun Medical Inc, Melsungen, Germany) is FDA approved for LDL removal from plasma.

Q. 2006 – Com.Tec® (Fresenius Hemocare Bad Homburg, Germany) is FDA approved as a cell separator, continuous flow, centrifugation device.

III. Devices used in therapeutic plasma exchange.

A. Centrifugation.
1. Continuous flow devices.
   a. The COBE Spectra®.
      (1) Can perform TPE as either a single-needle or a dual-needle procedure.
      (2) Using the single needle option lengthens the time to perform the treatment and is only used when the patient does not have vascular access to support two needles.
   b. The AS 104®.
      (1) No longer manufactured.
      (2) Has been replaced by the Com.Tec® device.
      (3) Single needle option is not available on this device in the United States.
   c. All of these devices use the continuous flow technology but differ in device specific ways.
      (1) These machines replaced the centrifuge bowl used in intermittent device machines with a spinning separation channel which uses centrifugal forces to separate the various elements of the blood according to their specific gravity.
      (2) Based on specific gravity, the heaviest elements, erythrocytes, pack along the outer wall of the channel while the lighter plasma moves to the inner wall.
      (3) The "buffy coat", a layer that consists of all the white blood cells and platelets, forms between the erythrocytes and plasma (see Table 3.39).
   d. Advantages of using continuous centrifugal flow devices compared to intermittent flow devices.
      (1) Higher blood flow rates.
      (2) Smaller extracorporeal blood volume.
      (3) Faster treatment times.
   e. Continuous flow centrifugation treatments are primarily performed for patients in acute care settings and an increasing number of nephrology departments.
2. Intermittent flow devices.
   a. Intermittent devices, or discontinuous flow devices, are used almost exclusively in blood banking and donation apheresis.
   b. The Haemonetics MCS® and PCS-2® (Haemonetics, Braintree, Massachusetts) are the few machines in the United States that use intermittent centrifuge systems for TPE.
   c. Whole blood is drawn from an access site into a spinning bowl-shaped device and processed as a set volume in cycles.

(1) As the bowl fills with whole blood, its components separate according to specific gravity.

(2) When the bowl is full, e.g., 125–375 mL, whole blood access pauses while plasma, the lightest component, is siphoned off from the other blood components similar to skimming of cream from raw milk.

(3) The remainder of the blood components are then returned to the patient along with a plasma replacement fluid through the same IV site used to access the patient's whole blood.

d. Advantages of intermittent flow devices.
   (1) Single-needle vascular access option.
   (2) Variable extracorporeal blood volumes.

e. Disadvantages of intermittent flow procedures.
   (1) Limited blood flow rates of 30–60 mL/min.
   (2) The extended length of time needed to process adequate amounts of whole blood in batches averaging 225 mL/cycle.
   (3) Hemodynamic instability in patients that can result from several cycles of whole blood volume depletion and fresh plasma infusion that is required with this type of device.
   (4) This potential for instability is a major reason intermittent flow devices are not the technology of choice for TPE.

B. Membrane filtration.
   1. Membrane filters separate plasma components according to their particle size.
   2. Membrane filtration used for plasma exchange follows the technological advances made within hemodialysis membranes.
   3. Membrane filtration therapies focus on the ability of solute and fluid to move across a semipermeable membrane, which is customarily encased in plastic using either a hollow fiber or parallel plate design.
   4. The membrane filtration device works on a balance of pressures within the filter, similar to a hemodialysis treatment.

Table 3.39

Specific Gravity of Blood Components

Component	Specific Gravity (g/ml)
Plasma	1.025–1.029
Platelets	1.040
B-lymphocytes	1.050–1.060
T-lymphocytes	1.050–1.061
Blasts/promyelocytes	1.058–1.066
Monocytes	1.065–1.066
Myelocytes/basophils	1.070
Reticulocytes	1.078
Metamyelocytes	1.080
Bands and segmented neutrophils	1.087–.092
Erythrocytes	1.078–1.114

Source: Zielinski, I. (2002). Principles of apheresis. In *Principles of Apheresis Technology* (3rd ed., p. 36). Vancouver, BC: American Society for Apheresis. Used with permission.

5. Filters.
   a. The hollow fiber filter is composed of a bundle of parallel single fibers, which resembles a straw with numerous holes in it, encased in a plastic cylinder.
   b. The patient's whole blood enters the filter under pressure and as it flows through, plasma is squeezed out through the holes in the "straw."
   c. A more concentrated cell suspension exits at the other end.
   d. Whole blood enters the bottom port, cells go up and exit from the top port, and plasma withdraws from a side port.
   e. An additional side port is used to monitor pressures.
   f. The Plasmaflo® membrane (Asahi Medical Co. Ltd., Tokyo, Japan) is a filter made by the same company that manufactures hemodialyzers.
   g. Plasauto®, Cascadeflo®, Plasorba®, and Immusorba® (Asahi Medical Co. Ltd., Tokyo, Japan) are all membrane filters by this same manufacturer.
      (1) These filters are not FDA approved in the United States but are widely used abroad.

(2) Information on these filters can be found at www.asahi-kasei.co.jp/medical/en.

(3) The filters can be used in conjunction with the Plasmaflo® to remove pathogenic substances from the separated plasma for a variety of diseases.

6. Membrane filtration devices enlist a highly porous plasma separator to strain plasma from whole blood.

7. Plasma membrane separators used in membrane filtration are capable of removing plasma and all of its dissolved elements up to 3 microns in size. The other elements of a patient's whole blood are larger and therefore do not pass through the porous walls of the membrane (see Table 3.40).

8. Clearance of plasma proteins will depend on where the particular protein is located, i.e., intravascular or extravascular. When antibody subclasses are the target for removal, it is important to note that approximately 76% of IgM is found in the intravascular space while only 45% of IgG is intravascular.

9. The advantage of using membrane filtration technology is that the equipment is very similar to other equipment that nephrology nurses use.
   a. Membrane technology has led nephrology nurses into the care of patients for whom TPE is prescribed.
   b. Similarity in the equipment is a primary reason for establishing TPE programs in dialysis units.

10. The disadvantage of using the plasma membrane filter is that it can only be used for plasma exchange since the membrane pore size is too small to allow for passage of any of the other blood components.

Table 3.40

Size of Blood Components

Component	Diameter in Microns
Plasma	2.8 microns
Platelet	3 microns
Erythrocyte	7 microns
Lymphocyte	10 microns
Granulocyte	13 microns

Source: Zielinski, I. (2002). Principles of apheresis. In *Principles of Apheresis Technology* (3rd ed., p. 36). Vancouver, BC: American Society for Apheresis. Used with permission.

C. Filtration-centrifugation combination.
   1. Fenwal Autopheresis C (Baxter-Fenwal Corporation, Deerfield, Illinois).
      a. This device is a combination of a centrifuge and a filter.
      b. It is a single-needle, intermittent flow device.
      c. The extracorporeal volume is 200 mL.
      d. Its use is limited to plasma collection from healthy donors in the United States.
   2. The mechanism of action.
      a. As the anticoagulated blood enters the separation chamber, a rotating filter causes the blood to rotate.
      b. This, in turn, sweeps the blood over the membrane surface and prevents cells from collecting there.
      c. The plasma passes through the filter and drains by the force of gravity into a collection container.
      d. A predetermined amount of plasma is collected and the remaining blood components are reinfused into the patient.
      e. This occurs in repeating cycles and, according to the manufacturer, extracts virtually cell-free plasma.

D. Plasma columns: LDL column systems.
   1. There are two column systems approved by the FDA for use in the United States for LDL apheresis to treat patients with familial hypercholesterolemia.
      a. The Liposorber® system.
         (1) Uses a hollow fiber plasma separator and two dextran sulfate LDL adsorption columns.
         (2) Device specific disposables.
      b. The HELP® system.
         (1) Uses a hollow-fiber membrane plasma separator.
         (2) Removes LDL from separated plasma via a heparin-induced precipitation filter.
         (3) Device specific disposables.
   2. Treatment specifics.
      a. Heparin is used as the anticoagulant.
      b. Patients requiring this therapy must continue treatment every 1–2 weeks for the duration of their lives.
      c. No replacement fluid is required.
      d. Treatment time is approximately 3 hours.
      e. The volume of plasma processed through these LDL removal devices varies from patient to patient.
   3. Indication for use.
      a. Heterozygous patients: LDL-C levels of

≥ 200 mg/dL who have a documented history of coronary heart disease (CHD).
b. Heterozygous patients: LDL-C levels of ≥ 300 mg/dL without CHD but refractory to cholesterol lowering medications.
c. Homozygous patients: LDL-C levels of ≥ 500 mg/dL.

IV. Pretreatment considerations.

A. Indications for treatment. Guidelines for indications of TPE were developed by the American Medical Association (AMA) in 1985. These guidelines have been further refined by the American Society for Apheresis (ASFA) and the American Association of Blood Banks (AABB). These guidelines divide the indications for TPE treatment into four categories:
1. Category I. Patients with conditions in this category should be treated with TPE. TPE is a standard and acceptable treatment and is used as a primary therapy or an essential first line adjunctive therapy. Evidence for use in this category is based on well-controlled clinical trials and a large base of published experience. An example of a category I condition is thrombotic thrombocytopenia purpura (TTP).
2. Category II. Patients with conditions in this category may be treated with TPE. TPE is generally beneficial and used as a supportive therapy. TPE is not the first-line therapy but has been found to be successful through a small number of randomized clinical trials and published case studies. An example of a category II condition is myeloma with acute kidney injury or cryoglobulinemia.
3. Category III. Patients with conditions in this category may or may not elect to be treated with TPE. The evidence to support using TPE is insufficient to establish efficacy and there is no clear documentation for a favorable benefit-to-risk ratio. The published controlled clinical trials have conflicting results or the cases are not numerous enough to elude any specific benefit for using TPE. The patients treated in this category have tried all other conventional therapies with little response or are part of an approved research protocol. An example of a category III condition is hemolytic uremic syndrome (HUS) or systemic lupus erythematosus (SLE).
4. Category IV. Patients with conditions in this category should not be treated with TPE.

The controlled trials or anecdotal evidence have failed to demonstrate a benefit to support the use of TPE. Treatments for diseases in this category are discouraged and should only be used in approved clinical trials. An example of a category IV condition is systemic amyloidosis (see Table 3.41).

B. Estimating total blood volume (TBV) and plasma volume (PV).
1. Importance of estimating TBV and PV.
a. These calculations are used to determine the dose or volume of plasma to be exchanged.
b. Used to estimate the length of a TPE procedure.
c. Typically, 1.0 to 1.5 times the patient's PV is exchanged.
d. The physician may decide to increase or decrease that amount for a variety of clinical reasons.
e. The larger the amount of plasma exchanged the longer the procedure will take, exposing the patient to more citrate anticoagulant, possible side effects, and potential adverse events.
f. The patient's clinical stability, severity of disease process, and the risk of exposure to blood products must be considered when determining the amount of plasma to be exchanged.
2. Calculation of estimated TBV and PV.
a. Centrifuge devices have software installed to calculate TBV and PV, but those calculations are dependent upon the correct input of the patient's gender, height, weight, and hematocrit (HCT).
b. The following formulas are based on actual patient weight. In very obese or edematous patients, the weight may need to be adjusted to the ideal body weight.
c. Formulas for estimated TBV.
(1) Estimated TBV by age and weight.

Patient ≥ 12 years	TBV = Weight (kg) x 70 mL/kg
Patient 1-12 years	TBV = Weight (kg) x 75 mL/kg
Patient 0-12 months	TBV = Weight (kg) x 80 mL/kg

(2) Nadler's formula is for adults only and is based on patient height in inches, actual patient weight in pounds and gender.

Males: TBV (mL) =
$(0.006012 \times \text{Height}^3 \text{ [in]}) + (14.6 \times \text{Weight [lb]}) + 604$
Females: TBV (mL) =
$(0.005835 \times \text{Height}^3 \text{ [in]}) + (15 \times \text{Weight [lb]}) + 183$

| Table 3.41 | Disease Listing by Specialty and Category |

Disease	Category
Renal, Metabolic Diseases, and Transplantation	
Antiglomerular basement membrane antibody disease	I
Phytanic acid storage disease	II
Rapidly progressive glomerulonephritis	II
Familial hypercholesterolemia	II
Hemolytic uremic syndrome	III
Renal transplantation; HLA desensitization	II
Recurrent focal glomerulosclerosis	III
Heart transplant rejection	III
Acute hepatic failure	III
Overdose/poisoning	III
Renal transplantation; antibody mediated rejection	II
Autoimmune and Rheumatic Diseases	
Cyroglobulinemia	I
Rheumatoid arthritis: Immunoadsorption	II
Scleroderma/progressive systemic sclerosis	III
Systemic lupus erythematosus	III
Hematologic Diseases	
Thrombotic thrombocytopenia purpura	I
Posttransfusion purpura	III
ABO incompatible marrow transplant	II
Idiopathic thrombocytopenia purpura	II
Myeloma/acute renal failure	III
Coagulation factor inhibitors	III
Aplastic anemia/pure red cell aplasia	III
Autoimmune hemolytic anemia	III

Disease	Category
Neurologic Disorders	
Chronic inflammatory demyelinating polyradiculoneuropathy	I
Acute inflammatory demyelinating polyradiculoneuropathy	I
Paraproteinemic polyneuropathies with IgG/IgA	I
Myasthenia gravis	I
Lambert-Eaton myasthenia syndrome	II
Sydenham's chorea	I
Waldenstrom's macroglobulinemia	II
PANDAS	I
Paraneoplastic neurologic syndromes	III
Multiple sclerosis: acute CNS inflammatory demyelinating disease	II
Multiple sclerosis: chronic progressive	III
Multiple myeloma with polyneuropathy	III
Rasmussen's encephalitis	II
Stiff-person syndrome	III

Adapted from Szczepiorkowski, Z. (2007). Clinical applications of therapeutic apheresis: An evidence based approach. *Journal of Clinical Apheresis, 22*(3), 101-103.

d. Formulas for estimated PV.
  (1) Calculation of estimated PV in adults using actual patient weight and an assumed normal HCT.
  PV (mL) = Weight (kg) x 40 mL/kg
  Example: Patient = 70 kg
  PV = 70 kg x 40 mL/kg = 2800 mL or 2.8 L
  (2) Calculation of estimated PV in adults using actual patient weight and HCT.

  PV (mL) = 0.65 x Weight (kg) x (100-HCT)
  Example: Patient = 70 kg, HCT = 42%
  PV = 0.65 x 70 kg x (100 – 42) = 2639 mL or 2.6 L
  (3) Calculation of estimated PV using TBV (above) and actual patient HCT.
  PV (mL) = TBV (mL) x (100 – HCT)
  Example: Patient = 70 kg, HCT = 42%
  TBV = 70 kg x 70 mL/kg = 4900 mL
  PV = 4900 ml x (100 - 42) = 2842 mL or 2.8 L

3. The number of PV exchanges during the TPE treatment is selected based on the protein and immunoglobulin clearance desired for a particular disease condition.
   a. Usually, 1.0–1.5 PV is exchanged.
   b. Removal of intravascular substances is estimated as follows.
      (1) 0.5 times the PV exchanged removes approximately 35%.
      (2) 1.0 times the PV exchanged removes approximately 65%.
      (3) 1.5 times the PV exchanged removes approximately 70%.
      (4) 2.0 times the PV exchanged removes approximately 75%.
   c. Some rebound effect may be observed within 24 to 48 hours of a TPE treatment.
   d. Recirculation in the TPE circuit, redistribution between intravascular and extravascular spaces and other factors may result in less than calculated clearances.

C. Treatment plan for plasmapheresis.
   1. Diagnosis.
      a. Proper diagnosis is critical to the successful incorporation of TPE into the treatment regimen.
      b. The timing of the initial TPE treatment course, the length of the treatment course, the target treatment parameters, the appropriate replacement fluids and the optimal vascular access option are all decisions that must be made by the ordering physician based on the patient's diagnosis and clinical picture.
   2. Amount of plasma to be removed.
      a. TPE is a treatment prescribed by volume not by time. Volume exchanged may range from 500–5000 mL, but typically is ordered as a multiple of the patient's PV.
      b. As noted above, the efficiency of plasma component removal decreases dramatically beyond one PV exchange.
      c. Additionally, effectiveness of TPE does not increase by performing TPE more than once in 24 hours.
   3. Frequency of treatments.
      a. The schedule for treatment is dictated by the patient's disease and may change depending on the patient's response to therapy.
      b. The physician, in deciding the number and frequency of the treatments, is guided by the American Society for Apheresis (ASFA) Guidelines for TPE. These published guidelines are based on clinical trials.

4. Replacement fluids.
   a. 5% albumin.
      (1) The preferred replacement fluid for patients without coagulation problems.
      (2) Blood volume expander, containing plasma proteins but not clotting factors.
      (3) Calcium gluconate may be added to albumin replacement fluid to replace patient calcium. There is no risk of clot formation.
      (4) Lower incidence of reactions and disease transmission compared to fresh frozen plasma (FFP) and it should be used whenever the replacement of clotting factors is not necessary.
      (5) If only 25% albumin is available, it must be diluted to a 5% albumin with 0.9% sodium chloride solution since mixing with any other solution can cause hemolysis when infused into patients.
   b. FFP.
      (1) FFP is the fluid portion of whole blood and contains all of the coagulation factors and plasma proteins present in whole blood.
      (2) FFP is used in diseases and situations requiring the immediate replacement of clotting factors such as reduced fibrinogen levels, decreased platelet counts, preoperatively, and post solid organ biopsy.
      (3) FFP is used as replacement fluid in TTP because there is platelet aggregation and an absence of effective von Willebrand Factor (vWF) cleaving metaloprotease.
      (4) There are a percentage of TTP patients who do not respond to the use of FFP, continuing to have active platelet aggregation related to the detrimental presence of the unusually large vWF multimers.
      (5) FFP is preserved with citrate to prevent clotting. Using FFP as a replacement fluid provides some of the citrate needed for anticoagulation during a TPE treatment.
      (6) Calcium gluconate should not be added to FFP, as it will bind with the citrate and allow clots to form with in the FFP.
   c. Cryoprecipitate-reduced plasma (CRP).
      (1) Also termed "cryo-poor plasma" and "cryoprecipitate-poor plasma." CRP is that fraction of plasma remaining after the removal of cryoprecipitable proteins.
      (2) The fibrinogen, factor VIII, fibronectin

and large multimers of vWF have been removed.

(3) In patients unresponsive to TPE with FFP, the physician may decide either to switch to CRP alone or a combination of FFP and CRP as replacement fluids.

d. Normal saline.

(1) Normal saline may be administered to wash or clear the plasma membrane of proteins, to treat hypotension with a fluid bolus, and to assist with reinfusion of the patient's blood at the end of treatment.

(2) Normal saline is used as an adjunct with other replacement fluids but not used as the primary replacement fluid since it does not provide any of the components of plasma.

e. Other solutions.

(1) A combination of any of these replacement fluids can be ordered depending on the patient's medical condition, fluid status and/or response to treatment.

(2) In situations where patients are, or chronically become, hypotensive early in a TPE treatment, a bolus of normal saline or a small amount of 25% albumin may be administered prior to the procedure to maintain hemodynamic stability during TPE.

5. An anticoagulation solution is used during the TPE treatment to prevent clotting in the extracorporeal circuit.

a. Anticoagulant citrate dextrose formula A (ACD-A®) (Baxter-Fenwal Corporation, Deerfield, Illinois).

(1) ACD-A is a citrate-based anticoagulant that contains dextrose, sodium citrate and citric acid.

(2) Citrate works as an anticoagulant by binding to calcium and thereby blocking the clotting cascade.

(3) Citrate is metabolized to bicarbonate by the liver.

(4) ACD-A is prescribed as a ratio infusion of whole blood to anticoagulant.

(5) The COBE Spectra® has a default ratio of 13:1 for TPE procedures which means for every 13 revolutions of the inlet flow pump the anticoagulant (AC) pump will turn once.

(a) Approximately 80% of the citrate anticoagulant solution goes into the plasma waste bag.

(b) The patient receives only 20% of the total amount of citrate administered during the TPE treatment.

(6) The Fresenius AS-104® has a default ratio of 12:1 for TPE procedures and the patient only receives approximately ten percent of the total amount of citrate administered during the TPE treatment.

(7) Patients with active bleeding problems, low platelet and HCT values and patients with liver or kidney dysfunction may need a blood flow to anticoagulant ratio of 18:1 to 22:1 to limit the exposure to citrate.

(8) Approximately 14% of the total volume of each unit of FFP used as replacement fluid is citrate. A higher blood flow to anticoagulant ratio is needed when using FFP as a replacement fluid.

(9) Citrate can temporarily lower the ionized calcium level causing symptoms as mild as perioral paresthesthia and as severe as complete body tetany and cardiac dysfunction, necessitating IV calcium replacement.

(10) Patients with liver or renal disease may have impaired citrate and calcium metabolism and are at an increased risk for citrate toxicity which may require a higher blood flow to citrate ratio and a slower over all blood flow rate.

b. Heparin (used with membrane filtration) in adult TPE treatments.

(1) At the start of a TPE treatment with membrane filtration, a heparin bolus is administered prefilter.

(a) Heparinization requirements vary according to the patient's platelet count.

(b) Those patients with a platelet count $\leq 70,000/mm^3$ or a blood dyscrasia may not require the heparin bolus.

(c) Patients with significant renal dysfunction and/or qualitative and possibly quantitative platelet defects may benefit from a small heparin bolus, < 40 units/kg.

(d) Those patients who do not have impairment of the hematologic system and/or do not have hepatic failure may require a heparin bolus dosage of 40–60 units/kg.

(e) Patients who have platelet counts ≥ 0.5 million/mm^3 may require additional heparin.

(2) After the initial heparin bolus, the blood flow is established between 100–150 mL/min and a heparin infusion may be started to maintain continuing anticoagulation. Orders may be similar to the following:

    (a) Heparin continuous infusion of 1,000 units/hour.

    (b) ACT goal = 180–220 seconds, when starting with a base ACT of 145 seconds.

    (c) For ACT < 180 seconds, increase heparin by 500 units/hour.

    (d) For ACT > 220 seconds, stop heparin infusion till ACT is back in range.

    (e) Monitor ACT every 20–30 minutes.

    (f) Stop heparin 30 minutes prior to treatment termination.

(3) On centrifuge equipment that normally uses only citrate as an anticoagulant, some heparin in combination with citrate may be required.

    (a) Patients acutely sensitive to citrate.

    (b) Some pediatric patients.

6. Fluid balance.

  a. The patient's condition determines the fluid balance parameters ordered for each TPE treatment.

  b. Adjustments to a patient's fluid balance of more than ± 5% should be avoided because the fluid being removed contains large amounts of plasma proteins.

  c. Unlike hemodialysis or ultrafiltration, which removes water and electrolytes, removal of a large quantity of plasma protein can seriously compromise the ability of a patient to maintain sufficient intravascular oncotic pressure to support blood pressure.

7. Premedications and medications used during TPE.

  a. Premedications are recommended before infusing large quantities of FFP or CRP as plasma replacement fluid.

    (1) To prevent or mitigate transfusion reactions.

    (2) To treat the signs and symptoms of transfusion reactions.

    (3) The medications can include:

      (a) Benadryl® (Warner Lambert Consumer Healthcare, Morris Plains, NJ), diphenhydramine hydrochloride.

      (b) Solu-Cortef® (Pfizer, New York, NY), hydrocortisone or Solu-Medrol®

(Pfizer, New York, NY), methylprednisolone.

      (c) Tylenol® (McNeil Consumer Healthcare, Guilph, Ontario), acetaminophen.

  b. Premedications are usually not needed when using albumin as the replacement fluid.

  c. Medications used to prevent and treat citrate side effects during the treatment are:

    (1) 10% calcium gluconate is the preferred medication since it is 1/3 the strength of calcium chloride and does not need dilution before administering.

    (2) It can be added directly to the 5% albumin bottles but not directly to the bags of FFP/CRP.

    (3) When using FFP/CRP, the 10% calcium gluconate can be given in small increments through a port, via a stopcock, or as a slow, continuous infusion piggybacked at the point on the tubing set close to reinfusion.

8. Laboratory tests.

  a. Specific lab test samples should be collected shortly before the initiation of TPE and/or 2–4 hours after the treatment is finished.

  b. Lab tests are ordered according to the patient's diagnosis and medical condition.

  c. A pretreatment HCT is critical in calculating an accurate PV or setting the equipment parameters.

  d. A pretreatment chemistry panel including calcium and magnesium, ensures what the patient's electrolyte values are.

  e. Citrate anticoagulation can affect serum calcium, potassium and magnesium levels.

9. Parameters for pretreatment vital signs:

  a. An elevated temperature may indicate a systemic infection or one related to central line placement.

    (1) Using an infected central catheter can circulate local pathogens throughout a patient's vascular system and cause sepsis that can be difficult and costly to treat.

    (2) TPE can cause immunosuppression as a result of the intended removal of antibodies and place the patient at risk for opportunistic infections.

    (3) Physician orders should indicate the threshold of change during TPE from the baseline vital signs that requires physician notification.

  b. Pretreatment blood pressure (BP) must be high enough to tolerate the expected BP drop at the start of the TPE treatment due to volume shifts.

(1) A bolus of normal saline or a small amount of 25% or 5% albumin may be infused to increase the patient's blood pressure to an acceptable starting range.

(2) Orders should include a limited number and/or volume of normal saline boluses for patient hypotension.

c. Respiratory assessment should be performed prior to a TPE treatment as changes in a patient's intraprocedure HCT can increase respiratory distress.

(1) Monitor deviations in HCT caused by the red cell volume depletion that occurs at the start of TPE.

(2) Critically ill or unstable patients may require oxygen to be ordered prior to treatment initiation for significant changes to the oxygen saturation levels that are related to respiratory distress.

V. Treatment considerations.

A. Patient assessment.
1. Initial patient assessment.
a. Before installing the disposable set, it is important to ensure that the vascular access is adequate and usable.

(1) Ensure that the central line has been medically cleared for use and that it is working well.

(2) If peripheral veins are to be used, perform a visual assessment of all potentially suitable vasculature.

b. A total body systems assessment should be completed with the patient's diagnosis used to focus on specific system-related abnormalities, e.g., renal, integument, cardiac, and neuromuscular.

c. The patient's and family's knowledge of the disease state, planned therapy, and planned course of therapy should be evaluated and education provided.

d. Monitor the patient's emotional and cognitive response to treatment.

e. Document the patient's weight and vital signs, i.e., blood pressure, pulse, respirations, temperature, and oxygen saturation. An assessment of a critically ill patient also may include hemodynamic parameters, e.g., central venous pressure, pulmonary capillary wedge pressure, and cardiac output.

f. Laboratory analyses should be reviewed with particular attention to complete blood count (CBC), protime (PT), electrolytes, albumin, fibrinogen and lactate dehydrogenase (LDH). There are a number of diagnoses and conditions treated that require close monitoring of specific labs.

(1) The patient with TTP should have daily CBC and LDH levels monitored to assist in evaluating response to TPE therapy.

(2) The patient with Waldenstrom's macroglobulinemia or multiple myeloma should have immunoglobulin levels monitored to assist in evaluating response to TPE therapy.

(3) Electrolyte abnormalities may need intervention before performing TPE, e.g., hyperkalemia, and hypokalemia, hypocalcemia, and hypomagnesemia.

g. Fluid balance assessment.

(1) If either volume deficit or excess are present, it may require hydration or ultrafiltration before commencing TPE.

(2) TPE is best delivered as an isovolemic procedure. If more plasma is removed than replaced the patient may become hypoalbuminemic, which can lead to undesirable extravascular fluid shifts.

(3) Administration of extra fluid during TPE to support blood pressure usually does not present problems unless the patient has renal dysfunction.

h. Review pertinent diagnostic tests or exams before starting TPE, e.g., pulmonary function test, electrocardiogram, peripheral nerve studies, and neuromuscular reflexes.

i. All medications should be reviewed, including PRN and IV medications.

(1) IV medications are not routinely administered before and during TPE because they may be removed with the plasma exchange.

(2) Confer with the patient's bedside nurse about scheduling specific medications in relation to TPE.

2. Pretreatment assessment.
a. Documentation of response to previous TPE treatments assists the clinician in determining the benefit the patient may be receiving in treating a particular disease state.

b. Laboratory analyses and diagnostic tests should be assessed to determine the patients continued need for TPE therapy.

c. A patient assessment is needed to find any changes to the patient's condition. The patient's current vital signs and historical tolerance to TPE should be reviewed along with other pertinent and available hemodynamic parameters.

    d. Fluid status should continuously be reevaluated as it pertains to the treatment goal to leave the patient either isovolemic, hypovolemic, or hypervolemic at the end of TPE.

    e. Medications should be reviewed and most are postponed until the treatment is completed.

B. Vascular access.
  1. Peripheral veins.
    a. Ideally both antecubital veins are used for blood access and return.
      (1) At times, other veins in the patient's forearms may have to be used.
      (2) The access, or draw needle, cannot be smaller than 17 gauge.
      (3) Most needles used for peripheral vein cannulation are 15–17 gauge steel needles with a back-eye for smoother blood flow.
      (4) The return site, if using a smaller vein in the arm, can be slightly smaller but anything smaller than a 19-gauge needle will cause lysis of red blood cells (RBC).
      (5) The needles must be able to sustain a blood flow rates of at least 40 mL/min and substantial positive or negative pressure.
    b. Using peripheral veins in the feet and legs are contraindicated due to the high risk of blood clots.
    c. Arteries are very rarely accessed due to the risk of complications secondary to infiltration.
    d. Risks associated with inserting peripheral catheters.
      (1) Hematoma.
      (2) Uncontrolled bleeding.
      (3) Infection at the insertion site.
      (4) Thrombi or emboli formation during the treatment that can travel and cause ischemic damage to other organs.
    e. When antecubital veins are used, pressure is held for several minutes after the needle is removed and a gauze pad secured over the site.
  2. Nontunneled central venous catheter (CVC).
    a. A double lumen, nontunneled CVC placed in the internal jugular, subclavian, or femoral vein may be used for a week, but should be monitored for signs and symptoms of infection.

      (1) Follow manufacturer's recommendation or facility policy for care and maintenance of catheter.
      (2) A femoral vein catheter is difficult to keep clean and is susceptible to kinking and infection. However, when infusing blood containing citrate into a CVC in the patient there is a lower incidence of arrhythmias associated with the femoral vein.
      (3) Frequently, a CVC must be removed because of kinking or clotting problems that inhibit adequate blood flow.
      (4) Double lumen dialysis catheters with a third smaller lumen for use as a central IV line are also available.
    b. Peripherally inserted central catheter (PICC) and "power PICC" lines are too small and flexible for use during a TPE procedure.
    c. Implanted ports cannot be used since the port can only accommodate one needle.
  3. Tunneled CVC.
    a. Long-term catheters are tunneled beneath the skin to increase patient comfort and reduce complications.
      (1) The double lumen tunneled catheter has a cuff. As the tissue grows into the cuff, it produces a barrier that prevents bacteria from invading the tunnel.
      (2) A tunneled CVC may be inserted into a jugular vein and tunneled into the upper chest near the collarbone.
    b. The tunneled, cuffed catheters are usually composed of silicone or polyurethane composites. These composites are softer than polyurethane but are stronger than silicone to allow larger lumen sizes able to withstand higher pressures from blood flow.
    c. Patients who require multiple treatments over a long period of time usually will have fewer complications with a tunneled catheter.
    d. Check with the individual catheter manufacturer to determine safe durations for each access device.
  4. Sites for placement.
    a. The CVC may be placed in the internal jugular, femoral, or subclavian veins.
    b. The internal jugular is the vein of choice. However, circumstances may dictate another vein is cannulated.
    c. Patients with peripheral neuropathy or cryoglobulinemia-induced vasculitis are poor choices for peripheral access. Pain and the lack of adequate venous blood vessels make

these patients candidates for a tunneled CVC.

    d. Patients needing both hemodialysis and apheresis on a long-term basis benefit from early placement of an arteriovenous (AV) graft or fistula.

5. CVC complications.

    a. Hemothorax, pneumothorax, and/or air embolisms can result from improper insertion of a CVC.

    b. Puncture of the femoral vein during insertion of a CVC may lead to a retroperitoneal hemorrhage.

    c. Bleeding at the insertion site may occur with any CVC.

        (1) Pressure applied at the CVC exit site to stop bleeding can kink the tubing and make the catheter unusable.

        (2) Special care should be taken when using sand bags to apply pressure to these fragile catheter insertion sites.

        (3) For an internal jugular or a subclavian vein catheter, position the patient with the head of the bed (HOB) elevated at least 45 degrees for the first 24 hours after catheter placement to decrease bleeding from intravascular pressure at the site.

        (4) An ice pack can be applied to the exit site to help stop oozing after line placement.

        (5) Patients with coagulopathy disorders may need platelet infusions due to the amount of oozing from the CVC site.

    d. An infected catheter can suspend or delay TPE treatments until the patient has completed a course of antibiotics and is able to receive a new vascular access device.

6. AV fistula/graft.

    a. The patient with maintenance TPE needs may benefit from a more permanent vascular access, i.e., AV fistula/graft.

    b. A native arterio-venous fistula or synthetic graft may be cannulated with the access needle pointing either with or against the direction of blood flow and the return needle pointing with the direction of blood flow in the vascular access.

    c. The needles ideally are placed at least 2 inches apart to reduce recirculation of blood.

    d. When accessing a fistula/graft the nurse must avoid aneurysms, curves and flat spots and the tip of the needle should be at least 1.5 inches away from an anastamosis.

    e. 17-gauge steel arteriovenous fistula needles can provide adequate blood flow when used

to access the fistula/graft for TPE to prevent excessive posttreatment bleeding.

    f. Complications include thrombosis, infection, aneurysms, venous hypertension, seromas, and local bleeding.

    g. When removing the needles from this type of access, gentle pressure, e.g., stops bleeding while not occluding blood flow, is held at the exact insertion site until hemostasis is achieved.

    h. After hemostasis occurs, a dressing is secured over the needle site.

C. Intraprocedure monitoring and patient care.

1. Vital signs, cardiac, and equipment monitoring.

    a. After the extracorporeal circuit is established, the patient's vital signs are measured within the first few minutes of treatment to assess the patient's response to the initiation of TPE.

    b. Vital signs are monitored and documented every 15–30 minutes, or as necessary during the treatment.

    c. Cardiac monitoring should accompany any TPE treatment using citrate anticoagulation.

    d. Pump flow rates, cumulative volumes, and system pressure readings should be monitored and documented every 15–30 minutes.

    e. The extracorporeal circuit is established with a blood flow rate of 45–50 mL/min for a centrifuge device and 100–150 mL/min for a plasma membrane filter device.

        (1) At these flow rates, the nurse expects a low resistance throughout the system, e.g., ± 70–150 mm Hg.

        (2) Pressure is monitored on the arterial blood inlet line and the venous pressure line.

        (3) For centrifuge equipment pressure this is monitored in the pressure display area.

        (4) Audible alarms indicate pressures outside the pressure window and require intervention by the nurse.

        (5) Pressure thresholds vary, depending on the TPE equipment used.

        (6) Manufacturer's recommendations should be followed.

    f. The initial access blood pump speed should be documented.

        (1) The pump speed can be increased by 5–10 mL/min every 15 minutes if the patient remains stable and there is adequate blood flow.

        (2) The maximum speed is determined by the device, the type of replacement fluid

infused, the equipment manufacturer's recommendations, and/or the prescription.

g. Membrane separation equipment.
  (1) The plasma filtrate pressure should be documented.
  (2) The plasma pump controls plasma removal.
  (3) The plasma flow rate varies depending upon what device or filter is used for the treatment. Often the plasma flow rate will run about 30% to 40% of the whole blood flow rate.
  (4) The plasma flow rate is also dependent on the patient's HCT.
     (a) The higher the HCT, i.e., > 40%, the faster the patient's plasma may be exchanged and the shorter the treatment will be.
     (b) For a very low HCT, i.e., < 30%, the plasma exchange may take longer.
  (5) When using FFP as a replacement fluid, plasma replacement flow rate should not exceed 40 mL/min.
  (6) During TPE with membrane filtration, monitor the patient's ACT every 20–30 minutes. Adjust heparin to maintain ACT in desired range.

2. Maintaining vascular access.
  a. It is important to maintain blood flow from the patient to prevent positive and negative system pressure alarms.
     (1) If alarms occur, the machine will pause and the reason for restricted flow should be corrected.
     (2) Flushing the access or return line with saline may correct the problem, but this dilutes the blood volume and gives the patient additional fluid.
  b. Access and return pressure changes, when using a central line, can be caused by a thrombus or a fibrin sheath around the tip of the catheter.
     (1) If a clot is present, infusion into the port may be possible, but aspiration may be compromised, leading to an increased chance of recirculation.
     (2) This can result in a less efficient plasma exchange.
  c. The fistula needles, whether using the antecubital vein or a fistula/graft, should be taped securely in place to prevent unintended removal or infiltration by patient movement.
     (1) Needle infiltration can lead to the

permanent damage or loss of the blood vessel or graft.
     (2) The insertion sites should always be visible to the nurse to ensure prompt action if an infiltration occurs or the needle is accidentally removed completely from the access.
  d. The patient should not feel constant pain at the insertion sites. "Buzzing" of the vein is common and can be alleviated by:
     (1) Having the patient squeeze and release a soft object in the hand.
     (2) Repositioning the needle of the accessed extremity to ensure proper alignment within the blood vessel.
  e. Keeping the extremity warm can dilate the vein, allowing good blood flow.

3. Fluid shifts.
  a. TPE may involve significant changes to the intravascular volume and hemodynamic changes may occur.
     (1) At the start of the TPE treatment some devices, such as the Cobe Spectra®, divert the prime saline into a waste bag leaving the patient with an initial fluid volume deficit of approximately 100–150 mL, which some patients cannot tolerate.
     (2) Those same devices often provide an option to allow the infusion of the saline prime from the disposable circuit to be given to the patient at the beginning of the treatment in order to prevent this deficit.
     (3) The decision to waste or administer the prime should be defined in the treatment order.
     (4) Other devices, such as the Fresenius AS 104®, always infuse the prime saline at the beginning of the procedure.
  b. Patients with heart disease and and/or renal failure are at a greater risk for hypervolemia.
     (1) In this situation it may be advantageous to leave the patient isovolemic by decreasing the fluid balance slightly.
     (2) The TPE machine is designed to remove pathogens and antibodies, not to perform ultrafiltration. Therefore, fluid volume removal is not routinely ordered as part of the TPE procedure.
  c. The concept of equilibration should be understood in order to prevent TPE treatments from being scheduled too closely together.
     (1) Equilibration occurs as the body attempts to restore a normal, physiologic

distribution of a particular substance in the intra and extravascular space.

(2) For example, fibrinogen is restored to its pre-apheresis level in approximately 72 hours. If a patient's fibrinogen is critically low and TPE treatments are scheduled closer than 72 hours the fibrinogen will not be able to equilibrate, leaving the patient at risk for bleeding.

4. Diagnosis related care.
   a. The nurse must take into account the mental status of the patient and provide patient care in light of this assessment.
      (1) A patient with TTP or a neurologic disorder may have an altered mental status. They may pull at or dislodge the vascular access.
      (2) It may be difficult for the patient to lie in bed for the length of time it takes to complete the TPE treatment.
      (3) The patient may need to be physically and/or chemically restrained while the treatment is taking place.
   b. Patients with cryoglobulinemia or cold-agglutinin disease cannot tolerate reduced blood temperatures. For these patients, and any patient receiving FFP as a replacement fluid, a blood warmer is added to the circuit.
   c. Certain medications and foods can affect the color of the plasma in the waste bag.
      (1) Patients with high fat or cholesterol levels may have opaque plasma.
      (2) Patients receiving antineoplastic medications may have green-tinged plasma.
      (3) Patients with disease-causing hemolysis can present with very dark-colored plasma, resembling cola or tea.
   d. It is customary to hold TPE treatments for 24 hours after a liver or renal biopsy is performed to prevent uncontrolled bleeding at the biopsy site. If TPE is necessary, adding FFP to the replacement fluid near the end of the procedure can replace lost clotting factors.
   e. TPE treatments should be timed to follow rather than precede the administration of infusions that are largely distributed to the plasma, e.g., immunoglobin, rituximab, other monoclonal antibody, or antineoplastic medications.
   f. TPE treatments typically precede rather than follow hemodialysis. The patient may present with a relatively low intravascular volume after hemodialysis related to ultrafiltration

requirements. The patient's relatively low intravascular volume makes it difficult for them to maintain adequate blood pressure during the TPE treatment.
   g. Patients with liver or renal disease may have impaired citrate metabolism and are at increased risk of citrate toxicity. These patients usually require more calcium gluconate during a treatment.
   h. Some hyperviscosity syndromes can cause significant hypotension near the end of the treatment due to the sudden change in oncotic pressure. Occasionally, they may require extra fluid boluses to safely complete the treatment.
   i. Patients receiving apheresis must have serial laboratory assessments to document improvement or decline in the patient's condition in response to the apheresis treatments.

D. TPE treatment termination.
   1. Reinfusion/rinseback of cells in extracorporeal circuit.
      a. Once the PV has been exchanged, the cells in the disposable circuit should be reinfused with a normal saline rinseback.
      b. In certain situations, rinseback/reinfusion is avoided. This must be clarified in the TPE orders and the patient's blood loss must be documented.
      c. The entire circuit, including the access and return lines and the blood warmer tubing, should be thoroughly flushed with normal saline to avoid loss of red cell volume.
   2. Disconnection from apheresis devices:
      a. The patient's access and return lines must be disconnected prior to removing the disposable circuit set from the apheresis equipment. A failure to do so can result in excess fluid or even air entering the patient's circulation.
      b. After disconnection, the patient should slowly go from a laying or sitting position to a standing position to allow for blood pressure equilibration and avoid hypotension with a potential patient fall.
   3. Care of vascular access.
      a. Peripheral access.
         (1) The needle sites must be held till hemostasis occurs.
         (2) Adequate pressure is held to prevent bleeding, but not occlude intravascular blood flow.
         (3) A dressing is then secured over the site.

(4) Patients should be instructed to resume direct pressure at the site if bleeding reoccurs spontaneously after the nurse has left.
b. CVC.
(1) Flush with normal saline.
(2) Fill with heparin or other anticoagulant. Fill volume is printed on the catheter.
(3) The concentration of the heparin fill is dictated by facility policy and varies from 1000–5000 units/mL.
(4) The exit site dressing on the catheter should be clean and dry at all times to prevent infection.
(5) Document catheter and exit site assessment and care.
(6) Educate the patient regarding catheter care and infection prevention, e.g., have the patient verbalize signs and symptoms of CVC infection.
(7) The CVC should be labeled to clarify the catheter must only be used for TPE and/or hemodialysis.
4. Disposing of the TPE circuit.
a. The patient's plasma is collected in a closed collection container, and it must be handled using standard precautions for blood products.
b. Disposable supplies are discarded in contaminated/biohazard waste receptacles with care to remove any needles that may be a part of the system.
c. Needles must be disposed of in an appropriate sharps container.
d. The machine is cleaned and stored in an area where it will not obstruct patient care or safety.

E. Adverse events (see Table 3.42).
1. Reaction to TPE with FFP or albumin.
a. Mild: reactions that can normally be anticipated and/or treated successfully without discontinuation of the procedure. Signs and symptoms include hypotension, parasthesia, hyperventilation, nausea, and lightheadedness.
b. Moderate: mild reactions persisting for ≥ 20 minutes.
c. Severe: moderate reactions along with any or all of the following:
(1) Respiratory insufficiency.
(2) Convulsions.
(3) Rigidity or tremor of the extremities.
(4) Cardiopulmonary arrest.
(5) Death.
2. Vasovagal reaction.

a. Hypotensive reaction in patients undergoing TPE procedures triggered by severe pain, anxiety, or other circumstances.
b. This reaction is caused by activation of the autonomic nervous system and can occur before, during, or after the procedure.
3. Citrate toxicity.
a. Citrate administration exceeds the rate of citrate metabolism, e.g., impaired liver or kidney function. Calcium binds to the citrate and symptoms of hypocalcaemia ensue.
b. Mild: perioral numbness and tingling. Pediatric patients may experience nausea and vomiting.
c. Moderate: muscle twitching.
d. Severe: tetany muscle spasm.
e. Treat by reducing the citrate infusion rate and providing IV calcium.

F. Pharmacology.
1. Few clinical studies have been done to assess medication removal during plasma exchange.
2. Medications distributed in the plasma.
a. If a medication has a low volume of distribution and a high affinity for plasma proteins, then the medication should not be administered before plasma exchange.
b. Medications included in this class are some antibiotics and immunoglobulins.
3. Medications distributed outside of the plasma.
a. Many of the medications routinely given to dialysis and apheresis patients are not bound to plasma proteins and have a higher volume of distribution, meaning that the medications migrate into the extravascular tissues and cells.
b. Any medication that is within a blood cell will not be eliminated with the plasma.
c. Medications in this class include prednisone and other steroids and a majority of antibiotics.
4. Frequency of administration.
a. The frequency of medication administration can influence how quickly a medication is distributed in the plasma volume and how effectively it is removed during TPE.
b. Medications taken once a day should be taken after a TPE procedure.
c. Medications taken at more frequent intervals have a better chance of being distributed into the extravascular tissues and are less likely to be removed during TPE.
d. Patients taking angiotensin-converting enzyme (ACE) inhibitors within a 24-hour period before TPE can develop bradykinin

Table 3.42

Adverse Events

Problem	Signs & Symptoms	Potential Cause	Treatment	Rationale
Allergic reaction (Mild)	Urticaria Itching Rhinitis Cough	Allergy to iodine	Cleanse skin with an alternative antimicrobial	Decrease amount of allergic substance to the patient
		Allergy to FFP	Pause procedure, consider Benadryl, continue procedure if symptoms subside	Decrease generation of allergic substances
		Allergy to albumin	Change albumin to Dextran 40 or HES and/or saline after consult with physician	Decrease amount of allergic substance to the patient
Allergic reaction/ Anaphylactic (Moderate/ Severe)	Widespread urticaria Itching Rhinitis Cough Tongue swelling Wheezing	Allergy to FFP	Stop procedure Change unit of FFP Consider Benadryl Consider short-acting steroid Consult with MD	Decrease amount of allergic substance to the patient May require further medical attention
Air embolus (rare)	Chest Pain SOB Shock Pallor Confusion Cold sweats Death	Air entering venous system via tubing Requires >15–25 mL in adults	Stop procedure and put patient on left side and Trendelenburg Consult with MD	Minimize effect on circulation Symptomatic treatment of SOB May require further medical treatment
Anxiety/ Apprehension	Restlessness Pallor Perspiration	Psychological (fear of procedure)	Reassure patient Be alert for signs of anxiety	Treat early symptoms Reverse possible causes Prevent further reaction
		Hypovolemia	Pause treatment Open IV lines to NS Consult with MD	Treat early symptoms Reverse possible causes Prevent further reaction
		Hypotension	Pause treatment Trendelenburg Open IV lines to NS Consult with MD	Treat early symptoms Reverse possible causes Prevent further reaction
		Allergic reaction	Consider drugs Consult with MD	Decrease generation of allergic substances
		Citrate toxicity	Decrease blood flow rates of blood return Warm with blanket or use blood warmer	Allow citrate to be metabolized Provide warmth to increase metabolism
		Hyperventilation	Have patient breathe into paper bag	Decrease respiratory alkalosis

Table continues

Table 3.42 (page 2 of 3) ———————— **Adverse Events**

Problem	Signs & Symptoms	Potential Cause	Treatment	Rationale
Arrhythmia	Pulse rate <60 or >100 Irregular pulse Both may cause: hypotension, dizziness, anxiety, perspiration, nausea or citrate toxicity	Vasovagal reaction Hypovolemia Hypotension Citrate toxicity Anaphylaxis	Stop procedure Identify cause Consult with MD	Maintain perfusion May require further medical attention
Cardiac arrest	Cessation of pulse and respiration	Citrate toxicity (rare) Severe hypotension or convulsion Related to primary disease	Stop procedure and initiate emergency resuscitation Initiate a CODE or call for emergency services Consult with MD	Must maintain oxygen perfusion
Chills/Tingling	Feeling cold especially in extremities, nose and ears Vibratory or tingling sensation of face and extremities	Cold blood return	Use blood warmer or warm blankets	Some replacement fluids are below room temperature
		Anxiety	Educate and reassure patient frequently	Patients who know what to expect have less fear of procedure
		Citrate effect	Slow blood return consider Administering oral calcium (TUMS) in adult patient	Allow citrate to be metabolized Source of non-prescription calcium
		Hyperventilation	Use paper bag for hyperventilation	Decrease respiratory alkalosis
Citrate toxicity (mild)	Circumoral paresthesia Chills Coldness Vibratory or tingling sensation in face and extremities	Decrease in circulating ionized calcium	Slow or stop procedure until symptoms subside	Allow citrate to be metabolized
			Cover with blanket or use blood warmer	Provide warmth to increase metabolism
			Consider TUMS in adult patient	Source of nonprescription calcium
Citrate toxicity (moderate to severe)	Heaviness in chest Nausea/vomiting Muscle cramps Cardiac arrhythmias (irregular pulse) Tetany Cardiac arrest	Decrease in circulating ionized calcium	Stop procedure Consult with MD Consider IV Calcium Gluconate Treat arrhythmias Call CODE or emergency services	Allow citrate to be metabolized Replace calcium Further medical attention may be necessary
Congestive heart failure	SOB Chest pain Shock Pallor Confusion Death	Fluid overload	Raise HOB Reduce fluid infusion to KVO to maintain patent IV access Consult with MD Initiate CODE or emergency services if patient loses consciousness	Prevent additional fluids from building around the heart Prevent exacerbation of CHF Allow for injection of medication if necessary May require further medical attention

Table continues

Table 3.42 (page 3 of 3) ———— **Adverse Events**

Problem	Signs & Symptoms	Potential Cause	Treatment	Rationale
Fever	Temperature increase >1 C during procedure May be accompanied by rigors	Incompatible blood transfusion Bacteremia: infected catheter Primary disease	Stop procedure and obtain blood sample as needed for lab Consult with MD	Stop infusion with potentially incompatible blood Obtain sample for workup and cultures May require further medical attention
Hemolysis	PINK or RED plasma Fever/chills Chest or back pain	Lysis of red blood cells May be caused by faulty disposable set May be caused by incompatible blood transfusion	Discontinue procedure immediately Consult with MD Notify manager	Do not return any additional hemolyzed cells to the patient Determination should be made as quickly as possible to determine cause in order to take appropriate corrective action Manager to notify manufacturer if equipment is suspected of being faulty
Hypotension	Restlessness Lightheadedness Dizziness Nausea/vomiting SOB	Vasovagal reaction Hypovolemia Citrate toxicity Anaphylaxis	Stop procedure Trendelenburg Consider saline infusion Rinseback blood if possible Consult with MD	Expand blood volume, restore blood pressure and normalize circulation May require further medical attention
Hypovolemia	Decrease in BP Increase in pulse Pallor Dizziness Weakness Syncope	Volume loss usually greater than 15% of patients estimated blood volume	Stop treatment Trendelenburg Rinseback blood Consider saline infusion Consult with MD	Stop volume loss Increase venous return Replacement of lost volume May require further medical treatment
Nausea/Vomiting	May be accompanied by lightheadedness, hyperventilation, bradycardia, tachycardia and/or hypotension	Hypotension Vasovagal reaction Hypovolemia Severe allergic reaction Citrate toxicity	As per potential cause	As per potential cause
Vasovagal reaction (mild)	Decrease in BP and pulse Pallor Dizziness Weakness Lightheadedness Hyperventilation Nausea Sweating	Anxiety Fear Pain Rapid blood removal from circulation Fatigue Hunger	Stop procedure Trendelenburg Open IVs to saline Instruction patient on procedure and reassure frequently throughout procedure Apply cold compress to forehead or back of neck For hyperventilation, have patient breathe into a paper bag Consult with MD	Increase venous return If patient has good understanding of procedure, their fears are more likely to be alleviated. The more comfortable a patient is, the less likely they will have this type of reaction Decrease respiratory alkalosis
Vasovagal (moderate to severe)	Bradycardia Hypotension Syncope	Anxiety Fear Pain Rapid blood removal from circulation Fatigue Hunger	Stop procedure Trendelenburg Open IVs to saline Consult with MD If pulse < 40 may require atropine with MD order	Improve perfusion May require further medical attention

reactions, exhibiting hypotensive, bradycardic episodes with accompanying symptoms of flushing, nausea and vomiting. ACE inhibitors must be held for 24–72 hours before a TPE procedure.

5. Medication used during TPE treatments.
  a. Citrate.
    (1) ACD-A is a 3% citrate solution and is used with the COBE centrifugal and membrane systems.
    (2) Citrate is added to the blood as it is drawn from the patient and prevents blood from clotting in the circuit.
    (3) Circuit anticoagulation, without citrate toxicity is the goal during a TPE treatment.
    (4) ACD-A or 3% sodium citrate solution can be instilled in the ports of a CVC at the end of a TPE treatment when a patient is allergic to heparin or has developed a heparin-induced thrombocytopenia.
    (5) Anticoagulant citrate dextrose formula B (ACD-B®) (Baxter-Fenwal Corporation, Deerfield, Illinois) has a much lower concentration of citrate and is used with the Haemonetics, centrifugal system. Care should be taken to select the desired ACD formula.
  b. Heparin.
    (1) Heparin is used as an anticoagulant during TPE to prevent clot formation in the TPE circuit.
    (2) Heparin, in a concentration of 1000–5000 units/mL, is used to fill the CVC. This assists in maintaining catheter patency between treatments.
    (3) This CVC heparin fill must be withdrawn prior to using the CVC for subsequent treatments.
  c. Calcium.
    (1) 10% calcium gluconate.
      (a) When using FFP/CRP as a replacement fluid, 10% calcium gluconate can be administered in small increments through an injection port on the return tubing, through a stopcock piggybacked into the return tubing, or as a slow continuous infusion in a separate IV line.
      (b) Critically ill patients and those patients sensitive to citrate may benefit from a continuous calcium infusion throughout the TPE treatment to prevent symptoms of hypocalcemia.
    (2) Calcium chloride.
      (a) This medication should not be

routinely used with TPE.
      (b) It is three times as potent as 10% calcium gluconate.
      (c) It must be diluted before administering to a patient.
    (3) Calcium carbonate.
      (a) Oral calcium in the form of chewable calcium tablets may be given to a patient receiving TPE with citrate anticoagulation. One tablet every 30 minutes will supplement the patient's calcium and may prevent symptoms of hypocalcemia.
      (b) Each TUMS® (GlaxoSmithKline, Brentford, Middlesex, United Kingdom) tablet contains 500 mg of calcium.
  d. Tylenol®, acetaminophen.
    (1) Premedications are given before using FFP or CRP as a replacement fluid to mitigate transfusion reactions.
    (2) Tylenol is used to suppress temperature spikes during the infusion of blood products.
  e. Benadryl®, diphenhydramine hydrochloride.
    (1) This medication may be administered before and/or midway through the treatment.
    (2) It is used to prevent histamine reactions to blood products that can lead to hives and rashes.
  f. Epinephrine.
    (1) Part of the adrenergic family of medications, it is used with TPE to relieve bronchospasms during respiratory distress and to relieve hypersensitivity reactions to medications and blood products.
    (2) It should be given cautiously and in emergencies.
  g. Steroids.
    (1) Solu-Cortef®, hydrocortisone is used as a premedication before using FFP/CRP as replacement fluid to suppress the immune system and therefore inhibit autoantibody and allergic responses to substances in the replacement fluid. The usual adult dosage is 50–100 mg IV.
    (2) Solu-Medrol®, methylprednisolone is used primarily in TPE as an antiinflammatory or immunosuppressant agent. The usual adult dose is 50–100 mg IV.
    (3) Patient allergies and pharmacy availability will determine which of these steroids is used during a plasma exchange treatment.

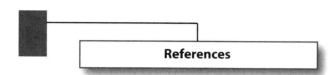

References

Abdelbasit, A., & Finlayson, M. (2004). Effect of cool temperature dialysate on the quality and patients' perception of haemodialysis. *Nephrology Dialysis Transplantation, 19*, 190-194.

Abernathy, V.E., & Lieberthal, W. (2002). Acute renal failure in the critically ill patient. *Critical Care Clinics, 18*, 203-222.

Acute dialysis quality initiative. (n.d.) Retrieved June 2, 2007, from http://www.adqi.net/

Agrawal, M., & Swartz, R. (2000). Acute renal failure. *American Family Physician, 61*, 2077-2088.

Allon, M., Dunlay, R., & Copkney, C. (1989). Nebulized albuterol for acute hyperkalemia in patients on hemodialysis. *Annals of Internal Medicine, 110*(6), 426-429.

Amgen, Inc. (1992). *Core curriculum for the dialysis technician.* Medical Media Publishing, Inc.

Aronoff, G., Berns, J., & Brier, M. (1999). *Drug prescribing in renal failure: Dosing guidelines for adults* (4th ed.). Philadelphia: American College of Physicians.

Asahi Kasei Medical Co., Ltd. (2001). *Plasmaflo AP-05H (L): Asahi plasma separator package insert.* Tokyo, Japan: Author.

Ascension Health. (2005). *Heatlhcare ethics.* Retrieved June 27, 2006, from http://www.ascensionhealth.org/ethics/public/issues/patient_self.asp

B. Braun Medical, Inc. (2007). *Diapact CRRT.* Retrieved June 2, 2007, from http://www.bbraunusa.com/

Baxter Healthcare Corporation. (2000). *Autopheresis-C system overview.* Deerfield, IL: Author.

Baxter International, Inc. (n.d.). *ACCURA: CRRT instrument.* Retrieved June 2, 2007, from http://www.baxter.com/products/renal/crrt/sub/accura.html

Bellomo, R., Ronco, C., Kellum, J.A., Mehta, R.L., Palevshy, P., & The ADQI Workgroup. (2004). Acute renal failure – definition, outcome measures, animal models, fluid therapy and information technology needs: The second international consensus conference of the acute dialysis quality initiative (ADQI) group. *Critical Care, 8*(4), R204-R212.

Berbece, A., & Richardson, R. (2006). Sustained low-efficiency dialysis in the ICU: Cost, anticoagulation, and solute removal. *Kidney International, 70*(5), 963-968.

Bergs, L. (2005). Goodpasture syndrome. *Critical Care Nurse, 25*, 50-58.

Block, C.A., & Manning, H.L. (2002). Prevention of acute renal failure in the critically ill. *American Journal of Respiratory Critical Care Medicine, 165*, 320-324.

Burgstaler, E.A. (1997). Current instrumentation for apheresis. In B.C. McLeod, T.H. Price, & J.J. Drew (Eds.), *Apheresis: Principles and practice* (1st ed., pp. 85-112). Bethesda, MD: AABB Press.

Burgstaler, E.A. (2002). Apheresis instrumentation. In I.D. Zielinski (Ed.), *Principles of apheresis technology* (3rd ed., pp. 41-55). Vancouver, B.C.: American Society for Apheresis.

Burrows-Hudson, S. (Ed.). (1993). *Standards of clinical practice for nephrology nursing.* Pitman, NJ: American Nephrology Nurses' Association.

Burrows-Hudson, S., & Prowant, B.F. (Eds.). (2005). *Nephrology nursing standards of practice and guidelines for care.* Pitman, NJ: American Nephrology Nurses' Association.

Cardiothoracic Care Guidelines. (2004). Physiological characteristics and clinical effects of commonly used intravenous solutions. *UpToDate Online.*

Chadha, V., Garg, U., Warady, B.A., & Alon, U.S. (2002). Citrate clearance in children receiving continuous venovenous renal replacement therapy. *Pediatric Nephrology, 17*, 819-824.

Chernecky, C.C., & Berger, B.J. (2001). *Laboratory tests and diagnostic procedures* (3rd ed.). Philadelphia: W.B. Saunders.

Christiansen, L. (2006). *Focus 11 class notes: Health law and ethics.* Omaha, NE: Clarkson College.

Clarkson, M.R., Giblin, L., O'Connell, F.P., O'Kelly, P., Walshe, J.J., Conlon, P., et al. (2004). Acute interstitial nephritis: Clinical features and response to corticosteroid therapy. *Nephrology Dialysis Transplantation, 19*, 2778-2783.

Clough, L.F. (2002). Pharmacology in apheresis. In I.D. Zielinski (Ed.), *Principles of apheresis technology* (3rd ed., pp. 41-55). Vancouver, B.C.: American Society for Apheresis.

Corbin, F., Cullis, H.M., Freireich, E.J., Ito, Y., Kellogg, R.M., Latham, A., et al. (1997). Development of apheresis instrumentation. In B.C. McLeod, T.H. Price, & J.J. Drew (Eds.), *Apheresis: Principles and practice* (1st ed., pp. 1-26). Bethesda, MD: AABB Press.

Crabtree, J.H., & Fishman, A. (2005). A laparoscopic method for optimal peritoneal dialysis access. *The American Surgeon, 2*(70), 135-143.

Crabtree, J.H., Kaiser, K.E., Huen, I.T., & Fishman, A. (2001). Cost-effectiveness of peritoneal dialysis catheter implantation by laparoscopy versus by open dissection. *Advances in Peritoneal Dialysis, 17*, 88-92.

Craig, M. (1998a). Applications in continuous venous to venous hemofiltration. Interactive case studies in the adult patient. *Critical Care Nursing Clinics of North America, 10*(2), 209-221.

Craig, M. (1998b). Continuous venous to venous hemofiltration: implementing and maintaining a program: Examples and alternatives. *Critical Care Nursing Clinics of North America, 10*(2), 219-233.

Craig, M.A., Depner, T.A., Chin, E., Tweedy, R.L., Hokana, L., & Newby-Lintz, M. (1996). Implementing a continuous renal replacement therapies program. *Advances in Renal Replacement Therapy, 3*(4), 348-350.

Culley, C., Bernardo, J., Gross, P.R., Guttendorf, S., Whiteman, K.A., Kowiatek, J.G., et al. (2006). Implementing a standardized safety procedure for continuous renal replacement therapy solutions. *American Journal of Health-System Pharmacy, 63*(8), 756-763.

Cwiertniewicz, M. (2001). The gerontologic patient with renal failure. In L.E. Lancaster (Ed.), *Core curriculum for nephrology nursing* (4th ed., pp. 430-433). Pitman, NJ: American Nephrology Nurses' Association.

Daugirdas, J.T., Blake, P.G., & Ing, T.S. (2001). *Handbook of dialysis* (3rd ed.). Philadelphia: Lippincott Williams & Wilkins.

Depner, T., Craig, M., Hu, K., Kumar, V., Tarne, J., & Yeun, J. (1999). Solute kinetics during extended daily hemodialysis in the intensive care unit (ICU) [Abstract]. *American Society for Artificial Internal Organs Journal, 45,* 185.

Dialysis Clinic, Inc. (DCI) Acute Service. (2006). *Acute education manual.* Omaha, NE: Author.

Dirkes, S. (2000). Continuous renal replacement therapy: Dialytic therapy for acute renal failure in intensive care. *Nephrology Nursing Journal, 27*(6), 581-592.

Dirkes, S., & Hodge, K. (2007). Continuous renal replacement therapy in the adult intensive care unit: History and trends. *Critical Care Nurse, 27*(2), 61-80.

Donauer, J., Kolblin, D., Bek, M., Krause, A., & Bohler, J. (2000). Ultrafiltration profiling and measurement of relative blood volume as strategies to reduce hemodialysis-related side effects. *American Journal of Kidney Diseases, 36*(1), 115-123.

Elhanan, N., Skippen, P., Nuthall, G., Krahn, G., & Seear, M. (2004). Citrate anticoagulation in pediatric continuous venovenous hemofiltration. *Pediatric Nephrology, 19,* 208-212.

Emili, S., Black, N.A., Paul, R.V., Rexing, C.J., & Ullian, M.E. (1999). A protocol-based treatment for intradialytic hypotension in hospitalized hemodialysis patients. *American Journal of Kidney Disease, 33*(6), 1107-1114.

Esson, M.L., & Schrier, R.W. (2002). Diagnosis and treatment of acute tubular necrosis. *Annals of Internal Medicine, 137,* 744-752.

Fernandes, N.M.S., Cendoroglo, M., Roque, A., Batista, P.B.P, Santos, O.F.P., Stella, R.S., et al. (2001). *Serial prognostic score indexes in acute renal failure (ARF): Best performance of scores obtained at the time of referral to the nephrologist.* Retrieved May 1, 2006, from http://ccforum.com/content/5/S3/P39

Fine, A., & Penner, B. (1996). The protective effect of cool dialysate is dependent on patients' predialysis temperature. *American Journal of Kidney Disease, 28*(2), 262-265.

Forum of End Stage Renal Disease Networks. (2006). *ESRD networks.* Retrieved April 7, 2006, from http://www.esrd networks.org

Fresenius, USA. (2002a). *2008K hemodialysis machine operator's manual.* Walnut Creek, CA: Author.

Fresenius, USA. (2002b). *Fresenius AS104 blood cell separator training manual.* Redmond, WA: Fresenius HemoCare.

Fry, A.C., & Farrington, K. (2006). Management of acute renal failure. *Postgraduate Medicine Journal, 82,* 106-116.

Gambro. (n.d.). *Prisma and Prismaflex.* Retrieved June 2, 2007, from http://www.USA-Gambro.com

Gambro BCT, Inc. (1996). *COBE spectra apheresis system operator's manual.* Lakewood, CO: Author.

Gardner, J. (2005). Managing preeclampsia buys time for a safe delivery. *Nursing 2005, 35,* 50-52.

Garrett, T., Baillie, H., & Garrett, R. (2001). *Health care ethics: Principles and problems* (4th ed.). Englewood Cliffs, NJ: Prentice Hall.

Gillum, D. (2005). *Vasopressors.* Lecture presented at Western Nephrology & Metabolic Bone Disease, Denver, Colorado.

Goldstein, S. (2003). Overview of pediatric renal replacement therapy in acute renal failure. *Artificial Organs, 27*(9), 781-785.

Goldstein, S., Currier, H., Graf, C., Cosio, C.C., Brewer, E.D., &

Sachdeva, R. (2001). Outcome in children receiving continuous venvenous hemofiltration, *Pediatrics, 107*(6), 1309-1312.

Golper, T. (2004). Hybrid renal replacement therapies for critically ill patients. Sepsis, kidney and multiple organ dysfunction. *Contributions to Nephrology, 144,* 278-283.

Golper, T. (2006a, May 8). Dialysis in acute renal failure: indications and dialysis dose. *UpToDate Online.*

Golper, T. (2006b, May 2). Use of peritoneal dialysis for the treatment of acute renal failure. *UpToDate Online.*

Greene, J.H., & Hoffart, N. (2001). Nutrition in renal failure, dialysis, and transplantation. In L.E. Lancaster (Ed.), *Core curriculum for nephrology nursing* (4th ed., pp. 213-215). Pitman, NJ: American Nephrology Nurses' Association.

Gutch, C.F., Stoner, M., & Corea, A. (Eds.). (1993). *Review of hemodialysis for nurses and dialysis personnel* (5th ed) St Louis: Mosby Year Book, Inc.

Halfman, M., & Reiner, S. (Ed.) (2001). *Quick guide to central venous access.* Irvine, CA: Edwards Lifesciences, L.L.C.

Henrich, W.L. (1999). *Principles and practice of dialysis* (2nd ed., pp. 32-33). Philadelphia: Lippincott Williams & Wilkins.

Henrich, W.L. (2006, April 27). Hemodynamic instability during hemodialysis: Overview. *UpToDate Online.*

Hodges, R.K., Garrett, K.M., Chernecky, C., & Schumacher, L. (2005). *Real-world nursing survival guide: Hemodynamic monitoring.* St. Louis: Elsevier Saunders.

Holley, J.L. (2005, August 28). Muscle cramps in dialysis patients. *UpToDate Online.*

Hotchkiss, R.S., & Karl, I.E. (2003). The pathophysiology and treatment of sepsis. *The New England Journal of Medicine, 348,* 138-148.

Johnson, R.J., & Feehally, J. (2003). *Comprehensive clinical nephrology* (2nd ed., p. 120). St. Louis: Mosby.

Kale-Pradham, P.B., & Woo, M.H. (1997). A review of the effects of plasmapheresis on drug clearance. *Pharmacotherapy, 17,* 684-695.

Kallstrom, T.J. (2002). American association of respiratory care clinical practice guideline: Oxygen therapy for adults in the acute care facility 2002 revision & update. *Respiratory Care, 47*(6), 717-720.

Kintzel, P., Eastlund, T., & Calis, K.A. (2004). Extracorporeal removal of antimicrobials during plasmapheresis. *Journal of Clinical Apheresis, 18,* 194-205.

Kiprov, D., Golden, P., Rohe, R., Smith, S., & Weaver, R. (2001). Adverse reactions associated with mobile therapeutic apheresis-analysis of 17,940 procedures. *Journal of Clinical Apheresis, 15,* 19-21.

Knaus, W.A., Draper, E.A., Wagner, D.P., & Zimmerman, J.E. (1985). APACHE II: A severity of disease classification system. *Critical Care Medicine, 13,* 818-829.

Koo, A.P. (2000). Therapeutic apheresis in autoimmune and rheumatic diseases. *Journal of Clinical Apheresis, 15,* 19-21.

Kumar, V., Craig, M., Depner, T., & Yeun, J. (2000). Extended daily dailysis: A new approach to renal replacement therapy for acute renal failure in the intensive care unit. *American Journal of Kidney Disease, 36,* 294-300.

Lameire, N., VanBiesen, W., & Vanholder, R. (2005). Acute renal failure. *The Lancet, 365,* 417-430.

Lancaster, L.E. (1990). Renal response to shock. *Critical Care Nursing Clinics of North America, 2,* 221-223.

Levin, N. (1998). Time on dialysis. *American Journal of Kidney Disease, 32*(6 Suppl. 4), S83-S85.

Levine, D.Z. (Ed). (1997). *Caring for the renal patient* (3rd ed.). Philadelphia: W.B. Saunders Co.

Lichtenthal, P.R. (1998). *Quick guide to cardiopulmonary care.* Irvine: Edwards Lifesciences L.L.C.

Lokhandwala, K.A. (2002). Clinical signs in medicine: Pulsus paradoxus. *Clinical Signs, 48*(1), 46-49.

Madison, J., Depner, T., & Chin, A. (2006). *Alternatives to heparin anticoagulation during slow extended daily dialysis in the ICU* [Abstract]. Retrieved June 2, 2007, from http://www.citrasate.com/pdf/nkfposter.pdf

Maggiore, Q. (2002). Isothermic dialysis for hypotension-prone patients. *Seminars in Dialysis, 15*(3), 187-190.

Martin, R. (2002). Who should manage continuous renal replacement in the intensive care setting? A nursing viewpoint. *The European Dialysis and Transplant Nurses Association/European Renal Care Association Journal,* (Suppl. 2), 43-45, 53.

McCormick, J.D. (1981, Nov/Dec). Care of the critically ill acute renal failure patient. *Critical Care Nurse,* 47-52.

Mehta, R. (1990). Regional citrate anticoagulation for continuous arteriovenous hemodialysis in critically ill patients. *Kidney International, 38,* 976-981.

Mehta, R., & Martin, R. (1996). Initiating and implementing a continuous renal replacement therapy program: Require-ments and guidelines. *Seminars in Dialysis, 9*(2), 80-87.

Mehta, R.L., Pascual, M.T., Soroko, S., Savage, B.R., Himmelfarb, J., Ikizler, T.A., et al. (2004). Spectrum of acute renal failure in the intensive care unit: The PICARD experience. *Kidney International, 66,* 1613-1621.

Mellwig, K.P., Baller, D., Gleichmann, U., & Moll, D. (1998). Improvement of coronary vasodilation capacity through single LD apheresis. *Atherosclerosis, 139,* 173-178.

Monahan, L. (2002). *A practical guide to health assessment.* Philadelphia: W.B. Saunders Co.

Mujias, S., Crabtree, J.H., Firanek, C.A., Piriano, B., & Abu-Alfa, A.K. (2006). *Access care and complications management: Care of the adult patient on peritoneal dialysis.* Baxter Health Care Corporation.

Myers, L. (2002). Thrombotic thrombocytopenic purpura-hemolytic uremic syndrome: Pathophysiology and management. *Nephrology Nursing Journal, 29,* 171-182.

Nissenson, A.R., & Fine, R. (1995). *Dialysis therapy* (3rd ed.). Norwalk, CT: Appleton & Lange.

NxStage Medical, Inc. (2007). *NxStage system one: Acute renal care.* Retrieved June 2, 2007, from http://www.nxstage.com/acute_renal_care

Owen, H.G., & Brecher, M.E. (1997). Management of the therapeutic apheresis patient. In B.C. McLeod (Ed.), *Apheresis: Principles and practice* (1st ed., pp. 223-238). Bethesda, MD: AABB Press.

Padden, M.O. (1999). HELLP syndrome: Recognition and perinatal management. *American Family Physician, 60,* 829-836.

Patel, V., James, P., & Smith, T. (2006). *Digitalis toxicity.* Retrieved Jun 16, 2006, from http://www.emedicine.com/med/topic568.htm

Pillitteri, A. (Ed.). (2002). *Maternal and child health nursing* (4th ed.). Philadelphia: Lippincott Williams & Wilkins.

Piraino, B., Bailie, G.R., Bernardini, J., Boeschoten, E., Gupta, A., Holmes, C., et al. (2005). *ISPD guidelines/recommendations peritoneal dialysis: Peritoneal dialysis-related infections.* Retrieved February 6, 2008, from http://www.ispd.org/guidelines/03Piraino4237ISPD%20with%20watermark.pdf

Price, C. (2001a). Continuous renal replacement therapy. In L.E. Lancaster (Ed.), *Core curriculum for nephrology nursing* (4th ed., pp. 452-477). Pitman, NJ: American Nephrology Nurses' Association.

Price, C. (2001b). Therapeutic plasma exchange. In L.E. Lancaster (Ed.), *Core curriculum for nephrology nursing* (4th ed., pp. 479-499). Pitman, NJ: American Nephrology Nurses' Association.

Price, C. (2003). Resources for planning palliative and end-of-life care for patients with kidney disease. *Nephrology Nursing Journal, 30*(6), 649-664.

Rabetoy, C.P. (2006). Acute renal failure. In A. Molzahn & E. Butera (Eds.), *Contemporary nephrology nursing: Principles and practice* (2nd ed., pp. 203-217). Pitman, NJ: American Nephrology Nurses' Association.

Richard, C.J. (2001). Renal disorders. In L.E. Lancaster (Ed.). *Core curriculum for nephrology nursing* (4th ed., pp. 85-95; 113-114). Pitman, NJ: American Nephrology Nurses' Association.

Rippe, B., & Levin, L. (2000). Computer simulations of ultrafiltration profiles for an Icodextrin-based peritoneal fluid in CAPD. *Kidney International, 47,* 2546-2556.

Ronco, C., & Bellomo, R. (2007). Dialysis in intensive care unit patients with acute kidney injury: Continuous therapy is superior. *Clinical Journal of the American Society of Nephrology, 2,* 597-600.

Ronco, C., Bellomo, R., Homel, P., Brendolan, A., Dan, M., Piccinni, P., et al. (2000). Effects of different doses in contin-uous veno-venous hemofiltration on outcomes of acute renal failure: A prospective randomised trial. *Lancet, 356,* 26-30.

Ronco, C., Bellomo, R., Homel, P., Brendolan, A., Dan, M., Piccinni, P., et al. (2002). Effects of different doses in continuous venovenous haemofiltration on outcomes of acute renal failure: A prospective randomised trial. *EDTNA ERCA Journal,* Suppl. 2, 7-12.

Russell, T.A. (2005). Acute renal failure related to rhabdomyolysis: pathophysiology, diagnosis, and collaborative management. *Nephrology Nursing Journal, 32,* 409-417.

Salvatori, G., Ricci, Z., Bonello, M., Ratanarat, R., D'Intini, V., Brendolan, A., et al. (2004). First clinical trial for a new CRRT machine: The Prismaflex. *International Journal of Artificial Organs, 27*(5), 404-409.

Sanderson, N.A., & Katx, M.A. (1994). The fate of hypertonic saline administered during hemodialysis. *American Nephrology Nursing Journal, 21*(4), 162-168.

Santos, P.W., Hartle, J.E. II, & Quarles, L.P. (2006). *Calciphylaxis.* Retrieved May 30, 2007, from http://www.utdol.com/utd/content/topic.do?topicKey=dialysis/45813&type=A&selectedTitle=1~9

Saudan, P., Niederberger, M., De Seigneux, S., Romand, J., Pugin, J., Perneger, T., et al. (2006). Adding a dialysis dose to continuous hemofiltration increases survival in patients with acute renal failure. *Kidney International, 70*(7), 1312-1317.

Sauret, J.M., & Marinides, G. (2002). Rhabdomyolysis. *American Family Physician, 65,* 907-912.

Schiffl, H., Lang, S., & Fischer, R. (2002). Daily hemodialysis and the outcome of acute renal failure. *New England Journal of Medicine, 346*(5), 305-310.

Schilling-McAnn, J.A. (2005). *Nursing 2005 drug handbook* (25th ed.) Philadelphia: Lippincott Williams & Wilkins.

Schmidt, R., Roeher, O., Hickstein, H., & Korth, S. (2001). Prevention of haemodialysis-induced hypotension by biofeedback control of ultrafiltration and infusion. *Nephrology Dialysis Transplant, 16,* 595-603.

Schwarz, A., Krause, P.H., Kunzendorf, U., Keller, F., & Distler, A. (2000). The outcome of acute interstitial nephritis: Risk factors for the transition from acute to chronic interstitial nephritis. *Clinical Nephrology, 54,* 179-190.

Shea, M., Hmiel, S.P., & Beck, A.M. (2001). Use of tissue plasminogen activator for thrombolysis in occluded peritoneal dialysis catheters in children. *Advances in Peritoneal Dialysis, 17,* 249-252.

Sink, B.L. (2002). History of the development of apheresis. In I.D. Zielinski (Ed.), *Principles of apheresis technology* (3rd ed., pp. 31-34). Vancouver, B.C.: American Society for Apheresis.

Smith, S., Smith, J., Leiva, J. Rohe-Penton, R., Stricker, R., & Kiprov, D. (1993). Quality assurance and improvement in therapeutic plasmapheresis-ACD reactions in patients with myasthenia Gravis. *Journal of Clinical Apheresis, 8,* 54.

Social Security Online. (n.d.). *Medicare coverage for end stage renal disease patients, section 1881 (42 U.S.C. 1395rr).* Retrieved April 6, 2006, from http://www.ssa.gov/OP_Home/ssact/title18/1881.htm

Springhouse Corporation. (1997). *Fluid and electrolytes made incredibly easy.* Philadelphia: Lippincott, Williams & Wilkins.

Szczepiorkowski, Z. (2007). Clinical applications of therapeutic apheresis: An evidence based approach. *Journal of Clinical Apheresis, 22*(3), 101-103.

Taipei Veterans General Hospital. (n.d.). *The sequential organ failure assessment score.* Retrieved May 1, 2006, from http://www.vghtpe.gov.tw/-icu/SOFA.htm

Terrone, D.A., Isler, C.M., May, W.L., Magann, E.F., Norman, P.F., & Martin, J.N. (2000). Cardiopulmonary morbidity as a complication of severe preeclampsia HELLP syndrome. *Journal of Perinatology, 2,* 78-81.

Traub, S.J. (2007). ASA intoxication overview. *UpToDate Online.*

U.S. Food and Drug Administration (FDA). (2005). *Important safety information on interference with blood glucose measurement following use of parenteral maltose/parenteral galactose/oral xylose-containing products.* Retrieved February 7, 2008, from http://www.fda.gov/Cber/safety/maltose110405.htm

U.S. Food and Drug Administration (FDA). (2006). *Updated public health notification: Gambro Prisma® continuous renal replacement system.* Retrieved June 2, 2007, from http://www.fda.gov/cdrh/safety/022706-gambro.html

Vriese, A.S. (2003). Prevention and treatment of acute renal failure in sepsis. *Journal of American Society of Nephrology, 14,* 792-805.

Wade, A., Arcuri, A., Hamiwka, L., Grisaru, S., Ross, B.C., Connors, M.R., et al. (2006). Use of the Freseinus 2008K hemodialysis (HD) machine for CRRT in children. *Pediatric Nephrology, 21*(3), 447-454.

Wallace, L.S. (2001). Rhabdomyolysis: A case study. *MEDSURG Nursing, 10,* 113-121.

Wilson, S. (2006, February). *Individualizing the management of intradialytic hypotension.* Educational presentation at the 12th International Symposium on Hemodialysis, San Francisco, CA.

Yagi, N., & Paganini, E. (1997). Acute dialysis and continuous renal replacement: The emergence of new technology involving the nephrologist in the intensive care setting. *Seminars in Nephrology, 17*(4) 306-320.

Zielinski, I.D. (2002). Principles of apheresis. In *Principles of apheresis technology* (3rd ed., pp. 35-38). Vancouver, B.C.: American Society for Apheresis.

Zorzanello, M.M., Fleming, W.J., & Prowant, B.F. (2004). Use of tissue plasminogen activator in peritoneal dialysis catheters: A literature review and one center's experience. *Nephrology Nursing Journal, 31*(5), 534-537.

Appendix Index

Appendix 3.1. Sample Patient Education Brochure

Source: Creighton Nephrology, Creighton University, Omaha, Nebraska.

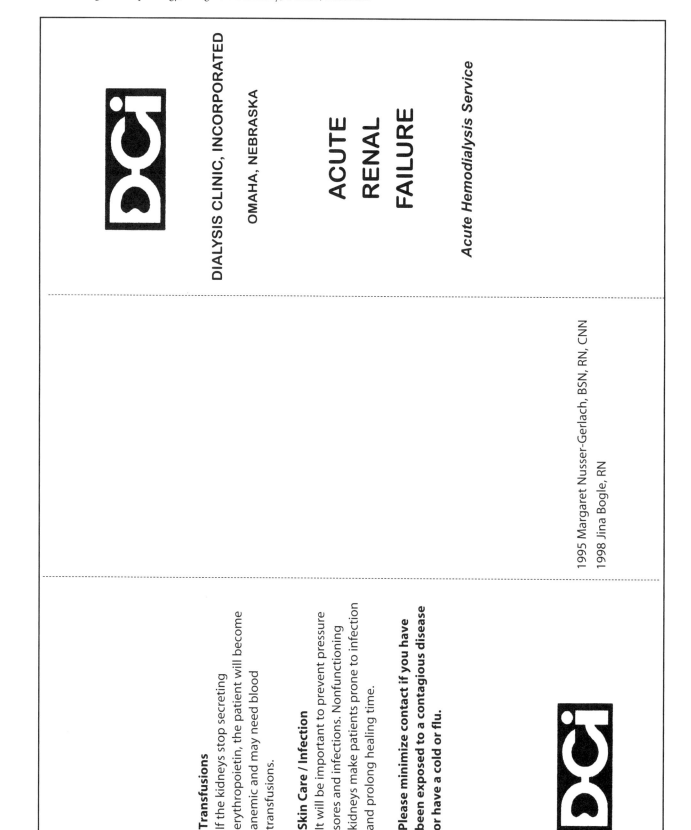

DIALYSIS CLINIC, INCORPORATED

OMAHA, NEBRASKA

ACUTE RENAL FAILURE

Acute Hemodialysis Service

1995 Margaret Nusser-Gerlach, BSN, RN, CNN

1998 Jina Bogle, RN

Transfusions
If the kidneys stop secreting erythropoietin, the patient will become anemic and may need blood transfusions.

Skin Care / Infection
It will be important to prevent pressure sores and infections. Nonfunctioning kidneys make patients prone to infection and prolong healing time.

Please minimize contact if you have been exposed to a contagious disease or have a cold or flu.

NORMAL KIDNEY FUNCTION
Healthy kidneys have many important functions:
- Filter waste products from metabolism (creatinine) and protein foods *blood urea nitrogen (BUN)
- Removal of excess fluids
- Regulate chemicals and minerals
- Regulate bone metabolism
- Regulate balance of acid/base in blood and lungs
- Regulate blood pressure and sodium
- Secrete erythropoiten, a hormone that tells the bone marrow to make new red blood cells

KIDNEY INJURY AND DAMAGE
Many situations can injure or damage kidneys:
- Trauma/crushing injury to organs and muscles
- Large blood loss
- Prolonged low blood pressure
- Burns
- Infections in the blood stream (sepsis)
- Heart or blood vessel operation
- Liver failure
- Diabetes
- Too much or any drug – prescription or street drugs
- Dyes or toxic chemicals

Acute Renal Failure
The kidneys have millions of microscopic blood vessels that need a large blood supply. Any problem that interferes with the blood supply may injure or damage the filtering part of the kidneys.

A sudden injury causing loss of kidney function is called **acute renal failure**. Acute renal failure can be temporary, and may be reversible if the kidneys are able to heal. During this time, waste products and extra fluid will build up in the blood stream. They are toxic and cause death unless filtered out another way. Special treatments called **Hemodialysis** or **Continuous Renal Replacement Therapy (CRRT)** can be done.

Vascular Access
Neither hemodialysis nor CRRT can be performed without a way to obtain a blood flow of 200-400 mls (about 6-13 ounces) a minute through a dialyzer. A vein cannot supply that much blood in one minute for three to four hours. There are several ways to obtain this blood supply. They are called vascular accesses.

A large intravenous catheter with a wall down the middle and holes on the end is called a **dual lumen hemodialysis catheter**. A physician inserts the catheter into the subclavian (under the collarbone), jugular (in the neck), or femoral (in the groin) vein. The physician decides the best place to insert the catheter. Local anesthetic is used, and the catheter is stitched into place. A chest x-ray makes sure the catheter is in the right place.

Special dressings will cover the insertion site and should not get wet. The lumens will be clamped while not being used for dialysis. The catheter may be used to infuse medications between dialysis treatments. The catheter is removed when dialysis is no longer needed.

Hemodialysis
A dialysis machine uses an artificial kidney called a dialyzer to filter the waste products and extra fluid from the blood. Tubing is attached to the vascular access for three to five hours. The patient cannot feel the actual dialysis treatment.

The treatment is monitored continuously by a specially trained RN who brings the machine and supplies to the ICU/CCU. The Dialysis RN may transfuse blood, proteins, or medications during the treatment, and works with ICU/CCU RN to manage patient care.

Patients who are not in ICU/CCU and are medically stable can be transported to the Inpatient Hemodialysis Unit 5316 on the 5th floor at Creighton University Medical Center. There, dialysis nurses work together to dialyze one to four patients at a time. Patients are dialyzed in their rooms in all other CDI contracted hospitals.

Continuous Renal Replacement Therapy
The Nephrologist may order a slower continuous waste and fluid removal system, using an automated pump-assisted machine and artificial kidney. This therapy requires a dual lumen catheter to be placed in a large vein to provide vascular access for blood purification. The dialysis RN will initiate the therapy and work with the Critical Care RN to manage the patient's care while receiving CRRT. After the CRRT machine is functioning and the system is working the Critical Care RN takes over monitoring the machine, system, and patient care. The Dialysis RN is available 24 hours a day for support and problem solving. The Dialysis RN checks the machine system twice daily and periodically changes the artificial kidney. Every 24 hours, the Nephrologist will instruct the Dialysis RN to make changes in the therapy, continue or end the therapy.

Treatment Schedule
There is no way to predict how long a patient will need hemodialysis. The Nephrologist will check lab value daily to determine how often dialysis is needed. The patient is monitored closely for signs of returning kidney function.

Nutrition
While the kidneys are functioning, dietary protein, potassium, sodium, and fluids will be restricted to decrease the kidneys' workload and to keep toxic levels as low as possible. A special IV mixture called hyperalimentation may be infused for food/calories. Tube feedings or supplements may be ordered. A special renal dietitian will work with the Nephrologist.

If you have any questions or concerns, please ask to talk to the Nephrologist or Dialysis Nurse. We want to help you understand Acute Renal Failure and the hemodialysis process.

Appendix 3.2. Acute Hemodialysis Flowsheet

Source: Western Nephrology Acute Dialysis, Denver, CO. Used with permission.

WESTERN ACUTE DIALYSIS, P.C.
HEMODIALYSIS RECORD

DATE _____ # of Setups _____
LOCATION: Dialysis Rm _____ Pt Rm _____
PT ROOM # _____ OP Unit _____
# of Pt's Run: 1   2   3
HOSPITAL: _____
PATIENT NAME: _____

MACHINE CHECKLIST
Bleach _____ Neg. _____ Pos. _____
Chloramines _____
Alarm Test _____
Pressure Test _____
Conductivity _____ pH _____

EDUCATION
Modality Training ☐
Family/Patient Education ☐
Printed Instructions ☐
Verbal Instructions ☐

HEMODIALYSIS ORDERS:
Dialyzer: _____ Total Tx Time: _____ Time On: _____
BFR: _____ Ultrafiltration: _____ Time Off: _____
Dialysate: K+ _____ CA** _____ HCO₃ _____ **Dialysate △s:**
Programmable Sodium: _____ Temp: _____ K+ _____ Ca+ _____
Heparin: HCO₃ _____
Bolus: _____ **LABS TO DRAW:** **LAB RESULTS**
Continuous: _____ Chem Screen _____ CA** _____ Mg** _____
Off At: _____ CBC _____ PO₄ _____
Total: _____ Coag _____ Albumin _____

Fluid To Remove:
Prime/RB _____
IV Fluids _____
Replacement Fluid _____
PO Fluids _____
PRBC _____
Machine Set To Remove: _____
Total Fluids Given During Tx _____
Liters Processed _____
Consent Signed _____ Yes _____ No

PATIENT ASSESSMENT: Diagnosis: _____

Pulmonary
Breath Sounds _____
Rate/Rhythm _____
O₂ Mode/Rate _____
SPO₂ _____
FIO₂ _____

Cardiovascular
Rhythm _____
Comments _____
Neuro AAO x _____
Responds to Sound _____
Pain No Response _____

Edema
None Ext
Slight Sacral
Moderate Abd
Pitting Orbital

Access
Type: R L
IJ SC
Fem AVG
Fistula

Bruit _____
Redness _____
Edema _____
Bruising _____
Drainage _____

Dr. _____
Insertion Date _____
Drsg. Chg'd Y N
Catheter Volume
A ___ ml V ___ ml

IV Medications/Amt
_____
_____

EPO _____
Total Hourly _____
I+O
INTAKE (Since last Rx) _____
OUTPUT (Since last Rx) _____

TIME	BP	APICAL bpm	TEMP °	RO Mach # PRE/WT	Dialysis Mach # GAIN	kg	DRY WT	kg	NURSING NOTES
PRE	BP								
POST	BP	bpm	°	POST/WT	LOSS	kg	LAST TX POST WT	kg	
	PULSE BLOOD FLOW		PRESSURES VEN Art/Neg	UFR FLUIDS GIVEN	ACT				Cartridge #
			TMP						

NURSING NOTES
Verified correct patient, procedure, site and equipment Initial _____ Timeout Performed _____

Staff Signature/Initials

Appendix 3.3. Sample Acute Hemodialysis Order

Source: Western Acute Dialysis in Denver, Colorado. Used with permission.

☐ **STAT**

Hemodialysis Orders
Meditech category: Hospitalist/Internal Medicine
Meditech Name:

◆M◆

Important: Pharmacy must receive a copy of all medication orders (new & change orders). Please scan to Pharmacy As Soon As Possible.

| A Therapeutic or generic equivalent drug approved by the Pharmacy may be substituted. ||
| Orders | Progress Notes |

Orders

Rev: 07/07   PPO.955
HEMODIALYSIS ORDERS
Treatment Date: _____ Allergies: _____
Dialyzer: ☐ F160NR   ☐ PF 14OH   ☐ Other: _____
Tx time: _____ BFR: _____ ml/min DFR _____ ml/min UFR: _____kg
PUF for _____time_____kg
☐ Calculate Kt/V   EDW _____ kg

Dialysate:
Temp: Normal (37C) or _____C
☐   Potassium _____ and adjust per protocol
☐   Potassium_____ do not adjust per protocol
       Serum Potassium   Dialysate Potassium
       > 5   mmol/L   2 mEq/L
       4 – 5   mmol/L   3 mEq/L
       3.5 – 3.9 mmol/L   3.5 mEq/L
       < 3.5   mmol/L   4 mEq/L

☐   Calcium _____ Notify MD of Calcium levels > 11 mg/dL or < 7.5 mg/dL
☐   Bicarb mEq per liter_____   Na_____
☐   Programmable Sodium   150____145____140____

☐ Profile 1: UF Custom step ▓▓▓   Na Progr Curve 150-140
☐ Profile 2: UF Constant   Na Progr Curve 148-138
☐ Profile 3: UF Step 1.5 / 1 / 0.5   Na Constant _____
☐ Profile 4: UF Progressive Curve   Na Constant _____
☐ Profile 5: UF Step 1.5 / 1 / 0.5   Na Step 14.8 / 14.5 / 13.8
☐ Profile 6: UF Progressive Curve   Na Progr Curve 148-138

Anticoagulation (for hemodialysis treatment only):
☐   Heparin bolus_____units; hourly_____units; off at _____min
☐   None
☐   Other; Specify: _____
☐   Review anticoagulation orders with MD if patient already on anti coag meds (Such
       as: Aggrastat, Alteplase, Aspirin, Coumadin, Fragmin, Heparin IV or Sub-Q, Hirudin,
       Lovenox, Plavix, ReoPro, Xigris)

Weights:
☐   Daily   ☐ Dialysis days only   ☐ Pre and post dialysis treatment

Labs:
☐   No labs
☐   Draw early to be on chart by 6am_____OR dialysis staff to draw pre-treatment_____
☐   Basic Metabolic/Chem Panel ☐ Comprehensive Metabolic/Chem Panel
☐   Renal   ☐ CBC   ☐ Albumin   ☐ Calcium   ☐ Phosphorus
☐   Magnesium   ☐ Vanco Random   ☐ Pt/PTT
☐   T& C for _____units Leuko poor RBC's   ☐ Give PRBC's_____# units

Signed: _____ MD Date/Time: _____

Progress Notes

Medications:
☐ **HYPOTENSION:**
   ☐ NS Bolus_____ml PRN to maximum of _____ml
   ☐ Albumin 25%____gm for SBP less than ____ max of ____gm
   ☐ Hypertonic Saline IV per protocol
   ☐ Pressors: _____
   ☐ Other: _____
☐   Mannitol _____gms Instructions: _____
☐   Epogen _____units IV/Sub-Q   M, W, F / T, T, S / Q dialysis day
                                                      / weekly on _____

Access:
☐   Fistula   ☐ Graft
       Special Instructions: _____
☐   Catheter   pack with:☐ Heparin   ☐ TPA   ☐ 4% Sodium Citrate
       Volume = A _____ ml   V _____ ml

Signed: _____ MD Date/Time: _____

Progress Notes

| FORM BARCODE LABEL HERE | PATIENT BARCODE LABEL MUST BE PLACED IN THIS SPACE |

Appendix 3.4. Catheter Instructions for the Patient

Source: Creighton Nephrology, Creighton University, Omaha, Nebraska. Used with permission.

Catheter Instructions for the Patient

Name:_____Date:_____

Catheter Type:_____Placement Date:_____

Catheter Placed by: Dr._____

Central Venous Access Devices (Catheters) may be:
  A. Temporary
  B. Permanent (Perm Cath)

A. Temporary
  1. Description: A device used on a temporary basis for vascular cannulation and circulatory access for hemodialysis until a permanent method can be prepared, or until a different mode of dialysis therapy can be instituted. These devices are currently made of carbothane, Teflon, polyurethane or silicone, all biocompatible materials.
  2. A hemodialysis catheter is needed when:
       a) Immediate access to the venous circulation is needed for in-patients experiencing acute renal failure
       b) While waiting for a graft or AV fistula to mature
       c) After removal of permanent access because of an infection
       d) Before initiation of peritoneal dialysis or during episodes of peritonitis

  3. Types (usually based on location of placement)
       a) Subclavian vein catheter (SVC)
       b) Jugular vein catheter (IJC)
       c) Femoral vein catheter (FVC)

B. Permanent Catheter
  1. Description: Operative placement of dual or single lumen catheter in the internal jugular or subclavian is tunneled subcutaneously to exit site on chest wall. The biocompatible cuff is designed to inhibit infection in tunnel and provide catheter immobilization in the chest keeping it place for months.

POSSIBLE COMPLICATIONS OF CATHETER PLACEMENT

  1. Immediate post-insertion complications as traumatic hemo or pneumothorax (air or blood in the chest cavity); inadvertent subclavian artery puncture; brachial plexus injury; air embolism (air entering the blood circulation). A chest x-ray is done post insertion, before the catheter is used, to assure proper placement/position of a catheter.
  2. Other complications include the following:
       a) Bleeding at insertion site during hemodialysis or after catheter removal.
       b) Hematoma (bruise) at insertion site.
       c) Thrombosis or clotting creating resultant poor blood flow.

d) Emboli (air or dislodged blood clots)

e) Cardiac arrhythmias (abnormal heart irregularity).

f) Infection and Sepsis (an infection in the blood). Commonly infection of insertion site especially when catheter left in place for longer periods of time.

g) Other complications may arise as kinked catheter, anchor suture removal, accidental removal of entire catheter, accidental unclamping, or uncapping of catheter.

CARE OF YOUR CATHETER

1. The catheter dressing is changed at each dialysis treatment by a Registered Nurse or a Licensed Practical Nurse under strict aseptic technique. It may be done at the start, during or after dialysis treatment. As a patient, you are not allowed to change the catheter dressing or to manipulate your catheter in any way. However, if there is a dire need to change dressing or manipulate catheter, please call the nurse for assessment of situation and to receive instructions. Never use scissors in handling catheters and dressings.

2. Keep your catheter exit site or dressing clean, sterile and dry. Do not get dressing wet when showering or bathing. If dressing accidentally gets wet, call clinic nurse.

3. Report immediately to the nurse (either by phone or during your clinic visit) the following signs or symptoms:

   a) Dressing soaked with any type of discharge from exit site

   b) Any foul smell from catheter site

   c) Blood soaked dressing

   d) Uncapped or unclamped catheter

   e) Fever of any cause and/or unknown cause

   f) Pain, redness, swelling around catheter site

EMERGENCY SITUATIONS

1. When bleeding from unclamped and uncapped catheter press with thumb and forefinger the two clamps until you hear it click or feel it snap. If you find it difficult to do pinching action, bend or kink catheter just below the caps, or if this is not possible for you to do, cover open ports with fingers. Call the clinic or physician office immediately. If blood loss from uncapped/unclamped catheter is great and/or you feel dizzy, lightheaded, shortness of breath or chest pain, call emergency 911, lie down, and limit ambulation.

2. When bleeding from accidental removal/yanking of catheter, immediately apply direct firm pressure over catheter site, lie down and limit movements and ambulation. If site continues to bleed for more than 15 minutes and/or you feel dizziness, lightheaded, shortness of breath or chest pain, call emergency 911. Continue to apply direct pressure until help arrives.

3. When there is continuous bleeding from the catheter exit or the dressing site a few days after catheter placement, call the physician office or dialysis unit for instruction. If site continues to bleed for more than 15 minutes and/or you feel dizziness, lightheaded shortness of breath, or chest pain, call emergency 911. Continue to apply direct firm pressure until help arrives.

4. When accidental removal of a new catheter dressing occurs, call the clinic.

Appendix 3.5. Patient Catheter Release Form

Source: Creighton Nephrology, Creighton University, Omaha, Nebraska. Used with permission.

Patient Catheter Release Form

I, _____, having a temporary/permanent catheter as a vascular access for hemodialysis have been advised and educated on the importance of catheter care and emergency procedures.

I have been shown and have returned demonstration on how to handle threatening situations involving catheters such as bleeding or leaking from exit site, bleeding from uncapped or unclamped catheter, and/or accidental removal of my catheter.

I have also been given a Catheter Instruction Sheet that I can take home and review or use as a referral when the need arises.

Outside the clinical setting, I agree to assume full responsibility for any actions I would take in case of catheter emergency and will not hold Dialysis Clinic, Inc. responsible for any outcomes of such actions.

Addendum: If the patient is unable to understand and/or perform the catheter procedures, a family member must be instructed on the above emergency care.

Nurse's Comments:

_____

_____

_____

_____   _____
Date   Patient/Legal Representative Signature

_____   _____
Date   Clinic Representative – Name and Title

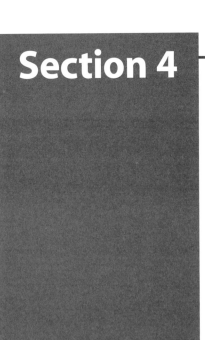

Section 4

The Individual with Kidney Disease

Section Editor

Donna Bednarski, MSN, ANP,BC, CNN, CNP

Authors

Donna Bednarski, MSN, ANP,BC, CNN, CNP

Molly Lillis Cahill, MSN, RN, ANP-C, APRN, BC, CNN

Debra Castner, MSN, RN, APRN-C, CNN

Caroline S. Counts, MSN, RN, CNN

Cheryl L. Groenhoff, MSN, MBA, RN, CNN

Lisa M. Hall, MSSW, LCSW

Glenda F. Harbert, ADN, RN, CNN, CPHQ

Patricia Painter, PhD

Beth Witten, MSW, ACSW, LSCSW

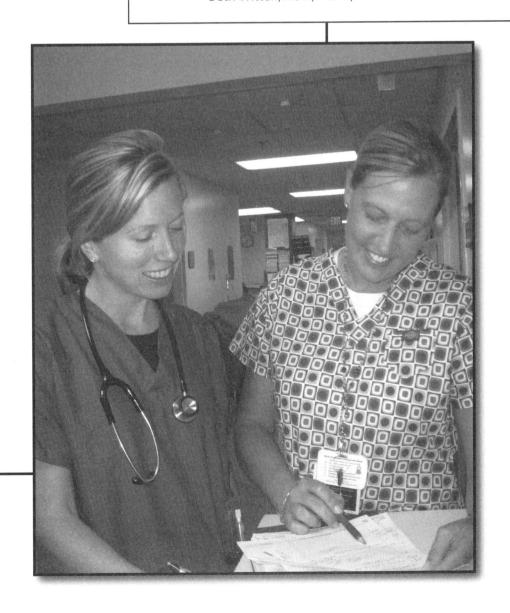

About the Authors

Donna Bednarski, MSN, ANP,BC, CNN, CNP, Section Editor and Author, is a Nurse Practitioner and Clinical Nurse Specialist, Nephrology, at Harper University Hospital in Detroit, Michigan.

Molly Lillis Cahill, MSN, RN, ANP-C, APRN, BC, CNN, is a Nurse Practitioner at Arms, Dodge, Robinson, Wilber, & Crouch in Kansas City, Missouri.

Debra Castner, MSN, RN, APRN-C, CNN, is a Supervisor in the CKD Health and Wellness Education Program at Horizon Blue Cross Blue Shield of New Jersey in Farmingdale, New Jersey.

Caroline S. Counts, MSN, RN, CNN, is Research Coordinator in the Division of Nephrology at the Medical University of South Carolina in Charleston, South Carolina.

Cheryl L. Groenhoff, MSN, MBA, RN, CNN, is a Kidney Patient Educator at Baxter Health Care in Plantation, Florida.

Lisa M. Hall, MSSW, LCSW, is Community Services Coordinator at FMQAI: The Florida ESRD Network (Network 7) in Tampa, Florida.

Glenda F. Harbert, ADN, RN, CNN, CPHQ, is Executive Director at ESRD Network of Texas, Inc., in Dallas, Texas.

Patricia Painter, PhD, is an Associate Professor in the Department of Medicine/Division of Renal Medicine at the University of Minnesota in Minneapolis, Minnesota.

Beth Witten, MSW, ACSW, LSCSW, is a Resource and Policy Associate at the Medical Education Institute, Inc., in Madison, Wisconsin.

Acknowledgment

Special thanks to the following people for their valuable contributions to Chapter 15:

Michael Janech, PhD, Assistant Professor, Associate Director Nephrology, Proteomics Facility, Medical University of South Carolina.

Kathleen Calzone, MSN, RN, APNG, Senior Nurse Specialist (Research), National Institute of Health, National Cancer Institute, Center for Cancer Research, Genetics Branch.

Elizabeth Ness, MS, RN, Director, Staff Development, National Institute of Health, National Cancer Institute, Center for Cancer Research.

Section 4

The Individual with Kidney Disease

Chapter

Chapter 15

Genetics and Genomics –
Perspectives in Nephrology Nursing

Purpose

The purpose of the section is to present information enabling the nephrology nurse to learn, understand, and deliver care to meet the individual needs of the patient with kidney disease.

The fundamental nature of every disease and condition has a genetic and genomic component; kidney disease is no exception. The development of the genomic infrastructure has accelerated the understanding of diseases and is helping to refine methods of disease prediction, diagnosis, and treatment. Targeted therapeutics will be tailored to individual genetic profiles.

In 2005, a Consensus Panel of nurse leaders established the "Essential Nursing Competencies and Curricula Guidelines for Genetics and Genomics." While these competencies are not meant to replace or recreate existing standards of practice, they are intended to assimilate the genetic and genomic perspective into all nursing education and practice. Regardless of academic preparation, role, or practice setting, the clinical application of genetic and genomic knowledge has major implications for the entire nursing profession. In 2006, ANNA endorsed this document and agreed to incorporate this central science into nephrology nursing education and practice.

While modern day genetics and genomics are still in their infancy, they will have a direct impact on nephrology in a variety of ways. With diabetes and hypertension being the leading causes of kidney disease, this in itself will have a tremendous effect. In addition, persons with kidney disease are not exempt from other diseases or conditions with a genetic link, for example, breast cancer, colon cancer, etc. The purpose of this chapter is to provide a foundation of knowledge for nephrology nurses to assist them with integrating genetics and genomics into clinical practice.

Objectives

Upon completion of this chapter, the learner will be able to:
1. Define genetics and genomics.
2. Describe the process of inheritance.
3. Explain the impact of cellular aging.
4. Discuss the ethical considerations regarding genetic testing, including the need for informed consent.
5. List at least three kidney diseases with a genetic component.
6. Recognize environmental risk factors that could endanger a person's health.
7. Discuss the importance of pharmacogenetics and pharmacogenomics to health care.
8. Recognize patients who are at risk for a heritable disease or condition based on their medical history, physical exam, or laboratory findings.
9. Perform a patient assessment from a genetic perspective and construct a family medical pedigree.
10. Locate resources for patient education and referral when needed.
11. Explain the general process of genetic counseling.

I. **Historical milestones. There is reason to believe that the concept of genetics was contemplated by the first human beings.** As specific traits were noted to be shared by parent and child, questions were raised about inheritance. The sharing of specific traits was then applied to other areas such as plant cultivation and animal husbandry. And thus, the foundation was laid for the modern genetics that is practiced today.

A. 1865 – Austrian monk, Gregor Mendel, first traced inheritance patterns in pea plants and is considered the founding father of modern genetics.

B. 1869 – Miescher studied extracts of cellular nucleic acid; 80 years later this material would be shown to be DNA.

C. 1889 – Weismann theorized that the material basis of heredity was located on the chromosomes.

D. 1905 – British biologist William Bateson coined the term *genetics*.

E. 1909 – Garrod described several inherited biochemical disorders and is now considered the founder of biochemical genetics.

F. 1910 – Thomas Hunt Morgan conducted experiments in fruit flies and established that some genetically determined traits were sex linked.

G. 1913 – Bridges, one of Morgan's students, showed that genes reside on chromosomes.

H. 1913 – Sturtevant, another of Morgan's students, showed that genes were arranged on chromosomes in a linear fashion and were in specific locations.

I. 1920 – Winkler coined the word *genome* and defined it as the haploid set of chromosomes and all the genes they contain.

J. 1941 – Edward Lawrie Tatum and George Wells Beadle showed that genes code for enzymes. Today it is known that genes code for protein in general.

K. 1944 – Oswald Avery, Colin McLeod, and Maclyn McCarty showed DNA was genetic material that carried genes.

L. 1953 – DNA structure was determined to be a double helix by James Watson and Francis Crick using data from Rosalind Franklin. Their discovery heralded a new age of discovery in genetics and laid the foundation for the sequencing of the human genome.

M. 1956 – Jo Hin Tjio and Albert Levan established the number of chromosomes in humans to be 46.

N. 1958 – Crick proposed what was to become the central dogma of molecular biology: DNA is transcribed into RNA, which is translated into protein.

O. Mid-1960s – Holley, Khorana, Nirenberg, and Leder crack the genetic code by determining the DNA sequence for each of the 20 most common amino acids.

P. 1977 – Fred Sanger, Walter Gilbert, and Allan Maxam working independently, developed techniques to determine the nucleic acid sequences for long sections of DNA.

Q. 1986 – The term *genomics* was coined by Thomas Roderick.

R. 1988 – The International Society of Nurses in Genetics (ISONG) began as a venue for nurses around the world to advance their knowledge and practice related to genomics.

S. 1989 – Francis Collins and Lap-Chee Tsui sequenced the first human gene. It encodes the CFTR protein; defects in this gene cause cystic fibrosis.

T. 1990 – The Human Genome Project was initiated. It is an international effort with scientists from 20 research centers in six countries: China, France, Germany, Japan, the United Kingdom, and the United States.

U. 1996 – The National Human Genome Research Institute, the American Nurses Association, and the American Medical Association form the National Coalition for Health Professional Education in Genetics (NCHPEG). The mission of NCHPEG is to promote health professional education and access to information about advances in human genetics to improve the health care of the nation.

V. 2001 – The first draft sequences of the human genome are released simultaneously by the Human Genome Project and Celera Genomics.

W. April 14, 2003 – Successful completion of the Human Genome Project with 99% of the genome sequenced to a 99.9% accuracy.

X. 2005 – An independent panel of nurse leaders from clinical, research, and academic settings developed the minimal amount of genetic and genomic competencies that are now expected of every nurse.

Y. 2006 – A wide variety of Nursing Organizations, including ANNA, endorsed these competencies.

II. Theoretical background.

A. Genetics is the study of gene variation and heredity which can be used to elucidate their impact on relatively rare single gene disorders.

B. Human genomics is the study of all genes in the human genome which includes genetic analysis and expression. It includes their interactions with each other, the environment, and the influences of other psychosocial factors and cultural factors.
   1. The Environmental Protection Agency (EPA) defines the environment as the sum of all external conditions affecting the life, development, and survival of an organism.
   2. Awareness of the individual's cultural values, beliefs, practices, norms, diversities, and the environment from which the person comes and may return to, is vital.

C. DNA, or deoxyribonucleic acid, is the hereditary material. Nearly every cell in the body has the same DNA. Most is located in the cell nucleus, but a small amount may be found in the mitochondria.
   1. Information in DNA is stored as a code made up of four nitrogenous bases: adenine (A), guanine (G), cytosine (C), and thymine (T) (see Figure 4.1).
   2. The order, or sequence, of these bases determines the information available for building and maintaining an organism.
   3. The DNA contains a specific set of instructions for making the proteins(s) needed by the body's cells for their proper functioning.
   4. DNA bases pair up with each other to form units called base pairs. Each base is also attached to a sugar molecule and a phosphate molecule.
   5. A nucleotide is the combination of this base, the sugar, and the phosphate. Nucleotides are arranged in two long strands that form a spiral called a double helix (see Figure 4.2).
   6. An important property of DNA is its ability to replicate. This is critical when cells divide as each new cell needs to have an exact copy of the DNA present in the old cell.
   7. Mitochondria are structures within cells that convert the energy from food into a form that cells can use. The genetic material in the mitochondria is known as mitochondrial DNA, or mtDNA. It contains 37 genes that are all necessary for normal mitochondria function.

D. RNA, or ribonucleic acid, is a chemical similar to a single strand of DNA.

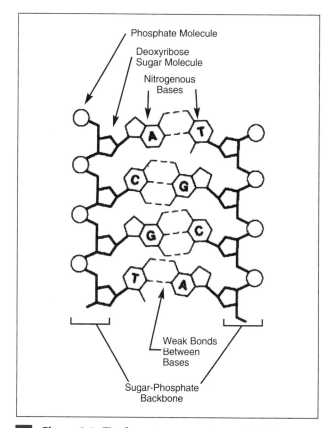

Figure 4.1. The four nitrogenous bases of DNA are arranged along the sugar-phosphate backbone in a particular order (the DNA sequence), encoding all genetic instructions for an organism. Adenine (A) pairs with thymine (T), while cytosine (C) pairs with guanine (G). The two DNA strands are held together by weak bonds between the bases.

Courtesy of U.S. Department of Energy Human Genome Program. Retrieved from http://www.ornl.gov/sci/techresources/Human_Genome/publicat/primer/fig2.html.

   1. RNA contains ribose rings and uracil, unlike DNA, which contains deoxyribose and thymine. It is primarily made up of four bases: uracil, adenine, guanine, and cytosine (see Figure 4.3).
   2. RNA is transcribed from DNA by enzymes called RNA polymerases and is further processed by other enzymes.
   3. RNA serves as a template for translation of genes into proteins. It delivers DNA's genetic message to the cytoplasm of a cell where proteins are made.

E. Genes are the basic physical and functional units of heredity. A gene is an ordered sequence of nucleotides located in a particular position on a particular chromosome that encodes for a specific

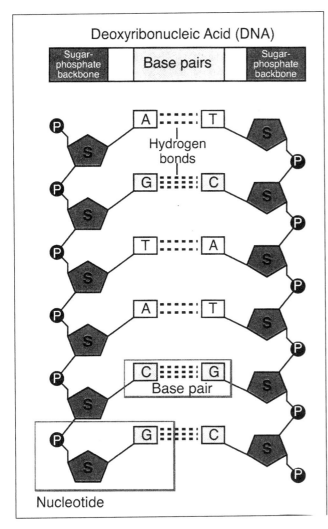

Figure 4.2. Nucleotide.

Courtesy of Talking Glossary of Genetics, http://www.genome.gov, National Human Genome Research Institute, National Institutes of Health.

functional product (i.e., a protein or RNA molecule) (see Figure 4.4).
1. Genes are made up of DNA, the code for a specific protein or RNA.
2. It is estimated that humans have between 20,000 and 25,000 genes.
3. Genes vary in size and range from a hundred DNA bases to more than 2 million bases.
4. Most genes are the same in all people. Less than 1% of the total is slightly different and account for each person's unique physical characteristics.
5. Alleles are variants of the same gene with slight differences in their sequence of DNA bases (e.g., at a locus for eye color, the allele might result in blue or brown eyes).

F. Chromosomes are the microscopic, thread-like structures in the cell nucleus into which the DNA molecule is packaged (see Figure 4.5).
1. Each chromosome is made up of DNA tightly coiled many times around proteins called histones that support its structure.
2. Distinct chromosomes are only visible under a microscope when the cell is dividing.
3. Each chromosome has a constriction point called a centromere that divides the chromosome into two sections or arms. The shorter arm is called p; the longer arm is called q. The centromere gives the chromosome its characteristic shape and can be used to help describe the location of specific genes.
4. The telomere is a repetitive segment of DNA found on the ends of the chromosomes. With each mitotic division, parts of the telomeres are lost. A theory of cellular aging proposes that the telomeres act as a biologic clock. When they are depleted, the cell dies or becomes less active.
5. Each human cell normally contains 23 pairs of chromosomes, for a total of 46. Twenty two of these pairs are known as autosomes and are the same in males and females. The 23rd pair differs between males and females and comprises the sex chromosomes. Females have two copies of the X chromosome; males have one copy of the X chromosome and one copy of the Y (see Figure 4.6).
6. The 22 autosomes are numbered by size from 1 to 22.

G. Genetic mapping is used to describe the location of a particular gene on a chromosome.
1. Cytogenetic location is based on a distinctive pattern of bands created when chromosomes are stained with certain chemicals. The combination of numbers and letters provide a gene's "address" on a chromosome.
2. Molecular location pinpoints the location of a gene in terms of base pairs. Researchers are now able to provide a gene's molecular address as a result of the Human Genome Project, the international effort completed in 2003 that determined the sequence of base pairs for each human chromosome.

H. Formation of protein.
1. Most genes contain the information to make proteins that are required for the structure, function, and regulation of the body's tissues and organs.
2. Twenty different amino acids can be combined to make a protein. The sequence of amino acids

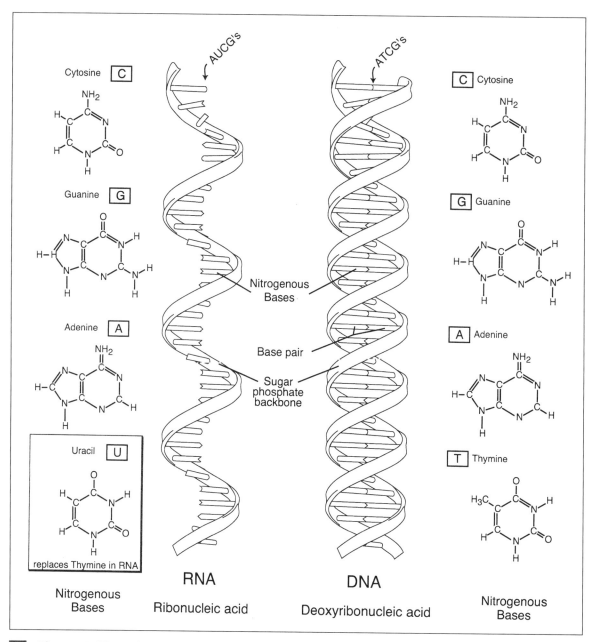

Figure 4.3. Ribonucleic acid.

Courtesy of Talking Glossary of Genetics, http://www.genome.gov, National Human Genome Research Institute, National Institutes of Health.

determines each protein's structure and function.
3. Examples of protein functions include antibody, enzyme, cell signaling messenger, receptor, structural component, transport/storage (see Figure 4.7 and Table 4.1).
4. Proteomics is the large scale study of proteins with particular emphasis placed on abundance and modifications. Unlike genomics, it attempts to look at the entirety of proteins in existence in an organism.

a. The term proteome is used to describe the entire complement of proteins encoded by the genome.
b. The proteome is complex and includes numerous modifications such as phosphorylation, glycosylation, and other posttranslation modifications.
c. Proteomic techniques are often used to investigate structure and functional interactions.

I. Gene expression requires two major steps: transcription and translation.

1. During transcription, the information in the gene's DNA is transferred to RNA. The type of RNA that contains the information for making protein is called messenger RNA (mRNA). It carries the "message" from the DNA out of the nucleus into the cytoplasm.

2. During translation, the mRNA interacts with a ribosome which reads the sequence of mRNA bases. Each sequence of three bases is called a codon and codes for one particular amino acid. A type of RNA called transfer RNA (tRNA) carries one amino acid to the ribosome where the protein is assembled one amino acid at a time.

3. The flow of information from DNA to RNA to proteins is one of the fundamental principles of molecular biology (see Figure 4.8).

J. Gene regulation is an important part of normal development.

1. Each cell expresses, or turns on, only a fraction of its genes. The rest of the genes are repressed, or turned off. This process is known as gene regulation.

2. Genes are turned on and off in different patterns, thus accounting for a muscle cell not looking or acting like a liver cell, for example.

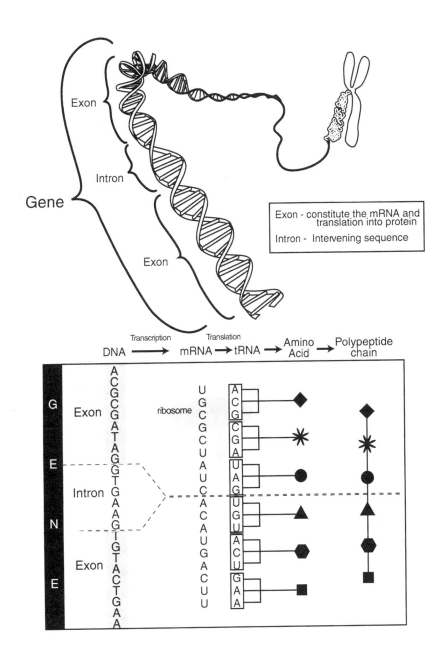

Figure 4.4. A gene can be defined as a region of DNA that controls hereditary characteristic. It usually corresponds to a sequence used in the production of a specific protein or RNA. The biological information that it carries must be copied and transmitted from each cell to all its progeny. This includes the entire functioning unit: coding DNA sequences, non-coding regulatory DNA sequences, and introns. National Human Genome Research Institute (NHGRI).

Courtesy of Talking Glossary of Genetics, http://www.genome.gov, National Human Genome Research Institute, National Institutes of Health. Artist: Darryl Leja

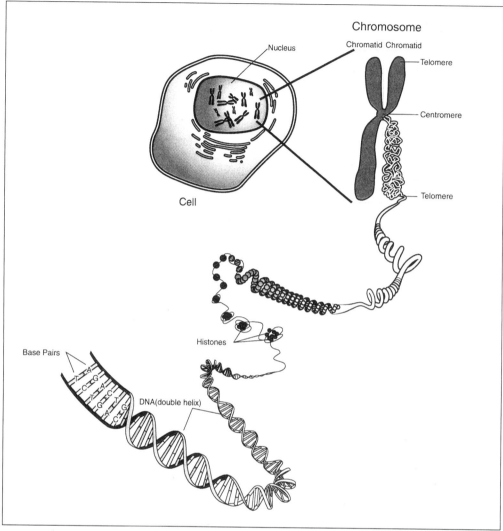

Figure 4.5. Each chromosome has a point of constriction called the centromere, which divides the chromosome into two sections or "arms." The short arm is the "p arm" and the long arm is the "q arm."

Courtesy of Talking Glossary of Genetics, http://www.genome.gov, National Human Genome Research Institute, National Institutes of Health.

3. Gene regulation allows cells to react quickly to changes in their environment. This complex process is not fully understood, but the usual result is changes in protein abundance over time.

K. The cell is the basic unit of any living organism. It contains a complete copy of the organism's genome (see Figure 4.9).

L. Cell division takes place via two different processes (see Figure 4.10).
   1. During mitosis a cell duplicates all of its contents and splits to form two identical daughter cells. Mitosis is a fundamental process for life and is

carefully controlled by a number of genes. When mitosis is not regulated correctly, health problems such as cancer can result.
   2. Meiosis ensures that humans have the same number of chromosomes in each generation. It is a two step process that reduces the number of chromosomes in half to form sperm and egg cells. At conception, each contributes 23 chromosomes, and the embryo has the usual 46. Meiosis also allows genetic variation through a process of DNA shuffling while the cells are dividing.
   3. This process is tightly regulated to ensure that a dividing cell's DNA is copied properly, any

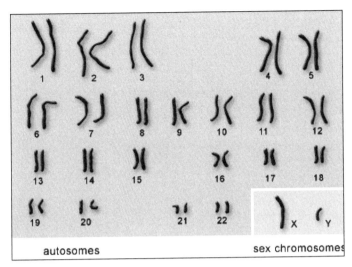

Figure 4.6. Chromosomes 1-22, X, and Y.
The 22 autosomes are numbered by size. The other two chromosomes, X and Y, are the sex chromosomes. This picture of the human chromosomes lined up in pairs is called a karyotype.

Courtesy of the U.S. National Library of Medicine, http://ghr.nlm.nih.gov/handbook/illustrations/chromosomes.

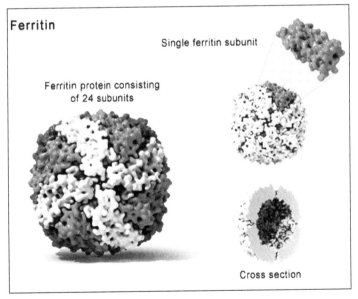

Figure 4.7. Ferritin.
Ferritin, a protein made up of 24 identical subunits, is involved in iron storage.

Courtesy of the U.S. National Library of Medicine, http://ghr.nlm.nih.gov/handbook/illustrations/ferritin.

errors in DNA are repaired, and each daughter cell receives a full set of chromosomes.

4. The cycle has check points that allow proteins to check for mistakes and halt the cycle for repairs.

5. If a cell has an error in its DNA that cannot be repaired, it may undergo apoptosis, or controlled cell death. Apoptosis is a common process throughout life that helps the body rid itself of cells it does not need. Macrophages consume the cell debris.

6. Cancer results from a disruption of the normal regulation of the cell cycle. Cells accumulate genetic errors and multiply without control.

M. Gene mutation is a permanent change in the DNA sequence that makes up a gene. Mutations range in size from a single DNA base to a large segment of a chromosome. Through natural selection advantageous mutations will be preserved and disadvantageous mutations will be eliminated. This is the process that drives evolutionary change. Most often mutations are thought to be deleterious.

1. Gene mutations can be inherited from a parent or acquired during a person's lifetime.

2. Hereditary mutations are present throughout a person's life in virtually all cells in the body.

   a. Mutations that occur only in an egg or a sperm or occur just after fertilization are called de novo (new) mutations.

   b. De novo mutations may explain genetic disorders that appear with no family history of the disorder.

3. Somatic mutations are acquired and can be caused by environmental factors such as ultraviolet radiation from the sun. These changes can also occur if a mistake is made during cell replication. Somatic mutations cannot be passed on to the next generation.

   a. Mitochondrial DNA (mtDNA) is prone to somatic mutations.

   b. Somatic mutations in mtDNA have been reported in some forms of cancer, including breast, colon, stomach, liver and kidney tumors, as

Table 4.1

Examples of Protein Functions

Function	Description	Example
Antibody	Antibodies bind to specific foreign particles, such as viruses and bacteria.	Immunoglobulin G
Enzyme	Enzymes carry out almost all of the thousands of chemical reactions that take place in cells. They also assist with the formation of new molecules by reading the genetic information stored in DNA.	Phenylalanine hydroxylase
Messenger	Messenger proteins, such as some types of hormones, transmit signals to coordinate biological processes between different cells, tissues, and organs.	Growth hormone
Structural Component	These proteins provide structure and support for cells. On a larger scale, they may also allow the body to move.	Actin
Transport/Storage	These proteins bind and carry atoms and small molecules within cellsand throughout the body.	Ferritin *See Figure 4.7.*

Source: Genetics Home Reference, http://ghr.nlm.nih.gov/handbook.

well as leukemia and lymphoma.

   c. mtDNA has limited ability to repair itself.

4. Germline mutations are inherited genetic mutations that are transmitted in the egg or sperm.

5. Polymorphisms are genetic variations that occur in all individuals. They are responsible for many of the normal differences among people such as eye color, blood type, etc. Some of the variations may influence the risk of developing certain disorders.

6. Gene mutations can prevent one or more of the thousands of proteins that are responsible for correct cell function from working properly. The mutation can cause the protein to malfunction or to be missing entirely. This can disrupt normal development or cause a medical condition – a genetic disorder.

7. Only a small percentage of mutations cause genetic disorders. Gene mutations are often repaired by certain enzymes before the gene is expressed as a protein. DNA repair is an important process by which the body protects itself from disease.

8. Gene mutations have varying effects on health depending on where they occur and whether they alter the function of essential proteins. The types of mutation include:

   a. Missense (one amino acid substituted for another).

   b. Onsense (a premature signal stops the process of building the protein).

   c. Insertion (a piece of DNA is added).

   d. Deletion (a piece of DNA is removed).

   e. Duplication (a piece of DNA is abnormally copied one or more times).

   f. Repeat expansion (short DNA sequences are repeated a number of times in a row).

   g. Frameshift (the addition or loss of DNA bases changes a gene's reading frame that codes for one amino acid). Insertions, deletions, and duplications can all result in frameshift mutations.

N. Chromosomal disorders are caused by a change in the number or structure of chromosomes. This can occur during the formation of reproductive cells, in early fetal development, or at other times during the life of an individual.

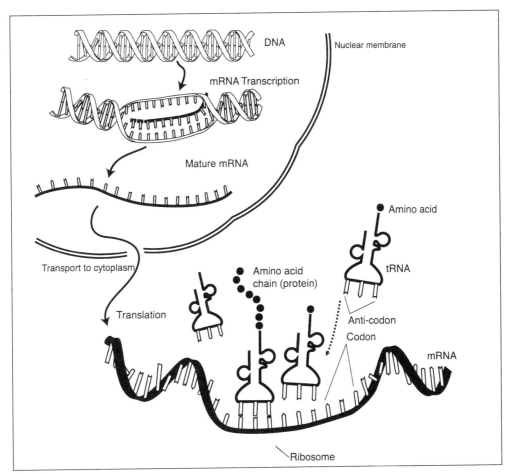

Figure 4.8. When genes are expressed, the genetic information (base sequence) on DNA is first transcribed (copied) to a molecule of messenger RNA (mRNA) in a process similar to DNA replication. The mRNA molecules then leave the cell nucleus and enter the cytoplasm, where triplets of DNA bases (codons) forming the genetic code specify the particular amino acids that make up an individual protein. This process, called translation, is accompanied by ribosomes (cellular components composed of proteins and another class of RNA) that read the genetic code from the mRNA, and transfer RNAs (tRNAs) that transport amino acids to the ribosomes for attachment to growing protein.

Courtesy of Talking Glossary of Genetics, http://www.genome.gov, National Human Genome Research Institute, National Institutes of Health.

1. Aneuploidy is the gain or loss of chromosomes from the normal 46.
   a. Trisomy is the most common form of aneuploidy and is the presence of an extra chromosome in each cell. Down syndrome is an example of a condition caused by trisomy.
   b. Monosomy is another form of aneuploidy and is the presence of one copy of a particular chromosome instead of two. Turner syndrome is a condition caused by monosomy.
2. Translocation is the breaking and removal of a large segment of DNA from one chromosome, followed by the segment's attachment to a different chromosome. This can potentially alter gene expression.
3. Loss of heterozygosity is the loss of one parent's contribution to the genome through the loss of a gene copy (or copies) due to chromosomal rearrangement or point mutations.

O. Researchers are discovering that nearly all conditions and diseases have a genetic component. Conditions caused by many contributing factors are called complex or multifactorial disorders.

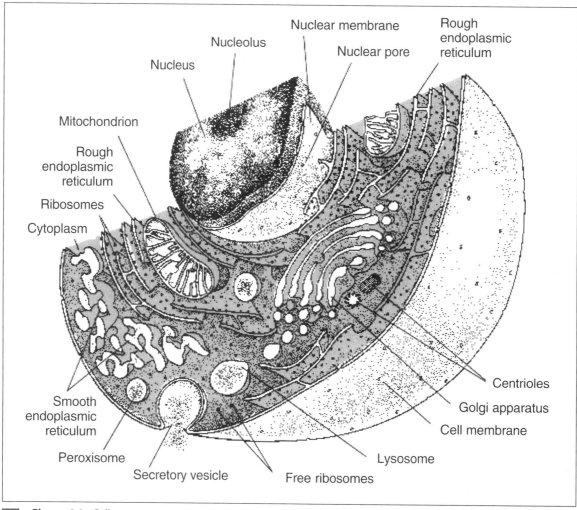

Figure 4.9. Cell.

Courtesy of Talking Glossary of Genetics, http://www.genome.gov, National Human Genome Research Institute, National Institutes of Health.

1. Diabetes, cardiovascular disease, and obesity are examples of complex or multifactorial disorders. They do not have a single genetic cause but are associated with the effects of multiple genes in combination with lifestyle and environmental factors.

2. While complex disorders often cluster in families, they do not have a clear-cut pattern of inheritance. With complex disorders it becomes difficult to determine the risk of inheriting or passing the disorder on as well as difficult to study and treat the disorders. This is because the specific factors that cause most of these disorders have not yet been identified.

3. It is predicted that by 2010, researchers will have found the major contributing genes for many common complex disorders.

P. A genome is an organism's complete set of DNA, including all of its genes. Each genome contains all of the information needed to build and maintain that organism. In humans, a copy of the entire genome, which includes more than 3 billion DNA base pairs, is contained in all cells that have a nucleus.

1. The term is derived from the words *gene* and *chromosome*.

2. Genomic researchers found that any two human beings are approximately 99.9% the same genetically.

3. The 0.1% difference represents about 3,000,000 differences between individuals' DNA.

4. A small fraction of these common variants (perhaps 200,000) are responsible for the genetic differences in health, behavior, and other human traits.

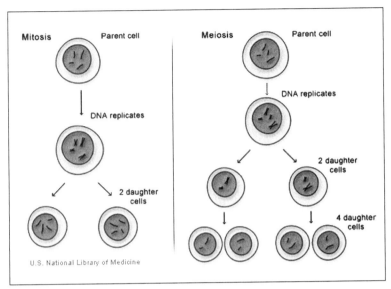

Figure 4.10. Mitosis and meiosis, the two types of cell division.

Courtesy of the U.S. National Library of Medicine,
http://ghr.nlm.nih.gov/handbook/illustrations/chromosomes.

5. The biologic concept of race that has been based on observable and measurable traits is now controversial.
6. Genetic markers exist to determine an individual's ancestry based on geographic origins. These ancestry markers are available for African, Asian, European, and Hispanic Americans and tend to be more reliable than self-reported ancestry in the United States.

III. Mendelian inheritance is defined as the manner in which genes and traits are passed from parents to children. Examples of Mendelian inheritance include autosomal dominant, autosomal recessive, and sex-linked genes.

A. Autosomal dominant is a pattern of inheritance whereby an affected individual possesses one copy of a mutant allele and one normal allele (see Figure 4.11).
1. Individuals with autosomal dominant diseases have a 50–50 chance, with each pregnancy, of passing the mutant allele and hence the disorder onto their children if one parent is heterozygous and the other is homozygous normal.
2. Paternal to male transmission can be observed.
3. An example of such a disease is autosomal polycystic kidney disease (ADPKD).

B. Autosomal recessive inheritance refers to disorders that appear only in persons who have received two copies of a mutant gene, one from each parent.
1. Autosomal recessive diseases are observed more frequently in consanguineous relationships because the individuals are descendants of the same ancestors and are more likely to carry the same genes.
2. Typically the parents of an affected individual are gene carriers and are not affected themselves.
3. With each pregnancy there is a 25% chance the offspring will inherit two copies of the disease allele and will have the disease: a 50% chance that one copy of the disease allele will be inherited and the person will become a carrier, and a 25% chance the offspring will inherit no copy of the disease allele and will not be at risk for passing the disorder on to the next generation (see Figure 4.12).

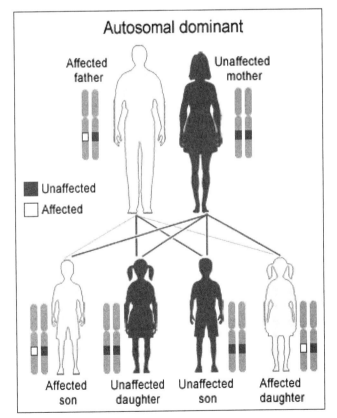

Figure 4.11. Autosomal dominant. In this example, a man with an autosomal dominant disorder has two affected children and two unaffected children.

Courtesy of the U.S. National Library of Medicine,
http://ghr.nlm.nih.gov/handbook/illustrations/chromosomes.

Autosomal recessive

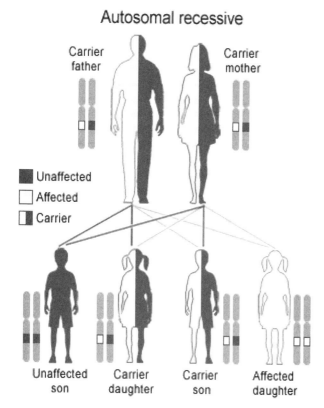

■ Unaffected
□ Affected
▨ Carrier

Figure 4.12. Autosomal recessive. In this example, two unaffected parents each carry one copy of a gene mutation for an autosomal recessive disorder. They have one affected child and three unaffected children, two of which carry one copy of the gene mutation.

Courtesy of the U.S. National Library of Medicine, http://ghr.nlm.nih.gov/handbook/illustrations/chromosomes.

4. Examples of such diseases include sickle cell anemia, cystic fibrosis, and autosomal recessive polycystic kidney disease (ARPKD).

C. Sex-linked inheritance (or X-linked) refers to those genes that reside on the X chromosome. Females have two X chromosomes; males have XY (see Figure 4.13).
1. If a girl has a defective trait on one of the X chromosomes, it will be suppressed by the dominant gene for the same trait on the other X chromosome. However, if she has identical defective genes on both of her X chromosomes, she will exhibit the condition and will have a 50% chance with each pregnancy of passing on the disease allele to her offspring.
2. Since males possess only one X chromosome, if a defective gene is on the X chromosome it will always be expressed because it is unopposed by

a normal gene on the other sex chromosome. For this reason, some inherited diseases are almost exclusively diseases of males and some X-linked disorders are lethal in males.
3. When a male is affected, all of his daughters will gain the diseased allele, but none of his sons.
4. Examples of X-linked diseases or conditions are hemophilia and color-blindness.

D. Additional terminology.
1. Penetrance: the degree in which a given trait will result in a phenotype. Some mutations can exist without showing a phenotype in every individual. Some conditions have age-related penetrance; i.e., the older a person is, the more likely he or she will develop the condition if carrying a susceptible genotype. Male pattern baldness is one such example.
2. Variable expression: many genetic disorders have a wide variety of signs and symptoms, but not all individuals with the disorder will manifest them to the same degree. Myotonic muscular dystrophy is one such example. The disease may manifest all of the associated symptoms, while others may have only mild symptoms or symptoms that go unrecognized.
3. Anticipation: genetic disease that increases in severity or appears at an earlier age with each successive generation. Huntington disease and fragile X disease are examples.
4. Codominance: a pattern of inheritance in which neither phenotype is dominant and the person expresses both phenotypes. For example, the Landsteiner blood types. The gene for blood types has three alleles: A, B, and i. The i allele causes O type and is recessive to both A and B.

IV. The impact of aging.

A. Three fundamental characteristics of the aging process.
1. It is an individual phenomenon and the issues of heterogeneity (unlike natures) and diversity within broad age-specific patterns must be taken into account.
2. It is a multidimensional and complex phenomenon. It involves multiple and diverse processes that lead to the gradual physical and cognitive deterioration of the person. No single variable can capture the full extent of the complexity.
3. It is dynamic as the nature and impact of aging changes as the individual gets older.

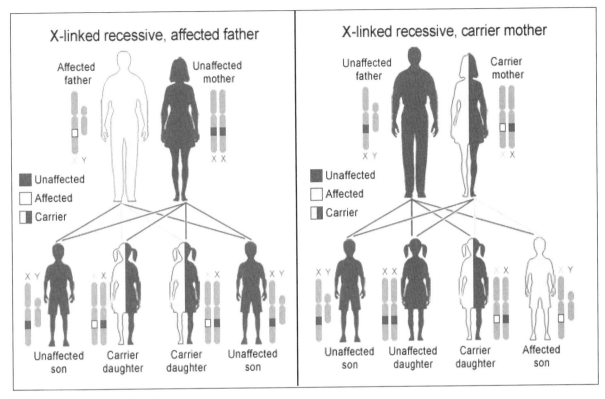

Figure 4.13. X-linked recessive.
Courtesy of the U.S. National Library of Medicine, http://ghr.nlm.nih.gov/handbook/illustrations/chromosomes.

B. Genetic and environmental factors.
1. Both genetic and environmental factors play a role in the aging process, although genetic factors seem to provide a more powerful effect.
2. The quality of health care received and living a healthy lifestyle are important environmental factors affecting aging.

C. Cellular changes associated with aging.
1. The rate at which cells multiply tends to slow down.
2. The T-cell lymphocytes decrease with age, having an effect on the immune system.
3. Age changes the response to environmental stresses such as ultraviolet rays, heat, inadequate oxygen, poor nutrition, and toxins.
4. Age interferes with apoptosis, resulting in cell death at the appropriate time. Diseases common in the elderly can affect the process in different ways. For example, cancer results in the loss of apoptosis, and the cells continue to multiply and invade surrounding tissue. In Alzheimer's disease and Parkinson's disease, cells die too early.

D. With advancing age, persons become less like each other biologically, and health care needs to be more individualized.

V. **Genetic testing is the analysis of human DNA, RNA, chromosomes, proteins, or certain metabolites** to detect alterations related to a heritable disease or condition. Genetic tests have the potential for broad public health impact.

A. Methods. Genetic tests are not equal. An optimal testing strategy for a specific condition may use one or more test methodologies and may include testing various specimens. Some tests are best used for specific patient groups.
1. Direct testing: directly examining the DNA or RNA that makes up a gene.
2. Linkage testing: looking at markers co-inherited with a disease-causing gene.
3. Biochemical testing: assaying certain metabolites.
4. Cytogenetic testing: examining the chromosomes.

B. Points to consider.
   1. Genetic test results usually apply to not only the patient but also to other family members.
   2. Other family members may need to be tested.
   3. Some genetic testing applies only to the individual. For example, the Oncotype DX test is used to determine the effects of treatment on breast cancer and the chance of its recurrence. This is quite different from genomic testing that could impact other family members and does not require an informed consent.
   4. Most genetic testing should include an informed consent, test interpretation, and follow-up care as determined.
      a. The purpose of the informed consent process is to provide people with sufficient information so they can make informed choices. It is a dynamic and continuing exchange of information.
      b. The informed consent document provides a summary of the information and is often considered the foundation of the process. It does not represent the entirety of the process of informing the patient.
      c. Because of the often profound impact of genetic testing, patients should be adequately counseled about the specifics of the test.
      d. There is a duty to inform the patient of the test's purpose, medical implications, alternatives, and possible risks and benefits. Patients should also be made aware of their rights to privacy, including if and where their DNA will be stored and who will have access to their personal information.
   5. Genetic testing is often done at specialized laboratories.
   6. Commercialization of tests must be prevented before safety, efficacy, and cost-effectiveness can be established.

C. Ethical considerations of genetic testing.
   1. Autonomy is synonymous with the right to choose. The patient must be given enough information to make an informed, reasonable, and independent decision on whether or not to proceed with testing (self-governance and respect for genetic privacy).
      a. Children and adolescents: the issues of consent and confidentiality are of concern. Particular attention is given to the implications of predictive testing for late onset disorders, carrier testing, and newborn screening.
      b. Prenatal testing: a diagnosis has the potential of providing early detection of abnormalities, reassuring and reducing anxiety, preparing for optimal management at birth, allowing for prenatal treatment in some cases, or allowing couples to make choices about continuation of pregnancies.
   2. Beneficence and nonmaleficence are the principles of "doing good" and "doing no harm." Within the informed consent and during the process of obtaining informed consent, the benefits and all possible risks must be disclosed to allow an informed decision by the patient.
   3. Justice relates to whether an individual is treated fairly and equitably in the context of society.
      a. Discrimination: there is public concern of potential loss of privacy and resulting insurance or employment discrimination if labeled with a "preexisting condition."
      b. Equitable access to resources: many people feel as though genetic testing is out of their reach.
   4. Confidentiality and privacy imply the assumption of nondisclosure of an individual's genetic information to third parties with the exception of certain situations that require protection of other persons ("duty to warn").
      a. Implications for family members.
         (1) A patient's genetic diagnosis always has to be interpreted in the context of family history.
         (2) A genetic diagnosis never has implications solely for the patient but instead reflects disease probability and risk factors in other blood relatives. There may be different reactions among family members. Some may not want the information, and healthy relatives who learn they have a predisposition to a disease may have significant changes in quality of life.
         (3) Issues on confidentiality may be raised when a person gives information on an affected family member without that individual's consent.
      b. A key assumption underlying the "duty to warn" is the availability of medical interventions to lessen the risk of developing disease or to lessen harm.
         (1) For some hereditary disorders, effective medical interventions are either minimal or just emerging.
         (2) For other hereditary disorders, there are clear interventions leading to prevention.

(3) For some syndromes, genetic risks may be incompletely defined and interventions may be ineffective.

(4) Less than 1% of clinicians surveyed believed that a breach of patient confidentiality would be warranted to warn at-risk relatives about a disease for which no medical intervention existed.

(5) The duty to warn is contrary to the Health Insurance Portability and Accountability Act (HIPPA) of 1996.

(6) Certain states have enacted statutes that prohibit the release of genetic information without the written consent of the individual.

(7) The American Medical Association (AMA), as well as the American Society of Clinical Oncology (ASCO), has taken a practical approach to the situation. They state that a physician's obligations (if any) to a family at risk are to communicate to the person being tested the risks that family members face. This information and communication should be carefully documented and should be a part of the Informed Consent and discussed again at the time of genetic counseling.

c. Nonpaternity issues.
(1) Detection of misattributed paternity is not a rare incidence in situations where DNA analysis is carried out.
(2) The situation can become complex (e.g., during testing to become a transplant donor for a sibling).

D. To request or decline genetic testing is ultimately the patient's choice. It is the patient who must consider the risks and benefits of a genetic test while considering his/her own personal and family situation. It is the patient who must make the decision based on his/her own beliefs, values, and priorities. Even though a health care provider may see direct benefit to a patient, providing the information regarding genetic testing should be done in a nondirective manner, not with the purpose of encouraging a particular course of action.

E. Evaluation of Genomic Applications in Practice and Prevention (EGAPP) is a model project initiated in 2004 by the Office of Genomics and Disease Prevention at the CDC.
1. Genetic tests for more than 1,200 diseases have been developed, with more than 950 currently available for clinical testing. These tests and other anticipated applications of genomic technologies for screening and prevention have the potential for broad public health impact.
2. There is the need to develop evidence to establish efficacy and cost-effectiveness before these tests are commercialized.
3. The project's goal is to support the first phases of a coordinated process for evaluating genetic tests and other genomic applications that are in transition from research to clinical and public health practice.

VI. The identification of mutations.

A. DNA sequencing: determining the exact order of the bases in a strand of DNA.

B. Microarray technology – studying which genes are "turned on" at a given time point and how the cell's regulatory networks control the vast numbers of genes simultaneously (see Figure 4.14).
1. This method uses a robot to precisely apply tiny droplets containing DNA or small complementary oligonucleotides to glass slides. Fluorescent labels are attached to modified RNA (complementary DNA) from the cells that are being studied. The slide is put into a scanning microscope where the brightness of each fluorescent dot is measured; the brightness reveals how much of a specific RNA or DNA is present which usually indicates whether or not a gene is active.

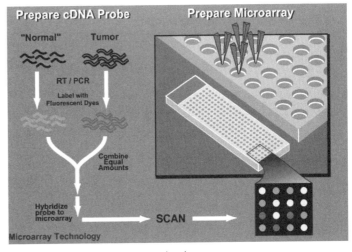

Figure 4.14. Microarray technology.

Courtesy of Talking Glossary of Genetics, http://www.genome.gov, National Human Genome Research Institute, National Institutes of Health.

2. Microarray technology is being used to try to understand gene expression, fundamental aspects of growth and development, and the underlying causes of the genetic relationship to many human diseases.

C. Allele-specific oligonucleotide testing (ASO) – detecting a specific mutation using a synthetic segment of DNA approximately 20 base pairs in length (an oligonucleotide) that binds to and identifies the complementary sequence in the DNA sample. An oligonucleotide is commonly called an oligo and is typically less than 50 nucleotides in length. This technology is often used in a microarray format.

D. Single-stranded conformational polymorphism (SSCP) uses gel electrophoresis to identify a segment of DNA containing a mutation.
   1. It can be used as the first step in mutation scanning.
   2. SSCP can be used when mutations are distributed throughout the gene and when mutations are rare as in family specific mutations.
   3. SSCP may cover the entire gene or select regions.

E. Protein truncation testing (PTT) – identifying the shortened (truncated) proteins that result from mutations which specifically cause premature termination of mRNA translation.

VII. Examples of kidney diseases with known genetic connection.

A. Anderson-Fabry disease (AFD) results from deficient activity of the enzyme alpha-galacto-sidase (alpha-Gal A) and progressive lysosomal deposition of globotriaosylceramide (GL-3).
   1. Deposition of glycolipids can be found in the glomerular cells, tubular epithelial cells, and vascular cells. Segmental and ultimately global sclerosis, tubular atrophy, and interstitial scarring lead to kidney dysfunction.
   2. The gene is mapped to the X-chromosome and contains 7 exons. Mutations have been described in every exon; 57% are missense mutations, 11% nonsense, 18% partial gene deletions, 6% insertions, and 6% RNA processing defects caused by abnormal processing.
   3. It affects more males than females. While 1 in 40,000 males has AFD disease, in the general population the figure is 1 in 117,000.
   4. Median survival is 50 years for affected males and 70 years for carrier females.

5. AFD disease is inherited in an X-linked recessive manner. In most cases, as de novo mutations are rare, the mother of an affected male is a carrier.
   6. A carrier female has a 50% chance of transmitting the mutation in each pregnancy.
   7. All daughters of affected males are obligate carriers.
   8. Prenatal testing is available.

B. Polycystic kidney disease (PKD) is a genetic disorder characterized by the growth of cysts in the kidneys.
   1. The fluid-filled cysts slowly replace much of the mass of the kidneys and compromise kidney function. The cysts originate in the nephrons but eventually separate and continue to enlarge. While roughly retaining its shape, the kidney also enlarges and can end up weighing as much as 22 pounds.
   2. In the United States, about 500,000 people have PKD.
   3. There are two major inherited forms of PKD and a noninherited form.
   4. Autosomal dominant PKD (ADPKD) is one of the most common inherited disorders and affects 1 in 400 to 1,000 live births. If one parent has the disease, there is a 50% chance of passing the mutation to every child conceived. However, de novo mutations occur in about 10% of affected families. In some rare cases the de novo mutation occurs spontaneously soon after conception, and the parents are not the source of the disease.
      a. It is important that parents are adequately screened by imaging methods.
      b. Mutations in the PKD1 gene account for approximately 85% of affected families. Mutations in PKD2 gene account for 15% of affected families.
      c. PKD1 and PKD2 mutations have different prognostic implications, with PKD2 patients developing kidney cysts, hypertension, and ESRD at a later age than PKD1 patients.
      d. Prenatal testing is possible if the mutation has been identified in an affected family member.
      e. Variability in the disease within families coupled with clustering of the disease's extrarenal manifestations suggest that environmental factors and modifier genes play a role in the clinical severity of ADPKD.
   5. Autosomal recessive PKD (ARPKD) affects 1/10,000 to 1/40,000 individuals. The disease is

caused by a particular genetic flaw that both parents must carry and both pass on to their baby. There is a 25% chance of this happening. If only one parent carries the abnormal gene, the baby cannot get the disease. Severity of the disease varies, but in the worst cases the baby can die hours or days after birth. Others may have sufficient kidney function for a few years.
  a. If there are other siblings, each child has a:
    (1) 25% chance of inheriting both the disease causing allele and being affected.
    (2) 50% chance of inheriting the disease causing allele and being a carrier.
    (3) 25% chance of inheriting neither the disease causing allele nor being a carrier.
  b. Mutations are in a single gene on the short arm of chromosome.
  c. Prenatal testing for pregnancies at 25% risk is available using molecular genetic testing if both disease causing alleles have been identified in an affected family member.
6. Acquired cystic kidney disease (ACKD) develops in persons with long-term kidney damage and scarring, especially in those who have been on dialysis for an extended period. About 90% of people on dialysis for 5 years develop ACKD.

C. Medullary cystic kidney disease (MCKD) is a hereditary disorder associated with familial juvenile nephrophthisis (NPH) and with familial juvenile hyperuricemia nephropathy (FJHN). MCKD and FJHN have an autosomal dominant pattern of inheritance. NPH has an autosomal recessive pattern of inheritance.
1. MCKD is characterized by functionally and morphologically abnormal tubules leading to interstitial inflammation and fibrosis.
  a. MCKD1 was mapped to chromosome 1 and accounts for the minority of cases. MCKD2 was mapped to chromosome 16 and accounts for mutations in most cases.
  b. MCKD occurs in older patients; patients reach end-stage renal disease between 30 and 50 years of age.
  c. When cysts are found, they are located at the corticomedullary junction and in the medulla. The presence of cysts is not universal.
2. FJHN has similar features and disease course with MCKD.
  a. FJHN gene has been identified on chromosome 16 in proximity to the MCKD gene locus, making these two disorders potentially allelic.

  b. Hyperuricemia caused by reduced fractional excretion of uric acid is the hallmark of FJHN and has also been described in some cases of MCKD.
3. NPH occurs in young children and may have associated extrarenal manifestations. The kidney problems begin at about 4 years of age leading to end stage usually by the second decade of life.
  a. The gene responsible for NPH has been mapped to chromosome 2, making this disease unrelated to MCKD.
  b. MCKD has been traditionally associated with NPH because of similar clinical features and pathologic findings.

D. Alport's syndrome or hereditary nephritis.
1. The prevalence of the genetic mutation is estimated to be 1 in 5,000 to 1 in 10,000.
2. In 85% of the cases there is an X-linked inheritance. Carrier mothers may have hematuria due to the random inactivation of one of the X chromosomes.
3. Of the non-X-linked cases, most are autosomal recessive.
4. Genetic mutation appears to result in a post-translational defect that prevents the assembly of protomers that are required for the formation of basement membranes.

E. Essential hypertension is by far the most common type of high blood pressure.
1. Essential hypertension is a multifactoral disease involving interactions among genetic, environmental, demographic, vascular, and neuroendocrine factors.
2. Molecular genetic studies have identified mutations in eight genes that cause hypertension. (They have also identified mutations in nine genes that cause hypotension.)
3. A number of polymorphisms have been associated with differences in blood pressure. Most prominent are the polymorphisms in the angiotensin-renin-aldosterone system. This system evolved millions of years ago to protect early humans during times of drought or stress. Today's high-salt diets and sedentary lifestyles can wreak havoc on this system.
4. Some studies suggest that some people with essential hypertension may inherit abnormalities of the sympathetic nervous system.
5. The complex nature of the hypertension phenotype makes large-scale studies indispensable.

VIII. Example of environmental exposure coupled with a genetic component and leading to kidney disease.

A. Identifying information.
   1. Nurses need to be able to locate credible and current resources to provide patient education (see Table 4.2).
   2. The Agency for Toxic Substances and Disease Registry (ATSDR) is directed by a congressional mandate to perform specific functions concerning the effect of public health of hazardous substances in the environment.
   3. Since 1970, the Environmental Protection Agency (EPA) has been working for a cleaner, healthier environment for the American people.

B. Exposure pathways explain how external conditions (exposures) relate to the development of disease. ATSDR defines an exposure pathway as the route a substance takes from its source (where it began) to its end point (where it ends) and how people can come into contact with it (or get exposed to it). There are 5 parts to the Exposure Disease Model:
   1. Environmental contamination of air, water, soil, or food with potential exposure.
   2. Biologic uptake leading to exposure. Primary routes of exposure are respiratory, oral, and dermal. Secondary routes of exposure are breast milk, transplacental, nonplacental/intrauterine, and parenteral (absorption > internal dose > distribution > metabolism > excretion).
   3. Target organ contact with a biologically effective dose.
   4. Biologic change with both repair and physiologic adaptation taking place or the threshold is exceeded.
   5. Clinical disease occurs.

C. While researchers are gaining a better understanding by identifying genes that influence the bioaccumulation and susceptibility of a person to an exposure, there are still unanswered questions as to why some people are more susceptible than others to develop the clinical disease.

D. Lead poisoning. At least three polymorphic genes have been identified that can potentially influence the bioaccumulation and toxicokinetics of lead in humans.
   1. Lead is a naturally occurring element that people have used almost since the beginning of civilization.
   2. Most human exposure to lead occurs through ingestion or inhalation. Almost all inhaled lead is absorbed into the body. From 20% to 70% is absorbed when ingested.
   3. Lead paint is the major source of exposure for children. Over 80% of the homes built before 1978 in the United States contain lead based paint.
   4. Certain folk remedies may also cause lead exposure.
      a. Mexican: azarcon and greta used to treat the colic-like illness empacho. Theses products are also known as liga, Maria Luisa, alacorn, coral, and rueda.
      b. Asian communities: chuifong tokuwan, ghasard, bali goli, and kandu.
      c. Middle Eastern: remedies and cosmetics include alkohl, saoott, and cebagin.
   5. Moonshine whiskey is another potential source of lead exposure.
   6. Acute, high-dose, lead-induced impairment of proximal tubular function manifests itself in aminoaciduria, glycosuria, and hyperphosphaturia. These effects appear to be reversible but can develop into chronic and irreversible lead nephropathy.

E. Acrodynia is a disease of infants and young children caused by chronic mercury poisoning. It is also known as pink disease.
   1. Clinical characteristics include proteinuria and nephrotic syndrome in progressing cases. Dialysis and plasma exchange may be needed.
   2. Fortunately this is now a rare disease as the use of mercury in different medications and products has been discontinued.

IX. Pharmacogenetics and pharmacogenomics involve the study of the role of inheritance in individual variation in drug response that can vary from potentially life-threatening adverse drug reactions to equally serious lack of therapeutic efficacy. These new and emerging fields evolved from the convergence of molecular pharmacology and genomics.

A. *Pharmacogenetics* focus on specific genes, such as drug-metabolizing enzymes. It dates back to the 1950s when researchers first noted an inherited tendency in the way people react to drugs.

B. *Pharmacogenomics* deals with the entire human genome, including genes for numerous proteins in the body, such as transporters, receptors, and the

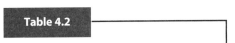

Genetic Resources for Nurses and/or Patients Found on the Web

Alliance of Genetic Support Groups http://www.geneticalliance.org	This is a coalition of genetic support groups that includes a list of genetic organizations.
American Nurses Association http://www.nursingworld.org	The "Essential Nursing Competencies and Curricula Guidelines for Genetics and Genomics" document created by the Consensus Panel in 2005 can be found here. Within the document is an 18-page appendix filled with additional resources that are broken down into categories.
Centers for Disease Control http://www.cdc.gov	The Office of Genetics and Disease Prevention not only provides a wealth of information regarding genetics and genomics, but it also provides many links to other valuable sites.
Cincinnati Children's Hospital Medical Center http://www.cincinnatichildrens.org/ed/clinical/gpnf	This site offers free continuing education modules for nurses on genetics.
Department of Health and Human Services http://www.os.dhhs.gov	Information can be found here on a wide variety of related topics, including the U.S. Surgeon General's Family History Initiative. There are also several links available.
Gene Tests http://www.genetests.org	This site provides information about genetic tests and laboratories performing them. It also has a very useful glossary of terms and illustrations.
Human Genome Project http://www.ornl.gov/hgmis/medicine/medicine.html	A large quantity of valuable information can be found here. It includes the Human Genome Project itself, research, education, ethics, and medicine.
International Society of Nurses in Genetics, Inc. (ISONG) http://www.isong.org	This site contains a variety of position statements, as well as a statement on the scope and standards of genetics clinical nursing practice.
March of Dimes http://www.marchofdimes.com	This site provides educational programs for nurses in genetics, as well as fact sheets on genetic conditions.
National Coalition for Health Professional Education in Genetics http://www.nchpeg.org	This site offers current information on educational initiatives and recommendations of core competencies in genetics for all health care professionals.
National Human Genome Research Institute http://www.genome.gov	This site contains an abundance of information on research, health, policy, ethics, education, and training.
National Institutes of Health http://www.nih.gov	This site also provides a plethora of information and multiple links.
PKD Foundation http://www.pkdcure.org	This site provides information about Polycystic Kidney Disease for patients, families, and health care providers.
U.S. Surgeon General Family History Initiative – "My Family Health Portrait" http://www.hhs.gov/familyhistory	The software for families to complete a pedigree drawing is found here.

entire signaling networks that respond to drugs and move them through the system.

C. This pharmacogenetics and pharmacogenomics combination hopes to form the road to

personalized medicine.

1. The products of this technology would replace the one-formula-fits-all drugs that typically work for only 60% of the population at best.
2. More worrisome and costly are the serious

adverse drug reactions that are responsible for 100,000 deaths a year in the United States and cost society approximately $100 billion a year.

D. Significant challenges remain to be overcome if pharmacogenetics and pharmacogenomics are to have a major medical impact. Research and policy changes are needed.
1. A key task for pharmacogenetics researchers is to pinpoint all of the proteins that medicine will encounter in the body and determine how these proteins vary from person to person.
2. The National Institute of General Medical Sciences (NIGMS) is leading a National Institute of Health (NIH) effort to encourage pharmacogenetics research. They are doing this by allocating funds to various research groups and developing a large public database of the results of the studies. The purpose of the database is to match up genetic variations (genotypes) with functional outcomes (phenotypcs).
3. The Pharmacogenetics and Pharmacogenomics Knowledge Base (PharmGKB) provides a shared online resource that contains information and analytic tools and is freely available to the scientific community. In addition, it helps researchers identify and fill in knowledge gaps. To protect the privacy of the study participants, names and other identifying information are not stored in this library.
4. An explosion of DNA testing will occur. Once drug sensitivity testing is available, it will become the standard against which negligence can be measured in cases of severe or fatal drug reactions.
5. Medical doctors (MDs) and advanced practice nurses (APNs) will have to work out means of educating patients about genetics and preserving confidentiality of the patient's records.
6. The cost of DNA testing and the high price for safer, more effective drug therapy will drive up expenses.

E. Application to clinical practice is currently limited, but the technology is steadily moving forward. For example, the Cincinnati Children's Hospital Medical Center launched a genetic pharmacology service that enables MDs and APNs to test 52 common medications against four well defined genes. This test, which only has to be done once in a lifetime, will help the clinicians to determine how patients will respond to these drugs and thereby improve patient safety.
1. Warfarin. Researchers have found that differ-

ences in a gene influence the dose of warfarin that is the most effective for each person. The genetic variation in drug metabolizing enzyme gene: CYP2C9, CYP1A2, CYP2C19, CYP3A4. This information could ultimately help in the determination of each patient's dose quickly and precisely and without trial and error.
2. Transporter proteins help control responses to antidepressants and other drugs. These proteins not only bring essential material into the cell, but also purge the cell of wastes, drugs, and other chemicals. Researchers have found more than 1,000 genetic differences in 40 of these transporters. The genetic changes may affect the way people respond to a wide variety of drugs.
3. Losartan: an angiotensin II receptor antagonist (ARB). There is a genetic variation in drug metabolizing enzyme gene(s): CYP2C9, CYP3A4, aldosterone synthase. There is also genetic variation in angiotensin II type 1 receptor gene.
4. Within nephrology, there is promise for improvement in the ability to individualize many drugs based on the patient's genetic profile; for example, control of hypertension, specific immunosuppressive therapy posttransplant, and individualized anticoagulation during hemodialysis.

X. **Nursing and required competencies.** Registered nurses are now required to incorporate genetic and genomic knowledge and skills into their nursing practice. The following information is from *Essential Nursing Competencies and Curricula Guidelines for Genetics and Genomics* that was established by the Consensus Panel September 21–22, 2005. The entire document can be viewed at www.nursingworld.org/ethics/genetics and www.genome.gov/17517037.

A. Professional responsibilities.
1. Recognize when one's own attitudes and values related to genetic and genomic science may affect care provided to clients.
2. Advocate for clients' access to desired genetic/genomic services and/or resources including support groups.
3. Examine competency of practice on a regular basis, identifying areas of strength, as well as areas in which professional development related to genetics and genomics would be beneficial.
4. Incorporate genetic and genomic technologies and information into registered nurse practice.
5. Demonstrate in practice the importance of tailoring genetic and genomic information and

services to clients based on their culture, religion, knowledge level, literacy, and preferred language.

6. Advocate for the rights of all clients for autonomous, informed genetic-related and genomic-related decision making and voluntary action.

B. Professional practice: applying and integrating genetic and genomic knowledge.

1. Assessment. The registered nurse:
    a. Demonstrates an understanding of the relationship of genetics and genomics to health, prevention, screening, diagnostics, prognostics, selection of treatment, and monitoring of treatment effectiveness.
    b. Demonstrates ability to elicit a minimum of three-generation family health history information.
    c. Constructs pedigree from collected family history information using standardized symbols and terminology.
    d. Collects personal, health, and developmental histories that consider genetic, environmental, and genomic influences and risks.
    e. Conducts comprehensive health and physical assessments that incorporate knowledge about genetic, environmental, and genomic influences and risk factors.
    f. Critically analyzes the history and physical assessment findings for genetic, environmental, and genomic influences and risk factors.
    g. Assesses clients' knowledge, perceptions, and responses to genetic and genomic information.
    h. Develops plan of care that incorporates genetic and genomic assessment information.

2. Identification. The registered nurse:
    a. Identifies clients who may benefit from specific genetic and genomic information and/or services based on assessment data.
    b. Identifies credible, accurate, appropriate and current genetic and genomic information, resources, services, and/or technologies specific to given clients.
    c. Identifies ethical, ethnic/ancestral, cultural, religious, legal, fiscal, and societal issues related to genetic and genomic information and technologies.
    d. Defines issues that undermine the rights of all clients for autonomous, informed, genetic and genomic related decision making and voluntary action.

3. Referral activities. The registered nurse:
    a. Facilitates referrals for specialized genetic and

genomic services for clients as needed.

4. Provision of education, care and support. The registered nurse:
    a. Provides clients with interpretation of selective genetic and genomic information or services.
    b. Provides clients with credible, accurate, appropriate and current genetic and genomic information, resources, services, and/or technologies that facilitate decision making.
    c. Uses health promotion and disease prevention practices that:
        (1) Consider genetic and genomic influences on personal and environmental risk factors.
        (2) Incorporates knowledge of genetic and/or genomic risk factors (e.g., a client with a genetic predisposition for high cholesterol who can benefit from a change in lifestyle that will decrease the likelihood that the genetic risk will be expressed).
    d. Uses genetic-based and genomic-based interventions and information to improve clients' outcomes.
    e. Collaborates with health care providers in providing genetic and genomic health care.
    f. Collaborates with insurance providers/payers to facilitate reimbursement for genetic and genomic health care services.
    g. Performs interventions/treatments appropriate to clients' genetic and genomic health care needs.
    h. Evaluates impact and effectiveness of genetic and genomic technology, information, interventions, and treatments on clients' outcomes.

XI. Applying genomics to nursing practice.

A. The application of genomics to nursing practice presents a challenge to nurses to evolve from the model of intervention after disease or loss of function to more predictive models of interventions, before the disease or loss of function occurs.

B. The understanding of genomics will lead to a better understanding of a disease and will in turn contribute to more targeted and individualized care.

C. Sufficient specialists will not be available to answer all questions related to genetics and genomics. Patients and families expect nurses to have this knowledge.

1. Nurses have a long tradition of being educators, being sensitive to emotional and psychological issues, and being advocates.

2. Nurses are ideally suited to address the emerging needs of patients, families, and communities.
3. There are several genetic resources for nurses and/or patients that can be found on the Internet.

D. Families will be faced with understanding the influence of genes, the environment, and behavior. The concept of "illness time" will need to be extended.
  1. The "pre-awareness or lack of knowledge about a genetic risk state" is the time before persons know they have a genetic risk factor. The risk might become known through awareness of a family history of disease or by having a genetic test.
  2. The "nonsymptomatic state" occurs when persons are aware of the genetic risk, but remain symptom free. This phase may last from years to decades to the end of life as the genetic risk may not result in the expression of the disease.
  3. The "knowledge of risk state" might require interventions for individuals and families in response to the increased awareness of the risk, new knowledge gained of genetic risk information, or early symptoms that may have been either previously been denied or be occurring for the first time. Family members may need to begin dealing with anticipatory loss, to accept increased surveillance, to adhere to changes in health behaviors, or to accept interventions that could potentially delay the onset or progression of the disease.

E. Nurses must understand that genetic information is not deterministic.
  1. Having a genetic mutation does not guarantee that the person has the disease or that the disease will develop.
  2. The lack of a demonstrated genetic mutation does not mean that a person does not have the disease present or is not at risk to develop the disease.
  3. Understanding genetic risks could lead to behaviors meant to reduce the risk (e.g., increased surveillance, changes in diet, increasing exercise, etc.).
  4. On the other hand, understanding genetic risks could lead to a fatalistic attitude with the thought that no matter what is done, the disease will present itself.
  5. Nurses should assure that genetic information is interpreted and used in the context of what is known about the person, the family, their sociocultural perspectives, and their other risk

factors. The information will then be likely to result in benefit and not harm to individuals and families.

XII. **The family health history, if detailed and accurate,** provides one of the most powerful "genetic/genomic tools" to identify individuals at risk for inherited disorders when laboratory tests are not available. It can capture the interactions of genetic susceptibility with the environmental, cultural, and behavioral factors shared by family members (see Figure 4.15).

A. Alison Whelan and others (2004) developed a mnemonic to help identify indicators that would send up a red flag that may raise a clinician's awareness of possible genetic influences on the patient. It is not 100% sensitive or specific. The mnemonic is Family Genes.
  1. Family history: multiple affected siblings or individuals in multiple generations. It must be remembered, however, lack of family history does not rule out genetic causes.
  2. **G**: group of congenital anomalies. Common anatomic variations are not unusual; two or more are more likely to indicate the presence of a syndrome with genetic implications.
  3. **E**: extreme or exceptional presentation of common conditions. Examples: early onset cardiovascular disease, cancer, or kidney failure; unusually severe reactions to infectious or metabolic stress; recurrent miscarriage; bilateral primary cancers in paired organs; multiple primary cancers of different tissues.
  4. **N**: neurodevelopmental delay or degeneration. Suspicion should be raised in developmental delay in the pediatric age group, or in developmental regression in children or early onset dementia in adults.
  5. **E**: extreme or exceptional pathology. Examples: unusual tissue histology, such as pheochromocytoma, acoustic neuroma, medullary thyroid cancer, multiple colon polyps, plexiform neurofibromas, most pediatric malignancies.
  6. **S**: surprising laboratory results. This may be thorny considering the nature of kidney disease.

B. Collection of family medical history should include:
  1. At least three generations.
  2. Ethnic background.
  3. Status of current pregnancies.
  4. Current and past health status on all family members.

Name	Family Disease Checklist							Date
Please start this family history by telling us about health problems that you may have in your family. Are you adopted? ☐ Yes. If so complete the following items only for any of your BIOLOGICAL family members. If you are filling this out for your child please indicate here – ☐ YES and fill it out as if "you" were your child.								
	You	Mother	Father	Children	Brothers or sisters	Uncle or Aunt	Father's Parents	Mother's Parents
Allergies	☐	☐	☐	☐	☐	☐	☐	☐
Alzeheimer's Disease or Dementia	☐	☐	☐	☐	☐	☐	☐	☐
Anemia	☐	☐	☐	☐	☐	☐	☐	☐
Asthma	☐	☐	☐	☐	☐	☐	☐	☐
Arthritis	☐	☐	☐	☐	☐	☐	☐	☐
Bleeding problems	☐	☐	☐	☐	☐	☐	☐	☐
Birth Defects	☐	☐	☐	☐	☐	☐	☐	☐
Any Cancer	☐	☐	☐	☐	☐	☐	☐	☐
Breast Cancer	☐	☐	☐	☐	☐	☐	☐	☐
Ovarian Cancer	☐	☐	☐	☐	☐	☐	☐	☐
Uterine (Uterus) Cancer	☐	☐	☐	☐	☐	☐	☐	☐
Lung Cancer	☐	☐	☐	☐	☐	☐	☐	☐
Colon or Rectal Cancer	☐	☐	☐	☐	☐	☐	☐	☐
Other Cancer	☐	☐	☐	☐	☐	☐	☐	☐
Other Cancer	☐	☐	☐	☐	☐	☐	☐	☐
High Cholesterol	☐	☐	☐	☐	☐	☐	☐	☐
Chronic Infections	☐	☐	☐	☐	☐	☐	☐	☐
Clotting Problems	☐	☐	☐	☐	☐	☐	☐	☐
Depression	☐	☐	☐	☐	☐	☐	☐	☐
Diabetes (type 1)	☐	☐	☐	☐	☐	☐	☐	☐
Diabetes (type 2)	☐	☐	☐	☐	☐	☐	☐	☐
Down Syndrome	☐	☐	☐	☐	☐	☐	☐	☐
Emphysema	☐	☐	☐	☐	☐	☐	☐	☐
Epilepsy/Seizures	☐	☐	☐	☐	☐	☐	☐	☐
Glaucoma	☐	☐	☐	☐	☐	☐	☐	☐
Hearing Loss	☐	☐	☐	☐	☐	☐	☐	☐
Heart Trouble	☐	☐	☐	☐	☐	☐	☐	☐
Hemochromatosis or "Iron Overload"	☐	☐	☐	☐	☐	☐	☐	☐
High Blood Pressure	☐	☐	☐	☐	☐	☐	☐	☐
Infertility	☐	☐	☐	☐	☐	☐	☐	☐
Kidney Trouble (Renal Dx)	☐	☐	☐	☐	☐	☐	☐	☐
Memory Loss/Alzheimer's	☐	☐	☐	☐	☐	☐	☐	☐
Mental Illness	☐	☐	☐	☐	☐	☐	☐	☐
Mental Retardation	☐	☐	☐	☐	☐	☐	☐	☐
Neurofibromatosis	☐	☐	☐	☐	☐	☐	☐	☐
Obesity	☐	☐	☐	☐	☐	☐	☐	☐
Osteoporosis or "Hip Fracture"	☐	☐	☐	☐	☐	☐	☐	☐
PKU or "Metabolic" Disease at Birth	☐	☐	☐	☐	☐	☐	☐	☐
Sickle Cell Anemia	☐	☐	☐	☐	☐	☐	☐	☐
Smoking	☐	☐	☐	☐	☐	☐	☐	☐
Stillborn/Infant Death	☐	☐	☐	☐	☐	☐	☐	☐
Stroke	☐	☐	☐	☐	☐	☐	☐	☐
Violence/Domestic Abuse	☐	☐	☐	☐	☐	☐	☐	☐
Alcohol Abuse	☐	☐	☐	☐	☐	☐	☐	☐
Drug Abuse	☐	☐	☐	☐	☐	☐	☐	☐

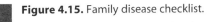

Figure 4.15. Family disease checklist.

Source: http://www.genetests.org/img/tools/famDisChecklist.gif

a. Age of onset.
b. Cause of death.
c. Age at death.

5. Inquiries about medical conditions with a known heritable component, presence of birth defects, mental retardation, and familial traits.

C. Consideration must be given to consanquinity, or genetic relatedness.

D. The family medical history should be depicted in a pedigree form using standard symbols (see Figure 4.16).
   1. First-degree relatives: parents, children, siblings (have approximately half of their genes in common).
   2. Second-degree relatives: grandparents, grandchildren, aunts, uncles, nieces, nephews.
   3. Further removed relatives as appropriate.

E. The family medical history is valuable for prevention and can influence the clinical management and prevention of disease. Prevention strategies include:
   1. Targeted lifestyle changes such as diet, exercise, and smoking cessation.
   2. Screening at earlier ages, more frequently, and with more intensive methods than might be used for average risk individuals.
   3. Use of chemoprevention such as aspirin.
   4. Referral to a specialist for assessment of genetic risk factors.

F. A research study conducted by the CDC has shown that 96.3% of respondents believed that their family history is important for their own health, yet few have actively collected health information from their relatives to develop a family history.

G. The United States Surgeon General launched a national public health campaign, called the U.S. Surgeon General's Family History Initiative to encourage all families to learn more about their family health history.
   1. The tool is "My Family Health Portrait" and is available in English or Spanish for free from the Web site www.hhs.gov/familyhistory. A free print version can be obtained by calling 1-888-275-4772. The English version is inventory #HRS00360; the Spanish version is inventory #HRS00361.
   2. The record can be shared with other family members and health care providers to help identify common diseases that may run in families.

XIII. **Genetic counseling is a communication process that deals with human problems** associated with the occurrence or risk of occurrence of a genetic disorder in a family. Due to the complexities involved with genetic testing and the far reaching effects that the results can have for both the patient and the family, genetic counseling is an integral part of the genetic testing process. Clinical genetic services may be located in a hospital, medical center, or private office. These services may be specialized by age group or by medical condition. Trained genetic practitioners can provide consultations that would include the services listed below.

A. Process includes information gathering, establishing, or verifying diagnosis, risk assessment, information giving, and psychosocial counseling. It typically takes place before and after the genetic testing is performed.

B. Assessment is gathering information from a variety of sources including:
   1. Exploring with the patient and family the reason for the referral, understanding of genetics, diagnoses under consideration, perception of disease status or risk, beliefs about the cause of the disease, and perception of disease burden.
   2. Documenting the patient's birth history, past medical history, and current status.
   3. Reviewing the family history, additional medical records on patient and affected family members, and family's social history, education, employment and social functioning.
   4. Assessing the family's sources of psychosocial support (e.g., community, religious, family, etc.).
   5. Identifying the potential ethical issues such as confidentiality, insurability, discrimination, and nonpaternity.

C. Evaluation.
   1. Consultation of relevant references.
   2. Comparison of the patient's history and exam to known diagnoses.
   3. Discussion of diagnostic impression:
      a. Clear diagnoses: information is shared about the condition.
      b. Differential diagnoses: further tests or evaluations are suggested.
      c. Unknown diagnoses: discussion focusing on

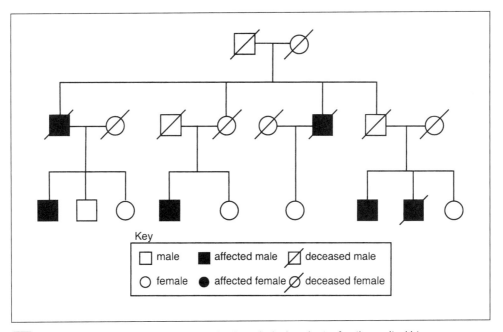

Figure 4.16. Pedigree form of standard symbols that depict family medical history.

Courtesy of Talking Glossary of Genetics, http://www.genome.gov, National Human Genome Research Institute, National Institutes of Health. Artist: Darryl Leja

what known diagnoses are ruled out; followed over time.

D. Communication involves sharing information about the condition within the family's ability to understand the information.
   1. The details about the disorder in question are reviewed, including:
      a. Expected course of the disease.
      b. Management issues and possible treatments and interventions.
      c. Underlying genetic cause if known including pattern of inheritance.
   2. Description of risks to family members compared to general population's risks.
   3. Discussion of reproductive options, if and when appropriate.
      a. Pregnancy with prenatal testing.
      b. Pregnancy without prenatal testing.
      c. Remaining childless.
      d. Parenting by adoption.
      e. Pregnancy by egg and sperm donation.
      f. Pregnancy following preimplantation genetic diagnosis.

E. Support includes helping the family cope.
   1. Recognition and discussion of the emotional responses of family members to the information given. This could include shock,

disbelief, relief, fear, guilt, sadness, shame, acceptance, etc.
   2. Review of the normal grief responses and signs that indicate further psychosocial support is needed.
   3. Listening to the whole story and hearing what the situation has meant to the family.
   4. Exploring strategies for communicating information to others, especially family members who might be at risk.
   5. Providing written materials and referrals to support groups, local and national service agencies, etc.

F. Follow-up means maintaining ongoing communication.
   1. Arranging for follow-up diagnostic testing or management appointments, or this information is communicated to the referring health care provider.
   2. Documentation of the content of the consultation for the referring health care provider and for the patient if appropriate.
   3. Contacting the patient to assess level of understanding and response to decisions made.
   4. Encouraging the family to recontact the clinic when considering pregnancy or for updated information.
   5. Being available for future questions.

Chapter 16

Cultural Diversity

Purpose

Our country has become a culturally and linguistically diverse nation, contributing to disparities in health care access, health outcomes, and health status. Nurses caring for patients from unfamiliar sociocultural backgrounds should consider a broad set of core cross-cultural issues important for these individuals. Efforts need to be made to avoid stereotyping or generalizing according to race and ethnicity. It is also important to recognize that some, but not all members, of a cultural group adhere to their traditional health beliefs or follow traditional health practices. The following information is offered to enhance the ability of nurses to understand and incorporate culturally competent care into their practice.

Objectives

Upon completion of this chapter, the learner will be able to:
1. Define culture and culturally competent services for patients with kidney disease.
2. Identify three challenges to providing culture and culturally competent services.
3. Identify the need to assess cultural needs for individual care plan development.
4. Provide culturally competent services to patients with kidney disease.

I. **Terminology.**

A. Ethnicity: human population whose members identify with each other, usually on the basis of a presumed common genealogy or ancestry (Smith, 1986).

B. Culture: a group of shared set of beliefs, norms, and values.
   1. External: physical appearance of an individual or what can be observed, which makes up 10% of culture.
   2. Internal: values, beliefs, world view, customs, traditions, language, kinship patterns, food, art and music, which makes up the other 90% of culture.

C. Race: describes populations or groups of people distinguished by different sets of characteristics and beliefs about common ancestry. The most widely used human racial categories are based on visible traits, e.g., skin color, facial features, and hair texture as well as self-identification.

D. Cultural competency: recognition and developing awareness of the patient's cultures and a set of skills, knowledge, and policies to deliver effective treatment.

E. Ethnocentrism: a person's belief in the inherent superiority of one's own culture over that of other cultures.

F. Cultural imposition: a situation where one culture forces their values and beliefs onto another culture or subculture.

G. Culture and nephrology nursing practice.
   1. When nurses recognize, understand, and incorporate cultural values of their patients into practice, patients are less apt to become dissatisfied, withdraw, and/or have unfavorable health outcomes.
   2. The nurse must first be aware of his/her own cultural values to understand another's culture in relationship to one's own. When there are identified shared meanings and common values, the patient-centered care plans are greatly facilitated. Where there are not, conscious efforts to incorporate the patient's unique values into the care plan will enhance effectiveness of the plan and patient adherence with the prescribed treatment regimen.
   3. Cultural diversity and variation occur among all humans. Professional, therapeutic care depends

on the nurse's knowledge and recognition of subtle or major differences among cultural groups. Culturally specific care leads to patient satisfaction and achievement of therapeutic outcomes.

4. Culturally competent care includes the recognition that successful adaptation for a patient will be measured and judged by his/her cultural beliefs and values, which may or may not be shared by health care professionals.

5. Other reasons to increase knowledge in cultural competency, include:
   a. Improved communication with patients and families.
   b. Increased ability in negotiating differences.
   c. Greater likelihood of disclosure of patient information to the health care provider.
   d. More effective use of time with patients.
   e. Enhanced patient adherence to treatment.
   f. Decrease in health care worker and patient stress.
   g. Higher degree of trust in a relationship.
   h. Increase in patient and provider satisfaction.
   i. Adherence to increasingly stringent government regulations and standards.
   j. Improved clinical outcomes.

H. Cultural knowledge.
   1. Obtaining information about patients' health beliefs and values to meet individual needs.
   2. Understanding disease incidence and prevalence among specific ethnic groups.

I. Cultural assessment.
   1. Gathering data about the culture of a patient.
   2. Giger and Davidhizer (1991) suggest that the culture assessment should include six domains: communication, space, social organizations, time, environmental control, and biologic variation.

J. Health.
   1. Absence of disease as defined by the patient's culture.
   2. Includes a state of complete physical, mental, and social well-being with the ability to function in activities of daily living to achieve self-fulfillment or realizing one's potential.

K. Disease.
   1. In contrast to health, disease is defined in terms of pathology and as defined by the patient's culture.
   2. Deviant behavior is determined by the culturally accepted value system to which one belongs, and therefore it is the culture, not the nature, that defines disease. Every society denotes what is normal and therefore healthy. What is considered normal is not universal.
   3. Pathology relates to the biologic structure and functioning of the human body and is described in terms of systems related to the cells, tissues, organs, fluids, and various chemicals.

L. Illness: a subjective description by a person relaying symptoms of disease or discomfort.

M. Sickness.
   1. Occurs when the person's state of illness becomes a social occurrence through either visibility or communication.
   2. Each condition can occur in the absence of any others.
   3. During the process of an illness, social roles change and behaviors are modified.
   4. A given biologic condition may or may not be considered a sickness depending on the cultural group in which it occurs.
   5. When a deviation is fairly prevalent or widespread, it is considered an everyday occurrence and therefore a normal state rather than a sickness.

N. Acculturation.
   1. The process by which a given cultural group adapts to or learns how to take on the behaviors of another group.
   2. An unconscious fusion of attitudes in order to coexist within a community. However, complete acculturation to values and beliefs rarely happens, particularly when they are in conflict with one's own values and beliefs.

O. Assimilation: the process by which individuals or groups are absorbed into and adopt the dominant culture and society of another group.

P. Cultural diversity.
   1. Variety of ethnic groups in a specific region or in the world as a whole with independent sets of norms.
   2. Considerable variations in health and illness practices.

II. **Prevalence and causation of CKD.**

A. Prevalence: According to the National Kidney Foundation (KDOQI, 2002), it is estimated that there are 20 million who have some degree of

kidney disease.
1. Stage 1, 2 (Normal or mildly reduced) 11.8 M.
2. Stage 3 (Moderate) 7.5 M.
3. Stage 4 (Severe) 400,000.
4. Stage 5 (Kidney failure and/or GFR < 15 mL/min) 300,000.

B. Causation. There are typical medical and social risk factors associated with CKD.
1. Medical risk factors include:
   a. Diabetes (30% of all patients diagnosed with CKD are diabetic).
   b. Hypertension.
   c. Autoimmune disease (e.g., lupus).
   d. Systemic infections.
   e. Frequent urinary tract infections.
   f. Recurring kidney stones.
   g. Malignancy.
   h. Family history.
   i. Trauma.
   j. Exposure to certain drugs during prolonged period of time e.g., nonsteroidal anti-inflammatory drugs.
   k. Hereditary or congenital defects.
2. Social risk factors.
   a. Age.
   b. Ethnicity.
   c. Exposure to certain chemicals and environmental conditions.
   d. Low income.
   e. Education < 12 years.
   f. Drug abuse.

C. Cultural risk factors.
1. African American (AA)/Black American. *Note*: Terminology was used based on a study in the Public Opinion Quarterly, 2005. Of all respondents, 50% preferred the term *African American* and 50% preferred the term *Black American.*
   a. Diabetes and hypertension. According to the National Institutes for Health (NIH), diabetes and hypertension account for about 70% of kidney failure in AA.
   b. Diabetes and obesity. It is estimated more than 750,000 AA have undiagnosed diabetes. Type 2 is most commonly caused by insulin resistance secondary to metabolic syndrome, obesity, hyperinsulinemia, gestational diabetes, and lack of physical exercise. Obesity is thought to play a role in 50-90% of type 2 diabetes. AA female obesity-related morbidity from diabetes has a relative risk of 2.5 deaths per 100,000 compared to whites.
   c. Cardiovascular disease, including coronary

artery disease and hypertension. The age adjusted prevalence for adults over 20 is 7.1 times higher for black men and 9 times higher for black women as compared to whites.
   d. Prostate cancer. Black males have the highest incidence and greatest mortality.
   e. HIV/AIDS is the leading cause of death in AA/Blacks between ages of 25 and 44. The death rate is higher among men than women but the trend for this is changing.
2. Hispanic.
   a. Diabetes. According to the NIH the prevalence of diabetes is 2–4 times greater in Latinos than non-Latino whites. Additionally, the incidence of type 2 diabetes in Mexican Americans is rising rapidly.
   b. Hypertension. The incidence of hypertension is equal in Hispanics and non-Latinos whites.
   c. Breast cancer. Although there is no increase in the number of Hispanics with breast cancer, there is an increase in the number who are diagnosed at a later stage of the disease.
   d. HIV/AIDs. Latinos represented 19% of the HIV/AIDS cases reported in the 1990s. There is a notable increase in the heterosexual cases of HIV among foreign born Latino men and women and of American born Latino IV drug users. Latinos and African-Americans have a higher death rate from HIV than whites.

III. Evidence-based treatment and minorities.

A. Treatment guidelines are often extrapolated from largely white populations, although applied to all, regardless of race or ethnicity.

B. The Minority Health Disparities Research and Education Act (2000) elevated the Office of Research on Minority Health to the National Center on Minority Health and Health Disparities.
1. Because of the above noted disparities, the NIH increased programmatic and budget authority for research on minority health issues and health disparities.
2. The law also promotes additional training and education for health care professionals, the evaluation of data collection systems, and a national public awareness campaign.

IV. Coping styles: those behaviors used in the management of an illness. There are cultural-specific behaviors viewed by various ethnic groups

as acceptable in certain circumstances.

A. Chinese have a need to maintain harmony and therefore will agree with everything the physician/provider or nurse is saying. Therefore, it may be difficult to ascertain if the treatment plan is understood and acceptable to the patient.

B. Vietnamese may hesitate to ask a question in group settings. Questioning an authority figure is viewed as a sign of disrespect. As a result, education in a group setting may not be effective and one on one care planning more appropriate with this cultural group.

C. Gender may also influence how persons within certain cultures cope with illness.
   1. Female AAs believe hypertension and stress are related and feel the need to discuss stress-related issues and not keep things inside.
   2. Male AAs believe stress should be dealt with through action and are not likely to express their feelings or seek help, as it is viewed as a sign of weakness.

V. Spirituality and religion in health care (refer to spirituality section for additional reading). Spirituality is a person's individual journey in finding purpose and meaning. Religion is an organized system of beliefs encompassing cause, nature, and the purpose of the universe, especially pertaining to the worshiping of a God and or gods.

A. Patient's attitudes are the key to the healing process and are essential for self-fulfillment.

B. Beliefs and attitudes need to be understood by the nurse for optimal physical and emotional health, including the patient's spiritual well-being. Spirituality is often neglected when providing nursing care. This can be attributed to nurses:
   1. Viewing religion as a private subject and belief that spirituality should be kept between the person and his/her maker.
   2. Being uncomfortable about own beliefs.
   3. Having a knowledge deficit related to spirituality and religious concerns of others.
   4. Mistaking spiritual needs for psychosocial needs.
   5. Considering spiritual needs as the job of spiritual leaders and not that of the nurse.

VI. Cultural assessment.

A. Spiritual/religious beliefs and values.
   1. Meaning of kidney disease.

   2. Preferred treatment.
   3. Preferred outcomes.
   4. Preferences about palliative care and advanced directives.
   5. Role of medications.
   6. Sources of cultural stigma and esteem.
   7. Preferred personal role on treatment team.

B. Role of significant others.
   1. Caretaker's role and effects of affiliations with cultural organizations.
   2. Types of support as defined by cultural and family networks.
   3. Preferred role for those networks (e.g., do not resuscitate orders).
   4. Role of family vs. individual in decision making.
   5. Role of the authority figure within family or social group.
   6. Role of the community or spiritual leaders in decision making.

C. Lifestyle and practices.
   1. Family and individual nutrition and dietary practices.
   2. Genetic risk patterns.
   3. Spiritual and religious practices.
   4. Substance use or nonuse.
   5. Activity levels.
   6. Stress generating or stress reduction practices.
   7. Practices affecting depression.
   8. Important cultural traditions.

D. Access to the health care system and other resources.
   1. Three high risk groups.
      a. Low socioeconomic status.
      b. Illegal immigrants for fear of deportation.
      c. Rural areas where logistics impede one's ability to seek or receive health care.
   2. Resources for transportation, medications, and nutritional requirements.
   3. Referrals to nephrologist, kidney education, kidney transplant evaluation, counseling for depression, loss, and grief, crisis management, transition planning (e.g., beginning dialysis), and translation and literacy support.

E. Adherence.
   1. The degree to which patients follow their medication and treatment regimen.
   2. Often, nonadherence is directly related to a knowledge deficit by the patient, and measures of a culturally competent teaching plan need to be implemented by the nurse (see Patient and Family Education chapter for additional infor-

mation). Therefore, the term *noncompliance* should not be used.

3. Adherence can also be impacted by lifestyle issues, values, medication side effects (cultural biology), and regimen complexity.

4. Adjust the plan of care based on culturally unique needs, resources, and beliefs.

5. Interventions to enhance adherence and service quality.

a. Identify effects of own cultural background on providing patient care.

b. Acknowledge cultural differences with patient and bridge similarities.

c. Complete a cultural assessment regarding adherence potential.

d. Use cultural validation statements to support cultural strengths, needs, and goals.

e. Use challenges, identified through assessment questions, to focus on meeting individualized needs.

f. Use cultural exception questions to enhance coping and lifestyle practices.

g. Increase patient and social network involvement in treatment.

h. Develop patient-centered behavioral contracts.

VII. Mistrust.

A. In a survey conducted for the Kaiser Family Foundation (Brown et al., 1999), 12% of AAs and 15% of Latinos, in comparison with 1% of whites, felt that a physician/provider judged them unfairly or treated them with disrespect because of their race or ethnic background.

B. Research indicates that some minority groups are more likely than whites to delay seeking treatment until symptoms are more severe.

C. Immigrants and refugees from many regions of the world, including Central and South America and Southeast Asia, feel extreme mistrust of government. This mistrust is based on atrocities committed in their country of origin and fear of deportation.

D. Tips for managing mistrust.
1. Recognizing prejudice and its effects.
2. Build trust and reassure your patient of your intentions.
3. Keep in perspective "what's at stake" for the patient; showing respect for patient's concerns.

VIII. Communication.

A. Human interaction: culture is transmitted and is both verbal and nonverbal.

B. Poor communication is one of the biggest challenges when working with patients from diverse cultures.

C. Misunderstandings lead to lack of respect for persons whose cultural values are different from one's own and may cause harm to those persons, sometimes culturally, psychologically, physically, or spiritually.

D. In some cultures, words are sacred, pauses are common, and interruptions are considered rude. Speaking too loudly may be a sign of disrespect.

E. Communication tools must include sensitivity, awareness, knowledge, and alternatives to written communication.

IX. Health care disparities.

A. Patient factors.
1. Patient choice or preference.
2. Cultural beliefs about health and medical care.
3. Minority mistrust of the health care system (based in part on high reported rates of perceived instances of past discrimination).
4. Language barriers.
5. Difficulties in cross-racial/ethnic provider-patient communication.
6. Alleged biologic differences in clinical presentation or responses to treatments and medications.
7. Unmeasured aspects of socioeconomic status assumed to be associated with race or ethnicity.

B. Provider factors.
1. Lack of cultural competency.
2. Professional practice styles.
3. Clinical uncertainty about the findings in assessment, medical history, or symptom presentation of patients from diverse cultures.
4. Both conscious and unconscious racial/ethnic bias and negative stereotyping that influence clinical decisions.
5. Groups of professionals can be said to have a "culture" in the sense that they have a shared set of beliefs, norms, and values.
6. Culture is reflected in the language and terms members of a cultural group use, emphasis in their textbooks, their mindset, or worldview.

X. Culture, society, and kidney disease.

A. With the range of effective treatments for kidney disease and the diversity of settings and sectors in which these treatments are offered, consumers can exercise choice in treatment.

B. Consumers can choose between treatment modalities, such as hemodialysis, peritoneal dialysis, kidney transplantation, and no treatment based on cultural beliefs or societal pressure.

XI. Cultural variances.

A. Family influences are important resources for effective prevention and behavior changes. The family is broadly defined to include relationships rooted in lineage, descent, or kinship.
   1. Within the AA culture, there is the frequent use of given titles such as Aunt, Uncle, Brother, or Sister. These individuals may be called upon during times of serious illness or to influence behavioral change.
   2. Also within the AA culture, there is a greater proportion of females that are the head of the household. On the average, AA women are the lowest wage earners of all race/gender groups; thus many live below poverty level.
   3. Within Asian cultures, often an individual puts the family's needs above his/her own. Extended families often live together as a single-family unit that includes grandparents, parents, children, and the families of paternal uncles. Family decision making usually includes extended family members. Children are expected to obey elders and to put the family's needs above their own.
   4. Within American Indians and Pacific Islanders, family is of paramount importance. The extended family structure of Indian communities reflects the importance to this socialization source. They may involve others who have experienced a disease or illness, outside the family, as well as the use of communal ceremony that involves both healing and prevention.

B. Communication and language.
   1. African Americans are a highly expressive people.
   2. African American language involves subtle patterns of verbal and body language that are often misunderstood by people unfamiliar with these patterns.
   3. Middle Easterner cultures consider it disrespectful to look directly into the eyes of an authoritative figure when speaking. This is in stark contrast to Western cultures who consider it disrespectful not to look in a person's eyes during conversation.

   4. Among Latinos, eye contact may not occur, especially among persons of low socioeconomic level, particularly if the patient does not agree with or understand the treatment plan.
   5. There are still a great many cultures such as Native Americans and Middle Easterners who require that a head of the household, most often males, communicate the wishes of the family. This can be challenging when attempting to maintain confidentiality and follow the Health Insurance Portability and Accountability Act (HIPAA) requirements.
   6. Nonverbal communication in the form of hugs, handshakes, and smiles are considered personal expressions of warmth and caring by Hispanics/Latinos and are important priorities. However, hand respect is valued, and handshakes may be seen as familiar or patronizing and experienced negatively.

C. Health beliefs.
   1. Traditional medicine in most Hispanic countries includes an extensive list of folk remedies.
      a. Using garlic to treat hypertension and cough.
      b. Chamomile to treat nausea, gas, colic, and anxiety.
      c. A purgative tea combined with stomach massage to cure lack of appetite, stomach pains, or diarrhea.
      d. Peppermint to treat dyspepsia and gas.
   2. Asian Americans believe that the universe is composed of opposing elements held in balance. Thus, health is a state of balance between these opposing forces, known as *am* and *duong* in Vietnam and *yin* and *yang* in China. Chinese medicine is complex with well established therapeutic tradition that uses acupuncture, acupressure, and herbs, often in combination with dietary therapy, Western medicine, and supernatural healing. Some Chinese may believe that illness is a result of moral retribution by ancestors due to a person's misdeeds or negligence. Other health beliefs, held by patients from this group, include cosmic disharmony due to a poor combination of year of birth, month of birth, day of birth, and time of birth, or poor Feng Shui such as improper placement of objects inside a room or orientation of the room or house itself.
   3. Among some Eastern religions, patients may feel that his/her illness is caused by karma (the law of cause and effect over countless lifetimes), even though the patient may understand that the actual illness has a biologic cause.
   4. Some Hispanic people believe that disease is

caused by an imbalance between hot and cold principles. Health is maintained by avoiding exposure to extreme temperatures and by consuming appropriate foods and beverages.

5. Some Cambodians may cup, pinch, coin, or rub an ill person's skin to treat a range of ailments. This may cause a skin alteration or scar so it is important that these techniques not be labeled as abuse without further cultural assessment.

6. American Indians often rely on traditional healers. Some Native Americans/American Indian/Alaska Natives believe that healing will result from sacred ceremonies that rely on having visions and using plants and/or objects symbolic of the individual, the illness, or the treatment. Native American herbal medicine is widely used by alternative medical practitioners. Examples include the use of echinacea, goldenseal, and burdock. Native Americans have a keen awareness of a sense of well-being, healing, and cultural context. To care for the Native American, the nephrology nurse must respect traditional healing practices that aim to restore balance and harmony to the mind, body, spirit, and community. Health care professionals must define and value health as they are defined and valued in traditional Native American communities.

D. Complementary alternative medicine (CAM).
1. Complementary medicine is used in conjunction with conventional medicine, for example, the use of aromatherapy to help lessen a patient's discomfort following surgery.
2. Alternative medicine is used in place of conventional medicine. For example, using a special diet to treat cancer instead of undergoing surgery, radiation, or chemotherapy that has been recommended by a conventional prescriber.
3. Five domains of CAM.
   a. Alternative medical systems are built upon complete systems of theory and practice. Examples of alternative medical systems that have developed in Western cultures include homeopathic and naturopathic medicine. Systems that have developed in non-Western cultures include traditional Chinese medicine and Ayurveda which is holistic Indian medicine.
   b. Mind-body interventions use a variety of techniques designed to enhance the mind's capacity to affect bodily function and symptoms. Some techniques that were considered CAM in the past have become mainstream (e.g., patient support groups and

cognitive-behavioral therapy). Other mind-body techniques, still considered CAM, include meditation, prayer, mental healing, and therapies that use creative outlets such as art, music, or dance.
   c. Biologically-based therapies use substances found in nature, such as herbs, foods, and vitamins. For example, dietary supplements, herbal products, and the use of other "so-called" natural, but as yet not scientifically proven, therapies (e.g., using shark cartilage to treat cancer).
   d. Manipulative and body-based methods are based on manipulation and/or movement of one or more parts of the body, including chiropractic or osteopathic manipulation and massage.
   e. Energy therapies involve the use of energy fields and include two types: biofield and bioelectromagnetic-based therapies. Biofield therapies are intended to affect energy fields that purportedly surround and penetrate the human body. The existence of such fields has not yet been scientifically proven. Some forms of energy therapy manipulate biofields by applying pressure and/or manipulating the body by placing the hands in, or through, these fields, including qi gong, Reiki, and therapeutic touch. Bioelectromagnetic-based therapies involve the unconventional use of electromagnetic fields, such as pulsed fields, magnetic fields, or alternating-current or direct-current fields.

E. Dietary considerations. Poor diet and exercise are modifiable risk factors to reduce cardiovascular morbidity and reduce obesity. Cultural impact on diet may alter the educational focus of care.
1. American-born AAs enjoy pork products high in salt content and fried meats with heavy gravies, as compared to immigrant AAs who have different dietary practices and preferences.
2. Kosher diets practiced by black Muslims exclude pork products.
3. Many Island cultures such as Haitians and Jamaicans have significant poverty. Therefore, obesity is a status symbol. It is considered a sign of health and wealth. Behavior modification with regard to calorie reduction and weight loss may be a challenge within this ethnic group.

F. Religion and spirituality.
1. Although many Asian Americans are Christian, Muslim, Hindu, Confucian, Taoist, and a host of other religions are practiced. Many follow

Buddhist concepts. Buddhism is a philosophy of life that has profound impact on health care beliefs and practices. Buddhism encourages respect for elders and those in authority, such as health care providers. Buddhism also teaches that life is a cycle of suffering and rebirth. Pain and illness are sometimes endured, and health-seeking remedies may be delayed. Healing is spiritual as well as scientific.

2. The Navajo Indians believe in the metaphysical premises of hozho/hochoo (hochxo), or beauty/harmony and ugliness/disharmony. While sometimes difficult for the nurse to understand, these are essential to conception of the "good life." Navajos, like many other Indians, are not a homogenous group, and beliefs about religion and healing vary.

3. American Indians believe there is a Supreme Creator. Humans have a body, mind, and spirit. Illness affects the mind, body, and spirit. Unwellness is the disharmony of body, mind, and spirit. Unnatural illness exists.
   a. Intertribalism is the exchanging of traits between different Indian nations.
   b. Pan-Indianism is a general sense of Indian cultural identity that unites members of different Indian nations.
   c. Religion and medicine are components of the Native North Americans that are inseparable.

4. Most Latinos are Roman Catholic, but an increasing number are Protestant. Additionally, a number of Jews settled in Latin America and have since immigrated to the United States. Many Catholics wear a crucifix as a symbol of faith and sometimes a protection against evil or illness. Arranging Last Rites or Sacrament of the Sick may be important to patients of Catholicism. Some Latinos, particularly those from the Caribbean, practice Santeria, which synthesizes African religion and Christianity. This belief system also includes healing practices.

5. The topic of withdrawing treatment for kidney disease is covered later in this section, but it is important for the nurse to understand that several religions or cultures associate this with suicide, and guidance is essential.

XII. Illegal immigrants.

A. Social patterns and family structure. Settlement patterns of illegal immigrants have been a barrier to acculturation into American society. These settlement patterns provide aid and comfort, a network of support, and common linguistic forms of communication. However, their illegal status makes the immigrant at higher risk for inadequate wages and economic resources as well as limited, if any, access to health care.

B. Health beliefs. As with other cultures, cultural-specific health beliefs and practices affect the health and well-being of individuals in this group. Therefore, it is important for the nurse to be aware of the individual practice patterns when providing care.

C. Communication and language. Communication is imperative to gaining access to health care services. Languages, such as Spanish, are becoming more prevalent. Ethnic groups such as Haitians who speak Creole have a linguistic disadvantage, as there are few health practitioners who are fluent in Creole. Inability to understand creates embarrassment, frustration, and stress. Many, therefore, choose not to seek health care or are unable to follow the prescribed treatment plan.

D. Barriers to care.
   1. Economic.
   2. Lack of health care insurance.
   3. Geographic disadvantage. Rural areas lack health care workers and facilities, putting migrant workers at high risk.
   4. Fear of deportation.

E. Major health issues. Poverty and poor living conditions are two major health risks facing illegal immigrants.

XIII. Patients as cultural consultants.

A. The patient is a teacher in disguise.

B. Allow patients to teach you about their culture and provide the necessary cultural resources for addressing their needs and enhancing adherence in their treatment.

XIV. Other resources.

A. www.culturediversity.org/cultcomp.htm

B. www.amsa.org/programs/gpit/cultural.cfm

C. www.ethnomed.org/

D. www.hrsa.gov/culturalcompetence/

E. www.diversityresources.com/rc21d/ sitemap.html

F. www.depts.washington.edu/pfes/cultureclues.html

Chapter 17

Psychosocial Impact and Spirituality

Purpose

To describe the psychosocial impact of chronic kidney disease (CKD) and end-stage renal disease (ESRD) on patients, identify implications for practice, and explore the influence of spirituality on adjustment to illness.

Objectives

Upon completion of this chapter, the learner will be able to:
1. Identify lifestyle changes experienced by patients diagnosed with CKD.
2. Identify five losses associated with initiation of dialysis.
3. Define the impact of CKD on caregivers.
4. Identify two psychosocial benefits of patient participation in self-care.
5. Identify three psychosocial factors to consider when a patient exhibits difficult behaviors.
6. Describe the benefits of screening, diagnosis, and treatment of depression.
7. Identify five interventions to address patient nonadherence.
8. Identify strategies for addressing patient anxiety.
9. Describe the role of spirituality in chronic illness.

I. Diagnosis of chronic illness: the patient's experience.

Illness can incapacitate people, damage lifelong values and commitments, destroy social relationships, produce role losses, generate discomfort and pain, result in repeated or continual loss of dignity, force a person to live with debilitating uncertainties, and threaten life itself. One has the sense that there is no refuge. The goal of effective intervention requires more sophisticated thought than currently exists and deep respect for the person who needs our help (Lazarus, 1983).

A. Lifestyle changes. CKD and ESRD patients experience multiple losses, disruptions in usual valued activities and routines, and psychosocial risks associated with diagnosis and treatment. They require comprehensive services at various stages throughout the course of their illness and treatment. Some of the losses and other lifestyle changes related to CKD and its treatment are listed below.
   1. Losses.
      a. Health.
      b. Libido, sexuality, and reproduction issues.
      c. Independence/autonomy (especially with in-center hemodialysis).
      d. Cognition.
      e. Physical strength.
      f. Body parts (amputation).
      g. Income/financial security.
         (1) Ability to pay for treatment.
         (2) Maintaining a job.
         (3) Managing reduction in income related to change in employment status.
         (4) Other financial stressors.
      h. Control over schedules, diet, fluid, and other lifestyle restrictions. A qualitative study by Ravenscroft (2005) found that the intrusion of hemodialysis on time was a major issue to participants. This included, not only time spent on actual treatment, but time spent on travel, waiting before and after treatments, preparing meals or snacks, and, in some instances, resting after treatments. The total time varied from approximately 6 hours to, for one participant, over 8 hours.
      i. Sleep.
   2. Vocational/economic.
   3. Social role. Changes in social status, loss of

familial role functions, feelings of isolation, decrease in social contacts, and loss of familiar role identities.
4. Somatic symptoms.
   a. Nausea.
   b. Restless leg syndrome.
   c. Insomnia.
   d. Uremia.
   e. Anemia.
5. Pain.
6. Lowered self-esteem. Any combination of the lifestyle changes mentioned in this section can result in lowered self-esteem.
7. Body image issues. Body image refers to the mental picture and attitudes one has toward his/her body and its structure and function. A unique kind of stressor in the population with ESRD that is not shared by others with different chronic diseases is the presence of a fistula, graft, or catheter used to provide access to the circulatory system during hemodialysis (Al-Arabi, 2006). Gokal and Hutchison (2002) found that some patients with ESRD worry about the integrity of the vascular access, fear that the access becomes damaged, and view it as an embarrassing disfigurement. Other aspects of kidney disease that may affect body image include ammonia breath, skin changes, hair changes, weight loss or gain, and surgical scars.
8. Tasked with decisions about treatment options.
9. Stress related to the disruption of homeostasis through the physical and psychologic changes of CKD. Manifestations may include:
   a. Physiologic.
      (1) Fatigue.
      (2) Weight loss/weight gain.
      (3) Changes in vital signs with increases in blood pressure, heart rate, and respirations.
      (4) Diaphoresis.
      (5) Cold hands and feet.
      (6) Increase in gastric secretions.
      (7) Bronchial dilation.
      (8) Pupil dilation.
      (9) Tremors.
      (10) Changes in blood hormone levels, especially ACTH and cortisol and an increase in catecholamine secretion.
   b. Behavioral: observable manifestations that may be a reflection of coping behaviors assumed by individuals.
      (1) Vomiting.
      (2) Fainting.
      (3) Trembling.
      (4) Tapping of fingers.
      (5) Kicking or swinging movement of lower extremities while sitting.
      (6) Clenched fists.
      (7) Other evidence of muscle tension.
      (8) Voice pitch.
      (9) Speed of talk.
      (10) Crying.
      (11) Pacing.
      (12) Immobilization.
      (13) Nonfunctional.
   c. Subjective: the feeling of being stressed is frequently attributed to job demands, treatment regimen demands, one's psychosocial environment, or one's state of physical health. These feelings may include:
      (1) Headache.
      (2) Nausea.
      (3) Anorexia.
      (4) Hunger.
      (5) Fatigue.
      (6) Problems with sleep.
      (7) Problems with concentration.
      (8) Sensations of uneasiness.
      (9) Gnawing or burning sensations in the gut.
      (10) Palpitations.
      (11) Angina.
      (12) Difficulty in breathing.

B. Coping.
   1. Coping is the constantly changing cognitive and behavioral efforts, both action oriented and intrapsychic, to manage specific external and/or internal demands that are appraised as taxing or exceeding the resources of the person.
   2. True coping requires a person to give up previously held secure states of mind and adapt to the changes in circumstances (Mazella, 2004). Following are common themes related to coping with CKD and its treatment.
      a. Denial regarding medical status is common among both CKD and new ESRD patients. Despite knowing about kidney failure, starting dialysis is frequently described as a surprise. Denial is one defense mechanism that can play an important role in the patient's ability to endure their illness (help them to cope). It may take time to let go of their past "ideal" state. However, denial must to be addressed when it interferes with the patient's life.
      b. Grief: bereavement over losses can be complicated by guilt or regret regarding health behaviors that may have led to progression of kidney disease.

c. Concerns about worsening health and facing issues of mortality.

d. Baseline coping prior to CKD diagnosis. CKD patients often have numerous comorbid conditions (such as diabetes, hypertension, cardiovascular disease, and lupus) and related social concerns. According to Ravenscroft (2005), review of the literature on diabetes and kidney failure indicates the psychosocial issues of chronic illness such as burden, fear, uncertainty, control, dependency, loss, depression, and guilt are considered compounded in these individuals due to the preexistence of diabetes.

e. Dependency issues, including a feeling of being a burden on loved ones, can be debilitating for patients, affecting their self-esteem. When patients go on dialysis, they see their lives becoming controlled by a dependence on medical technology. This dependency can carry over into the relationship with health care providers, particularly if the patients are not provided with the information and opportunity to have an active role in their treatment.

f. Stress.

g. Behavior changes. In response to the many lifestyle changes, many patients exhibit changes in behavior. Waiting to get on the dialysis machine, physical pain of cannulation, and other ESRD-related intrusions can cause unhappiness, lack of cooperation, and complaining. Staff tend to experience these patients as difficult, but their behaviors should be considered in the context of their adjustment phase.

3. Modes of coping.
   a. Information seeking.
   b. Direct action: to change the environment or oneself in some way to undo the injury, prevent the harm, or meet the challenge.
   c. Inhibition of action: the person resists acting because it is poorly grounded, dangerous, embarrassing, or morally reprehensible.
   d. Cognitive coping: a person manipulates his/her attention to change the way the event is comprehended to reduce the sense of injury.

C. Mood changes.
   1. Depression has been shown to be a considerable problem for patients with CKD and ESRD. Depression in this population is a legitimate, expectable, and understandable reaction to a dramatic lifestyle change. It is the most commonly encountered psychological complication of chronic dialysis patients. The patient new to dialysis may require an initial period of adjusting. However, for some patients, the depression becomes chronic. Patients may be depressed when they have the following symptoms lasting for more than 2 weeks or interfering with activities of daily life:
      a. Feeling sad or irritable most of the time.
      b. Feeling worthlessness or guilt.
      c. Feeling hopelessness or just giving up.
      d. Unable to enjoy things.
      e. Difficulty remembering things, indecisiveness, or problems with concentration.
      f. Irritable or angry feelings.
      g. Recurrent thoughts of suicide.
   2. Anxiety is often expressed by CKD patients about their level of functioning once they initiate dialysis. Common concerns include ability to care for self, ability to perform usual daily tasks, concerns about feeling ill all the time, the amount of time that dialysis takes from normal daily routines, decreased feelings of control, and financial status (bills, cost of treatment and medications, ability to work). Anxiety can be quite normal but problematic if protracted or excessive.

II. Impact on the caregiver.

A. Familial roles. When change occurs with one family member, the others have to step in and fill a role that they may not be comfortable with or feel equipped for. Usually with ESRD, the caregiver is expected to perform some supportive functions. The caregiver is burdened with:
   1. The daily demands of providing care and support.
   2. Assisting with planning and preparation of the kidney diet.
   3. Providing or arranging transportation.
   4. Coping with mood and behavior changes.

B. Lifestyle adjustments, losses, and stressors that affect patients are also observed by or experienced by the caregiver. The impact of this burden, or role demand, may result in feelings of guilt, hopelessness, isolation, a loss of freedom to pursue personal and recreational interests, and fatigue (Campbell, 1998). Caring for a person with a chronic illness impacts the caregiver's psychological and physical well-being, which is their quality of life, which often manifests itself in experiences of depression and fatigue (LoGiudice, Kerse, Brown, & Gibson, 1998).

C. Relationship changes in family dynamics and disruptions in usual routines can impact relationships. Participants in Ravenscroft's (2005) qualitative study talked about intrusion of kidney failure into intimate relationships (sexual) and family relationships, including with children.

III. Application to practice.

A. Psychosocial assessment. The purpose of the psychosocial assessment of the patient and family is to obtain data about the psychologic and social realms of function. A critical analysis of the significance of the data is essential for planning, implementing, and evaluating nursing care. The following assessment model is based on the work of Francis and Munjas (1976). This model represents a comprehensive approach, providing numerous and detailed parameters for assessment.
  1. Psychologic parameters include the variables that affect the patient's mind as they are manifested in the person's behavior. The following can be assessed:
    a. Cognition. The cognitive realm of behavior refers to intellectual activities, thinking processes, understanding, and problem solving. The following aspects within the cognitive domain can be assessed.
      (1) Consciousness.
      (2) Orientation.
      (3) Attention and concentration.
      (4) Memory.
      (5) Speech.
      (6) Thought processes.
      (7) Body image.
    b. Affect. The affective domain of behavior is the expression of feeling or emotion. Mood is frequently used to describe the person's subjective feelings. Several components of affect can be assessed.
      (1) Range: degree to which different emotions are displayed.
      (2) Intensity: quality of emotion expressed, e.g., flat, with great energy.
      (3) Type: the category of emotion. Common descriptors include angry, hopeful, elated, sad, fearful, and happy.
      (4) Appropriateness: congruency of the emotion being expressed with the content with which it is associated.
      (5) Level of anxiety.
    c. Conation refers to purposeful activity, the motor aspects of behavior, and the performance of acts by choice. Conation normally is congruent with cognition and affect, that is, motor activity logically relates to thoughts and feelings being experienced at the time. Conation is not usually assessed through interviewing, but rather is best performed with observation of the patient. The following aspects of conation can be assessed:
      (1) Appearance.
      (2) Psychomotor activity examined from three parameters.
        (a) Content: what the person is doing.
        (b) Purpose: relative to the person's frame of reference.
        (c) Appropriateness: relative to place and purpose.
      (3) Descriptors include very slow movement (psychomotor retardation), agitated, restless activity, and tremors.
  2. Social parameters. These aspects include those variables that affect the patient's role in society within the context of social systems. Familial, socioeconomic, cultural, developmental, and environmental concerns comprise the social realm. Assessment can include:
    a. Family systems.
    b. Socioeconomic status:
      (1) Refers to a combination of material worth along with social position indicating the person's prestige in the social system, e.g., occupation, education, geographic area of residence, and income.
      (2) Information obtained from assessing these variables can provide clues as to how the kidney failure will affect working status and what social resources might be available to the patient.
    c. Ethnicity and cultural values.
    d. Social habits.
      (1) Refers to behaviors that relate to one's interactions with others.
      (2) Observation as well as interviewing should be used when assessing social habits, e.g., eating patterns, alcohol and drug use, and response to stress.
    e. Sexual behavior.
      (1) Includes the feelings a person has about himself/herself and the ways in which the person interacts with others.
      (2) Refers to the ways in which a person chooses to express his/her sexuality.
      (3) Assessment variables include:
        (a) Age.
        (b) Values.
        (c) Culture.

(d) Emotional health.
(e) Physical health.

B. Family assessment. Family processes are usually disrupted when one of the members has a chronic illness. Changes in one family member lead to changes in the family system. Adaptation of the family must also be considered when planning care for the patient with kidney failure. The following aspects of family can be assessed:
1. Family composition/family members.
   a. Members and significant life events of each member.
   b. Number of persons living in household.
   c. Level of education.
   d. Health status and/or significant past medical and psychiatric history.
   e. Ethnic, religious, and cultural beliefs.
   f. Relationship with extended family.
2. Family structure.
   a. Coalitions and/or alliances.
   b. Delineation of boundaries.
   c. Roles and responsibilities.
   d. Decision making.
3. Communication patterns describe the relative openness or closedness of communication, e.g., who talks to whom, when, about what.
4. Health beliefs and related factors.
   a. Attitudes held by family regarding health, illness, disease prevention, choice, and responsibility.
   b. Health care practices.
   c. Understanding about family member's illness.
   d. Impact of illness on family's functioning.
5. Mood describes usual feeling of the family.
6. Financial status and environment.
   a. Housing.
   b. Food.
   c. Income and who earns it.
   d. Health maintenance.
   e. Relationship with the community.
   f. Strengths and weaknesses as identified by the family and as identified by the nurse.

C. Chronic illness management.
1. Prevention of medical crises and their management once they occur.
   a. Assessment of signs and symptoms of potential or impending crisis.
   b. Patient and families must be taught to recognize signs and symptoms and what to do in case of crisis.
2. Control of symptoms.

a. Assessment of symptoms and response to treatments.
b. Patients and families have to learn, in detail, about the symptoms of the illness and consequences of treatment.
3. Incorporate prescribed regimens and management of problems into daily living.
4. Prevention of, or living with, social isolation.
5. Adjustment to changes in the course of the disease, whether it moves downward or has remissions.

IV. Implications for practice.

A. Social/emotional.
1. Unaddressed, can manifest in numerous problems, including:
   a. Substance abuse problems.
   b. Thought, mood, and personality disturbances.
   c. Impaired functioning because of anxiety, depression, or mania.
   d. Somatic complaints with no organic basis.
   e. Suicidal ideation or attempt.
   f. Eating disorders.
   g. Sexual dysfunction.
   h. Persistent psychological distress (anxiety, depression, hopelessness).
   i. Behavior problems and nonadherence to treatment (or treatment drop-out).
2. Impact of psychosocial factors on the outcome of patients with kidney disease has been receiving more attention recently. The progressive increase in both the incidence and prevalence of patients with ESRD have focused research interest on those aspects of ESRD care that affect patient outcomes and are potentially amenable to modification to improve these outcomes (Finkelstein & Finkelstein, 2000). Treatment nonadherence and psychological distress are common and increasingly recognized as contributing to excess morbidity and mortality in dialysis patients.
3. General strategies for promoting adaptation.
   a. Nurse-patient relationships. The nurse traditionally has more frequent interactions with patients than other health care providers and as such has more opportunity to allow for thorough and up-to-date assessments and interventions, as well as for the development of an effective therapeutic relationship with the patient and family. The purpose of this interpersonal relationship is to facilitate the achievement of patient-focused outcomes.

The nurse-patient relationship can provide a strong basis for implementing other strategies to help the patient and family with adaptation/coping. The following are key aspects of the nurse-patient relationship to be considered:

(1) Therapeutic communication. Both verbal and nonverbal, several techniques are essential to effective therapeutic communication.
  (a) Conveying warmth and caring.
  (b) Respect.
  (c) Sensitivity.
  (d) Empathy.
  (e) Boundaries.
    [1] While encounters between nurse and patient can be described as friendly, the nurse-patient relationship needs to be defined in such a way that emphasizes patient outcomes to confine the relationship to a therapeutic, rather than a social one.
    [2] Boundaries and defining expectations also help to minimize excessive dependence on the part of the patient.
    [3] Mutual collaboration. Both the nurse and the patient bring personal abilities and qualities to the relationship, and each is accountable and responsible for outcomes.
  b. Patient-focused outcome goals.
  c. Patient and family education.
  d. Contracting is a means of facilitating behavioral change based upon the principle that a behavior is controlled by its consequences. Reinforcement helps to establish new habits and behaviors by providing positive consequences. Conversely, punishing or not rewarding a behavior would render that behavior extinct. Particularly with many new self-care practices required of kidney patients, contracting is a useful technique to help the patient learn and maintain new behaviors. Complex behavioral changes such as diet modification, access care, and medication therapy can be broken down into small steps, with each step being reinforced along the way. Thus, through a series of building blocks, the terminal or desired behavior is acquired.
  e. Social support.
  f. Emphasis on self-care. Organizing specific knowledge and skills related to kidney failure and its treatment is an essential aspect of adaptation. This provides the patient with an opportunity for increased power and control with less fear, anxiety, and uncertainty regarding unknowns. Further, the feelings of accomplishment in mastering new information and skills affirms the patient's personal abilities at a time in which meaningful and independent action may be scarce.
  g. Use of resources. Assistance with the economic and emotional demands faced by the patient with kidney failure may be found in a variety of community resources.
    (1) Financial assistance for treatment.
    (2) Transportation.
    (3) Lodging.
    (4) Social and recreational.
    (5) Rehabilitation.
    (6) Voluntary health agencies.

B. CKD.
  1. Early intervention and education before kidney disease progresses is critical. Patients who receive pre-ESRD education have higher mood scores, fewer mobility problems, fewer functional disabilities, a lower level of anxiety, and are enabled to make decisions regarding modality type (Klang, Bjorvell, & Clyne, 1999). Formal educational interventions in patients with CKD can delay the need for dialysis (Devins, Mendehssohn, Barre, & Harlow, 2003). It has also been noted to facilitate continued employment and aid in modality selection (Golper, 2001). Some clinics use formal classroom formats to educate patients, while others use one-to-one meetings. Tours of the dialysis unit can provide the opportunity for the patient to see the treatment process and to ask questions of staff and patients. Allowing them time to adjust to the eventual need for dialysis.
  2. Support for patients and their family is available through patient organizations, such as American Association of Kidney Patients (AAKP), National Kidney Foundation (NKF), American Kidney Fund (AKF), and Kidney Support Network (RSN). Peer support can help to alleviate stress. If there is not a local support group, providers should consider incorporating this into their CKD programs.

C. Transplantation.
  1. Education/referral. Provision of education about kidney replacement options, including transplantation, is recommended. Early referral for transplantation is optimal. The goal is to

ensure access to transplantation for every individual who may be eligible for such a procedure.

2. Coordination of process. Kidney transplantation requires teamwork and communication throughout the process, from initial referral to long-term care of the transplanted kidney. All disciplines should work together to provide optimal quality of life for the patient. Any barriers to the patient's transplant eligibility should be addressed with the patient by the team. Each transplant center has guidelines for selection of appropriate candidates. The health care team can assist kidney transplant candidates with factors that might affect their eligibility for transplant. These factors might include severe obesity, reinforcing adherence to prescribed medication or therapy, and social/emotional/financial factors related to ability to function posttransplant.

3. Organ donation. There is a national shortage of deceased donor organs. In spite of increased efforts at organ recovery and expanding acceptance guidelines, the number of patients waiting for a deceased donor kidney continues to grow. Living donor kidneys have a longer half-life than deceased donor kidneys, creating a significant benefit for the recipient without detriment to the donor. Therefore, all members of the health care team should make an effort to try to identify a suitable living donor for each recipient.

D. ESRD.

1. Participation in self-care and maintenance of an active lifestyle. Self-management has been defined as the positive efforts of patients to oversee and participate in their health care in order to optimize health, prevent complications, control symptoms, marshal medical resources, and minimize the intrusion of the disease into their preferred lifestyles (Curtin & Mapes, 2001).

a. Curtin, Sitter, Schatell, and Chewning (2004) propose that cooperative/participatory self-management behaviors can minimize the need for protective/proactive strategies. Further, increasing patients' knowledge of kidney disease may have long-term benefits.

b. Curtin and Mapes (2001) found that hemodialysis patients' ability to self-manage aspects of their disease and its treatment may be positively associated with their overall functioning and well-being.

c. Related research has shown that patients trained for self-care dialysis have higher role

function, social function, and emotional well-being then similar patients who received full care (Meers et al., 1996). Self-care modalities can include peritoneal dialysis, home hemodialysis, or in-center self-care including self-cannulation.

2. Focus on strengths. Reinforcement of any positive changes in patient adjustment, lifestyle, or behavior is recommended. In other words, catch them doing good. The strengths-based perspective makes several assumptions about the human condition. One assumption is that all people have strengths that enable them to move forward. Another assumption is that people are more motivated to move toward things they want than away from things they don't want. People are also more motivated to work toward a goal they have set for themselves than one that an expert has set on their behalf. This is self-determination, allowing individuals to determine their own destiny, is a very powerful thing. The strengths model also assumes that all people have the capacity to change. It does not promise, however, that all will (McFarlane, 2006).

3. Patient-centered care planning. To the extent possible, involve the patient in interdisciplinary team meetings. Allowing for the patient to share his/her perspective on care management and providing agreed upon goals for the patient and team to accomplish. Placing patients at the helm of the change process and letting them steer their own course has powerful ramifications and can lead to effectual treatment. Henry Ford said, "Whether you think you can or you think you can't, you're right." In addition, assist the staff with in-services in communication, professionalism, and patient sensitivity. Obtain training in the Dialysis Patient and Provider Conflict (DPPC) Tools by contacting your area ESRD Network, and use the tools when conflicts occur. To locate the ESRD Network in a particular area, go to www.esrdnetworks.org/.

E. Pediatric concerns.

1. Impact and significance of CKD on the child.

a. Factors influencing perception of illness.

(1) Age and developmental level.

(a) Infant: limited perceptions.

(b) Young child: inability to comprehend causality. Views illness as a punishment and questions parents' inability to provide protection from the illness.

(c) Older child: inaccurate perceptions; illness is poorly understood.

(d) Adolescent: focuses on body image, dependency related to illness, and separation from peers.

(2) Individual coping styles affected by:

    (a) Life experiences.

    (b) Emotional support from family.

    (c) Cognitive development.

    (d) Personality.

(3) Influence of family attitudes affected by:

    (a) Severity and prognosis of illness.

    (b) Congenital (increased feelings of guilt) versus acquired illness.

    (c) Age of child at onset, e.g., younger child more likely to be overprotected.

    (d) Presence of preexisting emotional problems in the family.

    (e) Nature of the disease and symptoms.

b. Confinement, restrictions, and immobility.

(1) Isolation of the child may result from confinement during treatment procedures and/or related to immunosuppression.

(2) Confinement imposed related to overprotectiveness of the child thwarts normal activities of exploration and social interaction.

(3) Restrictions in the form of diet, protection of access device, and treatment schedule may be perceived as punishment in the younger child, or as obstacles to independence in the older child/adolescent.

(4) Decreased mobility related to rickets, bone deformities, and abnormal gait diminishes the opportunities for play.

c. Pain related to needle sticks, fullness with peritoneal dialysis, etc.

2. Coping behaviors of children.

a. Release of emotions.

(1) Crying.

(2) Laughing.

(3) Temper tantrums.

b. Psychologic defenses.

c. Compensatory physical activities.

d. Use of cognitive functions.

(1) Learning about treatments and illness.

(2) Participating.

e. Ineffective coping manifested by:

(1) Extremely dependent behaviors.

    (a) Few outside interests.

    (b) Passive acceptance of treatments and procedures.

(c) Parental overprotectiveness.

(2) Overly independent behavior.

    (a) Daring noncompliance.

    (b) Defiance.

    (c) Repeated acting out episodes.

3. Coping behaviors of parents.

a. Initially will feel shock and disbelief upon learning of chronicity of child's condition. This may result in:

(1) Increased anxiety.

(2) Distortion of information.

(3) Difficulty in comprehending information.

b. Other emotional responses.

(1) Denial.

    (a) Decreases the anxiety and hurt felt by the parents.

    (b) Allows time for the parents to mobilize other resources.

(2) Guilt. Parents may accuse themselves of causing the child's illness.

    (a) Usually more pronounced if etiology of kidney failure is congenital.

    (b) Goal in assisting the parents to cope is to resolve the self-accusation.

(3) Anger.

    (a) Normal reaction to the loss of their child's health.

    (b) May be directed at health care team, God, spouse, and other healthy children.

    (c) Requires acceptance from health care team and assistance with grief resolution.

c. Overprotection.

(1) Usually results from feelings of guilt and need to punish self.

(2) Typical overprotective behaviors include:

    (a) Regulating all aspects of the child's life.

    (b) Monopolizing care giving functions.

    (c) Limited awareness of child's actual potential.

    (d) Restricting child from activities he/she is capable of mastering.

d. Control through knowledge (intellectualization).

(1) Response to feelings of helplessness.

(2) Learn all that they can to master the situation.

(3) May exhibit attitude of critical superiority toward health care team.

e. Peer support.

(1) Seek out other parents of children with kidney failure.

(2) Share knowledge of resources and coping strategies.

(3) Mutual expression of feelings.

(4) Involvement in voluntary health agencies.

f. Healthy adjustments of parents is demonstrated by:

(1) Awareness of normal growth and development patterns for ESRD patients.

(2) Consistent discipline of child and other siblings.

(3) Encouraging self-care of child and increasing independence.

(4) Focusing on achieving short-term goals.

(5) Maintaining relationships with friends, extended family, work colleagues, etc.

(6) Acknowledging frustrations and disappointments with appropriate expression of feelings.

F. Considerations for working with caregivers.

1. Treatment planning/education. Involvement of significant others in the care planning process and provision of education will serve to decrease the isolation the patient feels and bridge any gaps in knowledge about the patients' illness and treatment. Interactions with health care providers are perceived as more positive when there is mutual respect, trust, collaborative decision-making, and when health care providers share information with caregivers (Ravenscroft, 2005). Communication and coordination of care is also important when the patient is in a nursing home or other long-term care setting.

2. Provision of support. Involve the social worker in addressing family stressors and promote early intervention with identified caregiver and relationship concerns, including sexual intimacy. Participants in Ravenscroft's (2005) study recalled that there had been some discussion of sexual concerns with health care providers but that this had not been of assistance in resolving problems. Referral to appropriate resources to address sexual relationships and performance should not be overlooked. Additionally, caregivers should be encouraged to rest when able, use family or community resources, and reward themselves for their efforts. With the number of dialysis patients increasing each year, ESRD staff are interacting with a growing number of caregivers. It is essential that staff remain sensitive to the burden and demands of family care for dialysis patients. Proactive intervention can help to prevent conflict that can occur in the dialysis setting.

3. Tips for disruptive caregivers.

a. Be certain that facility policies and possible consequences of violation are clearly communicated to caregivers. Remember to equally enforce policies for all families.

b. Be sure to consider the patient's needs and behaviors separate from the caregiver's.

c. Refer to the social worker for assessment of the caregiver's emotional needs and intervene appropriately. Keep in mind that controlling behavior on the part of the caregiver is often related to fears and anxiety.

G. Illness behaviors and management.

1. Depression. Working with depressed patients can be draining. Some of these patients have a remarkable capacity for interpersonal insensitivity, manipulative behavior, and excessive demands. These patients are often labeled as difficult and staff often do everything possible to avoid them. Unless one has the capacity to step back and reflect on the patient's state of mind, a vicious cycle can develop where a patient's demand or need can lead to an inconsistent or irrational response by the worker who feels taken advantage of or manipulated (Mazella, 2004). Depression can result in diminished motivation and apathy and lead to a cascade effect of pervasive physical and mental deterioration. Often, when treating chronic illness, the mental components are lost within the context of multiple physiologic problems.

a. Prevalence. The kidney literature on depression has proven that depression is highly prevalent in the CKD population. Depression has been linked to increased hospitalization and mortality rates, an increased level of comorbid conditions, treatment nonadherence, and poor rehabilitation outcomes and overall patient adjustment. Its prevalence varies widely across studies, which may reflect variation in the criteria and methodology used to diagnose depression.

(1) Results from a study by Lopes et al. (2004) concluded that depression is highly prevalent among hemodialysis patients but is likely under diagnosed and undertreated. Higher scores on the quality of life (QOL) tool used in the study were significantly and independently associated with higher risk of all-cause death, hospitalization, and withdrawal from dialysis.

(2) Kimmel et al. (2000) also linked depression with increased risk of mortality.

(3) A national study of incident dialysis patients by Boulware et al. (2005) concluded that there is an increased risk for death and cardiovascular disease events in patients with depressive symptoms, particularly patients whose symptoms persisted for greater than 1 year.

b. Impact on outcomes.

(1) Depression is related closely to nutritional status and could be an independent risk factor for malnutrition (Koo et al., 2003).

(2) It is also associated with poor compliance of fluid restriction and higher weight gain between treatments (Garcia et al., 2002).

(3) Patients who are depressed and do not get treatment are also at a higher risk for hospitalization.

(4) Depression may manifest itself in behaviors such as ignoring treatment recommendations, not taking medicines, skipping treatments, or other self-defeating behaviors.

c. Diagnosis.

(1) Depression may be detected by staff based on observations/clinical suspicion. Indicators may include overt symptoms or subjective complaints of depression, failure to respond to treatment, nonadherence, apathy, prior history of depression, anxiety, behavioral changes (especially irritability) and substance abuse.

(2) The dialysis social worker can screen the patient for depression and assist with referral to available treatment. The following are some tools available online that can aid in the assessment of the depression.

(a) The Geriatric Depression Scale (short form). It is easy to score and scores can be prorated to remove the somatic components such as energy, appetite, etc. A Spanish version is also available on the Web site.

(b) The Beck Depression Inventory Fast Screen for medical patients. The BDI Fast Screen was constructed to reduce the number of false positives for depression in patients with known biologic, medical, or substance abuse problems.

(3) Quality of life assessment tools and resources. Because the dialysis patient suffers from a variety of physical symptoms, it is easy to confuse them with the somatic symptoms that are commonly associated with depression. Sleep, sexual dysfunction, appetite changes, and fatigue are not enough to warrant a diagnosis of depression. Use of QOL assessment tools can be an important step in improving patient health, decreasing hospitalization, increasing adherence, improving relationship potential, and decreasing mortality rates. The following are some tools available online that can aid in the assessment of the functional status of patients:

(a) The Kidney Disease Quality of Life survey (KDQOL) is a disease-specific survey that includes a generic functioning and well-being survey plus questions related to kidney disease like burden of illness, satisfaction with care, sexual functioning, and more. Several versions of the survey and associated scoring templates on the KDQOL Web site.

(b) The SF-36 is a Quality of Life (QOL).

d. Intervention. Depression is a treatable illness. Despite the prevalence of depression in dialysis patients, routine QOL assessments are not being conducted in facilities. The best way to address depression in this population is not yet clear. There is a paucity of data relating to the effectiveness of therapeutic interventions in the treatment of depression occurring in patients with ESRD. Many patients feel initially friendlier toward the medical management of their moods while other patients prefer to stay away from any sort of medication management. The social worker, patient, advanced practice nurse (APN), and nephrologist will find the combination that works best for each patient. Some barriers to treating depression can include the prescriber's comfort level with antidepressant medications and the patient's resistance to assessment, and/or treatment of depression. Patient resistance can be addressed with education, which details the benefits of working as a partner with the medical team to enhance adjustment to dialysis and quality of life. Some depressions do not require treatment and are limited to

sporadic feelings or moods that change as time goes on. With this type of depression, the focus can be on educating the patient about their kidney disease or connecting them to resources that help them to feel less isolated. Becoming involved with a support group or just talking to fellow patients may decrease their feelings of despair, loneliness, and isolation. Social support for persons with CKD increases the quality of their lives. Whatever the modality, treating depression can help patients with:
    (1) Relationships.
    (2) Work and other activities.
    (3) Transplant status.
    (4) Nutrition.
    (5) Ability to manage their illness.
    (6) Overall quality of life.
  2. Anxiety.
    a. There is limited research regarding the presence of anxiety in the CKD population. Predialysis anxiety was investigated in a study by Iacono (2005). Forty-four people who attended a predialysis educational class were evaluated for anxiety before and after attending the class. The class did appear to reduce the level of anxiety for most participants. Anxiety often occurs in CKD and ESRD patients due to:
      (1) Altered self-concept.
      (2) Threat to role functioning.
      (3) Uncertainty of outcomes.
      (4) Unfamiliar treatment regimen.
      (5) Restrictions of diet, medications, and treatment.
      (6) Decreased feelings of control.
      (7) An overload of stress related to chronic illness. Many hemodialysis patients have an anxious reaction to the prospect of cannulation due to a fear of needlesticks. This anxiety can interfere with their vascular access decisions (AV fistula vs. graft or catheter).
    b. Typical manifestations.
      (1) Nonadherence behaviors.
      (2) Denial.
      (3) Nervousness.
      (4) Irritability.
      (5) Increased heart rate, blood pressure, and respirations.
      (6) Inability to concentrate.
    c. Interventions for anxiety.
      (1) Assess for particular stressor versus generalized nonspecific threats.

  (2) Acknowledge the appropriateness of the feeling the patient is experiencing and convey understanding.
  (3) Determine usual coping mechanisms.
  (4) Reassurance and education. Talking through, explaining, or educating about the procedure in a calm, nonthreatening, and empathic manner can help to alleviate anxiety and help patients to feel like an active partner in their treatment. Allowing the patient to discuss their fears and concerns can offer reassurance. Assist the patient to assume control whenever possible.
  (5) Relaxation techniques can include deep breathing exercises, sighing, humming, and systematic relaxation of muscle groups.
  (6) Guided imagery is a mind-body intervention aimed at easing stress, promoting a sense of peace and tranquility, and changing physiology.
    (a) It involves taking conscious control over imagination and guiding it in a desired direction. Mental images are generated to evoke a psycho-physiologic state of relaxation or a specific outcome.
    (b) Some indicators for guided imagery include sleep, pain, grief, depression, anxiety, and side effects such as nausea and vomiting.
    (c) Use of guided imagery can also enhance self-confidence and decrease acting out behaviors such as substance abuse. A case study by Birnbaum & Birnbaum (2004) reported that spiritual concerns play a huge role among those who have attempted suicide, yet are poorly addressed, if addressed at all, by their psychotherapists. The researchers designed a therapeutic group/workshop to incorporate relaxation and mindfulness meditation, along with guided imagery to access inner wisdom. Many of the participants reported a significant positive experience, including connection to knowledge that was highly relevant to them in their current state of life. The authors concluded that whether such insights were experienced as coming from within (a deeper part of the

self) or from an external source (a guiding figure or divine presence), guided meditation appears to be a powerful resource.

    (d) Richardson et al. (1997) studied the effects of guided imagery versus group support with breast cancer survivors. After 6 weeks, the imagery group had less stress, more vigor, and better quality of life than the support group. Guided imagery is now used as a standard, complementary therapy to help reduce anxiety, pain, and length of stay among the cardiac surgery patients at Inova Fairfax (Halpin, Speir, CapaBianco, & Barnett, 2002).

    (e) A study from the National Institute on Aging (Liu & Park, 2004) found that guided imagery helps elderly patients remember to take their medicine (picturing an action improves likelihood of performing action).

    (7) Referral to MD for medications.

3. Powerlessness: Sensation of being out of control with no apparent solution to regain control.
   a. Usually related to:
      (1) Chronicity of disease.
      (2) Inability to perform role responsibilities.
      (3) Knowledge deficit.
      (4) Perceived loss of control.
   b. Typical manifestations.
      (1) Expressions of uncertainty.
      (2) Dependent behavior.
      (3) Apathy.
      (4) Depression.
      (5) Nonparticipation in care.
   c. Tips for managing powerlessness.
      (1) Assist patient in identifying feelings of powerlessness.
      (2) Identify factors contributing to the sense of powerlessness.
      (3) Assess usual level of control and decision making.
      (4) Help patient differentiate those situations that can be changed from those that cannot.
      (5) Encourage identification and use of strengths and potential.
      (6) Provide opportunities for patient to make decisions.
      (7) Patient education.
4. Grieving is a normal process of reacting to a loss.

   a. Usually related to:
      (1) Loss of kidney function.
      (2) Failure of access device.
      (3) Syndrome of impending loss.
      (4) Loss of roles and relationships.
   b. Typical manifestations.
      (1) May include the expressions of:
         (a) Anger.
         (b) Denial.
         (c) Guilt.
         (d) Anxiety.
         (e) Sadness.
         (f) Despair.
         (g) Crying.
      (2) Withdrawn behavior.
      (3) Physical reactions of grief can include sleeping problems, changes in appetite, physical problems, or illness.
   c. Managing the grieving patient.
      (1) Assist patient with engaging in grieving process.
         (a) Denial phase.
            [1] Be genuine and honest about loss.
            [2] Acknowledge normalcy of denial and feelings of loss.
         (b) Anger phase.
            [1] Be tolerant and patient. Avoid defensiveness.
            [2] Facilitate patient's expression of anger in constructive and acceptable ways.
            [3] Explore patient's feelings of guilt and depression.
         (c) Realization phase.
            [1] Offer support and acceptance.
            [2] Encourage patient to share feelings with significant others.
            [3] Convey to patient that behaviors such as crying are acceptable and healthy.
         (d) Acceptance phase. Assist patient in formulation new goals and making adjustments in lifestyle.
      (2) Explore the patient's perceptions of changes that illness has caused.
      (3) Encourage/provide for discussions with other patients with kidney failure about responses to illness.
      (4) Refer to social worker for further assessment and treatment.
5. Alterations in self-concept.
   a. Related to the composite of ideas, feelings, and attitudes that a person has about his/her own identity, worth, capabilities, and limitations.

(1) Loss of body function.
(2) Altered body image, e.g., access devices, etc.
(3) Role changes.
(4) Feelings of decreased control.
b. Typical manifestations.
(1) Dependent behaviors.
(2) Withdrawal.
(3) Self-criticism.
(4) Expressions of helplessness and/or disappointment.
(5) Preoccupation with body changes, e.g., hiding vascular access, not completing peritoneal exchanges due to abdominal distention.
c. Managing alterations of self-concept.
(1) Convey acceptance to patient that he/she is a worthwhile human being.
(2) Help the patient work through feelings of disappointment related to losses.
(3) Explore the meaning of illness and treatment with patient.
(4) Assist the patient in identifying major areas of concern related to body image. Use problem solving and role play with patient to explore ways of minimizing these concerns.
(5) Focus on patient's strengths, potential, and rehabilitation goal.
(6) Goal setting.
(7) Discourage use of poor self-esteem for secondary gains.
(8) Avoid false praise. Offer positive reinforcement for actual accomplishments and encouragement for attempting activity.
(9) Encourage social interaction.
(10) Refer to social worker for further assessment and treatment.
6. Effective coping to achieve and maintain effective coping:
(1) Support functional coping behaviors.
(2) Include patient and significant other in treatment planning.
(3) Encourage patient to communicate feelings and concerns to health care team and significant others.
(4) Convey acceptance that "bad days" can be expected but do not necessarily hinder effective coping.
(5) Encourage strategies for promoting mental health, such as stress management, importance of diversional/recreational activity, use of support systems, etc.

(6) Encourage continued rehabilitation, e.g., return to activities enjoyed before illness.
(7) Patient education.
(8) Refer to social worker for further assessment and treatment.
7. Alteration in family process.
a. Related to:
(1) Change in family member's ability to function and family's expectations.
(2) Disruption of family routines related to specific treatment modality.
(3) Change in family roles.
(4) Hospitalization of an ill family member.
(5) Financial crisis/change in employment status.
b. Typical manifestations.
(1) Emotional lability of family members.
(2) Verbalization of fear, anxiety, and anger.
(3) Over involved family member or absence of involvement.
(4) Family conflicts, e.g., bickering, arguing, etc.
(5) Inability to problem solve.
(6) If children are involved, change in school performance.
c. Managing alterations in family processes.
(1) Assess degree of family dysfunction and current coping methods of family members.
(2) Help family identify source of conflict.
(3) Set goals and identify alternatives.
(4) Support efforts made toward positive change.
(5) Promote separation and individuation and clear, functional boundaries between members.
(6) Identify patterns of communication.
(7) Patient education.
(8) Refer to social worker for further assessment and treatment and possible referral to outside resources.
8. Adherence with a prescribed therapeutic regimen has become a prime health care issue over the past few decades. It has coincided with advances in medical science, resulting in increased knowledge regarding etiology, treatment, and prevention of disease and other causes of impaired health. As knowledge increases about efficacy of treatment and/or prevention, so does frustration and concern increase when individuals fail to adhere with medical and nursing advice about the prevention and treatment.

a. Psychosocial barriers to adherence. Possible causes of nonadherence include lack of social support, lack of resources, feeling ineffective, low conscientiousness, high hostility and distrust, poor education about treatment, and untreated emotional or cognitive disorders.
b. Nonadherence behaviors can include anything from not taking prescribed medications to missing treatments.
c. Control issues. In Ravenscroft's (2005) study, participants indicated that they strove to find a balance between illness and their normal lives. Participants suggested that adherence to prescribed regimens was not always easy and described choosing, at times, to ignore treatment recommendations or making modifications to minimize the intrusive presence of these regimens. This moves away from the more traditional perspective on adherence as patient conformity to a prescribed regimen from a health care provider toward concepts such as choice, self-management, and alliance.
d. Major determinants of regimen adherence.
 (1) Degree of difficulty or ease to learn and carry out.
 (2) Takes much or little time.
 (3) Causes much or little discomfort or pain.
 (4) Does or does not cause side effects, especially if they are actual or perceived as high risk.
 (5) If known, might or might not cause others to stigmatize the person.
 (6) Is or is not expensive.
 (7) Does or does not lead to increasing social isolation.
e. Tips to maintaining adherence to treatment regimen.
 (1) Assess the patient's capacity to understand the risks of nonadherence.
 (2) Assess contributing factors to nonadherence.
 (3) Provide education to the patient and family regarding the risks and optimal outcomes.
 (4) Have the social worker address fears about treatment and social barriers to adherence.
 (5) Detect depression early and refer for treatment.
 (6) Ask team members to assist the patient in "staying on track."
 (7) Provide opportunity for the patient to make choices and maintain control.
 (8) Develop a partnership with the patient.
 (9) Use contracting as a means of facilitating behavioral change.
 (10) Minimize side effects of treatment.
 (11) Identify creative ways to motivate the patient.
 (12) If the patient's nonadherence is disrupting facility operations, adjust schedules or wait to set up until the patient arrives.
 (13) Reinforce patient achievements or successes, no matter how small.

Spirituality

The development of interventions that are relevant and sensitive to the client's world view is a foundational principle of cultural competence (Sue, Arrendondo, & McDavis, 1992). In other words, cultural competence is exhibited by designing interventions that incorporate beliefs and practices from the client's world view (including spiritual beliefs and practices) into the intervention. The incorporation of CKD and ESRD patients' spiritual beliefs and practices may foster increased patient investment in the healing process. Addressing the spiritual needs of patients can assist them in their suffering. The role of spirituality in health care, particularly in chronic illness and end-of-life care, should be recognized and addressed.

I. **Spirituality defined.** The dimension of a person who seeks to find meaning in his/her life; life as a spiritual journey. Many patients view their spiritual and religious strengths as essential assets that can be tapped to foster healing and growth. The practitioner can support patients in their suffering and in the midst of their existential pain. The George Washington Institute for Spirituality and Health (Puchalski, 2006) proposes that health care providers are entrusted with the care of the physical, the emotional, the social, and the spiritual aspects of their patients in all phases of patients' lives. Further, health care workers need to be aware of the importance of the spiritual needs of those who are ill and suffer; such awareness will lead to compassionate care. The Institute promotes inclusion of a spirituality component in medical education, research, policy decisions, and health care training for all disciplines.

II. Influence of spirituality on adjustment. Patients often suffer deeply in their lives, suffering that is both difficult to witness and ease.

A. A commitment to thinking positively has been noted to be an important activity in preparing oneself for dialysis. Mok, Lai, and Zhang (2004) observed this phenomenon as making an important contribution to ultimate acceptance of the treatment.

B. In 2006, Al-Arabi studied the quality of everyday life among dialysis patients, and identified a conceptual category that emerged from participants' descriptions of ways they coped with having ESRD. One theme that was revealed related to spirituality. Participants described: "trust in God," holding on to faith, and coming to terms with their illness through the knowledge and understanding they had gained by ESRD and dialysis. Some in the study found a sense of purpose in their lives, inner peace, and the ability to accept being on dialysis by holding onto faith. Prayer became more important to them at the onset of ESRD and gave them strength to keep going.

C. Patel, Shah, Peterson, and Kimmel (2002) studied psychosocial variables, quality of life, and religious beliefs in ESRD patients treated with hemodialysis. Psychosocial and medical variables included perception of importance of faith (spirituality), attendance at religious services (religious involvement), the Beck Depression Inventory, Illness Effects Questionnaire, Multidimensional Scale of Perceived Social Support, McGill QOL Questionnaire scores, Karnofsky scores, dialysis dose, and predialysis hemoglobin and albumin levels. The study concluded that religious beliefs are related to perception of depression, illness effects, social support, and QOL independent of medical aspects of illness. Further, religious beliefs may act as coping mechanisms for patients with ESRD.

III. Assessment. Spiritual values and beliefs can be assessed as part of the routine medical or psychosocial history. The George Washington Institute for Spirituality and Health uses the acronym FICA to help structure questions in taking a spiritual history by health care professionals.

A. F – Faith and Belief: "Do you consider yourself spiritual or religious?" or "Do you have spiritual beliefs that help you cope with stress?" If the patient responds "No," the practitioner might ask,

"What gives your life meaning?" Sometimes patients respond with answers such as family, career, or nature.

B. I – Importance: "What importance does your faith or belief have in your life? Have your beliefs influenced how you take care of yourself in this illness? What role do your beliefs play in regaining your health?"

C. C – Community: "Are you part of a spiritual or religious community? Is this of support to you and how? Is there a group of people you really love or who are important to you?" Communities such as churches, temples, mosques, or a group of like-minded friends can serve as strong support systems for some patients.

D. A – Address in care: "How would you like me, your health care provider, to address these issues in your health care?"

E. Further recommendations by the Institute in taking a spiritual history.
   1. Consider spirituality as a potentially important component of every patient's physical well being and mental health.
   2. Address spirituality at each complete physical examination and continue addressing it at follow-up visits if appropriate. Spirituality is an ongoing issue.
   3. Respect a patient's privacy regarding spiritual beliefs. Don't impose your beliefs on others.
   4. As appropriate, make referrals to chaplains, spiritual directors, or community resources.
   5. Be aware that your own spiritual beliefs will help you personally and will overflow in your encounters with those for whom you care to make the encounter a more humanistic one.

IV. Health care provider self-assessment. Recognize that as practitioners, your own spirituality plays a key role in our professional lives and affects how we interact with patients and colleagues. Self-examination is often helpful in respecting patient autonomy. In some cases, the most appropriate option is referral to another practitioner whose value system is more congruent with that of the patient's.

V. Collaboration and referral. Form collaborative partnerships with chaplains, clergy, and other spiritual care providers.

Chapter 18

Patient and Family Education

Purpose

To present the components of the teaching-learning process to assist the nurse in implementation of patient and family education. Patients with chronic kidney disease (CKD) need to comprehend all aspects of their disease and therapeutic treatment modalities to become active participants and decision makers in their care. The process of patient and family education is the primary mechanism for facilitating such understanding. In fact, patient and family education is so important that it alone has been cited by patients as being responsible for improving their quality of life. Therefore, as nurses, it is essential that we refine patient and family education so that it is effective and efficient for producing the desired patient outcomes.

Objectives

Upon completion of this chapter, the learner will be able to:
1. Define the teaching-learning process, differentiating between teaching and learning.
2. List three types of variables that will influence the teaching-learning process.
3. Identify the three major classifications of learning theories.
4. Describe a process, that can be, used to assess a patient's learning needs.
5. List the processes involved in developing a teaching plan.
6. List four types of learning methods and media that can be used in the process of patient and family education.
7. Identify at least five methods and media that are appropriate for learning according to Gagne's hierarchy.
8. List teaching activities that will enhance the retention of learning.
9. Describe ways to incorporate the family in the education process.
10. Discuss strategies to enhance the learning of patients and family affected by CKD.

I. The teaching-learning process.

A. Definition. The teaching-learning process involves the interaction of individuals and the environment for the purpose of achieving a specific goal.

B. Intervening variable. The nature of the teaching learning process changes in complexity based on the number of relationships of the intervening variables present. Intervening variables are introduced into the process by both the participants and the environment. Examples of those variables include:
   1. Teacher variables.
      a. Abilities.
      b. Skills.
      c. Motivation.
      d. Intelligence.
      e. Creativity.
      f. Personality.
      g. Culture and values.
      h. Age.
      i. Gender.
   2. Learner variables.
      a. Abilities.
      b. Knowledge.
      c. Attitude.
      d. Motivation.

e. Health state.
f. Values and culture.
g. Age.
h. Gender.
3. Environmental variables.
a. Degree of quietness.
b. Temperature of room.
c. Number of human, inanimate, and other distracters.
d. Schedule conflicts.
e. Furniture arrangement.

C. Components: Though related, two components of the teaching-learning process, teaching and learning, are independent of each other.
1. Teaching by definition is the intentional structuring of content to enhance human interactions to facilitate learning.
2. Learning is a change in behavior. In most instances, the degree of permanency of the behavior change is directly related to the amount of practiced reinforcement engaged in by the learner.

II. **Theories of learning.** One approach to understanding human learning is to begin with a review of the major theories of learning and then to examine the progression or order of learning.

A. Table 4.3 presents an overview of several major classifications of learning theories, including:
1. A definition.
2. The major tenets.
3. Some major theorists.
4. An example of the learning represented.

B. Table 4.4 presents Gagne's hierarchy of learning, including (a) the level of learning, (b) a definition, and (c) an example of the type of learning indicated for each level. The table can be used to assess and implement levels of learning required to meet specific objectives progressing toward mastery. Specific teaching strategies can be devised to produce the learning required to meet the objectives.

III. **Principles of learning.** Understanding the theory related to how people learn is beneficial in the education process. When translating theoretical perspectives into learning principles, their applicability increases tremendously. Use of the principles inpatient and family education enhances learning.

A. Perception is a prerequisite to learning.

B. Perception is relative, selective, organized, and influenced by what is expected to be perceived.

C. Attention is a prerequisite to learning.

D. Attention is directed and captured by creative, innovative change in stimuli.

E. A person's perceptual capacity is about seven items at one time.

F. A person processes perceived information in chunks or clusters.

G. Organized information is more easily perceived and processed.

H. Familiar information is more easily perceived and processed.

I. Using more than one sensory organ enhances learning.

J. Accurate perception of information enhances subsequent cognitive processes using that information.

K. Learning that is personally relevant or meaningful is more easily acquired and retained longer.

L. Consolidating information enhanced learning.

M. Repetition positively influences learning.

N. Concrete information is more easily learned and remembered than is abstract information.

O. Correcting wrong information immediately facilitates learning.

P. Learner maturity and motivation increases learning.

Q. Information given at the beginning and end of instruction will be retained longer.

R. Active learner involvement in the learning process enhances learning.

S. Practicing use of information in different context fosters the utility and retention of that information.

T. Demonstration and return demonstration enhance the learning of psychomotor skills.

U. Using examples facilitates learning.

V. A learner's readiness to learn, or need to know, will increase the effectiveness of the learning.

IV. **Adult learners.** The majority of our educational interaction occurs with adults, either the patient or family members. Those adults have specific characteristics that will influence the learning. Nurses must be cognizant of those needs as educational interactions are planned.

A. Ability. In general, learning ability decreases with

Table 4.3

An Overview of the Major Classifications of Learning Theories

Classification	Definition	Major Tenets	Major Theorists	Example of the Learning
Behaviorist or Connectionist	Interprets human behavior as connections between stimuli and responses under the influence of reinforcement.	Respondent behavior results from a specific stimulus (S-R). Operant behavior is emitted as an instrumental act (R-R). Reinforcement increases the possibility of operant behavior recurring. Most human behaviors are operant in nature. Punishment decreases the possibility of a response recurring. Continuous reinforcement leads to faster learning. Intermittent reinforcement leads to longer retention of that which is learned.	Skinner Watson Thorndike Guthrie	Programmed instruction for skill development such as administering an insulin injection.
Cognitive, Organismic, or Gestalt	Interprets human behavior in terms of cognitive processes, such as insight, intelligence, and organizational abilities.	Concerned with the process of decision making, cognitive structure, understanding, perception, and information processing. The emphasis is on the how of learning rather than what.	Bruner Piaget Ausubel	Exploring relationships such as those that exist between risk factors and the tendency to develop certain diseases.
Humanistic	Interprets human behavior as being self-centered and directly related to the process of self-actualization.	Learning is an individual internal process. People learn what they perceive to be helpful to maintaining their own structure. Self-actualization is the motivation for learning. Self-actualization and learning involve creative functioning. The organization of the self must not be threatened for new learning to occur.	Rogers Kohl	Exploring specific health promotion behaviors to stay healthy.

age, particularly in learning activities that are fast paced or complex. Adults in their 40s to 50s have a similar ability to when they were 20s to 30s if they are able to control the pace. There appears to be significant decline in learning ability after age 60, consistent with the decreases in internal cognitive processes related to aging. Additionally, the ability to reason and make effective, efficient decisions appears to decrease.

B. Experiential base. Adults approach learning based on their previous experiences. They come with a wide experiential base that influences their cognitive structure and how they encode information for storage and retrieval. Thus, the learning needs to be relevant to their past experiences.

C. Perception. Adults use selective perception to deal with "new" things. They try to make it meaningful to them within their perceptual context. When they are unable to incorporate the new information with existing cognitive structure they are prone to misperceptions and learning is hindered.

Table 4.4

Gagne's Hierarchy of Learning

Level of Learning	Definition	Example of the Learning
1. Signal learning	Learning to respond to a signal or developing a conditioned response.	Generating anxiety at the sight of a hypodermic needle.
2. Stimulus-response learning	Voluntary learning that involves making a specific response to a specified stimulus.	Responding "dialysis machine" when the stimulus of "artificial kidney" is given.
3. Chaining	Learning to connect sequentially two or more stimulus-response situations.	Performing each of the steps necessary for implementing home dialysis.
4. Verbal association	Learning to attach names or labels to objects or to translate words into other languages.	Translating medical terminology into lay terms for easy understanding.
5. Multiple discrimination	Learning an extensive series of simple chains and differentiating between similar stimuli.	Recalling the specific name of each medication when several different tablets or capsules are presented.
6. Concept learning	Learning to make a common response to a number of stimuli that may differ in appearance.	Recognizing that even though the substances presented are tablets, capsules, and elixirs, they are all medications.
7. Principle or rule learning	Learning a chain of two or more previously and separately learned concepts.	Recognizing that the concept of compliance represents a relationship between the concepts of adherence to a therapeutic regimen and feelings of being better.
8. Problem solving	Learning that requires considering previously learned principles to develop new, higher level principles.	Deciding how frequently to institute home dialysis based on previously agreed-upon parameters.

D. Memory. Memory includes the three phases of registration, retention, and recall. Registration includes exposure, acquisition and encoding of information in the brain. Registration process, particularly visual information, decreases with age. Retention is the persistence of the encoded information and it will decrease with age unless the information has direct meaning for the learner. Recall involves the search and retrieval processes used to remember information. Recall, particularly short-term recall, decreases with age.

E. Practice and repetition. Adults need repeated interactions with information coupled with, appropriate, immediate feedback to learn.

F. Learning effectiveness. Learning effectiveness is decreased in adults because of their wide experiential base and previous learning often interferes with their ability to cognitively organize new information. It requires time to sort through all of the old information to encode the new information. Therefore, learning usually takes longer for adults.

G. Self-pacing. Adults are self-directed and establish their own time lines for learning. They will learn more effectively if allowed to establish their own pace. Additionally, they need periodic breaks in the learning process.

H. Purposefulness. Adults engage in learning because they want to apply the information in their daily lives. The more practical and useful the information is to an adult, the easier it is for them to learn. They also learn to transfer the information to other situations more rapidly.

I. Resource interaction. The effectiveness of adult learning depends upon the availability, appropriateness, and utility of the resources for learning. Adults need easy access to and repeated opportunity to engage in interactions with educational resources.

J. Time perception. Adults tend to perceive time as being a valued, meaningful commodity. Their lives usually require them to manage their time appropriately to fulfill their responsibilities and meet their own needs. They recognize they take longer to learn, but they want their time spent doing so to be meaningful and useful.

IV. Activities of teaching.

A. Comparison to the nursing process. The process used in teaching patients is identical to the process used in delivering patient care.

B. The assessment/diagnosis phase. The teaching activities that occur during the assessment/diagnosis phase are determining the learning needs of the individual and assessing the individual's physical, psychologic, and maturational readiness to learn.
   1. Assessment of learning needs. The assessment of a patient's behavior, asking specific questions regarding physiology, pathology, or the treatment regimen, and listening carefully to the patient's responses and questions.
   2. Assessment of readiness and ability to learn. The first step in the assessment of a patient's readiness to learn is to establish a record of the patient's baseline knowledge, related health experiences, written or verbal communication problems, current lifestyle, and significant others. The second step is to assess the patient's physical, psychologic, and maturational readiness.
      a. Physical readiness.
         (1) Physiologic state.
         (2) Pharmacologic therapy.
      b. Psychologic readiness.
         (1) Mental status.
         (2) Previous knowledge.
         (3) Past experiences.
         (4) Motivation for learning.
         (5) Attitude toward learning and health care.
         (6) Coping mechanisms.
      c. Maturational readiness.
         (1) Life experiences.
         (2) Problem-solving ability.

C. The planning phase of the teaching process is critical to achieve a successful outcome. In most cases, this phase requires more time, energy, and deliberation than any other component of the entire process.
   1. Teaching activities. The teaching activities in the planning phase include:
      a. Determine the purpose of the teaching.
      b. Developing the teaching plan.
      c. Arranging the learning environment.
   2. Determine the purpose. In patient education, it is essential to be able to clearly articulate the precise nature of the learning to be accomplished. The purpose of the teaching serves as a broad guide for structuring the learning process, as well as for selecting the appropriate teaching strategy.
   3. Develop the teaching plan. Developing the teaching plan involves the following processes: identifying specific, measurable learning goals and behavioral objectives to meet specific learning activities. It is key to identifying alternative teaching strategies to meet the needs of all learner variables, such as auditory, tactile, and visual. Finally, establish measurable and validated tools that can be used in evaluating the effectiveness of both the teaching and learning processes.
      a. Develop behavioral objectives.
         (1) Definition. Behavioral objectives are statements of specific learner behaviors that are expected to occur as a result of the teaching-learning process.
         (2) Characteristics. A behavioral objective always contains the performance behavior, the condition under which it is to occur, and the acceptable standard for the performance. In other words, it specifies what the learner should do, under what conditions, and how well.
         (3) Classifications. Behavioral objectives are classified according to three domains depending upon the type and level of learning that is to be achieved.
            (a) Cognitive domain deals with intellectual abilities and includes the hierarchical levels of knowledge, comprehension, application, analysis, synthesis, and evaluation.
            (b) Affective domain deals with the expression of feelings and includes the hierarchical levels of attentiveness, responsiveness, acceptance of values, organization of values, and characterization by a value.
            (c) Psychomotor domain deals with

motor skills and includes the hierarchical levels of perception of a stimulus, preparation, guided response, mechanism (habit), complex overt response, adaptation, and organization of motor skills.

b. Develop a content outline by consulting various resources regarding the knowledge base essential for assisting the learner to achieve the desired behavioral objectives.

c. Identify specific learner activities.

(1) Definition. Learner activities are those specific behaviors that are completed by the learner as part of the educational process. These activities may occur before, during, or after the specific teaching-learning session, it is important that the evaluation of the learning not occur until they have been completed.

(2) Examples. Some examples of learning activities are reading specific items of information in preparation for the session, manipulating equipment, demonstrating a procedure, viewing various types of media, listening to audio tapes, and responding to practice situations.

d. Identify alternative teaching strategies.

(1) Definition. Teaching strategies are those methods and media used by the teacher to facilitate learning.

(2) Examples. Some examples of teaching methods are lecture, discussion, demonstration, and simulation. Educational media include regular printed materials, (such as textbooks), programmed instruction texts, still pictures, motion pictures, television, real objects, or models, audio tapes and records, teaching machines, and computers. The familiarity of most individuals with computers makes them a valuable asset in patient teaching especially when the learner lives in remote locations. There are many online teaching modules that provide simulated scenarios and allow for the learner to work at their own pace. These modules should be monitored, however, for levels of literacy and to ensure they are appropriate resource tools.

(3) Guidelines for use. As discussed, there are many methods of teaching methods and tools. The key to an effective learning process is assessing the needs of the

learner and using those tools, which will forester the greatest cognitive retention. Examples include:

(a) Using large colored pictures for older adult learners who may be visually impaired.

(b) Using dolls to locate where the kidneys are located for pediatric learners.

(c) The teaching tools should be age appropriate.

(d) Information that is current and accurate.

(e) Information needs to be presented in an interesting manner to maintain the attention of the learner.

(f) Tools should be adaptable to be used in a variety of settings such as one-on-one and group venues.

(g) In addition, Table 4.5 suggests those methods, tools, and media that are most appropriate for producing the various hierarchical levels of the learning as described by Gagne.

e. Plan for evaluation.

(1) Relationship to behavioral objectives. If the behavioral objectives are specific enough they can also be used as the evaluation criteria. However, if they are not specific enough, then additional criteria needs to be generated. For example, the objective, identify several foods that can be included on a low sodium diet, is not specific enough to provide criteria for evaluation. A more specific statement that would include the evaluation criteria would be: "After discussing sample menus, select in writing four foods that would be permitted on a 500 mg sodium diet and hand in at the end of the class." This objective states not only the behavior that is to be performed, but it also provides the conditions under which it must be performed and the degree of accuracy of the performance. These goals are SMART: specific, measurable, attainable, realistic and timely.

(2) Measurement tools. According to Redman, to evaluate educational processes effectiveness, there needs to be valid and reliable tools that will measure what is intended to measure. There are many types of evaluation tools. The most effective tool needs to be determined

when setting goals and objectives. Table 4.6 reviews the pros and cons to each to each of the following tools:

(a) Evaluation matrix.

(b) Anecdotal method.

(c) Focus groups.

(d) Questionnaire.

(e) Likert scale.

(f) Interval scale.

(g) Ratio scale.

4. Arrange the learning environment. The following factors are important when arranging the environment for learning.

a. Structured time: a definite time period.

b. Flexibility in both content and process.

c. Climate: an acceptable atmosphere.

d. Physical surroundings are comfortable and free of distraction.

D. The implementation phase.

1. Teaching activities. The implementation phase is devoted to the following teaching activities:

a. Teacher-learner mutual goals.

b. Carrying out the teaching plan.

c. Providing learning cues.

d. Providing appropriate stimuli and maintaining attentiveness with learner.

e. Fostering association of previously learned material.

f. Providing opportunities for practice and return demonstration.

g. Assisting the learner in associating new concepts with old ones.

2. Communication. Effective communication, both verbal and nonverbal, is essential in the process of patient education.

3. The evaluation phase. The evaluation phase is reserved for those activities needed to determine whether or not the objectives have been met and learning has occurred.

VI. Culturally sensitive approaches to patient education.

A. According to Price and Cordell there are four-steps that help nurses promote cultural sensitivity when creating patient teaching programs, titled Four Step Approach to Providing Culturally Sensitive Care.

1. Examine personal culture: Be aware of potential barriers to learning.

2. Familiarity with client culture: It is essential that minority issues be explored and professionals of similar backgrounds be

Table 4.5

Teaching Methods and Media Appropriate for Producing Specific Levels of Learning

Level of Learning	Appropriate Methods and Media
1. Signal learning	lecture, still pictures, motion pictures, television, audio recordings, texts
2. Stimulus-response learning	still pictures, motion pictures, models, television, demonstration
3. Chaining	motion pictures, programmed instruction, demonstration, still pictures, television
4. Verbal association	motion pictures, programmed instruction, demonstration, still pictures, television
5. Multiple discrimination	motion pictures, programmed instruction, still pictures, television, texts, lecture
6. Concept learning	motion pictures, television, still pictures, programmed instruction, texts, lecture
7. Principle learning	motion pictures, television, still pictures, programmed instruction, texts, lectures, simulation
8. Problem solving	lecture, motion pictures, television, texts, simulation

employed whenever possible to promote culturally sensitive care.

3. Identify adaptations made with client: Incorporate continuing education programs to increase the knowledge of staff nurses about their own culturally based values, beliefs and practices so that they can integrate the cultural-specific health related beliefs and practices of others into the nursing process within their specialty areas of practice such as kidney.

4. Modify client teaching based from earlier steps: Teaching must be based on culturological assessment, biocultural variations in health and illness, and cultural differences in communication, religious beliefs, nutrition, and aspects of the aging process. Literacy and age appropriate materials need to be incorporated to facilitate greater cognitive retention as well.

Table 4.6

Evaluation Tools Pros and Cons

Evaluation Tool	Pros	Cons
Evaluation matrix	Allows wide range of data to be collected.	Extra data not needed and may not be specific enough.
Anecdotal method	Narrative summation data.	Too subjective and difficult to validate.
Focus group	Information is easy to collect and open and honesty.	Kind and quality of information may not be relevant and may also may difficult to validate.
Questionnaires	Wealth of information can be obtained.	Questionnaires can be biased if not well-designed.
Likert Scale	Allows a respondent to rate a survey question at the level they agree or disagree: The categories represent an inherent order (more to less, stronger to weaker, bigger to smaller).	Numbers assigned to the categories do not indicate the magnitude of difference between the categories in the way that an interval or ratio scale would. Respondents, may misread 1 to be 5 and vice versa and the measurement may be altered.
Interval Scale	Numerical scales in which intervals have the same interpretation throughout.	Interval scales are not perfect, however. In particular, they do not have a true zero point even if one of the scaled values happens to carry the name "zero."
Ratio Scales	The ratio scale of measurement is the most informative scale. It is an interval scale with the additional property that its zero position indicates the absence of the quantity being measured.	None noted.

VII. Linguistic specific teaching strategies.

A. The most crucial element in the process of learning is the ability to understand language.

B. Linguistic-oriented theorists such as Cross and Brown specify there needs to be an association, reinforcement, and imitation. The most effective method of learning is first language learning. Therefore, an interpreter is critical if the educator is not language specific for the targeted patient population.

C. Pictures and visual aides are extremely effective when language is a potential barrier to learning.

VIII. Retention of learning.

A. Initial learning is only part of the process of patient education. The second part is that of cognitive retention. The learning, which is retained, produces the long-term rewards in terms of behavior modification and patient care. The retention of learning can be enhanced during the teaching-learning process through the use of the following specific types of learning activities or strategies:
1. Providing selective reinforcement immediately after the occurrence of an appropriate response.
2. Giving frequent, random reinforcement throughout the teaching-learning session.
3. Providing for repetitive practice of psychomotor skills and rote verbal learning.
4. Foster the application of meaningful learning to commonly encountered situations.
5. Maintaining a high learner motivation level.
6. Offering organizing elements for categorizing information.
7. Encouraging the review or rehearsal of the information to be retained.

IX. Incorporating family-centered education.

A. The concept of "family" is more than people who are biologically related. When viewed in the larger context "family" might include two people of the same or different sex living together with or without sexual attachment, single-parent families, remarried families with children and stepchildren, and many other forms of family as defined by the patient. When serious illness occurs the entire family is affected. Other family members alter their lifestyle and take on role functions of the patient. The extent of family disruption depends on the seriousness of the illness, the family's level of functioning before illness, socioeconomic considerations, and the extent to which family members can absorb the role of the patient.

1. No matter how the family is constructed, each is unique.
   a. Assess family function and style by talking with patient and family and observing their interactions.
   b. Gather information through their conversation about stressors, transition, family function, and expectations.
   c. Involve the family in teaching plan to avoid failure.
   d. As noted in theories of adult learning, use case studies of what other families have done in similar situations.
   e. Include pertinent information about disease process, focus on planning, care giving, and problem solving.
   f. If indicated, include education about planning for long term care, respite care, support, and other available resources.

X. Application to patients with CKD.

A. When implementing the teaching-learning process with patients diagnosed with CKD, it is important to remember that they have specific characteristics that occur as a result of their disease process that will influence their learning. In addition, it is important to recall some of the strategies that have been useful in assisting patients in their learning process.

1. Characteristics of patients with CKD. May process information differently depending on the stage of their CKD. Their variations in information processing are related to the following characteristics:
   a. Depressed mentation: requiring repetition of information.
      (1) Tell them what you are going to tell them (objectives).
      (2) Tell them (content).
      (3) Tell them what you told them (summary).
   b. Short attention spans: usually tolerating only 10–15 minute teaching sessions.
   c. Altered perceptual status: requires frequent clarification and reassurance.
   d. Altered sensory systems: thus respond better to ideas that are repetitively presented in different audio-visual forms.
   e. Decreased levels of concentration: requiring additional stimulation repetition, and positive reinforcement as part of the educational process.

B. Strategies for enhancing learning: It has been noted that patients tend to learn more effectively if the following principles are adhered to whenever possible:
   a. Brevity: Be brief in your educational interactions. About 50% of the statements made to a patient will be forgotten within 5 minutes of the interaction. This is particularly true if the other principles are not considered in the educational session.
   b. Organization: Information which is structured and clearly organized enhances learning by facilitating the encoding of information for the adult.
   c. Primacy: The items presented first are usually retained longer. This suggests that providing the patient with the specific purpose of the educational session and some brief, but essential, components at the initiation of the session will enhance retention of the information.
   d. Readability: Written or printed information that is given to a patient to supplement the educational process must be age specific and at an appropriate literacy level. Unfortunately, most educational tools are written at an 11th grade level; even though the research shows that the 8th grade level would be more appropriate for the majority of patients. Materials may need to be modified to accommodate the learner's characteristics.
   e. Repetition: Adults need repetition to enhance learning. Information that is repeated is more readily retained and recalled. Repetition may take many forms, including printed or other visual materials and audio or video tapes.
   f. Specificity: The more specific and useful the information is, the more powerful it is for the patient. In addition, specificity enhances retention and application of information.

Chapter 19

The Financial Impact

Purpose

This chapter is intended to provide basic information about financing the treatment for kidney disease and kidney failure, including financial burdens, and resources available to help people with kidney disease and kidney failure. Prior to Medicare coverage of kidney failure, patients with kidney failure often died. There were few dialysis clinics, and transplants were still experimental. Those chosen for kidney failure treatment were more likely to be young white males who were employed, insured, and not eligible for Medicare.

In October 1971, Shep Glazer, then Vice President of the National Association of Patients on Hemodialysis, now known as the American Association of Kidney Patients, appealed to Congress for funding for kidney failure while doing dialysis on the floor of Congress. Mr. Glazer and others testifying told legislators that the high cost of dialysis was limiting access to a treatment that would not just keep people alive but allow most to work. Congress passed and President Nixon signed H.R. 1 which became P.L. 92-603, the law extending Medicare coverage for dialysis and transplant treatment of kidney failure. Medicare started covering dialysis and transplants for kidney failure in July 1973.

Objectives

Upon completion of this chapter, the learner will be able to:
1. List three ways people become eligible for Medicare.
2. Explain Medicare benefits including eligibility, when it starts and ends, and coverage for dialysis and transplantation.
3. State how to determine eligibility for Medigap coverage and options.
4. Describe how benefits of employer group health plans (EGHP) and individual plans coordinate with Medicare.
5. Describe eligibility criteria for high risk health insurance.
6. Identify health insurance options for special populations including federal employees, military (active duty, retirees, or dependent), Native Americans, and youths under age 19.
7. Identify three sources of assistance to pay for prescribed drugs.
8. State two ways socioeconomic status can limit access to care and treatment options.
9. Describe ways that patients, providers, and payers benefit when patients work.
10. List three ways nurses can help patients retain employment.
11. State three ways social workers can help patients with financial and rehabilitation concerns.

I. Costs of treating kidney disease.

A. Costs and chronic kidney disease (CKD). In 2004, Medicare Part A paid an average of $257 per month and Part B paid an average of $198 per month for each Medicare beneficiary diagnosed with CKD in 2003. Costs were higher if the patient had hypertension or diabetes or both (USRDS, 2006).

B. Costs of dialysis and transplant: In 2004, as a primary payer, Medicare paid $67,733 per hemodialysis patient, $48,796 per peritoneal dialysis patient, and $23,840 per transplant recipient. That same year, as a primary payer, Medicare paid $98,968 per patient in the first year of transplant (USRDS, 2006).

C. Costs of ESRD care to employer group health plans (EGHPs). In 2003, employer group health plans (EGHPs) paid on average nearly $180,000 per dialysis patient, 2.7 times Medicare costs. EGHPs paid around $195,000 per transplant performed nearly twice as much as Medicare costs (USRDS, 2006).

II. Paying for treatment.

A. Medicare is health insurance for select groups of people.
1. Qualifications include people 65 and older, those who have received Social Security Disability Insurance (SSDI) checks for 24 months, and those who have ESRD requiring dialysis or transplant for survival.
2. To be eligible for ESRD Medicare, patients must be certified by a physician to have kidney failure requiring dialysis or transplant for survival. In addition, each patient must also have worked long enough to qualify on his/her own work record, his/her spouse's (or in some cases, an ex-spouse's) work record, or parent's work record if the patient is a child.
   a. Social Security can advise a patient if he/she is eligible for Medicare.
   b. Dialysis and transplant providers must complete the ESRD Medical Evidence Report Medicare Entitlement & Patient Registration form (CMS 2728). This registers the patient in the ESRD program and alerts Social Security that the patient may be eligible for Medicare. Applications are available at the local Social Security office and can be completed in person, by phone, or by mail.
3. Medicare Part A covers hospital room, board and care, transplant evaluation and surgery for recipients and donors, hospice care, and limited care in a skilled nursing facility. As a primary payer, Part A pays 100% for the first 60 days after the hospital deductible is paid. Medicare Part A hospital days are limited. After 60 days there is a copay for each hospital day. After a 90-day hospital stay, Medicare will only pay for 60 more days (called lifetime reserve days) and there is a higher copay. Although the first 90 Medicare Part A days can be renewed if someone stays out of the hospital at least 60 days, once used, lifetime reserve days are gone. If someone remains out of the hospital over 60 days, it starts a new benefit period with a new Part A deductible. Part A also pays up to 100 days in a skilled nursing facility. There is no daily charge for the first 20 days, but after that, there is a daily charge. Part A is premium free for anyone with enough work credits. Those 65 and older, without enough work credits, can purchase Part A. The cost is dependent upon how many credits have been earned.

4. Medicare Part B covers outpatient charges including doctors' and surgeons' fees, outpatient surgery, in-center and home dialysis, durable medical equipment, rehabilitation therapy, home health care, ambulance, and some prescription drugs. As a primary payer, Part B pays 80% of the allowed charge after the annual deductible is met. The Part B annual deductible increases every year. Starting in 2007, the Part B premium high for those earning over $80,000 for an individual or $160,000 a couple.
5. Patients with EGHP coverage may not want to pay the premium for Medicare Part B. If patients do not sign up for Part A or B, they can sign up at any time without penalty. However, if they sign up for Part A (free) and waive Part B (premium), they can only sign up for Part B, from January to March of each year, and Medicare would start the following July. Signing up late for Part B may also result in higher Part B premiums. Patients should talk with Social Security before deciding not to sign up for Medicare.
6. There are several Medicare plans available for patients to choose from. Original Medicare is provided by the government. In this plan, patients can choose their health care providers and know what percent or fees that will be owed. Patients who join Medicare Advantage (MA) plans purchase them through private insurance companies that contract with Medicare. In comparison to Original Medicare, MA plans may offer extra benefits, have different copays or coinsurance without any cap. Some plans offer a higher cost option to cover copays and coinsurance while others do not. Patients can stay in an MA plan when they start dialysis, but dialysis patients cannot sign up for an MA plan unless it is a "special needs plan" that has agreed to accept people on dialysis. Transplant patients who do not need dialysis can stay in or join an MA plan.
7. The type of treatment the patient chooses governs when Medicare can start. If the patient starts a home training program before the third full month of dialysis, Medicare coverage can be backdated to the first day of the month chronic

dialysis started, regardless of location (hospital or clinic) of initiation of dialysis. If in-center dialysis is the patient's choice of treatment, Medicare starts the first day of third full month of dialysis. If a patient receives a preemptive transplant, Medicare starts the month of the transplant or can be backdated up to 2 months if the patient was admitted for evaluation that month.

8. When Medicare ends is also dependent on the patient's type of treatment and whether or not he/she has Medicare for more than one reason. As long as someone is on dialysis he/she can receive Medicare indefinitely. If kidney function recovers and dialysis is no longer needed, Medicare coverage can continue for 12 months. If a patient is transplanted and has Medicare solely based on ESRD, Medicare coverage will end after 36 months. If someone is eligible for Medicare due to age or disability, as well as ESRD, even if he/she gets a transplant, Medicare continues indefinitely.

B. Medicare savings programs can help Medicare beneficiaries with limited income and assets to get state help to pay Medicare premiums and, in some cases, to pay secondary benefits for Medicare covered services. State medical assistance offices can screen patients for these programs.
   1. Qualified Medicare Beneficiary program (QMB) pays Medicare premiums and Medicare coinsurance or copays, but does not cover other Medicaid-only services.
   2. Specified Low-Income Medicare Beneficiary (SLMB) pays Medicare Part B premiums only, but does not cover Medicare copays or coinsurance or provide other Medicaid-only services.
   3. Qualified Individual program (QI), like SLMB, pays Medicare Part B premiums only.
   4. Qualified Working Disabled Individual (QWDI) program helps those with disabilities who would lose Medicare due to work pay Part A premiums. Those with Part A are eligible for Part B as well. Transplant patients who have a disability other than ESRD and continue to work may qualify for QWDI.

C. Every state has state medical assistance or Medicaid (Medi-Cal in California).
   1. To qualify for full Medicaid benefits, patients must meet eligibility criteria including state income and asset guidelines. Determining who is eligible for help and income requirements varies from state to state. Some states allow patients, with incomes above state Medicaid guidelines, to pay some of the costs of their medical care (called spend down or share of costs) with state Medicaid paying the remainder.
   2. The federal government mandates that states provide certain benefits and offers states the flexibility to cover additional services. Patients with limited income and assets may have Medicaid alone if they do not qualify for Medicare, usually because they have not earned enough work credits. Some states cover undocumented aliens on dialysis with 100% state funds. Most do not pay for transplants for these individuals.
   3. Some patients are "dual eligible." This means they have both Medicare and Medicaid. Medicare is considered the primary insurance and always pays first. Medicaid is considered secondary and therefore pays the deductible and coinsurance for Medicare covered services and services that are covered by Medicaid. Like Medicare, states have payment limits for covered services.

D. Medigap or Medicare supplement plans help to cover costs for Medicare covered services.
   1. Medigap plans are sold by private insurance companies and can pay all or part of Medicare deductibles and coinsurance for Part A and Part B covered services, including Part B covered drugs.
   2. Medigap plans in all but Massachusetts, Minnesota, and Wisconsin use the National Association of Insurance Commissioners (NAIC) model plan to structure benefits. In the NAIC model, plans are designated by letters A through L. All A plans offer the same benefits. All L plans offer the same benefits. This makes it easy to compare plans because the premium is the only difference.
   3. Under federal law, a Medigap plan must accept anyone 65 or older, even those with pre-existing conditions, during the first 6 months he/she has Medicare. Those with Medicare who are under 65 may be denied Medigap coverage or may have to wait for coverage for kidney disease. State insurance department health experts can advise patients about Medigap coverage in their state. For contacts to state insurance departments, see www.naic.org/state_web_map.htm.

E. Some patients have an Employer Group Health Plan (EGHPs) when their kidneys fail.
   1. An EGHP usually has more benefits and pays more than Medicare allows on Medicare covered services. An EGHP may also cover prescription drugs as well as or better than Medicare Prescription Drug Coverage (Part D).
   2. An EGHP is the primary payer for the first 30 months someone could have Medicare whether they enroll in Medicare or not. Providers can bill Medicare as a secondary payer for EGHP deductibles, copays and coinsurance, and for services that Medicare covers but the EGHP denies. Information about coordination of benefits and how to contact the Medicare coordination of benefits coordinator can be found at www.cms.hhs.gov/COBGeneralInformation.
   3. Having Medicare with an EGHP limits the amount a patient can be charged by providers that accept assignment to 100% of the Medicare allowable charge. Paying the Part B premium may save money as the EGHP pays at least 100% of Medicare's allowable because the patient is not liable for the difference between the charge and Medicare's allowable rate.

F. Some people have an individual (nongroup) health plan when their kidneys fail.
   1. Coverage varies and may not be as comprehensive as group plans. Premiums and cost shares may be higher.
   2. Medicare is always the primary insurance before a nongroup health plan.

G. High risk health insurance plans are available in some states.
   1. High risk health plans help people who have been denied coverage because of preexisting medical conditions. Although expensive, with possible waiting periods for pre-existing conditions coverage, they do, however, immediately cover any new health conditions.
   2. Some states do not have high risk plans and others do not allow those with Medicare to buy them. State insurance department health experts can advise patients about this coverage. For a list of states with high risk health insurance pools, refer to www.healthinsurance.org/riskpoolinfo.html.

H. Federal Employees Health Benefit (FEHB) Plans are available to federal employees.
   1. There are several choices of plans from managed care plans to fee-for-service.

2. Federal employees have an opportunity to change plans every year.
3. People can have both a FEHB plan and Medicare if they meet the qualifications for both.
4. FEHB plans may cover services that Medicare does not and Medicare can help to pay FEHB deductibles, copays, or coinsurance. For more information about FEHB, see www.opm.gov/insure/health/.

I. Veterans' health benefits are available for veterans.
   1. Those eligible for Veterans Administration (VA) health benefits include anyone who served on active duty without dishonorable discharge as well as those who were in the National Guard and called to active duty by executive order.
   2. VA provides care in VA health facilities or pays for the care of veterans at local health care facilities, including dialysis and transplant facilities.
   3. Veterans do not have to have service connected disabilities to receive certain health benefits. For more information about VA benefits, see www.va.gov/health.

J. TRICARE is the military health benefit for service members and dependents.
   1. Those eligible for TRICARE include active military duty, their dependents, and retirees and dependents.
   2. What is covered and where coverage must be received depends on the TRICARE plan selected: TRICARE Prime, TRICARE Extra, TRICARE Standard, and TRICARE for Life. The latter is for those 65 or older with Medicare.
   3. TRICARE applications are accepted at veterans health centers, by calling (877) 222-VETS or online at www.va.gov/101022.htm.

K. The Indian Health Service (IHS) funds health care for those who are members of American Indian tribes or Alaska Natives corporations.
   1. Health care is provided to American Indians or Alaska natives living on or near reservations as well as some care of those living in urban areas. For eligibility, see www.ihs.gov/GeneralWeb/HelpCenter/CustomerServices/elig.asp.
   2. IHS provides care for prevention and treatment of diseases, including kidney failure.
   3. Care is provided through IHS facilities or private providers through purchase of services. For general information on health benefits see www.ihs.gov.

L. State Child Health Insurance Program (SCHIP) is a program of services to children.
  1. SCHIP provides basic health care, physicians, hospitals, immunizations, and emergencies.
  2. To qualify, children must be under 19 and their families must meet eligibility requirements. In most states, families of 4 with no health insurance can earn up to $36,200 and still qualify for SCHIP. For more information, see www.insurekidsnow.gov/ or www.cms.hhs.gov/home/schip.asp.

M. Program of All-Inclusive Care for the Elderly (PACE) provides services to the elderly. The goal of this program is to allow the elderly to stay in their communities rather than in nursing facilities.
  1. PACE programs are not available in all states.
  2. Where available, people must be 55 years old or older to obtain PACE help.
  3. PACE programs provide comprehensive primary care services, social services, restorative therapies, personal care and supportive services, nutritional counseling, recreational therapy, and meals 24 hours a day, 7 days a week, 365 days a year in an adult day program or in-home. For more information about where PACE services are offered, see www.cms.hhs.gov/PACE/LPPO/list.asp.

N. State kidney programs are state-funded programs for people with kidney disease and kidney failure.
  1. All states do not have state kidney programs and in those states that do, eligibility guidelines vary.
  2. State kidney programs may help with such things as the cost of access surgery, treating kidney failure, medications, and treatment-related transportation. Covered services, in states with kidney programs, is determined by state funds and program guidelines.
  3. Most nephrology social workers know if their state has a state kidney program. To get a directory and/or to find out if your state has one, call Missouri Kidney Program at (800) 733-7345 or download the 2005 Directory of State Kidney Programs, www.muhealth.org/~mokp/FPub.htm.

O. Health Savings Accounts (HAS) allow people to set aside money, tax free, to pay for qualifying medical costs.
  1. HSAs are designed to help patients afford health care, particularly if they only qualify for high deductible health plans (HDHPs).
  2. Those with Medicare and those who can be claimed as a dependent on someone else's health plan are not eligible for a HSA.
  3. Those with cafeteria plans, set up by their employers, can save money on taxes by setting aside pre-tax dollars from their paycheck to pay their share of health insurance premiums, out-of-pocket medical or dental costs, and child care. In a traditional cafeteria plan, employees must spend the money they set aside for the year or lose what remains in the account at the end of the year. However, some HSAs do allow funds to carry over from year to year.
  4. Funds in an HSA are portable if the person changes jobs. For more information, see www.ustreas.gov/offices/public-affairs/hsa/pdf/HSA-Tri-fold-english-06.pdf.

III. Legal protections for health benefits.

A. Medigap. There are legal protections that allow patients with Medicare and Medigap plans, who return to work and obtain coverage through their job, to put their Medigap plan "on hold" and return if their employer plan coverage ends.

B. Consolidated Omnibus Budget Reconciliation Act (COBRA). Certain "events" grant continuation coverage if someone works for a company with 20 or more employees.
  1. If someone loses his/her job or experiences a reduction in hours/benefits, he/she is eligible for 18 months of COBRA coverage.
  2. In cases of separation or divorce, death, or the obtainment of Medicare from the employee, the spouse and dependent children are eligible for 36 months of COBRA coverage.
  3. If a child is no longer considered a dependent due to age, he/she is eligible for 36 months of COBRA coverage.
  4. The premium for COBRA is 102% of the full premium. The employee is responsible for paying the total premium and the employer pays nothing.
  5. Employees who are disabled before or within 60 days after the COBRA event can have an extra 11 months of coverage for a premium of 150% of the full premium. The employee is responsible for paying the total premium, while the employer pays nothing.
  6. Someone who has Medicare before he/she has COBRA must be offered COBRA coverage. An employer can terminate COBRA coverage if an employee signs up for Medicare after he/she has COBRA.

7. A COBRA plan is the primary payer for the first 30 months when patients have kidney failure and are eligible for Medicare.

C. Americans with Disabilities Act (ADA). The ADA applies to employers with 15 or more employees.
   1. The ADA does not require that any employer offer health insurance coverage to employees.
   2. If an employer has 15 or more employees and provides health benefits to others in the same job, the employer must provide health insurance to the person with a disability.
   3. It is legal for plans to have caps on coverage for certain diagnoses unless they do this for everyone within that group.

D. Health Insurance Portability and Accountability Act (HIPAA). This federal law allows those with pre-existing conditions to get group or individual health insurance on the commercial market.
   1. HIPAA applies to anyone losing Medicare, Medicaid, TRICARE, or VA benefits.
   2. Proof of coverage is needed and people must sign up for their new plan before 63 days elapse.
   3. When faced with the loss of health insurance, the plan must send a letter stating the loss coverage. This letter proves "creditable coverage" and when the clock is started for the open enrollment period.
   4. The new health plan must count time that the patient was covered in the previous plan, toward any pre-existing condition waiting period.
   5. HIPAA is the law that also protects the confidentiality of patients' personal health information.

IV. Paying for medications.

A. Insurance companies may offer coverage for prescription drugs.
   1. Out-of-pocket expenses vary by health plan.
   2. Some plans have formularies and coinsurance or copays.
   3. Plan enrollment packets and Web sites provide information on patient rights and responsibilities, including how to file an exception request to get a nonformulary drug covered.

B. Medicare Part D provides prescription drug coverage sold by private insurance companies.
   1. Anyone with Medicare Part A and/or Part B is eligible. Those who have current prescription coverage that is as good as or better than Part D coverage can wait to join Part D when needed.
   2. Anyone can enroll in Part D during the 3 months following their eligibility for Medicare. If they join after the 3-month period, they could have a higher premium when they join. In some cases, Medicare beneficiaries can join or switch outside the annual coordinated election period from November 15 to December 31. However, most can only join or switch during this period.
   3. Most drug coverage for patients with Medicare and Medicaid (dual eligible) is under Medicare Part D. Coverage depends on whether the patient's drugs are on the Part D formulary. Dual eligibles can switch plans any month to get the best coverage. Medicaid may still pay for drugs that are excluded under Part D.
   4. Drugs covered under Part A or Part B are still covered by Part A or Part B regardless of the patient's chosen Medicare plan: Original Medicare or Medicare Advantage.
   5. Those with limited income and assets are eligible for additional assistance called "extra help" to pay premiums and cost shares for covered drugs. Others pay premiums, deductibles, and coinsurance or copays. Social Security accepts applications for the low income subsidy (extra help).
   6. Unless someone qualifies for extra help, standard Part D plan have a coverage gap that is expected to grow larger every year. Once those with Medicare Part D have paid the annual "true out-of-pocket" (TrOOP) costs for Part D, they receive catastrophic coverage. Help from family, friends, qualified state pharmacy assistance programs, and charities to pay these TrOOP costs and can assist people in reaching the catastrophic benefit at which time the plan pays 95% of the cost of covered drugs. Some Part D plans do not have a coverage gap while others cover generic drugs or even brand name drugs during the gap. However these plans have a higher premium.
   7. Coverage estimates. Based on data on dialysis patients in the MedStat database, a database of EGHPs, it was estimated that over one-third of dialysis patients would spend enough on drugs to reach the coverage gap and another one-third will get help from Part D catastrophic coverage. There is no data available on what drugs cost or what patients, who signed up for Part D, paid out of pocket.
   8. Part D plans limit their costs by negotiating

prices with drug companies, limiting drug coverage, requiring prior authorization, step therapy, or limiting the number of pills a patient can obtain per month. If the patient's health or functioning may be harmed, patients or providers can request an expedited coverage determination and receive a response, from the plan, within 24 hours. There is a standard template that prescribers can use to request expedited coverage determination from the plan. However, Part D plans are not required to accept it. Medicare requires that Part D plans post their exception request forms online.

9. Nurses can encourage patients to take the time to compare plans every year and choose the one with the best coverage for their current medication regimen, taking into consideration future needs. Patients can call the Medicare Helpline at 1-800-MEDICARE or use the Prescription Drug Plan Finder at www.medicare.gov to compare plans offered in their state and even sign up for a plan during their initial enrollment or the annual enrollment period. The Formulary Finder on the Medicare Web site and Epocrates at www.epocrates.com can help nurse and other health care providers see what drugs are on a plan's formulary.

C. State Pharmacy Assistance Programs (SPAPs) are not available in every state. To determine which states offer these programs, refer to www.ncsl.org/programs/health/drugaid.htm.
1. Where available, these state funded programs are intended to help pay for certain drugs for patients meeting identified guidelines.
2. Help from qualified SPAPs for people with Medicare Part D counts toward the TrOOP costs patients must have before the Part D catastrophic benefit. Some state kidney programs are qualified SPAPs. For a list of qualified SPAPs, see www.cms.hhs.gov/States/Downloads/QualifiedSPAPList.pdf.

D. Pharmaceutical patient assistance programs (PAPs) are established by drug companies to help people without health or drug coverage get their drugs.
1. Each program has its own application form, eligibility guidelines, and frequency to reapply.
2. Some PAPs will not help those who have Part D. You can see which PAPs help people with Part D on www.rxassist.org/docs/medicare-and-paps.cfm.

3. For more information about what drugs have PAPs, see the Partnership for Prescription Assistance site at https://www.pparx.org/Intro.php.

E. Charities and foundations may help those who qualify to pay for drugs. For resources to help pay for drugs, see www.rxassist.org/ or www.needymeds.com.
1. Guidelines for eligibility vary. Some require that the patient has a certain diagnosis and is taking medications for that diagnosis.
2. Some obtain funds from pharmaceutical companies to run their PAP.
3. Because funding is limited, everyone who needs help to get their drugs may not get the help they need.
4. Help from charities can count toward the true out-of-pocket TrOOP costs patients must have before the Part D catastrophic benefit.

V. Income and income support.

A. Socioeconomic status and patient outcomes.
1. Low socioeconomic status is linked to premature births, diet, diabetes, hypertension, smoking, alcohol, and/or drug usage. All of these are risk factors for kidney disease.
2. Kidney function decline in diabetic African Americans is three times faster than in Caucasians and that 80% of the difference is explained by socioeconomic status, behaviors, and poor control of blood pressure and blood sugar.
3. For every $1,000 of higher income in black dialysis patients there was a 3.3% lower relative risk of dying.
4. Income less than 200% of the federal poverty level was associated with microalbuminuria, a factor in the progression of kidney disease.
5. Financial status affects access to transplantation.

B. Employment improves socioeconomic status and provides benefits for patients, providers, and the system.
1. Employment is one factor that predicts how well African American patients with hypertension and CKD function physically and emotionally.
2. For patients, employment provides a better standard of living, improved income, a sense of self-worth, socialization opportunities, and a better chance of having health insurance that covers preventive health care as well as

treatment for known illnesses. Working helps patients have the financial resources to overcome health care access barriers and assure early identification and treatment of kidney disease. Working patients have the money to afford lifestyle changes and treatments to prolong kidney function or keep someone with kidney failure healthy. Once kidneys fail, working improves the chances for transplant and for better dialysis. Even though Medicare will not routinely pay for more than three treatments a week, their EGHP may pay for more frequent dialysis treatments performed at home or in the dialysis clinic and ongoing prescription coverage.

3. For facilities, having working patients who can more easily afford their treatment plan reduces frustration that nurses and other health care providers often feel when they recommend treatments that patients do not follow. Staff working in dialysis clinics where patients function at a higher level, including working, have higher job satisfaction and lower turnover. Also, having a payer mix that includes patients with commercial payers that pay at a higher rate than Medicare allows clinics to offer more innovative treatments and higher quality care to all patients.

4. When patients work, they are taxpayers as well as recipients of government benefits. When a working patient has EGHP coverage, it saves Medicare money for 30 months when Medicare is the secondary payer.

5. It takes a team to keep patients working and to return patients who are not working to the workforce.
   a. The physician/provider and nurse play an important role in keeping CKD and ESRD patients working by assessing work-limiting symptoms and making sure that patients know they can work with kidney disease and kidney failure.
   b. The nurse and other dialysis team members can help assure that working patients are offered home dialysis and transplant and/or are assigned shift times that fit their work schedule.
   c. Nurses need to educate patients about what symptoms to report and to whom and advise the doctor about work-limiting symptoms as soon as the patient reports them.
   d. Nurses can assist with early referral for nutritional counseling. Dietitians can help patients learn how to eat healthy meals to stay strong and be physically able to work.
   e. Nurses can also refer patients expressing financial concerns to the social worker to help address financial issues and evaluate work ability. The social worker can help working patients and those seeking employment to understand their legal rights and advocate with an employer for workplace accommodations.
   f. Social workers can also offer emotional counseling and refer patients to physical and vocational rehabilitation services to help them keep their jobs or become job ready.

C. Government disability benefits are available for those with a disability that is expected to last a year or result in death. Social Security has a booklet that describes what conditions are considered potentially disabled. Some conditions that accompany kidney damage and ESRD are listed. For more information, refer to www.ssa.gov/disability/professionals/bluebook/ for adult and pediatric listings. Although government disability programs do not provide temporary disability benefits, there are work incentive programs to help people with disabilities return to work. For more information on work incentive programs, see www.socialsecurity.gov/work. Social Security can advise patients about disability benefits and work incentive programs.

1. Social Security Disability Insurance (SSDI) is a government funded disability program for people who meet work requirements. Other income doesn't affect eligibility for SSDI. However, there is a 5-month waiting period during which no checks are paid. On average SSDI pays an average of 35% of the patient's past earnings. SSDI replaces more of a low-income worker's wages than the wages of a high income worker. A spouse and children may be eligible for SSDI family benefits. Because someone receiving SSDI is eligible for Medicare after receiving SSDI checks for 24 months, some people with CKD may already have Medicare due to disability.

2. Supplemental Security Income (SSI) is a disability program for people who have limited income and assets, meet the disability qualifications, and have no or a limited work record. People who qualify can get SSI during the SSDI waiting period. SSI pays a very limited amount of income that is less than the federal poverty level. There are no family benefits with SSI. In most states, having SSI qualifies the patient for Medicaid.

D. Some people may receive private disability benefits through a job or private policy. These plans may provide short- or long-term benefits. To promote return to work, these plans usually pay only 60% of one's current income. When the patient also qualifies for Social Security benefits, these benefits reduce private disability benefits.

E. Other financial assistance programs may help those patients who qualify for programs to pay for housing, utilities, food, transportation, living expenses, etc. Programs may be funded by the federal or state government, by local agencies, or national kidney charities like the American Kidney Fund or local affiliates of the National Kidney Foundation. Patients must apply for assistance and meet the identified guidelines. Some programs assist patients as long as they qualify while others provide temporary assistance to meet emergency needs. Nephrology social workers often are aware of these programs and help patients access them.

VI. Resources to help nurses help patients.

A. Nurses can collaborate with social workers to help patients reach their maximum level of functioning.
  1. Nurses and technicians see patients every day. Nurses are one of the best referral sources for social workers to identify patients' concerns and target interventions to assist them.
  2. The social worker should assess patients' coping and offer counseling to patients and families, evaluate patients' psychosocial needs including financial concerns, assist patients to access helpful resources, provide directly or refer patients to agencies that can help them keep their jobs or find new ones, recommend care based on patients' individual psychosocial needs, and assess and address barriers that keep patients from following their treatment plan.

B. Other resources.
  1. Centers for Medicare and Medicaid Services. Medicare Coverage for Kidney Dialysis and Kidney Transplant Services, CMS Pub. No. 10128, www.medicare.gov/Publications/Pubs/pdf/10128.pdf.
  2. Centers for Medicare and Medicaid Services. Medicare for Children with Chronic Kidney Disease, CMS Pub. No. 11066, www.medicare.gov/Publications/Pubs/pdf/11066.pdf.
  3. Centers for Medicare and Medicaid Services. Your Guide to Medicare Prescription Drug Coverage, CMS Pub. No. 11109, www.medicare.gov/Publications/Pubs/pdf/11109.pdf.
  4. Centers for Medicare and Medicaid Services. A Physician's Guide to Medicare Coverage of Kidney Dialysis and Kidney Transplant Services, Publication ICN # 006558, www.cms.hhs.gov/MLNProducts/downloads/Book_Kidney_Dialysis-Final.pdf.
  5. Centers for Medicare and Medicaid Services. End Stage Kidney Disease (ESRD) Center, www.cms.hhs.gov/center/esrd.asp.
  6. Home Dialysis Central, www.homedialysis.org.
  7. Kidney School, www.kidneyschool.org.
  8. Life Options Rehabilitation Program, www.lifeoptions.org.
  9. Life Options, Employment: A Kidney Patient's Guide to Working and Paying for Treatment, www.lifeoptions.org/catalog/pdfs/booklets/employment.pdf.
  10. Health Well Foundation for help with premiums or prescription drug costs, www.healthwellfoundation.org.
  11. National Kidney Foundation. Taking Control: Money Matters for People with Chronic Kidney Disease, www.kidney.org/patients/pfc/control.cfm.
  12. National Organization for State Kidney Programs. Directory of State Kidney Programs, available from Missouri Kidney Program at (800) 733-7345.
  13. Social Security Administration. Disability Evaluation under Social Security, SSA Pub. No. 64-039, www.ssa.gov/disability/professionals/bluebook/.
  14. Social Security Administration. 2006 Red Book: A Summary Guide to Employment Support for Individuals with Disabilities under the Social Security Disability Insurance and Supplemental Security Income Programs, SSA Pub. No. 64-030, www.socialsecurity.gov/redbook/.

Chapter 20

Physical Rehabilitation

Purpose

This chapter will demonstrate how to incorporate physical rehabilitation as a component of care for all patients with chronic kidney disease (CKD). It is well documented in many studies that patients with CKD are limited in their ability to perform physical exercise, with levels of exercise capacity of dialysis patients reported to be 60–70% of age-expected levels (Johansen, 1999). Despite significant progress in technological aspects of renal replacement therapy and medical advances, patients remain limited physically, which negatively impacts overall health, quality of life and outcomes (i.e., hospitalizations, mortality). Since the publication of the first randomized clinical trial of exercise training in hemodialysis patients (Goldberg, Hagberg, et al., 1980), there have been some key studies that have demonstrated the importance of this neglected part of ESRD patient care.

Objectives

Upon completion of this chapter, the learner will be able to:
1. Define the differences between physical activity, physical fitness, cardiorespiratory fitness, physical functioning, and exercise training.
2. Describe measurement of physical functioning.
3. Identify the significance of low physical functioning in CKD patients.
4. Discuss the health benefits of increasing physical activity.
5. Describe the physical activity recommendations in the nephrology community.
6. Identify ways to reduce barriers to exercise in CKD.

I. **Clarifying terms.**

A. Physical activity: bodily movement that is produced by the contraction of skeletal muscle and that substantially increases energy expenditure.

B. Physical fitness: a set of attributes that people have or achieve that relates to the ability to perform physical activity. One of these attributes is cardiorespiratory fitness (often referred to as exercise capacity), which relates to the ability of the cardiac, circulatory, and respiratory systems to supply and use oxygen during sustained physical activity (Office of the U.S. Surgeon General, 1996).

C. Physical functioning: an individual's ability to perform activities required in their daily lives

(Painter, Stewart, et al., 1999; Stewart & Painter, 1997). Physical functioning is determined by many factors, including:
1. Physical fitness (cardiorespiratory fitness, strength, and flexibility).
2. Sensory function.
3. Clinical condition.
4. Environmental factors.
5. Behavioral factors.

D. Exercise training: the planned, structured, and repetitive bodily movement done to improve or maintain one or more components of physical fitness or other health benefits. Increased physical activity can be considered exercise training, although increased physical activity can also result from unstructured increases in movements throughout the day. This chapter will use exercise and physical activity interchangeably. The use of the term *physical activity* may be less intimidating to older, frailer individuals, whereas use of the term *exercise* with younger patients may be more motivating to them.

II. Measurement of functioning.

A. Given the multiple determinants of physical functioning, e.g., cardiorespiratory fitness, strength, sensory function, clinical status, environmental, and behavioral factors, it is clear that no one measure can cover all areas. Thus, the measurement is complicated and should be tailored to specific populations and specific characteristics of interest. Assessment of physical functioning (see Table 4.7) can range from objective laboratory measures of exercise capacity (stress testing) to questionnaires on self-report of physical functioning that include questions relating to the ability to perform activities that range from basic self-care to household activities and more strenuous tasks.

B. Cardiorespiratory fitness is objectively measured using laboratory measures of oxygen uptake

Table 4.7

Assessment of Physical Functioning

Type of Test	Description	Comment
Laboratory Exercise Testing (Stress testing)	• Treadmill or cycle testing with 12 lead ECG monitoring. • May involve analysis of respiratory gases to determine oxygen uptake (VO_2 peak).	• Physically challenging to maximal efforts. • Stress ECG has questionable diagnostic utility in dialysis patients. • Expensive. • Requires sophisticated equipment and trained technicians.
Physical Performance Testing	**Standardized Tasks That Simulate or Are Required in ADLs** • Gait speed (normal walking speed across 20 feet; fast walking speed across 20 feet). • 6 minute walk (distance covered on a standardized course in 6 minutes). • Sit-to-stand test (time it takes to stand up and sit down from a chair 5 or 10 times). • Stair climbing (time it takes to climb a flight of stairs, modified score depending on the manner in which the steps are climbed). • Timed balance test (standing in tandem position, semi-tandem position, and one foot). • Other specific task simulations (i.e., lift and reach).	• Easy to perform in the dialysis clinic. • Most appropriate for older and frail patients. • Predictive of hospitalizations, institutionalization, death in elderly.
Self-Reported Functioning (SF-36 Health Status Questionnaire)	**Physical Functioning Subscale** • Does your health limit you in these activities? If so, how much? • Vigorous activities, such as running, lifting heavy objects, participating in strenuous sports. • Moderate activities such as moving a table, pushing a vacuum cleaner, bowling, or playing golf. • Lifting or carrying groceries. • Climbing several flights of stairs. • Bending, kneeling, or stooping. • Walking more than one mile. • Walking several blocks. • Bathing or dressing yourself. *Responses are: no, not limited at all; yes, limited a little; yes, limited a lot.*	• Convenient to administer. • Reflects change in objective measures of functioning. • Widely used in CKD patients. • There are other questionnaires that provide similar assessment of physical functioning.

(VO$_2$ peak) during a maximal exercise test (stress testing) performed on a cycle ergometer or treadmill. This measurement is physically challenging for many patients and requires expensive equipment and specially trained personnel. For these reasons, maximal stress testing is not practical for assessment of physical functioning for part of routine care.

C. Physical performance testing. The growing interest in physical functioning in older and diseased populations has led to development of tests that measure physical performance of standardized tasks such as walking (6-minute walk, gait speed), balancing, reaching, rising from a chair and climbing stairs (Applegate, Blass, et al., 1990; Guralnik, Branch, et al., 1989). These tests are referred to as physical performance tests, and are not direct measures of cardiorespiratory fitness, strength or flexibility, but are indicators of these physical fitness measures.

D. Self-reported functioning can be assessed using questionnaires such as the physical functioning scale on the SF-36 Health Status Questionnaire, which assesses level of difficulty performing activities of daily living (ADL), instrumental activities of daily living (IADLs), and more strenuous activities (Ware, 1993; Ware & Sherbourne, 1992).

III. Physical functioning in dialysis patients.

A. No matter how physical functioning is measured (e.g., using objective laboratory measures, performance-based measures, or self-report) levels are low in patients with CKD.
1. In dialysis patients who are able to perform symptom-limited maximal exercise testing, the values for peak oxygen uptake (VO$_2$ peak) are severely reduced, averaging about 60% of age-predicted values ranging from 17.0 (Kouidi, Albani, et al., 1998) to 28.6 mL/kg/min (Lundin, Stein, et al., 1981).
2. The specific limitations to VO$_2$ peak in patients treated with dialysis have not been identified and are potentially numerous, and may be due to cardiac dysfunction, vascular endothelial dysfunction, autonomic dysfunction, and/or metabolic or structural abnormalities within the skeletal muscles (Painter, Moore, et al., 2002). Any of these abnormalities alone or in combination could reduce transport of oxygen from the atmosphere to the working muscles

and/or utilization of oxygen for energy production within the skeletal muscle for sustaining muscle contraction.
3. Anemia is not considered to be a limiting factor as long as patients are adequately treated with r-huErythropoeitin (Painter & Johanson, 2006; Painter, Moore, et al., 2002).
4. Exercise capacity improves with the removal of uremia following a successful transplantation (Painter, Hanson, et al., 1987).

B. The reported values for VO$_2$ peak are for those patients who are physically capable to perform the test. It is probable that over 50% of patients are physically not capable of performing a symptom-limited exercise test. Most research studies have only included patients at the highest functional levels and have excluded patients with comorbidities such as diabetes or cardiovascular disease. To put these levels of VO$_2$ peak in perspective, patients with congestive heart failure (CHF) are classified as moderate severity if the VO$_2$ peak levels are between 16–20 mL/kg/min (Weber, Kinasewitz, et al., 1982). Although there are many patients who have comorbid medical conditions that may contribute to limited exercise capacity, the markedly low functioning in the best of the patients indicates that there is a need to intervene to increase functioning.

C. In patients who may not be able to perform symptom-limited exercise testing, physical performance testing may provide an indication of levels of functioning. Physical performance testing results are also low in dialysis patients.
1. Johansen et al. (2002) reported that, compared to age-matched healthy controls, gait speed was significantly lower in hemodialysis patients.
2. In a group of kidney transplant candidates, gait speed was reported to be 77% of normal age-expected values (Bohannon, Smith, et al., 1995) and in a group of 131 hemodialysis patients who were more representative of the general dialysis population, gait speed was reported to be 66.1% of normal age-expected values.
3. Lower extremity function as measured by sit-to-stand testing was found to be severely limited in 111 patients, averaging less than 25% of normal age-predicted values (Painter, Carlson, et al., 2000a, 2000b).

D. Self-reported physical functioning is the most commonly reported assessment in dialysis patients.

1. Self-reported physical functioning (as measured by the SF-36 Health Status Questionnaire) is also severely limited in dialysis patients (DeOreo 1997; Johansen, Kaysen, et al., 2002; Painter, Carlson et al., 2000a, 2000b).
2. The Physical Function (PF) Scale is reported to be between 30 and 56, averaging around 44 (on a scale of 0–100), all significantly below reported age-norms (Ware, 1993). Figure 4.17 demonstrates how limited dialysis patients' reported physical functioning is compared to documented levels in other chronic disease populations.
3. The Physical Component Scale (PCS) is a combined measure of all the "physical" scales on the full questionnaire (including the PF scale). PCS in dialysis patients is consistently reported to be 35 (DeOreo, 1997; Painter, Carlson, et al., 2000a, 2000b; Tawney, Tawney, et al., 2000) well below the age norm.
4. Other self-report instruments used in dialysis patients also report levels of physical functioning that are significantly lower than age predicted norms (Parkerson & Gutman, 2001).

IV. Significance of low physical functioning.

A. As early as 1997, DeOreo reported that the self-reported physical functioning scores were predictive of outcomes. They reported in a historical prospective analysis of a large sample (n=1,000) of hemodialysis patients. Those patients who scored below the median (< 34) on the physical component scale on the SF-36 questionnaire were twice as likely to die and 1.5 times more likely to be hospitalized. This

measure was as predictive of mortality as protein catabolic rate or Kt/V. They concluded that for every 5-point increase in the physical composite score (PCS), there was a corresponding 10% increase in the probability of survival.

B. Knight et al. (2003) reported the predictive values (hazard ratio for 1-year mortality) of the self-reported functioning (PCS on the SF-36) in 15,000 dialysis patients. They showed that compared to patients with a PCS score > 50:
1. Those with PCS score < 20 had a hazard ratio of 1.97 (97% greater chance of death in 1 year).
2. Those with PCS = 20–29 had a hazard ratio of 1.62 (62% greater chance of death in 1 year).
3. Those with a PCS score = 30–39 had a hazard ratio of 1.32 (32% greater risk of death in 1 year).
4. Those who had a decline in PCS over 1 year had additional increase risk in mortality as evidenced by a hazard ratio of 1.25 per 10-point decline in PCS score.

C. Low exercise capacity as measured by treadmill testing is also predictive of outcomes. Seitsema et al. (2004) reported the prognostic value of exercise capacity as measured by VO_2 peak in 175 ambulatory hemodialysis patients over a 3.5-year follow-up period. They also reported that exercise capacity was the strongest predictor of survival over the 3.5 year follow-up, even when corrected for other contributing variables.

D. Although there is no data relating physical function test scores to outcomes in dialysis patients, there is a significant amount of observational data in the elderly that clearly document that the loss of mobility and lower extremity function results in higher rates of institutionalization, hospitalization, morbidity, and mortality (Branch & Jette, 1982; Guralnik, Ferrucci, et al., 1995). The Established Populations for Epidemiologic Studies of the Elderly (EPESE), a very large study (n > 5,000) sponsored by the National Institute on Aging (NIA), has established a large database of functional measures of lower extremity function, e.g., gait speed, standing balance, sit-to-stand, which have been shown to be highly predictive of morbidity, mortality, hospitalization, and institutionalization in elders with arthritis, cardiovascular disease, peripheral artery disease, and general aging (Hirsch, Fried, et al., 1997; McDermott, Greenland, et al., 2002; Messier, Royer, et al., 2000; Simonsick, Newman, et al., 2001).

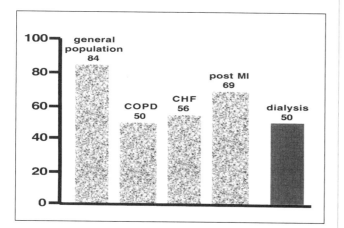

Figure 4.17. SF-36 Physical function scale scores in dialysis and other chronic conditions (Ware, 2003).

V. Physical activity levels in ESRD.

A. Most dialysis patients are sedentary:
1. Data from the Kidney Exercise Demonstration Project showed that 59% of 286 hemodialysis patients participated in no physical activity beyond basic activities of daily living (ADLs) (Painter, Carlson, et al., 2000a, 2000b).
2. Johansen et al. (2000) reported that physical activity as measured by accelerometry (activity monitor) was significantly low in 39 hemodialysis patients compared to age-matched sedentary healthy controls. In this study, physical activity declined in the dialysis patients at a rate of 3.4% per month over a 12-month period (Johansen, Kaysen, et al., 2002).
3. Data from the USRDS Dialysis Morbidity and Mortality Study survey was used by O'Hare et al. (2003) to dichotomize patients into sedentary (never, or almost never participate in physical activity during leisure time) and non-sedentary (participation in some physical activity during leisure time). Out of a total sample of 4,024 patients, 12.4% were unable to ambulate or transfer. Of the 2,264 who had physical activity data, 35% were categorized as sedentary. Eleven percent of the sedentary patients died over the 1-year follow-up period compared to 5% of the nonsedentary patients (p < .001). The patients classified as sedentary at study initiation showed a 62% greater risk of mortality over 1 year compared with non-sedentary patients with adjustment for other variables associated with survival in this group (perception of general health, cardiac disease, peripheral vascular disease, creatinine, hematocrit, dialysis modality, education level, male sex, diabetes, phosphorous level).

B. The Kidney Exercise Demonstration Project (Painter, Carlson, et al., 2000a, 2000b) was a study that was designed to provide physical activity information and encouragement to a group of 286 patients who were representative of the general dialysis population. There was an average of three comorbid conditions, including cardiovascular disease and other common conditions. Physical activity levels were categorized into four levels:
1. Activities of daily living only.
2. Calisthenics (stretching/strengthening exercises).
3. Some cardiovascular exercise (< 20 minutes/session and/or 3 times per week).
4. Recommended cardiovascular exercise (> 20 minutes/session and > 3 times/week). At baseline nearly 60% did only activities of daily living. This decreased to 6.4% at the end of the intervention. Those reporting the recommended levels of cardiovascular exercise were 12% at baseline and increased to 45% at the end of the intervention. The frequency and duration of exercise in those categorized as recommended cardiovascular exercise increased from 23.7 min/session 3.2 days/week of participation to an average of 4.1 days/week for 38.4 min/session at the end of the study. This clearly demonstrates that dialysis patients will increase their physical activity if given specific information and encouragement to do so. There was an effort to include documentation of activity as a routine part of the predialysis assessment by the dialysis staff, and patient participation was greater in those clinics where this was accomplished.

VI. Exercise training in dialysis patients.

A. There are many exercise training studies in hemodialysis patients, and several in peritoneal dialysis.
1. Cardiovascular exercise training has conclusively been shown to result in increased exercise capacity ranging from 5% to 42% increases in VO_2 peak (Akiba, Matsui, et al., 1995; Goldberg, Geltman, et al., 1983; Goldberg, Hagberg, et al., 1980; Kouidi, 1998; Moore, Parsons, et al., 1993; Painter, Moore, et al., 2002; Painter, Nelson-Worel, et al., 1986; Ross, Grabeau, et al., 1989; Shalom, Blumenthal, et al., 1984; Zabetakis, Gleim, et al., 1982).
2. Physical inactivity is one of the strongest predictors of physical disability in older persons (Buchner, Beresford, et al., 1992; Carlson, Fried, et al., 1999).
3. Although there are no data on elderly dialysis patients, the increasing age of patients on dialysis makes the data in the general population of older persons relevant to the nephrology community. Regular physical exercise has been shown in longitudinal observational studies to extend longevity and to reduce risk of physical disability in later life (Ferrucci, Izmirlian, et al., 1999; LaCroix, Guralnik, et al., 1993; Leveille, Guralnik, et al., 1999; Strawbridge, Cohen, et al., 1996; Wu, Leu, et al., 1999).
   a. In the EPESE studies of 6,200 older persons free of baseline disability, those with a low level (lower tertile) of regular physical activity were 1.8 times more likely to develop

disability in activities of daily living (ADLs) or mobility over 6 years than those with a high level (upper tertile) of physical activity.

b. The benefit of cardiovascular exercise on physical function in older populations may be through direct effect on impairments such as muscle strength low cardiorespiratory fitness and impaired balance, or through prevention of disabling diseases such as cardiovascular disease (Huang, Maceera, et al. 1998; Perrin, Gauchard, et al. 1999; Rantanen, Era, et al. 1994).

c. There have been several randomized clinical trials that have demonstrated beneficial effects of physical exercise programs in diseased and/or frail older adults.

(1) The Fitness and Arthritis in Seniors Trial (FAST) studied 439 community-dwelling older adults with knee osteoarthritis. Self-reported physical function was significantly improved in those participating in an 18-month cardiovascular exercise training or resistance exercise training program compared to those participating in a health education program. The FAST programs also resulted in improved walking speed and balance (Messier, Royer, et al., 2000).

(2) Frail older adults have shown significant improvements from resistance exercise programs, and structured exercise programs, specifically in improved mobility, gait speed and muscle strength (Fiatarone, Marks, et al., 1990; Fiatarone, O'Neill, et al., 1994).

B. Cardiovascular exercise training has also been shown to result in significant improvement on physical performance tests in dialysis patients (Mercer, Crawford, et al., 2002; Painter, Carlson, et al., 2000a, 2000b). In the Kidney Exercise Demonstration Project, there were significant differences in the change over time in normal and fast gait speed and sit-to-stand tests between the exercise intervention group and no intervention group (see Figure 4.18). The changes were most pronounced in patients who had low self-reported physical function scores (SF-36 PCS scale). This demonstration project clearly indicates that the natural course is for deterioration of physical functioning over time. Thus, maintenance of functioning is a positive outcome that can

certainly be obtained with increasing physical activity.

C. The Kidney Exercise Demonstration Project also resulted in significant improvements in self-reported physical functioning in the exercise intervention group (see Figure 4.19). All four physical scales on the SF-36 improved in the exercise intervention group and either showed no change or deterioration in the no-intervention group. Thus the PCS score (a composite of the individual scale scores) was significantly improved as a result of the exercise intervention. It is not known whether changes in self-reported functioning resulting from exercise training results in improved outcomes. However, if the relationship between the PCS score and probability of survival and/or odds of death holds, the average increase in PCS score of 7 points in the demonstration project in the low-functioning patients would translate to an increase in the probability of survival by 14% (using Deoreo et al. [1997] data) or an improvement in the odds of death of 24.5% (using Lowrie et al. [1994] data).

VII. Health benefits of increasing physical activity.

A. Many studies have shown positive health benefits from increased physical activity without structured exercise training. Regular physical activity may benefit a number of conditions that affect survival in the general population, many of which have been outlined in the document, *Physical Activity and Health: A Report of the Surgeon General*, 1996. Benefits of physical activity outlined in this report that are relevant to dialysis patients are shown in Table 4.8. There may be other benefits of regular physical activity that could positively impact other factors that are of concern in dialysis patients, specifically muscle wasting, cardiovascular risk, oxidative stress, and chronic inflammation.

B. Muscle wasting and muscle strength.
1. Skeletal muscle atrophy is a significant problem in hemodialysis patients and is a significant predictor of morbidity and mortality in these patients and may be a significant contributor to limitations in physical functioning (Lowrie, Huang, et al., 1994).

a. Johansen et al. reported that contractile mass is reduced in hemodialysis patients compared to healthy age-matched controls. The reduction was associated with the reduced muscle strength.

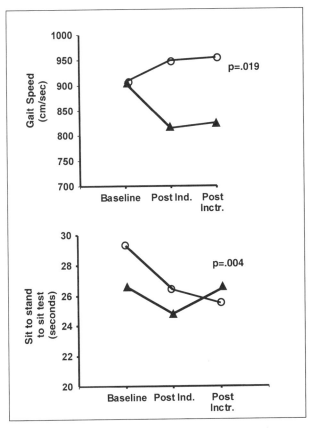

Figure 4.18. Changes in physical function tests in kidney exercise demonstration project (Painter, Carlson, et al., 2000).

Key: open circles = intervention group; triangles = no intervention group; ind = independent exercise; inctr = in-center exercise. Sit-to-stand is the time it takes to stand up and sit down 10 times. Gait speed is over 20 feet.

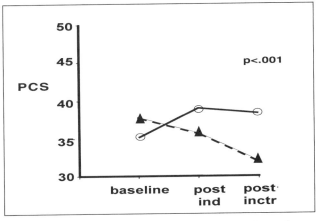

Figure 4.19. Changes in the physical composite scale on the SF-36 in the Kidney Exercise Demonstration Project (Painter, Carlson, et al., 2000).

Key: open circles = intervention group; triangles = no intervention group; ind = independent exercise; inctr = in-center exercise.

b. Kouidi et al. (1998) reported impressive reversal in muscle atrophy assessed by morphometric analysis of muscle fibers obtained from muscle biopsy. The exercise training program was fairly intensive and involved combined cardiovascular and strengthening (through calisthenics and low weight resistance exercises) 90 minutes per session 3 times per week for 6 months in a supervised setting. They observed a 29% increase in fiber area, as well as favorable changes in ultrastructure and capillary and mitochondrial density.

c. Headley et al. (2002) report that muscle strength can be increased with resistance training in hemodialysis. After 12 weeks of resistance training, there was an increase in quadriceps peak torque (measure of strength) of 12.7% and improvements in 6-minute walk distance, maximal walking speed, and the sit-to-stand test.

2. Muscle wasting is both dialysis and nondialysis related. Decreased dietary intake, sedentary lifestyle, and hemodialysis-associated

Table 4.8

Benefits of Regular Physical Activity as Reported in the Surgeon General's Report on Physical Activity and Health

(Office of the U.S. Surgeon General, 1996)

■ Reduction in cardiovascular disease risk.

■ Prevention or delay in the development of hypertension and improvement of blood pressure in those with hypertension.

■ Reduction of the risk of developing diabetes.

■ Maintenance of muscle strength and joint structure and function.

■ Preservation of strength in older adults, and help to maintain independent living status and reduction of the risk of falling.

■ Relief of symptoms of depression and anxiety.

■ Enhancement of psychological well-being by improving physical functioning in people compromised by poor health.

catabolism are all important. Pupim et al. (2004) demonstrated that cycling exercise during dialysis enhances the anabolic effects of intradialytic parenteral nutrition (IDPN). Exercise for 15 minutes initiated 15 minutes after initiation of the dialysis session resulted in increased uptake of amino acids and net muscle protein accretion by twofold compared to IDPN alone. These results are consistent with well documented anabolic effects of cardiovascular exercise in healthy subjects, in which increased muscle amino acid uptake and muscle protein accretion in healthy subjects has been observed following an acute bout of exercise and following exercise training of the cardiovascular type (Levenhagen, Gresham, et al., 2002; Tipton, Wolfe, 1998).

C. Cardiovascular risk.
1. Regular cardiovascular exercise also has a positive influence on cardiovascular risk profile. In hemodialysis patients, early studies showed improvements in fasting glucose, insulin levels, and blood pressure with exercise training. Reductions in blood pressure have been reported with cardiovascular exercise training by Hagberg et al. (1983) and Painter et al. (1986), with reductions in antihypertensive medication requirements. With the use of erythropoietin for treatment of anemia, it is not known whether exercise training can override the vasoconstrictive side effects of EPO therapy. Miller, Cress, et al. (2002) reported a careful assessment of blood pressure responses to a program of 6 months of cycling exercise during hemodialysis in 40 patients, with 35 non-exercising controls. There were no statistical differences in predialysis or postdialysis blood pressures between the two groups at baseline or at 6 months. However, 13 (54%) of the exercise group had a reduction in antihypertensive medication use over the 6 months compared to 4 patients in the control group. The average relative benefit of exercise was a 36% reduction in antihypertensive medications with an average annual cost savings of $885/patient/year (p = .005) in the exercise group.
2. There have been no randomized trials to study the effects of exercise training on cardiovascular risk profile in dialysis patients. The very high prevalence of risk factors for cardiovascular disease and the high rates of cardiovascular disease would certainly justify such an intervention trial or trial of multiple risk factor

interventions which have been proven effective in reducing cardiovascular risk in other high-risk populations. The cardiovascular KDOQI guidelines specifically recommend that all dialysis patients should be counseled and regularly encouraged by nephrology and dialysis staff to increase their level of physical activity. This guideline is based on the abundant data in other high risk populations of the positive impact of regular physical activity on cardiovascular disease risk.

VIII. Intradialytic exercise.

A. Cheema et al. (2005) have made an elegant argument for incorporation of regular intradialytic exercise into the routine dialysis care. They argue that the practice of using stationary cycles during the hemodialysis treatment is safe, in that there have been no reported untoward events in any of the reported studies. The experience of the author using cycling during dialysis is extensive, with exercise training in over 400 hemodialysis patients. There have been no untoward events, and it is clear that there is no negative hemodynamic; in fact systolic blood pressure stabilizes during the exercise time and patients typically experience less cramping and hypotensive episodes. Cycling during dialysis has been shown to be effective in improving exercise capacity in several controlled studies and in a randomized controlled trial. Exercise training during dialysis has also been shown to reduce antihypertensive medication requirements (Miller, Cress, et al., 2002; Painter, Nelson-Worel, et al., 1986).

B. For many years, it was thought that exercise had no effect on the dialysis treatment, however, recent studies have demonstrated that cycling exercise during the treatment results in increased solute removal.
1. Vaithilingam et al. (2004) reported statistically greater weekly phosphate removal in 12 patients who exercised during dialysis compared to those who did not exercise. Exercise also increased midweek URR. However, this did not prove to be statistically significant. The phosphate removal with exercise was similar to increasing dialysis time by 1 hour per session.
2. Kong et al. (1999) studied 11 patients who were on paired dialysis session: one with exercise and the other as a control. The rebound of urea, creatinine, and potassium were reduced significantly with the exercise treatment. The

rebound of urea dropped from 12.4 to 10.9%, creatinine from 21.2 to 17.2%, and potassium from 62 to 44%. Kt/V and reduction ratios of all three solutes also increased significantly.

3. These authors concluded that the improvement in dialysis adequacy with exercise training was equivalent to extending the length of the hemodialysis treatment by 30 minutes. The mechanism of these increases in clearance with exercise is thought to be dilation of vasculature within the skeletal muscles. At rest, muscle blood flow is minimal, rendering a very large percent of the body tissue unexposed to dialysis. During exercise, muscle blood flow increases in proportion to the relative intensity of the exercise effort, thus increasing the tissue mass that is exposed to the dialysis treatment.

4. The improved clearances that are achieved with cardiovascular exercise during the treatment plus the increases in physical functioning and other possible benefits certainly make the recommendations of incorporation of intra-dialytic exercise as a part of the routine treatment proposed by Cheema worth considering.

IX. Physical activity recommendations in the nephrology community.

A. The Life Options Kidney Rehabilitation Advisory Council was established in 1993 with the goal of identifying barriers to rehabilitation in patients with ESRD treated with dialysis. Rehabilitation was defined as a coordinated program of medical treatment, education, counseling, and dietary and exercise regimens designed to maximize the vocational potential, functional status, and quality of life of dialysis patients (Oberly, 1994). The focus of the Life Options Initiative is to develop "bridges" to the barriers to kidney rehabilitation. The bridges (core principles) identified are:
1. Encouragement to adopt a positive bias toward rehabilitation on the part of the patient, dialysis team members, and families.
2. Education for all patients and families about kidney disease, treatment options, self-care, and employment.
3. Exercise to prevent physical deterioration resulting from reduced activity.
4. Employment goals to maintain their current jobs whenever possible and assuring access to vocational rehabilitation when needed.
5. Evaluation of rehabilitation outcomes to guide treatment and policy decisions. This group is committed to developing educational materials

and promoting changes in practice within the dialysis and nephrology community in regards to rehabilitation. One of the first educational initiatives was to develop an educational program for exercise for the dialysis patient, titled *Exercise for the Dialysis Patient: A Comprehensive Guide* (Painter, Blagg, et al., 1995).

B. The Life Options *Exercise for the Dialysis Patient: A Comprehensive Program* was published and distributed to all dialysis clinics in the United States in 1995. Since that time, two surveys have been published that reveal practices related to exercise in dialysis clinics.
1. In June 2000, the Rehabilitation Committee of the ESRD Network of New York (Network 2) surveyed the 200 dialysis clinics in the Network to learn about their exercise programs, to identify units with successful programs, and to identify factors that may be barriers to developing successful programs. Of the 91% of the units (n = 182) who returned the survey, 14% (26 units) offered an exercise program. On average, 20 patients per unit participated, most while dialyzing. There was approximately a 25% patient dropout rate due primarily to medical problems, loss of interest, and staff shortages. The major barriers identified included:
   a. Nephrologists were either not interested or not convinced of the benefits of exercise for their patients.
   b. Nephrologists were concerned about the safety of exercise.
   c. Staffing issues were of concern, including funding and lack of time.
   d. Patients lack information about the benefits of exercise.
2. A second survey was performed by the Life Options Advisory Council staff in cooperation with the ESRD Network of Texas and Council of Nephrology Social Workers of North Texas. The survey used the Unit Self Assessment Tool (USAT), which was developed to quantify and catalog ongoing rehabilitation efforts within dialysis clinics. The exercise category consisted of 20 activities divided into levels of difficulty or complexity, each of which was given 1 point for scoring with a total possible score of 20. The survey was completed by 169 centers (68% response rate). Exercise practice was the lowest of all rehabilitation practices, with an average of 3.7 ± 2.9 activities in the units. Only 21% of facilities had advanced exercise activities, e.g., support of local fitness events among kidney

patients, providing for exercise programming outside of the unit, providing in-center, or organized fitness activities during dialysis.

C. Painter, Carlson, et al. (2004) confirmed that staff within the dialysis clinics are not routinely encouraging patients to participate in regular physical activity. One hundred dialysis staff with direct patient care responsibilities (nursing staff, patient care technicians, dietitians, or social workers) in five clinics completed questionnaires to assess encouragement for physical activity practices. Results included:
   1. 31% of staff rated the levels of physical functioning of their patients as "excellent" or "very good" with only 17% rating functioning "poor" or "very poor."
   2. 44% stated that at least half of their patients would benefit from increasing physical activity.
   3. 34% never ask about physical limitations.
   4. 24% never or rarely encourage patients to be more physically active, with only 32% stating that they regularly encourage patients to be active.
   5. Predictors of low physical activity encouragement among dialysis staff were:
      a. Job position (e.g., not professionally trained).
      b. Agreement with the statement, "It is not my responsibility to help patients increase their physical functioning."
      c. A perception of a lack of skills for motivating patients to exercise.
      d. Agreement with the statement, "Dialysis patients lack motivation to exercise."
   6. It is clear from this data that, although patient care staff think exercise is important and they want their patients to improve their levels of functioning, no consistent training is provided or policies/responsibilities are in place within the units for staff to either assess functioning or encourage exercise.

D. Exercise counseling practices among nephrologists caring for patients on dialysis were the topic of a survey reported by Johansen et al. (2003). The investigators surveyed a total 505 nephrologists attending the meeting of the American Society of Nephrology, 277 of who were from the United States. Although 98.6% of the U.S. nephrologists stated that physical activity is beneficial for patients on dialysis, only 48.9% often ask about physical activity, and only 28.5% routinely prescribe exercise for their patients. Additionally, only 4.3% of the nephrologists provide written material about exercise to their patients. Characteristics that were significantly associated with noncounseling behavior in multivariate analysis were:
   1. No time for physical activity counseling.
   2. Not confident in counseling ability.
   3. Physical activity not as important as other medical concerns.
   4. Younger age of physician.
   5. Male sex.
   6. Lower percentage of practice that was primary care.

X. **Existing recommendations for exercise.** Several national guidelines in the United States recommend increased physical activity as the first line of treatment of several medical concerns that are important in dialysis patients.

A. For the general population, increased physical activity is included in published guidelines for the treatment of hypertension, hyperlipidemia, and patients with known cardiac disease or at high risk for developing cardiac disease, including:
   1. The Seventh Report of the Joint National Committee on Prevention (JNC 7), 2003.
   2. National Cholesterol Education Project, 2000.
   3. National Institutes of Health, 1995.
   4. Office of the U.S. Surgeon General, 1996.

B. There are also specific recommendations for patients with kidney failure, including:
   1. The Renal Physician's Association Clinical Practice Guidelines *Preparing Patients for Renal Replacement Therapy* states: "If a patient has GFR < 30 mL/min/1.73m^2 and does not engage in regular physical activity, then s/he should receive counseling and encouragement to increase physical activity."
   2. The K/DOQI Clinical Practice Guidelines for Cardiovascular Disease state: "All dialysis patients should be counseled and regularly encouraged by nephrology and dialysis staff to increase their level of physical activity." Thus it appears that there are sufficient guidelines to recommend increased levels of physical activity for this patient group based on the high risk for cardiovascular disease. The relationship of low functioning and outcomes should also be a compelling reason for the nephrology community to incorporate increased physical activity as a routine part of the patient care.

XI. Reducing barriers to exercise in CKD.

A. Barriers to adopting exercise are well documented in the general population and include time commitment, lack of interest, lack of support from family members, etc. In addition to all of these, individuals with a chronic illness have much more to deal with. Obviously the illness and symptoms, clinical status, and physical limitations resulting from the disease make it difficult to contemplate physical activity.

B. One of the main barriers to exercise for patients with CKD is that physical functioning is not routinely assessed and physical activity recommendations and follow-up are not part of the routine care provided to patients. This results in a situation in which interventions such as physical therapy are incorporated only when the patient becomes nonambulatory or when it is too late. The lack of routine assessment, recommendations, and follow-up also sets up a situation where there is significant misunderstanding about what the patient can and cannot do.

C. Physical activity is not mentioned by the physician, and reinforced regularly, the patient and family will most likely become (or remain) sedentary. There is a justifiable fear of exertion on the part of the patient and family members. There is a very real fear that exertion will make the condition worse, will make the individual tired/fatigued and/or is just not OK for someone with CKD. Thus, just as it takes very specific instructions and encouragement to get apparently healthy people to increase their physical activity, it takes even more specific instructions and encouragement for those who have a medical condition to get them to adopt physical activity.

D. In addition to the message sent by providing No Information on physical activity, there are many other messages that are inadvertently transmitted to patients by health care providers.
   1. "Take it easy" is easily interpreted to mean "Don't do anything strenuous." "Taking it easy" means different things to different people. Thus, the health care provider should be very specific in what is meant by "take it easy." Say instead: "Why don't you cut back your walking to 20 minutes instead of 60 minutes?" or "When you go out for your walk, don't push yourself until a given <clinical situation> is taken care of."

   2. "Don't overdo it." We must remember that an individual with a chronic disease probably does not know how much he/she can do, and has probably experienced severe fatigue and malaise. Thus it is justifiable for them to think that anything may be "overdoing" it. Again, specific recommendations on how to start out with physical activity and how to progress gradually so they will experience benefits and enjoy it.

E. Contradictory messages from various health care providers also present a barrier to adoption of physical activity. Thus, all individuals involved in the care of a patient must consistently understand what is recommended for a patient and encourage and support the patient in adopting those recommendations. Everyone taking care of a patient knows what medications are prescribed and thus are able to encourage the patient to take their medications. Likewise, including assessment of activity and recommendations for adoption and participation in physical activity into the routine care and follow-up will assure consistent messages from all health care providers. Consistent recommendations and encouragement may alleviate misunderstanding on the part of the patient and families regarding physical activity, and possibly reduce future disability. The ongoing opportunity of encouraging physical activity for patients seen regularly for dialysis should be capitalized on.

F. Another barrier to adoption of physical activity by patients with chronic illness may be the low expectations for physical functioning, as if the inability to be physically active is an inevitable consequence of the disease. In the nephrology community, this expectation is held by many physicians, nurses, and technicians as well as family members. It is not surprising that patients adapt to this low level of functioning by modifying what they do and how they do it and by enlisting assistance from others for their activities. Once this low level of functioning is accepted by patients, their family, and the health care professionals working with them, the expectation is fulfilled. In practice, the result of this acceptance is that there is no assessment of physical functioning and no attempt at interventions to improve physical functioning. Although the general population of the United States understands that regular physical activity is important to health, patients with chronic illness depend on physicians and health care professionals to provide guidance on what they can and cannot do. Thus, health care workers have an enormous influence on whether patients become physically active and try to maintain, and possibly improve, their level of functioning or they accept the low functioning that is expected to accompany their chronic illness. This responsibility should not be taken lightly, and every effort should be made to look beyond the disease and/or treatment to how it is impacting the patient's life and functioning.

G. Suggested changes in practice to facilitate increased physical activity are listed in Table 4.9.

XII. Assessment of physical functioning.

A. Just as the patient's nutrition, medications, and other clinical factors are routinely monitored, baseline and subsequent physical functioning assessments allow physicians and providers to monitor the patient's clinical course as it relates to their physical ability. The KDOQI Practice Guidelines for Cardiovascular Disease Management identify that physical functioning should be assessed every 6 months and included in the routine patient care assessment (see Figure 4.20).

Table 4.9

Suggested Changes in Practice to Facilitate Increased Physical Activity

■ Be aware of messages such as:
  1. Providing NO information on physical activity.
  2. "Take it easy."
  3. "Don't overdo it."

■ Work to change expectations for physical activity.
  1. Of staff.
  2. Of family members.
  3. Of patients.

■ Incorporate physical activity participation as a part of the routine care.
  1. Include as a medical order.
  2. Include participation as an assessment made at every patient contact point.
  3. Include in short-term and long-term care plan.
  4. Include inpatient review.

■ Develop a referral system for:
  1. Physical therapy.
  2. Cardiac rehabilitation.
  3. Exercise physiology counseling.
  4. Community-based programs for participation.

■ Include assessment of physical functioning on a regular basis.
  1. To assess progress.
  2. To assess any changes in functioning that may be medically relevant.

■ Include education on the importance of regular physical activity in all training.
  1. Staff training.
  2. Patient and family training.
  3. Staff training on how to positively encourage participation.

■ Provide regular follow-up and assessment of progress.

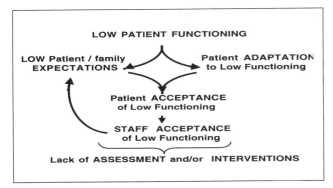

Figure 4.20. Cycle of feedback that reinforces low expectations and acceptance of low physical functioning in CKD patients (Painter, 2003).

B. In determining whether laboratory stress testing is necessary, the provider should determine:
   1. The risk associated with the disease in question and individual patient.
   2. The diagnostic utility of the results of the test.
   3. The current level of activity that is tolerated by the individual.
   4. The level of intensity that will be recommended to the patient. Keeping in mind that requiring exercise testing presents a significant barrier to adopting a program of increased physical activity, less rigid guidelines for pre-participation exercise testing have been suggested for dialysis patients (Copley, Lindberg, et al., 1999).

C. The diagnostic utility of standard exercise testing in ESRD patients is limited for several reasons, including inability to achieve adequate stress due to blunted heart rate responses to exercise and skeletal muscle limitations, long standing hypertension with LVH strain patterns on the ECG, and electrolyte abnormalities that alter the baseline ECG.

D. The goal of most recommendations is to increase the frequency and duration of activity to maintain functioning and prevent deterioration rather than to elevate the patient to an arbitrary fitness or activity level. Obviously, appropriate cardiac risk stratification must be assessed, and the requirement for exercise testing must be individualized based on cardiac risk stratification and the intensity of the anticipated exercise program.

E. Less strenuous, more practical assessments of physical functioning are possible using simple physical performance testing. In most patients it is easy to identify those with lower extremity function that would benefit from physical therapy or other form of exercise intervention, thereby attenuating or halting the progression of disability. There are many individuals who report no or minimal limitations in functioning. However, have modified tasks in ways that reduce limitations. Task modification is described as "preclinical disability" and is strong predictor of future disability. Identification of task modification can identify individuals for targeted interventions, e.g., physical therapy or supervised physical activity programs. Identification of task modification can be done using questions about regular everyday activities that indicate whether:
   1. The patient has any difficulty in doing a task (e.g., getting out of a car).
   2. The patient has modified the way the task is performed.
   3. The patient has changed the frequency of doing the task.
   4. Any changes in the way or frequency of doing the task is related to health or physical problem or symptom.

F. Changes in physical function detected through follow-up assessments may alert providers to a change in medical status, which may not have been detected until later without the testing results (Painter, Stewart, et al., 1999). This surveillance of physical functioning is commonly cited by physicians as a benefit of the structured cardiac rehabilitation programs for patients with cardiac disease. A change in the responses and/or tolerance to a routine bout of exercise (or in the performance of a specific task) can be an early warning of a change in medical status.

G. Assessment of physical activity participation can be done using questionnaires or just screening questions or using more technical methods such as accelerometers or pedometers. The patient should be asked to be as specific as possible about the type of exercise, frequency of participation, length of participation each session, and a rating of the exertion or effort during the session. Typically, individuals will say they exercise regularly. However, when questioned about specifics, it is determined that they participate in activity at frequency, duration, and effort levels less than the level recommended for health benefits as described by the Surgeon General's Report on Physical Activity and Health, 1996.

XIII. Activity recommendations.

A. A starting, sample program for exercise for patients on dialysis can be found on the following Web site: www.lifeoptions.org in the free materials "Exercise for the Dialysis Patient." A common-sense, gradually progressing approach for starting activity, which is individualized and considers the symptoms, clinical status, medications, and treatments of each patient is recommended. Basically the recommendation should be for an increase in physical activity which is gradual, for most, if not all days of the week, working up to 30 minutes per session at an exertion level that is easily tolerated (and may be limited by symptoms). Recommendations for cardiovascular exercise, resistance exercise, and flexibility are shown in Table 4.10. Age of the patient, cultural considerations, and identification of barriers (perceived and real) to adopt and maintain physical activity must also be addressed. The patient should also be given clear information on how to monitor their activity in terms of the symptoms experienced. Participation should be assessed and encouraged at every patient encounter, either at dialysis treatments, clinic, or physician visits. It is critical to be positive and encouraging, even if the patient is making very slow progress. If they have any increased participation at all at follow-up, they should be praised and encouraged to continue.

XIV. Implementation.

A. The challenge for the kidney community is finding the resources to provide counseling and encouragement as a routine part of the patient care, whether it is in the provider's office or at the dialysis clinic.
   1. Intradialytic exercise is an ideal setting to provide the opportunity for increased physical activity, since patients are there 3 times/week using their time quite unproductively. With training and commitment from the leadership of the clinic, the environment could become a supportive and encouraging place to provide motivation for regular activity and the clinical supervision may put the concerns of medical risk (which are minimal) at bay.
   2. Providing exercise at the dialysis location (either prior to the treatment or during the treatment) will facilitate participation because it is convenient, supported as part of the routine care, and an expectation of the treatment of the kidney disease.

   3. Missing the opportunity for productive use of the dialysis treatment time is disappointing. However, the Kidney Exercise Demonstration project clearly showed that patients can significantly improve functioning through an independent home exercise prescription. Thus, many patients can increase physical activity in their homes and/or participate in programs in the community.

B. No matter what programming is decided upon for exercise (predialysis, intradialysis, postdialysis, or independent exercise at home), several changes in the routine care may enhance physical activity participation.
   1. Medical order for exercise. If there is an order for exercise participation, then the patient should receive information/education about how to start a program and how to progress. Providing this information could be in the form of educational materials or referral to a physical therapist or exercise specialist. Patients who qualify for cardiac rehabilitation (e.g. post MI, bypass surgery, angioplasty) should be referred to cardiac rehabilitation.
   2. Regular follow-up and documentation of participation. This can be done on several levels.
      a. Ask about exercise participation at the time of every patient encounter, e.g., as a part of the assessment done before putting the patient on dialysis or at every clinic visit or phone contact.
      b. Incorporating physical functioning assessment and participation into the routine short and long-term care plans to facilitate regular review of participation at the time of the patient review. If, at the time of patient review, there is a change in participation, it should be addressed to identify problems and concerns with participation or the program.
   3. Dialysis staff education on the benefits of regular physical activity for their patients and how to encourage patient participation in regular physical activity. This should be a part of the staff training for new employees and could become a part of the unit quality assurance program.

XV. Summary.

Patients with CKD have very low levels of physical functioning that negatively affect overall health, quality of life, and outcomes. Incorporation of regular assessment and encouragement of physical

Table 4.10

Basics of Exercise Recommendations

Type of Exercise	Frequency	Starting Level	Goal	Progression
Resistance or strengthening	3 times per week	Using amount of resistance that can comfortably be lifted 10–12 times, perform one set of 10–12 repetitions of exercises for all major muscle groups.	3 sets of 10–12 repetitions of exercises for major muscle groups.	Start with low weights (or Thera-bands®) at 1 set of 10–12 repetitions and increase the number of sets to 3 sets, then increase the weight.
Flexibility	4 times per week	■ Perform stretching around each major groups ■ Hold each stretch for 10–15 seconds.		■ Move into stretch position gradually until a stretch is felt. ■ Do not bounce. ■ Be sure to breathe throughout the stretch.
Cardiovascular exercise	4–7 times per week	5–10 minutes as tolerated ■ May be intervals of work/rest ■ Low level intensity 30–45 minutes per session, includes warm-up, conditioning time, and cooldown ■ Duration: • warm-up 3–5 minutes • conditioning 20–35 minutes • cooldown 3–5 minutes ■ Intensity: • warm-up: RPE of 9–10 • conditioning: RPE of 12–15 • cooldown: RPE 9–10	Increase duration by 2–5 minutes per session each week. ■ Once 30 is achieved, increase intensity to 12–15. ■ For intervals, gradually decrease the rest interval.	

activity and exercise as a part of the routine care of CKD patients is needed to facilitate increased physical activity. This will be a challenge within the existing system of dialysis care and will necessitate a change in the mindset on the part of nephrology health care providers. It will require a change in administrative procedures, staff training, as well as patient and family training and education. There is ample evidence that increasing physical functioning through increased physical activity, will improve quality of life, may improve outcomes, and could improve survival through improvement in overall health and cardiovascular risk profile.

Chapter 21

Ethical Considerations and Dilemmas

Purpose

To review basic ethical principles and the multitude of factors associated with appropriate initiation and withdrawal of renal replacement therapy (RRT). The nephrology nurse encounters ethical dilemmas in daily practice that arise in all treatment settings with all patient populations and modalities. These dilemmas begin with considerations regarding appropriate initiation of RRT and continue through the life cycle of a person with chronic kidney disease (CKD) and through the approach to and decisions about end-of-life care. The nephrology nurse is often in a unique position to serve as advocate and advisor. In all cases the duty of the nurse is to advocate for the patients autonomy, protect human dignity, ensure informed consent, and privacy of those we serve (ANA, 2001).

Objectives

Upon completion of this chapter, the learner will be able to:
1. Describe the basic ethical principles underlying initiation of dialysis.
2. List three considerations in determining appropriate initiation of therapy.
3. Explain options to resolve conflicts.
4. Describe the principles of informed consent.

I. Basic ethical principles.

A. Respect for autonomy: based on the concept that people are free to make their own decisions to the extent that they are able to understand and decide and that one ought not to interfere with the autonomous beliefs and actions of another in the pursuit of their goals. The legal right of self-determination is based on this principle.

B. Beneficence: obliges persons to benefit or help others with positive actions to prevent or remove what is harmful and to promote benefit.

C. Nonmaleficence: requires persons to refrain from harming others and to exercise due care to prevent harm to others.

D. Professional integrity: compels health care professionals to practice in a manner consistent with the shared values of their profession such as doing no harm and benefiting others.

II. Appropriate initiation of therapy.

A. While RRT is almost universally available in the United States for all in need, treatment for all with kidney failure is neither compassionate nor appropriate.

B. Generally, the goal of RRT is, by definition, replacement of kidney function to prolong life that would otherwise end prematurely.

C. Primary questions that should be contemplated when considering the appropriateness of RRT.
1. What are the goals of the treatment?
2. Can the desired benefit be achieved or delivered?

D. Withholding and withdrawing treatment is appropriate if:
1. The care would be futile. In clinical settings, futility designates an effort to provide a benefit to the patient (through treatment), which reason and experience suggest is highly likely to

fail and whose rare exceptions cannot be systematically produced (Jonsen, Siegler, & Winslade, 2002).

2. Quality of life is poor. Treatment should be considered in cases when RRT will indeed prolong life but cannot restore other serious comorbidities such as multiorgan failure, dementia, end-stage heart, liver, or pulmonary diseases, the effects of a massive CVA. In these instances perhaps the goal (replacing kidney function) can be attained but may not be worthwhile (Jonsen, Siegler, & Winslade, 2002).

3. The patient is permanently incapable of purposefully relating to others (RPA & ASN, 2000).
   a. Severe irreversible dementia.
   b. Persistent vegetative state.

4. The care is unwanted (RPA & ASN, 2000).
   a. Competent, informed patients who have refused dialysis or request withdrawal.
   b. Patients without decision-making capacity and:
      (1) Who have previously indicated refusal of dialysis.
      (2) Whose legal agents decline dialysis or request withdrawal.

5. Other conditions for which RRT may be inappropriate (RPA & ASN, 2000):
   a. End-stage vascular access.
   b. Those who may be harmful to themselves and others.

E. Referral for hospice care should be made whenever treatment is withheld or withdrawn.

III. Shared decision making between professionals, patient, and patients' decision makers should be employed to:

A. Examine the patient's condition.

B. Explore the potential risks and benefits of treatment.

C. Ensure that the patient's wishes are known and followed.

D. Establish agreed goals for treatment.

E. In cases where the benefit of treatment is unknown or dubious, a time-limited trial may be suggested.

F. Timing.
   1. Prior to initiation of RRT therapy.
   2. After each significant change or deterioration in condition.

G. Participants.

1. Patient with decision-making capacity.
2. Interdisciplinary nephrology professionals.
3. Decision makers for those who lack decision-making capacity.
4. Family of patient with decision-making capacity if requested. "Support of autonomy in the broadest sense also includes recognition that people of some cultures place less weight on individualism and choose to defer to family or community values in decision making" (ANA, 2001).

H. Considerations.
   1. Prior advance directives.
   2. Known wishes of patient.
   3. Data based prognostic indicators on life expectancy.

I. Conflict resolution when disagreements arise regarding appropriateness of RRT, goals of treatment, and between duly appointed decision makers and/or other family members.
   1. Ensure a systematic approach for conflict resolution.
   2. Review shared decision-making process for:
      a. Miscommunication or misunderstanding.
      b. About prognosis.
      c. Intrapersonal or interpersonal issues.
      d. Values.
   3. Involve clergy.
   4. Use ethnic consultants when appropriate.
   5. Use Ethics Committees when possible. The ANA Code of Ethics requires that for nurses practicing in the hospital setting, nurse administrators must ensure that all nurses have access to hospital ethics committees and that ethics committees have nurse representation.

IV. Conflicts between institutional policies and duly executed advanced directives (ADs) that prohibit CPR.

A. The health professional's duty is to honor the AD. The ANA Code of Ethics reminds nurses that they are "leaders and vigilant advocates for the delivery of dignified and humane care."

B. State laws.
   1. Professionals can be charged with medical battery in some states if ADs are not followed.
   2. Right to self-determination is recognized in all states.

V. Informed consent.

A. Fundamentally based on respect for the individual and for each individual's capacity and right to define his or her own goals and to make choices designed to achieve those goals.

B. "Each nurse has an obligation to be knowledgeable about the moral and legal rights of all patients to self-determination" (ANA, 2001).

C. Full explanation.
1. Available dialysis modality.
2. Not starting dialysis: continuing conservative management/end-of-life care.
3. Time limited trial of dialysis.
4. Stopping dialysis and end-of-life care.

D. Use of prognostic data based on patient condition may expand understanding of life expectancy, the treatment path ahead, and thus increase preparation for informed consent.

E. Information should be provided on all treatment modalities that includes time limited trials and no treatment (RPA & ASN, 2000).

VI. Decisional capacity.

A. *Competent* and *incompetent* are legal terms.

B. Decisional capacity is a medical term for one who can comprehend, evaluate, and choose among realistic options (Jonsen, Siegler, & Winslade, 2002). Patients are noted to have or not have decisional capacity.

C. Surrogate decision makers.

VII. Patient behaviors.

A. Nonadherence, threatening, and violent.
1. Risk is the possibility of harm or injury as determined by:
   a. Degree of harm (type and seriousness).
   b. Probability of harm (frequency and duration of exposure).
2. Risks of behavior (DPC, 2005).
   a. Risk to self, nonadherence relative to patient autonomy.
   b. Risk to facility.
   c. Risk to others: threatening and violent behaviors.

3. Patients who pose a risk only to themselves have a right to continued treatment (DPC, 2005).
4. Patient autonomy allows for acceptance or refusal of some or all of a recommended treatment. As stated in the ANA Code of Ethics "limitation of individual rights must always be considered a serious deviation from the usual standard of care" so that nurses are obligated to honor the patients right to autonomy except in cases where there is a threat of harm to others.

B. Disturbing to other patients.
1. Loud verbalizations and moaning of patients without decisional capacity.
2. Difficult to distinguish disruptive patients from those who are challenging or frustrating.

VIII. Adverse events and medical errors. In its landmark 1999 report, To Err Is Human, the Institute of Medicine (IOM) declared that medical injury is a major cause of preventable deaths and called on health care to make reduction of medical errors a priority.

A. Response to and disclosure of medical errors may present an ethical dilemma for professionals. While fear of litigation may drive secrecy, research has shown that less litigation occurs when patients and families are told the truth regarding medical errors and their effects. When errors occur, the ethical obligation is twofold:
1. Our commitment to care for the patient harmed.
2. Our responsibility to change our systems to prevent future error.

B. Truth telling. Patients and families are entitled to the truth, to know the details of adverse events and medicals errors and their impact. Communication should be open, prompt, and ongoing so that openness and collaboration with patients and families are the forefront of the response of the medical team.

C. Organizational ethics. Each organization must establish an organizational culture around honest and open acknowledgment of adverse events and medical errors that includes no fault reporting mechanisms, communications, root cause analysis investigation, and follow-up. Implementation of a Patient Safety Program should include staff education and policy and procedure development supportive of this culture.

Chapter 22

Advance Care Planning and Palliative/End-of-Life Care

Purpose and Background

The final components of this section include advance care planning and end-of-life issues. End-of-life care includes evidenced-based predictors of morbidity and mortality and ethical considerations. Hospice will be defined with a review of Medicare hospice benefits as well as a review of symptoms seen at the end of life for the patient with CKD. Treatment options will be shared.

Objectives

Upon completion of this chapter, the learner will be able to:
1. Describe advance care planning as it relates to the nephrology patient.
2. Explain the differences between a health care proxy, living will, and DNR.
3. Recall statistics on CKD stage 5 survival rates.
4. List the predictors of morbidity and mortality in CKD stage 5.
5. Summarize the basic guiding principles of ethics.
6. Compare and contrast hospice care to palliative care.
7. Explain the hospice benefit under Medicare and specific considerations as it relates to nephrology patients.
8. List common symptoms and treatment strategies seen at End of Life (EOL) in nephrology patients and treatment.
9. Describe how to assist family members and professional colleagues in the bereavement and grief period after a nephrology patient dies.

Advance Care Planning (ACP)

I. Patient Self-Determination Act (PSDA), 1991.

A. A federal mandate for facilities who receive Medicare of Medicaid funding says that each state should address the issue of identifying care wishes of all patients on admission to acute care facilities, nursing homes, home health agencies, and hospice programs, including:
1. Providing each incoming patient with a statement of rights regarding making health care decisions.
2. Asking patients if they have an advance directive and, if one is available, this fact must be documented in the medical record.
3. Providing the patient an explanation of the facility's policy regarding advance directives.
4. Ensuring compliance with the requirements of state law.

B. Dialysis centers often have the nephrology social work or registered nurse ask about medical directives during admission process to the outpatient center.

II. Advance care planning process.

A. Not a form, but a process of communication to identify patient wishes related to medical decisions and care.

B. ACP evolves over many conversations with the patient.

C. It helps identify and formulate the patient's plan related to medical decision making when they may no longer be able to do so for themselves.

D. Predicting what patients may want at the end of life is complicated by:
1. The patient's age.
2. The status of the chronic illness.

3. The ability to sustain life with the medications and treatment regimens available.
4. The emotions of the family and/or significant others when the patient disease progresses and end of life approaches.

E. Families may find it difficult to make decisions on whether to continue medical treatment, and if so, how much and for how long.

F. The nurse is often the facilitator of the conversation. Patients rely on trusted health care professionals for guidance. Therefore it is important to discuss, not only for those who are terminally ill or whose death is imminent, but for those with chronic illness, including CKD. With chronic illness, the disease trajectory is more uncertain, and the patient has an increased likelihood of a shortened life span with a slow progressive decline in health with sudden episodes of disease exacerbation, possibly requiring hospitalization. This pattern usually repeats itself with the patient's overall health steadily declining, until the patient dies. It is also important in situations where patients have experienced comorbid complications or a new terminal diagnosis, in addition to kidney disease.
1. Discussions should include:
   a. Treatment options, including:
      (1) Length of time the treatment may be required.
      (2) Invasiveness of the treatment.
      (3) Consideration for the benefits and burdens of treatment options including what the patient would regard as worthwhile and what treatments as overly burdensome.
      (4) Chance of success.
   b. Overall prognosis.
   c. Reflection on patient's values, beliefs, and goals in life.
   d. Quality of life during and after the treatment.
2. Prepare the environment. Attempts should be made to create a supportive environment that would facilitate discussions, including:
   a. Adequate privacy.
   b. Ensuring patient comfort.
      (1) Timing of discussion. Ensure adequate time so the patient and family do not feel hurried or rushed.
      (2) Adequate space for all participants.
      (3) Proper position of all participants. Health care providers should be relaxed and comfortable. Avoid standing and looking down on the patient.
   c. Maintaining therapeutic communication. Convey warmth and caring, respect,

sensitivity, active listening, and empathy.
   d. Ensuring discussions are at the patient's level of understanding.

G. A formal process for ACP is helpful.
1. Should be a team effort including not only the nurse but the nephrology social worker, physician/provider, technician, and dietitian, in addition to those persons identified by the patient as important to the process.
2. Initiate guided discussions when initiating care, whether in the clinic, dialysis center, or hospital setting.
3. Introduce the subject of ACP. Inform the patient that these conversations occur with all patients, and provide education and information to clarify any misconceptions.
4. Have ACP documents ready and available.
5. Review the patient's preferences on a regular basis and update documentation. Discussions should be held at regular intervals as well as when there is a change in patient condition.

H. Pediatric ACP.
1. The pediatric population needs to be included in ACP. Children/adolescents can participate in planning and decision making.
2. They should have the same rights as adults to information and involvement in discussions, which are age appropriate and suited to the child's stage of development.
3. In pediatric palliative care, there is usually time for these discussions as death is rarely sudden.
4. Parents often try to protect their child from knowledge regarding the severity of their illness. However, children usually know and want to talk about it.
5. Children are often more ready to talk about death than their parents. They are more able to face the truth about illness and death. The child may, in fact, guide the parents in the process by talking about their condition and asking questions.
6. There are a variety of therapies that can be used to help children express their feelings and desires including play, music, and art therapy.

III. Advance medical directive (AMD).

A. The AMD is a form that asks under what circumstances the patient would or would not want care initiated related to medical/emergent health needs. There are two types of AMD (advance medical directive): health care proxy and living will. A lawyer is not necessarily needed to complete either one. They are usually written but could be given verbally if patient is still able to do so.

1. Health care proxy is also known as a *medical power of attorney* or *durable power of attorney for health care;* assigns a surrogate to make health decisions if the patient cannot. This legal document overrides the "next of kin" decision-making power. It does not allow for proxy to make legal or financial decisions.
2. Living will is a legal document also called an *instructive directive;* expresses the treatment of the patient related to end-of-life care. The patient specifies what is to be done and in what situations.
3. State by state considerations.
   a. All 50 states have passed laws related to AMD.
   b. Each state has specific requirements of what makes up an AMD.
   c. It is crucial, as a nurse, that you become familiar with your state's specific requirements which cover terminology used, appropriate forms to use, and any special circumstances.
4. Do not resuscitate (DNR).
   a. Laws regarding DNR include the process for obtaining, recording, and recognizing that status varies across states.
   b. The DNR process allows patients to not receive cardiopulmonary resuscitation (CPR) in the event of cardiac arrest and relieves emergency services staff, other health professionals, or good Samaritans from the responsibility of "not treating."
   c. Allow a Natural Death (AND) is a term being used to describe DNR. Some believe this term better reflects what is trying to be accomplished and does not imply that you are not "treating" or caring for a patient at the time of their death.

Palliative Care/End-of-Life Care

I. Predictors of morbidity and mortality.

A. Statistics related to survival rates and end of life in CKD stage 5 population.
   1. 1 out of 5 patients withdraw from dialysis each year.
   2. Patients with CKD stage 5 have a 30–50% shorter life span.
   3. Overall average survival on dialysis is 5 years.
   4. Survival rate to discharge from hospital after CPR:
      a. Patient without CKD is 10–15%.
      b. Patient with CKD stage 5 less than 5%.
B. Evidence-based predictors in CKD stage 5.
   1. 50% survival first year of dialysis if albumin level < 3.5mg/dL.

2. 40–72% increased risk of death if amputation in last year.
3. 50% survival rate if acute myocardial infarction in last year.
4. Late referral to start of dialysis.
5. Race, sex, and age.
   a. African-Americans have longer survival than Caucasians on dialysis but higher incidence.
   b. Older age at start of dialysis gives higher morbidity.
   c. Women in age bracket 20–54 years old have higher death rates than males (USRDS, 2002).

II. Ethical considerations.

A. Guiding principles.
   1. Beneficence: to do good or receive benefit from something rendered.
   2. Nonmalificence: to prevent harm.
   3. Autonomy: patient right to self-govern his/her care; respect of patient wishes.
B. Guidelines and standards for care guiding nursing practice related to end-of-life care include:
   1. American Nurses Association Code of Ethics for Nurses with Interpretive Statements.
   2. ANNA Nephrology Nursing Standards of Practice and Guidelines for Care.
   3. Clinical Practice Guideline – "Shared Decision-Making in the Appropriate Initiation and Withdrawal from Dialysis."
   4. Clinical Practice Guidelines for Quality Palliative Care.
C. Ethical issues at end of life.
   1. Futile care. Medical futility can be considered care that serves no useful purpose and provides no immediate or long-term benefit, or treatment which, even though having physiologic effects, is nonbeneficial to the patient as a person. Aspects of futile care include:
      a. There is no hope for improvement and no treatment to improve an incapacitating condition. It is dissimilar to the idea of euthanasia or assisted suicide because assisted suicide involves active intervention to end life, while withholding futile medical care does not encourage the natural onset of death.
      b. Serves only to prolong death.
      c. There are no physical or spiritual benefits.
      d. Prolongs the grieving process and frequently raises false hope.
   2. The issue of cost in medical futility involves the expenditure of resources that could be used for those with a greater likelihood of achieving a

positive outcome. Traditionally, discussions about medical futility do not include the ability of the patient to pay for treatment.

3. Assisted suicide is the practice of providing a means to terminate the life of a person. Usually the person has an incurable disease, intolerable suffering, or a possibly undignified death with the purpose to limit suffering. Laws regarding assisted suicide vary greatly.
   a. Physician-assisted suicide generally refers to the practice in which the physician provides a patient with a lethal dose of medication, upon the patient's request to end his/her own life. The significant difference is whether a lethal dose of medication is administered by the patient or by the physician.
   b. Passive-assisted suicide is the withdrawal or withholding of life-sustaining medical treatment in accordance with a competent patient who has made an informed decision to refuse treatment.
   c. Often terminally ill patients require dosages of pain medication that impair respiration or have other effects that may hasten death. Administering pain medications to achieve the desired patient comfort, even if the medication may compromise vital functions is generally held by most professional societies, and supported in court decisions, justifiable as long as the intent is to relieve suffering.
   d. Providers are faced with balancing these concerns with their legal duty and moral obligation to treat pain in the suffering patient.

4. Informed consent is the process that fully informed patients can make choices in their health care. There are four general standards to informed consent including the ability of the patient to:
   a. Express a choice.
   b. Understand information relevant to the decision about treatment.
   c. Understand the significance of the information provided.
   d. Analyze the relevant information and to weigh the treatment options.

III. Personal considerations.

A. Your personal past experience and values associated with death affect how you will care for patients. You need to have a clear understanding of situations in which you, ethically, are unable to assist in patient care and refer the care to a colleague who is able to work with the patient.

B. Cultural diversity. As discussed in a previous section, reviewing cultural impact related to death customs, traditions, and beliefs specific to individual populations is critical in developing the patient focused plan of care. Clarify and ask the patient or family member about any preferences.
   1. Research has identified three basic dimensions in end-of-life treatment that vary culturally:
      a. Communication of "bad news."
      b. Views regarding decision making.
      c. Attitudes toward advance directives and end-of-life care.
   2. Cultural considerations.
      a. By assessing the patient's values, spirituality, and relationship dynamics, health care providers can incorporate and follow cultural preferences.
      b. It is not uncommon for health care professionals from outside the United States to conceal serious diagnoses from patients as disclosure may be viewed as disrespectful, impolite, or even harmful to the patient.
      c. Among some cultures, emphasizing patient autonomy in decision making may contrast with preferences for more family or physician based decision making.
      d. Completion of advance directives is lower among patients of various ethnic backgrounds. This may be due to the distrust of the health care system, health care disparities, cultural perspectives on death and suffering, and family dynamics.

IV. Palliative care definition: The World Health Organization defines it as "an approach which improves quality of life of patients and their families facing life-threatening illness through prevention, assessment, and treatment of pain and other physical, psychosocial, and spiritual problems." It begins when the patient is diagnosed with a serious illness and the start of a life-prolonging therapy. The goal for the patient may still include remission or cure with a focus on relief of symptoms.

V. Hospice definition: A subset of palliative care, where patient comfort takes precedence over other goals and treatments are simplified. The goals are the same as in palliative care, but the patient is in the terminal phase of disease. The focus is on providing for a "good" death.

VI. Hospice benefit.

A. Medicare enacted the hospice benefit in 1982. Hospice services may also be covered by private insurance.

B. Physician certification is required to document patient life expectancy of 6 months or less and it is not limited to cancer diagnoses.

C. If hospice benefit is based on a nonkidney diagnosis, such as cancer or late stage emphysema, the patient may stay on dialysis while in hospice, if that is their wish and it meets the individual hospice program requirements.

D. Patients with kidney disease are also entitled to hospice benefit. Hospice programs may ask that they stop all life-sustaining treatments, including dialysis, to enroll. In certain circumstances patients can stay on dialysis while they adjust to the hospice option.

E. The hospice referral process requires a physician order for hospice evaluation. The nursing role is to expedite patient requests for information about hospice and to keep the lines of interdisciplinary communication open.

VIII. Symptoms seen at end of life in kidney patient.

A. Fatigue, pruritis, anorexia, dyspnea, difficulty concentrating.

B. Nausea, vomiting.

C. Myoclonic movements, convulsions, coma.

D. Pain is usually related to nonkidney cause of death such as cancer diagnosis or neuropathic pain.

E. Most have few symptoms: usually more fatigue, lengthening sleep cycle, then coma.

VII. Treatment of symptoms.

A Pain.
1. Be mindful of the method of excretion for medications used and the effects of metabolites from the breakdown of medications, especially narcotics and hypnotics.
2. Methadone, hydromorphone (Dilaudid), or fentanyl are excreted by the liver, making them a better choice for pain control in late kidney failure.
3. Morphine products can cause symptoms due to metabolites produced in long-term use and may cause confusion.
4. Refer to available drug tables to adjust dosing or schedule appropriate for kidney failure.
5. Always provide for bowel hygiene when using pain medication by adding a daily stool softener or other agent. The goal is to treat prophylactically versus waiting until constipation occurs.
6. As with many other medications used in patients with kidney failure, they may have side effects not commonly seen in the typical population.

Frequent patient assessment of response to medications is important, as well as dictating the direction of the treatment of symptoms based on the patient's individual response.

B. Other.
1. Simple measures can give relief, such as using fans for patients with feeling of dyspnea or using a clear liquid diet for nausea and vomiting.
2. Food and fluids. It is best to avoid force feeding or fluids; let the patient guide you. A decrease in appetite is common in later stages of impending death. It is also an area where families and friends feel the need to "feed" the patient so they can "maintain their strength." Food is symbolic of health, family, and pleasurable memories. Yet feeding or offering fluids may be detrimental as gag reflex becomes suppressed or as the level of consciousness changes.
3. Relaxation. Guided meditation techniques or massage can be helpful in coping with symptoms such as anxiety, pain, or nausea.
4. Treating symptoms should be on an individual basis as they occur, using simplest measures first and progress based on patient feedback.
5. Depression. Be aware that many terminal patients may have depression and can benefit from treatment.

IX. Grief counseling and bereavement period.

A. Nephrology nursing allows for a unique connection to the patients.

B. Following patient from diagnosis to death can be emotionally straining.

C. Nephrology nurses need to develop support systems within their work, personal, or professional environments to assist with coping with these feelings.

D. Hospice programs offer bereavement counseling to family survivors for the first year following the death of a patient.

E. There are grief/bereavement groups available in most counties.

F. Though patients have a serious illness, death may come as a surprise to families and even nephrology staff.

G. Do not forget to anticipate the grief response of other patients who have known the deceased, and support their needs for sharing their feelings or referral for counseling.

H. Some dialysis centers offer memorial services to recognize patients who have died, allowing for staff and families to participate.

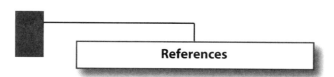

References

Chapter 15

Agency for Toxic Substances & Disease Registry (ATSDR). (n.d.). *About ATSDR*. Retrieved February 6, 2008, from http://www.atsdr.cdc.gov/about.html

Agency for Toxic Substances & Disease Registry (ATSDR). (n.d.). *Pediatric environmental health: Exposure-disease model*. Retrieved February 6, 2008, from http://www.atsdr.cdc.gov/HEC/CSEM/pediatric/appendixa.html

AGS Foundation for Health and Aging. (n.d.). *The aging process*. Retrieved February 6, 2008, from http://www.healthinaging.org/agingintheknow/chapters_print_ch_trial.asp?ch=1

Altman, R.B. (2005). *The PharmGKB: Catalyzing research in pharmacogenetics*. Retrieved February 6, 2008, from http://www.pharmgkb.org/

Bonham, V.L., Warshauer-Baker, E., & Collins, F.S. (2005). Race and ethnicity in the genome era the complexity of the constructs. *American Psychologist, 60*(1), 9-15.

Centers for Disease Control and Prevention (CDC). (2004). *Awareness of family health history as a risk factor for disease – United States, 2004*. Retrieved February 6, 2008, from http://www.cdc.gov/mmwr/preview/mmwrhtml/mm5344a5.htm

Centers for Disease Control and Prevention (CDC). (2006). *Evaluation of genomic applications in practice and prevention (EGAPP): Implementation and evaluation of a model approach*. Retrieved February 6, 2008, from http://www.cdc.gov/genomics/gtesting.htm

Consensus Panel. (2005, September 21-25). *Essential nursing competencies and curricula guidelines for genetics and genomics*. Retrieved February 6, 2008, from http://www.nursingworld.org/ethics/

Coy, V. (2005). Genetics of essential hypertension. *Journal of the American Academy of Nurse Practitioners, 17*, 219.

Cultural Diversity. (1997). *The basic concepts of trancultural nursing*. Retrieved February 6, 2008, from http://www.culturediversity.org/basic.htm

Dell, K.M., & Avner, E.D. (2006). *Autosomal recessive polycystic kidney disease*. Retrieved February 6, 2008, from http://www.genetests.org

Desnick, R.J., & Astrin, K.H. (2004). *Fabry disease*. University of Washington, Seattle. Retrieved February 6, 2008, from http://www.genetests.org

Emory University School of Medicine. (2004). *Multifactoral health conditions*. Retrieved February 6, 2008, from http://www.genetics.emory.edu

Ensenauer, R.E., Michels, V.V., & Reinke, S.S. (2005). Genetic testing: Practical, ethical, and counseling considerations. *Mayo Clinics Proceedings*. Retrieved February 6, 2008, from http://www.mayoclinicproceedings.com/inside.asp?AID=815&UID=

Feetham, S., Thomson, E.J., & Hinshaw, A.S. (2005). Nursing leadership in genomics for health and society. *Journal of Nursing Scholarship, 37*(2), 102-110.

Genzyme Therapeutics. (2003). *Fabry community*. Retrieved February 6, 2008, from http://www.fabrycommunity.com

Glauser, T.A. (2006). *Genetic pharmacology service for adult and pediatric patients*. Retrieved February 6, 2008, from http://www.cincinnatichildrens.org/svc/alpha/g/gps/

Gwinn, M., Bedrosian, S., Ottmann, D., & Khoury, M.J. (Eds.). (2004). *Genomics and population health: United States 2003*.

Retrieved February 6, 2008, from http://www.cdc.gov/genomics/activities/ogdp/2003.htm

Hadley, D. (2006). *Performing an assessment from a genetic perspective*. Paper presented at Cancer Genetics and Genomics: A Workshop for Oncology Nurses, Bethesda, MD.

Harris, P.C., & Torres, V.E. (2004). *Autosomal dominant polycystic kidney disease*. Retrieved February 6, 2008, from http://www.genetests.org

Jenkins, J. (2006). *Relevance of genetics and genomics to oncology nursing practice*. Paper presented at Cancer Genetics and Genomics: A Workshop for Oncology Nurses, Bethesda, MD.

Jenkins, J., Grady, P.A., & Collins, F. (2005). Nurses and the genomic revolution. *Journal of Nursing Scholarship, 37*(2), 98-101.

Lagay, F. (2006). *Pharmacogenomics: A revolution in a bottle?* Retrieved February 6, 2008, from http://www.ama-assn.org/

Lalouel, J., Rohrwasser, A., Terreros, D., Morgan, T., & Ward, K. (2001). Angiotensinogen in essential hypertension: From genetics to nephrology. *Journal of the American Society of Nephrology, 12*, 606-615.

Levy, D., DeStefano, A., Larson, M., O'Donnell, C., Lifton, R., Gavras, H., et al. (2000). Evidence for a gene influencing blood pressure on chromosome 17: Genome scan linkage results for longitudinal blood pressure phenotypes in subjects from the Framingham heart study. *Hypertension, 36*, 477-483.

Lister Hill National Center for Biomedical Communications, U.S. Library of Medicine National Institutes of Health Department of Health & Human Services. (2006). *Handbook: Help me understand genetics*. Retrieved February 6, 2008, from http://www.ghr.nlm.nih.gov/handbook

Loescher, L.J., & Merkle, C.J. (2005). The interface of genomic technologies and nursing. *Journal of Nursing Scholarship, 37*(2), 111-119.

Lorentz, C.P., Wieben, E.D., Tefferi, A., Whiteman, D.A.H., & Dewald, G.W. (2002). *Primer on medical genomics Part I: History of genetics and sequencing of the human genome*. Retrieved February 6, 2008, from http://www.mayoclinicproceedings.com/inside.asp?a=1&ref=7708mg1

Medline Plus. (2006). *Medical encyclopedia: Medullary cystic kidney disease*. Retrieved February 6, 2008, from http://www.nlm.nih.gov/medlineplus/ency/article/000465.htm

Minois, N. (2005). How should we assess the impact of genetic changes on ageing in model species? *Ageing Research Reviews, 5*(1), 52-59.

Monsen, R.B. (2005). *Genetics nursing portfolios: A new model for the profession*. Silver Spring, MD: American Nurses Association.

National Cancer Institute. (2006). *Simplification of informed consent documents*. Retrieved February 6, 2008, from http://www.cancer.gov/clinicaltrials

National Human Genome Research Institute. (2006). *A brief guide to genomics*. Retrieved February 6, 2008, from http://www.genome.gov/18016863

National Institute of General Medical Sciences. (2007). *Fact sheet: What is pharmacogenetics?* Retrieved February 6, 2008, from http://www.nigms.nih.gov/Publications/FactSheet_Pharmacogenetics.htm

National Kidney & Urologic Diseases Information Clearinghouse. (2004). *Polycystic kidney disease*. Retrieved February 6, 2008, from http://kidney.niddk.nih.gov/kudiseases/pubs/polycystic/index.htm

Offit, K., Groeger, E., Turner, S., Wadsworth, E., & Weiser, M. (2004). The "duty to warn" a patient's family members about hereditary disease risks. *Journal of the American Medical Association, 292*(12), 1469-1473.

Onalaja, A.O., & Claudio, L. (2000). Genetic susceptibility to lead poisoning. *Environmental health perspectives supplements, 108*(S1), 23-28.

Padlewska, K.K., & Schwartz, R.A. (2005). *Acrodynia. eMedicine from WebMD.* Retrieved February 6, 2008, from http://www.emedicine.com/derm/topic592.htm

Paik, S. (2004, December 30). New genetic test predicts recurrence in women with node-negative, estrogen-receptor-positive breast cancer. *New England Journal of Medicine.*

Pestka, E.L., & Williams, J.K. (2005). International collaboration on genomics education for nurses. *Journal of Continuing Education for Nurses, 36*(4), 180-184.

PKD Foundation. (n.d.). *Learning about polycystic kidney disease.* Retrieved February 6, 2008, from http://www.pdkcure.org

Rizk, D., & Chapman, A.B. (2003). Core curriculum in nephrology. *American Journal of Kidney Disease, 42*(6), 1305-1317.

Ruppert, V., & Maisch, B. (2003). Genetics of human hypertension. *Herz, 28*(8), 655-662.

Tefferi, A., Wieben, E.D., Dewald, G.W., Whiteman, D.A.H., Bernard, M.E., & Spelsberg, T.C. (2002). *Primer on medical genomics Part II: Background principles and methods in molecular genetics.* Retrieved February 6, 2008, from http://www.mayoclinicproceedings.com/inside.asp?a=1&ref=7708mg2

United States Environmental Protection Agency. (2006). *About EPA.* Retrieved February 6, 2008, from http://www.epa.gov/epahome/aboutepa.htm

University of Maryland. (2002). *Essential hypertension.* Retrieved February 6, 2008, from http://www.umm.edu/ency/article/000153.htm

University of Washington, Seattle. (2004). *About genetic services.* Retrieved February 6, 2008, from http://www.geneclinics.org

Vinks, A.S. (2006). *Developing computer models for personalized drug dosing.* Retrieved February 6, 2008, from http://www.cincinnatichildrens.org/research/about/horizons/2005-1/vinks.htm?GOSEARCH.X=0\&GOSEARCH.Y=0

Weinshilboum, R.M., & Wang, L. (2006). Pharmacogenetics and pharmacogenomics: Development, science, and translation. *Annual Review of Genomics and Human Genetics, 7,* 223-245.

Whelan, A.J., Ball, S., Best, L., Best, R.G., Echiverri, S.C., Ganschow, P., et al. (2004). Genetic red flags: Clues to thinking genetically in primary care practice. *Primary Care, 31*(7), 497-508.

Williams, J.K., Skirton, H., & Masny, A. (2006). Ethics, policy, and educational issues in genetic testing. *Journal of Nursing Scholarship, 38*(2), 119-125.

Chapter 16

Andrews, M.M., & Boyle, J.S. (2002). Transcultural concepts of nursing care. *Journal of Transcultural Nursing, 13*(3), 178-180.

Antai-Otong, D. (2006). *Nurse-client communication: A life span approach.* Sudbury, MA: Jones and Bartlett Publishers.

Bastable, S.B. (2003). *Nurse as educator: Principles of teaching and learning for nursing practice* (2nd ed.). Sudbury, MA: Jones and Bartlett Publishers.

Boyle, J.S., & Andrews, M.M. (1989). *Transcultural concepts in nursing care.* Glenview, IL: Scott, Foresman/Little, Brown College Division.

Brown, H.D. (1980). *Principles of language learning and teaching.*

Retrieved February 6, 2008, from http://tip.psychology.org/language.html

Cross, K.P. (1990). *Adult learning.* Retrieved February 6, 2008, from http://tip.psychology.org/cross.html

DDHS. (2004). National Center for Health Statistics. *Monthly vital statistics report, 47*(25).

Giger, J.N., & Davidhizar, R.E. (1991). *Transcultural nursing: Assessment and intervention.* St. Louis: Mosby.

Hudson, S., & Prowant, B. (2005). *Nephrology nurse standards and guidelines for care.* Pitman, NJ: American Nephrology Nurses' Association.

McFarlane, C.D. (2006). My strength: A look outside the box at the strengths perspective. *Social Work: A Journal of the National Association of Social Workers, 51*(2), 175-176.

Nápoles-Springer, A.M., Santoyo, J., Houston, J., Pérez-Stable, E J., & Stewart, A.L. (2005). Patients' perceptions of cultural factors affecting the quality of their medical encounters. *Health Expectations, 8*(1), 4.

Chapter 17

Al-Arabi, S. (2006). Quality of life: Subjective descriptions of challenges to patients with end stage kidney disease. *Nephrology Nursing Journal, 33*(3), 285-293.

Birnbaum, L., & Birnbaum, A. (2004). In search of inner wisdom: Guided mindfulness meditation in the context of suicide. *Scientific World Journal,* 216-217.

Boulware, L.E., Liu, Y., Fink, N.E., Coresh, J., Ford, D.E., Klag, M.J., et al. (2006). Temporal relation among depression symptoms, cardiovascular disease events, and mortality in end-stage kidney disease: Contribution of reverse causality. *Clinical Journal of the American Society of Nephrology,* 1-9.

Campbell, A. (1998). Family caregivers: Caring for aging ESRD partners. *Advances in Kidney Replacement Therapy,* 98-108.

Curtin, R.B., Bultman Sitter, D.C., Schatell, D., & Chewning, B.A. (2004). Self-management, knowledge, and functioning and well-being of patients on hemodialysis. *Nephrology Nursing Journal, 31*(4), 378-387.

Curtin, R.B., & Mapes, D.L. (2001). Health care management strategies of long-term dialysis survivors. *Nephrology Nursing Journal, 28*(4), 385-394.

Devins, G.M., Mendelssohn, D.C., Barre, P.E., & Binik, Y.M. (2003). Predialysis psychoeducational intervention and coping style influence time to dialysis in chronic kidney disease. *American Journal of Kidney Diseases, 42*(4), 693-703.

Finkelstein, F.O., & Finkelstein, S.H. (2000). Depression in chronic dialysis patients: Assessment and treatment. *Nephrology Dialysis & Transplantation, 15,* 1911-1913.

Francis, G.M., & Munjas, B.A. (1976). *Manual of social psychologic assessment.* New York: Appleton-Century-Crofts.

Garcia Vladerrama, F.W., Fajardo, C., Guevara, R., Gonzales Perez, V., & Hurtado, A. (2002). Poor adherence to diet in hemodialysis: Role of anxiety and depression symptoms. *Nefrologia, 22,* 244-52.

Gokal, R., & Hutchison, A. (2002). Dialysis therapies for end stage kidney disease. *Seminars in Dialysis, 15*(4), 220-226.

Golper, T. (2001). Patient education: Can it maximize the success of therapy? *Nephrology Dialysis & Transplantation, 16*(7), 20-24.

Halpin, L.S., Speir, A.M., CapoBianco, P., & Barnett, S.D. (2002). Guided imagery in cardiac surgery. *Outcomes in Management & Nursing Practice, 6*(3), 132-137.

Harwood, L., Locking-Cusolito, H., Spittal, J., Wilson, B., & White, S. (2005). Preparing for hemodialysis: Patient stressors and responses. *Nephrology Nursing Journal, 32*(3), 295-302.

Hodge, D.R. (2006). Spiritually modified cognitive therapy: A review of the literature. *Social Work: A Journal of the National Association of Social Workers, 51*(2), 157-165.

Iacono, S.A. (2005). Predialysis anxiety: What are the concerns of patients? *The Journal of Nephrology Social Work, 24,* 21-24.

Klang, B., Bjorvell, H., & Clyne, N. (1999). Predialysis education helps patients choose dialysis modality and increases disease-specific knowledge. *Journal of Advanced Nursing, 29*(4), 869-876.

Koo, J.R., Yoon, J.Y., Joo, M.H., Lee, H.S., Oh, J.E., Kim, S.G., et al. (2005). Treatment of depression and effect of antidepression treatment on nutritional status in chronic hemodialysis patients. *The American Journal of the Medical Sciences, 329*(1), 1-5.

Lazarus, R.S. (1983). The trivialization of distress. In J.C. Rosen & L.J. Solomon (Eds.), *Preventing health risk behaviors and promoting coping with illness* (Volume 8). Hanover, NH: University Press of New England.

Liu, L., & Park, D. (2004). Aging and medical adherence: The use of automatic processes to achieve effortful things. *Psychology and Aging, 19*(2), 318-325.

LoGiudice, D., Kerse, N., Brown, K., & Gibson, S.J. (1998). The psychosocial health status of caregivers of persons with dementia: A comparison with the chronically ill. *Quality of Life Research, 7,* 345-351.

Lopes, A.A., Albert, J.M., Young, E.W., Satayathum, S., Pisoni, R.L., Andreucci, V.E., et al. (2004). Screening for depression in hemo-dialysis patients: Associations with diagnosis, treatment, and outcomes in the DOPPS. *Kidney International, 66,* 2047-2053.

Mapes, D.L., Callahan, M.B., & Richie, M.F. (2001). Psychosocial and rehabilitative aspects of kidney failure and its treatment. In L. Lancaster (Ed.), *Core curriculum for nephrology nursing* (4th ed.). Pitman, NJ: American Nephrology Nurses' Assocation.

Mazella, A. (2004). Psychosocial factors in treating the depressed kidney patient. *The Journal of Nephrology Social Work, 23,* 40-47.

McFarlane, C.D. (2006). My strength: A look outside the box at the strengths perspective. *Social Work: A Journal of the National Association of Social Workers, 51*(2), 175-176.

Meers, C., Singer, M.A., Toffelmire, E.B., Hopman, W., McMurray, M., Morton, A.R., et al. (1996). Self-delivery of hemodialysis care: A therapy in itself. *American Journal of Kidney Diseases, 27*(6), 844-847.

Mok, E., Lai, C., & Zhang, Z. (2004). Coping with chronic kidney failure in Hong Kong. *International Journal of Nursing Studies, 41*(2), 205-213.

Patel, S.S., Shah, V.S., Peterson, R.A., & Kimmel, P.L. (2002). Psychosocial variables, quality of life, and religious beliefs in ESRD patients treated with hemodialysis. *American Journal of Kidney Disease, 40*(5), 1013-1022.

Puchalski, C. (2006). *The George Washington Institute for Spirituality and Health (GWish).* Retrieved February 6, 2008, from http://www.gwish.org

Ravenscroft, E.F. (2005). Diabetes and kidney failure: How individuals with diabetes experience kidney failure. *Nephrology Nursing Journal, 32*(4), 502-509.

Richardson, M.A., Post-White, J., Grimm, E.A., Moye, L.A., Singletary, S.E., & Justice, B. (1997). Coping, life attitudes, and the immune responses to imagery and group support after breast cancer treatment. *Alternative Therapy Health Medicine, 3*(5), 62-70.

Sue, D.W., Arrendondo, P., & McDavis, R.J. (1992). Multicultural counseling competencies and standards: A call to the profession. *Journal of Counseling and Development,* 477-486.

Chapter 18

Adsit, K.I. (1996). Multimedia in nursing and patient education. *Orthopaedic Nursing, 15*(4), 59-63.

Aldrige, M. (2004). Writing and designing readable patient education materials. *Nephrology Nursing Journal, 31*(4), 373-377.

Andrews, M.M., & Boyle, J.S. (2002). Transcultural concepts of nursing care. *Journal of Transcultural Nursing, 13*(3), 178-180.

Antai-Otong, D. (2006). *Nurse-client communication: A life span approach.* Sudbury, MA: Jones and Bartlett Publishers.

Baer, C. (2001). Principles of patient education. In L. Lancaster (Ed.), *Core curriculum for nephrology nursing* (4th ed.). Pitman, NJ: American Nephrology Nurses' Assocation.

Bastable, S.B. (2003). *Nurse as educator: Principles of teaching and learning for nursing practice* (2nd ed.). Sudbury, MA: Jones and Bartlett Publishers.

Bastable, S.B. (2006). *Essentials of patient education.* Sudbury, MA: Jones and Bartlett Publishers.

Blanchard, W.A. (1998). Teaching an illiterate transplant patient. *ANNA Journal, 25*(1), 69, 70, 76.

Boyd, M.D., Gleit, C.J., Graham, B.A., & Whitman, N.J. (1998). *Teaching in nursing practice: A professional model* (3rd ed.). Norwolk, CT: Appleton-Century-Crofts.

Brown, H.D. (1980). *Principles of language learning and teaching.* Retrieved February 6, 2008, from http://tip.psychology.org/language.html

Brundage, D.J., & Swearengen, P.A. (1994). Chronic kidney failure: Evaluation and teaching tool. *ANNA Journal, 21*(5), 165-270.

Cross, K.P. (1990). *Adult learning.* Retrieved February 6, 2008, from http://tip.psychology.org/cross.html

Deccache, A. (1995). Teaching, training, or educating patients? Influence of contexts and models of education and care on practice in patient education. *Patient Education and Counseling, 26*(1-3), 119-129.

Eble, K.E. (1988). *The craft of teaching* (2nd ed.). San Francisco: Jossey-Bass Publishers.

Gagne, R. (1985). *The conditions of learning* (4th ed.). Retrieved February 6, 2008, from http://tip.psychology.org/gagne.html

Gerstle, D.S. (1999). Grab their attention! Make your point! *MCN, 24*(5), 257-261.

Giacome, T., Ingersoll, G.L., & Williams, M. (1999). Teaching video effect on kidney transplant patient outcomes. *ANNA Journal, 26*(1), 29-33, 81.

Hansen, M., & Fisher, J.C. (1998). Patient-centered teaching from theory to practice. *American Journal of Nursing, 98*(1), 56, 58, 60.

Hilgard, R.R., & Bower, G. H. (1966). *Theories of learning.* New York: Appleton-Century-Crofts.

Hudson, S.B., & Prowant, B. (2005). *Nephrology nursing standards of practice and guidelines for care.* Pitman, NJ: American Nephrology Nurses' Association.

Knox, A.B. (1986). *Helping adults learn.* San Francisco: Jossey-Bass Publishers.

Lane, D. (2003). *Levels of measurement: Connexions module.* Retrieved February 6, 2008, from http://cnx.org/content/m10809/latest/

Maynard, A.M. (1999). Preparing readable patient education handouts. *Journal for Nurses in Staff Development, 15*(1), 11-18.

Molzahn, A.E. (1996). Changing to a teaching paradigm for teaching and learning. *ANNA Journal, 23*(2), 217-221.

Ramsdell, R., & Annis, C. (1996). Patient education: A continuing repetitive process. *ANNA Journal, 23*(2), 217-221.

Redman, B. (1997). *The process of patient education* (8th ed.). St Louis: Mosby.

Redman, B.K. (2003). *Measurement tools in patient education* (2nd ed.). New York: Springer Publishing Company.

Ross, P.E., Groenhoff, C., & Zin, P. (2004). Chronic kidney disease, now what! *American Association of Occupational Health Nurses Journal, 52*(7), 287-297.

Sandrick, K. (1998). Teach your patients well. *Health Management Technology, 19*(3), 16-18.

Swartzendruber, D. (1994). Gaming: A creative strategy for staff education. *ANNA Journal, 21*(1), 21-25.

Tang, P.C., & Newcomb, C. (1998). Informing patients: A guide for providing patient health information. *Journal of the American Medical Informatics Association, 5*(6), 563-570.

Tattersall, R. (1995). Patient education 2000: Take-home messages from this congress. *Patient Education and Counseling, 26*(1-3), 373-377.

Van den Borne, H.W. (1998). The patient from receiver of information to informed decision-maker. *Patient Education and Counseling, 34*(2), 89-102.

Wingard, R. (2005). Patient education and the nursing process: Meeting the patient's needs. *Nephrology Nursing Journal, 32*(2), 211-215.

Chapter 19

Centers for Medicare & Medicaid Services (CMS). (n.d.). *Excluded drug coverage by state Medicaid program.* Retrieved February 6, 2008, from http://www.cms.hhs.gov/States/EDC/list.asp

Krop, J.S., Coresh, J., Chambless, L.E., Shahar, E., Watson, R.L., Szklo, M., et al. (1999). A community-based study of explanatory factors for the excess risk for early kidney function decline in blacks vs. whites with diabetes: The atherosclerosis risk in communities study. *Archives of Internal Medicine, 159*(15), 1777-1783.

Kusek, J.W., Greene, P., Wang, S.R., Beck, G., West, D., Jamerson, K., et al. (2002). Cross-sectional study of health-related quality of life in African Americans with chronic kidney insufficiency: The African American study of kidney disease and hypertension trial. *American Journal of Kidney Diseases, 39*(3), 513-524.

Martins, D., Tareen, N., Zadshir, A., Pan, D., Vargas, R., Nissenson, A., et al. (2006). The association of poverty with the prevalence of albuminuria: Data from the Third National Health and Nutrition Examination Survey (NHANES III). *American Journal of Kidney Diseases, 47*(6), 965-971.

Port, F.K., Wolfe, R.A., Levin, N.W., Guire, K.E., & Ferguson, C.W. (1990). Income and survival in chronic dialysis patients. *ASAIO Transplantation, 36*(3), M154-157.

Robinson, K., & Ricca, L. (2002). AAKP reviews 30 years of the Medicare ESRD Program. *Kidney Life, 17*(6).

Satayathum, S., Pisoni, R.L., McCullough, K.P., Merion, R.M., Wikstrom, B., Levin, N., et al. (2005). Kidney transplantation and wait-listing rates from the international Dialysis Outcomes and Practice Patterns Study (DOPPS). *Kidney International, 68*(1), 330-337.

Shoham, D.A., Vupputuri, S., & Kshirsagar, A.V. (2005). Chronic kidney disease and life course socioeconomic status: A review. *Advances in Chronic Kidney Disease, 12*(1), 56-63.

St. Peter, W. (2005). *United States Kidney Data System.* Presentation by the American Society of Nephrology.

U.S. Renal Data System. (2006). *USRDS 2006 annual data report: Atlas of chronic kidney disease & end-stage renal disease in the United States.* Bethesda, MD: National Institutes of Health, National Institute of Diabetes and Digestive and Kidney Disease.

Chapter 20

Akiba, T., Matsui, N., Shinohara, S., Fujiwara, H., Nomura, T., & Marumo, F. (1995). Effects of recombinant human erythropoietin and exercise training on exercise capacity in hemodialysis patients. *Artificial Organs, 19*, 1262-1268.

Applegate, W.B., Blass, J.P., & Williams, T.F. (1990). Instruments for the functional assessment of older patients. *New England Journal of Medicine, 322*, 1207-1214.

Barnea, N., Drory, Y., Iaina, A., Lapidot, C., Resin, E., Eliahou, H., et al. (1980). Exercise tolerance in patients on chronic hemodialysis. *Israel Journal of Medical Sciences, 16*, 17-21.

Beasley, C.R., Smith, D.A., & Neale, T.J. (1986). Exercise capacity in chronic kidney failure patients managed by continuous ambulatory peritoneal dialysis. *Australian & New Zealand Journal of Medicine, 16*, 5-10.

Berry, M.J., Rejeski, W.J., Adair, N.E., & Zaccaro, D. (1999). Exercise rehabilitation and chronic obstructive pulmonary disease. *American Journal of Respiratory Critical Care Medicine, 160*, 1248-1253.

Bluestone, P.A., Rasmussen, G., & Rogers, T. (2002). *Exercise programs at Network 2 dialysis units.* CMS Forum of ESRD Networks Annual Meeting.

Bohannon, R.W., Smith, J., Hull, D., Palmeri, D., & Barnhard, R. (1995). Deficits in lower extremity muscle and gait performance among kidney transplant candidates. *Archives of Physical and Medical Rehabilitation, 76*, 547-551.

Branch, L.G., & Jette, A.M. (1982). A prospective study of long-term care institutionalization among the aged. *American Journal of Public Health, 76*, 1373-1379.

Braun-Curtin, R., Klag, M.J., Bultman, D.C., & Schatell, D. (2002). Renal rehabilitation and improved patient outcomes in Texas dialysis facilities. *American Journal of Kidney Diseases, 40*, 331-338.

Buchner, D.M., Beresford, S.A., Larson, E.B., LaCroix, A.Z., & Wagner, E.H. (1992). Effects of physical activity on health status in older adults II: Intervention studies. *Annual Review of Public Health, 13*, 469-488.

Carlson, M.C., Fried, L.P., Xue, Q.L., Bandeen-Roche, K., Zeger, S.L., & Brandt, J. (1999). Association between executive attention and physical functional performance in community dwelling older women. *Journals of Gerontology Series B: Psychological Sciences and Social Sciences, 54*, S262-S270.

Cheema, B.S.B., Smith, B.C.F., & Singh, M.A. (2005). A rationale for intradialytic exercise training as standard clinical practice in ESRD. *American Journal of Kidney Diseases, 45*, 912-916.

Chobanian, A.V., Bakis, G.L., Black, H.R., Cushman, W.C., Green, L.A., Izzo, J.L., et al., & the National High Blood Pressure Education Programming Coordinating Committee. (2003). The seventh report of the Joint National Committee on Prevention, Detection, Evaluation, and Treatment of High Blood Pressure. *JAMA, 289*, 2560-2572.

Copley, J.B., & Lindberg, J.S. (1999). The risks of exercise. *Advances in Kidney Replacement Therapy, 6*(2), 165-171.

DeOreo, P.B. (1997). Hemodialysis patient-assessed functional health status predicts continued survival, hospitalization and dialysis-attendance compliance. *American Journal of Kidney Diseases, 30*, 204-212.

Ferrucci, L., Izmirlian, G., Leveille, S., Phillips, C.L., Corti, M.C., Brock, D.B., et al. (1999). Smoking, physical activity, and active life expectancy. *American Journal of Epidemiology, 149*, 645-653.

Fiatarone, M.A., Marks, E.C., Ryan, N.D., Meredith, C.N., Lipsitz, L.A., & Evans, W.J. (1990). High intensity strength training in nonagenarians: Effects on skeletal muscle. *JAMA, 263,* 3029-3034.

Fiatarone, M.A., O'Neill, E.F., Ryan, N.D., Clements, K.M., Solares, G.R., Nelson, M.E., et al. (1994). Exercise training and nutritional supplementation for physical frailty in very elderly people. *New England Journal of Medicine, 330,* 1769-1775.

Goldberg, A.P., Geltman, E.M., Gavin, J.R. III, Carney, R.M., Hagberg, J.M., Delmez, J.A., et al. (1986). Exercise training reduces coronary risk and effectively rehabilitates hemodialysis patients. *Nephron, 42,* 311-316.

Goldberg, A.P., Geltman, E.M., Hagberg, J.M., Gavin, J.R. III, Delmez, J.A., Carney, R.M., et al. (1983). Therapeutic benefits of exercise training for hemodialysis patients. *Kidney International, S16,* S303-S309.

Goldberg, A.P., Hagberg, J.M., Delmez, J.A., Carney, R.M., McKevitt, P.M., Ehsani, A.A., et al. (1980). The metabolic and psychological effects of exercise training in hemodialysis patients. *American Journal of Clinical Nutrition, 33,* 1620-1628.

Goldberg, A.P., Hagberg, J.M., Delmez, J.A., Florman, R.W., & Harter, H.R. (1979). Effects of exercise training on coronary risk factors in hemodialysis patients. *Proc Dialysis Transplant Forum,* 39-42.

Guralnik, J.M., Branch, L.G., Cummings, S.R., & Curb, J.D. (1989). Physical performance measures in aging research. *Journal of Gerontology, 44,* M141-146.

Guralnik, J.M., Ferrucci, L., Simonsick, E.M., Salive, M.E., & Wallace, R.B. (1995). Lower-extremity function in persons over the age of 70 as a predictor of subsequent disability. *New England Journal of Medicine, 43,* 845-854.

Hagberg, J.M., Goldberg, A.P., Ehsani, A.A., Heath, G.W., Delmez, J.A., & Harter, H.R. (1983). Exercise training improves hypertension in hemodialysis patients. *American Journal of Nephrology, 3,* 209-212.

Haskell, W.L., Alderman, E.L., Fair, J.M., Maron, D.J., Mackey, S.F., Superko, H.R., et al. (1994). Effects of intensive multiple risk factor reduction on coronary atherosclerosis and clinical cardiac events in men and women with coronary artery disease: The Stanford Coronary Risk Intervention Project (SCRIP). *Circulation, 89,* 975-990.

Headley, S., Germain, M., Mailloux, P., Mulhern, J., Ashworth, B., Burris, J., et al. (2002). Resistance training improves strength and functional measures in patients with end stage kidney disease. *American Journal of Kidney Diseases, 40,* 355-364.

Hirsch, C.H., Fried, L.P., Harris, T., Fitzpatrick, A., Enright, P., & Schulz, R. (1997). Correlates of performance-based measures of muscle function in the elderly: The cardiovascular health study. *Journal of Gerontology: Medical Sciences, 52A,* M192-M200.

Huang, Y., Macera, C.A., Blair, S.N., Brill, P.A., Kohl, H.W. III, Kronenfeld, J.J. (1998). Physical fitness, physical activity, and functional limitation in adults aged 40 and older. *Medicine and Science in Sports and Exercise, 30,* 1430-1435.

Johansen, K.L. (1999). Physical functioning and exercise capacity in patients on dialysis. *Advances in Kidney Replacement Therapy, 6*(2), 141-148.

Johansen, K.L., Chertow, G.M., Ng, A.V., Mulligan, K., Carey, S., Schoenfeld, P.Y., et al. (2000). Physical activity levels in patients on hemodialysis and healthy controls. *Kidney International, 57,* 2564-2570.

Johansen, K.L., Kaysen, G., Young, B.S., Hung, A.M., da Silva, M., & Chertow, G.M. (2003). Longitudinal study of nutritional status, body composition, and physical function in hemodialysis patients. *American Journal of Clinical Nutrition, 77*(4), 760-761.

Johansen, K.L., Sakkas, G.K., Doyle, J., Shubert, T., & Dudley, R.A.

(2003). Exercise counseling practices among nephrologists caring for patients on dialysis. *American Journal of Kidney Diseases, 41,* 171-178.

Knight, E., Ofsthun, N., Teng, M., Lazarus, J.M., & Curhan, G.C. (2003). The association between mental health, physical function and hemodialysis mortality. *Kidney International, 63,* 1843-1851.

Kong, C., Tattersall, J., Greenwood, R.N., & Farrington, K. (1999). The effect of exercise during hemodialysis on solute removal. *Nephrology, Dialysis and Transplantation, 14,* 2927-2931.

Kouidi, E., Albani, M., Natsis, K., Megalopoulos, A., Gigis, P., Guiba-Tziampiri, O., et al. (1998). The effects of exercise training on muscle atrophy in haemodialysis patients. *Nephrology, Dialysis and Transplantation, 13,* 685-699.

LaCroix, A.Z., Guralnik, J.M., Berkman, L.F., Wallace, R.B., & Satterfield, S. (1993). Maintaining mobility in late life II: Smoking, alcohol consumption, physical activity and body mass index. *American Journal of Epidemiology, 137,* 858-869.

Latos, D.L., Strimel, D., Drews, M.H., & Allison, T.G. (1987). Acid-base and electrolyte changes following maximal and submaximal exercise in hemodialysis patients. *American Journal of Kidney Diseases, 10,* 439-445.

Leveille, S.G., Guralnik, J.M., Ferrucci, L., & Langlois, J.A. (1999). Aging successfully until death in old age: Opportunities for increasing active life expectancy. *American Journal of Epidemiology, 149,* 654 653.

Levenhagen, D.K., Carr, C., Carlson, M.G., Maron, D.J., Borel, M.J., & Flakoll, P.J. (2002). Postexercise protein intake enhances whole-body and leg protein accretion in humans. *Medicine & Science in Sports & Exercise, 34,* 828-837.

Lowrie, E.G., Huang, W.H., Lew, N.L., & Liu, Y. (1994). The relative contribution of measured variables to death risk among hemodialysis patients. In E.A. Friedman (Ed.), *Death on hemodialysis: Preventable or inevitable?* (pp. 121-141). Amsterdam: Kluwer Academic.

Lowrie, E.G., Zhang, H., Lefaine, N., Lew, N.L., & Lazarus, J.M. (1998). Health related quality of life among dialysis patients: Associations with contemporaneous measures and future mortality (abstract). *Journal of the American Society of Nephrology, 9,* 219A.

Lundin, A.P., Stein, R.A., Frank, F., LaBelle, P., Berlyne, G.M., Krasnow, N., et al. (1981). Cardiovascular status in long-term hemodialysis patients: An exercise and echocardiographic study. *Nephron, 28,* 234-238.

McDermott, M., Greenland, P., Ferrucci, L., Criqui, M.H., Liu, K., Sharma, L., et al. (2002). Lower extremity performance is associated with daily life physical activity in individuals with and without peripheral arterial disease. *Journal of American Geriatrics Society, 50*(2), 247-255.

Mercer, T.H., Crawford, C., Gleeson, N.P., & Naish, P.F. (2002). Low-volume exercise rehabilitation improves functional capacity and self-reported functional status of dialysis patients. *American Journal of Physical Medicine and Rehabilitation, 81,* 162-167.

Mercer, T.H, Naish, P.F., Gleeson, N.P., Wilcock, J.E., & Crawford, C. (1998). Development of a walking test for the assessment of functional capacity in non-anemic maintenance dialysis patients. *Nephrology, Dialysis and Transplantation, 13*(8), 2023-2026.

Messier, S.P., Royer, T.D., Craven, T.E., O'Toole, M.L., Burns, R., & Ettinger, W.H. Jr. (2000). Long-term exercise and its effect on balance in older, osteoarthritic adults: Results from the Fitness, Arthritis, and Seniors Trial (FAST). *Journal of the American Geriatric Society, 48,* 131-138.

Meyer, K., Schwaibold, M., Westbrook, S., Beneke, R., Hajric, R., Lehmann, M., et al.(1997). Effects of exercise training and activity restriction on 6-minute walking test performance in patients with chronic heart failure. *American Heart Journal, 133*(4), 447-453.

Miller, B.W., Cress, C.L., Johnson, M.E., Nichols, D.H., & Schnitzler, M.A. (2002). Exercise during hemodialysis decreases the use of antihypertensive medications. *American Journal of Kidney Diseases, 39*(4), 828-833.

Moore, G.E., Brinker, K.R., Stray-Gundersen, J., & Mitchell, J.H. (1993). Determinants of VO2 peak in patients with end stage kidney disease: On and off dialysis. *Medicine and Science in Sports and Exercise, 25*(1), 18-23.

Moore, G.E., Parsons, D.B., Stray-Gundersen, J., Painter, P.L., Brinker, K.R., & Mitchell, J.H. (1993). Uremic myopathy limits aerobic capacity in hemodialysis patients. *American Journal of Kidney Diseases, 22*(2), 277-287.

National Institutes of Health (NIH). (1995). *NIH Consensus Conference statement. Physical activity and cardiovascular health.* Bethesda, MD: Author.

National Kidney Foundation (NKF). (2005). KDOQI clinical practice guidelines: Cardiovascular disease in dialysis patients. *American Journal of Kidney Diseases, 45.*

Oberly, E. (Ed.). (1994). *Kidney rehabilitation: Bridging the barriers.* Medical Education Institute: Madison, WI.

Office of the U.S. Surgeon General. (1996). *Physical activity and health: A report of the surgeon general.* U.S. Department of Health and Human Services, Public Health Service.

O'Hare, A.M., Tawney, K., Bacchetti, P., & Johansen, K.L. (2003). Decreased survival among sedentary patients undergoing dialysis: results from the dialysis morbidity and mortality study wave 2. *American Journal of Kidney Diseases, 41*, 447-454.

Painter, P.L. (2003). Exercise in chronic disease: The responsibility of the primary care physician. *Current Sports Medicine, 2*(3), 173-180.

Painter, P., Blagg, C., & Moore, G.E. (1995). *Exercise for the dialysis patient: A comprehensive program.* Madison: Medical Education Institute.

Painter, P.L., Carlson, L., Carey, S., Myll, J., & Paul, S. (2004). Determinants of exercise encouragement practices in dialysis staff. *Nephrology Nursing Journal, 31*(1), 67-74.

Painter, P.L., Carlson, L., Carey, S., Paul, S.M., & Myll, J. (2000a). Low functioning patients improve with exercise training. *American Journal of Kidney Diseases, 36(3)*, 600-608.

Painter, P.L., Carlson, L., Carey, S., Paul, S.M., & Myll, J. (2000b). Physical functioning and health related quality of life changes with exercise training in hemodialysis patients. *American Journal of Kidney Diseases, 35*(3), 482-492.

Painter, P., Hanson, P., Messer-Rehak, D., Zimmerman, S.W., & Glass, N.R. (1987). Exercise tolerance changes following kidney transplantation. *American Journal of Kidney Diseases, 10*(6), 452-456.

Painter, P., & Johanson, K.L. (2006). Improving physical functioning: Time to become a part of the routine care. *American Journal of Kidney Diseases.*

Painter, P.L., Messer-Rehak, D., Hanson, P., Zimmerman, S.W., & Glass, N.R. (1986). Exercise capacity in hemodialysis, CAPD and kidney transplant patients. *Nephron, 42*, 47-51.

Painter, P.L., Moore, G.E., Carlson, L., Paul, S., Myll, J., Phillips, W., et al. (2002). The effects of exercise training plus normalization of hematocrit on exercise capacity and health-related quality of life. *American Journal of Kidney Diseases, 39*(2), 257-265.

Painter, P.L., Nelson-Worel, J.N., Hill, M.M., Thornberry, D.R., Shelp, W.R., Harrington, A.R., et al. (1986). Effects of exercise training during hemodialysis. *Nephron, 43*, 87-92.

Painter, P.L., Stewart, A.L., & Carey, S. (1999). Physical functioning: Definitions, measurement, and expectations. *Advances in Kidney Replacement Therapy, 6*(2), 110-123.

Parkerson, G.R., & Gutman, R.A. (2001). Health-related quality of life predictors of survival and hospital utilization. *Health Care Financing Review, 21*, 171-184.

Perrin, P.P., Gauchard, G.C., Perrot, C., & Jeandel, C. (1999). Effects of physical and sporting activities on balance control in elderly people. British *Journal of Sports Medicine, 33*(2), 121-126.

Project, N.C.E. (2000). *Third report of the expert panel on detection, evaluation and treatment of high blood cholesterol in adult* (Adult Treatment Panel III). Bethesda, NIH-NHLBI.

Pupim, L.B., Flakoll, P.J., Levenhagen, D.K., & Ikizler, T.A. (2004). Exercise augments the acute anabolic effects of intradialytic parenteral nutrition in chronic hemodialysis patients. *American Journal of Physiology-Endocrinology and Metabolism, 286*(4), 589-597.

Rantanen, R., Era, P., & Heikkinen, E. (1994). Maximal isometric strength and mobility among 75-year-old men and women. *Age and Ageing, 23*(2), 132-137.

Ross, D.L., Grabeau, G.M., Smith, S., Seymour, M., Knierim, N., & Pitetti, K.H. (1989). Efficacy of exercise for end-stage kidney disease patients immediately following high-efficiency hemodialysis: A pilot study. *American Journal of Nephrology, 9*(5), 376-383.

Rowell, L.B. (1974). Human cardiovascular adjustments to exercise and thermal stress. *Physiological Reviews, 54*, 75-159.

Sallis, J.F., & Hovell, M.F. (1990). Determinants of exercise behavior. *Exercise and Sports Sciences Review, 18*, 307-327.

Shalom, R., Blumenthal, J.A., Williams, R.S., McMurray, R.G., & Dennis, V.W. (1984). Feasibility and benefits of exercise training in patients on maintenance dialysis. *Kidney International, 25*(6), 958-963.

Sietsema, K.E., Amato, A., Adler, S.G., & Brass, E.P. (2004). Exercise capacity as a prognostic indicator among ambulatory patients with end stage kidney disease. *Kidney International, 65*(2), 719-724.

Simonsick, E.M., Newman, A.B., Nevitt, M.C., Kritchevsky, S.B., Ferrucci, L., Guralnik, J.M., et al. (2001). Measuring higher level physical functioning well-functioning older adults: Expanding familiar approaches in the Health ABC study. *Medical Sciences, 56*(10), M644-M649.

Stewart, A.L., & Painter, P.L. (1997). Issues in measuring physical functioning and disability in arthritis patients. *Arthritis Care and Research, 10*, 395-405.

Strawbridge, W.J., Cohen, R.D., Shema, S.J., & Kaplan, G.A. (1996). Successful aging: Predictors and associated activities. *American Journal of Epidemiology, 144*(2), 135-141.

Tawney, K.W., Tawney, P.J.W., Hladik, G., Hogan, S.L., Falk, R.J., Weaver, C., et al. (2000). The Life Readiness Program: A physical rehabilitation program for patients on hemodialysis. *American Journal of Kidney Diseases, 36*(3), 581-591.

Tipton, K.D., & Wolfe, R.R. (1998). Exercise-induced changes in protein metabolism. *Acta Physiologica Scandinavica, 162*, 377-387.

Vaithilingam, I., Polkinghorne, K.R., Atkins, R.C., & Kerr, P.G. (2004). Time and exercise improve phosphate removal in hemodialysis patients. *American Journal of Kidney Diseases, 43*(1), 85-89.

Ware, J. (1993). *SF-36 health survey: Manual and interpretation guide.* Boston: The Health Institute.

Ware, J.E., Kosinski, M., & Keller, S.K. (1994). *SF-36 physical and mental health summary scales: A user's manual* (2nd ed). Boston: The Health Institute.

Ware, J.E., & Sherbourne, C.D. (1992). The MOS 36-item short-form health survey (SF-36): I. Conceptual framework and item selection. *Medical Care, 30,* 473-483.

Weber, K.T., Kinasewitz, G.T., Janicki, J.S., & Fishman, A.P. (1982). Oxygen utilization and ventilation during exercise in patients with chronic cardiac failure. *Circulation, 65*(6), 1213-1223.

Wu, S.C., Leu, S.Y., & Li, C.Y. (1999). Incidence of and predictors for chronic disability in activities of daily living among older people in Taiwan. *Journal of American Geriatric Society, 47*(9), 1082-1086.

Zabetakis, P.M., Gleim, G.W., Pasternack, F.L., Saraniti, A., Nicholas, J.A., & Michelis, M.F. (1982). Long-duration submaximal exercise conditioning in hemodialysis patients. *Clinical Nephrology, 18*(1), 17-22.

Chapter 21

American Nurses Association (ANA). (2001). *Code of ethics for nurses with interpretative statements.* Washington, DC: Author.

Forum of ESRD Networks. (2005). *Decreasing patient-provider conflict* (DPC), 90-100.

Jonsen, A., Siegler, M., & Winslade, W. (2002). *Clinical ethics* (5th ed.). New York: McGraw-Hill Medical Publishing Division.

Renal Physicians Association (RPA) & American Society of Nephrology (ASN). (2000). *Clinical practice guideline on shared decision-making in the appropriate initiation and withdrawal form dialysis.* Washington, DC: Author.

Chapter 22

American Medical Association (AMA). (2006). *AMA code of medical ethics.* Retrieved February 8, 2008, from http://www.ama-assn.org/ama/pub/category/2498.html

American Nurses Association (AMA). (1994). *Ethics and human rights position statements: Assisted suicide.* Retrieved February 8, 2008, from http://nursingworld.org/MainMenuCategories/HealthcareandPolicyIssues/ANAPositionStatements/Ethicsand HumanRights/prtetsuic14456.aspx

American Nurses Association (AMA). (2001). *Code of ethics for nurses with interpretive statements.* Washington, DC: Author.

Briggs, L. (2004). Shifting the focus of advance care planning: Using an in-depth interview to build and strengthen relationships. *Journal of Palliative Medicine, 7*(2), 341-349.

Briggs, L., Kirchhoff, K.T., Hammes, B.J., Song, M.K., & Colvin, E.R. (2004). Patient centered advance care planning in special populations: A pilot study. *Journal of Professional Nursing, 20*(1), 47-58.

Centers for Medicare & Medicaid Services (CMS). (2005). Rules and regulations. Medicare program; hospice care amendments. *Federal Register, 70*(224).

Chambers, J., Germain, M., & Brown, E. (2005). *Supportive care for the renal patient.* New York: Oxford.

City of Hope National Medical Center. (1999). City of Hope end of life care content guidelines. Duarte, CA: Author.

Dinwiddie, L., & Colvin, E., (2002). End of life care in the chronic kidney disease population. In A. Molzahn & E. Butera (Eds.), *Contemporary nephrology nursing: Principles and practice* (2nd ed., pp. 361-367). Pitman, NJ: American Nephrology Nurses' Association.

Ferell, B., & Coyle, N., (2005). *Textbook of palliative care nursing* (2nd ed.). New York: Oxford Press.

Hospice and Palliative Nurses Association. (2002). *Competencies for advanced practice hospice and palliative care nurses.* Dubuque, IA: Kendall/Hunt.

Hospice and Palliative Nurses Association. (2005). *Compendium of treatment of end stage non-cancer diagnoses: Renal.* Dubuque, IA: Kendall/Hunt.

Hudson, S., & Prowant, B., (2005). *Nephrology nurse standards of practice and guidelines for care.* Pitman, NJ: American Nephrology Nurses' Association.

Jecker, N.S. (2000). *Futility.* Retrieved February 8, 2008, from http://depts.washington.edu/bioethx/topics/futil.html

Joishy, S. (1999). *Palliative medicine secrets.* Philadelphia: Hanley & Belfus.

Kinzbrunner, B., Weinreb, N.J., & Policzer, J.S. (2002). *20 common problems: End-of-life care.* New York: McGraw-Hill.

Kuebler, K., Berry, P., & Heidrich, D. (2002). *End of life care clinical practice guidelines.* Philadelphia: Saunders.

National Cancer Institute (NCI). (2006). A guide to understanding informed consent. Retrieved February 8, 2008, from http://www.cancer.gov/ClinicalTrials/AGuidetoUnderstandingInformed Consent/page2

National Consensus Project. (2004). *Clinical practice guidelines for quality palliative care.* Retrieved February 8, 2008, from http://www.nationalconsensusproject.org

Nuland, S.B. (2000). Physician-assisted suicide and euthanasia in practice. *New England Journal of Medicine, 342,* 583-584.

Price, C.A. (2003). Resources for planning palliative and end-of-life care for patients with kidney disease. *Nephrology Nursing Journal, 30*(6), 649-56, 664.

Renal Physicians Association (RPA) and American Society of Nephrology (ASN). (2000). *Clinical practice guideline: Shared decision-making in the appropriate initiation of and withdrawal from dialysis.* Washington, DC: Author.

Robert Wood Johnson Foundation End-Stage Renal Disease Workgroup. (2003). *Completing the continuum of nephrology care recommendations to the field.* Retrieved February 8, 2008, from http://www.promotingexcellence.org

Watson, M., Lucas, C.F., Hoy, A.M., & Back, I.N. (Eds.). (2005). *Oxford handbook of palliative care.* New York: Oxford University Press.

Internet Resources

- www.annanurse.org (End of Life Decision Making and the Role of the Nephrology Nurse, CD-ROM, ANNA, 2004)
- www.kidneyeol.org (ESRD-specific End of Life Care)
- www.abcd-caring.com (Americans for Better Care of the Dying)
- www.abhpm.org (American Board of Hospice and Palliative Medicine)
- www.adec.org (Association of Death Education and Counseling)
- www.aacn.nche.edu/ELNEC (End of Life Nursing Education Consortium)
- www.hpna.org (Hospice and Palliative Nurses Association)
- www.lastacts.com (Robert Wood Johnson "Last Acts Movement")
- www.WSJ.com (Wall Street Journal AMD information)
- www.Medicinenet.com (AMD information)
- www.Medlawplus.com (AMD information)

Section 5

The Role of the Advanced Practice Nurse in Nephrology

Section Editor

Troy A. Russell, MSN, RN, APRN, BC, CNN-NP

Authors

Kim Alleman, MS, RN, FNP-C, APRN, CNN

Deborah H. Brooks, MSN, RN, ANP, CNN-NP

Sally Campoy, MS, APRN, BC, CNN

Lesley C. Dinwiddie, MSN, RN, FNP, CNN

Andrea Easom, MA, MNSc, APN, BC, CNN-NP

Katherine Healy Houle, MSN, C-FNP, CNN-NP

Carol L. Kinzner, MSN, ARNP, GNP, CNN-NP

Carrie N. May, MS, RN, ANP, CNN

Patricia Merenda, MN, ARNP, CNN-NP, CCTC

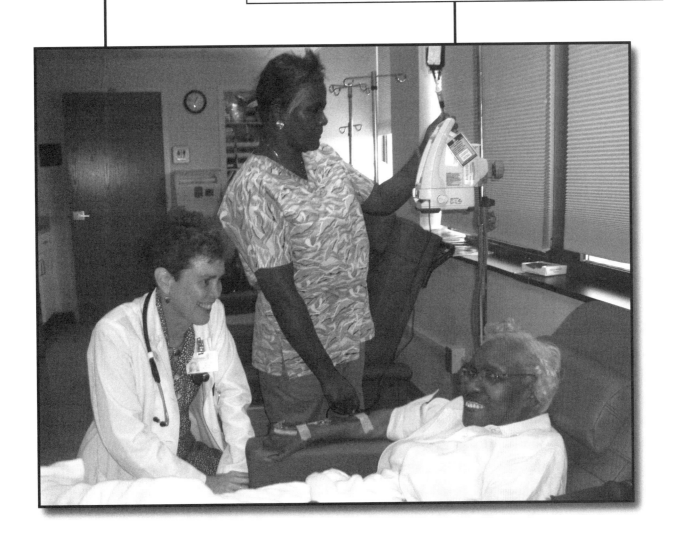

About the Authors

Troy A. Russell, MSN, RN, APRN, BC, CNN-NP, Section Editor, is a Nephrology Nurse Practitioner with the VA-TN Valley Healthcare System in Nashville, Tennessee.

Kim Alleman, MS, RN, FNP-C, APRN, CNN, is a Nurse Practitioner at the Hartford Hospital Transplant Program in Hartford, Connecticut.

Deborah H. Brooks, MSN, RN, ANP, CNN-NP, is a Nurse Practitioner and Research Coordinator at the Medical University of South Carolina in Charleston, South Carolina.

Sally Campoy, MS, APRN, BC, CNN, is a Nurse Practitioner at the Denver VA Medical Center, Renal Section, in Denver, Colorado.

Lesley C. Dinwiddie, MSN, RN, FNP, CNN, is a Nephrology Nurse Consultant at Vascular Access Education and Research in Cary, North Carolina, and the Executive Director for the Institute of Excellence, Education and Research (ICEER).

Andrea Easom, MA, MNSc, APN, BC, CNN-NP, is an Instructor in the College of Medicine, Nephrology Division, at the University of Arkansas for Medical Sciences in Little Rock, Arkansas.

Katherine Healy Houle, MSN, C-FNP, CNN-NP, is a Nephrology Nurse Practitioner at Marquette General Health Systems in Marquette, Michigan.

Carol L. Kinzner, MSN, ARNP, GNP, CNN-NP, is a Nurse Practitioner at Evergreen Nephrology Associates in Tacoma, Washington.

Carrie N. May, MS, RN, ANP, CNN, is an Adult Nurse Practitioner and Nephrology Care Manager at Lutheran General Hospital in Park Ridge, Illinois.

Patricia Merenda, MN, ARNP, CNN-NP, CCTC, is a Nurse Practitioner at the Polyclinic Swedish Medical Center in Seattle, Washington.

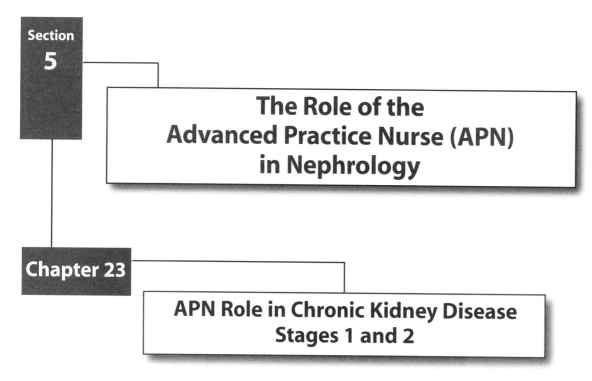

Purpose

Discuss how to prevent or slow progression of kidney disease as an advanced practice nurse (APN).

Objectives

Upon completion of this chapter, the learner will be able to:
1. Identify patients who are at risk or already in stages 1 and 2 of chronic kidney disease (CKD).
2. Discuss diagnostic procedures to evaluate people who may be at risk for CKD.
3. Outline management strategies, both short-term and long-term, for people with CKD stages 1 and 2.
4. Differentiate management plans for patients depending on their underlying pathology.

I. Definition.

A. CKD is kidney damage OR estimated glomerular filtration rate (eGFR) < 60 mL/min/1.73 m^2 > 3 months.

B. Kidney damage is defined as pathologic abnormalities in urine, serum, or imaging studies. The eGFR may remain normal due to an adaptive increase in glomerular blood flow and pressure.
1. Stage 1.
   a. eGFR > 90 mL/min/1.73 m^2.
   b. Kidney damage with normal or increased eGFR.
   c. People with normal eGFR but with kidney damage are at increased risk of losing more kidney function and of developing cardiovascular disease.
2. Stage 2.
   a. eGFR 60–89 mL/min/1.73 m^2.
   b. Kidney damage with mildly decreased eGFR.
   c. The NKF-KDOQI Workgroup concluded that there is insufficient evidence to label eGFR 60–89 mL/min/1.73 m^2 and no evidence of kidney damage as having CKD.
3. Examples of decreased eGFR but no kidney damage include:
   a. Normal for age, e.g., elderly or infants.

b. Other causes: vegetarians, unilateral nephrectomy, fluid volume depletion, decreased kidney perfusion.

II. Identification of at-risk population.

A. Assess for potential risk. Goal is to detect kidney disease at the highest level of kidney function to reduce the rate of decline.
   1. Age over 60 years; may be normal aging.
   2. Race and ethnicity: African American, American Indian, Hispanic, Asian Pacific.
   3. Cardiovascular disease: hypertension can be both a cause and consequence of kidney disease. Everyone with hypertension should be evaluated for CKD.
   4. Diabetes mellitus.
   5. Autoimmune diseases, e.g., systemic lupus erythematous (SLE).
   6. Infections (streptococcus, HIV).
   7. Exposure to drugs or procedures associated with decreased kidney function.
   8. Family history of kidney disease.
   9. Hereditary and acquired diseases, e.g., polycystic kidney disease (PKD), acquired cystic kidney disease (ACKD), Alport's syndrome.
   10. History of acute kidney injury with recovery.
   11. Organ transplant.
   12. Kidney donor.

B. Identify patients at risk and categorize as low, high, or very high risk.
   1. Low risk example: 70-year-old woman with no other risk factors.
   2. High risk example: 70-year-old African American woman with hypertension.
   3. Very high risk example: 70-year-old African American woman with hypertension, diabetes, and family history of kidney disease.

III. Screening.

A. Minimum evaluation. An abnormal finding needs to be verified within a 3-month time period.
   1. Serum creatinine.
   2. Proteinuria. Albuminuria is a marker for both the progression of CKD and for the development of cardiovascular disease.
   3. Urine sediment for RBC/WBC.
   4. Blood pressure evaluation.
   5. Calculate eGFR using Modified Diet In Renal Disease (MDRD) or Cockcroft-Gault equation. Estimated GFR equations are less accurate in higher range eGFRs. However, they are still

clinically useful to 90 mL/min/1.73 m². There is insufficient validity of accuracy in higher ranges.
   6. Look for other risk factors.

B. Elderly evaluation.
   1. Assess for CKD risk.
   2. Blood pressure check.
   3. CMP, CBC, lipid panel.
   4. Spot urine for protein to creatinine ratio.
   5. Urine for WBC/RBC.
   6. Medication review.
   7. Imaging studies as indicated.

C. Diabetic evaluation.
   1. Assess for CKD risk.
   2. Blood pressure check.
   3. CMP, CBC, lipid panel.
   4. Urine for microalbuminuria.
   5. Medication review.
   6. Imaging studies as indicated.

D. Proteinuria evaluation.
   1. First morning specimen corresponds with 24-hour protein excretion and helps exclude a diagnosis of orthostatic proteinuria. Overnight protein excretion.
   2. Midmorning specimen is acceptable if a first morning specimen is not available. A 24-hour urine or first morning specimen may be necessary if orthostatic proteinuria is suspected. Corresponds with 24-hour protein excretion.
   3. Urine for microalbuminuria.
      a. > 3 mg/dL with spot urine albuminuria dipstick.
      b. > 300 mg/day in 24-hour urine.
      c. > 250 mg/g (men), > 355 mg/g (women) spot urine albuminuria to creatinine ratio.
   4. Urine for proteinuria.
      a. > 30 mg/dL spot urine dipstick.
      b. > 300 mg/day in 24-hour urine.
      c. > 200 mg/g spot urine for protein to creatinine ratio.

E. Urine sediment evaluation.
   1. Fresh specimen with early morning specimen preferred.
   2. Casts are formed only in the kidney, cells can originate outside the GU tract.
   3. Urine dipstick useful for identifying RBC, neutrophils and eosinophils (leukocyte esterase), and bacteria (nitrites).
   4. Sediment exam needed for tubular epithelial cells, fat, casts, crystals, fungi, and parasites.

F. Imaging studies.
1. Renal ultrasound: size, stones, obstruction, cysts.
2. Computed tomography scan: obstruction, tumors, cysts, stones. If contrast is used, renal artery stenosis may be seen.
3. Magnetic resonance imaging: lesions, cysts, renal vein thrombosis.
4. Nuclear scan: asymmetry of size or function, functional evidence of renal artery stenosis, acute pyelonephritis, scars.

G. Diabetic clinical features.
1. 5–10 year history of diabetes: microalbuminuria, retinopathy, hypertension.
2. 10–15 year history of diabetes: albuminuria, retinopathy, hypertension (see Tables 5.1 and 5.2).

IV. Prevention and treatment.

A. Treat comorbid conditions, e.g., diabetes, dyslipidemia.

B. Treat cardiovascular disease aggressively. CKD is a risk factor for development and progression of CVD.

C. Blood pressure.
1. Strict blood pressure control: < 130/80 for nondiabetics, < 125/75 diabetics.
2. Hypertension.
   a. Follow established guidelines, e.g., JNC 7.
   b. Use multiple drugs as needed to control blood pressure to goal.
   c. Drug doses do not usually need adjusting at these stages.
   d. Check labs 7–10 days after starting ACE or ARB for increased serum creatinine and potassium.
3. Essential hypertension without proteinuria. Thiazide diuretics are first choice; combine with ACEi, ARB, or CCB.
4. Coronary artery disease and hypertension. Beta blockers first line.
5. Proteinuria.
   a. Type 1 diabetes: angiotension-converting enzyme inhibitors (ACEi) or angiotensin receptor blockers (ARB), sometimes combined.
   b. Type 2 diabetes: angiotensin receptor blockers (ARB) or ACEi, sometimes combined.
   c. Nondiabetic: ACEi and/or ARB, combining with nondihydropridine calcium channel blocker (diltiazem or verapamil) can lower proteinuria more.
6. Lifestyle changes including increased exercise, dietary adjustments for weight loss, decreased salt and fat intake, e.g., DASH (Dietary Approaches to Stop Hypertension).

D. Nutrition: general guidelines, modify as needed for special populations, e.g., diabetes, obesity.
1. Protein: 0.6–0.75 g protein/kg body weight/day to maintain neutral or positive nitrogen balance.
2. Energy intake 35 kcal/kg ideal body weight/day.

Table 5.1

Nondiabetic Kidney Diseases: Clinical Features and Risk Factors

Nondiabetic Disease	Clinical Features	Risk Factors
Glomerular	Proteinuria and RBCs	Autoimmune disease, systemic infection, drug exposure, family history, cancer
Vascular	Microalbuminuria, hematuria, hypertension	Family history, hypertension
Tubulointerstitial	WBCs and hydronephrosis, electrolyte abnormalities depending on tubular defect	Infections, obstructions, stones, drug exposure
Cystic	Cysts and RBCs	Family history

Table 5.2		

Transplant Related Kidney Diseases: Clinical Features and Risk Factors

Transplant Disease	Clinical Features	Risk Factors
Rejection	Hypertension	
Drug toxicity	Hypertension	Cyclosporine and tacrolimus
Recurrent disease	Proteinuria	Glomerulonephritis
Transplant glomerulonephritis	Proteinuria, hypertension	

3. Carbohydrate: 50–60% of calories.
4. Fat: 25–30% of calories with saturated fatty acids at < 10% of calories.
5. Sodium 2.4 g/day.
6. Potassium: no restriction unless indicated.
7. Calcium and phosphorus: use age-appropriate dietary guidelines.

E. Vaccinations.
1. Influenza annually.
2. Pneumococcal polysaccharide vaccine (Pneumovax 23) administration depends on age and health factors.
3. Tetanus toxoid, reduced diphtheria toxoid, acellular pertussis vaccine adsorbed.
   a. (Tdap) ADACEL™ booster vaccine for ages 19–64.
   b. BOOSTRIX® for ages 10–18. Replaces the former Td (tetanus/diphtheria booster). Given every 10 years but can be given up to 2 years after last Td to protect against pertussis.
4. Hepatitis B: Recombivax HB™ or Engerix-B® if < 19 years of age or in high risk category.
5. Zostavax® to prevent shingles (for age > 60, previous history of chickenpox, no immunosuppressive therapy, e.g., transplant, no HIV).

V. **Monitoring.**

A. Laboratory values (e.g. CMP, CBC, urinalysis, urine for protein to creatinine or albumin to creatinine ratio) annually or more often depending on values and abnormalities.

B. Blood pressure every 3 months if elevated or more often if medications adjusted.

C. Screen for other risk factors, e.g., proteinuria, diabetes, dyslipidemia.

D. Indicators of worsening CKD: new onset hypertension or worsening hypertension, metabolic acidosis, calcium/phosphorus/iPTH abnormality, anemia, new onset proteinuria/albuminuria.

VI. **Education.**

A. Progression of CKD.

B. Smoking cessation.

C. Blood pressure control.

D. Weight loss or maintenance.

E. Exercise.

F. Dietary recommendations.

G. Glycemic control.

H. Lipid control.

I. Limiting or eliminating use of NSAIDs, alternate therapy for chronic pain.

Chapter 24

APN Role in Chronic Kidney Disease Stages 3 and 4

Purpose

Discuss the concepts and management of patients with chronic kidney disease (CKD) stages 3 and 4 from an advanced practice nurse perspective.

Objectives

Upon completion of this chapter, the learner will be able to:
1. Estimate progression of CKD.
2. Prevent or slow the progression of CKD.
3. Diagnose and treat comorbid conditions and complications that commonly occur in these stages (see Table 5.1).
4. Educate and prepare patients and their families for kidney replacement therapy, as appropriate.

I. Definition and prevalence.

A. Stage 3.
   1. Moderate decrease in estimated glomerular filtration rate (eGFR), range 30-59 mL/min.
   2. Note this is regardless of any evidence of kidney damage (see Figure 5.1).
   3. Estimated 7.4 million persons in the United States have CKD stage 3.

B. Stage 4.
   1. Severe decrease in eGFR, range 15–29 mL/min.
   2. Estimated 300,000 Americans have CKD stage 4.
      a. Dramatic drop in prevalence.
      b. Thought to be due to cardiovascular death in CKD stage 3.

II. Prevention and treatment.

A Everything that is done in CKD stages 1 and 2.

B. Estimate progression.
   1. Teach "Know your number." Provide eGFR as the key measure of kidney function.
      a. Based on a percentage (0–100%).
      b. Dialysis generally, but not always, needed when function decreases to 10–15% (see Chapter 25).

c. Provide a handout or flow chart for tracking.
   2. Use rate of progression as a guide for response to therapy and preparation for kidney replacement therapy education.

III. Proteinuria.

A. May develop as kidney function declines or needs continued monitoring of previously identified proteinuria by:
   1. Urine albumin: creatinine (Cr) ratio *or*
   2. Urine protein: Cr ratio *or*
   3. 24-hour urine collection.
   4. Serum albumin.
      a. Increased risk for hypoalbuminemia and malnutrition as level declines.
      b. Increased risk of thrombotic events if serum albumin falls to less than or equal to 2.5 g/dL.

B. The greater the amount of proteinuria, the more rapid progression of kidney loss.

C. Continue treatment with an angiotensin-converting enzyme inhibitor (ACE-I) and/or an angiotensin-receptor blocker (ARB).
   1. Can reduce proteinuria by 40–50%.
   2. Monitor for hyperkalemia. If uncontrollable, discontinue ACE-I and/or ARB.

3. Monitor for elevated serum creatinine (SCr). If greater than 20% increase present, discontinue ACE-I and/or ARB.
4. Monitor for cough. If present, discontinue ACE-I and start an ARB.
5. Unless contraindicated, JNC 7 recommends use of ACE-I usually with a diuretic to control hypertension.
6. An ACE-I and ARB can be combined to reduce proteinuria and possibly protect against greater loss of kidney function.

D. Diet.
1. Maintain patient on salt restriction.
2. Cautious use of low protein diet as increases risk of malnutrition.

E. Medical nephrectomy.
1. Only in cases of severe proteinuria (generally in children).
2. Patient at risk of dying from the protein malnutrition.

V. Hypertension.

A. Treat to goal (< 130/80). See Sections 1 and 2.

B. Average number of antihypertensives required to meet goal is usually three to four.

C. Use an agent that inhibits the renin-angiotensin system (RAS) whenever possible (examples: lisinopril, monopril, ramipril, valsartan, irbesartan).
1. They protect the kidney by relaxing the efferent arteriole of the nephron, hence decreasing intraglomerular pressure.
   a. Decrease proteinuria.
   b. Drug of choice for congestive heart failure.
2. Monitor for hyperkalemia.
3. Monitor for decreasing eGFR.
   a. Expect a small (< 20%) decrease when starting an ACE-I or ARB from the drop in intraglomerular pressure.
   b. This is not a true decrease in eGFR but a hemodynamic effect and is reversible with drug discontinuation (shows the drug is working).
   c. Be cautious and consider a different agent if decrease is larger than 20%.
4. These agents should not be used during pregnancy (most are Category D).

D. The dihydropyridine calcium channel blockers, such as felodipine and nifedipine, can cause edema and may require an increase in diuretic therapy.

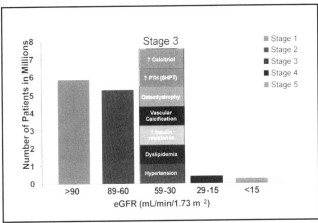

Figure 5.1. Metabolic and pathologic comorbidities as they begin to apear in CKD Stage 3.

Source: Andress, 2005; Becker et al., 2005; Elder, 2002; Kramer et al., 2005.

E. The nondihydropyridine calcium channel blockers, such as diltiazem and verapamil, are indicated to lower proteinuria if an ACE-I or ARB is contraindicated.

F. Direct vasodilators such as hydralazine and minoxidil can cause compensatory reactions including tachycardia, edema, flushing, and headaches.
1. Concomitant use of a beta-blocker or clonidine and a diuretic may reduce these side effects.
2. Minoxidil is usually reserved for patients with severe hypertension that have not responded to other therapies.
   a. Monitor for pericardial effusions.
   b. Hirsutism may preclude use in women who are unwilling to deal with this condition.

H. Diuretics.
1. Thiazides are not generally effective when the eGFR is less than 30 mL/min.
2. Thiazides, such as metolazone, may have some effect at lower eGFRs if used in combination with a loop diuretic.
3. Use caution when using a potassium-sparing diuretic, especially in combination with an ACE-I or an ARB.

VI. Diabetes and insulin resistance.

A. Treat to goal. See Chapter 29.

B. Insulin is excreted by the kidney. As eGFR decreases, patients are at increased risk of hypoglycemia.

C. Beta-blockers may mask symptoms of hypo-glycemia, also placing patients at increased risk.

D. Glyburide can cause increased hypoglycemia when eGFR is < 50 mL/min due to a build up of active metabolites and is therefore not recommended for patients with CKD stages 3 and 4.

E. Metformin is contraindicated when the SCr is > 1.5 mg/dL in males and > 1.4 mg/dL in females or the eGFR is < 60–70 mL/min due to the increased risk of lactic acidosis.

F. Increased renal insulin resistance and hyperinsulinemia have been reported in CKD patients that are neither diabetic nor hypertensive.

VII. Monitor and manage dyslipidemias.

A. Measure lipid panel at presentation, 3 months after change in status and annually thereafter.

B. If dyslipidemia is present, evaluate and/or treat secondary causes.
1. Comorbidities such as hypothyroidism, diabetes mellitus, nephrotic syndrome, alcoholism, and chronic liver disease.
2. Medications such as beta-blockers, diuretics, corticosteroids, calcineurin inhibitors, sirolimus, oral contraceptives, anticonvulsants, and antiretroviral therapy.

C. Treat the dyslipidemia.
1. Use the same initial treatment guidelines as for the general population.
2. Some agents such as fluvastatin, simvastatin, and lovastatin should not be dosed higher than 50% of the usual dose when the eGFR is < 30 mL/min. Only pravastatin and atorvastatin can be safely administered at higher doses for these patients.
3. Monitor labs as recommended for any agent selected.
4. There is an increased risk of rhabdomyolysis with the use of HMG CoA reductase inhibitors (statins) and/or fibrates. The risk is higher for a combination of both.

VIII. Cardiovascular disease (CVD).

A. Use research-based knowledge to educate and motivate patients to adhere to their plan of care.
1. Decreased eGFR is a risk factor for CVD.
2. CVD is thought to be the leading cause of death in patients with CKD stage 3.

3. Albuminuria is associated with increased risk for CVD.

B. Regardless of blood pressure, treatment with an agent that inhibits the renin-angiotensin-aldosterone system (RAAS) should be considered.
1. Drugs of choice for treatment of congestive heart failure.
2. Drugs of choice for treatment of proteinuria.
3. Preferred agents for slowing eGFR decline.

C. If patient is on digoxin, note that the dose adjustment for CKD begins at an eGFR of less than 50 mL/min.
1. Reduce dose by 25–75% depending on the eGFR.
2. Monitor for digoxin toxicity.

IX. Anemia of chronic kidney disease.

A. CKD anemia management programs.
1. Excellent initial program for CKD management clinics.
2. APN managed.
3. Model after dialysis anemia management programs.
4. Protocol driven for erythropoietic stimulating agents (ESA) and IV iron titrations done by office staff nurse, when possible.
5. Outliers reviewed by APN for further orders.
6. Medicare and other payor reimbursement generally available.
   a. Varies by state and payor.
   b. General Medicare guidelines: An SCr 2.0 mg/dL or above or eGFR less than 45 mL/min and a hemoglobin less than 11.0 g/dL with symptoms of anemia.

B. Anemia of CKD should be normocytic and normochromic. If not:
1. Check for iron deficiency and, if found, correct.
2. Check for obvious blood losses. If diagnosed, treat.
3. If other, refer to hematology for workup. Obtain vitamin B12 and folate levels.

C. Testing for all patients with CKD regardless of stage or cause.
1. Measure hemoglobin (Hb) at least annually.
2. Diagnose at Hb concentrations of
   a. < 13.5 g/dL in adult males.
   b. < 12.0 g/dL in adult females.
3. Frequently begins in CKD stage 3.

D. Initial assessment includes the following tests:
 1. Complete blood count.
 2. Absolute reticulocyte count.
 3. Serum ferritin.
 4. Transferrin saturation (TSAT) or content of hemoglobin in reticulocytes (CHr).

E. Target Hb is generally in the 11–12 g/dL range.
 1. There is insufficient evidence to recommend routine maintenance of a Hb above 13 g/dL.
 2. Quality of life benefits have been associated with sustained Hb levels above 13 g/dL.
 3. Serious adverse events have been seen with Hb >13 g/dL including:
  a. Cerebrovascular accidents.
  b. Thrombosis.
  c. Myocardial infarctions.

F. Treat with (ESAs) at least monthly.
 1. Available ESAs.
  a. Epoetin alfa (Epogen, Procrit).
   (1) Half-life is 4–13 hours when given IV.
   (2) Half-life is 20% longer in CKD patients when compared to healthy subjects.
   (3) Peak plasma levels are achieved 5–24 hours after subcutaneous administration.
  b. Darbepoetin alfa (Aranesp).
   (1) Half-life is about 3 times as long as epoetin alfa.
   (2) Currently used mainly in CKD clinics.
  c. Micera is a long-acting ESA that was recently FDA approved for use in the United States.
 2. Trending of Hb with dose adjustments as needed.
  a. Decreasing the dose but not necessarily withholding it is preferred.
  b. Scheduled doses that have been missed may be administered as soon as possible.
  c. Due to the length of time for erythropoiesis, a clinically significant rise in Hb is usually not seen in less than 2 weeks and can require up to 6 weeks in some patients.
 3. Recommended route of administration is subcutaneous for CKD stage 5 patients not on hemodialysis.

G. The patient must have adequate iron stores.
 1. Target transferrin saturation (TSAT) is 20–50%. When the total iron binding capacity (TIBC) is less than 200 ug/dL, the TSAT may be falsely elevated and not reflective of true iron status.
 2. If the content of hemoglobin in reticulocytes (CHr) is above 29 pg/cell, this denotes sufficient

available iron. There is no CHr value that denotes iron overload.
  a. There has been considerable controversy over the appropriate CHr level.
  b. In one study, patients with baseline CHr ≥ 31.2 pg/cell were 5.3 times more likely to respond to ESA and iron than patients with lower CHr levels.
 3. Target ferritin is 100 ng/mL or above.
  a. No upper limit of ferritin is recommended.
  b. When ferritin is above 500 ng/mL, the patient's clinical status, ESA responsiveness, and Hb and TSAT levels should be considered.
  c. When ferritins are above 500 ng/mL or below 100 ng/mL, the clinical status of the patient should be evaluated.
   (1) History and physical.
   (2) Laboratory workup includes C-reactive protein, WBC, and CHr (if not routinely done).
   (3) Differentiate between:
    (a) Absolute iron deficiency: insufficient iron for effective erythropoiesis (low TSAT and ferritin).
    (b) Inflammatory iron blockade: iron is blocked from leaving the reticulo-endothelial system (RES) usually from infection or inflammation. (Total iron binding capacity (TIBC) may be reduced.) IV iron should not be given during an active infection.
    (c) Functional iron deficiency: iron is mobilized too slowly from the RES to keep up with the demands of EPO-driven erythropoiesis (TIBC is generally normal to elevated). IV iron will correct.
    (d) Patients with high ferritins should be evaluated for secondary causes such as infection and inflammatory states, including malignancies that need to be diagnosed and treated.
    (e) A trial of intravenous iron may be helpful in patients without active infection. If hemoglobin does not increase or ESA dose does not decrease after 1 month, then discontinue.
 4. Treat with iron supplementation, as needed.
  a. Oral iron, once to three times daily depending on the product.
  b. Intravenous iron may still be necessary to attain or maintain targets.
 5. Monitor iron indices every 1–3 months

depending on iron status, ESA responsiveness, and the stability of the patient.

H. Other agents used as adjunctive anemia therapy, but not recommended by the NKF-KDOQI work group, include:
   1. Insufficient evidence to recommend.
      a. L-carnitine.
      b. Vitamin C.
   2. Strong recommendation NOT to use androgens.
   3. Discussed but not addressed in guidelines:
      a. HMG Co-A reductase inhibitors (statins).
      b. Pentoxifylline.
      c. Folate, B12, and other B vitamins.

X. Mineral and bone metabolism disturbances.

A. Common disturbances in mineral and bone metabolism in CKD.
   1. Secondary hyperparathyroidism (SHPT) (see Figure 5.2).
   2. Hypocalcemia.
   3. Hyperphosphatemia.
   4. Altered vitamin D metabolism.
   5. Defective intestinal absorption of calcium.
   6. Bone disease.
   7. Soft tissue calcifications including vascular calcifications.
   8. Altered handling of phosphate, calcium, and magnesium by the kidney.
   9. Proximal myopathy.
   10. Skin ulcerations and soft-tissue necrosis.

B. CKD BMD management programs.
   1. Excellent addition for CKD management clinics.
   2. APN managed.
   3. Modeled after dialysis renal osteodystrophy management programs.
   4. Protocol driven for both vitamin D and binder, titrations done by office staff nurse or renal dietitian, when possible.
   5. Outliers reviewed by APN for further orders.

C. Secondary hyperparathyroidism (SHPT).
   1. As eGFR decreases, 1,25-dihydroxycholecalciferol production decreases (see Figure 5.3), serum calcium decreases, and phosphate retention develops, resulting in secondary hyperplasia of the parathyroid glands.
   2. A decrease in the number of vitamin D receptors (VDR) develops and they become more resistant to the action of vitamin D and calcium.

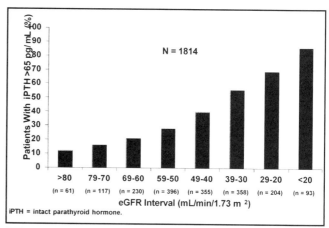

Figure 5.2. Prevalence of elevated iPTH by eGFR intervals.

Source: Bakris et al., 2005.

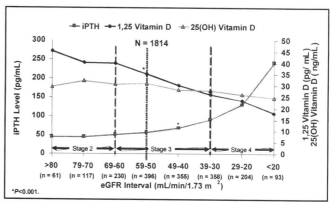

Figure 5.3. Mean values of iPTH, 1,25(OH)$_2$D$_3$, and 25(OH)D$_3$ by eGFR.

Source: Bakris et al. 2005.

   3. Progressive parathyroid gland hyperplasia and nodularity are associated with declining levels of vitamin D.
   4. Need to screen for SHPT based on CKD stage 3 and not wait for a change in calcium and phosphorus levels. These changes occur later (see Figure 5.4).
   5. Intact parathyroid hormone (iPTH) targets.
      a. Stage 3: iPTH 35–70 pg/mL.
      b. Stage 4: iPTH 70–110 pg/mL.
      c. If PTH is elevated, 25(OH)D$_3$ levels should be measured and if low, corrected.
      d. Also see XI.C. Vitamin D.
   6. iPTH monitoring.
      a. Annually in CKD stage 3.
      b. Quarterly in CKD stage 4.

c. More frequently when vitamin D therapy initiated or titrated.
   (1) Some vitamin D therapies recommend weekly to every 2-week initial monitoring.
   (2) Quarterly monitoring after being on a stable dose for 6 months.

7. Mineral goals and management.
   a. Serum calcium.
      (1) Goal: total corrected calcium should be maintained in the "normal" range for the laboratory used, preferably at the lower end of "normal."
      (2) Monitor at least every 3 months and more frequently if initiating or titrating vitamin D therapies.
      (3) Hypocalcemia can cause SHPT, have adverse effects on bone mineralization, and is associated with increased mortality.
      (4) Hypercalcemia can occur with use of calcium-containing phosphate binders and/or active vitamin D sterols. Can occur spontaneously in CKD patients. Also consider other causes, such as primary hyperparathyroidism and malignancies such as multiple myeloma.
      (5) If low, treat with calcium salts such as calcium acetate or calcium carbonate and/or oral vitamin D sterols.
      (6) If high, change to a noncalcium-based binder or reduce binder and/or stop or reduce vitamin D.
      (7) Also see XI.D.4. Calcium.
   b. Serum phosphorous.
      (1) Goal: maintain at or above 2.7 mg/dL and no higher than 4.6 mg/dL.
      (2) Monitor at least every 3 months and more frequently if initiating or titrating vitamin D therapies.
      (3) Low levels are associated with osteomalacia and malnutrition.
      (4) High levels.
         (a) Directly induce SHPT.
         (b) Indirectly contribute to SHPT by reducing conversion of $25(OH)D_3$ to $1,25(OH)_2D_3$.
         (c) Decreases ionized calcium.
         (d) Can facilitate extraskeletal calcification.
         (e) Associated with increased mortality.
      (5) Treat with dietary restriction or supplementation and phosphate binders, as needed. Calcium-based binders may be used as initial therapy.

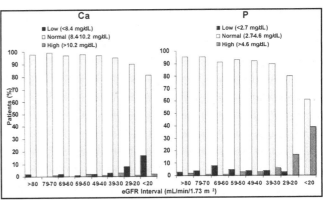

Figure 5.4. Prevalence of abnormal corrected Ca and P levels.

Source: Bakris et al., 2005.

   (6) See XI.D.3. Phosphorus.
8. Active vitamin D therapy.
   a. Start when iPTH is above goal for CKD stage and repletion of $25(OH)D_3$ and phosphate restriction have not brought iPTH into target range.
   b. Regular monitoring required, so patient should be adherent.
   c. Active vitamin D therapies.
      (1) Calcitriol (Rocaltrol®).
         (a) Active form of vitamin D3 (animal source).
         (b) Increases gut absorption of calcium and phosphorus, especially at higher doses.
         (c) Approved in the 1970s with the purpose to correct hypocalcemia.
         (d) Increases urinary calcium excretion over 100%, still in normal range.
         (e) Elimination half-life 3–8 hours.
      (2) Doxercalciferol (Hectorol®).
         (a) Inactive vitamin D2 (plant source).
         (b) Must be hydroxylated in the liver to become active.
         (c) Pivotal study showed an increased need for phosphate binders to maintain targets (patients requiring binders increased from 22% to 44% over the 24-week study).
         (d) Elimination half-life is 32–37 hours with a range up to 96 hours.
         (e) Increases urinary calcium excretion over 42%, still in normal range.
         (f) Pivotal study showed 74% of patients achieved a >/= 30% reduction in

their iPTH from baseline at weeks 20–24.

   (3) Paricalcitol (Zemplar®).
     (a) Active vitamin D2 (plant source).
     (b) Minimal calcemic and phosphatemic effects on the intestines as shown in preclinical studies.
     (c) Urinary calcium excretion nonsignifcant.
     (d) Elimination half-life is 17 hours.
     (e) In a pivotal 24-week study, 91% of the patients obtained two consecutive >/= 30% reductions in iPTH.
   (4) No head-to-head studies have been performed comparing agents.
   (5) Goals of therapy.
     (a) Efficacy: reduce/maintain iPTH in target range.
     (b) Minimal or no effect on calcium, phosphorus, and urinary calcium levels.
     (c) Prevent hyperplasia/hypertrophy and nodularity of the parathyroid gland.
     (d) Minimize bone resorption; promote bone formation; prevent bone loss.

D. Early, optimal management of SHPT can prevent and minimize the risks associated with the majority of common MBDs associated with CKD.

XI. Nutritional concerns.

A. Protein calorie malnutrition (PCM).
  1. Factors associated with PCM.
    a. Proteinuria.
    b. Anorexia.
    c. Uremia (nausea and vomiting).
    d. Depression.
    e. Socioeconomic issues.
    f. Comorbid conditions.
  2. Dietary protein intake.
    a. Though the Modification of Diet and Renal Disease (MDRD) study did not conclusively show that protein restriction slows progression of kidney disease, ad hoc analyses indicated it may retard the progression or delay the onset of kidney replacement therapy in individuals with severe CKD stage 4.
    b. Frequently, patients have spontaneous decrease in protein and energy intake when eGFR falls below 50 mL/min and even more so when eGFR falls below 25 mL/min.
    c. A positive correlation between energy intake and eGFR has been found regardless of prescribed diet.
    d. Malnutrition is linked to poor clinical outcomes.
    e. Caution should be used when instructing patients to decrease protein. NKF-KDOQI recommends considering 0.60 g/protein/kg body weight/day when eGFR is < 25 mL/min.
    f. The majority of the protein should come from high-biologic-value (HBV) sources such as meat and egg whites.
    g. Caloric intake should be 35 kcal/kg/d for adults younger than 60 years old and 30–35 kcal/kg/d above 60 years old.
    h. Monitoring should be done at regular intervals and should include both anthropometric and biochemical evaluation such as albumin, edema free actual body weight, percent standard (NHANES II) body weight, or subjective global assessment and normalized protein nitrogen appearance (nPNA) or dietary interviews and diaries.
  3. Support from a renal dietitian is invaluable.

B. Obesity.
  1. Obesity-related disorders that cause CKD.
    a. Focal segmental glomerulosclerosis (FSGS).
    b. Stone disease.
    c. Obesity-related glomerulopathy (ORG).
    d. Metabolic syndrome.
    e. Diabetes mellitus (type 2) leading to diabetic nephropathy.
  2. Persons most at risk.
    a. Those with central adiposity.
    b. Those with high waist-to-hip ratios.
  3. Dietary modifications for weight loss.
    a. Must be individualized and appropriate for their specific stage of CKD.
    b. Goal is to lighten the kidney's load of the end products of metabolism while helping the kidney maintain normal equilibrium.
    c. Weight loss of 5–10% lowers blood pressure and cholesterol levels.
    d. Healthy eating habits and exercise are essential.
    e. If no renal dietitian is available, the Dietary Approaches to Stop Hypertension (DASH) diet is appropriate for earlier stages of CKD but needs modification for protein and phosphorus as eGFR decreases.

C. Vitamin D.
  1. Vitamin D levels start to fall early in CKD (Figure 5.3).

2. Serum levels of 25-hydroxyvitamin D – 25(OH)D$_3$ – should be measured at the first visit. If normal (> 30), repeat annually.
3. If 25(OH)D$_3$ is less than 30, supplement with vitamin D2 (ergocalciferol).
4. Dicontinue use of ergocalciferol if the total corrected calcium is above 10.2 mg/dL.
5. See X. Bone Metabolism and Disease.

D. Minerals.
   1. Potassium.
      a. May be hyperkalemic or hypokalemic depending on underlying medical condition and medications.
      b. Recommended intake is 40–70 mEq/day if hyperkalemic.
      c. If hyperkalemic, avoid salt substitutes.
      d. Should be monitored closely for hyperkalemia if patient is on an ACE-I or ARB or a potassium-sparing diuretic such as spironolactone.
      e. Should be monitored closely for hypokalemia if patients on other diuretics, particularly loop diuretics.
   2. Sodium.
      a. Recommended intake is 1000–3000 mg/day.
      b. Some patients are salt sensitive and limiting sodium intake may decrease both their blood pressure and any edema they may be experiencing.
   3. Phosphorus.
      a. Generally not elevated until CKD stages 4–5, yet bones are being demineralized.
      b. Limiting phosphorus intake early (e.g., when eGFR ~50 mL/min) can in itself reduce iPTH levels.
      c. The goal for phosphorus is between 2.7 mg/dL and 4.6 mg/dL. If above goal, limit dietary phosphorus to 800–1000 mg/day adjusted for dietary protein needs.
   4. Calcium.
      a. Generally not low until CKD stages 3 and 4, yet bones are being demineralized.
      b. The goal for corrected calcium should be in the normal range for the laboratory used, preferably toward the lower end.
      c. Total elemental calcium intake including both diet and medications should not exceed 2,000 mg/day (1500 mg from binders and 500 mg from diet).
      d. If serum albumin is low, calcium will need to be corrected.
         (4-serum albumin) x 0.8 + serum calcium = corrected calcium

XII. Miscellaneous drug issues.

A. Polypharmacy is a common problem in every stage of CKD. A review of the patient's medications for any drug that could be discontinued should be done at each clinic visit.
B. Nonsteroidal antiinflammatory drugs (NSAIDs) should be avoided.
   1. NSAIDs affect prostaglandins, causing a relaxation of the afferent arteriole of the nephron.
      a. May cause a decrease in eGFR, especially with concomitant use of ACE-I or ARBs.
      b. May cause or worsen hypertension.
      c. May cause gastrointestinal bleeding.
C. Many drugs are excreted by the kidneys and require dose adjustments as eGFR declines.
D. Bisphosphonates such as alendronate should be avoided when the eGFR is less than 35 mL/min.
E. Antihistamines such as cetirizine and hydroxyzine should be decreased by 50% when the eGFR is less than 50 mL/min.
F. Antibiotics such as gentamicin and vancomycin should be decreased according to eGFR and levels monitored, as appropriate.
G. Avoid magnesium-containing drugs such as milk of magnesium (MOM), Mylanta, and Maalox. As eGFR decreases, so does the ability of the kidney to excrete magnesium.
H. Avoid enemas and laxatives that contain phosphorus.
I. Herbals, especially those obtained from foreign sources, have been associated with kidney injury and most should be avoided.
J. Check reliable sources to see if dose adjustments are needed or agent is contraindicated before prescribing drugs or herbals.

XIII. Education and preparation for kidney replacement modalities.

A. Consult published guidelines.
   1. American Nephrology Nurses' Association (ANNA).
   2. Renal Physicians Association (RPA).
   3. National Kidney Foundation (NKF).
   4. American Society of Nephrology (ASN).

B. Earlier initiation of therapy promotes better long-range outcomes. Start dialysis when subjective symptoms of uremia manifest (see stage 5).

C. Patient and family psychosocial preparation.
   1. Introduce kidney replacement therapy options early.
   2. Will require multiple repeated conversations.
   3. Encourage participation in multidisciplinary educational offerings.
   4. Patients and families need time to adjust to change in lifestyle.
   5. Focus on positives and provide constant encouragement and hope.
   6. Acknowledge fear, anxiety, and sense of loss.
   7. Refer to social worker for assessment, coping strategies. and financial assistance.
   8. Be cognizant of possible spousal abandonment.
   9. Identification and treatment of depression.

D. Peritoneal dialysis (PD).
   1. Preferred therapy on initiation of dialysis when there is residual kidney function.
   2. Requires peritoneal catheter placement.
   3. Normal serum albumin desired.
   4. May require transfer to another modality if adequacy is not achieved.
   5. Challenge to achieve adequacy of dialysis in a person with excessive body mass index and no residual kidney function.
   6. Possibility of peritonitis if sterile technique broken.
   7. Patient desires home therapy and unable to do home hemodialysis.
   8. Allows freedom in schedule.
      a. Continuous ambulatory peritoneal dialysis (CAPD).
         (1) Usually four manual exchanges of dialysis fluid daily requiring ~ 30 minutes each to complete.
         (2) Generally 4–6 hours between exchanges.
      b. Automated peritoneal dialysis (APD).
         (1) Uses a machine (cycler) to deliver dialysate through the night and then leaves fluid in for a daytime exchange.
         (2) Varied, but generally connected to the cycler 8–10 hours nightly.
      c. Times for either CAPD or APD can be adjusted to meet scheduling needs.
   9. PD contraindicated/not recommended in:
      a. Severe malnutrition or morbid obesity.
      b. Fresh intraabdominal foreign body.
      c. Bowel disease or other sources of chronic infection.

   10. Cost-effective.
   11. Fosters independence, no partner needed.
   12. Easier to arrange backup travel support.

E. In-center hemodialysis.
   1. Requires an available spot in a dialysis center and placed on a set schedule of days and time.
   2. Usually 4 hours, three times per week to achieve desired kinetics.
   3. May require additional treatments for fluid management.
   4. Childcare issues.
   5. Requires transportation to and from dialysis center.
   6. Access to the blood circulation is required and involves surgery to create an arteriovenous (AV) fistula (preferred) or AV graft.

F. Home hemodialysis.
   1. Requires space for equipment and supplies.
   2. A trained support person available during treatments is preferred.
   3. Requires specialized training.
   4. Medical adherence.
   5. Costs less than in center but more than PD.
   6. Allows greater freedom with schedule.

G. Transplantation.
   1. Performed preemptive or after initiation of dialysis.
   2. Surgically acceptable candidate.
      a. Cardiac stability.
      b. Infection free.
      c. Cancer free (usually for 2 years, but varies dependent on the type of cancer and by transplant program).
      d. Medically adherent.
      e. Financial resources available for surgery and medications.
   3. Consider age, family support, lifestyle, cognitive ability, and substance abuse.
   4. Start conversation about living donors.
   5. Refer to Medicare-approved transplant center for formal evaluation.
      a. Medical evaluation by transplant nephrologists and/or APN.
      b. Surgical evaluation by transplant surgeon.
      c. Psychosocial evaluation by social worker.
      d. Nutritional evaluation by dietitian.

H. Nondialysis management and palliative care.
   1. Patients may choose no kidney replacement therapy. Need to respect this decision.

2. Advance directive obtained. Patient has option to change mind even at the last second.
3. Involve family, clergy.
4. Involve primary care health provider and nurses caring for patient.
5. Provide education and assistance to make process as comfortable as possible.
6. Provide palliative care and/or referral to hospice care.

I. Access for dialysis.
1. Save an arm when eGFR approaches < 30 mL/min. This means no phlebotomy, IV access, or PICC lines in chosen extremity. Be aware of magnitude of possible complications, e.g., significant subclavian vein stenosis caused by subclavian vein catheterization.
2. Arrange hemodialysis access 6 months in advance when AV fistula placement is planned or 3–6 weeks in advance for AV grafts.
   a. AV fistula preferred. PTFE grafts are the next preferred type of vascular access.
   b. Timely placement obviates need for temporary catheters.
   c. Order vein mapping.
   d. Refer to vascular access surgeon.
3. Refer for peritoneal catheter placement if doing PD at least 2 weeks in advance.
4. Prepare patient psychologically for body image changes.
5. Monitor access for development, stenosis, patency, steal syndrome, and infection at every clinic visit. Refer back to surgeon immediately for any problems.
6. Lack of advance planning or late presentation can create emergency situations that may require vascular catheters. Temporary or tunneled dialysis catheters are generally considered short-term and are prone to infection. They also can increase cost, discomfort, venous stenosis, and thrombosis.

J. Patient and family education.
1. Identify resources and encourage patients and family members to be proactive in seeking out resources.
   a. Community resources are available in nephrology offices, kidney centers, and universities.
   b. Internet Web sites such as:
      (1) Home Dialysis Central www.homedialysis.org
      (2) American Kidney Fund www.akfinc.org

(3) American Association of Kidney Patients www.aakp.org
(4) Kidney Care partners www.kidneycarepartners.org
(5) Renal Support Network www.RSUhope.org
(6) National Kidney Foundation www.kidney.org
   c. Audiovisual materials.
2. Providers give education with every visit. Keep teaching sessions short and try to introduce only one new topic each visit as well as reinforce previous teachings.
3. Family expectations need to change.
   a. Patient often has decreased energy and increased difficulty in maintaining same level of activities of daily living (ADLs) due to the onset of uremic symptoms.
   b. Initiation of disability or increased absence from work and possible reduction in financial income.
   c. Encourage continued contact with renal social worker as lifestyle changes occur.
4. Follow-up nephrology clinic visits are essential and increase in frequency for monitoring of kidney function and ESA injections.
5. As eGFR drops below 30 mL/min, there is infertility but birth control and prevention of pregnancy are strongly advised.
6. Continue to reinforce taking prescribed medications and review rationale. If income drops or insurance becomes a problem, be cognizant of the costs of medications.
7. Encourage patient to maintain ongoing health care visits with primary care, diabetologist, cardiologist, dentist, and others deemed necessary to maintain optimal health.
8. Encourage and teach importance of continued exercise.
9. Encourage the patient to keep up appearances and hygiene.

K. Education for hospitals and primary care providers. Referral to nephrology specialty clinic is essential in CKD stages 3 and 4. Patients are managed by nephrologist and/or nephrology APNs, depending upon the individual state's practice laws.
1. Nephrologist and/or APN to evaluate kidney function when SCr elevates or eGFR declines from baseline.
2. Establishes diagnosis and/or performs kidney biopsy if not done earlier.

3. Initiation of any mode of dialysis requires an order from a nephrologist and/or qualified APN.
4. Surveillance of polypharmacy and potential drug interactions, especially with multiple providers such as primary care provider (PCP), cardiologists, etc.
5. Drug dose adjustment or avoidance of certain drugs as eGFR declines.

6. Early management delays progression of CKD and comorbidities.
7. Plots progression of renal disease and implements care for prevention of progression of renal disease, e.g., hypertension management and difficult to control hypertension.

<hr>

Chapter 25

APN Role in Chronic Kidney Disease Stage 5 and Hemodialysis

Purpose

Discuss ways to maintain optimal health for the patient who is in stage 5 of chronic kidney disease (CKD) and/or on hemodialysis from the perspective of the advanced practice nurse.

Objectives

Upon completion of this chapter, the learner will be able to:
1. Discuss management of the patient with CKD stage 5 not on dialysis by the APN.
2. Outline a detailed hemodialysis prescription that can be written by the APN.
3. Discuss the ongoing management and care by the APN of the patient who is on hemodialysis as appropriate.

CKD stage 5 is defined by the National Kidney Foundation – Kidney Dialysis Outcomes Quality Initiative (NKF-KDOQI) Guidelines as kidney failure with a severely decreased eGFR or < 15 mL/min/1.73 m².

I. CKD Stage 5 – not on dialysis.

A. Continuous assessment of signs and symptoms of uremia.

B. Education of patient and family regarding the disease process.

C. Continuing management of comorbid conditions as outlined in CKD stages 1–4.

1. Hypertension (HTN).
2. Diabetes mellitus.
3. Dyslipidemia and reduction of cardiovascular risk factors (see Table 5.3).

D. Continuing management of complications, as outlined for CKD stages 1–4.
1. Anemia.
2. Renal osteodystrophy/secondary hyperparathyroidism.
3. Bowel dysfunction: constipation or diarrhea.
4. Coping mechanisms of patient and family.
5. Fluid balance abnormalities.

6. Acid-base imbalances.
7. Integrity of skin and mucous membranes.
8. Neuropathy.
9. Malnutrition.
10. Sleep disorders.

E. Prepare for initiation of kidney replacement therapy or conservative therapy.
   1. Refer for access placement if not already initiated.
   2. Transplant center referral if not contraindicated.
   3. Referral to hospice if indicated.

II. CKD Stage 5 – to initiate hemodialysis treatments.

A. Initial prescription for hemodialysis to include the following:
   1. Dialyzer: considerations for prescription.
      a. NKF-KDOQI target for Kt/V$_{urea}$: minimum of 1.3 (opinion-based).
      b. Availability of dialyzers.
      c. Patient characteristics.
      d. Dialyzer characteristics (solute removal and ultrafiltration characteristics) as reviewed in Section 11.
      e. Type of delivery system to be used.
   2. Dialysis bath: interpret patient's current laboratory values to prescribe.
      a. See Section 11 for general dialysate composition.
      b. Potassium content.
      c. Calcium content.
      d. Sodium content.
   3. Dry weight.
      a. See Section 11 for fluid removal.
      b. Assess patient for volume status to include but not be limited to:
         (1) Edema.
         (2) Blood pressure.
         (3) Cardiovascular status.
         (4) Breath sounds.
   4. Flow rates.
      a. Blood flow rates to achieve target NKF-KDOQI Kt/V$_{urea}$ and appropriate for access to be used. See Section 12: Vascular Access.
      b. Dialysate flow rate to achieve target NKF-KDOQI Kt/V$_{urea}$.
      c. See Section 11 for solute removal/water removal/blood pump.
   5. Anticoagulation.
      a. Assessment.
         (1) See Section 11.

Table 5.3

Managing Cardiovascular Risk Factors

Risk Factor	Primary Prevention
Hypertension	Antihypertensive agents, ACE, ARBs suggested for all with CKD
Dyslipidemia	Lipid-lowering diet and drugs
Diabetes	Glycemic control
Tobacco use	Cessation
Physical inactivity	Exercise
Menopause	HRT
Elevated homocysteine levels	B vitamins/Folate
Thrombogenic factors	Antiplatelet therapy – ASA

         (2) Comorbid conditions that may affect bleeding.
         (3) Type of access to be used. See Section 12.
         (4) Review medications for interactions.
         (5) Allergies.
      b. Prescribe.
         (1) Type of anticoagulation to be used.
         (2) Bolus.
         (3) Hourly infusion rate.
         (4) Time to discontinue before end of hemodialysis treatment.
   6. Duration of treatment based on assessment of:
      a. The NKF-KDOQI target Kt/V$_{urea}$ – See Section 11 and NKF-KDOQI Clinical Guidelines for Hemodialysis Adequacy.
      b. Patient characteristics.
      c. Current laboratory values.
      d. Dialyzer characteristics.
      e. Type of delivery system to be used.
      f. Patient's fluid and cardiovascular status.
   7. Medications to be given during hemodialysis dialysis treatment.
      a. Erythropoietic stimulating agents such as erythropoietin alfa or darbepoeitin alfa.
         (1) NKF-KDOQI guidelines and goals of therapy: hemoglobin 11–12 g/dL (evidence-based).

(2) Assess current hemoglobin/hematocrit (Hgb/Hct).

(3) Manufacturer's product insert for dosing guidelines.

(4) Medicare guidelines for maximum dosing.

b. Vitamin D analogs: considerations.

(1) NKF-KDOQI guidelines and goals for therapy.

(a) iPTH – 150–300 mg (opinion-based).

(b) Ca++ - 8.4–9.5 mg/dL (opinion-based).

(c) PO_4 – 3.5–5.5 mg/dL (evidence-based).

(d) Ca/PO_4 product (Ca++ x PO_4) – < 55 mg^2/dL^2 (evidence-based).

(2) Intact PTH results.

(3) Serum corrected calcium level.

(4) Serum phosphorous level.

(5) Manufacturer's product insert for dosing guidelines.

c. Iron replacement therapy: considerations.

(1) NKF-KDOQI guidelines and goals for therapy: TSAT > 20% and ferritin > 100 ng/dL (evidence-based).

(2) Iron, transferrin saturation (TSAT), and ferritin levels.

(3) Signs/symptoms of inflammatory or infectious processes.

(4) Type of iron infusion product available.

(5) Manufacturer's product insert for dosing guidelines.

8. Interventions for interdialytic complications to include the following but not limited to.

a. See Section 11 for complications related to hemodialysis.

b. Pruritis.

(1) Antihistamines.

(2) Lotions.

(3) Evaluate for serum phosphorous control and educate as needed.

c. Nausea and vomiting.

(1) Antiemetics.

(2) Normal saline if indicated.

d. Hypotension.

(1) Normal saline bolus.

(2) Hypertonic normal saline.

(3) Salt poor albumin (if available).

(4) Decrease ultrafiltration.

(5) Medication review of hypertensive medications and assess patient's adherence. Educate if necessary.

(6) Cramping.

(a) Normal saline bolus.

(b) Hypertonic normal saline.

(c) Decrease ultrafiltration.

9. Ongoing laboratory values to be ordered.

a. Unit specific.

b. Guideline specific.

c. Patient specific, e.g., drug levels for digoxin or protimes/INR.

B. Ongoing assessment and management of the hemodialysis patient.

1. Access. Monitor for vascular access function as outlined in Section 12: Vascular Access.

2. Adequacy of treatments.

a. Assessment.

(1) Interpret results of kinetic modeling.

(2) Monitor prescribed and delivered dose of treatment.

(3) Monitor patient's response to treatments.

(4) Assess for signs and symptoms of dialysis inadequacy.

(5) Monitor patients adherence to dialysis prescription.

(6) Assess patient's residual urine output.

(7) Monitor vascular access function.

(8) Review patient's nutritional status.

(9) Assess patient's cardiovascular status.

(10) Monitor anemia status.

(11) Evaluate for technical difficulties with treatment.

(12) See Section 11.

(13) Review NKF-KDOQI Clinical Guidelines for Hemodialysis Adequacy.

b. Interventions.

(1) Adjust dialysis prescription to achieve the NKF-KDOQI target Kt/V_{urea}.

(2) Adjust dialysis prescription based on patient's response to treatment and kinetic modeling data.

(3) Order additional laboratory tests or diagnostic studies as appropriate.

(4) Initiate consults or referrals as necessary.

(5) If indicated educate patient regarding adherence to dialysis prescription.

3. Anemia.

a. Assessment.

(1) Interpret current laboratory values to include Hgb/Hct and iron panel.

(2) Monitor patient's response to therapy.

(3) Monitor for causes of hyporesponse.

(a) Inflammation or infection.

(b) Blood loss.

(c) Secondary hyperparathyroidism.

(d) Vitamin deficiency.

(e) Neoplasia.

(f) Malnutrition.

(g) Inadequate dialysis dose.

(h) Medication interactions.

b. Interventions.

(1) Treat anemia according to the NKF-KDOQI guidelines.

(2) Adjust medication dosage based on patient response.

(3) Order laboratory or diagnostic tests as indicated to rule out causes of hyporesponse.

(4) Consult hematology if cause of hyporesponse not easily identified.

4. Complications: interdialytic.

a. See Section 11 for possible complications.

b. Adjust therapy and prescribe interventions to correct if not already addressed in initial dialysis prescription as listed in II.A.8 in this section.

5. Diabetes mellitus if a comorbid illness.

a. Assessment.

(1) Response to prescribed therapy.

(2) Review patient-reported blood sugars.

(3) Interpret Hemoglobin A1C results and blood glucose levels.

(4) Assess for diabetic complications.

(5) Assess patient's knowledge of disease and the management of their diabetes.

b. Interventions.

(1) Educate patient regarding the disease and management. Refer to diabetes educator if further education needed.

(2) Adjust medications to achieve American Diabetes Association (ADA) goals for therapy: Hemoglobin A1C – as close to < 6% as possible without significant hypoglycemia.

(3) Refer to endocrinologist, diabetologist, or primary provider if management of the patient's diabetes is provided in those practices.

(4) Order additional laboratory tests or diagnostic tests as indicated.

(5) If indicated, initiate consults and referrals to treat complications.

(6) Prescribe therapies to alleviate or treat complications such as these listed for neuropathy.

(a) Tricyclic antidepressants.

(b) Antiseizure medications.

(c) Anti-Parkinson's medications.

6. Dry weight/volume and fluid status.

a. Assessment.

(1) Monitor patient's response to therapy.

(2) Interpret results of diagnostic studies and laboratory tests.

(3) Assess patient's understanding of fluid control.

(4) Monitor patient's adherence to therapy.

(5) See Section 11.

b. Interventions.

(1) Adjust hemodialysis prescription to achieve goal.

(2) Educate regarding benefits of fluid control.

(3) Initiate consult with interdisplinary team to provide further education as indicated.

(4) Order additional diagnostic studies and laboratory tests as indicated.

7. Dyslipidemia and reduction of cardiovascular risk factors.

a. Assessment.

(1) Interpret current laboratory values.

(2) Assess patient's cardiovascular risk status.

(3) Assess patient's knowledge of lipid control and other lifestyle changes to reduce cardiovascular risk.

b. Intervention.

(1) Order further laboratory tests as indicated.

(2) Educate regarding lipid control and lifestyle changes.

(3) Refer to dietitian for further education if indicated.

(4) Prescribe therapies to achieve the Adult Treatment Panel III (ATP III)/NKF-KDOQI guidelines for dyslipidemia.

(a) LDL < 100.

[1] Therapeutic lifestyle changes (TLC).

[2] HMG-Co A reductase inhibitors (statins).

(b) Triglycerides < 180.

[1] Fibrates.

[2] Omega 3 fatty acids.

[3] Niacin.

8. Functional status.

a. Assessment: baseline functional status to current status.

b. Intervention: initiate referrals to interdisplinary team to ensure optimal status obtained.

9. HTN: continue to monitor, educate, and adjust therapies to achieve the Seventh Report of the Joint National Committee on Prevention, Detection, Evaluation, and Treatment of High Blood Pressure (JNC 7 and NKF-KDOQI Guidelines).

10. Nutrition.
    a. Assessment.
        (1) Interpret current laboratory values.
        (2) Assess patient response to current prescribed diet.
        (3) Assess patient's knowledge regarding diet.
        (4) Assess patient's functional status that might impact nutrition.
        (5) See Section 8.
    b. Intervention.
        (1) Order further laboratory tests as indicated.
        (2) Educate patient regarding dietary needs.
        (3) Initiate referrals to interdisciplinary team.
        (4) Prescribe nutritional supplements as indicated.
11. Renal osteodystrophy/bone metabolism.
    a. Assessment.
        (1) Interpret current laboratory values.
        (2) Monitor patient's response to therapy.
        (3) Assess patient's knowledge regarding the therapies.
        (4) Monitor patient's adherence to therapy.
        (5) Monitor for financial considerations to therapy.
    b. Intervention.
        (1) Treat disorders based on the NKF-KDOQI guidelines.
        (2) Add or adjust phosphorous binder doses.
        (3) Adjust vitamin D analog doses.
        (4) Add or adjust calcimemetic doses.
        (5) Educate regarding bone metabolism and expected results and benefits of the therapies.
12. Psychosocial.
    a. Assessment.
        (1) Patient coping mechanisms.
        (2) Family coping mechanisms.
    b. Interventions.
        (1) Provide support.
        (2) Initiate referrals to the interdisciplinary team as indicated.

Chapter 26

APN Role in Acute Care

Purpose

Discuss the management of hospitalized patients diagnosed with kidney failure from the advanced practice nurse perspective.

Objectives

Upon completion of this chapter, the learner will be able to:
1. Identify roles of the nephrology advanced practice nurse in the inpatient/acute care setting.
2. Describe management strategies of the hospitalized patient diagnosed with acute kidney injury (AKI).
3. Describe management strategies of the hospitalized patient diagnosed with chronic kidney disease receiving dialysis.
4. Describe management strategies of the hospitalized patient diagnosed with chronic kidney disease not on dialysis.
5. Discuss components of the acute hemodialysis, acute peritoneal dialysis, and continuous kidney replacement therapy prescriptions.
6. Highlight complications of kidney replacement therapy in the inpatient arena.

I. **Roles of the nephrology advanced practice nurse in the inpatient setting.**

A. Assess, diagnose, and manage hospitalized patients with kidney disease in collaboration with the nephrologist.

B. Communicate hospital course and update hemodialysis (HD) orders upon discharge with outpatient HD clinic or extended care facility.

C. Counsel and educate patients regarding disease process and treatment options.

D. Serve as a resource, consultant, and mentor to the health care team.

E. Initiate and revise hospital protocols to reflect evidenced-based practice.

F. Integrate current scientific knowledge into advanced nursing practice.

G. Promote nursing research at the bedside level.

II. **The hospitalized patient with acute kidney failure.**

A. Acute kidney injury occurs in 5% of all hospitalized patients, and up to 30% of intensive care unit admissions.

B. Acute kidney injury is defined as an acute increase of the serum creatinine level from baseline (an increase of at least 0.5 mg per dL).

C. Determine etiology of acute kidney injury.
1. Prerenal is a condition causing hypoperfusion to the kidneys.
2. Intrinsic renal is actual damage to the renal parenchyma.
   a. Categorized as:
      (1) Tubular disease.
      (2) Glomerular disease.
      (3) Vascular disease.
      (4) Interstitial disease.
   b. Acute tubular necrosis (ATN), ischemic and nephrotoxic, accounts for 90% cases of intrinsic acute kidney injury.

3. Postrenal occurs if both urinary outflow tracts are obstructed or if a solitary kidney is obstructed.

D. Workup as indicated.
   1. History and physical exam.
   2. Chemistry panel and CBC.
   3. Urinalysis with urine sediment examination.
   4. Urine chemistry studies.
   5. Fractional excretion of sodium (FeNa).
   6. Autoimmune studies.
   7. Radiologic studies.
   8. Percutaneous renal biopsy.

E. General management of the patient with acute kidney injury.
   1. Support the patient while investigating the precipitating event.
   2. Correct fluid volume disturbances.
      a. Volume depletion.
         (1) Restore volume with isotonic saline.
         (2) Limit intake to output + 300–500 cc/day.
         (3) Restrict salt intake to 2 g/day.
      b. Volume overload.
         (1) Limit intake to less than output.
         (2) Diurese with loop diuretics.
         (3) Restrict salt intake to less than 2 g/day.
   3. Correct acid-base disturbances (most common is metabolic acidosis).
      a. Search for cause of acidosis by interpreting arterial blood gas.
      b. Limit protein intake to < 0.6 mEq/day.
      c. Determine amount of bicarbonate needed based on bicarbonate deficit equation. Administer bicarbonate orally or parentally.
      d. Initiate hemodialysis for severe acidosis.
   4. Correct electrolyte disturbances, most common and most dangerous is hyperkalemia.
      a. Obtain and interpret electrocardiogram (ECG).
      b. Depending on severity, the following approaches may be taken to treat hyperkalemia.
         (1) Calcium gluconate (temporary correction).
         (2) Insulin and glucose (temporary correction).
         (3) Intravenous sodium bicarbonate.
         (4) Sodium polystyrene sulfonate (Kaexylate).
      c. For severe or refractory hyperkalemia, initiate hemodialysis.
   5. Review medications daily.
      a. Adjust dosages according to kidney function and serum drug levels.

b. Discontinue all nephrotoxic agents.
   (1) Nonsteroidal antiinflammatory drugs (NSAIDs).
   (2) ACE inhibitors.
   (3) Aminoglycosides.
   (4) Avoid radiocontrast material.
6. Support nutritional needs.
   a. Patients with AKI have high energy and nitrogen needs.
   b. Consult with a dietitian.
   c. Most patients with AKI requiring dialysis have energy needs between 30 and 40 kcal/kg.
   d. Frequent dialysis or CRRT may be required to support the patient's nutritional needs and control elevations in blood urea nitrogen (BUN).
7. Focus management based on etiology once identified.
   a. Prerenal.
      (1) Correct underlying cause and remove any offending nephrotoxic agents.
      (2) Restore kidney perfusion.
      (3) Aggressively manage cardiac failure.
      (4) Consider invasive hemodynamic monitoring.
   b. Renal.
      (1) Optimize cardiovascular function and volume status.
      (2) Specific therapy based on etiology of intrinsic renal disease.
   c. Postrenal: early urologic consultation.
8. Indications to initiate hemodialysis.
   a. Blood urea nitrogen > 100 mg/dL.
   b. Serum creatinine > 10 mg/dL.
   c. Uremic signs (pericarditis, encephalopathy).
   d. Refractory or severe hyperkalemia.
   e. Refractory or severe acidosis.
   f. Severe volume overload.
9. Order insertion of dialysis catheter. If temporary access is required, a cuffed catheter is favored over a noncuffed catheter if the catheter is expected to stay in > 3 weeks.
10. Prevent complications and remove all unnecessary lines promptly.

III. ATN is the most common hospital-acquired type of acute kidney injury. Usually preceded by a prerenal condition causing hypoperfusion to the tubules.

A. Classified as ischemic or nephrotoxic ATN.
   1. Risk factors for ischemic ATN: hypotension, obstetric complications, prolonged prerenal state, sepsis, and surgery.

2. Risk factors for nephrotoxic ATN: exposure to nephrotoxic agents (aminoglycosides, amphotericin B, cisplatin, and contrast dye) or certain molecules (myoglobin released by muscle cells as seen in rhabdomyolysis).
3. Four stages of ATN.
   a. Initiating or onset.
   b. Oliguric.
   c. Diuretic.
   d. Recovery.

B. Management focuses on eliminating the cause and supporting the patient.
   1. Specific examples of management.
      a. Rhabdomyolysis: aggressive hydration, forced diuresis.
      b. Risk for contrast induced nephropathy: hydrate prior to procedure, consider acetylcysteine (Mucomyst).
C. Renal recovery from ATN typically occurs in 7–21 days.

IV. Acute HD prescription.

A. Type of dialyzer. Be familiar with the specifications on the dialyzers available in your institution.

B. Length of session (Qt).
   1. With initial treatments and when serum blood urea nitrogen > 130 mg/dL, reduce length of session.
   2. Typically 2 hours for initial treatments, 3–4 hours for subsequent treatments (usually guided by unit or hospital protocols).

C. Blood flow rate (Qb).
   1. Reduce blood flow rate with initial treatments and when serum urea nitrogen > 130 mg/dL.
   2. Typically three times the body weight in kilograms for initial treatments.

D. Dialysis frequency.
   1. Determine frequency. For example, a patient starting dialysis may dialyze 3 consecutive days and then transition to every other day.
   2. More frequent dialysis may be needed to correct extreme volume overload and/or azotemia.

E. Dialysate: customize dialysis bath to patient's needs.
   1. Base: bicarbonate (HCO_3) recommended over acetate, as the use of acetate is associated with hemodynamic instability, usual concentration of bicarbonate is 30–35 mEq/L.
      a. HCO_3 concentrations exceeding 35 mEq/L may result in metabolic alkalosis.
      b. If acetate is used (when bicarbonate not available), avoid the use of dialyzers with large surface areas and dialyzers with high efficiency and high-flux capabilities. The use of these dialyzers with an acetate bath would cause too great of an acetate accumulation.
   2. Sodium level. Usual range is 140–145 mEq/L.
      a. Higher levels may predispose the patient to increased thirst and weight gain.
      b. Lower levels enhance intradialytic hypotension, cramps, headaches, nausea, vomiting, and dialysis disequilibrium syndrome.
   3. Potassium level usually ranges from 1 to 4 mEq/L.
      a. Lower concentrations (0–1 mEq/L) may be needed for patients with excessive dietary potassium (K+) loads, hemolysis, trauma, or gastrointestinal bleeding.
      b. Higher concentrations may be needed for patients with severe cardiac disease who are at increased risk for developing dysrhythmias.
      c. Keep in mind if acidosis is being corrected this will cause a shift of potassium into the cells lowering the serum potassium.
      d. A potassium rebound occurs 1–2 hours postdialysis. Do not supplement if the patient is hypokalemic during this time frame.
   4. Calcium level usually ranges from 2.5 to 3.5 mEq/L.
      a. A positive calcium balance is desired as additional control of metabolic bone disease.
      b. Use of lower levels in the acute setting is not recommended as this will lower ionized calcium levels.
   5. Magnesium level usually ranges from 0.75 to 1.5 mEq/L.
   6. Glucose level. Usual level is 200 mg/dL (nearly normoglycemic).
      a. Dextrose is needed to prevent hypoglycemia.
      b. Sepsis, diabetes, and the use of beta-blockers are all predisposing factors for developing hypoglycemia during a HD session.
   7. Phosphorus level.
      a. Normally absent in the bath.
      b. Can be added to the bicarbonate concentrate.

F. Dialysate solution flow rate is usually 500 mL/min.

G. Dialysis solution temperature is usually 35°–37° C.

H. Ultrafiltration may range from 0 to 5 kg/session.
   1. Use ultrafiltration and/or sodium modeling to accommodate fluid removal.
   2. Avoid extreme hypotension in the acute patient as this may aggravate kidney injury (hypoperfusion) and delay recovery.

I. Anticoagulation.
   1. Standard heparin protocol.
      a. Heparin bolus followed by a continuous infusion.
      b. Heparin bolus followed by repeated boluses.
   2. Tight heparin protocol for patients at slight risk for bleeding: tighter dose of heparin bolus followed by a continuous infusion.
   3. Heparin-free for patients who are actively bleeding, have a high risk of bleeding, or in which heparin is contraindicated.
      a. Saline rinses used to minimize filter clotting.
      b. Increased blood flow rates used to minimize filter clotting.
   4. Regional citrate is an alternative to heparin-free dialysis.

J. Hyperosmolar agent is usually prescribed for first few treatments.
   1. Mannitol or dextrose.
   2. Prevents dialysis disequilibrium syndrome (rare).

V. Acute peritoneal dialysis (PD).

A. PD is a nonvascular approach to treating acute kidney injury. The use of acute peritoneal dialysis is most appropriate in patients who are hemodynamically unsuitable for HD and continuous kidney replacement therapy is not available, and in patients without functional vascular access.

B. Order insertion of peritoneal catheter.
   1. A temporary stylet catheter can be inserted if a longer dwelling peritoneal catheter cannot be placed.
   2. The temporary catheter should not stay in longer than 3 days.

C. Postop care after insertion of a new PD catheter.
   1. Minimize bacterial colonization of the exit site and tunnel.
   2. Immobilize catheter to prevent trauma to exit site and traction on catheter.
   3. Minimize intraabdominal pressure.
   4. Until healed, sterile dressing changes should be performed by trained staff only.

   5. Exit site should be kept dry (no showers or baths).
   6. Teach patient how to do self-care after healing completed, usually 2 weeks postinsertion.

D. Acute peritoneal dialysis prescription. Order for 24 hours. Review and update daily. Hourly exchanges may be required for the patient with acute kidney injury for the first few days.
   1. Choose type of therapy: continuous ambulatory peritoneal dialysis (CAPD – manual exchanges) vs. automated peritoneal dialysis (APD – cycler).
   2. Session length.
   3. Cycle fill volume.
   4. Exchange time.
      a. Inflow.
      b. Dwell.
      c. Drain.
   5. Dialysis solution (1.5%, 2.5%, 4.25%, 7.25%).
   6. Dialysis solution additives.
      a. Potassium.
      b. Heparin.
      c. Insulin.
      d. Antibiotics.

E. Order I/Os and daily weights.

F. Review total ultrafiltration daily.

G. Monitor volume status.

H. Monitor and manage uremic symptoms.

I. Monitor clearance daily.
   1. Goal of therapy is blood urea nitrogen should be < 80 mg/dL.
   2. Increase clearance by increasing dwell times or by decreasing exchange times.

J. Monitor for complications of acute PD.
   1. Incomplete drainage/abdominal complications.
   2. Infection (peritonitis, tunnel infection, exit site infection).
   3. Catheter malfunction.
   4. Hypovolemia/hypervolemia.
   5. Hypotension.
   6. Hyperglycemia.
   7. Hypokalemia.
   8. Hypernatremia.
   9. Hypoalbuminemia.

VI. The hospitalized patient with acute or chronic kidney injury.

A. Perform comprehensive health history with patient.

B. Determine etiology of acute decline in kidney function.

C. Avoid nephrotoxic agents.

D. Maintain adequate hydration.

E. Control blood pressure.

F. Monitor urine output.

G. Prepare for kidney replacement therapy, if indicated.

H. Renal biopsy if indicated.
   1. Order serial hemograms (hemoglobin/hematocrit) after biopsy.
   2. Monitor urine output.

VII. The hospitalized patient with chronic kidney disease stage 5 – not on dialysis.

A. Avoid nephrotoxic agents.

B. Maintain adequate hydration.

C. Maintain adequate blood pressure.

D. Adjust dosing of medications.

E. Monitor urine output.

F. Monitor kidney function.

G. Continue outpatient medications (erythropoietic-stimulating agents, iron replacement agents, phosphate binders, vitamin D analogs, calcimimetics, and vitamins).

H. Save arm for future access placement.

I. Early vascular referral for access.

J. Transplant referral.

VIII. The hospitalized patient with CKD stage 5 on dialysis.

A. If patient's access is a temporary dialysis catheter, activate plan for permanent access.
   1. Educate the patient and family about permanent access.
   2. Save nondominant arm.
      a. Place sign above bed: *No IVs, phlebotomy, BPs in chosen arm.*
      b. Indicate in chart that arm is being saved for future vascular access creation.
      c. Educate patient, family, and staff that arm is being saved.
   3. Obtain venous mapping of bilateral extremities.
   4. Vascular consult either while hospitalized or have patient follow up as outpatient.

B. Protect patient's AVF/AVG while hospitalized.
   1. Educate patient and staff about protecting AVF/AVG.
   2. Place sign above patient's bed: *No IVs, phlebotomy, or BPs in right or left arm.*
   3. Make note in the chart alerting other health care personnel that the patient has an AVF/AVG.
   4. Assess access with every patient encounter. Monitor for any complications or signs of infection.
   5. AVF/AVG should only be used for hemodialysis and accessed by trained dialysis staff.
   6. AVF/AVG should be cannulated according to technique outlined by NKF-KDOQI guidelines.
   7. Educate patient, family, and staff to remove compression bandages (TipStops, gauze dressings) after 2 hours.

C. Protect patient's hemodialysis catheter while hospitalized.
   1. Use catheter for hemodialysis or plasmapheresis ONLY.
   2. Hemodialysis catheters should only be accessed by trained dialysis staff.
   3. Hemodialysis catheters should be accessed according to NKF-KDOQI guidelines.
   4. Hemodialysis catheter dressing changes and catheter manipulation should be performed by dialysis-trained staff.
   5. Assess dialysis catheter exit site for signs of infection with every patient encounter.

D. Medications.
   1. Continue outpatient meds (erythropoietic-stimulating agents, iron replacement agents, phosphate binders, vitamin D analogs, calcimimetics, and renal vitamins).
   2. Review medication list daily and adjust dosages accordingly.

E. Diet.
   1. Order renal diet with appropriate fluid restriction.
   2. Consult dietitian if patient needs further instruction regarding diet or fluid restriction.
   3. Protein supplements with meals, if appropriate.
   4. Liberalize diet if patient is malnourished or not eating well.

F. Nursing care.
  1. Daily weights.
  2. I/Os.
  3. Hold medications, if appropriate, prior to dialysis.
  4. Administer appropriate medications immediately after dialysis.
  5. Feed patient prior to dialysis, order early tray if needed.
  6. Administer phosphate binders with meals.
  7. Enforce fluid restriction.
  8. Protect patient's access.

G. Minimize risk of infection.
  1. Promote meticulous hand hygiene among caregivers.
  2. Discontinue all unnecessary lines promptly (Foley catheters, IVs, etc.).
  3. Staff and patient should be masked when accessing the dialysis catheter.
  4. Give influenzae/pneumococcal vaccines prior to discharge.
  5. Give hepatitis B vaccine prior to discharge.

H. Avoid daily blood draws if unnecessary and obtain labs with dialysis.

IX. The hospitalized patient with CKD stage 5 who chooses hospice.

A. Provide the option to withdraw dialysis or not initiate dialysis.

B. Educate the patient and family of the consequences of withdrawing dialysis or not initiating dialysis.

C. Support patient's decision to withdraw from dialysis or not initiate dialysis.

D. Collaborate with social services and chaplain, if appropriate.

E. Hospice referral.

X. The hospitalized patient after kidney transplant.

A. Prescribe antirejection medications upon admission.

B. Avoid nephrotoxic agents.

C. Maintain adequate hydration.

D. Closely monitor kidney function while hospitalized.

E. Assess for allograft rejection.

F. Aggressively treat hypertension.

G. Review medication list daily.

H. Reinforce importance of continuing to take medications daily.

I. Consult social services if any financial issues arise regarding paying for medications.

XI. Hemodialysis access complications while hospitalized.

A. Catheter malfunction. Take action prior to discharging patient. May be due to catheter malposition or formation of a thrombus or fibrin sleeve.
  1. Try to run with patient's lines reversed.
  2. Order thrombolytic lock.
  3. Order thrombolytic infusion.
  4. Order catheter venogram.
  5. Exchange the catheter over a guide wire (interventional radiology).
  6. Insert new catheter in another site (consult interventional radiology).

B. Suspected catheter infection.
  1. Use of catheters for hemodialysis is the most common risk factor for bacteremia.
  2. Obtain blood cultures.
  3. *Staph aureus* is the leading cause of exit site infections and bacteremia in hemodialysis patients.
  4. Order appropriate antibiotic coverage.
  5. Consult with infectious disease.
  6. Remove dialysis catheter, if indicated.
  7. If dialysis catheter is removed, coordinate insertion of a new catheter. Criteria:
    a. Surveillance blood cultures negative.
    b. Afebrile for 48 hours.

C. Poor blood flow rates (Qb) with AVF/AVG.
  1. Shuntogram to evaluate patency.
  2. Vascular consult.
  3. Angioplasty/stent placement.
  4. Thrombolytic infusion.

D. Suspected steal syndrome.
  1. Shuntogram to evaluate patency.
  2. Vascular consult.
  3. Coordinate insertion of dialysis catheter with dialysis schedule, if indicated.

E. Hemorrhage.

F. Vascular or visceral organ injury.

XII. Most common patient complications during hemodialyis.

A. Hypotension (20–30%).

B. Cramps (5–20%).

C. Nausea and vomiting (5–15%).

D. Headache (5%).

E. Chest pain (2–5%).

F. Back pain (2–5%).

G. Itching (5%).

H. Fever and chills (less than 1%).

XIII. Measures to minimize intradialytic hypotension while hospitalized.

A. Ensure patients eat prior to their hemodialysis session and not during hemodialysis session.

B. Order antihypertensive medications to be held prior to dialysis (as appropriate depending on patient and timing of dialysis).

C. Minimize hyptotension by avoiding excessive ultrafiltration.

D. Slow the ultrafiltration rate.

E. Perform isolated ultrafiltration.

F. Increase the dialysate sodium concentration as appropriate.

G. Switch from acetate to bicarbonate-buffered dialysate.

H. Proper positioning of patient during HD session.

I. Reduce the dialysate temperature.

J. Administer Amantine (midodrine) predialysis.

K. Correct anemia.

L. Administer supplemental oxygen.

M. Reevaluate dry weight systematically after each hemodialysis session.

XIV. The hospitalized patient on chronic PD.

A. Assess volume status and labs.

B. Order peritoneal dialysis prescription. Refer to aforementioned components of the peritoneal dialysis prescription.
  1. Tailor chronic prescription based on assessment.
  2. Update prescription daily.

C. Protect patient's catheter while hospitalized.
  1. Care of the PD catheter should be performed by staff trained in PD or trained patients.
  2. Aseptic technique should be used.
  3. Educate and insure that catheter is anchored/secured to abdomen.

D. Exit site care.
  1. Evaluate the organisms causing exit site infections at your institution.
  2. Institute an appropriate protocol to minimize risk (exit site application of mupirocin or gentamicin, or intranasal mupirocin).

E. Surgical procedures may increase risk for peritonitis.
  1. Consider prophylactic antibiotics prior to certain procedures.
  2. Drain the peritoneal cavity prior to any procedures involving the abdomen or pelvis.

F. Bowel program. Constipation predisposes peritoneal dialysis patients to bowel sources of infection.
  1. Assess patient's bowel patterns.
  2. Ensure patient is adequately hydrated.
  3. Order agents to reduce constipation while hospitalized.
  4. Treat hypokalemia.

G. Prevent infection.
  1. Meticulous hand hygiene among all caregivers.
  2. Remove all unnecessary lines promptly (e.g., Foley catheters).
  3. Administer appropriate vaccinations prior to discharge (influenza, pneumoccocal, hepatitis B).

XV. Infectious peritoneal catheter complications while hospitalized.

A. Peritonitis.
  1. Symptoms include cloudy effluent, abdominal pain, and fever.
  2. Obtain stat cell count and differential.
  3. Obtain gram stain and culture on initial drain.
  4. Obtain abdominal film if bowel source suspected.
  5. Diagnosis of peritonitis is supported by an elevated effluent count of white blood cells (WBC) of more than 100/mm^3, of which at least 50% are polymorphonuclear neutrophils (PMNs).
  6. Initiate empiric therapy covering both gram-positive and gram-negative organisms.
     a. Empiric therapy should target organisms that

are causing peritonitis at your institution and the patient's history of previous organisms.

b. Gram-positive may be covered by vancomycin or a cephalosporin. Gram-negative may be covered by a third-generation cephalosporin or aminoglycoside.

7. Narrow antibiotic coverage once sensitivities are obtained. Refer to the International Society for Peritoneal Dialysis (ISPD) Peritonitis Guidelines to guide therapy (see Table 5.4).

8. Clinical improvement should be seen within 72 hours after therapy is initiated.

9. Patients who fail to improve within 72 hours should be evaluated closely on a day-to-day basis.
   a. Consider catheter removal if symptoms persist after appropriate antibiotic therapy.
   b. Continue antibiotics for 1 week after catheter removal.
   c. Consider CT to evaluate for abscess formation.
   d. Consider surgical consult.

10. Duration of treatment is determined based on organism.
    a. Gram-positive peritonitis and culture-negative peritonitis should be treated for at least 1 week after a clear dialysate (< 100 leukocytes/mm³) and negative cultures have been obtained (total length of therapy typically 10–14 days).
    b. Uncomplicated peritonitis due to a gram negative organism should be treated for 21 days.

c. Multi gram-negative organism peritonitis has high relapsing rates, so catheter removal should be considered. If catheter is not removed, antibiotic therapy should continue for 21 days. CT scan should be considered to evaluate for abscess formation.
    d. Fungal peritonitis should be treated for 4 weeks.

11. Order pain medications.
12. Promote protein intake.
13. If patient unable to continue peritoneal dialysis, transition patient to hemodialysis.

B. Exit site infection (ESI).
   1. An ESI is defined by the "presence of purulent drainage with or without erythema of the skin at the catheter epidermal interface."
   2. Obtain gram stain and culture of drainage.
   3. *S. aureus* and *P. aeruginosa* are the most common exit site pathogens.
   4. Initiate empiric antibiotic therapy based on gram stain if condition warrants, or delay therapy until sensitivities available.
   5. Avoid the use of vancomycin in routine treatment of exit site infections due to the threat of vancomycin-resistant enterococcus (VRE).
   6. Oral therapy is as effective as intraperitoneal, with the exception of methicillin-resistant *S. aureus*.
   7. Order appropriate antibiotic coverage.
      a. Gram-positive organism: oral penicillinase-

Table 5.4

Empiric Initial Therapy for Peritoneal Dialysis-Related Peritonitis Stratified for Residual Urine Volume

Antibiotic	Residual urine output	
	< 100 mL/day	> 100 mL/day
Cefazolin or cephalothin	1 g/bag, qd or 15 mg/kg BW/bag, qd	20 mg/kg BW/bag, qd
Ceftazidime	1 g/bag, qd	20 mg/kg BW/bag, qd
Gentamicin, tobramycin, netilmycin	0.6 mg/kg BW/bag, qd	Not recommended
Amikacin	2 mg/kg BW/bag, qd	Not recommended

qd = daily   BW = body weight

Source: International Society for Peritoneal Dialysis (ISPD) Peritonitis Guidelines.

resistant penicillin, cephalexin, or sulfa-methoxazole trimethoprim. Add rifampin 600 mg if slow to respond or severe case of *Staph aureus*. Avoid the use of vancomycin.
   b. Gram-negative organism: oral fluoroquinolone.
8. Continue therapy until exit site appears normal. Minimum length of treatment is 2 weeks.
9. Increase exit site care to twice daily.
10. If infection persists after 3–4 weeks of appropriate antibiotic therapy, catheter removal should be considered.

C. Tunnel infection.
   1. A tunnel infection is defined by erythema, edema, and/or tenderness over the sub-cutaneous pathway, and may be characterized by intermittent or chronic, purulent, or bloody drainage, which discharges spontaneously or after pressure is placed on the cuff.
   2. Usually occurs in the presence of a exit site infection.
   3. Most common organisms are *S. aureus* and *P. aeruginosa*.
   4. Diagnosis is made based on ultrasound findings of fluid around the subcutaneous tunnel.
   5. Tunnel infections usually require catheter removal.

XVI. Drug dosing.

A. Measure kidney function.

B. Dose drugs accordingly with decreased kidney function.

C. Dose drugs accordingly based on type of kidney replacement therapy.
   1. CAPD.
   2. APD.
   3. HD.
   4. CRRT.

D. Monitor closely for adverse drug reactions.

E. Measure plasma drug concentrations/drug levels (e.g., digoxin, vancomycin).

XVII. The critically ill patient requiring continuous kidney replacement therapy (CRRT).

A. Perform comprehensive patient assessment.

B. Order insertion of dialysis catheter.
   1. Cuffed, longer dwelling dialysis catheter.
   2. Temporary nontunneled, noncuffed dialysis catheters.
      a. Associated with high rates of infection.
      b. Should not be left in place longer than 7 days.
         (1) Track time of insertion.
         (2) Order new catheter insertion as indicated.
      c. Femoral temporary catheters.
         (1) Easier technique insertion; however, associated with higher rates of infection.
         (2) Order strict bed rest and knee immobilizer to prevent kinking of the catheter.

C. Educate patient and family regarding the goals of CRRT.

D. Order CRRT prescription.

E. Evaluate patient's status daily and adjust prescription accordingly.

F. Manage electrolyte replacements and parental nutrition orders while patient is on CRRT.

G. When patient is stable, coordinate transition to HD if needed.

H. Prepare patient and family regarding transition to HD.

XVIII. Continuous kidney replacement therapy (CRRT) prescription.

A. Type of therapy to be delivered: SCUF, CVVH, CVVHD, CVVHDF.

B. Blood flow rate.

C. Replacement flow rate.

D. Dialysate flow rate.

E. Patient hourly fluid removal rate.

F. Anticoagulation.

G. Labs are frequency based on patient's condition, typically between every 6 and 12 hours.
   1. Chemistry panel including phosphorus, magnesium, and ionized calcium.
   2. Coagulation profile.
   3. CBC.

H. Specific parameters in which to be notified (e.g., filter clotting, hemodynamic changes).

I. Strict bed rest.

J. I/Os.

K. Daily weights.

XIX. Kidney replacement therapy complications while hospitalized.

A. Intradialytic hypotension/hemodynamic compromise.
   1. Volume depletion.
   2. Solute disequilibrium.
   3. Vasodilation.

B. Extracorporeal circuit associated complications.
   1. Bioincompatibility.
   2. Mechanical dysfunction.
   3. Microbiologic or chemical contamination.
   4. Anticoagulation.

C. Electrolyte and metabolic complications.
   1. Electrolyte depletion states (hypophosphatemia, hypokalemia, hypomagnesemia).
   2. Acid base imbalances.
   3. Vitamin and micronutrient depletion.
   4. Glycemic control (hyperglycemia, hypoglycemia).
   5. Amino acid depeletion.
   6. Thermal balance.

D. Human error.

Chapter 27

APN Role in Transplantation

Purpose

Discuss the concepts of kidney and pancreas transplantation from an advanced practice nurse perspective.

Objectives

Upon completion of this chapter, the learner will be able to:
1. Discuss the role of the advanced practice nurse in the transplant setting.
2. Describe the evaluation process of the transplant recipient from an advanced practice perspective.
3. Discuss the advanced practice nurse's role during the perioperative care of a transplant recipient.
4. Outline management strategies used by the advanced practice nurse in managing short-term and long-term complications.
5. Discuss the health maintenance strategies in the transplant recipient.

I. Role of the Advanced Practice Nurse (APN) in the transplant setting.

The advanced practice nurse "must be able to assess, conceptualize, diagnose, and analyze complex clinical and nonclinical problems" related to the transplant patient. This care can be delivered through the role of direct caregiver, coordination of care, consultative, educator, researcher, or administrative.

In the transplant patient, this includes assessment and management of acute and chronic conditions, management of immunosuppression, preoperative and postoperative care, perioperative and ongoing patient education, detection and treatment of allograft dysfunction, and management of long-term complications. The care of the transplant recipient is usually in collaboration with other health care providers, depending on state practice laws and the individual practice setting.

II. Evaluation of the patient for candidacy for transplantation.

A. Comprehensive history and physical of potential transplant recipient.
1. Determine cause of chronic kidney disease.
2. Assessment of indications for transplant.
3. Determine if any absolute contraindications to transplant exist.
4. Comprehensive assessment of all body systems.
5. Comprehensive assessment of all positive findings and comorbidities.
6. Assessment of potential for infection.
7. Psychosocial screening.
8. Review dietitian evaluation.

B. Interpretation and review of all diagnostic studies.
1. Comprehensive review of serologies, tissue typing, ABO.
2. Comprehensive review of all laboratory studies including chemistries, CBC, urinalysis, PSA, etc., as indicated.
3. Comprehensive review and interpretation of all radiologic studies including chest x-ray, ultrasonography, cardiac stress test, mammography, and others as indicated.
4. Review of all screening studies including colonoscopy, PAP smear, dental screening, and others as indicated.

C. Patient education.
1. Determination of patient's ability to learn.
2. Evaluation process.
3. Transplant process.
4. Risks and benefits of transplant procedure.
5. The waiting time for transplant, when to notify the transplant center, what to do when called.
6. Risks and benefits of long-term immunosuppression.
7. Signs, symptoms, implication of rejection.
8. Signs and symptoms of infection.

III. Perioperative care of the living donor.

A. Comprehensive history and physical of potential donor.
1. Review health history and physical assessment.
2. Determine if any contraindications to donation.
3. Comprehensive assessment of all body systems.
4. Assessment of potential for current infection.
5. Psychosocial screening.

B. Interpretation and review of all diagnostic studies.
1. Comprehensive review of serologies, tissue typing, ABO.

2. Comprehensive review of all laboratory studies including chemistries, CBC, urinalysis, PSA, 24-hour urine, etc., as indicated.
3. Comprehensive review and interpretation of all radiologic studies including chest x-ray, EKG, spiral CT, or MRI/MRA to document anatomy of kidneys, ureters, bladder, and others as indicated.

C. Patient education.
1. Determination of patient's ability to learn.
2. Evaluation process.
3. Risks and benefits of donation procedure.
4. Review recovery time and activity level after donation.
5. Follow-up care.

D. Additional preparation for surgery.
1. Shower and skin preparation.
2. Order antibiotics as indicated.
3. Final patient and family education regarding the procedure, timing, and postoperative care.

E. Postoperative management.
1. Comprehensive physical assessment.
   a. Pulmonary function.
   b. Cardiovascular function.
   c. Urine output.
   d. Fluid balance.
   e. Electrolytes.
   f. Infection.
2. Assess for complications.
   a. Kidney function.
   b. Bleeding.
   c. Fluid and electrolyte balance.
   d. Infection.
      (1) Pulmonary.
      (2) Wound.
3. Pain control.
4. Emotional support.
5. Patient education.

IV. Perioperative care of the transplant recipient.

A. Admission history and physical.
1. Review all of previous workup in addition to any recent and current illnesses that may impact ability to receive transplant.
2. Assess timing of last dialysis treatment and determine if an additional treatment is needed prior to surgery.
3. Review current laboratory values to detect any abnormalities that may preclude transplant.
4. Interpret current chest x-ray and EKG.

B. Additional preparation for surgery.
 1. Shower and skin preparation.
 2. Order antibiotics as indicated.
 3. Order induction immunosuppression, if indicated.
 4. Determine results of final cytotoxic crossmatch.
 5. Final patient and family education regarding the procedure, timing, and postoperative care.

C. Postoperative management.
 1. Comprehensive physical assessment.
    a. Pulmonary function.
    b. Cardiovascular function.
    c. Urine output.
    d. Fluid balance.
    e. Electrolytes.
    f. Infection.
 2. Evaluate kidney function.
    a. Monitor for signs of delayed graft function.
    b. Assess need for dialysis: hyperkalemia, fluid overload, etc.
    c. Assess for possible complications and order diagnostic studies as appropriate.
       (1) Renal artery thrombosis.
       (2) Renal vein thrombosis.
       (3) Ureteral leak.
    d. Monitor for possible rejection. Follow closely for signs and symptoms of rejection.
       (1) Hyperacute.
          (a) Onset is minutes to hours.
          (b) Results of preformed antibodies from antidonor antibodies and complement.
          (c) Signs and symptoms: sudden loss of urine output, fever, systemic toxicity, and pain in the area of graft placement.
          (d) Ischemia, acidosis, hypoxia occur in transplanted tissue.
          (e) Transplant nephrectomy necessary for treatment.
       (2) Acute.
          (a) Onset is days to weeks.
          (b) Caused by activation of T lymphocytes.
          (c) Signs and symptoms: increased creatinine and BUN, decreased urine output, electrolyte imbalances, edema, graft tenderness, fever, elevated leukocyte count, malaise.
          (d) Usually treated with increased immunosuppression.
       (3) Chronic rejection/chronic allograft nephropathy.
          (a) Onset is months to years.
          (b) Cause is unclear, but is likely a

combination of T lymphocyte and B lymphocyte mediated rejection.
          (c) Signs and symptoms can be asymptomatic but usually there is a slow rise in serum creatinine and onset of proteinuria.
          (d) There is no successful treatment.
    e. Order kidney transplant biopsy as appropriate.
 3. Order immunosuppression.
    a. Follow response to medications.
    b. Monitor for side effects.
    c. Adjust medications based on kidney function, drug trough levels.
 4. Assess wound for complications.
    a. Nonhealing.
    b. Infection.
    c. Drainage.
    d. Lymphocele.
    e. Hematoma.
 5. Assess for complications.
    a. Posttransplant diabetes mellitus.
    b. Hypophosphatemia.
    c. Hyperkalemia.
    d. Hypomagnesemia.
 6. Order prophylactic medications.
    a. Antivirals.
    b. Antibiotics.
    c. Proton pump inhibitor/H_2 antagonist.
 7. Continue postoperative teaching.
    a. Assess patient's ability to learn and understand medications.
    b. Assess understanding of home treatment regimen and follow-up.
    c. Continue patient education as appropriate.
    d. Collaborate with other members of health care team.

V. Long-term management of transplant recipient.

A. Periodic visits for assessment and management of health problems related to transplant.
 1. Renal dysfunction.
    a. Determine if patient is taking nephrotoxic medications (angiotensin-converting enzyme inhibitors [ACE-I], angiotensin receptor blockers [ARBS], nonsteroidal inflammatory drugs [NSAIDs], aminoglycosides, etc.).
    b. Determine if recent changes in health (diarrhea, nausea, vomiting, edema, etc.).
    c. Determine if acute or chronic change.
    d. Check drug trough levels.
    e. Evaluate for proteinuria and edema.
    f. Order appropriate diagnostic studies, as indicated.

(1) Ultrasound.
(2) CT scan.
(3) MRI/MRA.
g. Order biopsy and treat accordingly.
(1) Acute rejection.
(2) Calcineurin inhibitor toxicity.
(3) Chronic allograft nephropathy.
(4) BK virus.
(5) Recurrent disease.
2. Management of immunosuppression.
a. Wean immunosuppression per individual transplant center protocol.
b. Adjust immunosuppression based on side effects, toxicity, or patient's response to treatment.
3. Evaluate for signs and symptoms of infection, particularly opportunistic infections. Treat accordingly.
a. CMV.
b. BK virus.
c. Bacterial infections.
d. Viral infections.
e. Fungal infections.
f. *Pneumocystis carinii.*
g. *Nocardia.*
h. *Aspergillus.*
i. Administer vaccines as appropriate (live vaccines are contraindicated).
4. Evaluate for malignancy.
a. Routine health screenings.
(1) Colonoscopy.
(2) PAP smear.
(3) Mammography.
(4) PSA.
(5) Yearly complete physical exam.
b. Posttransplant lymphoproliferative disorders (PTLD).
(1) Linked to Epstein-Barr virus.
(2) Suspect with any weight loss, night sweats, unexplained fevers.
5. Diabetes.
a. Tight glycemic control using oral agents and/or insulin.
b. Follow guidelines for general population (DCCT, 1993).
6. Hypertension.
a. Control of blood pressure < 130/80 as per JNC 7 guidelines.
b. Use of multiple agents to control blood pressure is common.
7. Hyperlipidemia.
a. Follow lipid profiles at least quarterly.
b. Lifestyle modifications.
c. Follow ATP III treatment guidelines.

d. Treatment with HMG-coenzyme A inhibitors (statins) and other agents as needed.
e. Careful monitoring for drug interactions.
(1) Monitor liver function and creatine kinase (CK) levels.
(2) Mild: myositis, increased liver function tests.
(3) Severe: rhabdomyolysis with cyclosporine and possibly sirolimus (rare).
(4) Symptoms usually resolve quickly with cessation of medication.
8. Osteoporosis.
a. Bone density scan (DEXA) screening every 1–2 years.
b. Weight-bearing exercise and calcium supplementation as appropriate.
c. If normocalcemic, consider bisphosphonate or calcitonin.
9. Chronic kidney disease.
a. Nearly all kidney transplant recipients have some degree of renal insufficiency.
b. Treatment dependent on stage as per NKF-KDOQI guidelines.
10. Cardiovascular disease.
a. Lifestyle modifications.
b. Control of blood pressure, diabetes, hyperlipidemia.
c. Smoking cessation.
d. Weight control.
e. Consider yearly stress test and follow-up care with cardiology.
11. Health maintenance.
a. Encourage follow-up with local nephrologist and primary care provider.
b. Yearly complete physical exam.
c. Surveillance studies (age-appropriate).
(1) Colonoscopy.
(2) Mammography.
(3) Pap smear.
(4) PSA.
d. Immunizations (no live vaccines).
(1) Flu vaccine.
(2) Pneumococcal.
(3) Tetanus.
(4) Others, as appropriate.
e. Maintain a healthy weight.
f. Exercise.
12. General principles of management of long-term complications (Danovitch, 2005).
a. Minimize immunosuppression.
b. Be alert for nonadherence.
c. Monitor kidney function closely.
d. Encourage a healthy lifestyle.

Exemplar

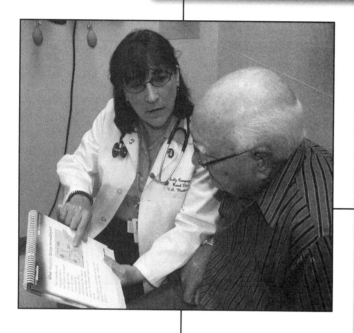

The advanced practice nurse (APN) in the nephrology specialty, by virtue of education, training, certification, state regulations, and documented competencies, is able to provide safe, competent, high-quality care in a cost-effective manner, according to the American Nephrology Nurses' Association (ANNA) APN Position Statement (2005).

The APN, not only addresses the disease process, but also health promotion and disease prevention, while minimizing complications along the continuum of chronic kidney disease (CKD).

ANNA recognizes the Nurse Practitioner (NP) and Clinical Nurse Specialist (CNS) as two of the APN roles that work in nephrology. It is important to stress that in each title of the APN role is the word "nurse." It is the nurse who integrates the disease process with the total person, encompassing all aspects of the individual, including their social, psychological, spiritual, and physical well-being.

The nurse incorporates the family into the health care regimen as the patient will allow. With skills in education, the nurse can assess for learning readiness, barriers to learning, and implement an individual education program to meet each patient's needs.

In 2000, the renal physicians and I collaborated on the development of a CKD clinic, which would be implemented by me, a Nurse Practitioner. The doctors recognized, with the increasing numbers of patients needing kidney replacement therapy, that the Nurse Practitioner was a cost-effective alternative that would allow them more time to handle acute cases and new consults. They understood that the patients with estimated glomerular filtration rate (eGFR) less than 30 mL/min, needed more time, education, and planning for future options, than they could provide.

Using Pereira's article (2000) as our reference, I developed a clinic structure that included education of treatment options and referrals to appropriate services, such as vascular surgery, interventional radiology, nutrition, and social services. From the onset, I wanted my clinic to be based upon outcomes measures. The measures identified were completion of at least one formal education session; laboratory parameters such as hemoglobin and hematocrit, calcium, phosphorus, albumin; initiation of hepatitis B vaccination series before the patient went to his first dialysis, and placement of arterial venous fistula (AVF) before the first dialysis.

Throughout the years, these outcomes still form the basis of my CKD clinic. Use of NKF-KDOQI guidelines provided the baseline for the outcomes. While I adhered to the guidelines as much as possible, I recognized individual issues did not always fit the guidelines and modified my approach to fit that person's individualized needs.

As a nurse, my strengths are assessment of the total person and integration of the medical issues into a holistic approach that is individualized for each person. I work to form a partnership with each patient and to work with that person from his level of acceptance and understanding, not mine.

My clinic has the luxury of 30-minute appointment

Continues on next page

times. Most of the clinic time is devoted to listening to the patient, checking for understanding of previous education, medication regimen, concerns about his/her disease process and its effects on his relationships, and ongoing education about the person's stage of CKD, what to expect, medications changes, and laboratory results.

Each patient receives a report card when the lab results come back. The report card includes the eGFR, stage of CKD, anemia and iron parameters, calcium, phosphorus, vitamin D-25, intact parathyroid hormone level, albumin, and potassium. Along with each laboratory test is an explanation of the test and an action plan. Patients want to know, "What's my kidney number?" Often, a family member attends the clinic and actively participates in the action plan.

The outcomes of my clinic were summarized in an article published in 2007 (Lee et al., 2007). A retrospective review of all patients who started dialysis over a 5-year period was done on the quality-of-care indicators at the initiation of dialysis and all-cause hospitalization for the first year after dialysis. The patients were divided into two groups based upon which clinic they attended — the nephrologist-in-training vs. the nurse practitioner clinics. There were no differences between the cohort groups in demographics or the length of time followed in clinic before dialysis.

At the initiation of dialysis, patients in the NP CKD clinic had statistically significant higher hemoglobin and serum albumin levels, higher percentage of functioning AVF, and lower all-cause hospitalizations in the first year on dialysis.

As a Nurse Practitioner, I am proud of what I have accomplished to improve the care of persons with CKD. I could not have done this without the collaboration of the medical team, who have offered their time, expertise, and support of my role and participation in the renal clinics. Their respect of my unique contributions and willingness to expand my responsibilities make this job truly fulfilling and rewarding.

Sally Campoy

References

American Nephrology Nurses' Association (ANNA). (2005). *APN position statement* (Revised and reaffirmed, 2005). Pitman, NJ: Author.

Lee, W., Campoy, S., Smits, G., Vu Tran, Z., & Chonchol, M. (2007). Effectiveness of a chronic kidney disease clinic in achieving K/DOQI guideline targets at initiation of dialysis – A single centre experience. *Nephrology Dialysis Transplantation, 22*(3), 833-838.

Pereira, B.J.G. (2000). Optimization of pre-ESRD care: The key to improved dialysis outcomes. *Kidney International, 57,* 351-365.

Photo courtesy of Sally Campoy

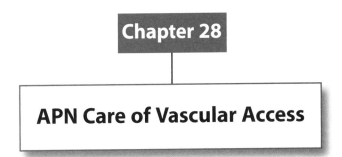

Chapter 28

APN Care of Vascular Access

Purpose

The purpose of this chapter is to augment the nursing process detailed in the general section on vascular access with those actions that require the educational preparation and licensure of an APN and that are in accordance with the clinical guidelines for advanced practice nursing care .

Objectives

Upon completion of this chapter, the learner will be able to:
1. Discuss the role of the advanced practice nurse in the comprehensive assessment and management of vascular access.
2. Describe the augmented role that the advanced practice nurse fulfills as a vascular access coordinator.
3. Discuss the advanced practice nurse's role as a mentor to staff nurses in the hemodialysis unit in the use of the nursing process to care for vascular access.
4. State the components of the leadership role that the advanced practice nurse could take in the CQI process with the vascular access team (VAT).

Introduction

Two distinct roles have evolved for the APN in the care of the hemodialysis vascular access in collaboration with a nephrologist. The more common is as a provider of the comprehensive patient medical/nursing management for a defined caseload. The second role is as dedicated vascular access coordinator with the expanded role to assess, diagnose, treat, and refer for both the creation and maintenance of vascular access for hemodialysis. The added benefit of having an APN as part of the vascular access team (VAT) is the potential for mentoring less experienced nurses in the day-to-day management of vascular access.

I. Assessment.

A. Assess the CKD patient's peripheral vascular and cardiovascular system for immediate and future access interventions:
   1. Perform history and physical examination.
   2. Calculate eGFR to stage CKD.
   3. Project time to initiation of dialysis.
   4. For the patient who is already on dialysis and has a functioning forearm graft in place, observe for AVG outflow vein that could be converted to fistula (FFBI change concept known as "sleeves up").

B. Monitor the patient's vascular access function.
   1. Perform thorough evaluation of new fistula creation within 2 weeks postop to assess maturation (see Rule of 6's in Table 12.2 in Section 12).
      a. Increased flow.
      b. Vein expansion.
      c. Wall thickening.
      d. Stenosis-free outflow vein.
   2. Perform periodic access monitoring and surveillance on established functional access.
      a. Interdialytic physical exam including:
         (1) Hemodynamic compromise, especially in high flow AVFs.
         (2) Neurologic dysfunction secondary to:
            (a) Access surgery as evidenced by pain, tingling, numbness, or diminished function.
            (b) Pressure on the recurrent laryngeal nerve by swelling from superior vena cava syndrome as evidenced by hoarseness.
            (c) Pressure on the optic nerve by swelling from superior vena cava syndrome as evidenced by visual disturbances.
      b. Review dialysis adequacy laboratory results and resulting trend.
      c. Review mechanical surveillance results.

II. Intervention.

A. Collaborate with the nephrologist to formulate a plan for hemodialysis access.
   1. Order vein mapping/evaluation to identify prospective fistula sites with artery > 2mm and vein >2.5 mm.
   2. Educate patient about vein preservation for future access creation.
   3. Give patient a card with your contact information and the prescription for vein preservation when referred to other health care personnel.
   4. Teach patient weight-bearing exercises to increase venous flow and build muscle to support and define veins.
   5. Determine patient's risk for fistula failure to mature using the REDUCE FTM I rule, which describes a preoperative, clinical prediction rule to determine fistulas that are likely to fail to mature (FTM) if created (see Table 5.5).
   6. Refer to vascular surgeon for "fistula only" creation if patient will need hemodialysis within 12 months.
   7. Monitor PD patients for adequacy of dialysis and refer for AVF evaluation should HD be the potential KRT in less than 12 months.
   8. Plan for AVG within 6 weeks for HD initiation if no AVF possibility.
   9. CVC will not be placed till initiation if no other options available. A tunneled, cuffed catheter is preferred (over a short-term non-cuffed catheter) to minimize risk for infection, dislodgement, and a replacement procedure.

B. Refer for echocardiogram to further evaluate hemodynamic complications related to the fistula that has flows > 1.5 L.

C. Order laboratory tests (hypercoagulable testing) and diagnostic studies as appropriate to assessment findings.

D. Collaborate with nurses and technicians for initiation and/or complications of cannulation.

E. Modify intradialytic heparinization orders to prevent extracorporeal clotting and minimize postdialysis bleeding.

F. Initiate evaluation and treatment of fistula or graft complications:
   1. Hemodynamically significant venous stenosis (one that reduces the intraluminal diameter > 50% and is symptomatic, e.g., significantly reduces flow to 400–500 mL/min in an AVF and < 600 mL/min in an AVG or increases intragraft pressures).
   2. Thrombosis.
   3. Infection.
   4. Graft degeneration and pseudoaneurysm formation if risk of rupture or evidence of spontaneous bleeding, thinning of skin overlying pseudoaneurysm if compromised, or available puncture sites are limited.
   5. Ischemia in limb.

Table 5.5

Reduce FTM I Prediction Rule

The four categories and associated score that predict risk of failure to mature are:

a. Age > 65 years	+2.0
b. White race (has a protective effect)	-3.0
c. Peripheral vascular disease	+3.0
d. Coronary artery disease	+2.5
e. Baseline risk	+3.0

There is a possible total of 10.5 for nonwhite patients and the risk and suggested clinical application associated with the score is:

Score	Risk Category	Clinical Application
< 2	Low risk: 25%	Do physical exam with or without duplex ultrasound; create AV.
2.0 to 3.0	Moderate risk: 35%	Physical exam with duplex ultrasound, with or without venogram; create AVF.
3.1 to 6.9	High Risk: 50%	Arteriogram and venogram; any necessary preop procedure. Create AVF with very close post op monitoring anticipating need for aggressive intervention to facilitate maturation.
> 6.9	Very high risk: 70%	Consider another form of long-term access (e.g., graft): continue to avoid catheter use.

The utility of this rule is to provide objective information for the vascular access decision-making process and the associated risk/benefit to the patient.

Source: Lok, C.E., Allon, M., Moist, L., Oliver, M.J., Shah, H., & Zimmerman, D. (2006). Risk equation determining unsuccessful cannulation events and failure to maturation in arteriovenous fistulas (Reduce FMT I). *Journal of the American Society of Nephrology, 17*(11), 3204-3212.

6. Loss of normal function.
7. Unacceptable body image.
8. Pediatric patients with AVG and AVF: < 650 mL/min/1.73 m^2 refer for balloon angioplasty within 48 hours.

G. Initiate evaluation and treatment of complications of the dialysis catheter or port/catheter system:
1. Inadequate flow.
2. Infection.
   a. All catheter-related infections, except for exit site infections should be treated with IV antibiotics appropriate for the suspected organism.
   b. Catheters should be exchanged as soon as possible and within 72 hours of starting antibiotics if they do not require a negative blood culture first.
   c. If the patient with bacteremia is afebrile within 48 hours and is clinically stable, catheter salvage might be considered using an interdialytic antibiotic lock solution (see Table 5.6) and 3 weeks of parenteral antibiotics in appropriate situations. A follow-up blood culture 1 week after completion of the course of antibiotics should be performed.
   d. Antibiotic lock to which the organism is sensitive is indicated when follow-up cultures indicate reinfection with the same organism in a patient with limited catheter sites.
3. Loss of integrity of catheter.
4. Facial or neck edema, visual disturbances, hoarseness, dysphagia, or dysphasia.
5. Pain or discomfort of percutaneous catheter.
6. Buttonhole and/or surrounding tissue erosion.
7. Unacceptable body image.

Table 5.6

Sample Protocol for Antibiotic Lock for Catheter Salvage

1. Initiate systemic IV antibiotics using vancomycin and ceftazidime .

2. After each dialysis, lock catheter with a mixture of vancomycin (1 mL of 5 mg/mL), ceftazidime (0.5 mL of 10 mg/mL), and heparin (0.5 mL of 10,000 u/s).

3. After cultures are received, modify both the systemic and lock antibiotics to the appropriate sensitivity.

4. Treat for 3 weeks with systemic and catheter lock antibiotics.

5. Resume heparin lock as per facility protocol.

6. Get surveillance cultures for bacteria and yeast 1 week after antibiotics.

7. Exchange catheter in any patient who remains febrile after 48 hours or has a positive surveillance culture.

Adapted from Allon et al., 2004, and
University of Alabama at Birmingham protocol, 2007.

H. Assume a leadership role in the CQI process for the VAT.
  1. Document interventions appropriately to assure efficient data collection.
  2. Collaborate with nephrologist to select a data collection tool appropriate for trend analysis that includes the following information and data points.
    a. Type and location of access.
    b. Date of insertion/creation.
    c. Date of first use.
    d. Average flow rates per treatment.
    e. Blood volume processed (BVP) per treatment.
    f. Average arterial and venous pressures.
    g. Adequacy labs.
    h. Cannulation events including:
      (1) Failure to cannulate successfully requiring new needle and site.
      (2) Infiltration.
      (3) Needle dislodgement.
      (4) Surveillance data with flows and pressures.
      (5) Thrombosed AVG or AVF.

    i. Number and type of catheter dysfunction events.
    j. Number and type of interventions to correct any type of access dysfunction, including:
      (1) Referral for ultrasound mapping and flows.
      (2) Referrals to interventionalist or surgeon.
      (3) Bacteremias (with cultures and sensitivities).
      (4) Antibiotic therapy including antibiotic locks.
  3. Assure that each patient has a "next step/next access" plan in place to minimize the risk of short-term catheter placement. Catheter prevalence figures frequently include patients who have had a previous functional AVF or AVG.
  4. Institute a "catheter appropriateness" plan that assures that only those patients with no other options for vascular access have long-term catheters.
  5. Mentor dialysis staff in appropriate documentation for data collection.
  6. Stay current with the vascular access literature, standards of practice, and guidelines for care and share significant findings with VAT and dialysis staff.
  7. Initiate and participate in vascular access research.
  8. Disseminate CQI findings and goal setting to staff and patients.

I. Assume a leadership role in staff and patient vascular access education.
  1. Explain the need for both central and peripheral vein preservation.
  2. Demonstrate fistula maturation exercises.
  3. Explain fistula maturation using the Rule of 6's as the model.
  4. Demonstrate the techniques of physical examination of the vascular access.
  5. Encourage self-cannulation when appropriate.
  6. Share journal articles and other sources of new information about the care of vascular access.
  7. Explain the importance of the CQI process.
  8. Disseminate, in a timely fashion, outcomes of vascular access events and procedures and subsequent changes in dialysis orders.

J. Exemplify the incorporation of the Nephrology Nursing Standards for Clinical Practice and Professional Performance into all aspects of care for the patient and his/her vascular access.

Chapter 29

APN Role in Patients with Chronic Kidney Disease and Diabetes Mellitus

Purpose

Discuss the management of the patient with chronic kidney disease (CKD) and diabetes mellitus (DM) from an advanced practice nurse perspective.

Objectives

Upon completion of this chapter, the learner will be able to:
1. Discuss the role of the APN in the management of the patient with CKD and DM.
2. Discuss assessment of the patient with CKD and DM by the APN.
3. Describe management of complication and treatment plan adjustment from an APN perspective.
4. Discuss types of kidney replacement therapy as they relate to the patient with CKD and DM.

A team approach is often used in managing the CKD patient with diabetes. The team usually consists of the primary care provider, nephrologist, nephrology nurse, endocrinologist, APN, dietitian, social worker, diabetes educator, and transplant coordinator. Assessment and treatment of the patient with CKD and DM consists of a comprehensive history and physical examination.

I. Access.

A. Vascular.
   1. Assessment.
      a. Assess for native arteriovenous fistula (AVF) placement.
      b. Vein mapping.
      c. Signs and symptoms of infection if access in place.
      d. Signs and symptoms of distal ischemia, arterial steal syndrome, and stenosis.
      e. Assess patient's knowledge of need to preserve the vascular access.
      f. See Vascular Access (Section 12) for further assessment.
   2. Interventions
      a. Preservation of vasculature for access placement.
      b. No cannulation of the extremity intended to be used for vascular access.

   c. Instruct patient in ways to preserve arm for access or access if in place.
   d. See the previous chapter and Section 12 for further interventions.

B. Peritoneal.
   1. Assessment.
      a. Evaluate patient's prior abdominal surgical history.
      b. Assess patients ability to perform procedure.
      c. Assess patients knowledge of peritoneal dialysis and requirements.
      d. See Peritoneal Dialysis (Section 13) for further assessment.
   2. Interventions.
      a. Consult with surgeon regarding catheter placement.
      b. Educate patient regarding care of catheter and exit site.
      c. See Peritoneal Dialysis (Section 13) for further interventions.

II. Glycemic control.

A. Assessment.
   1. Review home glucose monitoring log.
   2. Monitor fasting serum glucose levels.

3. Monitor HbA1c levels on admission and as indicated.
4. Monitor albumin and catabolic rate (PCR).
   a. Albumin goal: 4.0 g/dL.
   b. PCR goal: at least 0.8 g/kg/day.
5. Monitor fasting lipid levels.
6. Determine body mass index (BMI).
7. Evaluate patients knowledge of diabetes and need for glycemic control.
8. Assess financial concerns.
9. If on peritoneal dialysis control may be more problematic due to glucose from dialysate – assess the following.
   a. Increased daily caloric intake.
   b. Increased blood glucose.
   c. Increased lipids.
   d. Weight gain.
10. Assess for complications of poor glycemic control.
    a. Hypervolemia due to increased thirst.

b. Hypertension.
c. Severe hyperkalemia.
d. Diabetic ketoacidosis.
e. Anorexia, nausea, vomiting, and weakness.
f. Increased risk of infection.

B. Interventions.
   1. Coordinate with primary care provider, endinocrinologist, or diabetologist for diabetic medication management.
   2. Follow the American Diabetes Association Guidelines for goal of treatment.
   3. Dietitian and/or diabetes education referral to aid in education.
   4. Social work referral for financial issues.
   5. Prescribe medications for DM (see Tables 5.7 and 5.8).
   6. If modality of treatment is peritoneal dialysis then intraperitoneal insulin can provide more consistent insulin absorption.

Table 5.7

Types of Insulin Used in the Management of Diabetes Mellitus

Insulin Type	Color	Approximate Length of Action		
		Onset	Peak	End
Rapid-acting Lispro (Humalog) Aspart (Novalog) Glulisine (Apidra)	Clear	5 minutes	1–2 hours	3–4 hours
Short-acting Regular (Humulin R) (Novolin R)	Clear	$\frac{1}{2}$–1 hour	2–3 hours	3–6 hours
Intermediate-acting NPH (Humulin N) (Novolin N)	Milky white when mixed	2–4 hours	4–10 hours	10–16 hours
Long-acting Glargine (Lantus) Detemir (Levemir)	Clear Clear	2–4 hours 1–2 hours	peakless relatively flat	20–24 hours 6–23 hours (low dose – high dose)
Mixtures Humulin 70/30 Novolin 70/30	Milky white when mixed	$\frac{1}{2}$–1 hour	2–6 hours	16–24 hours
Novolog 70/30	Milky white when mixed	5 minutes	1–3 hours	16–22 hours
Humalog 75/25	Milky white when mixed	5 minutes	1–3 hours	16–22 hours
Humalog 50/50	Milky white when mixed	5 minutes	1–3 hours	16–22 hours

| Table 5.8 | Oral Medications Used in the Management of Diabetes Mellitus |

Medication	Class and Mode of Action	Dosage Range	Comments
Diabeta & Micronase glyburide	**Sulfonylureas** Works on pancreas to make more insulin	2.5-20 mg/day	• All forms of glyburide can be taken once or twice daily. • Most common side effect is low blood sugar. • Caution in elderly, due to risk of low blood sugar. • Glucotrol XL is controlled release, take once daily. • When dose of Glucotrol exceeds 15mg, divide and take twice a day. • Weight gain possible.
Glynase PresTab glyburide (micronized)		1.5-12 mg/day	
Glucotrol, Glucotrol XL glipizide		5-40 mg/day 5–20 mg/day	
Amaryl glimepiride		1–8 mg/day	
Avandia rosiglitazone	**Thiazolidinediones** Decreases insulin resistance in muscle and fat cells	4–8 mg /day	• When Actos is used in combination therapy, max dose is 30mg/day. • When Avandia is used with insulin, max dose is 4mg/day. • Avandia can be taken once or twice daily. • Liver enzymes (ALT) should be done at start of therapy and every 2 months for 1 year and periodically thereafter. • May cause weight gain.
Actos pioglitazone		15–45 mg/day	
Prandin repaglinide	**Meglitinides** Works on pancreas to make more insulin	0.5–4 mg/meal	• Works more quickly than sulfonylureas. • Taken with each meal, only if eating. • Low blood sugar may occur. • Interacts with some drugs for treating fungal and bacterial infections. • May cause weight gain. • Good option for individuals with irregular schedules.
Starlix nateglinide		60–120 mg/meal	
Glucophage & Glucophage XR metformin	**Biguanides** Decreases liver glucose output and decreases insulin resistance in muscle and fat cells	500–2,550 mg/day	• Glucophage should be taken twice daily. Glucophage XR should be taken once daily. • Not advised for those with liver or kidney problems, excessive alcohol use or over the age of 80. • Does not cause low blood sugar when used alone. • Does not cause weight gain. • GI side effects possible – start on 500 mg dose and increase gradually.
Precose acarbose	**25–100 mg/meal**	Alpha-glucosidase Inhibitors – slow the digestion of some carbohydrates	• Take with first bite of meal, generally 3x per day. • Do not cause low blood sugar when used alone. • If low blood sugar occurs, must treat with pure glucose. • Not advised in those with bowel disease. • Side effects include abdominal pain, diarrhea, and/or gas. GI side effects may lessen over time.
Glyset miglitol	**25-100 mg/meal**		
Glucovance glyburide & metformin	**Combinations** See mode of action for each drug	See dose ranges for each drug	• See comments for each drug, listed above.
Avandemet rosiglitazone & metformin			
Metaglip glipizide & metformin			
Actoplus met pioglitazone & metformin			
Avandaryl rosiglitazone & glimepiride			
Januvia sitagliptin phosphate	**DPP-4 Inhibitor** Increases and prolongs the actions of incretin hormones (see below)	100 mg/day	• Can be used with metformin and/or thiazolidinediones. • Take once daily, with or without food. • May need lower than recommended dose with renal insufficiency. • Does not cause low blood sugar when used alone.
Byetta exenitide	**Incretine Mimetic** Increases insulin, decreases glucagon, and promotes satiety by regulating gastric emptying	5–10 mcg with a.m. & p.m. meals	• Not advised in those with severe renal impairment or with severe GI disease. • Given by SQ injection – comes in a prefilled pen – 1 month supply. • Take 60 minutes before a.m. and p.m. meals. • For use with metformin, sulfonylureas and/or thiazolidinediones. • Most common side effect is nausea.
Symlin pramlintide acetate	**Synthetic form of the hormone amylin** Amylin slows gastric emptying, suppresses glucagon secretion, and promotes satiety and regulates appetite	60–120 mcg/meal 60 mcg = 10 u 120 mcg = 20 u	• Only for use in insulin dependant type 2 diabetes. • Take at all meals containing > 250 calories or > 30 g carbohydrates. • Most common side effect – nausea. • Given by SQ injection – supplied in vial. • Not advised in those with an A1c >9%, hypoglycemic unawareness, or a diagnosis of gastroparesis. • Reduce mealtime insulin by 50%.

III. Cardiac status.

A. Assessment.
  1. Identify coronary risk factors.
  2. Review need for further cardiac evaluation to include:
     a. Cardiac stress test.
     b. Echocardiogram.
     c. Cardiac catheterization.
  3. Evaluate patient's knowledge regarding coronary disease risk and prevention of complications.

B. Interventions.
  1. Review results of cardiac testing.
  2. Cardiology referral if indicated.
  3. Dietary modifications.
  4. Instruct patient in dietary modification and other risk modifying behaviors to decrease risk of heart disease.
  5. Avoid intravenous contrast studies whenever possible to minimize the risk of IV contrast nephropathy.

IV. Vision.

A. Assess for complications.
  1. Glaucoma.
  2. Cataracts.
  3. Retinopathy.
     a. Nonproliferative retinopathy is most common.
     b. Proliferative can cause retinal detachment.
  4. Vitreous hemorrhage.
  5. Assess for knowledge about vision complications.

B. Interventions.
  1. Ophthalmology referral for yearly examination.
     a. Panretinal photocoagulation.
     b. Focal photocoagulation.
     c. Retinal reattachment.
  2. Instruct patient in ways to prevent visual complications.

V. Peripheral vascular occlusive disease (PVD).

A. Assessment.
  1. Lower extremity Doppler ultrasound evaluation.
  2. Lower extremity MRA evaluation.
  3. Lower extremity physical examination for:
     a. Absent pulses.
     b. Poor hair growth.
     c. Atrophic skin changes.
     d. Cool temperature.
     e. Ulcers.
     f. Ingrown nails.
     g. Calluses.
  4. Assess for patient's knowledge regarding prevention of PVD and modifiable risk factors.

B. Intervention.
  1. Podiatry referral for yearly examination.
  2. Interventional radiologist referral as indicated to further assess vascular status. Avoid contrast studies whenever possible to minimize the risk of IV contrast nephropathy.
  3. Vascular surgery referral as indicated.
  4. Wound care team referral as indicated.
  5. Exercise program.
  6. Protective footwear.
  7. Smoking cessation.
  8. Instruction in modifiable risk factors and disease process.

VI. Gastroparesis.

A. Assessment for signs and symptoms to include nausea and vomiting or delayed gastric emptying.

B. Intervention.
  1. Prescribe Reglan (metoclopramide) or other prokinetic drugs.
  2. Prescribe proton pump inhibitors.
  3. Gastric emptying study.
  4. Gastroenterology referral as indicated.

VII. Neuropathy.

A. Assessment.
  1. Electromyogram and/or nerve conduction study.
  2. Check sensations in lower extremities.
  3. Assess knowledge of disease process and prevention of injury.

B. Intervention.
  1. Exercise program.
  2. Prescribe medications to alleviate symptoms – i.e. neuroleptics, tricyclic medications.
  3. Neurology consult as indicated.
  4. Instruct in ways to prevent injury.

VIII. Nutrition.

A. Assessment.
  1. Follow serum albumin and prealbumin levels.
  2. Monthly albumin and protein catabolic rate (PCR) monitoring. Clarify method of albumin measurement.
     a. Bromcresol purple dye-binding measurement most closely agrees with the gold standard of

immunonephelometry. Range 3.4–4.9 g/dL.
   b. Bromcresol green dye-binding measurement is less accurate as it tends to overestimate the albumin level. Range 3.5–5.2 g/dL.
3. Subjective global assessment.
4. Assess understanding of dietary concerns.

B. Interventions.
1. Prescribe high protein supplements for CKD stage 5 patients.
2. Prescribe Megace (megestrol).
3. Dietitian referral.
4. Obesity management if indicated.
5. Instruct in renal diet and protein needs.

IX. Hypertension.

A. Assessment.
1. Measure blood pressure. Goal: less than 125/75 for patients with CKD and DM and a systolic BP of < 130 mm Hg for CKD patients (refer to NKF-KDOQI & JNC 7 Guidelines).
2. Review home blood pressure logs.
3. Assess knowledge regarding diet modifications, medication adherence, and consequences of continual high blood pressure.

B. Interventions.
1. Recommend low sodium diet.
2. Prescribe the following either alone or in combination.
   a. Angiotension converting enzyme inhibitors (ACE-I).
   b. Angiotension receptor blockers (ARBs).
   c. Calcium channel blockers.
   d. Diuretics if not on kidney replacement therapy or if still indicated.
3. Review JNC 7 and NKF-KDOQI Guidelines.
   a. Provide information regarding low sodium diet.
   b. Refer to dietician if indicated.
   c. Instruct regarding purpose and desired results of prescribed therapy.

X. Infectious processes. Incidence is increased related to alteration in patient's immunity due to uremic toxins, skin breakdown, foreign material (catheter, graft) and malnutrition.

A. Assessment.
1. Evaluate skin integrity.
2. Review vital signs to include temperature. Bacteremia should always be suspected in febrile patients with CKD and DM; however, the patient may be afebrile and/or confused.
3. Obtain blood cultures and CBC.

4. If on peritoneal dialysis:
   a. Peritonitis.
      (1) Observe effluent – cloudy.
      (2) Obtain effluent sample for gram stain and cell count with a culture and sensitivity.
   b. Exit site.
      (1) Inspect site for erythema, drainage.
      (2) Obtain culture of exit site for culture and sensitivity.
   c. Tunnel of catheter. Inspect along tunnel for erythema, and drainage.
   d. See Peritoneal Dialysis section for further assessment.
5. Assess knowledge regarding prevention of infection.

B. Interventions.
1. Order IV antibiotics (gentamicin and vancomycin if access infection is suspected).
   a. Use vancomycin cautiously as there is a risk of developing vancomycin-resistant enterococcus (VRE).
   b. Follow peak and trough antibiotic levels if on vancomycin to ensure adequate dosing.
2. Once sensitivities are available, narrow antibiotic coverage and treat for 3–4 weeks.
3. Meticulous follow up including graft, hemodialysis or peritoneal dialysis catheter removal if indicated.
4. Transesophageal echocardiogram to assess for valvular vegetations.
5. Instruct patient in skin care and other measures to prevent infections.

XI. Hyperkalemia. More common in patients with diabetes due to insulin deficiency or resistance. Potassium increases with severe hyperglycemia.

A. Assessment.
1. Evaluate laboratory data including blood glucose level and potassium.
2. If on kidney replacement therapy evaluate adherence to treatments and potassium bath.
3. Evaluate patient's knowledge regarding diet and high potassium foods and relationship to hyperglycemia.

B. Interventions.
1. Start Kayexalate (sodium polystyrene sulfonate).
2. In more severe cases where hospitalization is required, IV insulin without added glucose may be indicated.

C. Transplantation: see previous chapter focusing on the APN role in transplantation.

Chapter 30

APN Role in Patients with Chronic Kidney Disease and Dyslipidemia

Purpose
Discuss the management of the patient with CKD and dyslipidemia.

Objectives
Upon completion of this chapter, the learner will be able to:
1. Discuss the overview of dyslipidemia.
2. Discuss the pathogenesis of dyslipidemia.
3. Discuss the signs and symptoms of dyslipidemia.
4. Discuss the role of the APN in the management of the CKD patient with dyslipidemia.
5. Discuss lipid management in kidney transplant patients.

I. **Overview.** Total cholesterol (goal: less than 200 mg/dL).

A. High density lipoprotein (HDL).
   1. Protective, "good cholesterol."
   2. Goal: greater than or equal to 60 mg/dL (females); greater than or equal to 55 mg/dL (males).

B. Low density lipoprotein (LDL).
   1. Atherogenic, "bad cholesterol."
   2. Goal: less than 100 mg/dL.

C. Triglycerides (very low density and intermediate density lipoproteins).
   1. Chemical form in which most fat exists.
   2. Goal: less than 180 mg/dL.

II. **Pathogenesis of dyslipidemia.**

A. Causes of primary hypercholesterolemia.
   1. Diet.
   2. Heredity.
   3. Obesity.
   4. Sedentary lifestyle.
   5. Stress.

B. Causes of secondary hypercholesterolemia.
   1. Hypothyroidism.
   2. Diabetes mellitus.
   3. Nephrotic syndrome.
   4. Liver obstruction.

   5. Medications such as progestins, anabolic steroids, diuretics (except indapamide), beta-blockers, immunosuppressants.

III. **Signs and symptoms that dyslipidemia may be present.**

A. May be asymptomatic.

B. Arterial bruits.

C. Claudication.

D. Angina pectoris.

E. Cardiovascular accident.

F. Corneal (senilis) arcus.

G. Xanthomas (lipid deposits) (for illustration, see www.nlm.nih.gov).

H. Xanthelasmas (lipid deposits on eyelids).

I. Myocardial infarction.

IV. **Management of CKD patients with dyslipidemia.**

A. Perform comprehensive history and physical examination.
   1. Determine onset and duration of symptoms (if any).
   2. Obtain complete family history.
   3. Assess comorbid conditions (DM, SHPT, CAD).
   4. Assess risk factors associated with CKD.
      a. High calcium intake from diet and/or medications.

b. Increased serum phosphorus levels.
c. Increased intact parathyroid levels.
d. Increased homocysteine levels.
e. Inflammatory processes.
5. Assess physical findings (if any).
a. Claudication.
b. Arterial bruits.
c. Xanthomas.
(1) Tendons.
(2) Buttocks.
(3) Elbows and knees.
(4) Trunk.
(5) Skin folds.
d. Xanthelasma.
6. Note treatment modality. Peritoneal dialysis patients are more likely to develop dyslipidemia due to absorption of glucose from the dialysis solution in the peritoneal cavity.

B. Order and evaluate lab work.
1. Draw fasting lipid panel.
a. Serum cholesterol level including HDL and LDL. Draw 2–3 months after modality change and annually thereafter.
b. Triglyceride level. Must be drawn after a 9–12-hour fast.
2. Serum glucose level.

3. Thyroid studies.
a. TSH.
b. T3 and free T4 if TSH is abnormal.

C. Assess patient's knowledge regarding dyslipidemia.

V. **Treatment of dyslipidemia.** Prescribe therapies to achieve the Adult Treatment Panel III (ATP III)/NKF-KDOQI guidelines for dyslipidemia.

A. Therapeutic lifestyle changes: diet. Instruct the patient in the following:
1. Low saturated fat and cholesterol.
2. Decrease use of transaturated fatty acids since they can raise LDL cholesterol.
3. Use plant stanols and sterols.
4. Increase soluble fiber.
5. Exercise program.
6. Dietary counseling if indicated.

B. Medications.
1. Assess for medications that might adversely influence lipid profile.
2. Prescribe medications to treat dyslipidemia (see Table 5.9).
a. HMG CoA reductase inhibitors (statins)are drug of choice for elevation of LDL.

Table 5.9

Medications to Treat Dyslipidemia

Classes	Drugs	LDL	HDL	TG
HMG Co-A reductase inhibitors (statins)	atorvastatin (Lipitor) fluvastatin (Lescol) lovastatin (Mevacor) pravastatin (Pravachol) rosuvastatin (Crestor) simvastatin (Zocor)	↓18–55%	↑5–15%	↓7–30%
Resins	cholestyramine (Questran) calestipol (Colestid) colesevelam (Welchol)	↓15–30%	↑3–5%	0–30%
Cholesterol absorption inhibitors	ezetimibe (Zetia, Vytorin)	↓18%	↑1%	↓8%
Niacin or nicotinic acid	Extended-release niacin (Niaspan)	↓5–25%	↑15–35%	↑20–50%
Fibrates	clofibrate (Atromid-S) fenofibrate (Tricor) gemfibrozil (Lopid	↑↓5–20%	↑10–20%	↓20–50%

(1) Inhibit cholesterol synthesis.
(2) Side effects.
  (a) Myopathy.
  (b) Elevated transaminases.
  (c) Pravastatin (Pravachol) and atorvastatin (Lipitor) require no dose adjustment for patients with CKD.
b. Bile acid sequestrants.
(1) Bind with bile acids in the intestine.
(2) Side effects.
  (a) Constipation.
  (b) Nausea and vomiting.
  (c) Anorexia.
  (d) Can increase triglycerides.
c. Cholesterol absorption inhibitors (ezetimibe [Zetia]).
(1) Decrease triglycerides.
(2) Increase HDL concentrations.
(3) Used when greater LDL lowering is needed.
(4) No dose adjustment needed for CKD patients.
d. Niacin or nicotinic acid.
(1) Interferes with synthesis of cholesterol and lipoproteins.
(2) Side effects.
  (a) Severe hepatic toxicity.
  (b) Flushing.
  (c) Cardiac arrhythmias.
  (d) Peptic ulceration.
e. Fibrates.
(1) Lower triglycerides.
(2) Increase HDL (to lesser extent).

(3) Side effects.
  (a) Nausea and vomiting.
  (b) Development of cholesterol gallstones.
  (c) Increase the effect of anticoagulants.
f. Omega-3 fish oil used as adjunct to diet for reduction of triglycerides.

VI. Lipid management in transplant patients.

A. See NKF-KDOQI Clinical Practice Guidelines for Managing Dyslipidemias in Kidney Transplant Patients (see Figure 5. 5).

B. Insulin resistance.
1. Glucocorticosteroids cause an increase in insulin resistance.
  a. Increased hyperglycemia.
  b. Increased triglycerides.
  c. Variable changes in HDL.
2. Cyclosporin and tacrolimus.
  a. Induce insulin resistance.
  b. Impair insulin secretion.
3. Cyclosporin can have major drug interactions with some statins.
  a. Atorvastatin (Lipitor): increased risk of myopathy and rhabdomyolysis.
  b. Fluvastatin (Lescol): no major adverse effects (ALERT study).
  c. Pravastatin (Pravachol): can increase cyclosporin levels.
  d. Simvastatin (Zocor): increased risk of rhabdomyolysis.

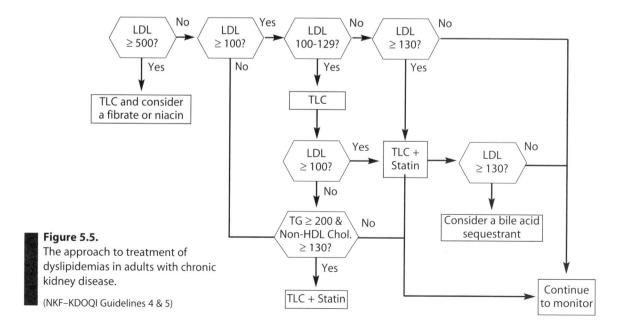

Figure 5.5.
The approach to treatment of dyslipidemias in adults with chronic kidney disease.

(NKF–KDOQI Guidelines 4 & 5)

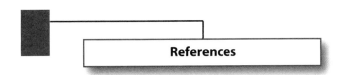

References

Chapter 23

Centers for Disease Control and Prevention (CDC). (n.d.). *CDC Web site: Your online source for credible health information.* Retrieved February 8, 2008, from http://www.cdc.gov

Mitch, W.E., & Klahr, S. (Eds.). (2005). *Handbook of nutrition and the kidney* (5th ed.). Philadelphia: Lippincott Williams & Wilkins.

Molzahn, A., & Butera, E. (Eds.). (2006). *Contemporary nephrology nursing: Principles and practice* (2nd ed.). Pitman, NJ: American Nephrology Nurses' Association.

National Institutes of Health (NIH). (2004). *The seventh report of the Joint National Committee on Prevention, Detection, Evaluation, and Treatment of High Blood Pressure – Complete report.* Retrieved February 8, 2008, from http://www.nhlbi.nih.gov/guidelines/hypertension/jnc7full.htm

National Institutes of Health (NIH). (2006). *Your guide to lowering your blood pressure with DASH.* Retrieved February 8, 2008, from http://www.nhlbi.nih.gov/health/public/heart/hbp/dash/

National Kidney Foundation (NKF). (n.d.). *Kidney Dialysis Outcome Quality Initiative (NKF/KDOQI).* Retrieved February 8, 2008, from http://www.kidney.org/professionals/KDOQI/

Wilcox, C.S., & Tisher, C.C. (Eds.). 2005. *Handbook of nephrology and hypertension* (5th ed.). Philadelphia: Lippincott Williams & Wilkins.

Chapter 24

Andress, D.L. (2005).Vitamin D treatment in chronic kidney disease. *Seminars in Dialysis, 8*(4), 315-321.

Aronoff, G.R. (Ed.). (1999). *Drug prescribing in renal failure: Dosing guidelines for adults* (4th ed.). Philadelphia: American College of Physicians.

Aw, T.J., Haas, S.J., Liew, D., & Krum, H. (2005). Meta-analysis of cyclooxygenase-2 inhibitors and their effects on blood pressure. *Archives in Internal Medicine, 165*, 490.

Becker, B., Kronenberg, F., Kielstein, J., Haller, H., Morath, C., Ritz, E., & Fliser, D. (2005). Renal insulin resistance syndrome, adiponectin and cardiovascular events in patients with kidney disease: The mild and moderate kidney disease study. *Journal of the American Society of Nephrology, 16*(4), 1091-1098.

Bakris, G.L., Levin, A., Molitch, M., Griff, S., Smulders, M., Tian, J., et al. (2005, November). *Disturbances of serum 1,25 dihydroxyvitamin D3 [1,25OH)2 D3] in patients with chronic kidney disease.* Poster presented at American Society of Nephrology Renal Week 2005, Philadelphia, PA.

Chikotas, N., Gunderman, A., & Oman, T. (2006). Uremic syndrome and end-stage renal disease: Physical manifestations and beyond. *Journal of the American Academy of Nurse Practitioners, 18*(5), 195-202.

Coburn, J., Maung, H., Elangovan, L., Germain, M., Lindberg, J., Sprague, S., et al. (2004). Doxercalciferol safely suppresses PTH levels in patients with secondary hyperparathyroidism associated with chronic kidney disease stages 3 and 4. *American Journal of Kidney Diseases, 43*(5), 877-890.

Coresh, J., Byrd-Holt, D., Astor, B., Briggs, J., Eggers, P., Lacher, D., et al. (2005). United States Renal Data System (USRDS) 2005 annual data report. *Journal of the American Society of Nephrology, 16*, 180-188.

Curtain, R.B., Mapes, D., Schatell, D., & Burrows-Hudson, S. (2005). Self-management in patients with end stage renal disease: Exploring domains and dimensions. *Nephrology Nursing Journal, 32*(4), 389-395.

DeFronzo, R.A. (1999) Pharmacologic therapy for type 2 diabetes mellitus. *Annals of Internal Medicine, 131*, 281.

Easom, A. (2006). The challenges of using serum ferritin to guide IV iron treatment practices in patients on hemodialysis with anemia. *Nephrology Nursing Journal, 33*(5) 543-553.

Elder, G.J. (2002). Pathophysiology and recent advances in the management of renal osteodystrophy. *Journal of Bone and Mineral Research, 17*(12), 2094-2105.

Foley, R.N., Parfrey, P.S., & Sarnak, M.J. (1998). Clinical epidemiology of cardiovascular disease in chronic renal disease. *American Journal of Kidney Diseases, 32*(5)(Suppl. 3), S112-119.

Hillege, H.L., Fidler, V., Diercks, G.F., van Gilst, W.H., de Zeeuw, D., van Veldhuisen, D.J., et al. (2002). Urinary albumin excretion predicts cardiovascular and non-cardiovascular mortality in general population. *Circulation, 106*(14), 1777-1782.

Johnson, R.J., & Freehally, J. (2003). *Comprehensive clinical nephrology* (2nd ed.). Edinburgh: Mosby.

Kramer, H., Toto, R., Peshock, R., Cooper, R., & Victor, R. (2005). Association between chronic kidney disease and coronary artery calcification: The Dallas heart study. *Journal of the American Society of Nephrology, 16*(2), 507-513.

McCarthy, J. (1999). A practical approach to the management of patients with chronic renal failure. *Mayo Clinical Proceedings, 74*, 269-273.

National Kidney Foundation (NKF). (2000). K/DOQI clinical practice guidelines for nutrition in chronic kidney disease. *American Journal of Kidney Diseases, 35*(6)(Suppl. 1), 1-140.

National Kidney Foundation (NKF). (2003). K/DOQI clinical practice guidelines for bone metabolism and disease in chronic kidney disease. *American Journal of Kidney Diseases, 42*(4)(Suppl. 3), 1-202.

National Kidney Foundation (NKF). (2004). K/DOQI clinical practice guidelines on hypertension and antihypertensive agents in chronic kidney disease. *American Journal of Kidney Diseases, 43*(5)(Suppl. 1), 1-290.

National Kidney Foundation (NKF). (2006). K/DOQI clinical practice guidelines and clinical practice recommendations for vascular access. *American Journal of Kidney Diseases, 48*(1)(Suppl. 1), 177-322.

Obrador, G., & Pereira, B. (1999). Referral to the nephrologist and timely initiation of renal replacement therapy: A paradigm shift in the management of patients with chronic renal failure. *American Journal of Kidney Diseases, 31*, 398-417.

Parving, H., Lehnert, H., Brochner-Mortensen, J., Gomis, R., Andersen, S., & Arner, P. (2001). The effect of irbesartan on the development of diabetic nephropathy in patients with type 2 diabetes. *New England Journal of Medicine, 345*, 870-878.

Pereira, B. (2000). Optimization of pre-ESRD care: The key to improved dialysis outcomes. *Kidney International, 57*, 351-365.

Ross, W., & McGill, J. (2006). Epidemiology of obesity and chronic kidney disease. *Advances in Chronic Kidney Disease, 13*(4),325-335.

Singh, A.K., Shapiro, W., Rizkala, A.R., Coyne, D.W., & the DRIVE Study Group. (2006, November). *High reticulocyte hemoglobin content predicts response to IV iron in hemodialysis patients with high ferritin: Lessons from the DRIVE study*. Presented at American Society of Nephrology Convention, San Diego, CA.

Chapter 25

American Diabetes Association. (2006). Summary of revisions for the 2006 clinical practice recommendations. (2006). *Diabetes Care, 29*(S3).

Burrows-Hudson, S., & Prowant, B. (Eds.). (2005). *Nephrology nursing standards of practice and guidelines for care*. Pitman, NJ: American Nephrology Nurses' Association.

National Cholesterol Education Program Expert Panel. (2001, May). *Detection, evaluation, and treatment of high cholesterol in adults (Adult Treatment Panel III)*. NIH Publication No. 01-3670.

National Institutes of Health (NIH). (2003). *The seventh report of the Joint National Committee for Prevention, Detection, Evaluation, and Treatment of High Blood Pressure – Complete report*. NIH Publication No. 04-5230.

National Kidney Foundation (NKF). (2001a). K/DOQI clinical practice guidelines for hemodialysis adequacy. *American Journal of Kidney Diseases, 37*(Suppl. 1), 7-64.

National Kidney Foundation (NKF). (2001b). K/DOQI clinical practice guidelines for treating anemia in chronic renal failure. *American Journal of Kidney Diseases, 37*(Suppl. 1), 182-238.

National Kidney Foundation (NKF). (2003a). K/DOQI clinical practice guidelines for bone metabolism and disease in chronic kidney disease. *American Journal of Kidney Diseases, 42*(Suppl. 3), 1-201.

National Kidney Foundation (NKF). (2003b). K/DOQI clinical practice guidelines for managing dyslipidemias in chronic kidney disease. *American Journal of Kidney Diseases, 41*(3), 1-91.

National Kidney Foundation (NKF). (2004). K/DOQI clinical practice guidelines on hypertension and antihypertensive agents in chronic kidney disease. *American Journal of Kidney Diseases, 43*(Suppl. 1), 1-290.

Chapter 26

Agrawal, M., & Schwartz, R. (2001). *Acute renal failure*. Retrieved June 8, 2006, from http://www.aafp.org/afp/20000401/2077.html

American Nephrology Nurses' Association (ANNA). (2002). *Scope and standards of advanced practice in nephrology nursing*. Pitman, NJ: Author.

Baldwin, I., Davenport, A., Goldstein, S., Paganini, & Palevsky, P. (2005). *Acute dialysis quality initiative: Minimizing impact of renal replacement therapy on recovery of acute renal failure*. Retrieved June 8, 2006, from http://www.ccm.upmc.edu/adqi/adqi04.html

Bregman, H., Daugirdas, J.T., & Ing, T.S. (2001). Complications during hemodialysis. In J.T. Daugirdas, P.G. Blake, & T.S. Ing

(Eds.), *Handbook of dialysis* (p. 148). Philadelphia: Lippincott Williams & Wilkins.

Daugirdas, J.T., Blake, P.G., & Ing, T.S. (Eds.). *Handbook of dialysis*. Philadelphia: Lippincott Williams & Wilkins.

Daugirdas, J., Ross, E.A., & Nissenson, A.R. (2001). Acute hemodialysis prescription. In J.T. Daugirdas, P.G. Blake, & T.S. Ing (Eds.), *Handbook of dialysis* (pp. 102-120). Philadelphia: Lippincott Williams & Wilkins.

Keane, W.F., Bailie, G., Boeschoten, E., Gokal, R., Golper, T., Holmes, C., et al. (2000). *Adult peritoneal dialysis-related peritonitis treatment recommendations: 2000 update*. Retrieved June 8, 2006, from http://www.ispd.org/2000_treatment_recommendations.html

National Kidney Foundation (NKF). (2001). K/DOQI clinical practice guidelines for hemodialysis adequacy. *American Journal of Kidney Diseases, 37*(Suppl. 1), 7-64.

National Kidney Foundation (NKF). (2006). K/DOQI clinical practice guidelines for vascular access. *American Journal of Kidney Diseases, 48*(Suppl. 1), 176-307.

Piraino, B., Baile, G.R., Bernardini, J., Boeschoten, E., Gupta, A., Holmes, C., et al. (2005). Peritoneal dialysis-related infections. Recommendations: 2005 update. *Peritoneal Dialysis International, 25*, 107-131.

Chapter 27

Ader, J., & Rostaing, L. (1998). Cyclosporin nephrotoxicity: Pathophysiology and comparison with FK-506. *Current Opinion in Nephrology and Hypertension, 7*(5), 539-545.

American Nephrology Nurses' Association (ANNA). (2002). *Scope and standards of advanced practice in nephrology nursing*. Pitman, NJ: Author.

Barone, C., Martin-Watson, A., & Barone, G. (2004). The postoperative care of the adult renal transplant recipient. *MEDSURG Nursing, 13*(5), 296-302.

Burrows-Hudson, S., & Prowant, B.F. (Eds.). (2005). *Nephrology nursing standards of practice and guidelines for care*. Pitman, NJ: American Nephrology Nurses' Association.

Chobanian, A.V., Bakris, G.L., Black, H.R., Cushman, W.C., Green, L.A., Izzo, J.L, et al. & National High Blood Pressure Education Coordinating Committee. (2003). The seventh report of the Joint National Committee on Prevention, Detection, Evaluation, and Treatment of High Blood Pressure: The JNC 7 Report. *JAMA, 289*, 2560-2572.

Cupples, S.A., & Ohler, L. (2003). *Transplantation nursing secrets*. Philadelphia: Hanley & Belfus, Inc.

Danovitch, G.M. (2005). *Handbook of kidney transplantation* (4th ed.). Philadelphia: Lippincott Williams & Wilkins.

Davis, C.L. (2004). Transplant: Immunology and treatment of rejection. *American Journal of Kidney Diseases, 43*(6), 1116-1134.

Diabetes Control and Complications Trial Research Group, The. (1993). The effect of intensive treatment of diabetes on the development and progression of long-term complications in insulin-dependent diabetes mellitus. *New England Journal of Medicine, 30*, 329(14), 977-986.

Fishman, J.A., & Rubin, R.H. (1998). Infection in organ-transplant recipients. *The New England Journal of Medicine, 338*(24), 1741-1751.

Friedman, A., Miskulin, D., Rosenberg, I., & Levey, A. (2003). Demographics and trends in overweight and obesity in patients at time of kidney transplantation. *American Journal of Kidney Diseases, 41*(2), 480-487.

Hoffman, F.M., Nelson, B.J., Drangstveit, M.B., Flynn, B.M., Watercott, E.A., & Zirbes, J.M. (2006). Caring for transplant recipients in a nontransplant setting. *Critical Care Nurse, 26*(2), 53-73.

Jindal, R., & Zawada, E. (2004). obesity and kidney transplantation. *American Journal of Kidney Diseases, 43*(6), 943-952.

Kasiske, B.L., Heim-Duthoy, K.L., Tortorice, K.L., & Rao, K.V. (1991). The variable nature of chronic declines in renal allograft function. *Transplantation, 51*(2), 330-334.

Miller, B., & Brennan, D. (2006). Maintenance immunosuppressive therapy in renal transplantation in adults [Electronic version]. *UpToDate.*

Molzahn, A., & Butera, E. (Eds.). (2006). *Contemporary nephrology nursing: Principles and practice* (2nd ed.). Pitman, NJ: American Nephrology Nurses' Association.

Mylonakis, E., Goes, N., Rubin, R., Cosimi, A.B., Colvin, R.B., & Fishman, J.A. (2001). BK virus in solid organ transplant recipients: An emerging syndrome. *Transplantation 72*(10), 1587-1592.

Pascual, M., Theruvath, T., Kawai, T., Tolkoff-Rubin, N., & Cosimi, A.B. (2002). Stategies to improve long-term outcomes after renal transplantation. *The New England Journal of Medicine, 346*(8), 580-590.

Paul, L.C. (1999). Chronic allograft nephropathy: An update. *Kidney International, 56*, 783-793.

Penn, I. (1993). Incidence and treatment of neoplasia after transplantation. *The Journal of Heart and Lung Transplantation, 12*(6), S328-S336.

Schrier, R.W. (Ed.). (1995). *Manual of nephrology* (4th ed.). Boston: Little, Brown and Company.

Vella, J., & Brennan, D. (2006). Induction immunosuppressive therapy in renal transplantation [Electronic version]. *UpToDate.*

Wallace, M. (2003). What is new with renal transplantation? *AORN Journal, 77*(5), 945-970.

Wilcox, C.S., & Tisher, C.C. (Eds.). (2005). *Handbook of nephrology and hypertension* (5th ed.). Philadelphia: Lippincott Williams & Wilkins.

Zand, M.S. (Ed.). (2001). Care of the well transplant patient. *Graft, 4*(4), 230-231.

Chapter 28

Allon, M. (2004). Dialysis catheter-related bacteremias: Treatment and prophylaxis. *American Journal of Kidney Disease, 44*(5), 779-791.

Arteriovenous Fistual First. (n.d.) *Change concepts of the Fistula First Breakthrough Initiative.* Retrieved October 3, 2006, from http://www.fistulafirst.org/professionals/change_concepts.php

Burrows-Hudson, S., & Prowant, B. (2005). *Nephrology nursing standards of practice and guidelines for care.* Pitman, NJ: American Nephrology Nurses' Association.

Danese, M.D., Liu, Z., Griffiths, R.I., Dylan, M., Yu, H-T., Dubois, R., et al. (2006). Catheter use is high even among hemodialysis patients with a fistula or graft. *Kidney International, 70*(8), 1482-1485.

Lok, C.E., Allon, M., Moist, L., Oliver, M.J., Shah, H., & Zimmerman, D. (2006). Risk equation determining unsuccessful cannulation events and failure to maturation in arteriovenous fistulas (Reduce FMT I). *Journal of the American Society of Nephrology, 17*(11), 3204-3212.

MacRae, J.M., Levin, A., & Belenkie, I. (2006).The cardiovascular effects of arteriovenous fistulas in chronic kidney disease: A cause for concern? *Seminars in Dialysis, 19*(5), 349-352.

Mitchell, D. (2003). Tertiary vascular access. In A.H. Davies & C.P. Gibbons (Eds.), *Vascular access simplified* (p. 110). Worcester, UK: Trinity Press.

National Kidney Foundation (NKF). (2006). K/DOQI clinical practice guidelines for vascular access. *American Journal of Kidney Diseases, 48*(Suppl. 1), 176-307.

Silva, M.B., Hobson, R.W. II, Pappas, P.J., Jamil, A., Aracki, C.T., Goldberg, M.C., et al. (1998). A strategy for increasing use of autogenous hemodialysis access procedures: Impact of preoperative noninvasive evaluation. *Journal of Vascular Surgery, 27*(2), 302-307.

Chapters 29 & 30

American Diabetes Association (ADA). (n.d.). *American Diabetes Association home page.* Retrieved February 8, 2008, from http://www.diabetes.org

American Nephrology Nurses' Association (ANNA). (2002). *Scope and standards of advanced practice in nephrology nursing.* Pitman, NJ: Author.

Burrows-Hudson, S., & Prowant, B. (Eds.). (2005). *Nephrology nursing standards of practice and guidelines for care.* Pitman, NJ: American Nephrology Nurses' Association.

Henrich, W.C. (Ed.). (2004). *Principles and practice of dialysis* (3rd ed.). Philadelphia: Lippincott, Williams & Wilkins.

Kaiser Permanente Care Management Institute. (2005). *Adult diabetes clinical practice guidelines.* Retrieved February 8, 2008, from http://www.guideline.gov

McKenney, J.M. (2007). Prescription omega-3 fatty acids for the treatment of hypertriglyceridemia. *American Journal of Health-System Pharmacists, 64*(6), 595-605.

Molitch, M.E. (2006). Management of dyslipidemias in patients with diabetes and chronic kidney disease. *Clinical Journal of the American Society of Nephrology, 1*, 1090-1099.

National Kidney Foundation (NKF). (n.d.). *Kidney Dialysis Outcome Quality Initiative (NKF/KDOQI).* Retrieved February 8, 2008, from http://www.kidney.org/professionals/KDOQI/

National Kidney Foundation (NKF). (2008). *A to Z health guide.* Retrieved January 1, 2008, from http://www.kidney.org/atoz/index.cfm

Nissenson, A.R., & Fine, R.N. (Eds.). (2005). *Clinical dialysis* (4th ed.). New York: McGraw-Hill.

Pereira, B.J.G., Sayegh, M.H., & Blake, P. (Eds.). (2005). *Chronic kidney disease, dialysis, and transplantation: A companion to Brenner and Rector's the kidney.* Philadelphia: Elsevier Saunders.

University of Wisconsin School of Medicine. (n.d.). *Lipid guidelines.* Retrieved February 8, 2008, from http://www.med.wisc.edu/

Weiner, D.E., & Sarnak, M.J. (2004). Managing dyslipidemia in chronic kidney disease. *Journal of General Internal Medicine, 19*(10), 1045-1052.

Section 6

Evidence-Based Practice

Section Editor
Janet L. Welch, DNS, RN, CNS

Authors
Sally Burrows-Hudson, MSN, RN, CNN

Margie A. Hull, MEd, MSN, RN, APRN-BC, CDE

Marjorie J. Kurt, MSN, RN

Donna Mapes, DNSc, MS, RN

Terran R. Mathers, DNS, RN

Mildred Sue McManus, MSN, RN, APRN (FNP)-BC, CNN

Charlotte Thomas-Hawkins, PhD, RN

Janet L. Welch, DNS, RN, CNS

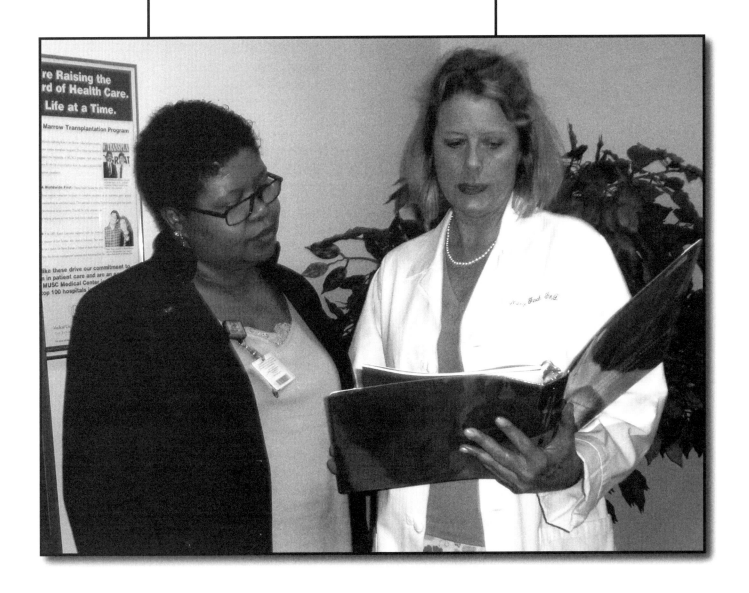

About the Authors

Janet L. Welch, DNS, RN, CNS, Section Editor, is an Associate Professor and Chair of Adult Health at Indiana University School of Nursing in Indianapolis, Indiana.

Sally Burrows-Hudson, MSN, RN, CNN, is President of the Nephrology Management Group in Sunnyvale, California.

Margie A. Hull, MEd, MSN, RN, APRN-BC, CDE, is a Visiting Lecturer at Indiana University School of Nursing in Indianapolis, Indiana.

Marjorie J. Kurt, MSN, RN, is an Assistant Clinical Professor at Indiana University School of Nursing in Indianapolis, Indiana.

Donna Mapes, DNSc, MS, RN, is an Adjunct Senior Researcher at the University Renal Research & Education Association, and President of Donna L. Mapes & Associates, as well as an Assistant Clinical Professor (Adjunct) at the USCF School of Nursing in Moorpark, California.

Terran R. Mathers, DNS, RN, is an Associate Professor at Spring Hill College in Mobile, Alabama.

Mildred Sue McManus, MSN, RN, APRN (FNP)-BC, CNN, is a Nephrology Nurse Practitioner and Kidney Transplant Coordinator at Richard L. Roudebush Medical Center in Indianapolis, Indiana.

Charlotte Thomas-Hawkins, PhD, RN, is an Assistant Professor at the College of Nursing at Rutgers University in Newark, New Jersey.

Section 6

Evidence-Based Practice

Section 6

Evidence-Based Practice

Purpose

Using the available evidence to make clinical decisions in nephrology nursing practice is essential for effective, efficient, and safe care delivery. This section begins with an introduction to evidence-based practice and its importance. The evolution and existing standards for nephrology nursing practice are also introduced. The section concludes with the KDOQI guidelines, results from the DOPPS I and DOPPS II studies, and an introduction to the USRDS database.

Objectives

Upon completion of this section, the learner will be able to:
1. Describe the process used in establishing evidence-based practice.
2. Incorporate standards for care into clinical practice.
3. Compare KDOQI guidelines to actual clinical findings.
4. Identify outcomes associated with the DOPPS studies.
5. Describe data available on the USRDS Web site.

Chapter 31

Evidence-Based Practice

I. What is evidence-based practice (EBP)?

A. Historical background.
   1. Dates back to 1837 in Paris.
      a. EBP Started by Pierre Louis.
      b. Statistical data used to support medical therapies.
   2. EBP movement: founded by Archie Cochrane.
      a. Encouraged public to pay only for empirically supported care.
      b. Criticized medical profession for not doing rigorous reviews of randomized controlled trials (RCTs) to assist others in making decisions about health care (e.g., policy makers and organizations).

   c. Laid foundation for initiation of the Cochran Center, 1992 and Cochrane Collaboration, 1993.
      (1) Cochrane Library produced by world-wide virtual Cochrane Collaboration.
      (2) Develops, maintains, updates systematic reviews.
      (3) Ensures that reviews are accessible to the public.
   3. The Brigg's Report published in 1970s through Department of Health and Social Security recommended that nursing become evidence-based.

B. Terminology commonly used in EBP resources.
1. Bias is a distortion in study design, conduction of the study, or the outcomes that may cause a deviation from the truth.
2. Clinical practice guidelines are statements used as a guide to one's practice arena.
3. Cost-benefit analyses are the costs and benefits assessed to determine whether the benefit of an intervention is worth the cost.
4. Evidence summary is a single conclusion/summarization and synthesis of the knowledge gained from a review of research studies obtained through a scientific, rigorous approach. It is an all inclusive term for a systematic review (which is synonymous with evidence synthesis used by the Agency for Health care Research and Quality [AHRQ] and integrative reviews [used by the Online Journal of Knowledge Synthesis]).
5. Evidence-based practice.
   a. The conscientious, explicit, judicious use of current best evidence in making decisions about patient care (Dicenso, Guyatt, & Ciliska, 2005).
   b. A problem-solving approach to clinical practice.
6. Meta-analysis is a systematic review of multiple research studies that uses statistical methods to quantitatively measure the same outcomes and summarize the results of the studies.
7. A Randomized Control Trial (RCT) is the random assignment of two of more groups, one to a treatment or other strategy (i.e., diagnostic procedure) and the other to a placebo or another type of strategy. A comparison of outcomes is then made between the groups. Commonly used by the Cochran Collaboration as evidence of valid and reliable research.
8. Systematic review is a critical assessment and evaluation of research studies focusing on a specific clinical question through the use of identified methods to limit bias.
9. Validity is reference made to a study's results/findings which have been obtained by sound scientific methods.
10. Reliability is a reference made to a study's effects on practice regarding consistency and dependability.
11. Research utilization is applying knowledge gained from a single research study within the clinical setting.

II. Gathering the evidence.

A. Identifying the right databases (Dicenso et al., 2005).
1. Types of databases.
   a. Bibliographic database describes the article in an abstract or synopsis. The title, author, journal name, and publisher are provided.
   b. Full-text database provides the full text of the article as well as the abstract, title, author, journal name, publisher, and citations.
2. Systematic approach to using appropriate literature.
   a. Determine the quality of the study.
   b. Identify the findings/results of the study.
   c. Consider how to put the evidence into practice.
   d. Obtain organizational support to implement findings.
   e. Initiate, monitor, and evaluate changes.
3. Quantitative vs. qualitative research.
   a. Quantitative data is collected in numeric form, then statistical analyses are conducted. Consideration for use in practice should include evaluation of the:
      (1) Validity and reliability of the results.
      (2) Application of the results to one's personal clinical practice.
      (3) Reason for the study.
      (4) Decision for the sample size.
      (5) Validity and reliability of the instruments.
      (6) Data analysis.
      (7) Limitations or unusual occurrences during the study.
      (8) Congruency of the results with previous research.
   b. Qualitative data is collected in nonnumeric form through the use of methods such as interviews (indepth interviews, focus groups), journals, photographs, observations (participant observations, naturalistic observations, field experiments), life histories, and documents. Consideration for use in practice should include evaluation of the:
      (1) Credibility (validity) or rigor (reliability) of the results.
      (2) Interpretation of the human experience (conscious lived experience as seen by the individual [phenomenology] or group/cultural experience by the researcher immersing oneself [ethnography]).
      (3) Application of the results to one's personal clinical practice.
      (4) Reason for the study with the approach fitting the purpose.

Table 6.1

Suggested Guideline Databases

Source	Web Site
National Guideline Clearinghouse (NGC)	http://www.guideline.gov
CMA InfoBase	http://mdm.ca/cpgsnew/cpgs/index.asp
Health Services/Technology Assessment Text (HSTAT)	http://hstat.nlm.nih.gov
Guidelines Advisory Committee	http://www.gacguidelines.ca
Scottish Intercollegiate Guideline Network (SIGN)	http://www.sign.ac.uk/guidelines/index.html
National Institute for Clinical Excellence (NICE)	http://www.nice.org.uk/catcg2.asp?c=20034
Guidelines International Network	http://www.G-I-N.net
American College of Physicians	http://www.acponline.org/clinical/guidelines
American Academy of Pediatrics	http://aappolicy.aappublications.org/practice_guidelines/index.dtl
American Nephrology Nurses' Association Standards of Practice	http://www.annanurse.org
National Kidney Foundation KDOQI Guidelines	http://www.kidney.org/professionals/doqi/guidelineindex.cfm

(5) Selection of study participants. Is it controlled by the researcher for composition and size?

(6) Techniques for the data collection and analysis.

(7) Congruency of the results with previous research.

4. Guideline databases. Finding guidelines can be an overwhelming process, and three specific concerns should guide the user: validity of the recommendations, identification of the recommendations, and the usefulness of the recommendations (see Table 6.1 for sample guidelines).

B. Steps toward EBP (Melnyk & Fineout-Overholt, 2005).

1. Identify the clinical question.

a. A focused clinical question is the driving force of the steps that follow in the EBP process (Cochran Collaboration, 2003).

b. Form question in PICO format.

(1) P = patient population information, setting, or disorder; includes age, gender, ethnicity as well as specification of disorder of concern.

(2) I = intervention of interest: exposure to disease, diagnostic factors, risk behaviors.

(3) C = comparison against something else: treatment medication vs. placebo, new intervention against the standard of care.

(4) O = identification of an outcome variable.

2. Find the best evidence to answer the question.

a. Determine the review criteria to select only those research studies that will answer the question. A rating system offered by Melnyk and Fineout-Overholt (2005) is located in Table 6.2.

b. Select appropriate searchable databases (see II. A. *Identifying the right databases*).

c. Understand setup of the database to specify the search.

d. Use database language to search. Put in appropriate symbols, words/combination of words, spacing, etc., to obtain information being requested.

3. Appraise the evidence.

a. Does the study demonstrate validity?

b. Determine if the results are reliable by assessing the size (number of participants) and the strength of the effect (difference between groups).

Table 6.2

Rating System for the Hierarchy of Evidence

Level I	Evidence from a systematic review or meta-analysis of all relevant randomized controlled trials (RTCs), or evidence-based clinical practice guidelines based on systematic reviews of RTCs.
Level II	Evidence obtained from at least one well-designed RTC.
Level III	Evidence obtained from well-designed controlled trials without randomization.
Level IV	Evidence from well-designed controlled trials without randomization.
Level V	Evidence from systematic reviews of descriptive and qualitative studies.
Level VI	Evidence from a single descriptive or qualitative study.
Level VII	Evidence from the opinion of authorities and/or reports of expert committees.

Source: Melnyk, B., & Fineout-Overholt, E. (2005). *Evidence-based practice in nursing & healthcare.* Philadelphia: Lippincott Williams & Wilkins. Used with permission.

c. Are the results applicable to the current clinical issue/question, and facilitate patient care?

4. Integrate the evidence into clinical practice, taking into account the current condition of the patient, resources available, clinician expertise, and patient preference and values.

5. Evaluate the changes and outcomes as a result of evidence implementation.

III. Barriers to EBP.

A. Personal perspective.
   1. Lack of skills finding and then perusing databases.
   2. Knowledge deficit regarding critiquing the quality of research.
   3. Overwhelming experience to review the evidence.
   4. Lack of confidence to implement change.
   5. Negative attitude toward research.

B. Organizational characteristics.
   1. Dedicated time unavailable to find evidence.
   2. Inadequate access to databases.
   3. Lack of support, incentives, and peer pressure.

IV. Facilitating EBP.

A. Question clinical practice.
   1. Prioritize clinical issues and problems.
   2. Incorporate research findings to include clinical practice guidelines, clinical pathways, and systematic reviews.
   3. Promote a culture of organizational acceptance for EBP (see Table 6.3).
      a. Transferability.
      b. Feasibility.
      c. Cost-benefit ratio.

B. Promote acceptance among colleagues.
   1. Access with surveys; focus groups.
   2. Identify baseline knowledge.
   3. Identify real case scenarios and how EBP would address the situations better.

C. Correct misperceptions.
   1. Key leaders should be educated at EBP nursing centers.
   2. Teach the basics of EBP through online tutorials. Tutorials are easy to access at any time of day that fits with one's personal schedule.
   3. Expose nurses to useful databases.

Table 6.3

Criteria for Evaluating the Implementation Potential of an Innovation Under Scrutiny

Transferability of the Findings	1. Will the innovation "fit" in the proposed setting?
	2. How similar are the target populations in the research and in your setting?
	3. Is the philosophy of care underlying the innovation fundamentally different from the philosophy prevailing in your setting? How entrenched is the prevailing philosophy?
	4. Is there a sufficiently large number of clients in your setting who could benefit from the innovation?
	5. Will the innovation take too long to implement and evaluate?
Feasibility	1. Will nurses have the freedom to carry out the innovation? Will they have the freedom to terminate the innovation if it is considered undesirable?
	2. Will the implementation of the innovation interfere inordinately with current staff functions?
	3. Does the administration support the innovation? Is the organizational climate conducive to research utilization?
	4. Is there a fair degree of consensus among the staff and among the administrators that the innovation could be beneficial and should be tested? Are there major pockets of resistance or uncooperativeness that could undermine efforts to implement and evaluate the innovation?
	5. To what extent will the implementation of the innovation cause friction within your organization? Does the utilization project have the support and cooperation of departments outside the nursing department?
	6. Are the skills needed to carry out the utilization project (both the implementation and the clinical evaluation) available in the nursing staff? If not, how difficult will it be to collaborate with or to secure the assistance of others with the necessary skills?
	7. Does your organization have the equipment and facilities necessary for the innovation? If not, is there a way to obtain the needed resources?
	8. If nursing staff need to be released from other practice activities to learn about and implement the innovation, what is the likelihood that this will happen?
	9. Are appropriate measuring tools available for a clinical evaluation of the innovation?
Cost/benefit ratio of the Innovation	1. What are the risks to which clients would be exposed during the implementation of the innovation and what are the potential benefits to clients?
	2. What are the risks of maintaining current practices (i.e., risks of trying the innovation)?
	3. What are the material costs of implementing the innovation? What are the costs in the short term during utilization, and what are the costs in the long run, if the change is to be institutionalized?
	4. What are the material costs of not implementing the innovation (e.g., could the new procedure result in some efficiencies that could lower the cost of providing service)?
	5. What are the potential nonmaterial costs and benefits of implementing the innovation to the organization (e.g., in terms of lower staff morale, staff turnover, absenteeism)?

Source: Polit, D., & Beck, C. (2006). *Essentials of nursing research: Methods, appraisal, and utilization* (6th ed.). Philadelphia: Lippincott Williams & Wilkins. Used with permission.

Chapter 32

Standards for Care

I. Standards.

A. Definition: Standards are authoritative statements by which the nursing profession describes the responsibilities for which its practitioners are accountable (ANA, 2004).

B. Describes competent level nursing practice (standards of practice) and professional performance (standards of professional performance).

C. Common to all registered nurses regardless of clinical specialty, practice setting, patient population, or educational preparation and experience.

D. Reflects the values and priorities of the profession.

E. Provides direction for professional practice.

F. Provides a framework for the evaluation of the professional.

G. Assumptions.
   1. There is a link between the professional, the work environment, and the registered nurse's ability to practice. It is assumed that employers will provide an environment supportive of nursing practice.
   2. Nursing practice is individualized to meet patient's unique needs, including patient/family goals and preferences.
   3. The nurse establishes partnerships with patient, family, and other health care providers.

H. Development.
   1. Process initiated by American Nurses' Association (ANA).
   2. Draft and review provided by ANA councils, specialty nursing organization, and others.
   3. Final standards reviewed and adopted by individual specialty nursing organizations. Since 1991, the American Nephrology Nurses' Association (ANNA) has acknowledged and adapted the ANA Standards of Practice and all revisions.

II. Standards of practice.

A. Describe a competent level of nursing care.

B. Uses the critical thinking model known as the nursing process.
   1. Assessment.
   2. Diagnosis.
   3. Outcome identification.
   4. Planning.
   5. Implementation.
      a. Coordination of care.
      b. Health teaching and health promotion.
      c. Consultation.
      d. Prescriptive authority and treatment.
   6. Evaluation.

C. Provides a framework for nurse's decision making.

D. Underlying principles that influence nursing practice.
   1. Provide age appropriate and culturally and ethnically sensitive care.
   2. Maintain a safe environment.
   3. Educate patients.
   4. Assure continuity of care.
   5. Coordinate care across settings and among caregivers.
   6. Manage information.
   7. Communicate effectively.
   8. Use technology.

III. Standards of professional performance.

A. Describe a competent level of behavior in professional role.
   1. Quality of practice.
   2. Education.
   3. Professional practice evaluation.
   4. Collegiality.
   5. Collaboration.
   6. Ethics.
   7. Research.
   8. Resource utilization.
   9. Leadership.

B. Expectation that all registered nurses engage in professional role activities appropriate to education and position.

C. Underlying principle is that registered nurses are accountable for professional action to themselves, their peers, patients, and ultimately to society.

IV. Nephrology nursing guidelines for care.

A. Definition: Guidelines are systematically developed statements that address the care of specific populations or phenomena and are based on the best scientific evidence and expert opinion.

B. Guidelines describe a process of care that has the potential to improve patient and provider decision-making and outcomes.

C. Guidelines address areas where there is:
1. High degree of variability in practice.
2. Significant number of patients affected by practice.
3. Significant benefits or risks associated with the practice.
4. Availability of sufficient information.

D. Nephrology nursing guidelines for care incorporate the evidence support recommendations or clinical practice guidelines from National Kidney Foundation Kidney Disease Outcomes Quality Initiative (NKF-KDOQI), American Heart Association, American Diabetes Association, Centers for Disease Control, Association for the Advancement of Medical Instrumentation, and others.

E. Where no published evidence exists, expert clinical opinion is considered.

F. Format designed to guide nursing care: Area of clinical concern or concept, patient outcome statement in the form of an ideal desired outcome, followed by nursing assessment, intervention, and patient education.

V. History of nephrology nursing standards and guidelines.

A. 1972 – American Association of Nephrology Nurses and Technicians (AANNT) published *Standards of Clinical Practice* – focus on hemodialysis.

B. 1975 – AANNT published *Standards of Clinical Practice for Transplantation.*

C. 1976 – AANNT published *Standards of Clinical Practice for Peritoneal Dialysis.*

D. 1977 – AANNT published *Standards of Clinical Practice for the Nephrology Patient*; included hemodialysis, peritoneal dialysis, transplantation, and acute renal failure.

E. 1982 – AANNT published *Nephrology Nursing Standards of Clinical Practice.*
1. Focused on nursing process.
   a. Standard 1. Nursing assessment of the adult and child.
   b. Standard 2. Nursing diagnosis.
   c. Standard 3. Plan and intervention.
2. Expanded to include conservative management, hemoperfusion, and pediatrics.

F. 1984 – *Nephrology Nursing Standards of Clinical Practice* reprinted without revision to reflect organizational name change: *ANNA Standards of Clinical Practice.*

G. 1988 – *ANNA Standards of Clinical Practice* revision.
1. Structure standards introduced.
   a. Professionalism.
   b. Practice.
   c. Research.
2. Initiates concept of clinical problem or label.
3. Introduces patient outcome statements.
4. Describes process as nursing management.
   a. Assessment.
   b. Intervention.
   c. Patient teaching.
5. Acute patient included in each modality.

H. 1993 – *Standards of Clinical Practice for Nephrology Nursing* (revision).
1. Introduced newly written standards of practice (ANA, 1991) developed in collaboration with specialty nursing organizations and American Nurses' Association.
2. Combined common clinical problems or labels into universal nursing standards of care.
3. Added:
   a. Therapeutic plasma exchange.
   b. Continuous renal replacement therapy (endorsed by American Association of Critical Care Nurses).

I. 1999 – *ANNA Standards and Guidelines of Clinical Practice for Nephrology Nursing.*
 1. Expanded edition included:
    a. Disease management.
    b. Pancreas transplantation.
    c. Sleep.
    d. Infection.
    e. Tuberculosis.
 2. Introduced the concept of clinical practice guidelines by incorporating the NKF Dialysis Outcome Quality Initiative (DOQI), 1997 CPG for anemia, adequacy of hemodialysis, adequacy of peritoneal dialysis, and vascular access.
 3. Updated standards of practice, accepting ANA's 1998 revision.

J. 2002 – *Advanced Practice Nurse Standards of Professional Performance.*
 1. Focus on professional performance.
 2. Used ANA's *Scope of Practice and Standards of Advanced Practice Registered Nursing.*

K. 2005 – *Nephrology Nursing Standards of Practice and Guidelines for Care.*
 1. Updated standards of practice, adapting ANA's 2004 revision; additional standards introduced.
    a. Coordination of care.
    b. Health teaching and health promotion.
    c. Consultation.

 d. Prescriptive authority and treatment.
 e. Leadership.
 2. Introduced standards of practice measurement criteria that includes the registered nurse and the advanced practice nurse.
 3. Described the nursing care of the advanced practice nurse for most guidelines.
 4. Expanded Universal Guidelines for Care by incorporating clinical practice guidelines from NKF Kidney Disease Outcomes Quality Initiative (KDOQI), American Heart Association (JNC-VII), American Diabetes Association, and others.
    a. Hypertension.
    b. Glycemic control.
    c. Nutrition and metabolic control.
    d. Bone metabolism and disease.
    e. Dyslipidemia and reduction of cardiovascular disease risk factors.
 5. Added new nephrology nursing care guidelines.
    a. Chronic kidney disease, stages 1–4.
    b. Self-care and home dialysis.
    c. Palliative care and end-of-life care.
    d. Self-management.
    e. Rehabilitation.

VI. Practical application. Table 6.4 provides standards and guidelines for care and relevant clinical applications.

Table 6.4

Standards and Guidelines for Care and Relevant Clinical Applications

Standards and Guidelines for Care	Applications
Standards of Practice	Nursing practice Care delivery
Standards of Professional Performance	Role descriptions Performance reviews Professional development

Nephrology Nursing Guidelines for Care	Policies
	Procedures
	Clinical pathways, plan of care
	Patient education
	Staff education and training
	Documentation guidelines
	Quality improvement
	    Outcome assessment
	    Process review
	Research questions
	Database development

Chapter 33

The National Kidney Foundation Disease Outcomes Quality Initiative

I. Definition (NKF, 2006e).

A. The National Kidney Foundation Kidney Disease Outcomes Quality Initiative (KDOQI) guidelines provide clinical practice guidelines to improve outcomes in individuals across the stages of kidney disease.

B. The KDOQI guidelines provide evidence-based information to aid in clinical decision making.

C. The KDOQI guidelines are not standards of care.

II. History (NKF, 2006c).

A. Dialysis Outcomes Quality Initiative (DOQI).
1. The initiative began in 1995.
2. The initial focus was only on dialysis patients.
3. The first guidelines were released in 1997.

B. The Kidney Disease Outcomes Quality Initiative (KDOQI).
1. The scope of the initiative changed in 1999.
2. The name changed to KDOQI.
3. The focus changed to include all stages of chronic kidney disease: goals to define and classify stages of chronic kidney disease.
   a. Prevent loss of kidney function.
   b. Slow progression to kidney failure.
   c. Lessen organ dysfunction and comorbid condition in those individuals with chronic kidney failure.

III. Development of the guidelines (NKF, 2006d).

A. Development of each guideline takes 2 to 3 years.
B. Members of multidisciplinary work groups are chosen based on leadership, commitment to quality care, and clinical expertise.
C. Each work group critically reviews the available literature using the approach based on the Agency for Healthcare Research and Quality procedure (NKF, 2006e).
D. The rationale and evidence for the guidelines are provided.
E. Each guideline has a time for open review before publication.

F. Comments provided during the open review are considered by each work group.
G. Final guidelines are published.
H. Updates are considered 3 years after publication if a sufficient body of evidence is available.
I. Updates undergo the same development process, but it takes 1 to 2 years to publish an updated guideline.
J. Guidelines have been translated into more than a dozen languages.
K. Guidelines have provided the basis of clinical performance measures developed and put into effect by the Center for Medicare and Medicaid Services (CMS).

IV. Components of the KDOQI guidelines (NKF, 2006a).

A. Introduction.
B. Summary.
C. Introduction and rationale.
D. Process and methods.
E. Guideline statements.
F. Rationale statements.
G. Evidence base for the guidelines.
H. Tables of the evidence.
I. Limitations of the current guidelines.
J. Clinical considerations.
K. Recommendations for research.
L. Guidelines that could be used to assess clinical performance.

V. Current guidelines.

A. Most KDOQI guidelines are available on the Web.

B. KDOQI guidelines are kept in dialysis units and clinics.

C. There are several published guidelines, and the Web site for each is located in the reference list.
1. Cardiovascular Disease in Dialysis Patients (NKF, 2005b).
2. Hypertension and Antihypertensive Agents in Chronic Kidney Disease (NKF, 2004).

3. Bone Metabolism and Disease in Chronic Kidney Disease (NKF, 2003a).
4. Bone Metabolism and Disease in Children with Chronic Kidney Disease (NKF, 2005a).
5. Chronic Kidney Disease: Evaluation, Classification, and Stratification (NKF, 2002).
6. Managing Dyslipidemias in Chronic Kidney Disease (NKF, 2003b).
7. Hemodialysis Adequacy (NKF, 2006a).
8. Peritoneal Dialysis Adequacy (NKF, 2006a).
9. Anemia in Chronic Renal Disease (NKF, 2006b).
10. Vascular Access (NKF, 2006a).
11. Nutrition in Chronic Renal Failure (NKF, 2000).
12. Diabetes and Chronic Kidney Disease (NFK, 2007).

VI. Use of KDOQI in practice.

A. Use KDOQI guidelines to make informed decisions about managing CKD patients at specific stages of the disease process.
B. Use KDOQI guidelines in assessment of CKD patient with comorbid conditions.
C. Use KDOQI guidelines to translate complexities of CKD stages and interventions.
D. Use KDOQI guidelines in context of caring and respect for patients and their families.
E. Use KDOQI guidelines with consideration for age, gender, environment, and cultural sensitivity.

Chapter 34

The Dialysis Outcomes and Practice Patterns Study (DOPPS)

I. The Dialysis Outcomes and Practice Patterns Study (DOPPS) is a prospective, longitudinal study designed to explain relationships between practice patterns and patient outcomes (Pisoni, Gillespie, et al., 2004).

A. Background.
1. In 1990, Held et al. published data suggesting that mortality rates for patients with end-stage renal disease (ESRD) in the United States were significantly higher than those in Europe and Japan (Held, Brunner, et al., 1990).
2. While very complete data were available in the United States, thanks to the U.S. Renal Data System, data registries in other countries relied heavily on volunteer participation, precluding significant comparison between patient case mix (age and comorbidity differences) and outcomes.
3. There was a strong opinion within the U.S. renal community that the mortality rates were due to older age and greater comorbidity. It was felt that differences in mortality rates were largely because of selection bias.
4. The DOPPS was designed to answer two major research questions.

a. Is the difference in mortality between the United States and other countries a result of case mix?
b. If case mix does not explain all of the mortality difference, do practice patterns explain differences in patient outcomes?

B. Research design.
1. The DOPPS is a prospective, longitudinal, observational study begun in 1996. Two phases have been completed, and the third phase is ongoing.
a. Phase I included 308 hemodialysis facilities from seven countries – United States: 145 facilities (1996–2001); Japan: 62 facilities (1999–2001); Europe: 20 facilities each in France, Italy, Spain, and the United Kingdom; and 21 in Germany (1998–2000).
b. Phase II (modified protocol from Phase I), included 320 hemodialysis units and more than 12,400 patients from the DOPPS I countries, plus facilities in Australia, Belgium, Canada, New Zealand, and Sweden (2002–2004) (see Figure 6.1).

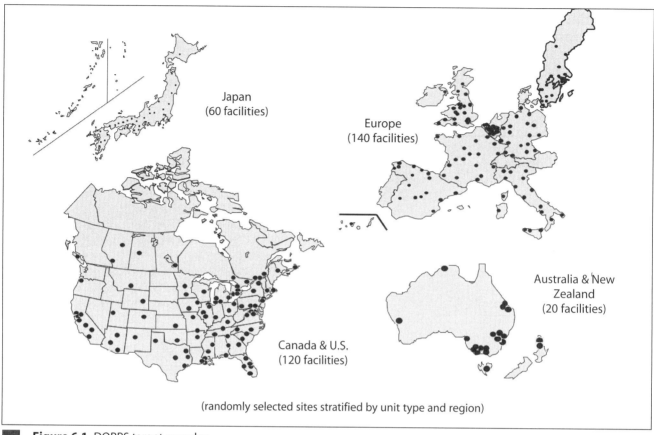

Figure 6.1. DOPPS target samples.

Figures 6.1 and 6.2 reprinted from Pisoni et al. (2004). Dialysis outcomes and practice patterns study (DOPPS): Design, data elements, and methodology. *American Journal of Kidney Diseases, 44*(5 Suppl. 2), S7-S15. Used with permission from The National Kidney Foundation, Inc.

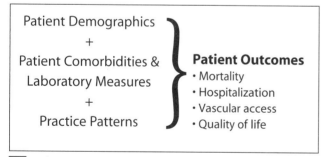

Figure 6.2. DOPPS Framework for hypothesis.

c. Phase III was begun in late 2005 in the same 12 countries as Phase II and will include up to 340 facilities.

2. The unique study design of the DOPPS allows examination of relationships between many types of outcomes and patient or facility-level characteristics (see Figure 6.2), while allowing numerous adjustments for potentially confounding factors.

a. Within each country, dialysis facilities are randomly selected and stratified by type and geographic region, with facility sampling proportional to size within each stratum.

b. Cumulative census data are collected on all patients including demographics, diabetes as cause of ESRD, and mortality.

c. Additional detailed medical data are collected on a random sample of 20–40 patients in each facility at study entry and every four months for the study duration.

d. Data in DOPPS II was collected on both prevalent and incident patients.

(1) Data includes demographics, more than 70 individual measures of comorbidity, plus information on socioeconomic status, insurance coverage, lab values, medication use, hospitalization and outpatients events, vascular access use and procedures, dialysis treatment information, residual renal function, nutritional measures, aspects of care before ESRD, and kidney transplant status.

Table 6.5

Facility-Level Data Collection Items

Anemia and iron therapy	Facility staffing practices	Patient turnover
Antihypertensive therapy	Health care maintenance	Physician practices
Continuing education policies/practice	Hospital and outpatient practices	Pre-ESRD practices
Dialysate processing and composition	Immunizations	Quality assurance and improvement
Dialysis dose	Information systems	practices
Dialysis machines	Initiation and discontinuation of dialysis	Scheduling practices
Dialysis practices	Insurance policies	Social service practices
Dialyzer reuse	Laboratory testing	Vascular access
Dialyzers	Local dialysis market	Water treatment and surveillance
Dietitian and nutrition practices	Mineral metabolism	
Facility characteristics	Nurse and technician practices	

Source: Pisoni et al. (2004). Dialysis outcomes and practice patterns study (DOPPS): Design, data elements, and methodology. *American Journal of Kidney Diseases, 44*(5 Suppl. 2), S7-S15. Used with permission from the National Kidney Foundation, Inc.

Table 6.6

Examples of Methods

Type of Question	Sample Used	Analytic Technique
Characterization (e.g., prevalence of patient conditions or facility practices, patient characteristics)	Prevalent cross-sectional sample (initial sample) or incidence sample	Descriptive statistics (mean, variance, proportion)
Cross-sectional associations (no temporality)	Cross-section of enrolled patients (prevalent or incident)	Linear, logistic, other regression models
Prospective associations (baseline conditions predict future event)	Initial sample and replacement patients with follow up	Cox regression (time to event with censoring); repeated measures models

Source: Pisoni et al. (2004). Dialysis outcomes and practice patterns study (DOPPS): Design, data elements, and methodology. *American Journal of Kidney Diseases, 44*(5 Suppl. 2), S7-S15. Used with permission from the National Kidney Foundation, Inc.

(2) Patients also complete questionnaires on kidney disease quality of life and other medical care issues at study entry and annually thereafter.

(3) Detailed facility practice information is assessed from patient data and from questionnaires completed annually by the medical director and the facility's nurse manager or designee (see Table 6.5).

(4) A variety of statistical analytical methods are employed and examples are given in Table 6.6.

(5) Statistical adjustments for confounding are required to make "all else equal," since causality cannot be confirmed, only inferred in observational studies.

II. **Case mix and mortality outcomes** — the first research question (Goodkin, Young, Kurokawa, Prütz, & Levin, 2004).

A. Case mix and practice patterns vary widely in dialysis facilities, both within nations and globally.

B. Any conclusions require careful correction for the effects of demographic differences and comorbid conditions (case mix).

1. The DOPPS analyzed the relationship between case mix and mortality in 16,720 patients followed up to 5 years in France, Germany, Italy, Japan, Spain, the United Kingdom, and the United States (see Table 6.7).

2. In a cross-sectional analysis, the U.S. mean age

Table 6.7

Prevalence of Comorbid Conditions by Region and Association between Case-Mix Variables and Mortality

	Prevalence (%)			
	EUR	Japan	U.S.	Relative Risk of Mortality†
Coronary artery disease	29	19*	50*	1.13
Congestive heart failure	25	6*	46*	1.22
Diabetes mellitus	20	26*	46*	1.27
Other cardiac disease	37	24*	36	1.15
Left ventricular hypertrophy	55	28*	34*	0.92
Hypertension	73	56*	83*	0.74
Vision problems	31	18*	28*	0.91
Peripheral vascular disease	23	12*	26*	1.21
Psychiatric disease	25	3*	24	1.30
Cerebrovascular disease	14	13	18*	1.21
		Age (per year)		1.03
		Black (vs. all other)		0.80

*P < 0.05 vs. Europe; † P < 0.03 for all.

† For comorbidity present versus absent, unless otherwise specified. Adjustments include continent, age, sex, race, coronary artery disease, congestive heart failure, other cardiac disease, left ventricular hypertrophy, cardiomegaly by x-ray, hypertension, cerebrovascular disease, peripheral vascular disease, diabetes mellitus, lung disease, dyspnea, smoking, cancer, HIV/AIDS, gastrointestinal bleed, peptic ulcer disease, hepatitis B, hepatitis C, neurological disorder, psychiatric disease, recurrent cellulitis or gangrene, and vision problems.

Source: Goodkin, D.A., et al. (2004). Mortality among hemodialysis patients in Europe, Japan, and the United States: Case mix effects. *American Journal of Kidney Diseases, 44*(5 Suppl. 2), S16-S21. Used with permission from the National Kidney Foundation, Inc.

was the oldest at 60.5 ± 15.5 years, Europe close at 60.2 ± 15.2 years, and Japan the youngest at 58.6 ± 12.5 years. The U.S. population was 53% male compared with 58% in Europe and 62% in Japan. More than 95% of European patients were white and more than 99% of Japanese patients were Asian, but the United States was mixed with 54% white, 38% black, and 4% Asian.

3. The 10 most common comorbid conditions associated with mortality in the U.S. are shown in Table 6.7. Each year of increasing age was associated with a 3% increase in mortality.

Black race was associated with a decrease in mortality, and sex was not associated with significant mortality differences. However, in a recently published paper, additional analyses of DOPPS data suggest the survival advantages for racial and ethnic minority groups are largely explainable by measurable case-mix and treatment characteristics (Robinson, Joffe, Pisoni, Port, & Feldman, 2006).

The relative risk values (RR) in Table 6.7 are from a multivariate model and include 15 additional comorbid factors (cancer, HIV, AIDS, GI bleeding, peptic ulcers, HBV, HCV, neurologic disease, recurrent cellulitis or gangrene, DVT, carpal tunnel syndrome, beta-2-microglobulin disease, cardiomegaly by x-ray, dyspnea, and smoking).

4. Survival curves for the three regions (see Figure 6.3) are first shown unadjusted (A) and then adjusted for case mix (B). Crude U.S. mortality (22%) is considerably higher than Europe (16%) and Japan (7%), and crude RR of mortality was significantly higher (P<0.0001) in both Europe (RR=3.12) and the United States (RR=5.34) than Japan.

5. Figure 6.3 then illustrates the change in splay of the curves when adjusted for case mix; the adjusted RR values were also significantly higher in the U.S. compared with both Europe and Japan (RR=3.78 for the United States vs. Japan, p<0.0001; RR=1.33 for United States vs. Europe, p<0.0001).

C. Conclusions.
1. The crude rate of U.S. mortality is almost approximately 1.7 times that of Europe and five times that of Japan, suggesting the need for improvement in patient outcomes.
2. Accounting for case mix and comorbidities reduces the differences in mortality; however death rates remain significantly different between nations and across dialysis facilities.
3. While case mix and comorbid conditions (older and sicker) explain some of the differences in mortality outcomes, it is clear they do not explain all the differences in outcomes.
4. The data strongly suggest that practice patterns explain some of the variation in outcomes.
5. The goal of the DOPPS is to explore and clarify those practice patterns associated with improved patient outcomes.

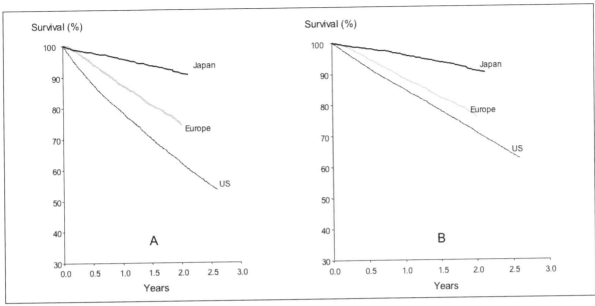

Figure 6.3. Cox survival curves for dialysis patients by continent: (A) unadjusted and (B) adjusted for patient demographics and comorbidities.

Source: Goodkin et al. (2003). Association of comorbid conditions and mortality in hemodialysis patients in Europe, Japan, and the United States: The Dialysis Outcomes and Practice Patterns Study (DOPPS). *Journal of the American Society of Nephrology, 14*(12), 3270-3277. Used with permission from Lippincott Williams & Wilkins.

III. **Relationship between practice patterns** and patient outcomes using the Kidney Disease Outcomes Quality Initiative (KDOQI) clinical practice patterns as a framework.

A. Anemia (Locatelli, Pisoni, Akizawa, et al., 2004).
1. Data from DOPPS I and II suggest large variation in anemia management, as observed among the countries. As illustrated in Table 6.8, mean Hgb in prevalent hemodialysis patients ranged from 10.1 g/dL to 12.0 g/dL.
   a. Percentage of patients below the target of 11 g/dL set by both the National Kidney Foundation Kidney Disease Outcome Quality Initiative (NKF KDOQI) and the European Best Practice Guidelines (EBPG) ranged from 23% to 77% (see Table 6.8).
   b. In the five European countries participating in DOPPS I, overall median Hgb increased from 10.8 in 1998–99 to 11.1 in 2000, nicely demonstrating the influence of clinical practice guidelines.
   c. While the percentage of prevalent hemodialysis patients receiving rHuEpo has increased overall and the majority of such patients now receive rHuEpo, only 21–65% of incident patients received rHuEpo during the pre-ESRD period. As a result, their mean Hgb was lower and fewer patients achieved the KDOQI target (see Table 6.8). While data demonstrate that both mean Hgb concentration and rHuEpo use increase after patients start dialysis, 3 to 6 months typically are required for patients to reach the KDOQI target (see Figure 6.4). Given that the DOPPS and other studies have suggested improved patient outcomes when target Hgb is achieved, it is of serious concern to note that even after 12 months of dialysis therapy, the mean Hgb of 10.8 remains below target.
   d. Anemia has been shown to both cause and worsen cardiovascular disease in patients with chronic kidney disease (Silverberg, Wexler, et al., 2006), and one of the goals of the KDOQI anemia clinical practice guideline is to prevent cardiovascular problems through good anemia management. Clearly, if patients have not achieved the target after 12 months of dialysis, they are at greater risk for poor outcomes and poor quality of life. Guideline-directed anemia management must be an imperative for every nephrology nurse.
2. Anemia and outcomes.
   a. The DOPPS has shown that in spite of anemia clinical practice guidelines, wide variation in anemia management still exists, resulting in a gap between guideline targets

Table 6.8

Mean Hemoglobin (Hgb) Concentrations for Hemodialysis Patients on Dialysis >180 Days and at Time of Starting Dialysis, Percentage of Patients with Hgb <11 g/dL, and Percentage Epo Use for Hemodialysis Patients on Dialysis >180 Days and During the Pre-ESRD Period, by Country: DOPPS II

Country	Among Patients on Dialysis > 180 Days				Among Patients New to ESRD, At Start of Dialysis*			
	n_1	Epo Use (% of pts)	Mean Hgb (g/dL)	Hgb < 11 g/dL (% of pts)	n_2	Epo Use Prior to ESRD (% of pts)	Mean Hgb (g/dL)	Hgb < 11 g/dL (% of pts)
Sweden (SW)	466	94	12.0	23	168	65	10.7	55
United States (US)	1690	91	11.7	27	458	27	10.4	65
Spain (SP)	513	93	11.7	31	170	56	10.6	61
Belgium (BE)	442	94	11.6	29	213	33	10.3	66
Canada (CA)	479	91	11.6	29	150	43	10.1	70
Australia/New Zealand (ANZ)	423	86	11.5	36	108	50	10.1	70
Germany (GE)	459	86	11.4	35	142	46	10.5	61
Italy (IT)	447	87	11.3	38	167	59	10.2	68
United Kingdom (UK)	436	94	11.2	40	93	44	10.2	67
France (FR)	341	83	11.1	45	86	43	10.1	65
Japan (JA)	1210	84	10.1	77	131	62	8.3	95

* Includes patients who were new to ESRD and entered the DOPPS within 7 days of first-ever chronic dialysis treatment. Those receiving Epo prior to ESRD had a 0.35 g/dL higher Hgb at time of starting dialysis compared with patients not receiving Epo during the pre-ESRD period (p<0.001).

Source: Goodkin, D.A., et al. (2004). Mortality among hemodialysis patients in Europe, Japan, and the United States: Case mix effects. *American Journal of Kidney Diseases, 44*(5 Suppl. 2), S16-S21. Used with permission from the National Kidney Foundation, Inc.

and what is achieved in everyday practice.
b. Data from the DOPPS have found strong associations between higher Hgb concentrations and improved outcomes.
c. DOPPS is one of the few studies providing data with detailed adjustment for case mix and comorbid conditions that support the guideline targets in achievement of better patient outcomes.

d. Data analyses from both DOPPS I and II have shown that the adjusted risk for mortality and hospitalization is 4–5% and 5–6% lower, respectively, for every 1 g/dL higher Hgb concentration (see Figure 6.5) (Locatelli, Pisoni, Akizawa, et al., 2004; Locatelli, F., Pisoni, R.L., Combe, et al., 2004; Pisoni, Bragg-Gresham et al., 2004).

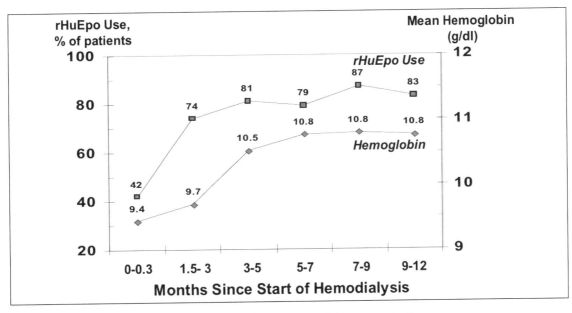

Figure 6.4. Time trend in rHuEpo use and mean hemoglobin concentration for new ESRD patients after initiating hemodialysis.

Source: Locatelli et al. (2004). Anaemia and associated morbidity and mortality among haemodialysis patients in five European countries: Results from the Dialysis Outcomes and Practice Patterns Study. *Nephrology Dialysis Transplantation, 19*,121-132. Used with permission from Oxford University Press.

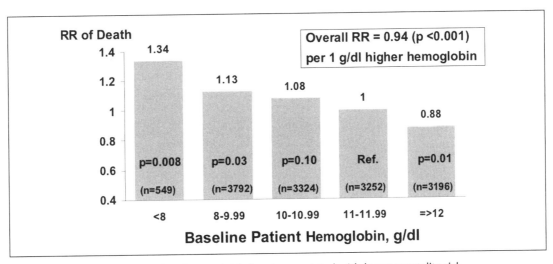

Figure 6.5. Higher baseline hemoglobin levels associated with lower mortality risk.

Souce: Port et al. (2006). Improving outcomes for dialysis patients in the International Dialysis Outcomes and Practice Patterns Study. *Clinical Journal of the American Society of Nephrology, 1*, 246-255. Used with permission from Lippincott Williams & Wilkins.

e. Although this observational data cannot prove causality, they do provide additional evidence of improved patient outcomes with guideline-directed anemia management.
3. Focus on the patients.
    a. DOPPS demonstrates the potential gain to patients, should the KDOQI guidelines be achieved.

b. Analysis of the anemia data (assumes causality for purposes of the analysis) estimates that if all patients in the United States whose Hgb is below 11 g/dL were treated to achieve 11 g/dL or higher, it would result in a potential gain of 23,910 life years over a 5-year period (Port, Pisoni, Bragg-Gresham, et al., 2004).
c. DOPPS indicates that implementation and

Table 6.9

Percentage of Patients with Lab Values Within KDOQI Guideline Range, by Country and Year*

Lab Measure:	PTH		S. Phosphorus		S. Calcium$_{Alb}$		Ca x P	
Country (n^1/n^2)	DOPPS I	DOPPS II	DOPPS I	DOPPS II	DOPPS I	DOPPS II	DOPPS I	DOPPS II
France (540/512)	23.1	20.5	44.2	39.1	35.2	35.4	61.9	64.5
Germany (505/571)	24.0	28.6	26.0	39.5	54.9	52.0	43.6	57.8
Italy (561/576)	21.7	29.6	48.8	46.8	35.9	47.8	65.2	68.2
Japan (2168/1802)	21.4	27.5	40.6	45.9	42.7	45.7	56.8	61.2
Spain (491/613)	21.4	25.9	43.8	48.6	37.1	26.3	56.9	59.3
UK (493/544)	20.7	16.4	38.0	39.6	32.7	31.5	55.0	60.1
US (3853/2246)	20.7	26.9	41.2	44.4	41.1	46.1	56.3	60.8
Overall 7 countries (8611/6864)	21.4	26.2	40.8	44.4	40.5	42.5	56.6	61.4

* Among prevalent cross sections in each region:
DOPPS I: US = 1996, Europe = 1998, Japan = 1999; DOPPS II: 2002
Includes data from France, Germany, Italy, Japan, Spain, UK, and US only.
n_1/n_2 = sample size from DOPPS I/DOPPS II
KDOQI guideline ranges: PTH 150–300 pg/mL, S. Phosphorus 3.5–5.5 mg/dL, S. Calcium$_{Alb}$ 8.4–9.5 mg/dL, Ca x P <55 mg^2/dL^2.

Source: Young, E.W., et al. (2004). Magnitude and impact of abnormal mineral metabolism in hemodialysis patients in the Dialysis Outcomes and Practice Patterns Study (DOPPS). *American Journal of Kidney Diseases, 44*(5 Suppl. 2), S34-S38. Used with permission from the National Kidney Foundation, Inc.

achievement of guidelines can lead to a significant increase in patient outcomes.

B. Mineral metabolism (Young et al., 2004).
1. Growing evidence supports a strong relationship between mortality and abnormal mineral metabolism, probably the result of vascular calcification and atherosclerotic occlusive disease.
2. Changes in mineral metabolism lead to clinical problems such as bone disease, musculoskeletal symptoms, and growth retardation.
3. The potential vascular morbidity and mortality associated with abnormal mineral metabolism led to the development of KDOQI and EBPG clinical practice guidelines.
4. DOPPS provides data on guideline achievement and on the associations between outcomes and clinical lab markers of mineral metabolism.
   a. Lab markers include PTH concentration, serum phosphorous, serum calcium correct-ed for serum albumin, and the calcium-phosphorous product (CaxP).
   b. The majority of PTH measurements now are based on the "intact" PTH assay used before 2005, known to recognize the 1-84 whole PTH and 7-84 fragment of PTH.
   c. Patient and all-cause mortality were modeled by Cox regression with case mix and comorbid conditions adjustment.
   d. Cardiovascular deaths included acute myocardial infarction (MI), cardiac arrhythmia, cardiac arrest, and atherosclerotic heart disease (ASHD).
5. The percentages of patients within KDOQI guidelines during both DOPPS I versus II are shown in Table 6.9. A large fraction of patients fell outside the guidelines for parathyroid hormone (PTH), calcium, phosphorous, and calcium phosphorus CaxP product guidelines.
   a. In patients falling outside the range (see

Table 6.10

Overall Distribution of Mineral Metabolism Lab Values by Time (DOPPS I and DOPPS II)*

Measurement (n1/n2)	Range	Patients (%)		
		DOPPS I	DOPPS II	p-value
PTH (pg/mL) (n¹/n² = 5439/4261)	< 150	52.9	47.5	< 0.001
	150–300	21.4	26.2	
	> 300	25.7	26.3	
S. calcium_Alb (mg/dL) (n¹/n² = 6892/5780)	< 8.4	9.4	8.9	0.06
	8.4–9.5	40.5	42.5	
	> 9.5	50.1	48.6	
S. phosphorus (mg/dL) (n¹/n² = 8263/6383)	< 3.5	7.6	9.0	< 0.001
	3.5-5.5	40.8	44.4	
	> 5.5	51.6	46.7	

* Among prevalent cross sections in each region:
DOPPS I: US = 1996, Europe = 1998, Japan = 1999; DOPPS II: 2002
Includes data from France, Germany, Italy, Japan, Spain, UK, and US only.
n_1/n_2 = sample size from DOPPS I/DOPPS II

Table 6.11

Percentage of Patients Within Guidelines for Varying Numbers of Laboratory Values

Number of measurements in guideline range	DOPPS I	DOPPS II	p-value*
0	20.7	17.8	<0.001
At least 1	79.3	82.2	
At least 2	54.0	57.6	
At least 3	23.1	27.5	
All 4	4.6	5.5	

* P-value is X^2 for overall distribution of number of target values met by each stage of DOPPS (*n*=4679/3565).

Tables 6.10 and 6.11 reprinted from Young et al. (2004). Magnitude and impact of abnormal mineral metabolism in hemodialysis patients in the Dialysis Outcomes and Practice Patterns Study (DOPPS). *American Journal of Kidney Diseases, 44*(5 Suppl. 2), S34-S38. Used with permission from the National Kidney Foundation, Inc.

Table 6.10) for PTH, more than twice as many fell in the low (<150 pg/mL) rather than the higher range of >300 pg/mL. By DOPPS II, fewer patients fell in the low range and the percentage in the higher range increased.

b. Most patients outside the phosphorous target range were in the high phosphorous category; the number of patients decreased slightly by DOPPS II.

c. Most patients out of range were in the high calcium category (> 9.5 mg/dL), but no overall change between DOPPS I and II was seen in the percentage of patients meeting the serum calcium KDOQI guideline (Albert et al., 2006).

d. Table 6.11 shows the difficulty in achieving all four guideline targets. Only 4.6% of patients in DOPPS I and 5.5% in DOPPS II achieved all four targets.

6. The DOPPS has shown associations between nonachievement of guideline targets and all-cause and cardiovascular mortality risks.

a. Table 6.12 shows the increasing relative risk of mortality as the four lab markers for mineral metabolism rise.

b. The relative risk (RR) for both all-cause and cardiovascular mortality is statistically significant for all four lab markers.

c. Careful assessment of mineral metabolism markers and appropriate interventions to reduce mortality risk must be incorporated into all nephrology nurse assessments.

7. Focus on the patients.

a. DOPPS demonstrates the potential gain to patients should the KDOQI guidelines be achieved.

b. Analysis of the phosphorous data (again assuming causality for purposes of the analysis) estimates that if all U.S. hemodialysis patients above a phosphorous level of 5.5 mg/dL were treated to the guideline target of < 5.5 mg/dL, it would lead to a significant gain of 33,793 life years if 100% of patients achieved target, and to 16,322 life years if 50% of patients achieved target.

Table 6.12

Association between Study Outcomes (All-Cause and Cardiovascular Mortality) and Markers of Mineral Metabolism

Predictor	Outcome Measure*	
	All-Cause Mortality **RR** **(95% CI)** *p-value*	**Cardiovascular Mortality** **RR** **(95% CI)** *p-value*
Phosphorus (per 1mg/dL)	1.04 (1.023–1.059) < 0.0001	1.10 (1.067–1.128) < 0.0001
Albumin-Corrected Calcium (per 1 mg/dL)	1.12 (1.079–1.160) < 0.0001	1.13 (1.065–1.196) < 0.0001
Calcium-Phosphorus Product (per 5 mg^2/dL^2)	1.03 (1.015–1.035) < 0.0001	1.06 (1.041–1.072) < 0.0001
PTH (per 100 pg/mL)	1.01 (1.001–1.018) 0.03	1.02 (1.005–1.030) 0.007

* DOPPS I (1996–2001) & II (2002–2004) data; Models stratified by country and adjusted for age, sex, black race, duration of ESRD, prior parathyroidectomy, serum albumin, hemoglobin, dialysis dose (spKt/V), 14 summary comorbid conditions, and predictors listed in Table 6.14, and year of enrollment in DOPPS, controlling for effects of facility clustering.

Source: Young, E.W., et al. (2004). Magnitude and impact of abnormal mineral metabolism in hemodialysis patients in the Dialysis Outcomes and Practice Patterns Study (DOPPS). *American Journal of Kidney Diseases, 44*(5 Suppl. 2), S34-S38. Used with permission from the National Kidney Foundation, Inc.

C. Nutrition (Combe, McCullough, et al., 2002).
1. The latest KDOQI nutrition clinical practice guidelines were published in 2000 and again focused on the importance of nutritional markers as predictors of mortality and morbidity.
2. Data from the DOPPS have demonstrated that changes in nutritional indicators are associated with survival.
    a. The usefulness of serum albumin in the assessment of nutritional status and patient outcomes is supported by several DOPPS studies. Table 6.13 demonstrates the differences in countries for baseline albumin concentration.
    b. The U.S. value for serum albumin was significantly lower than all of Europe (3.60 vs. 3.72 g/dL); within Europe, the United Kingdom had the lowest value.
    c. Japan, in a separate analysis, had significantly higher albumin than the United States when adjusted for age, sex, and day of blood draw.
    d. In DOPPS II, the United States had 20.5% of patients with albumin values below 3.5 g/dL.
    e. In the United States (see Figure 6.6) there is a strong inverse relationship between mortality and albumin, with a 2.12 increase in the relative risk of death for the lowest quartile (<3.3 g/dL) compared with the highest (>4.0) (Pifer et al., 2002).
    f. Compared with the KDOQI target of 3.5 g/dL, the mortality risk for U.S. patients below target was 1.38 times greater than those above target.
    g. Also important, change in serum albumin is also predictive, with an increasing mortality risk as albumin declines over a 6-month period.
    h. Subjective global assessment (modified) (Combe et al., 2004) data was also collected. (see Table 6.14).

Table 6.13

Nutritional Indicators in the United States and Five European Countries

Measure	US	France	Germany	Italy	Spain	UK	All Euro-DOPPS
Predialysis serum albumin (g/dL)	3.6	3.87	4.17§	3.98	3.98	3.72#	3.92
Predialysis serum creatinine (mg/dL)	8.8	9.5	8.7*	9.8§	9.1	9.2	9.3
nPCR (g/kg/day)	1.0	1.12*	0.97*	1.14§	1.09	1.03§	1.09
Weight (kg)	73.1	63.6§	69.7#	63.9§	63.5#	68.1§	65.6
BMI (kg/m²)	25.4	23.2§	24.5§	23.5	23.9	24.2	23.8
mSGA score (%)							
Moderately malnourished	7.6	18.0	14.1	16.1	11.2*	15.4	15.1
Severely malnourished	11.0	4.5	2.6	2.3	3.2	6.5§	3.8

Patients entering the study within 90 days of their first dialysis treatment were excluded from this analysis. In Germany, albumin commonly is measured using total protein and serum protein electrophoresis, which may overestimate albumin compared with the direct method. BUN, blood urea nitrogen; nPCR, normalized protein catabolic rate; IDWG, interdialytic weight gain; BMI, body mass index; mSGA, subjective global assessment, modified to adapt to available DOPPS data.

* P<0.05; §P<0.01; #P<0.0001 vs. All Euro-DOPPS, accounting for facility clustering.

Source: Combe, C., et al. (2004). Kidney Disease Outcomes Quality Initiative (K/DOQI) and the Dialysis Outcomes and Practice Patterns Study (DOPPS): Nutrition guidelines, indicators, and practices. *American Journal of Kidney Diseases, 44*(5 Suppl 2), S39-S46. Used with permission from the National Kidney Foundation, Inc.

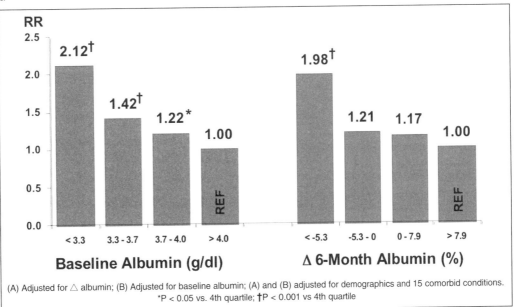

(A) Adjusted for △ albumin; (B) Adjusted for baseline albumin; (A) and (B) adjusted for demographics and 15 comorbid conditions.
*P < 0.05 vs. 4th quartile; †P < 0.001 vs 4th quartile

Figure 6.6. Relative risk of mortality and quartiles of serum albumin.

Source: Pifer, T.B., et al. (2002). Mortality risk in hemodialysis patients and changes in nutritional indicators: DOPPS. *Kidney International, 62*, 2238-2245. Used with permission.

Table 6.14

Adjusted Relative Risk (RR) for Mortality by Nutritional Indicators as Continuous Variables

Nutritional indicator (vs. reference group or per one SD increase)	Isolated models [a]	Overall multivariate model [a]
Severe SGA *vs. normal*	1.33 [b]	1.25 [b]
Moderate SGA *vs. normal*	1.05	0.97
BMI *per 5.9 kg/m²*	0.81 [c]	0.88 [c]
△ BMI *per 10%*	0.89	1.02
Albumin *per 0.56 g/dL*	0.74 [c]	0.78 [c]
△ Albumin *per 20%*	0.75 [c]	0.76 [c]
Creatinine *per 3.7 mg/dL*	0.78 [c]	0.85 [c]
△ Creatinine *per 39%*	0.88	0.92
nPCR *per 0.28 units*	1.02	NA
△ nPCR *per 34%*	0.98	NA
Lymphocyte count *per 1300 cells/mm³*	0.98	0.95
△ Lymphocyte count *per 34%*	0.99	0.93
Bicarbonate *per 4.2 mEq/liter*	0.97	NA
△ Bicarbonate *per 25%*	0.97	NA
Neutrophil count *per 2800 cells/mm³*	1.26 [c]	1.09 [b]
△ Neutrophil count *per 27%*	1.00	1.0

NA – did not significantly predict mortality in Overall Model.

[a] All models adjusted for age, race, sex, duration of ESRD, and 15 comorbid factors.

[b] $P < 0.05$

[c] $P < 0.001$

Source: Pifer et al. (2002). Mortality risk in hemodialysis patients and changes in nutritional indicators: DOPPS. *Kidney International, 62*, 2238-2245.

(1) Moderately malnourished patients ranged from 7.6% in the United States to 18% in France.
(2) Severely malnourished patients ranged from 2.3% in Italy to 11% in the United States.
(3) Japan had significantly fewer moderately or severely malnourished patients than either the United States or Europe.

(4) Severely malnourished U.S. patients had a 33% higher mortality risk and moderately malnourished patients had a 5% higher risk.
i. Serum creatinine.
(1) Hemodialysis patients with little residual renal function on a steady dose of dialysis have a predialysis creatinine proportional to dietary protein intake and skeletal

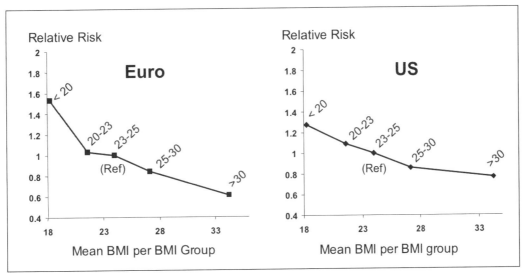

Figure 6.7. Mortality versus BMI, Euro-DOPPS and U.S.-DOPPS.

Source: Leavey et al. (2001). Body mass index and mortality in "healthier" as compared with "sicker" haemodialysis patients: Results from the Dialysis Outcomes and Practice Patterns Study (DOPPS). *Nephrology Dialysis Transplantation, 16*, 2386-2394. Used with permission from Oxford University Press.

muscle mass. Thus, low or stabilized creatinine is an indicator of decreasing muscle mass and/or low protein intake.

(2) Mortality risk was inversely related to baseline creatinine and independently with a decrease in creatinine over time (U.S. patients); risk was 60–70% higher in the lowest quartile compared with the highest for both cases (Pifer et al., 2002).

j. Mortality risk (see Figure 6.7), adjusted for demographics and comorbidities, is lower for U.S. and Europe hemodialysis patients with higher BMI, thereby suggesting a protective effect for larger patients.

k. Inflammation.

(1) Studies have addressed the negative impact of inflammation on nutritional status and survival (Kalantar-Zadeh, Kopple, Block, & Humphreys, 2001).

(2) The DOPPS has collected data regarding some of the traditional inflammation markers. A Malnutrition Inflammation Score (MIS) based on the work of Kalantar-Zadeh et al. (2001) was designed using DOPPS I data, with a higher score representing worse nutrition/inflammation status (Combe, Bragg-Gresham et al., 2004).

(3) For every 1 unit higher of modified MIS score, patients were found to have an 8% higher mortality risk (P<0.0001) and a

6% higher risk of hospitalization (Combe, Bragg-Gresham et al., 2004).

3. Focus on the patients.

a. The DOPPS data demonstrate that assessing nutritional status of hemodialysis patients according to clinical practice guidelines is a challenging and sometimes difficult process.

b. The data also provide evidence of the critical need to assess nutritional status regularly and to design and implement appropriate interventions.

c. Practices vary widely between facilities and between countries and there are those who achieve positive outcomes for a greater number of patients, even after adjusting for case mix and comorbidity.

d. Analysis of the data (assuming causality for purposes of the analysis) (Port, Pisoni, Bragg-Gresham, 2004), estimates that if 100% of patients had an albumin > 3.5 g/dL, the patient years could potentially be increased by 50,079 yrs and 24,188 yrs if only 50% of patients achieved the target.

D. Dialysis dose (Saran et al., 2004).

1. Guideline 4 of the KDOQI indicates that the minimum delivered dose of hemodialysis for both adult and pediatric hemodialysis patients should be equivalent to a Kt/V of at least 1.2. For those using urea reduction ratios (URR), the delivered dose should be equivalent to a

single pool (sp) Kt/V of 1.2 (i.e., an average URR of 65%). Guideline 5 of the KDOQI indicates that, to prevent the delivered dose from falling below the recommended minimum dose, the prescribed dose of hemodialysis should be equivalent to a spKt/V of 1.3 and a URR of 70%.

2. An analysis of DOPPS I data for 1997–1999 indicated that in Europe between 14% of patients (France) and 42% (Germany) had a spKt/V of <1.2; the percentages of patients in Japan and the United States were 27% and 24%, respectively. An analysis of DOPPS II data for 2002–2003 revealed an improvement in the percentage of patients with a spKt/V of <1.2. The range for Europe was 13% (France) to 31% (Germany), and the percentages were 23% and 10%, respectively, for Japan and the United States (Port et al., 2006).

3. Dialysis dose and mortality.
   a. Findings from the DOPPS show a significant relationship between dialysis dose and mortality risk in adult hemodialysis patients (Goodkin et al., 2004; Port, Pisoni et al., 2004). The relative risk of mortality in patients with a Kt/V less than 1.2 was 16% higher compared to patients with a Kt/V greater than 1.2.
   b. DOPPS findings suggest that sex differences explain some of the differences in mortality rates associated with dialysis dose (Goodkin et al., 2004; Port, Wolfe et al., 2004). The survival benefit (i.e., lower mortality rates) related to high dialysis doses (i.e., URR greater than 75%) is seen in women but not men, despite adjustment for size.
   c. DOPPS data suggest that, after adjustments for multiple comorbidities, patient demographics, and Kt/V, a treatment time of less than 3.5 hours is associated with significantly higher mortality risk compared with a treatment time of greater than 3.5 hours.
   d. Higher rates of ultrafiltration (UFR) may be responsible, in large part, for intradialytic hypotension and unstable treatments (Saran et al., 2006). In turn, unstable treatments may lead to the delivery of inadequate doses of dialysis. DOPPS data reveals that, compared with patients with a UFR less than 8 mL removed/kg/hour, patients with a UFR greater than 8 mL removed/kg/hour are twice as likely to experience intradialytic hypotension (i.e., a blood pressure drop of >30 mmHg with postdialysis blood pressure of <100 mmHg systolic), have a 16% higher

chance of an unstable treatment (i.e., treatment requiring extra nurse attention), and have a 10% higher chance of mortality. These results suggest that if fluid is removed too quickly, patients are at an increased risk for negative outcomes, including intradialytic and postdialysis hypotension, unstable treatments, and higher mortality. The findings also suggest that patients with large interdialytic weight gains should be dialyzed for longer periods of time to avoid these adverse outcomes.
   e. It is estimated that 12,446 patient years would be gained if 100% of patients not meeting KDOQI minimum dialysis dose targets achieved the recommended dose, and 6,011 patients years would be gained if 50% of patients out of the KDOQI range were brought within the range (Port, Pisoni, Bragg-Gresham, et al., 2004). This analysis presents an opportunity to improve dialysis dose outcomes and lower the percentage of patients outside of dialysis dose targets.

E. Vascular access.
   1. Vascular access use among prevalent hemodialysis patients (see Table 6.15).
      a. The KDOQI Clinical Practice Guidelines for Vascular Access state that the preferred permanent vascular access for hemodialysis patients is a native arteriovenous fistula (AVF).
      b. A comparison of vascular access use in Phase I of the DOPPS in Japan, Europe, and the United States reveals that the use of AVF among prevalent hemodialysis patients in Europe and Japan is much higher compared with the United States (Pisoni et al., 2002; Pisoni, Young, Mapes, Keen, & Port, 2003). In Europe and Japan, more than 80% of all accesses were AVFs and 10% were grafts. In the United States, grafts were the predominant access, making up 58% of all accesses, with 24% of patients using an AVF. Preliminary data from DOPPS II indicates that AVF use among hemodialysis patients in the United States has increased by several percentage points. Almost 31% of prevalent hemodialysis patients in the United States have an AVF and 41% have a graft (Rayner et al., 2004).
      c. Pisoni et al. (2002) also analyzed patient characteristics significantly associated with AVF use, and they included younger age, male sex, nondiabetic status, lower body mass

Table 6.15

Vascular Access Use, DOPPS I (1997–1999) and DOPPS II (2002–2003)

Country	Fistula (%)		Graft (%)		Catheter (%)	
	DOPPS I	DOPPS II	DOPPS I	DOPPS II	DOPPS I	DOPPS II
France	79.6	79.4	12.3	9.0	6.9	11.3
Germany	86.2	85.1	11.0	9.4	2.8	5.4
Italy	90.3	85.8	4.2	3.7	4.6	10.1
Japan	91.3	90.8	3.6	6.5	2.3	1.3
Spain	82.5	79.5	11.1	10.5	6.0	9.9
UK	68.3	68.6	6.6	6.2	23.4	24.9
US	20.7	26.5	62.8	44.6	15.2	28.2

Among prevalent cross-section of patients, restricted to dialysis units participating in both DOPPS I and DOPPS II (DOPPS II data as of June 2003). Percentages do not always add to 100 due to missing data.

Source: Rayner et al. (2004). Vascular access results from the the Dialysis Outcomes and Practice Patterns Study (DOPPS): Performance against Kidney Disease Outcomes Quality Initative (K/DOQI) clinical practice guidelines. *American Journal of Kidney Diseases, 44*(5 Suppl. 2), S22-S26. Used with permission from the National Kidney Foundation, Inc.

index, no history of angina, and absence of peripheral vascular disease. The likelihood of AVF use was also much greater in Europe compared with the United States. These findings indicate that particular patient characteristics are associated with AVF versus AVG use, but large differences remain between Europe and the United States in vascular access that are not accounted for by different patient characteristics.

d. A comparison of AVF in two prevalent hemodialysis patient subgroups in Europe and the United States with different levels of comorbidity was also done in the DOPPS (Pisoni et al., 2002). The first subgroup consisted of patients who were 18 to 54 years of age and without diabetes, peripheral vascular disease, and coronary artery disease. The second subgroup consisted of diabetic patients who were greater than 54 years of age and who had peripheral vascular disease and/or coronary artery disease. In the first subgroup, AVF use was high in Europe, with 76% of women and 89% of men using AVFs compared with 41% of U.S. men and 22% of U.S. women. In the second subgroup, 64% of women and 82% of men in Europe had an AVF compared with only 22% of men and 10% of women in the United States. This subpopulation analysis demonstrates a high use of AVFs in Europe in patients with both low and high levels of comorbidity. On the

other hand, AVF use in the United States is substantially lower than Europe, even for relatively young, nondiabetic patients without coronary artery disease.

e. The percentage of AVF use in different dialysis units also was analyzed in the DOPPS (Pisoni et al., 2002). Dialysis units in Europe displayed a range of AVF use varying from 39% in some facilities to 100% in others, with a median facility value of 83% AVF use. U.S. dialysis units displayed AVF use rates as low as 0% and as high as 87%, with a median facility value of 21% AVF use. These results indicate that despite a low overall use of AVF in the United States, some U.S. dialysis units achieve an AVF use rate similar to Europe. However, one fourth of U.S. dialysis units had a very low AVF use rate (0–12%).

f. The pattern of arteriovenous graft (AVG) use varies widely from country to country. An analysis of DOPPS I data (1997–1999) reveals that an average of 9% of patients in Europe (country range 4.2% to 12.3) used an AVG. While 62.8% of U.S. patients used an AVG, only 3.6% of patients in Japan used an AVG. DOPPS II data for 2002 to 2003 indicates a decrease in AVG use in Europe to 7.8% of patients, an increase in Japan to 6.5% of patients, and a decrease in the United States to 44.6% of patients.

g. DOPPS I analyses indicate that central vein catheters are used by 15% of prevalent

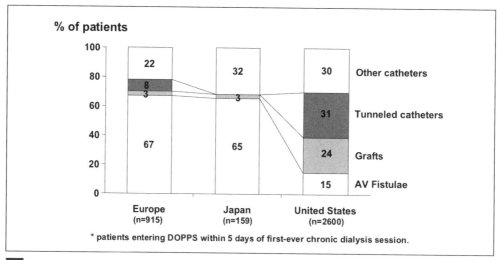

Figure 6.8. Vascular access use among incident hemodialysis patients in Europe, Japan, and the United States.

Reprinted with permission from Pisoni et al. (2003, May). Vascular access use and outcomes in the U.S., Europe, and Japan, *Nephrology News & Issues, 17*, 38-43, 47.

hemodialysis patients in the United States compared with 3–9% in Europe and Japan (Rayner et al., 2004). DOPPS II analyses for the years 2002 to 2003 reveal an increase in catheter use in Europe and the United States, and a decrease in catheter use in Japan. An average of 12% of patients in Europe used a catheter (country range 5% to 25%). Only 1.3% of patients in Japan used a catheter, while 28% of patients used a catheter in the United States during the same time period (Rayner et al., 2004). Thus, catheter use is especially high in the United States among prevalent hemodialysis patients.

2. Vascular access use among new hemodialysis patients.
   a. KDOQI guidelines indicate that AVFs should be constructed in at least 50% of all new kidney disease patients starting hemodialysis as their initial form of renal replacement therapy (see Figure 6.8).
   b. A comparison of vascular access use in Phase I of DOPPS in Japan, Europe, and the United States reveals that the use of AVF among incident hemodialysis patients in Europe and Japan is much higher compared with the United States (Pisoni et al., 2002; Pisoni et al., 2003). In Japan and Europe, 65–67% of new patients initiate hemodialysis with an AVF compared with 15% in the United States. On the other hand, AVGs made up 24% of new accesses in the United States compared with

only 3% in Europe and Japan. These findings indicate that Europe and Japan rarely choose synthetic grafts for new ESRD patients who initiate hemodialysis treatments.
   c. Combe et al. (2001) described the use of tunneled (cuffed) and untunneled catheters for new hemodialysis patients in Europe and the United States. In Europe, 8% of patients used a tunneled catheter and 23% an untunneled catheter at the start of hemodialysis. In the United States, 31% of patients used a tunneled catheter and 29% an untunneled catheter at the start of hemodialysis. These findings indicate that catheter use, particularly tunneled catheter use, is especially high in the United States at the time patients newly diagnosed with ESRD first start hemodialysis. High catheter use is seen in the United States despite the U.S. practice of using more AVGs than AVFs with grafts typically cannulated sooner after creation compared with AVF.

3. Factors that affect vascular access placement.
   a. The effect of predialysis care (i.e., length of time that nephrologic care is received prior to starting dialysis) on vascular access placement was evaluated in the DOPPS (Pisoni et al., 2002). Patients who received nephrologic care more than 30 days prior to starting hemodialysis were six times more likely to initiate hemodialysis with a permanent vascular access and almost twice as likely to initiate hemodialysis with an AVF versus an AVG (see Figure 6.9) (Pisoni et al., 2002).

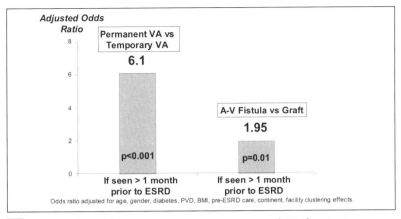

Figure 6.9. Odds of access type used at start of HD if patient sees nephrologist > 1 month before ESRD.

Reprinted with permission from Pisoni et al. (2002). Vascular access use in Europe and the United States: Results from the DOPPS. *Kidney International, 61,* 305-316.

b. Predialysis care was also compared between Europe and the United States in the DOPPS to determine its effect on vascular access use in new hemodialysis patients (Pisoni et al., 2002). DOPPS data indicate that 84% of patients in Europe and 74% of U.S. patients received nephrologic care greater than 30 days before starting dialysis.

c. Various relationships between early nephrologic care and type of access used at start of hemodialysis were examined. For patients receiving nephrologic care more than 30 days prior to the start of dialysis, 79% of European patients and 48% of U.S. patients used a permanent vascular access for their first dialysis treatment. These data indicate that European pre-dialysis practice is more successful than U.S. predialysis practice in placing permanent accesses that are functional at the start of dialysis. Moreover, 46% of U.S. incident patients and 25% of European incident patients did not have a permanent access placed prior to starting dialysis, even though 55% of these patients had received nephrologic care greater than 30 days prior to dialysis.

d. DOPPS I data also reveal an association between medical director and nurse preferences for vascular access and type of access placed (Young et al., 2002). AVG was the preference for permanent vascular access among 21% of U.S. DOPPS dialysis facility medical directors and 40% of U.S. DOPPS dialysis facility nurse study coordinators. On the other hand, 100% of Europe and Japan DOPPS facilities preferred the AVF for permanent vascular access. In the United States, patients in facilities in which the medical director and nurse manager preferred an AVG were twice as likely to have an AVG compared with facilities that did not prefer grafts. These data suggest that a dialysis unit's preference for vascular access may influence the type of vascular access placed in patients in the unit. However, opinions among hemodialysis facility nurse managers have since shifted, from 40% preferring grafts in 1996 to 1999 to only 7% in 2003 (Rayner et al., 2004).

e. Another factor that seems to influence access placement is the involvement of surgical trainees (Pisoni et al., 2002). Surgery trainees participate in vascular access placement in one third of DOPPS dialysis facilities in Europe and the United States. In dialysis facilities where surgery trainees participated in placement, the likelihood of patients receiving an AVF was 40% lower compared with dialysis units that did not use surgery trainees. These results suggest that graft placement is higher in surgical training settings or that trainees are not adequately prepared for AVF placement.

f. KDOQI guidelines recommend referral for vascular access surgery within 1 year of starting dialysis or when creatinine clearance is less than 25 mL/min. An analysis of DOPPS I data for incident patients reveals variations in time from *referral for* to *creation of* vascular access. Rayner et al. (2003) indicated that, in a majority of dialysis facilities (65–95%) in France, Germany, Italy, Japan, and the United

States, time from referral to creation of vascular access was ≤ 2 weeks. On the other hand, a majority of facilities in the United Kingdom (60%) reported intervals of greater than 4 weeks between referral for and creation of a vascular access. New hemodialysis patients had a 1.8-fold greater chance of starting hemodialysis with a permanent access if time from referral to access placement was ≤ 2 weeks.

4. Permanent vascular access survival.

a. Permanent vascular access survival was analyzed for incident patients in DOPPS I who used an AVF or AVG for their first hemodialysis treatment (Pisoni et al., 2002). Survival was defined as the amount of time an access functioned until first failure. Survival analysis, which was adjusted for patient age, sex, body mass index, and continent of residence, demonstrated a nearly twofold higher rate of failure for AVGs compared with AVFs. In the United States, 68% of AVFs survived for 1 year compared with 49% of AVGs. In Europe, 83% of AVFs survived for 1 year. The low number of AVGs in Europe precluded a survival analysis for AVGs. After accounting for patient mix differences, DOPPS analyses suggest that the substantially higher mortality risk for hemodialysis patients in the United States versus Europe may be explained by difference in vascular access use (Pisoni, Mapes, & Port, 2006).

b. The pattern of better survival for AVFs compared with AVGs is more complex when a temporary catheter was used for the first hemodialysis treatment and then the survival of a subsequently used AVF or AVG was determined. In this instance, no significant survival advantage between AVF and AVG was observed in the United States during the first 240 days of use, but after this time period AVF survival was substantially better than AVG survival.

c. A patient's prior use of a central venous catheter was associated with AVF failure in the DOPPS. AVF survival was substantially better in Europe and the United States when AVFs were used for the first hemodialysis treatment compared with AVF first used after starting hemodialysis with a catheter. A similar detrimental effect is seen with AVGs. AVG survival was also better in the United States if used for the first hemodialy-sis treatment versus AVG use after starting hemodialysis with a catheter.

d. One practice pattern that is important for whether a new patient starts hemodialysis with a permanent vascular access is the amount of time before the newly created access can be cannulated. An analysis of AVF survival according to the time between creation and first cannulation for a random DOPPS I sample of incident patients in Europe, Japan, and the United States revealed the median time to first AVF cannulation varied greatly between countries: Japan and Italy (25 and 27 days); Germany (42 days); Spain and France (80 and 86 days); United Kingdom and United States (96 and 98 days) (Pisoni et al., 2006).

e. This variation in practice patterns provided the opportunity in the DOPPS to investigate any associations between time to first cannulation and AVF survival (Pisoni et al., 2006). AVF cannulation ≤14 days after creation was associated with a twofold increase of subsequent fistula failure compared with cannulation ≥14 days following creation. No significant difference in AVF failure was observed for fistulae cannulated in 15 to 28 days after creation compared with 43 to 84 days. Even though these analyses were adjusted for patient characteristics, comorbidities, and country of residence, it is possible that the good AVF survival observed in accesses cannulated after 14 days could be due, in part, to more favorable vasculature or more rapid development of AVF, which was not adjusted for in the analyses (Pisoni et al., 2003). Thus, these findings may not apply to all hemodialysis patients. Nonetheless, these findings suggest that first cannulation of AVF may be feasible as early as 15–28 days after creation for certain types of patients if this helps to avoid the use of central venous catheters.

f. Various medications have been considered in the DOPPS for their potential effect on vascular access survival. Saran et al. (2002) studied the effects of certain cardioprotective and antithrombotic drugs on graft and fistula survival in hemodialysis patients. In this analysis, there was the assumption that these drugs were prescribed for reasons unrelated to vascular access preservation. Analyses were adjusted for patient characteristics and other factors shown to be associated with access survival. The findings indicated a substantially lower risk of AVF failure for patients prescribed angiotensin-converting enzyme (ACE) inhibitors. In addition, the risk of primary AVG failure was lower for patients on calcium channel blockers and aspirin therapy. The use of warfarin was associated with a higher risk of primary graft failure. This finding was not surprising since warfarin is sometimes prescribed for patients with a poorly functioning access or patients believed to be at higher risk for access thrombosis. These results can help to guide the research community in the design of future clinical trials to evaluate the effect of various pharmacotherapeutic agents on vascular access outcomes.

5. Outcomes of catheter use.
   a. The DOPPS has quantified a number of adverse outcomes associated with the use of hemodialysis catheters. After adjusting for patient characteristics and comorbidities, a significant relationship has been shown between an increasing percentage of patients within a dialysis facility receiving hemodialysis with a catheter and lower average hemoglobin levels and higher rates of hospitalization and mortality (Pisoni, Bragg-Gresham, et al., 2004; Pisoni et al., 2002).
   b. Combe et al. (2001) also showed that patients newly diagnosed with ESRD starting hemodialysis with a tunneled catheter had a 25–30% higher mortality rate compared with new ESRD patients who started hemodialysis with a permanent access, even after adjusting for patient characteristics and comorbidities. Starting dialysis with a tunneled catheter was associated with a relative risk of mortality of 1.31 compared with starting dialysis with a permanent access. The risk of vascular access infection was five times higher for tunneled catheters and seven times higher for untunneled catheters compared with AVFs.
   c. Facility level analyses were also done in the Combe et al. study, and the range of catheter use in DOPPS facilities was 0–50% of patients. Facilities with greater than 28% catheter use had 60% higher rates for infectious complications, 30% higher rates for hospitalization due to any cause, and higher mortality rates.
   d. Catheter use is also associated with an increased risk of failure of subsequent AVF.

DOPPS I data indicated that the relative risk of fistula failure was twice as high if a catheter was used before the first AVF cannulation compared with the use of the AVF for the first hemodialysis treatment. Similarly, the relative risk of AVG failure in the United States was 43% higher in patients with prior catheter use compared to patients without a prior catheter (Pisoni et al., 2002).

6. Performance against KDOQI Clinical Practice Guidelines.
   a. DOPPS data have been collected since the publication of the NKF-KDOQI Clinical Practice Guidelines for Vascular Access. This allows an assessment of the impact of these guidelines on vascular access practices worldwide.
   b. KDOQI has set the following vascular access targets:
      (1) Constructing an AVF in at least 50% of all new ESRD patients initiating hemodialysis.
      (2) Achieving 40% AVF use among prevalent hemodialysis patients.
      (3) Limiting the use of catheters as permanent vascular access to 10% of chronic hemodialysis patients.
   c. Within the United States, opinion among nurse managers has shown a substantial decrease in those preferring grafts. The percentage of prevalent patients using AVFs has increased over time in the United States with a fall in the percentage of patients using grafts. However, there is a disturbing trend toward an increase in prevalent patients in the United States and other countries that use central venous catheters.
   d. These mixed results, particularly the worsening trend for using catheters as vascular accesses, will require collaboration among multiple disciplines including vascular access surgeons, nephrologists, nurses in dialysis units, and interventional radiologists. There needs to be greater emphasis in surgical training programs on skills required to create AVFs. Similarly, nurses in hemodialysis units must become more proficient in and confident about cannulating AVFs rather than AVGs.

IV. Health-related quality of life (HRQOL)
(Mapes et al., 2004).

A. Background.
1. What matters most to patients is how well they are able to function and how they feel about their day-to-day life. This defines health-related quality of life for the patient. Capturing the impact of chronic illness and its associated treatment on functioning and well-being in physical, mental, and social dimension of life is the goal of health-related quality of life instruments (Hays et al., 1994).
2. In addition to the high mortality rate in the ESRD population, the level of health-related quality of life remains significantly lower.
3. The DOPPS has provided important evidence for the renal community in demonstrating a wide variation in practice patterns, patient outcomes, and the achievement of clinical practice guidelines.
4. In 1997, the Institute of Medicine recommended patients be routinely assessed for functional status and well-being at routine intervals.
5. The KDOQI Clinical Practice Guidelines for Chronic Kidney Disease (2002) include regular assessment of functioning and well-being in patients with chronic kidney disease and call for assessing the effect of interventions on these outcomes.
6. Health-related quality of life has been extensively studied over a 35-year period, both as an outcome and as a predictor. It was included as a primary outcome in the DOPPS original research design, as well as in analytic plans for using it as a predictor.

B. DOPPS design.
1. DOPPS used the Kidney Disease Quality of Life Short Form (KDQOL-SF) (Lopes et al., 2002) to measure patient assessment of functioning and well-being. The instrument was developed as a self-report measure for hemodialysis patients. The SF-36 generic core yields an 8-scale profile of functional health and well-being scores as well as psychometrically-based health utility index. It also includes multi-item scales targeted at quality of life concerns of special relevance for patients with kidney disease (Hays et al., 1994).
2. Patients' responses determined scores of the kidney disease component summary (KDCS), the mental component summary (MCS), and the physical component summary (PCS).

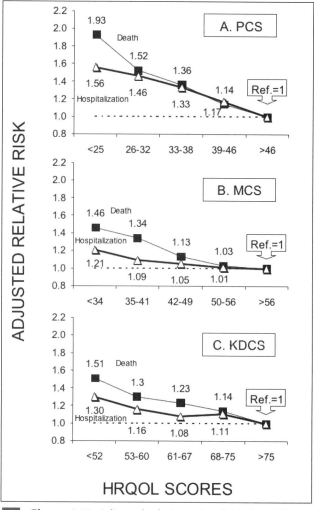

Figure 6.10. Adjusted relative risks of death and first hospitalization by quintile of scores for HRQOL component summary scores.

Source: Mapes et al. (2003). Health-related quality of life as a predictor of mortality and hospitalization: The Dialysis Outcomes and Practice Patterns Study (DOPPS). *Kidney International, 64*, 339-349. Used with permission.

3. Patients completed the questionnaire at entry into the study and annually thereafter.
4. Three studies were conducted to provide additional evidence of relationships between HRQOL and hemodialysis outcomes (HRQOL as predictor) (Lopes et al., 2002; Lopes et al., 2004; Mapes et al., 2004).
5. The first study was designed to verify whether different components of HRQOL are associated with mortality and hospitalization and also compared the predictive power of HRQOL and serum albumin.
6. The second study investigated the predictive power of depression on mortality and hospitalization.

7. Both studies used the standard DOPPS adjustments for case mix and comorbid conditions.

C. Study 1: HRQOL.
   1. Quintiles of HRQOL component scores, using the highest quintile as a referent, were compared using Cox models adjusted for relative risk of death and hospitalization. The association of serum albumin with the same outcomes was assessed using similar models.
   2. Both mortality and hospitalization increased significantly from the highest to the lowest component scores, even after adjustment (see Figure 6.10).
   3. The associations were similar across subgroups defined by age, albumin levels, and time on dialysis.
   4. The association between HRQOL and death was much stronger than the one for hospitalization, but both remained statistically significant.
   5. PCS was the component most strongly significant with both outcomes. The adjusted risk of death was 93% higher for patients at the lowest quintile compared with the highest.
   6. Risk of death was 29% higher (RR=1.29, P<0.001) per 10 points of lower PCS score.
   7. The effects of MCS on the two outcomes were independent of PCS and vice versa. In other words, both MCS and PCS scores were independent predictors (including albumin and KDCS) of death and hospitalization and were as strong as albumin, the strongest known predictor of mortality in hemodialysis patients for over 30 years.
   8. Also, lower scores in all subscales of the MCS and PCS were associated with higher risk of death and hospitalization.
   9. While the KDCS also predicted death and hospitalization independent of albumin, it did not add to the model when MCS and PCS were included, suggesting that measuring MCS and PCS alone are sufficient predictors.
   10. This study strongly suggests that regular assessment of HRQOL is just as important as clinical lab measures and provides opportunities for interventions designed to improve functioning and well-being.

D. Study 2: Depression.
   1. Depression is an integral component of quality of life; the predictive power of depression on death and hospitalization was assessed by the depression-related questions on the KDQOL-SF and a medical record diagnosis by the physician (Lopes et al., 2004).

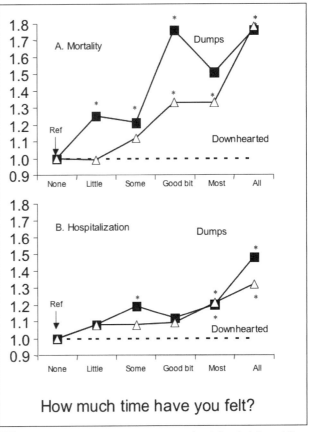

Figure 6.11. Adjusted relative risk of death (A) and first hospitalization (B) according to level of depression.

Source: Lopes et al. (2002). Depression as a predictor of mortality and hospitalization among hemodialysis patients in the United States and Europe. *Kidney International, 62,* 199-207.

2. The two relevant KDQOL questions were, "Have you felt so down in the dumps that nothing can cheer you up?" and "Have you felt downhearted and blue?" Responses considered indicative of depression included "a good bit of the time," "most of the time," and "all of the time" over the previous four weeks.
3. The adjusted RRs of death and first hospitalization are shown in Figure 6.11. An increased risk of death was suggested (P<0.001) from "none of the time" to "all of the time."
4. Patients with physician diagnosed depression had a 27% higher mortality risk and 14% higher risk of hospitalization.
5. Findings suggest that patient-reported depression is easily assessed and offers opportunities for intervention that may reduce risk for death and hospitalization and should be studied in clinical trials.
6. Findings also support the essential need for routine assessment of depression in hemodialysis patients by nephrology nurses. Simply using

the two questions from the KDQOL-SF™ as described in the DOPPS can yield useful information from the patient's perspective.

V. Medications (Andreucci et al., 2004).

A. Background.
1. Medications, including patient adherence to medications, play a very important role in the achievement of positive patient outcomes.
2. KDOQI clinical practice guidelines are integrating some recommendations for medications within existing guidelines.
   a. The KDOQI guidelines suggest that more than 60% of hemodialysis patients require treatment for hyperlipidemia.
   b. KDOQI guidelines recommend all hemodialysis patients be prescribed a water soluble vitamin.
3. DOPPS data provide comprehensive information on hemodialysis patient medications along with comprehensive case mix, comorbidity, and medical information.

B. Statins: hydroxymethylglutaryl-coenzyme A (HMG-CoA) reductase inhibitors.
1. The most frequent cause of mortality in hemodialysis patients is cardiovascular.
2. Statins have been shown to affect mortality in the general population, but minimal data have been available in ESRD patients in terms of effect on patient outcomes.
3. The DOPPS has studied the relationship between prescribed statins and clinical outcomes.
   a. Wide variation occurred between countries with an average of 16.6% use in the United States, 15.7% in France, 11.9% in Germany, 8.1% in the United Kingdom, 7.1% in Japan, 4.9% in Spain, and only 3.5% in Italy (Mason et al., 2005).
   b. By multivariate analysis, patients less likely to be prescribed statins were older, male, and on dialysis longer; patients more likely to be prescribed statins had coronary artery disease (CAD, 45% higher), peripheral vascular disease (PVD; 48% higher), and diabetes (61% higher).
   c. Even in patients considered high risk (cholesterol >200 mg/dL, CAD, history of myocardial infarction), only 27.5% of patients in the United States were prescribed statins, and the percentage was much lower in other countries.
   d. Patients prescribed statins had an overall 31% lower risk of death compared with those

who were not prescribed statins.
   e. Prescribed statins were associated with a 23% lower risk of cardiac causes of death (P = 0.03).
   f. Prescribed statins were associated with a 44% lower risk of noncardiac mortality, suggesting a statin effect beyond lipids.

C. Water soluble vitamins.
1. Since chronic hemodialysis therapy became available, replacement of water soluble vitamins (WSV) removed by dialysis therapy, particularly with high-flux, high efficiency dialyzers, has been recognized (Fissell et al., 2004).
2. Data have shown that ESRD patients have high levels of homocysteine, a cardiovascular risk factor; these levels are reduced by WSV, particularly folic acid.
3. In the absence of randomized, controlled clinical trials, the DOPPS working hypothesis is that WSV are associated with patient outcomes.
   a. Wide variation occurred among countries. Surprisingly, 27.8% of patients in the United States were not prescribed WSV. The range of patients prescribed WSV in Europe was much lower, ranging from 6.4% in Italy to 37.9% in Spain; only 5.6% of Japanese were prescribed WSV.
   b. Analyses showed those patients more likely to have WSV prescriptions were older, male, and longer on dialysis therapy; those less likely to be prescribed WSV were black and had diabetes.
   c. Patients prescribed WSV had a mortality risk 16% lower than those who did not and a 6% lower risk of hospitalization.

D. Conclusions.
1. These observational studies suggest significant associations between prescribing statins and water soluble vitamins for hemodialysis patients.
2. Until randomized, controlled clinical trials are conducted, specific evidence-based clinical practice guidelines cannot be developed, but recommendations can be suggested. Risks must be balanced against potential gains.
3. Especially with water soluble vitamins, the risk appears to be negligible, leading to the conclusion that all patients should at least be prescribed a WSV.

E. Implications for nursing practice.
1. Routine nursing assessment must include monitoring prescriptions for water soluble vitamins for every dialysis patient.
2. Indications for statin therapy also should be assessed for each dialysis patient and discussed with the patient's physician.

Chapter 35

United States Renal Data System (USRDS)

I. Goals defining the mission of USRDS.

A. Prevalence and incidence with trends in mortality and disease rates.
B. Investigation of relationships among patient demographics, treatment modalities, and morbidity.
C. Identification of new areas for special renal studies and support of investigator-initiated research.
D. Provision of data to support research.

II. Administrative oversight.

A. Oversight of Coordinating and Special Studies Center.
B. Input and feedback by ESRD networks.

III. Responsibilities of the Steering Committee, the governing body of the USRDS.

A. Coordination among the centers.
B. Assurance of data availability.
C. Oversight of Annual Data Report production.

IV. USRDS Advisory Committee.

A. Advisement on appropriate and special studies and analyses.
B. Review of annual data reports and manuscripts.

V. Data Management Advisory committee (DMAC).

A. Addresses the accuracy and completeness of the data provided to USRDS.
B. DMAC ensures timely fulfillment of data requests.

VI. Annual Data Report Committee (ADRC) reviews.

A. Past data reports.
B. Proposals for future editions.
C. Ideas for expanded date availability on USRDS Web site.

VII. Information Systems Committee (ISC) reviews.

A. Planned hardware requirements.
B. Systems configuration.
C. Documentation and performance.
D. Evaluates new technologies.

VIII. Special Studies Review Committee (DRRC).

A. Operation committee for proposals.
B. Projects support.

IX. Data Request Review Committee (DRRC).

A. Reviews data requests.
B. Makes recommendations to the Project Officers.

X. Renal Community Council (RCC) – Liaison between USRDS and the ESRD community.

XI. Implications for nursing practice.

A. Awareness of USRDS system and the data it provides to guide practice and inform policy.
B. Facilitation of information (atlas with graphs, maps, and reference tables).
C. Availability of PDF and Excel files of data.
D. Advocacy group interested in ESRD.
E. Compilation of information from professional and scientific groups.
F. Interest in future publications.

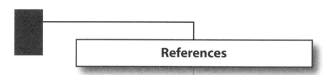

References

Albert, J., Akiba, T., Akizawa, T., Goodkin, D., Jacobson, S., Jadoul, M., et al. (2006). Baseline and time-varying measures of serum calcium and mortality in the Dialysis Outcomes and Practice Patterns Study (DOPPS). *Nephrology Dialysis Transplantation, 21*(Suppl. 4), 288.

American Nurses' Association (ANA). (2004). *Nursing: Scope and standards of practice.* Washington, DC: Author.

Andreucci, V.E., Fissell, R.B., Bragg-Gresham, J.L., Ethier, J., Greenwood, R., Pauly, M., et al. (2004). DOPPS data on medications in hemodialysis patients. *American Journal of Kidney Diseases, 44*(Suppl. 2), S61-S67.

Burrows-Hudson, S., & Prowant, B. (Eds.). (2005). *Nephrology nursing standards of practice and guidelines for care.* Pitman, NJ: American Nephrology Nurses' Association.

Cochran Collaboration, The. (2003). *Cochran reviewer's handbook.* Retrieved February 11, 2008, from http://www.cochrane.org/

Combe, C., Bragg-Gresham, J.L., Pifer, T.B., Bommer, J., Cruz, J.M., Asano, Y., et al. (2004, May). *Validation of a malnutrition-inflammation score (MIS) to predict mortality and hospitalisation in the DOPPS* [abstract]. Proceedings of the XLI Congress of the European Renal Association/European Dialysis and Transplant Association, Lisbon, Portugal.

Combe, C., McCullough, K.P., Asano, Y., Ginsberg, N., Maroni, B., & Pifer, T. (2004). K/DOQI and the DOPPS: Nutrition guidelines, indicators, and practices. *American Journal of Kidney Diseases, 44*(Suppl. 2), S39-S46.

Combe, C.H., Pisoni, R.L., Port, F.K., Young, E.W., Canaud, B., Mapes, D.L., et al. (2001). Dialysis outcomes and practice patterns study: Données sur l'utilisation des cathéters veineux centraux en hémodialyse chronique. *Nephrologie, 22*, 379-384.

Counts, C.S., & Ulrich, B. (Eds.). (2005). *Application to the American Nurses Association for recognition of nephrology nursing as a specialty in nursing.* Pitman, NJ: American Nephrology Nurses' Association.

Dicenso, A., Guyatt, G., & Ciliska, D. (2005). *Evidence-based nursing: A guide to clinical practice.* St. Louis: Elsevier/Mosby.

Fissell, R.B., Bragg-Gresham, J.L., Gillespie, B.W., Goodkin, D.A., Bommer, J., Saito, A., et al. (2004). International variation in vitamin prescription and association with mortality in the Dialysis Outcomes and Practice Patterns Study (DOPPS). *American Journal of Kidney Diseases, 44*(2), 293-299.

Goodkin, D.A., Young, E.W., Kurokawa, K., Prütz, K.G., & Levin, N.W. (2004). Mortality among hemodialysis patients in Europe, Japan, and the United States: Case-mix effects. *American Journal of Kidney Diseases, 44*(Suppl. 2), S16-S21.

Hays, R.D., Kallich, J.D., Mapes, D.L., Coons, S.J., & Carter, W.B. (1994). *Development of the Kidney Disease Quality of Life (KDQOL) Instrument. Quality of Life Research.* Santa Monica, CA: Rand Corporation.

Held, P.J., Brunner, F., Odaka, M., Garcia, J., Port, F.K., & Gaylin, D.S. (1990). Five-year survival for end stage renal disease patients in the U.S., Europe, and Japan 1982-87. *American Journal of Kidney Diseases, 15*, 451-457.

Jordan, P.S. (Ed.). (1993). *Nephrology nursing: A guide to professional development.* Pitman, NJ: American Nephrology Nurses' Association.

Kalantar-Zadeh, K., Kopple, J.D., Block, G., & Humphreys, M.H. (2001). A malnutrition-inflammation score is correlated with morbidity and mortality in maintenance hemodialysis patients. *American Journal of Kidney Diseases, 38*(6), 1251-1263.

Locatelli, F., Pisoni, R.L., Akizawa, T., Cruz, J.M., DeOreo, P., Lameire, N., et al. (2004). Anemia management for hemodialysis patients: KDOQI guidelines and DOPPS findings. *American Journal of Kidney Diseases, 44*(Suppl. 2), S27-S33.

Locatelli, F., Pisoni, R.L., Combe, C., Bommer, J., Andreucci, V.E., Piera, L., et al. (2004). Anaemia and associated morbidity and mortality among haemodialysis patients in five European countries. Results from the Dialysis Outcomes and Practice Patterns Study (DOPPS). *Nephrology Dialysis Transplantation, 19*(1), 121-132.

Lopes, A.A., Albert, J.M., Young, E.W., Satayathum, S., Pisoni, R.L., Andreucci, V.E., et al. (2004). Screening for depression in hemodialysis patients: Association with diagnosis, treatment, and outcomes in the DOPPS. *Kidney International, 66*, 2047-2053.

Lopes, A.A., Bragg, J., Young, E., Goodkin, D., Mapes, D., Combe, C., et al. (2002). Depression as a predictor of mortality and hospitalization among hemodialysis patients in the United States and Europe. Results from the Dialysis Outcomes and Practice Patterns Study (DOPPS). *Kidney International, 62*, 199-207.

Mapes, D.L., Bragg-Gresham, J.L., Bommer, J., Fukuhara, S., McKevitt, P., Wikstrom, B., et al. (2004). Health-related quality of life in the DOPPS. *American Journal of Kidney Diseases, 44*(Suppl. 2), S54-S60.

Mason, N.A., Bailie, G.R., Satayathum, S., Bragg-Gresham, J.L., Akiba, T., Akizawa, T., et al. (2005). HMG-coenzyme A reductase inhibitor use is associated with mortality reduction in hemodialysis patients. *American Journal of Kidney Diseases, 45*(1), 119-126.

Melnyk, B., & Fineout-Overholt, E. (2005). *Evidence-based practice in nursing and healthcare.* Philadelphia: Lippincott Williams & Wilkins.

National Institute of Diabetes and Digestive and Kidney Diseases (NIDDK). (2006). *United States renal data system.* Retrieved February 11, 2008, from http://www.usrds.org

National Kidney Foundation (NKF). (2000). *Clinical practice guidelines for nutrition in chronic renal failure.* Retrieved November 2, 2007, from http://www.kidney.org/professionals/kdoqi/guidelines_updates/doqi_nut.html

National Kidney Foundation (NKF). (2002). *Clinical practice guidelines for chronic kidney disease: Evaluation, classification, and stratification.* Retrieved November 2, 2007, from http://www.kidney.org/professionals/kdoqi/guidelines_ckd/toc.htm

National Kidney Foundation (NKF). (2003a). *Clinical practice guidelines for bone metabolism and disease in chronic kidney disease.* Retrieved November 2, 2007, from http://www.kidney .org/professionals/kdoqi/guidelines_bone/index.htm

National Kidney Foundation (NKF). (2003b). *Clinical practice guidelines for managing dyslipidemias in chronic kidney disease.* Retrieved November 2, 2007, from http://www.kidney.org/ professionals/kdoqi/guidelines_lipids/index.htm

National Kidney Foundation (NKF). (2004). *Clinical practice guidelines on hypertension and antihypertensive agents in chronic kidney disease.* Retrieved November 2, 2007, from http://www .kidney.org/professionals/kdoqi/guidelines_bp/index.htm

National Kidney Foundation (NKF). (2005a). *Clinical practice guidelines for bone metabolism and disease in children with chronic kidney disease.* Retrieved November 2, 2007, from http://www.kidney.org/professionals/kdoqi/guidelines_ped bone/index.htm

National Kidney Foundation (NKF). (2005b). *Clinical practice guidelines for cardiovascular disease in dialysis patients.* Retrieved November 2, 2007, from http://www.kidney.org/ professionals/kdoqi/guidelines_cvd/index.htm

National Kidney Foundation (NKF). (2006a). *Clinical practice guidelines and clinical practice recommendations: 2006 updates – Hemodialysis adequacy, peritoneal dialysis adequacy, and vascular access.* Retrieved November 2, 2007, from http://www. kidney.org/professionals/kdoqi/guideline_upHD_PD_VA/ index.htm

National Kidney Foundation (NKF). (2006b). *Clinical practice guidelines and clinical practice recommendations for anemia in chronic kidney disease.* Retrieved November 2, 2007, from http://www.kidney.org/professionals/kdoqi/guidelines_ anemia/index.htm

National Kidney Foundation (NKF). (2006c). *KDOQI history.* Retrieved July 10, 2006, from http://www.kidney.org/ professionals/kdoqi/aboutHistory.cfm

National Kidney Foundation (NKF). (2006d). *NKF KDOQI guidelines.* Retrieved July 10, 2006, from http://www.kidney. org/professionals/kdoqi/guidelines.cfm

National Kidney Foundation (NKF). (2006e). *Executive summary.* Retrieved July 10, 2006, from http://www.kidney.org/ professionals/kdoqi/guidelines ckd/p1exec.htm

National Kidney Foundation (NKF). (2007). *Clinical practice guidelines and clinical practice recommendations for diabetes and chronic kidney disease.* Retrieved November 2, 2007, from http://www.kidney.org/professionals/KDOQI/guideline_ diabetes/pdf/Diabetes_AJKD_linked.pdf

Pifer, T.B., McCullough, K.P., Port, F.K., Goodkin, D.A., Maroni, B.J., Held, P.J., et al. (2002). Mortality risk in hemodialysis patients and changes in nutritional indicators: DOPPS. *Kidney International, 62*(6), 2238-2245.

Pisoni, R.L., Bragg-Gresham, J.L., Young, E.W., Akizawa, T., Asano, Y., Locatelli, F., et al. (2004). Anemia management outcomes from 12 countries in the Dialysis Outcomes and Practice Patterns Study (DOPPS). *American Journal of Kidney Diseases, 44*(1), 94-111.

Pisoni, R.L., Gillespie, B.W., Dickinson, D.M., Chen, K., Kutner, M., & Wolfe, R.A. (2004). The Dialysis Outcomes and Practice Patterns Study: Design, data elements, and methodology. *American Journal of Kidney Diseases, 44*(Suppl. 2), S7-S15.

Pisoni, R.L., Mapes, D.L., & Port, F.K. (2006). Higher mortality and hospitalization risks in facilities with greater catheter use:

The search for practices to reverse the trend towards higher catheter use – International results from the DOPPS (abstract). *Nephrology News & Issues, 20*(12), 81-82.

Pisoni, R.L., Young, E.W., Dykstra, D.M., Greenwood, R.N., Hecking, E., Gillespie, B., et al. (2002). Vascular access use in Europe and the United States: Results from the DOPPS. *Kidney International, 61*, 305-316.

Pisoni, R.L., Young, E.W., Mapes, D.L., Keen, M.L., & Port, F.K. (2003, May). Vascular access use and outcomes in the U.S., Europe, and Japan. *Nephrology News and Issues,* 38-45.

Port, F.K., Pisoni, R.L., Bommer, J., Locatelli, F., Jadoul, M., Eknoyan, G., et al. (2006). Improving outcomes for dialysis patients in the International Dialysis Outcomes and Practice Patterns Study. *Clinical Journal of the American Society of Nephrology, 1*, 246-255.

Port, F.K., Pisoni, R.L., Bragg-Gresham, J.L., Satayathum, S.S., Young, E.W., Wolfe, R.A., et al. (2004). DOPPS estimate of patient life years attributable to modifiable hemodialysis practices in the United States. *Blood Purification, 22*, 175-180.

Port, F.K., Wolfe, R.A., Hulbert-Shearon, T.E., McCullough, K.P., Ashby, V.B., & Held, P.J. (2004). High dialysis dose is associated lower mortality among women but not among men. *American Journal of Kidney Diseases, 43*, 1014-1023.

Rayner, H.C., Besarab, A., Brown, W., Disney, A., Saito, A., & Pisoni, R.L. (2004). Vascular access results from the Dialysis Outcomes and Practice Patterns Study (DOPPS): Performance against Kidney Disease Outcomes Quality Initiative (K/DOQI) clinical practice guidelines. *American Journal of Kidney Diseases, 44*(Suppl. 2), S22-S26.

Rayner, H.C., Pisoni, R.L., Gillespie, B.W., Goodkin, D.A., Akiba, T., Akizawa, T., et al. (2003). Creation, cannulation, and survival of arteriovenous fistulae: Data from the Dialysis Outcomes and Practice Patterns Study. *Kidney International, 63*, 323-330.

Robinson, B.M., Joffe, M.M., Pisoni, R.L., Port, F.K., & Feldman, H.I. (2006). Revisiting survival differences by race and ethnicity among hemodialysis patients: The Dialysis Outcomes and Practice Patterns Study. *Journal of the American Society of Nephrology,* 17, 2910-2918.

Saran, R., Bragg-Gresham, J.L., Levin, N.W., Twardowski, Z.J., Wizemann, V., Saito, A., et al. (2006). Longer treatment time and slower ultrafiltration in hemodialysis: Associations with reduced mortality in the DOPPS. *Kidney International, 69*, 1222-1228.

Saran, R., Canaud, B., Depner, T., Keen, M., McCullough, K.P., Marshall, M.R., et al. (2004). Dose of dialysis: Key lessons from major observational studies and clinical trials. *American Journal of Kidney Diseases, 44*(Suppl. 2), S47-S53.

Saran, R., Dykstra, D.M., Wolfe, R.A, Gillespie, B., Held, P.J., & Young, E.W. (2002). Association between vascular access failure and the use of specific drugs: The Dialysis Outcomes and Practice Patterns Study (DOPPS). *American Journal of Kidney Diseases, 40*, 1255-1263.

Silverberg, D.S., Wexler, D., Iaina, A., Steinbruch, S., Wollman, Y., & Schwartz, D. (2006). Anemia, chronic renal disease and congestive heart failure – The cardio renal anemia syndrome: The need for cooperation between cardiologists and nephrologists. *International Urology Nephrology, 38*(2), 295-310.

Young, E.W., Akiba, T., M.D., Albert, J.M., McCarthy, J.T., Kerr, P.G., Mendelssohn, D.C., et al. (2004). Magnitude and impact of abnormal mineral metabolism in hemodialysis patients in the Dialysis Outcomes and Practice Patterns Study. *American Journal of Kidney Diseases, 44*(Suppl. 2), S34-S38.

Young, E.W., Dykstra, D.M., Goodkin, D.A., Mapes, D.L., Wolfe, R.A., & Held, P.J. (2002). Hemodialysis vascular access preferences and outcomes in the Dialysis Outcomes and Practice Patterns Study (DOPPS). *Kidney International, 61*, 2266-2271.

Suggested Readings

Burns, N., & Grove, S. (2005). *The practice of nursing research: Conduct, critique, and utilization* (5th ed.). St. Louis: Elsevier/Saunders.

Malloch, K., & Porter-O'Grady, T. (2006). *Evidence-based practice in nursing and health care.* Boston: Jones & Bartlett.

Netting the Evidence. (n.d.). *Introduction to evidence-based practice on the Internet.* Retrieved February 11, 2008, from http://www.shef.ac.uk/~scharr/ir/netting/

Polit, D., & Beck, C. (2006). *Essentials of nursing research: Methods, appraisal, and utilization* (6th ed.). Philadelphia: Lippincott Williams & Wilkins.

Wood, G., & Haber, J. (2006). *Nursing research: Methods and critical appraisal for evidence-based practice* (6th ed.). St. Louis: Elsevier/Mosby.

Section 7

Health Policy

Section Editor

Donna Bednarski, MSN, ANP,BC, CNN, CNP

Authors

Donna Bednarski, MSN, ANP,BC, CNN, CNP

Kristin Larson, MSN, RN, ANP, GNP, CNN

Gail Wick, MHSA, BSN, RN, CNN

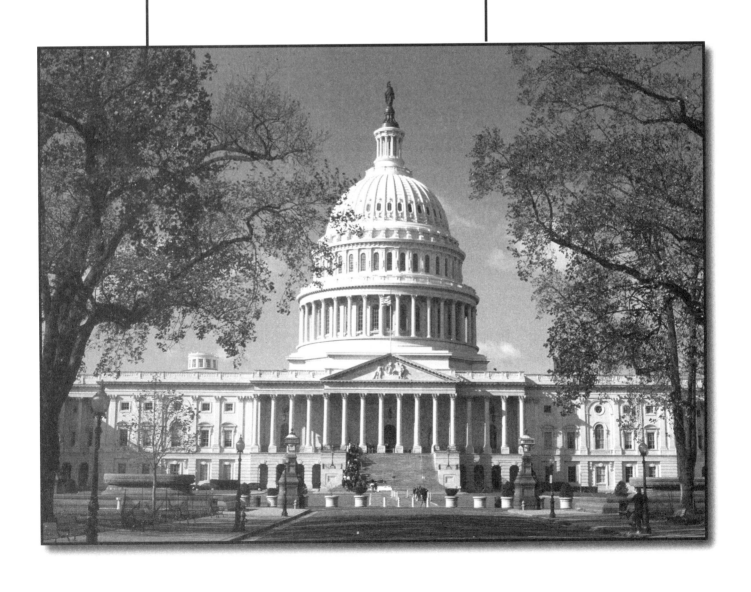

About the Authors

Donna Bednarski, MSN, ANP,BC, CNN, CNP, Section Editor and Author, is a Nurse Practitioner and Clinical Nurse Specialist, Nephrology, at Harper University Hospital in Detroit, Michigan.

Kristin Larson, MSN, RN, ANP, GNP, CNN, is a Nurse Practitioner at Nephrology Associates in Salt Lake City, Utah.

Gail Wick, MHSA, BSN, RN, CNN, is a consultant.

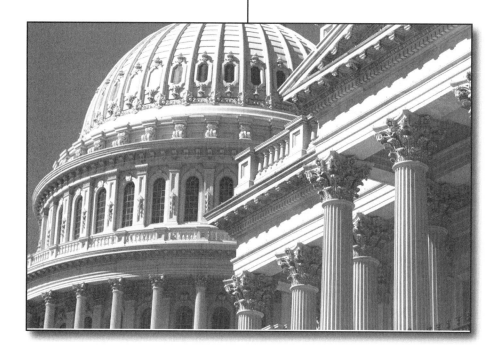

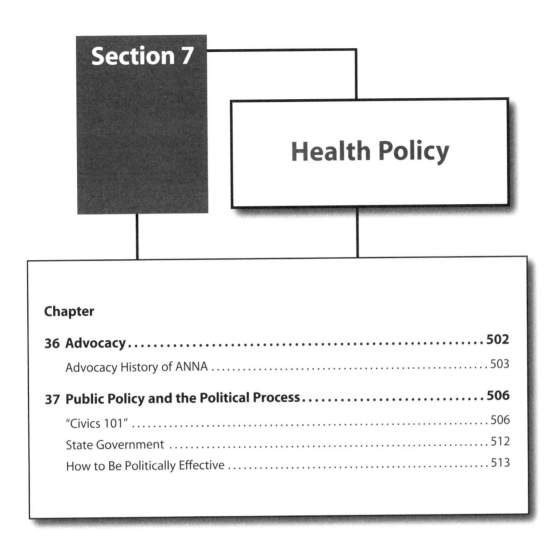

Section 7

Health Policy

Health Policy

Purpose and Background

The purpose of this section is to familiarize the reader with the importance of being proactive in the political and legislative arenas. This section will also provide an overview of the legislative process, communicating with members of Congress, and ANNA's involvement in health policy. As a core value of the organization's strategic plan, ANNA is a leader in advocacy for nephrology nursing and patients with kidney disease and their families. Through collaborative work with Congress, government agencies, and organizations, nephrology nurses have demonstrated their ability to impact patients and families and will continue to do so through their expertise as leaders in the kidney community.

Objectives

Upon completion of this section, the learner will be able to:
1. Describe what constitutes advocacy.
2. Define basic terms used in the legislative process.
3. Identify the characteristics of members of Congress.
4. Describe how a bill becomes a law.
5. Describe methods of communication with a member of Congress.
6. Verbalize the process to schedule an appointment with an elected official.
7. Review how to conduct an interview with a congressional staffer or a member of Congress.
8. Outline the history of ANNA's advocacy over the past 3 decades.
9. Review the purpose and preparation for Kidney Disease Awareness and Education Week.
10. Verbalize the process to obtain a proclamation from an elected official.

Chapter 36

Advocacy

I. Facets of advocacy.

A. Advocacy is a term used for organized activism related to a particular set of issues. Advocacy, therefore, supports a cause.

B. Advocacy requires an understanding of the issue, identifying goals, and communicating them to others.

C. It is every nurse's professional responsibility to act as a patient advocate. Political advocacy is an important component of patient advocacy.

D. The purpose of being a political advocate includes:
1. To provide representation on an issue.
2. To ensure the facts are presented in a manner that enables legislators to make informed decisions.
3. To promote good legislation on the state and federal levels.

II. Reasons to get involved.

A. Much of the professional lives of nurses is and will continue to be influenced by legislation and regulation at both the state and national levels.

B. Often Congress makes decisions that affect the health care of the nation. Members of Congress are not particularly knowledgeable about health care. Nurses can play key roles in educating and influencing policymakers. Nurses who work in nephrology possess expert knowledge in the care and needs of persons with kidney disease.

C. Nurses are the largest group of health care providers and as such have tremendous power to influence legislation.

D. Nurses can provide valid information on the needs of the health care system and methods to improve patient care.

E. Gallup's annual poll (2005), reflecting the opinion of the general public, found that nurses top the honesty and ethics list.

F. It is critical that nurses speak up about health care issues such as quality patient care, adequate staffing, safe workplaces, environments, etc.

G. The formation of health care policy is a process that offers many opportunities for active participation and making an impact.

Advocacy History of ANNA

I. 1980s.

A. ANNA was known as the American Association of Nephrology Nurses and Technicians.

B. The first position statements were published in 1983. Position statements represent succinct summaries of the organization's stand on an issue for the purpose of influence, advocacy, and/or clar-

ification. The first position statements supported:
1. The use of advanced practice nurses.
2. Cost containment efforts.
3. Efforts to increase organ donation.

C. Initiation of the Legislative Committee, 1987.

D. Establishment of the Legislative Consultant role, 1988.

II. 1990s.

A. The initiation of ANNA legislative workshops, which were held every other year.

B. The first legislative handbook was published.

C. The Legislative Representative was added to the roster of chapter officers.

D. The State Director role was instituted.

E. The Legislative Advisors were added to the roster of regional officers.

F. Development of the ANNA Health Policy Statement and Health Policy Agenda. Both documents are reviewed and updated annually and can be found on the ANNA Web site.

III. 2000s.

A. Establishment of the State Legislative Consultant, 2000.

B. ANNA purchased and began maintaining Cap Wiz, in 2003, which can be found on the ANNA Web site. ANNA maintains the Cap Wiz Legislative Action Center so members can communicate quickly and easily with their elected representatives about issues that have an impact on nephrology nursing practice.

C. Education for state and federal lawmakers.
1. In August 2003, the first ESRD Education Day was held. This initiative was dedicated to educate lawmakers about kidney disease, treatment options, and legislative issues facing the kidney community. Members are encouraged to invite Congressional delegations, Centers for Medicare and Medicaid Services (CMS) staff, ESRD regional office staff, and local and regulatory agency staff to visit a local dialysis facility, transplant center, or KEEP program.

2. Allows all willing nephrology nurses, from bedside to administration, to share their knowledge of patient care and participate in political advocacy.

3. Since the initial ESRD Education Day, hundreds of federal, state, and city officials and their staffs, have toured dialysis facilities nationwide.

4. ESRD Education Day grew to ESRD Education Week by August 2005 with other organizations and associations participating in the educational endeavor.

5. Name changed to Kidney Disease Awareness and Education Week in 2008. The focus continues to be dedicated to educating policymakers and their staff members about the needs of patients suffering from or at risk for ESRD.

D. Terminology changes, 2004.
   1. ANNA Legislative Committee became the Health Policy Committee.
   2. Legislative Consultant became Health Policy Consultant.
   3. State Legislative Consultant became State Health Policy Consultant.
   4. Legislative Advisors became Health Policy Advisors.
   5. State Directors became Health Policy State Directors.
   6. Legislative Representatives became Health Policy Representatives.

E. Updates to Health Policy Committee. The addition of the following volunteer roles:
   1. Advisor for Position Statements.
   2. Advisor for Kidney Disease Awareness and Education Week.
   3. Advisor for Cap Wiz.

F. The initiation of the ANNA Capitol Gang. The ANNA Capitol Gang is a group of ANNA volunteer nurses who have experience speaking with legislators and the ability to get to Washington D.C. in a "moment's notice" to discuss issues on behalf of ANNA.

G. Increased ANNA health policy activities. Refer to ANNA Web site: www.annanurse.org. For a list of recent activities, choose Legislative Activities, then Activities/Endorsements. Sample activities include:
   1. Contribution by ANNA to regulatory language with formation of task forces to review legislative documents, e.g. revised Conditions for Coverage for ESRD facilities to formulate a

collective response.

2. Support for federal legislative initiatives.
   a. Kidney Care Quality and Improvement Act of 2005.
   b. The Kidney Care Quality and Education Act of 2007.
   c. Written testimony to support funding for nursing and nephrology-related program in fiscal year 2008.
   d. Nursing education, such as the appropriation of funds for the Nurse Reinvestment Act.

3. Support for state legislative initiatives.
   a. Letter was sent to the National Council of State Boards of Nursing in support of State Licensure Compacts.
   b. In 2004, letter was sent to the Indiana State Board of Nursing regarding the role of unlicensed personnel in dialysis and the legitimate role of registered nurses in delegating to and supervising such personnel.
   c. In 2004, letter was sent to the West Virginia Board of Registered Professional Nurses regarding emergency rule 19CSR13, "Dialysis Technicians."
   d. In 2005, letter was sent to the Montana State Board of Nursing regarding the January 13 MAR Notice No. 8-32-64, proposed adoption of New Rules I-IX pertaining to delegation (specifically New Rule IX, Advance Delegation to a dialysis technician).

4. Input into regulatory agencies' activities, e.g., response to the Joint Commission Field Review: Organ Transplant Center Certification, 2006.

5. Endorsements of nursing organization standards, e.g., endorsement of AACN Standards for Establishing and Sustaining Healthy Work Environments, 2006.

6. Member of Kidney Care Partners (KCP).
   a. Founded in May of 2003 and located in Washington, D.C., KCP is a coalition of patient advocates, dialysis professionals, providers, and suppliers working together to improve the quality of care for individuals with chronic kidney disease (CKD).
   b. Their mission, individually and collectively, is to ensure:
      (1) CKD patients receive optimal care.
      (2) CKD patients are able to live quality lives.
      (3) Dialysis care is readily accessible to all those in need.
      (4) Research and development leads to enhanced therapies and innovative products.
   c. Partners include organizations from the

nephrology community, including patient advocate organizations (National Kidney Foundation, National Kidney Fund, Davita Patient Citizens, etc.), professional organizations (e.g., ANNA, Renal Physician Association), dialysis providers (e.g., Davita Inc., Fresenius Renal Care North America), dialysis suppliers (e.g., Amgen, Genzyme), and other related organizations (e.g., Medical Education Institute).
   d. More information can be found on their Web site: http://www.kidneycarepartners.org.

H. Second week of September established as Nephrology Nurses Week.

  1. Initiated in 2005 to honor the dedicated nephrology nurses who care for patients with kidney disease.
  2. ANNA launched Nephrology Nurses Week to give employers, patients, and others the opportunity to thank nephrology nurses for their life-saving work.
  3. Celebrates the many skills of the nephrology nurse at the bedside and in patient advocacy.
  4. Sample activities.
    a. ANNA chapter-sponsored educational sessions.
    b. Structured recognitions and awards.
    c. Distribution of Nephrology Nurses Week pins or other ANNA items.
    d. Thank-you notes to nephrology nurses.
    e. Games and prizes.
    f. Ice cream socials.
  5. Additional resources can be found on the ANNA Web site, including:
    a. ANNA Health Policy Toolkit: created to educate, inform, and encourage people interested in health care issues to become knowledgeable about the legislative process and become involved in health policy advocacy.
    b. Nephrology Nurses Week Online Toolkit.
     (1) Nephrology Nurses Week logo.
     (2) Nephrology Nurses Week poster.
     (3) Nephrology Nurses Week press release.
     (4) Nephrology Nurses Week newsletter article.
     (5) Nephrology Nurses Week proclamation.
    c. Nephrology Nurses Week pins.
    d. Nephrology Nurses Week report and evaluation form.

I. In December 2005, Gardner, Carton & Douglas was retained as the legislative consulting firm for ANNA.
  1. In 2007, Gardner, Carton & Douglas merged with Drinker Biddle to become Drinker Biddle & Reath LLP.
  2. Activities.
    a. Helps increase ANNA member involvement, understanding, and appreciation by explaining the need to engage in advocacy at the grassroots level.
    b. Engages in activities on ANNA's behalf with KCP.
    c. Monitors legislative and regulatory activities that are perceived to have a direct impact on the practice of nephrology nursing and the ESRD program, CKD, transplantation, and related therapies.
    d. Reviews, analyzes, and evaluates proposed legislation that affects ANNA and its interests and make recommendations regarding courses of action.
    e. Represents ANNA before Congress, federal agencies, and the nursing and nephrology communities.
    f. Assists in the development of position statements and revision of ANNA's legislative platform.
    g. Serves as a member of the Health Policy Committee.

Chapter 37

Public Policy and the Political Process

"Civics 101"

I. Basic terminology.

A. Constituent – an individual who appoints or elects another as their representative or agent.

B. Bill – legislation introduced in either the House or Senate.

C. Authorization bill – legislation that formally establishes a program or activity and obligates funding that program or activity. An authorization may be effective for 1 year, a fixed number of years, or an indefinite period. An authorization may be for a specified amount of funds or for "such sums as may be necessary."

D. Appropriations bill – legislation that formally approves the provision of funds from the United States Treasury for an authorized program or activity.

E. Resolutions – formal statements of decisions or expressions of opinions, put before or accepted measures passed by either the House or Senate.

F. Sponsor – the original member who introduced a bill.

G. Cosponsor – a member (or members) that formally add his/her name in support of another member's bill.

H. Amendment – to change a bill by adding, deleting, or substituting portions of it.

I. Committee – a group of members assigned to review certain bills.

J. Act – legislation that has been passed into law by both houses of Congress.

K. Veto – power to say no or forbid.

II. Characteristics of members of Congress.
Bicameral – consists of two chambers or houses of government, the Senate and the House of Representatives. See Table 7.1.

III. Enacting legislation.

A. There are three branches of government.
  1. The executive branch includes the president, vice president, federal departments, and agencies.
  2. The judicial branch is a court system for the interpretation of laws.
  3. The legislative branch is Congress with the primary purpose to make laws.

B. Introducing legislation.
  1. There are two main types of legislation: authorizing bill and appropriations bill.
    a. How a bill becomes law (refer below) generally applies to both authorizing and appropriations legislation.
    b. For a law to be enacted, it must be authorized and funds appropriated.
    c. Before money can be spent, Congress must authorize the expenditure and then appropriate the funds to do so. This formal process consists of two sequential steps.
      (1) Enactment of authorization of a program or activity. Legislative committees from both chambers are responsible for authorizing legislation related to agencies and programs under their jurisdiction.
      (2) Enactment of appropriations to provide funds for the authorized program or activity. The Appropriations committees of the House and Senate have jurisdiction over appropriations measures.
  2. Bills are drafts of a proposed legislation that are introduced in either the House or Senate.
    a. They create public policies.
    b. Ideas can come from any citizen.
    c. Can be introduced by any member of Congress.
    d. Bills introduced in the House are labeled with "HR" and followed by a number.

Table 7.1

Bicameral Legislative System

	U.S. House of Representatives	U.S. Senate
Referred to as	1. Representative 2. Congressman or Congresswoman	1. Senator 2. Member of Congress
Numbers	1. 435 individuals determined by the Federal Census and reviewed every 10 years. 2. The District of Columbia and U.S. territories (Guam, Puerto Rico, Samoa, Virgin Islands) each have a single delegate. 3. All states have at least one representative.	1. 100 individuals, 2 from each state. 2. No senator from U. S. territories or the District of Columbia.
Term	1. 2 years. 2. All members elected every 2 years.	1. 6 years. 2. One third elected every 2 years.
Eligibility	1. Age 25 or older. 2. U.S. citizen for 7 years. 3. Reside in the district representing.	1. Age 30 or older. 2. U.S. citizen for 9 years. 3. Reside in the district representing.

e. Bills introduced in the Senate are labeled with an "S" and followed by a number.

f. While thousands of bills are introduced into congressional session, fewer than 5% are enacted into law.

g. If a bill is not acted upon over the course of the 2-year session of Congress, it dies at the end of the session and must be reintroduced in the next session.

C. How a bill becomes law.

1. After being introduced, bills are assigned a number and labeled with a sponsor's name. The bill may have a cosponsor or cosponsors, but they are not required.

2. The Speaker of the House or the presiding officer in the Senate will then assign the bill to the committee with jurisdiction over the subject.

   a. Bills may be referred to more than one committee and may be split so that parts are sent to different committees and subsequently to subcommittees.

   b. The major work of reviewing and modifying bills is done in committee.

   c. If there is failure of the committee to act on a bill, the bill will "die in committee." This happens frequently if grassroots and member support is not highly visible.

3. Activities within the committee.

   a. Subcommittee hearings and markups.

      (1) Hearings. Subcommittees have the option to hold hearings on a bill and invite testimony from public and private witnesses.

      (2) Markups. Once hearings are complete, subcommittee members go through the measure line-by-line, marking up adopted changes.

      (3) Subcommittee members vote on whether to report the bill favorably to the full committee. If the vote is not favorably reported, the bill usually dies.

   b. Full committee hearings and markups.

      (1) The full committee may repeat any or all

of the subcommittee's procedures: hearings, markups, and a vote.

(2) If there are substantial revisions, the committee can introduce a "clean bill." The new bill will be assigned a new number.

(3) If the full committee votes favorably, it is reported to the whole chamber, House, or Senate.

4. Floor action.
   a. The bill is brought to the Senate or House floor for debate.
      (1) The bill may be amended.
      (2) Voted up or down.
      (3) Referred back to committee or tabled. If these options occur, the bill usually dies.
   b. The bill is then voted on and passed by majority vote. It is sent to the other chamber unless the other chamber has already had a similar bill being considered. If it fails, then the bill usually dies.
   c. If both chambers, the House and Senate, pass the same bill, then it is sent to the president. However if the bills are not the same, and they both pass, they are sent to a conference committee. Most major legislation goes to a conference committee.
      (1) The bills move to conference committee for further review and amending.
      (2) The conference committee is made up of members from each chamber.
      (3) If the conference committee is unable to reach an agreement with changes or amendments, the bill usually dies.
      (4) If the conference committee reaches a compromise, it completes a conference report, which is sent back to each chamber. Both the House and the Senate must approve the conference report or the bill usually dies.
   d. After the bill has been approved by both the House and Senate, it is sent to the president.

5. Presidential and congressional actions.
   a. The president can sign the bill into law.
   b. If the president takes no action within 10 days, while Congress is in session, the bill dies.
   c. If the president takes no action within 10 days, after Congress has adjourned, the bill does not become law and is called a "pocket veto."
   d. The president can veto the bill and send it back to Congress with recommendations.
   e. Congress can override a veto with two-thirds vote.

D. After a law is passed.
   1. It is referred to the appropriate executive branch agency for the development of regulations. These regulations implement the law.
      a. Agencies issue proposed rules in advance of regulatory action.
      b. The draft is then circulated for review.
      c. Once cleared, the proposed rule is printed in the Federal Register, a document used to notify the public of all proposed rules, administrative matters, and selected presidential activities.
         (1) The Federal Register lists:
            (a) The regulating agency.
            (b) The name of the proposed rule.
            (c) The summary of the regulatory action.
            (d) Any needed background information.
            (e) A contact person at the agency.
      d. The public usually has 30–60 days to respond to a proposed rule, allowing another opportunity for grassroots/member involvement.
      e. Each of the comments is reviewed, and a final rule is developed.
      f. The final rule is published in the Federal Registry, specifying an effective date for implementation. A summary of public comments to the proposed rule is included.

   Tables 7.2 and 7.3 delineate events in legislative history and regulatory history that have impacted the kidney patient.

IV. Federal budget.

A. Budgets are prepared by each federal agency and submitted to the Office of Management and Budget (OMB). OMB then finalizes the proposed funding levels based on the priorities of the president.
   1. Three main components.
      a. How much the federal government should spend on public purposes.
      b. How much it should take in as tax revenue.
      c. Identification of the deficit or surplus the federal government should run.
   2. The president's budget spells out how much funding is recommended for each "discretionary" or "appropriated" program.
      a. These programs fall under the jurisdiction of the House and Senate Appropriations committees.
      b. To continue operating, any discretionary program must have funding renewed each year, or at the previously defined interval.

Table 7.2 ———— **Events in Legislative History That Have Impacted the Kidney Patient**

Title of Legislation	Important Dates	Key Points
Gottschalk Committee	1967	■ Responsible for considering all aspects of the problems posed by CKD and making recommendations toward managing them. ■ Recommendations. 1. Initiate a national program for the treatment of ESRD. 2. Finance the program by amending the Social Security Act to "cover the permanently disabled regardless of age." 3. Deem persons with CKD as disabled, thereby entitling ESRD patients to Medicare benefits.
HR-1: Social Security Amendments of 1972	1. ESRD amendment introduced September 30, 1972. 2. House-Senate conference report issued October 14, 1972. 3. HR-1 became Public Law 92-603 when signed by President Nixon on October 30, 1972. 4. Effective date for Medicare coverage for chronic kidney failure was July 1, 1973.	■ Intent of Medicare coverage. 1. Provide equitable access for all ESRD patients. 2. Patients who were certified to have chronic kidney failure and require dialysis or transplantation by a physician were deemed disabled. 3. Entitled to Medicare Part A and Part B benefits via Medicare disability program. 4. Premium paid by beneficiary for Part B benefits.

National Organ Transplant Act of 1984	1984	■ Public Law 98-507.
		1. Created task force on organ transplantation.
		2. Amended the Public Health Service Act to authorize the Secretary of HHS to make grants for the establishment, initial operation, and expansion planning of qualified organ procurement organizations (OPOs).
		3. Directed the Secretary of the Health and Human Services to:
		  a. Establish an Organ Procurement and Transplantation Network (OPTN) to provide a central registry linking donors and potential recipients.
		  b. Establish a scientific registry of organ recipients.
		  c. Designate and maintain an identifiable unit in the Public Health service to coordinate federal organ transplant programs and policies.
		  d. Publish an annual report on the scientific and clinical status of organ transplantation.
		4. Prohibited the purchase or sale of human organs if such transfer affects interstate commerce and established criminal penalties for such violations.

Omnibus Budget Reconciliation Act (OBRA) of 1986 (ESRD provisions)	1986	■ Legislated via Public Law 99-609. 1. Amended section 1881 of the Social Security Act. 2. Authorized Secretary of HHS to set composite rate for dialysis services provided between October 1, 1986 and October 1, 1988 at a level equal to the rate in effect as of May 13, 1986, reduced by $2.00. 3. Reduced the composite payment rate by an additional $0.50 to finance the Network administrative organization. 4. Required a study to evaluate the effects of the payment reductions on access and quality of care (due January 1, 1988). 5. Established a national ESRD registry to assemble and analyze data, known as U.S. Renal Data System (USRDS). 6. Modified/reorganized the Network Administration Organization. 7. Extended coverage of immunosuppressive drugs. 8. Established protocols or standards and conditions for safe and effective dialyzer reuse. 9. Established organ procurement protocols as a requirement for hospitals and organizations involved in procuring organs for transplantations.

Table 7.3 ——— **Events in Regulatory History That Have Impacted the Care of the Kidney Patient**

Title of Regulation	Important Dates	Key Points
Conditions of participation	Interim regulations: June 29, 1973	1. Interim conditions of participation and payment rates for dialysis and transplant services.
	Interim regulations: April 22, 1975	1. Minor modifications to and republication of initial interim regulations concerning coverage of services.
	NPRM: July 1, 1975	1. Specified conditions of coverage that facilities must meet to qualify for Medicare reimbursement. 2. Included health and safety requirements. 3. Directed the organization of the ESRD Network System.
	Final rule: June 3, 1976	1. Finalized condition of participation as ESRD provider/supplies and coverage.
	Final rule: August 11, 1978	1. Authorized temporary approval as kidney transplantation centers for pediatric hospitals. 2. Allowed for Medicare approval/reimbursement without meeting the required minimal utilization for number of kidney transplants performed.
Prospective composite rate payment system	NPRM: February 12, 1982 Final rule: May 11, 1983	1. Established a payment rate per treatment adjusted for geographic wage differences. 2. Separate rates for hospital-based and independent dialysis facilities. 3. Exception process developed based on atypical patient mix, extraordinary circumstances, education costs, or as an isolated essential facility. 4. Physician payment modified to a single monthly prospective capitation payment (MCP).
Final rule: ESRD Networks	August 26, 1986	1. Authorized the Secretary of HHS to designate the ESRD Network areas. 2. Delineated 14 network areas and criteria used to determine these areas. 3. OBRA of 1986 required modification to at least 17 Network organizations.
Final rule: Reuse	October 1, 1987	1. Standards for the reuse of hemodialyzers, filters, and other dialysis supplies.

Notice for Proposed Rule Making (NPRM): Occupational exposure to bloodborne pathogens	May 30, 1989	1. Infection control plan must be designed and implemented by each employer to minimize or eliminate employee exposure.
		2. Plan shall be reviewed and updated as needed.
		3. Universal precautions shall be observed inclusive of:
		   a. Hand washing as frequently as needed.
		   b. Use of personal protective equipment.
		     • Gloves.
		     • Masks, eye protection, and face shields.

Table 7.3 (contd.) — Events in Regulatory History That Have Impacted the Care of the Kidney Patient

Title of Regulation	Important Dates	Key Points

Medicare Program; Conditions for Coverage for End Stage Renal Disease (ESRD) Facilities; Proposed Rule; CMS-3818-P	NPRM: February 4, 2005	1. This proposed rule would revise the requirements that ESRD dialysis facilities must meet to be certified under the Medicare program.
		2. The revised requirements focus on the patient, including:
		  a. The results of the care provided to the patient.
		  b. Establish performance expectations for facilities.
		  c. Encourage patients to participate in their care plan and treatment.
		  d. Eliminate many procedural requirements from the current conditions for coverage.
		  e. Preserve strong process measures when necessary to promote patient well being and continuous quality improvement.
		3. Changes are necessary to reflect the advances in dialysis technology and standard care practices since the requirements were last revised in their entirety in 1976.

Medicare Program; Hospital Conditions of Participation: Requirements for Approval and Re-approval of Transplant Centers to Perform Organ Transplants; Proposed Rule; CMS-3835-P	NPRM: February 4, 2005 Final: March 30, 2007 Effective: June 28, 2007	1. Establishes, for the first time, Medicare conditions of participation for heart, heart-lung, intestine, kidney, liver, lung, and pancreas transplant centers. 2. Sets forth clear expectations for minimal health and safety rules to provide safe, high quality transplant service delivery in all Medicare-participating facilities.
Proposed Rule for Revisions to Payment Policies Under the Physician Fee Schedule for Calendar Year (CY) 2006	Federal Register: September 1, 2005	This document corrects errors in the proposed rule that appeared in the Federal Register on August 8, 2005 entitled "Medicare Program; Revisions to Payment Policies Under the Physician Fee Schedule for Calendar Year 2006."

c. Discretionary programs make up about one third of all federal spending and include programs such as defense spending, health research, and housing.

3. The president's budget can also include changes to "mandatory" or "entitlement" programs (e.g., Social Security, Medicare, Medicaid, food stamps, military retirement benefits, unemployment insurance). Entitlement programs are not controlled by annual appropriations.

4. The president's budget can also include changes to the tax code. Any proposal to increase or decrease taxes should be reflected in the change in federal revenue over the following and future years.

B. On the first Monday in February, the president submits this budget to the House and the Senate budget committees.

1. The House and Senate Budget committees are to draft the budget resolution.

2. Once completed, the resolution goes to the House and Senate where it can be amended.

3. Once both houses pass the resolution, it goes to the House-Senate conference to reconcile any differences, and a conference report is developed.

4. Once approved, it does not go to the president for signature or veto. It requires only a majority vote to pass. As a result, no funds are appropriated. The budget resolution serves as a template for the actual appropriation process.

5. The budget resolution is to be passed by April 15, but it often takes longer. The fiscal year begins on October 1.

6. If Congress does not pass a budget resolution, a "continuing resolution" is passed. The continuing resolution temporarily funds federal programs at some agreed upon rate or previous year's level, until the appropriations bills are passed.

7. The budget committees are required by law to issue two budget resolutions each year.
   a. The initial resolution defines revenue and spending.
   b. Later in the year, this resolution is updated to reflect actual economic data.

C. If government spending exceeds the parameters of the budget resolution, budget reconciliation is needed to balance the budget.
   1. Historically, health programs are dramatically affected by this activity.
   2. Each authorizing committee targets specific areas of "savings." Often program changes are voted on as well as legislation passed to authorize spending.

D. Budget reconciliation.
   1. An optional process that Congress may use to assure compliance with direct spending, revenue, and debt limit levels set forth in the budget resolution.
   2. If Congress decides to use the reconciliation process, language known as a "reconciliation directive" must be included in the budget resolution. The reconciliation directive instructs various committees to produce legislation by a specified date to achieve the goals in budget resolution.

V. **Other resources.**
   http://www.annanurse.org
   http://www.firstgov.org
   http://www.congress.org
   http://thomas.loc.gov
   http://vote-smart.org/index.htm

State Government

I. **Powers under the state government.**

A. States must take responsibility for:
   1. Ownership of property.
   2. Education of inhabitants.
   3. Implementation of welfare and other benefits programs and distribution of aid.
   4. Protection of people from local threats.
   5. Maintenance of a justice system.
   6. Establishment of local governments (counties and municipalities).
   7. Maintenance of state highways and establishment of a means for administration of local roads.
   8. Regulation of industry.
   9. Procurement of funds to support these required activities.
   10. Administration of mandates set forth by the federal government.

B. Each state must have its own constitution to use as the basis for laws with a means for amending.

II. **State variations.**

A. Each state has variations in the operation of its government.

B. Legislative salaries range from nothing to large salaries.

C. Health policy sessions also vary among states, ranging from very short sessions (3–4 months) to longer sessions (6–12 months).

D. There are other elected positions that may include:
   1. Lieutenant governor.
   2. Secretary of state.
   3. Attorney general.
   4. Auditor.
   5. Treasurer.
   6. Superintendent of public instruction.

C. State similarities.
   1. Each state has a governor, lieutenant governor, and other appointed or elected officials.
   2. All states except Nebraska are composed of two chambers – a Senate and General Assembly or House of Representatives.
      a. Nebraska is the only state with a unicameral legislature, having only one chamber, the House, and is nonpartisan.

b. Nonpartisan refers to government officials who do not identify a formal party affiliation or formal alignment with a political party.

3. Leaders of each house are responsible for referring bills to committee, recognizing speakers in debate, and presiding over deliberations.

D. Nurse practice acts (NPAs).
1. Nursing practice is governed by state agencies, which vary from state to state.
2. NPAs are the most important legal documents for the nursing profession and the individual nurse. NPAs are created with the purpose of protecting the public.
3. NPAs define what the functions of nursing shall be and set standards for licensure.
4. Each state has a local board authorized to formulate and enforce the rules and regulations governing the nursing profession.

E. Nurse Licensure Compact (NLC).
1. The Nurse Licensure Compact is a mutual recognition model of nurse licensure allowing a nurse to have one license (in their state of residency) and to practice in multiple states, unless otherwise restricted.
2. The nurse is subject to each state's practice laws and regulations.
3. To achieve mutual recognition, each state must enact legislation authorizing the Nurse Licensure Compact.
4. States entering the compact must also adopt administrative rules and regulations for implementation of the compact.
5. More information, including participating states, can be found on the National Council of State Boards of Nursing Web site: https://www.ncsbn.org/index.htm.

How to Be Politically Effective

I. Register and vote in elections.

A. Primary elections are held prior to the general elections and enable voters to select the candidates who will run on each party's ticket.

B. General elections are held to fill public offices.

II. Keep your eyes and ears open.
Learn more about state and federal issues that affect your practice and daily life.

A. State level.
1. Obtain a copy of your nurse practice act through your state board of nursing. A copy can be found on http://www.ncsbn.org.
   a. Read it.
   b. Learn how to advise your state board of nursing regarding changes needed to improve nephrology nursing.
2. Contact your state board of nursing and offer your assistance.
3. Understand your state legislature. Check your state Web site often to keep in touch with issues pending in the state legislature.
4. Get to your know representatives. Invite them to participate in Kidney Disease Awareness and Education Week (see "Participate in Kidney Disease Awareness and Education Week").

B. Federal level.
1. Get to know your representatives.
2. Invite them to participate in Kidney Disease Awareness and Education Week.

III. Take advantage of the CapWiz Legislation Center
to identify issues important to nephrology nurses.

A. E-mail elected officials, including the president, members of Congress, and more, by using ZIP codes.
1. Type in your ZIP code (identifies your representatives) or search by last name.
2. Create a message to send to the representatives.
3. There are optional prewritten e-mail templates that ANNA develops on various issues of importance to nephrology nurses or a person with kidney disease.

B. Identify issues and legislation. ANNA scans legislation and provides a listing of the key legislation and initiatives underway that impact your day-to-day practice in nephrology nursing.
1. Legislative alerts and updates – news and information about important issues.
   a. Use prewritten e-mail templates developed by ANNA.
   b. Click on the topic of interest and complete the required information. The prewritten template will be sent to the representatives.
2. Current legislation – summaries and status information about key bills.
3. Key votes – key Congressional roll call votes.

4. Capitol Hill basics – tips about communicating with members as well as general information about Hill staffers, the legislative process, and more.

C. Elections and candidates. To find election results, enter your ZIP code or search by state.

D. Media guide.
   1. Find and contact national and local media.
   2. This can be done by using a member's ZIP code, individual search, by entering the name of editors, reporters, or producers, or by organization search by entering the organization name, e.g., newspaper, TV, radio, etc.

IV. Participate in Kidney Disease Awareness and Education Week. Tools are available to assist in this educational week and can be found on the ANNA Web site, www.annanurse.org.

A. *Planning and Orientation Guide.* A step-by-step guide to assist with all the activities associated with setting up a tour, including instructions for sending tour invitations, how to schedule a tour, how to conduct a tour with a Congressional member, and how to follow up the tour to ensure long-term success.

B. *ESRD Briefing Book for State and Federal Policymakers: A Guide to Kidney Disease Awareness and Education.* The booklet presents in lay terms the basics of ESRD and includes information on underlying conditions such as diabetes and hypertension, incidence, and treatment costs.

V. Soliciting for a proclamation.

A. Tips for getting an official proclamation from your community or state can be found on the ANNA Web site.

B. Proclamations can be issued by a governor or a mayor. In many areas, a mayor or governor can issue a proclamation without action from the city council or state legislature.

C. A letter requesting a proclamation should follow the same format used to write a federal official (see VI. Communicating with elected officials).
   1. Within the text of the letter, include:
      a. The reason for the proclamation, e.g., Kidney Disease Awareness and Education Week, Nephrology Nurses Week.

b. How the issue affects local citizens.
      c. A fact sheet with statistics and trends for your state or city that relate to the issue (these statistics can provide the text of the proclamation). For example: The number of patients with ESRD in the state, the number of new cases each year, the number of nurses caring for these patients.
      d. Dates of the proclamation.

D. Always follow up with a written thank-you note.

E. Inform the ANNA National Office of the proclamation.

VI. Communicating with elected officials.

A. Can it make a difference?
   1. The offices of elected officials count all calls, e-mails, faxes, and mail received.
   2. The staffers log each opinion that is expressed.
   3. The information is then reported to the member of Congress.

B. Effective communication with legislators is the backbone of every successful legislative initiative.

C. Legislators rely on informed citizens to help them identify key issues and positions on those issues. Nephrology nurses are the experts who have personally seen the devastating effects of kidney disease on patients and their families.

D. Phone calls.
   1. Plan what you want to say before you call.
   2. Always be polite.
   3. Ask to speak to the staff member who handles the issue you wish to discuss.
   4. Begin by identifying yourself by name and as a registered nurse.
   5. Find out the member's position on an issue. It can be a waste of time for the member if they already support your position.
   6. Keep the call brief; make a few brief points.
      a. State your position.
      b. Be clear and specific as to what you are asking your representative to do (e.g., support or cosponsor the legislation).
   7. Be prepared to answer questions and leave a telephone number where you can be contacted to provide additional information.
   8. Offer assistance to the member or staff.
   9. Express appreciation.
   10. Always send a follow-up letter.

E. Sending a letter or e-mail.
1. Guidelines are the same for state and federal officials.
2. Standard mail takes quite a while longer. Since the anthrax attacks in 2001, the U.S. Postal Service mail has been handled differently by Congress. If your message is time sensitive, consider e-mail, fax, or phone communication.
3. Addressing the letter or e-mail.
   a. Senator.
      (1) The Honorable (full name)
          United States Senate
          Washington, D.C. 20510
      (2) Dear Senator:
   b. House of Representatives.
      (1) The Honorable (full name)
          United States House of Representatives
          Washington, D.C. 20515
      (2) Dear Congressman/Congresswoman:
          or
          Dear Representative:
   c. Committee chair.
      (1) Use examples above for address.
      (2) Dear Mr. Chairman/Dear Madam Chairwoman:
4. Text of the letter.
   a. Concisely state purpose of letter in first paragraph.
   b. State your name and identify yourself as a registered nurse.
   c. Include your area of work and define the patients you care for.
   d. Give your full home mailing address so the office can verify you are a constituent and send you a response. If you are not a constituent, identify any connection with the recipient's district (e.g., working in the district).
   e. Identify legislation by HR____ or S____.
   f. Be very specific as to what you would like your representative to do.
   g. Include vital pieces of information such as how this issue affects the member's constituents. If applicable, make it personal. Relay personal testimony or experiences.
   h. Offer assistance to serve as a resource to the member or the staff.
   i. Express appreciation for the time and effort the member has spent or will spend on the issue or bill.
   j. Request a response from the member.
   k. Overall tips.
      (1) Keep text to one page.
      (2) Address only one issue per letter.
      (3) Be honest and accurate.
      (4) Be brief and to the point.
5. Be sure to follow up.
   a. By phone or with another letter.
   b. If you receive an unsatisfactory response, write or call again.
      (1) Express appreciation for the time and effort.
      (2) Be firm and polite in communicating your position.
      (3) Review the vital pieces of information.
6. Keep in regular contact.

F. Scheduling a visit with a representative.
1. Guidelines are the same for Washington, D.C., or your local district.
   a. Remember you do not need to go to Washington, D.C., to see your representatives.
   b. Visit the district office; it is probably very near your home.
   c. Plan your visit carefully.
2. Contact the representative's scheduler or secretary by phone or e-mail.
   a. Washington, D.C., switchboard.
      (1) House (202) 225-3121
      (2) Senate (202) 224-3121
   b. The district office will be listed in the blue pages of your local telephone book.
   c. State your name and where you live.
   d. State that you are a registered nurse.
   e. Relay the reason for requesting a visit to speak with the member.
   f. The scheduler may ask for a faxed request. In that case, create a concise letter with all the necessary information (refer to previous information on composing the letter).
   g. Include a list of those who would like to attend the meeting.
   h. You will be notified by phone or e-mail of the appointment time.
   i. Be polite and persistent.
   j. Call or re-fax a request if there is no response from the scheduler within a week of your initial contact.

G. Meeting your elected official.
1. The visit may be with the member or his/her staff.
2. Role playing is a good method to prepare for the visit.
3. Be on time, preferably early, for your appointment.
4. Be prepared to wait for the member or staff.
   a. It is not uncommon for a member to be late.

b. If you are interrupted, take the opportunity to continue your meeting with the staff.

5. Introduce yourself with confidence.
   a. For example: "Hello, I'm Jane Doe, and I'm a registered nurse in your district."
   b. Hand the member your business card and deliver a firm handshake.
6. Be flexible; the meeting may have to take place in a hallway or common area.
7. Organize objectives for the visit.
   a. Be clear what you want to achieve.
   b. Clarify your key points.
   c. Bring any materials that support your position.
      (1) Members are required to take positions on many issues.
      (2) Members may lack the information about the pros and cons of an issue.
      (3) Handouts also provide useful information for review after you leave.
8. Assign a spokesperson if multiple people are attending.
9. Explain how the issue impacts the member's constituency. Provide a personal story or example.
10. Provide concise information on a one-page document or have a packet of information to leave with the member.
11. Always be polite and listen carefully.
12. Be prepared to answer questions. If you do not know the answer to a question, be honest and say so. Offer to supply the information.
13. Offer to assist the member regarding your issue.
    a. Become a resource on kidney disease for your elected official.
    b. If requested, be prepared to supply additional information.
14. Express appreciation.
15. Enjoy the visit!
    a. Do not be nervous. You are the expert in the care of patients with kidney disease.
    b. You are building a long-term relationship with your elected official.
16. After the visit.
    a. Keep notes as a reference for the next time you visit your member.
    b. Send a thank-you note either written or faxed.
       (1) Be sure to briefly review the key points of your issue.
       (2) Send any additional information that was requested.
    c. Share the result of the meeting with the local ANNA chapter.
17. Maintain communication with the member both in Washington and the home district.

H. Locating your members of Congress
   1. http://www.annanurse.org
      Tab to CapWiz Legislative Action Center
   2. http://www.firstgov.org
   3. http://www.congress.org
   4. http://thomas.loc.gov

Learning Opportunities for Nurses in Health Policy
Organizational and National Programs for Nurses

ANNA's Health Policy Workshop

Sponsored by ANNA and held every other year in Washington, D.C.

Attended by chapter health policy representatives. Chapters without health policy representation may recommend a member who is interested and willing to assume the role of chapter health policy representative for the chapter after the workshop. Also attended by state health policy directors, committee chairs and Special Interest Group leaders, Board of Directors, and other interested ANNA members.

Nurse in Washington Internship

Sponsored by Nursing Organizations Alliance, held annually in Washington, D.C.

ANNA has supported, provided representation, and provided faculty since the first program in 1985.

Robert Wood Johnson Health Policy Fellowship Program

Sponsored by the Institute of Medicine of the National Academies.

These hands-on internships offer experience in policy making in Washington, D.C., with a member of Congress.

White House Fellowship Program

Hands-on experience for young professionals to experience policy making in the highest levels of the federal government.

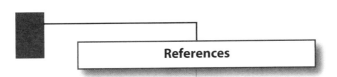

References

American Nephrology Nurses' Association (ANNA). (2006a). *ANNA health policy toolkit.* Retrieved February 15, 2008, from http://www.annanurse.org

American Nephrology Nurses' Association (ANNA). (2006b). *ANNA legislative handbook.* Pitman, NJ: Author.

American Nephrology Nurses' Association (ANNA). (2006c). *ESRD education week: Planning and orientation guide.* Pitman, NJ: Author.

Bodenheimer, T.   S., & Grumbach, K. (2005). *Understanding health policy: A clinical approach* (4th ed.). New York: McGraw Hill.

Congress at your fingertips, 109th Congress, 1st session. (2005). Merrifield, VA: Capitol Advantage Publishing.

Eckard, P., & Pearce, S. (2003, November). Are politics and nursing strange bedfellows? *Nursing Spectrum.*

Gurney, D. (2005). Impressions: An emergency nurse goes to Washington: Felling legislative power at the U.S. Capitol. *Journal of Emergency Nursing, 31*(6), 574-576.

Halpern, I.M. (2005). Advocacy and health policy. In M. Gullate (Ed.), *Nursing management: Principles and practice* (pp. 601-620). Philadelphia: Oncology Nursing Society.

Jones, J. (2005). *Nurses remain at top of honesty and ethics poll.* Retrieved Feburary 15, 2008, from http://www.galluppoll.com/

Keepnews, D. (2006). Policy and politics. *Policy Politics and Nursing Practice, 7*(83).

Kitchen, L. (2004). Legal checkpoints. To impact political policy, first prepare. *Nursing Management, 35*(1), 14-15, 53.

Kuchta, K., Gilbreth, A., Gilman. C, & Wieler, A. (2006). The legislative process and the kidney care quality and improvement act of 2005. *Nephrology Nursing Journal, 2*(33), 229-232.

Mason, D., Leavitt, J.K., & Chaffee, M.W. (2002). *Policy and politics in nursing and health care* (4th ed.). St. Louis: Mosby.

National Council of State Boards of Nursing. (2006). *Nursing licensure compact.* Retrieved February 15, 2008, from https://www.ncsbn.org/nlc.htm

PKD Foundation. (n.d.). *Learning about polycystic kidney disease.* Retrieved February 15, 2008, from http://www.pkdcure.org

Russell, G., & Fawcett, J. (2006). Conceptual model for nursing and health policy: What role for history? *Policy Politics and Nursing Practice, 7*(119).

Smith, K. (2006a). Public policy issues and legislative process. In A. Molzahn & E. Butera (Eds.), *Contemporary nephrology nursing: Principles and practice* (2nd ed., pp. 833-850). Pitman, NJ: American Nephrology Nurses' Association.

Smith, K. (2006b). Public policy issues and legislative process. *Nephrology Nursing Journal, 2*(33), 201-205.

Section 8

Nutrition in Kidney Disease, Dialysis, and Transplantation

Section Editor

Deborah Brommage, MS, RD, CSR, CDN

Authors

Kay Atkins, MS, RD

Louise Clement, MS, RD, CSR, LD

Ann Beemer Cotton, MS, RD, CNSD

Maria Karalis, MBA, RD, LDN

Chhaya Patel, MA, RD, CSR

Jean Stover, RD, LDN

Cynthia J. Terrill, RD, CSR, CD

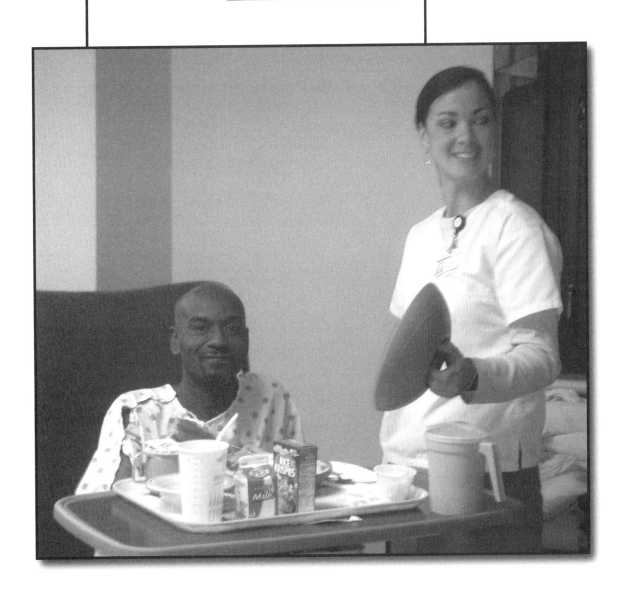

About the Authors

Deborah Brommage, MS, RD, CSR, CDN, Section Editor, is a Renal Clinical Consultant for Genzyme Renal in Long Island, New York.
Topics: chronic kidney disease, dialysis

Kay Atkins, MS, RD, is a Transplant Nutrition Specialist at Banner Good Samaritan Transplant Services in Phoenix, Arizona.
Topic: transplant

Louise Clement, MS, RD, CSR, LD, is a Renal Dietitian at South Plains Kidney Disease Center in Lubbock, Texas.
Topics: nutrients important in kidney disease, diabetes

Ann Beemer Cotton, MS, RD, CNSD, is a Clinical Dietitian Specialist in Critical Care and Transplant at Methodist Hospital in Indianapolis, Indiana.
Topics: malnutrition, acute kidney injury

Maria Karalis, MBA, RD, LDN, is Regional Scientific Manager at Abbott Renal Care in Abbott Park, Illinois.
Topics: nutrition screening and assessment, education strategies and behavior modification

Chhaya Patel, MA, RD, CSR, is Area 1 Divisional Dietitian at DaVita, Inc., in Walnut Creek, California.
Topic: cultural diversity

Jean Stover, RD, LDN, is a Renal Dietitian at DaVita, Inc., in Philadelphia, Pennsylvania.
Topics: pregnancy, geriatrics

Cynthia J. Terrill, RD, CSR, CD, is a Pediatric Renal Dietitian at University Healthcare/University Hospitals and Clinics in Salt Lake City, Utah.
Topic: pediatrics

Acknowledgment

Thanks to Jane H. Greene, RD, CSR, LDN, and Nancy Hoffart, PhD, RN, authors of the fourth edition of the *Core Curriculum*, for their contributions to this section.

Section

8

Nutrition in Kidney Disease, Dialysis, and Transplantation

Purpose

The focus of this section is to examine nutrition issues related to kidney disease and kidney replacement modalities. This review will look at the nutrition care process in managing kidney disease, including nutrition assessment, nutrition diagnosis, nutrition intervention, and nutrition monitoring and evaluation.

Nutrition assessment encompasses interpretation of anthropometric, biochemical and clinical data, and evaluation of medications.

Nutrition diagnosis involves recognizing complications such as malnutrition, bone disease, and anemia. This identification of nutrition problems is necessary for determining nutritional needs for acute vs. chronic kidney disease, for different types of kidney replacement therapy, and for special life stages such as pregnancy and early childhood.

Nutrition intervention includes strategies for patient education and behavior modification to meet the special needs of adults, young children, the elderly, patients with diabetes, and culturally diverse populations.

Nutrition monitoring and evaluation uses selected outcome indicators such as biochemical markers and clinical data to ensure that nutrition goals are being met for patients with kidney disease.

Objectives

Upon completion of this section, the learner will be able to:
1. Interpret the results of procedures and biochemical tests used for assessing nutritional status in patients with kidney disease.
2. Identify signs, symptoms, and indices of malnutrition in patients with kidney disease.
3. Identify physiologic functions of protein, carbohydrates, fat, vitamins, selected minerals and water.
4. Perform a nutrition-focused physical examination on patients with kidney disorders.
5. State at least five reasons patients with kidney failure are at risk for malnutrition.
6. Explain nutritional recommendations for patients with acute kidney injury (AKI).
7. Explain nutritional recommendations for patients with chronic kidney disease (CKD).
8. Explain nutritional recommendations for patients receiving hemodialysis (HD) and peritoneal dialysis (PD).
9. Explain nutritional recommendations and potential nutritional problems for patients who have undergone kidney transplantation.
10. State dietary considerations for patients with diabetes and kidney disease.
11. Outline goals of nutrition care for geriatric patients with kidney disease.
12. Outline goals of nutrition care for pediatric patients with kidney disease.
13. Discuss how to meet increased nutritional needs of pregnant patients receiving dialysis or kidney transplant.
14. Identify cultural factors that impact food practices and the implications for nutrition care of patients with kidney disease.
15. Outline stages of behavioral change that influence patients with kidney disease to adjust to the renal nutrition regimen.

Chapter 38

Nutrition Screening and Assessment

I. Nutrition screening is a process used to identify nutrition-related problems.

A. Patients identified as either high risk or currently malnourished should be referred to the renal dietitian for a comprehensive nutritional assessment, including subjective global assessment (SGA).

B. No single measure can diagnose malnutrition or identify the different aspects of protein-energy malnutrition (PEM).

II. Nurses may be the first to notice signs of malnutrition in CKD patients.

A. Simple clinical signs include loose fitting clothes, rings, or dentures as a result of weight loss secondary to inadequate caloric intake.

B. Loss of muscle mass can be evident when taking blood pressure.

C. Decreased strength and endurance may be noted in assisting the patient with mobilization.

D. Identification of nutrition-related problems and intervention to resolve them involves the entire health care team.

III. Identifying patients at risk for poor nutritional status from a nursing perspective.

A. Medical history.
1. Chronic disease that affects ingestion, digestion, or absorption of nutrients (e.g. scleroderma, Crohn's disease, amyloidosis, diabetic gastroparesis, GI bleeding, bowel obstruction).
2. Significant change in usual body weight or weight when patient started kidney replacement therapy (was weight change intentional and over what period of time?).
3. Increased metabolic needs related to dialysis, sepsis, fever, infection, inflammation or medications.
4. Increased nutrient losses from open wounds, draining fistulas, chronic blood loss, or peritonitis.
5. Recent major surgery or hospitalization with clear liquid diet or NPO status for extended period of time.
6. Neurologic impairment or presence of dysphagia.

B. Social history.
1. Lives alone.
2. Depression.
3. Limited financial resources.
4. Physical or psychologic disabilities that limit ability to prepare meals or shop for food.
5. Alcoholism or drug and/or tobacco abuse.
6. Behavioral barriers.
7. Limited literacy skills that affect the ability to follow oral/written instructions.

C. Food and nutrition history.
1. Dietary interviews and/or diaries that indicate adequacy of intake are less than estimated nutrient needs.
2. Multiple dietary restrictions or modifications that make diet more difficult to follow.
3. Anorexia, nausea, vomiting, or change in bowel habits.
4. Impaired sense of taste or smell.
5. Poor dentition.
6. Religious, ethnic, or cultural beliefs that influence intake.
7. Food allergies, preferences, or intolerances.
8. Medications/food-drug interactions.
9. Dietary supplements or alternative therapies.

IV. Identifying nutritional risk from laboratory data.

A. Serum albumin less than 4.0 g/dL predialysis using the bromcresol green method laboratory assay (BCG).
1. Readily available and widely accepted nutritional parameter in most patient groups; strongest laboratory predictor of outcome in dialysis patients.
2. Slow response to depletion or repletion; altered by factors other than malnutrition since it is a negative acute phase reactant (may be a reflection

of illness or inflammation rather than visceral protein stores).
3. Low levels may be secondary to infection, inflammation, trauma, decreased synthesis related to liver disease, peritoneal/urinary albumin losses, hydration status, and/or acidemia.
4. High levels may be secondary to severe dehydration and albumin infusion.
5. Clinical status must be considered when evaluating changes in serum albumin concentration.

B. Cholesterol less than 150 mg/dL (nonfasting state).
1. Low levels may be secondary to acute infection, starvation, and PEM.
2. Maintenance hemodialysis patients with a low normal serum cholesterol level have a higher mortality rate than hemodialysis patients with higher cholesterol.
3. Serum cholesterol should be used only for nutrition screening purposes. Patients with low levels should be evaluated for other comorbidities in addition to nutrition deficits.

C. Prealbumin less than 30 mg/dL predialysis.
1. Marker of protein energy malnutrition.
2. Low levels have been associated with increased mortality risk and correlates with other markers of malnutrition in dialysis patients.
3. High levels may be secondary to administration of corticoids.
4. May be falsely elevated in patients with significantly decreased kidney function secondary to impaired degradation by the kidney.
5. Negative acute-phase reactant; levels can decline as a response to inflammation or infection.

D. Serum bicarbonate less than 22 mEq/dL.
1. Metabolic acidosis is associated with increased oxidation of branch chain amino acids.
2. Metabolic acidosis decreases albumin synthesis and increases muscle protein catabolism.
3. Acidosis affects bone mineral content, increases osteoclast activity, and decreases osteoblast activity.

E. Predialysis BUN less than 60 mg/dL. Serum creatinine less than 10 mg/dL (anuric).
1. BUN is the end product of dietary protein intake whereas creatinine is a reflection of skeletal muscle mass and protein (muscle) intake.
2. Residual kidney function and dose of dialysis must be considered when using BUN and serum creatinine as markers of nutritional intake.

3. High levels of BUN may be secondary to excessive protein intake, inadequate dialysis, GI bleeding, dehydration, and hypercatabolism.
4. Low levels of BUN may be secondary to overhydration, acute low protein intake, malabsorption, and increased secretion of anabolic hormones.

V. Nutrition-focused physical examination (also see Section 1, Chapter 3, for further guide to physical assessment of patients with kidney disease).

A. Using a systems approach, a nutrition-focused physical exam can be integrated into the complete physical assessment of kidney patients.

B. General survey.
1. Nutrition focus.
a. Body weight and height compared with normal height-weight chart.
b. General wasting of muscle and/or loss of adipose tissue.
c. Alertness, orientation.
d. Any deviation from normal growth or development.
e. Note skin condition throughout exam. Check for signs of dryness/scaling and overall skin pigmentation.
2. Nutrition implications.
a. Insufficient calories and protein.
b. Inability to feed self.
c. Food preparation.
d. Other activities of daily living.
e. Poor wound healing and pressure ulcers associated with protein, vitamin C, and zinc deficiencies; purpura associated with vitamins C and K deficiencies.

C. Vital signs.
1. Temperature. Fever increases energy and fluid needs.
2. Respirations. Increased rate or work of breathing can impact calorie and protein requirements, quantity of food eaten, and acid-base status.
3. Pulse. Heart rate may increase with anemia.
4. Blood pressure. May indicate need for diet modification, such as weight reduction and sodium or fluid restriction.

D. Head and face.
1. Nutrition focus.
a. Inspect and palpate shape and symmetry.
b. Note texture, distribution, and quantity of

hair (check for signs of thin, sparse hair with easy pluckability).

   c. Palpate temporomandibular joint (TMJ) while patient opens and closes mouth.

   d. Assess CN V (trigeminal) and CN VII (facial).

2. Nutrition implications.

   a. Bilateral temporal wasting may reflect protein-calorie deficiency.

   b. Problems with TMJ may influence the ability to eat.

   c. Weakness, asymmetry, or pain related to CN V and CN VII problems can affect chewing or may result in holding food in mouth.

   d. May suggest protein, biotin or zinc deficiencies.

E. Eyes.

1. Nutrition focus.

   a. Inspect appearance of sclerae, conjunctivae, and corneae. Is the eye drying or tearing (photographphobia)?

   b. Inquire about problems with adjustments to darkness or visual impairment.

2. Nutrition implications.

   a. May suggest vitamin A deficiency or B-carotene deficit, though very rare in dialysis-dependent patients:

     (1) Dull, rough appearance to inner lids (conjunctival xerosis).

     (2) Softening of cornea (keratomalacia).

     (3) Foamy or cheesy raised lesions noted on the temporal side of the sclera (bitot's spots).

     (4) Dull, milky, hazy/opaque appearance of cornea (corneal xerosis) or night blindness.

   b. Vision impairment can affect ability to cook, shop, eat, or follow written dietary guidelines.

F. Nose.

1. Nutrition focus.

   a. Determine patency of each nostril; inspect mucosa, septum, and turbinates.

   b. Test CN I (olfactory).

2. Nutrition implications.

   a. Patency of nostrils may influence decision on feeding tube placement.

   b. Sense of smell influences foods eaten and may alter appetite.

G. Mouth and pharynx.

1. Nutrition focus.

   a. Inspect lips, buccal mucosa, gums, hard and soft palates, and floor of mouth for color and surface characteristics.

   b. Inspect teeth for color, number, surface characteristics.

   c. Inspect and palpate tongue, noting color, characteristics, symmetry, and movement.

   d. Test CN IX (glossopharyngeal), CN X (vagus), and CN XII (hypoglossal).

2. Nutrition implications.

   a. Bilateral cracks and redness of lips (angular stomatitis) or vertical cracks of lips (cheilosis) may suggest riboflavin, niacin, and pyridoxine deficiency.

   b. Dryness of mucosa can reflect hydration status.

   c. Condition of teeth influences ability to chew.

   d. Spongy, swollen, bleeding gums may be secondary to vitamin C deficiency.

   e. Slick or beefy-red tongue (glossitis) suggests riboflavin, niacin, folate, iron, or B_{12} deficiency.

   f. Note any evidence of dysphagia or risk for aspiration.

H. Neck.

1. Nutrition focus.

   a. Inspect symmetry and smoothness of neck.

   b. Palpate thyroid and parotid glands.

2. Nutrition implications.

   a. Enlarged thyroid may reflect iodine deficiency.

   b. Bilateral enlargement of parotids may reflect protein deficiency. Consider bulimia.

I. Upper extremities.

1. Nutrition focus.

   a. Inspect skin and nail characteristics.

   b. Palpate hands, arms, and shoulders.

   c. Assess amount of subcutaneous fat in triceps and biceps and any evidence of interosseous wasting.

   d. Check range of motion in wrists, elbows, and shoulders.

   e. Assess muscle and grip strength bilaterally.

2. Nutrition implications.

   a. Fat and muscle wasting reflect protein and calorie deficiency.

   b. Swollen painful joints may suggest vitamin C deficiency.

   c. Range of motion in upper extremities affects ability to feed independently.

   d. Muscle and grip strength may indicate need for assistive devices or assistance with food preparation.

J. Chest and lungs.

1. Nutrition focus. Inspect, palpate, percuss, auscultate.

2. Nutrition implications.
   a. Prominent bony skeleton with muscle and fat wasting reflect inadequate calorie and protein intake.
   b. Crackles and wheezes suggest fluid overload and may influence fluid requirements and nutrition regimen.
   c. Increased work of breathing increases energy needs.

K. Cardiovascular.
   1. Nutrition focus. Inspect, palpate, auscultate.
   2. Nutrition implications.
      a. Jugular venous distention (JVD) and edema will influence fluid requirements.
      b. Edema may be related to protein deficiency.
      c. Dysrhythmias may be related to potassium, calcium, magnesium, or phosphorus imbalances.
      d. Tachycardia and heart failure have been associated with thiamin deficiency.
      e. Cardiac cachexia is associated with inability to eat and digest adequate quantities of food; loss of lean body mass may not be detected if hidden by fluid overload.

L. Abdomen.
   1. Nutrition focus.
      a. Inspect skin, contour, muscle development.
      b. Auscultate for bowel sounds.
      c. Percuss for tone.
      d. Palpate all quadrants.
   2. Nutrition implications.
      a. Poor wound healing may reflect inadequate calories, protein, zinc, or vitamin C.
      b. Presence of ascites may impact fluid, sodium, and protein requirements.
      c. Absent or hypoactive bowel sounds will influence feeding route.
      d. Hepatomegaly may reflect protein deficiency or excessive vitamin A intake.

M. Lower extremities.
   1. Nutrition focus.
      a. Inspect skin and nails.
      b. Palpate thigh, calf, feet bilaterally.
      c. Evaluate range of motion (ROM) and muscle strength of lower extremities.
      d. Test deep tendon relfexes (DTRs) bilaterally.
      e. Sensory exam in three dermatomes.
   2. Nutrition implications.
      a. Muscle wasting and prominent skeleton suggest inadequate calorie and protein intake.
      b. Poor wound healing associated with inade-

quate calorie, protein, zinc, and vitamin C intake.
      c. Motor weakness in lower extremities associated with thiamin deficiency.
      d. Hypoactive reflexes may reflect thiamin or B_{12} deficiency.
      e. Peripheral neuropathy associated with thiamin, B_{12}, and pyridoxine deficiency.

VI. Anthropometric data.

A. Determine percentage of usual body weight (UBW). Unintentional weight loss greater than 10% is clinically significant.

B. Determine percentage of standard body weight (SBW) determined from NHANES II data (average 50th percentile weights for men and women by age, height, and frame size in the U.S.).

C. Determine body mass index (BMI).
   1. BMI = wt in kg/ht in m^2.
   2. BMI of 14 to 15 kg/m^2 is associated with significant mortality in general populations.
   3. Upper 50th percentile BMI may be best for survival in dialysis patients. NKF KDOQI suggests 23.6 for women and 24.0 for men.

D. Determine adjusted edema-free body weight (aBWef) for assessing or prescribing calorie and protein intake for patients less than 95% or greater than 115% of the median standard weight as determined from NHANES II data.

E. Patients whose edema-free body weight is between 95% and 115% of the median standard weight should have calorie and protein needs assessed or prescribed based on actual edema-free body weight.

F. Determine triceps skinfold thickness (TSF), mid-arm circumference (MAC), mid-arm muscle circumference (MAMC), and mid-upper arm muscle area (MAMA).

G. Dual energy x-ray absorptiometry (DEXA) suggested by NKF KDOQI is a validated method to assess body composition in patients with CKD. DEXA is affected by hydration and tissue density.

H. Other measures of body composition not typically done include hydrodensitometry or underwater weighing, BIA or bioelectric impedence, and near infrared interactance.

Chapter 39

Kidney Disease and Kidney Replacement Therapies

Acute Kidney Injury

I. **Acute kidney injury (AKI) is a clinical syndrome** hallmarked by a rapid decline in kidney function with the failure to excrete nitrogenous wastes and inability to regulate fluid and electrolyte balance.

II. **Mortality rates for AKI can be as high as 60–80%** depending on the cause of AKI and the presence of comorbid conditions.

III. **Acute malnutrition is prevalent in AKI and may** be compounded by pre-AKI chronic malnutrition with the potential to further complicate outcome.

IV. **Causes** (Liano & Pascual, 1999).

A. Prerenal injury to include loss of extracellular volume with decrease kidney perfusion, decreased cardiac output, peripheral vasodilation, or kidney vasoconstriction.

B. Postrenal injury to include acute tubular necrosis (also considered with prerenal causes), drug toxicity, intratubular deposition of uric acid or oxalate, myoglobin rhadomylosis, bilateral renal artery/vein thrombosis.

C. Tubulointerstitial injury to include congenital abnormalities, malignancy causing obstruction or urinary catheter occlusion.

V. **Clinical manifestations.**

A. Biochemical.
   1. An elevating blood urea nitrogen (BUN) and creatinine.
   2. Often increased urea generation is noted from catabolism related to sepsis, gastrointestinal bleeding, excessive intake of amino acids/protein, infusion of albumin/fresh frozen platelets, and/or costicosteroid administration.
   3. Important to identify pre-AKI or baseline creatinine and trend this parameter over the course of AKI.

4. Conditions that increased urea generation are also likely to elevate serum potassium and phosphorus.

B. Urine volume.
   1. Anuric AKI: urine output (UOP) < 100 mL/24 hr. Aggressive RRT therapy is required and permits adequate nutrition support while innate clearance of excessive volume and nitrogenous wastes is low to nonexistent.
   2. Oliguric AKI: UOP < 400 mL/24 hr and > 100 mL/24 hr provided.
   3. Nonoliguric AKI: UOP > 400 mL/24 hr. Higher creatinine clearance is noted with increased removal of nitrogenous wastes, fluid, and electrolytes. RRT is often not necessary, and nutrition support is more liberal in fluid and electrolytes.
   4. Diuretic phase of AKI: UOP increases significantly with a decline in BUN and creatinine. During diuresis, following anuric/oliguric AKI, kidneys often lack the ability to concentrate urine, and volume depletion may result if fluid and volume replacement is inadequate. Nutrition support should be adjusted accordingly.

VI. **Medical nutrition therapy (MNT) requirements and support.**

A. Nutrition support in AKI considers the underlying reason for AKI, degree of catabolism, type and frequency of RRT, pre-AKI nutritional status, and any other contributing comorbidities.

B. Some prerenal and many postrenal causes of AKI when corrected in a timely manner may not require any specific MNT.

C. Goals of medical nutrition therapy.
   1. Provide supportive MNT which minimizes wasting and prevents further AKI injury.
   2. Control uremic toxicity and any potential for fluid and electrolyte excess.
   3. Avoid overfeeding of substrates.

D. Mild catabolism in AKI.
1. Urea nitrogen appearance (UNA) < 5 g/24 hr.
2. RRT usually not required or limited to one to two treatments.
3. Occurs with volume depletion/dehydration, drug toxicity, or urinary catheter/ureter obstruction.
4. Adequate nutrition support maintained via oral and/or enteral route(s).
5. Provide 30 to 35 kcal/kg of edema free body weight and 0.8 to 1.0 g protein/kg as both essential and nonessential amino acids.
6. Fluid and electrolyte restrictions not often indicated.

E. Moderate catabolism in AKI.
1. UNA 5 to 10 g/24 hr.
2. RRT provided as needed to control fluid and waste product accumulation.
3. Occurs following abdominal vascular surgery or with a combination of simultaneous injuries such as volume depletion, drug toxicity, hypotension, and/or preexisting nondialysis-dependent chronic kidney disease (CKD).
4. Nutrition support may be oral, enteral, and/or parenteral.
5. Feed 25 to 35 kcal/kg edema free body weight. Provide 1.0 to 1.2 g /protein/kg without RRT and minimum 1.2 g/kg protein with RRT provided as both essential and nonessential amino acids.
6. Fluid requirement adjusted for intake versus output including dialysis losses. Electrolytes usually limited unless biochemical results indicate otherwise.
7. If RRT is initiated, a kidney-specific vitamin should be prescribed to replace water soluble vitamin losses. Total intake of vitamin C should not exceed 200 mg to avoid oxalate accumulation in the renal tubules at low glomerular filtration rates with the potential to make the AKI irreversible.

F. Severe catabolism in AKI.
1. UNA > 10 g/24 hr.
2. Intermittent hemodialysis is required to control nitrogenous waste production and electrolyte abnormalities from hypercatabolism as well as permit adequate nutrition support.
3. Occurs in severe trauma, multiorgan dysfunction syndrome, sepsis, extensive body surface area thermal injury with infection.
4. Enteral and/or parenteral nutrition support used most often depending on presence of gastrointestinal dysfunction. Attempt early enteral nutrition within 48 hr of injury if possible, maintaining at least trophic feeds to support gut integrity.
5. Feed 20 to 25 kcal/kg edema free body weight. Hypocaloric feeding may improve outcome by alleviating the additional stress of feeding with concurrent hypercatabolism. Provide 1.5 to 2.0 g of protein/kg both of essential and nonessential amino acids.
6. Fluid requirement adjusted for input and output including dialysis losses. Electrolytes limited as hypercatabolism can further exacerbate impaired excretion of potassium and phosphorus.
7. A kidney-specific vitamin should be prescribed to replace water soluble vitamin losses. Total intake of vitamin C should not exceed 200 mg/day to avoid oxalate accumulation in the renal tubules at low glomerular filtration rates with the potential to make the AKI irreversible.

VII. Continuous kidney replacement therapy.

A. CRRT is a 24/7 therapy that uses diffusive and/or convective clearance to remove nitrogenous wastes, volume excess, and control acid-base and electrolytes in the hemodynamically unstable patient. The slow, continuous solute and volume removal provided by CRRT protects injured kidneys from a RRT-associated hypotensive event and related ischemic reperfusion injury (IRI).

B. Used in severe trauma, multiorgan dysfunction syndrome, sepsis, extensive body surface area thermal injury with infection.

C. The continuous nature of CRRT as well as the use of convective and/or diffusive clearances incurs nutrient loss over the hemofilter.
1. Convective clearance permits the loss of proteins up to at least a molecular weight (MW) of 20K, the pore size of many hemofilters.
2. Diffusive clearance removes smaller solutes up to a MW of 500 which includes the MW of all amino acids.
3. Effluent volume directly impacts amino acid losses which occur over a range of 13 to 30 g/day.

D. Medical nutrition therapy requirements and support.
1. Provide 2.0 to 2.5 g/kg of protein/day and up to 25 kcal/kg day of edema free body weight.
2. Parenteral and/or enteral nutrition should be maximally concentrated and electrolytes restricted. Serum electrolytes are controlled by

their prescribed concentrations in the dialysate/replacement fluid.
3. A kidney-specific vitamin should be provided to replace water soluble vitamin losses. Total intake of vitamin C should not exceed 200 mg/day. Accumulation of oxalate, a precursor of vitamin C, can occur in the renal tubules at low glomerular filtration rates and has the potential to make AKI irreversible.
4. Continuous removal of phosphorus results in hypophosphatemia requiring 20 to 40 mmol/day of bolus sodium phosphate replacement.

Nutrition as a Component of Conservative Management of the Patient with CKD

I. **Goal of therapy:** Achieve or maintain optimal nutritional status and preserve remaining kidney function through alterations in protein and electrolyte intake, blood glucose, and blood pressure control.

II. **Nutritional interventions.**

A. Protein restriction.
1. Protein-restricted diets reduce the symptoms of uremia, and may postpone the need for kidney replacement therapy.
2. The Modification of Diet in Renal Disease (MDRD) study did not show conclusively that protein restriction slows the progression of kidney disease.
3. Recommended protein restriction for patients with a GFR < 25 mL/min who are not on dialysis is 0.6 g protein/kg body weight.
4. Patients who cannot tolerate this low level of protein may be prescribed a protein intake of 0.75 g protein/kg body weight.
5. At least 50% of the protein should be from high biologic value sources, such as meat, fish, poultry, and eggs.
6. Because there is a spontaneous decline in protein intake as GFR falls, patients should be carefully selected, and the indices of malnutrition should be followed closely.
7. With the increased incidence of malnutrition at initiation of kidney replacement therapy, low protein diets should not be generalized for all patients.
8. Low protein diets should only be planned and implemented by dietitians with experience and expertise in nephrology care.

B. Energy intake.
1. A prescribed low protein diet for patients not yet on dialysis must provide adequate calories to maintain neutral nitrogen balance and prevent a decline in nutritional status.
2. Recommended caloric intake for patients with CKD.
   a. 35 calories/kg for those < 60 years of age.
   b. 30–35 calories/kg for those ≥ 60 years of age.

C. Prevention of CKD mineral bone disorder.
1. Control of calcium and phosphate metabolism should be considered when CrCl is < 60 mL/min.
2. Dietary phosphate restriction of < 10 mg/kg/day and the use of phosphate binders help prevent secondary hyperprathyroidism.
3. The addition of calcitriol should be considered in patients with mild to moderate CKD, controlled serum phosphate levels, but less than adequate serum calcium levels.
4. Goals of therapy (CKD stages 3 and 4).
   a. Serum phosphorus levels 2.7–4.6 mg/dL.
   b. Corrected serum calcium level within the normal range for the laboratory used.
   c. Intact PTH levels.
      (1) CKD Stage 3 = 35–70 pg/mL.
      (2) CKD Stage 4 = 70–110 pg/mL.

D. Control of metabolic acidosis.
1. Dietary protein restriction reduces hydrogen ion generation.
2. Correction of metabolic acidosis is necessary because acidosis increases muscle protein catabolism, reduces albumin synthesis, and can lead to negative nitrogen balance.
3. Goal of therapy: serum CO_2 ≥ 22 mEq/L, prescribing sodium bicarbonate as needed.

III. **Other interventions to slow progression of CKD.**

A. Tight blood glucose control in patients with diabetes has been shown to slow progression of diabetic nephropathy.

B. Use of angiotensin-converting enzyme inhibitors slows progression of CKD in patients with and without diabetes independent of blood pressure control. Monitor serum potassium with the use of ACE and ARBS; may need dietary potassium restriction.

C. Strict blood pressure control. BP goal for patients with CKD is ≤ 130/80.

Nutrition Care for the Patient Receiving Dialysis

I. **Goal of therapy.** Meet nutritional requirements, prevent malnutrition, maintain acceptable blood chemistries, blood pressure, and fluid status through consumption of prescribed diet and prescribed medications.

II. **Hemodialysis.**

A. Amino acid and peptide losses average 10 to 13 g/dialysis session.

B. Recommended protein intake for stable hemodialysis patients is 1.2 g/kg/day; at least 50% of the protein should be from high biologic value sources.

C. Protein requirements for acutely ill maintenance hemodialysis patients is at least 1.2 to 1.3 g/kg/day.

D. Protein intake can be monitored in the stable hemodialysis patient by assessing protein catabolic rate (PCR) or protein equivalent of total nitrogen appearance (PNA).
  1. PCR is the amount of protein catabolized in g/day. Urea kinetic modeling (UKM) allows for a direct calculation of PCR.
  2. PNA expresses total nitrogen appearance in terms of protein in g/day; nitrogen content of mixed proteins is approximately 16%.
    a. PNA = PCR, if the patient has no kidney function and no significant protein losses.
    b. PNA = PCR + protein losses in the patient that has urine output or protein losses.

E. Recommended caloric intake for hemodialysis patients < 60 years of age is 35 cal/kg/day; or patients ≥ 60 years of age, 30 to 35 cal/kg/day.

F. The adjusted edema free body weight (aBWef) should be used to calculate calorie and protein needs, and the weight should be obtained postdialysis.

III. **Peritoneal dialysis.**

A. Average protein loss is 9 g/day for CAPD; 4 to 6 g of amino acids and peptides are lost each day. Protein losses can double with peritonitis.

B. Recommended protein intake for stable peritoneal dialysis patients is 1.2 to 1.3 g/kg/day; at least 50% of the protein should be from high biologic value sources.

C. Protein requirements for acutely ill peritoneal dialysis patients is at least 1.3 g/kg/day.

D. Protein intake can be monitored in the stable PD patient by assessing the Protein Equivalent of Nitrogen Appearance (PNA).

E. Recommended caloric intake for PD patients is 35 cal/kg/day for patients < 60 years of age and 30–35 cal/kg/day for patients ≥ 60 years of age.

F. The adjusted edema free body weight (aBWef) should be used to calculate calorie and protein needs and should be obtained after draining dialysate fluid.

G. PD patients with normal peritoneal transport capacity absorb approximately 60% of the dextrose calories on CAPD and 40% of dextrose calories on ADP from their PD exchanges.

H. 1.5% dextrose solution contains 15 grams of monohydrous dextrose per liter. 2.5% dextrose solution contains 25 grams of monohydrous dextrose per liter. 4.25% dextrose solution contains 42.5 grams of monohydrous dextrose per liter.

I. To estimate calories absorbed from PD fluid.
  1. Total the grams of dextrose from all exchanges for 24 hr.
  2. Multiply by 3.4 calories/gram (conversion factor for monohydrous dextrose).
  3. Multiply total calories by 60% for CAPD and 40% for APD (average absorption) to estimate calories patient receives from dialysate fluid.

IV. **Daily and nocturnal hemodialysis.**

A. Fewer dietary restrictions and increased energy and protein intake which may result in an increase in dry weight and improved serum albumin levels.

B. Lower serum phosphorus levels with nocturnal hemodialysis.
  1. May require less need for phosphate binding medications and phosphorus supplementation.
  2. Normalized Ca x Phos product has the potential to reverse vascular calcification.

C. Dietary potassium needs may be increased, resulting in more liberal dietary potassium intake and possible need for 3 K dialysate.

D. Improved blood pressure, fluid control, anemia management, and quality of life.

V. Survival skills for new patients on dialysis.

A. Two important elements of the kidney diet to implement immediately until the patient can be seen by the dietitian.
   1. Potassium. Limit servings of fruits, vegetables, and juices to a total of 4 to 6 half-cup servings per day. Avoid salt substitutes and any other form of potassium chloride.
   2. Fluid. Allow 4 cups of fluid plus the amount equal to urine output. Fluids are any foods or beverages that are liquid at room temperature.

B. Protein. If the patient was on a low protein diet prior to dialysis, more protein foods can now be consumed (unsalted meats, fish, poultry, eggs). Limit dairy products to ½ cup per day until needs are determined.

C. Sodium. Avoid the salt shaker, convenience foods, "fast foods," and cured or processed meats.

VI. Frequent problems for patients on dialysis.

A. Thirst.
   1. Suck on cold sliced fruit, lemon wedges, mints, or sour candy.
   2. Use spray mouth wash, sports gum, or rinse mouth with chilled mouthwash.
   3. Add lemon juice to drinking water.
   4. Use small cups and glasses for beverages.
   5. Limit high sodium foods.
   6. Keep blood glucose under good control if diabetic.

B. Constipation.
   1. Increase dietary fiber with allowed fruits, vegetables, grains, and cellulose fiber (bran and whole grains are high in phosphorus).
   2. Stool softeners or bulk laxatives.
   3. Increase exercise/activity as tolerated.

C. Poor appetite.
   1. Assess adequacy of dialysis.
   2. Small, frequent meals (adjust binders accordingly).
   3. Maintain good oral care to improve tastes.
   4. Appetite stimulant such as megesterol acetate.

D. Diabetic gastroparesis (see Diabetes and Kidney Disease, VII. Gastroparesis).

E. Hyperkalemia related to causes other than diet.
   1. Inadequate dialysis.
   2. Dialysis bath too high in potassium.
   3. Hemolysis of lab specimen.
   4. Metabolic acidosis.
   5. Hyperglycemia.
   6. Tissue destruction.
   7. Drug interactions.
   8. Severe constipation.
   9. GI bleeding.

F. Wound healing.
   1. Vitamin A. Should only be supplemented if usual intake is inadequate or deficiency is present; then supplement 900 mcg per day for 7–10 days.
   2. Vitamin C. Supplementation should not exceed 250 mg per day to prevent the risk of oxalosis and soft tissue calcification.
   3. Zinc. Supplement 50 mg of elemental zinc provided by 220 mg of zinc sulfate.
   4. Arginine. A safe dose of the amino acid arginine is 20 mg per day and may be achieved through arginine-enhanced enteral formulas.
   5. Calories. Energy intake of 30 to 35 kcal/kg to achieve protein-sparing effect and positive nitrogen balance.
   6. Protein. Intake of 1.2 to 2.0 grams per day to meet the nitrogen needs of wound healing. Higher protein intake appropriate for stage 3 and 4 wounds.

Kidney Transplant

I. Pretransplant nutrition.

A. Patients should attempt to maintain optimal nutritional status. A serum albumin less than 4.0 g/dL could put patients at risk for potential problems with wound healing and infection posttransplant.

B. Nutritional status including underweight or obesity can affect kidney transplant outcomes. Weight criteria are used in some transplant programs but are controversial.
   1. Body mass index less than 18.5 kg/m^2 or greater than 35 kg/m^2 has been shown to cause complications.
   2. Body mass index of the donor has been shown to affect graft function.
   3. Problems secondary to immunosuppression and malnutrition may arise when underweight

patients are transplanted. The results can lead to decreased graft survival.

4. Obese kidney recipients appear to be at risk for decreased graft survival marked by:
   a. Increased risk of delayed graft function.
   b. Increased length of hospital stay.
   c. More wound infections.
   d. Increased chance for acute rejection and graft loss; surmised to be an immunologic problem.

5. Morbidly obese patients who desire kidney transplantation may opt for surgery.
   a. The two surgical procedures are gastric banding and gastric bypass (Roux-en-Y).
   b. There are reports of successful kidney transplants after both procedures.

II. Posttransplant nutrition.

A. Initial recovery period, 2-3 months.
   1. Transplant recipients are adjusting to their new medication regimen, healing the transplant wound, and beginning the new phase of their life without dialysis.
   2. See Table 8.1 for recommendations for nutrition for kidney transplant patients.
   3. Initially the protein allowance is greater for wound healing.
      a. The transplant wound must granulate from bottom up.
      b. Immunosuppresive medications and obesity can complicate healing.
   4. Potassium.
      a. Serum potassium can be elevated secondary to tacrolimus level elevation. This medication can cause potassium retention if the blood trough level is high.
      b. Low potassium diet of 2–4 g may be indicated.
      c. Kayexalate may be used depending on the potassium level.
   5. Phosphorus.
      a. Serum phosphorus levels may be low due to wasting in the renal tubule. Glucocorticosteroids cause phosphorus wasting This can also contribute to hypercalcemia.
      b. Patients are usually willing to increase intake of high phosphorus foods like milk, dairy products, nuts, and beans.
      c. A phosphorus supplement may be used but can cause diarrhea.
   6. Magnesium.
      a. Cyclosporine A and tacrolimus promote magnesium-wasting by the kidney. This may be because of cyclosporine A and tacrolimus toxicity.
      b. Selected foods such as peanuts, tofu, and broccoli are high in magnesium.
      c. A magnesium supplement may be necessary if increasing dietary sources is not successful.
   7. Blood glucose.
      a. Blood glucose may be elevated from the transplant surgery, infection, transplant medications; especially prednisone, tacrolimus, and cyclosporine A, older age, obesity, genetics, and prior type 1 or type 2 diabetes mellitus.
      b. Depending on the level of blood glucose and other factors will determine whether the recipient is placed on an oral agent or insulin.
      c. Carbohydrate-counting is usually taught to patients with diabetes.
      d. Blood glucose checks three to four times per day are usual practice.
   8. Hypertension.
      a. Both cyclosporine A and tacrolimus can exacerbate high blood pressure.
      b. Blood pressure medications may be discontinued as the kidney begins to regulate blood pressure through the renin-angiotensin system.
      c. Sodium should be limited to 2–4 grams per day if the kidney transplant patient is retaining fluid and taking several blood pressure medications.
   9. Excessive weight gain.
      a. Patients consume the foods that have been severely restricted while on dialysis.
      b. Most dialysis patients lead sedentary lifestyles so becoming active will be a challenge.
      c. Patients gain weight even though prednisone is not used as much. With stronger immunosuppressant medications, there is less need for methylprednisolone sodium succinate (Solu-Medrol).
   10. Hyperlipidemia.
       a. Medications that contribute to hyperlipidemia are cyclosporine A, sirolimus, and prednisone.
       b. Total cholesterol and triglycerides may be elevated.
       c. Patients are instructed to consume low fat, low concentrated carbohydrate diets.
       d. Statins may be used to help decrease lipid levels.
   11. Food safety.
       a. Hand washing and surface cleaning should occur often.
       b. Avoidance of cross contamination is imperative. For example, keep raw meats, poultry,

Table 8.1

Daily Nutrient Recommendations for Adult Kidney Transplantation

Nutrient	Acute Period	Chronic Period
Protein	1.3–2.0 g/kg*	0.8–1.0 g/kg; limit with chronic graft dysfunction.
Calories	30–35 kcal/kg* or BEE x 1.3; may increase with postoperative complications.	Maintain desirable body weight.
Carbohydrate	Limit simple carbohydrate intake if intolerance is apparent.	Emphasize complex carbohydrate intake and distribution.
Fat	Remainder of calories; emphasize PUFA and MUFA.	Emphasize PUFA and MUFA.
Sodium	2–4 g	2–4 g with hypertension.
Potassium	2–4 g if hyperkalemic.	Unrestricted unless hyperkalemic.
Calcium	1200–1500 mg	1200–1500 mg
Phosphorus	DRI; may need supplementation to normalize serum levels.	DRI †
Other vitamins	DRI †	DRI †
Other minerals	DRI †	DRI †
Trace elements	DRI †	DRI †
Fluid	Limited only by graft function.	Limited only by graft function; generally unrestricted.

Abbreviations: BEE, basal energy expenditure; MUFA, monounsaturated fatty acids; PUFA, polyunsaturated fatty acids; DRI (dietary reference intake)

*Based on standard or adjusted body weight.

†Due to lack of research, no specific recommendations are available for this population. Currently the DRI is used as the guideline.

Source: American Dietetic Association. (2004). Reprinted with permission.

and seafood away from already cooked foods.
  c. Raw protein foods like eggs, sushi, steak tartar, and oysters must be avoided. This includes raw cake batter and cookie dough.
  d. Patients must use proper food temperatures; safety occurs below 40 or above 140 degrees F.

B. Long-term nutrition concerns, after the initial period to the end of the transplanted kidney's function.
  1. The major goal for this period is to maintain graft function.
  2. From Table 8.1 the nutrient needs can be viewed for the chronic period. Needs are closer to those of normal adults.
  3. Physical activity continues to be important.
  4. Hypertension may still be a concern.
    a. Following a 2-4 gram sodium diet is recommended if the patient is hypertensive.
    b. Most patients are used to having less sodium in their diets so do not necessarily mind this modification.
  5. Obesity continues to be a problem.
    a. Weight-bearing joints can suffer.
    b. Hypertension may worsen.
    c. Diabetes mellitus may occur.
    d. Some patients gain weight with every visit.
      (1) Nutrition counseling and physical activity remain the hallmarks of weight loss and maintenance.

    (2) Keeping a food diary can be a helpful tool.
  6. Diabetes mellitus can occur at any phase of kidney transplant.
    a. Age, obesity, and transplant medications contribute to the development of diabetes.
    b. Glucose monitoring and medication compliance are imperative to retain graft function.
  7. Cardiovascular disease is the number one cause of death for kidney transplant patients.
    a. Keep hyperlipidemia in check with medication or diet.
    b. Control hyperhomocysteinemia.
      (1) Discontinuing prednisone.
      (2) Add folic acid and vitamin B_6 supplement.
      (3) Reducing weight for obese patients.
  8. Long-term bone problems.
    a. Osteoporosis can occur.
    b. Hyperparathyroidism may still be a problem.
    c. The kidney should be able to convert vitamin D to the active metabolite.
    d. Some of the transplant medications like prednisone contribute to calcium loss from bone.
    e. Calcium supplement should be taken if the patient does not consume dairy products (see Table 8.1 for amount).

Chapter 40

Special Considerations in Kidney Disease

Malnutrition in Kidney Disease

I. Incidence.

A. The incidence of protein-calorie malnutrition (PCM) in chronic kidney disease (CKD) has not been well defined but studies suggest decline in glomerular filtration rate (GFR) coincides with a decrease in calorie and protein intake as well as a fall in markers of nutritional status.

B. The prevalence of PCM among individuals receiving renal replacement therapy (RRT) is high, ranging from 23% to 73% across various studies.

C. PCM in kidney transplant recipients has not been studied but may relate to level of GFR and/or the presence of comorbidities such as cardiovascular disease(CVD) and diabetes mellitus (DM).

II. Morbidity and mortality.

A. Nutritional status at the initiation of RRT is a strong predictor of clinical outcome and mortality risk. Mortality after 36 months of hemodialysis (HD) reaches 75% when PCM, inflammation, and CVD are all observed at initiation of HD.

B. There appears to be a significant link between PCM, inflammation, and comorbidities such as CVD and DM with morbidity and mortality risk.

C. PCM is associated with a higher frequency of hospitalization, longer length of stay, and threefold increase in hospital cost.

D. Impaired wound healing and increased susceptibility to infection occurs in the presence of PCM.

E. A poorer quality of life is linked with PCM in both HD and peritoneal dialysis patients.

III. Indices of malnutrition (NKF KDOQI, 2000).

A. Serum albumin less than 4.0 g/dL by the bromocresol green method.
B. Serum prealbumin less than 30 mg/dL.
C. Serum cholesterol less than 150 mg/dL.
D. Predialysis serum creatinine less than 10 mg/dL in patients without residual kidney function.
E. Continued decline in body weight or body weight less than 90% of standard body weight.
F. Hand grip strength, as measured by a hand dynamometer, less than 85% of the age adjusted standard.
G. Decreased skinfold thickness and/or mid-arm muscle circumference.
H. Low spontaneous dietary protein intake as measured by 24-hour urea nitrogen excretion in patients with CKD not on dialysis, <0.7 g/kg/day, or by protein catabolic rate (PCR) in patients on chronic dialysis, <1.0 g/kg/day.

IV. Contributing factors to protein-calorie malnutrition.

A. An inadequate dose of dialysis, Kt/V < 1.2 in HD, Kt/V <1.7 per week in PD.
B. Bioincompatible membranes increase protein catabolism.
C. Loss of amino acids, proteins, glucose and water-soluble vitamins into the dialysate.
D. Peritonitis in PD patients potentially doubling their usual protein losses.
E. Use of acetate containing dialysate which is associated with an increased incidence of nausea, vomiting, and hypotension.
F. Use of high calcium dialysate with associated nausea, vomiting, and confusion from hypercalcemia.
G. Glucose absorption and abdominal distention resulting in early satiety in PD patients.
H. Pica.

V. Metabolic factors.

A. Chronic activation of the systemic inflammatory response.
B. Acidosis contributing to increased muscle protein catabolism.
C. Elevated parathyroid levels which decrease insulin secretion adversely affecting glucose metabolism, protein synthesis, and amino acid transport into cells.
D. Anemia.
E. Insulin resistance with increased gluconeogenesis contributing to muscle wasting and decreased glycogen stores.
F. Accumulation of nitrogenous wastes as uremia progresses from CKD 4 to 5 verging on the need for dialytic intervention.

VI. Gastrointestinal factors.

A. Anorexia.
B. Difficulty chewing, swallowing, and/or altered taste sensation.
C. Periodontal disease with related inflammatory effects.
D. Gastroparesis, related to uremia or diabetes mellitus.
E. Malabsorption from gastrointestinal comorbidities.
F. Gastroesophageal reflux disease (GERD).
G. Upper gastrointestinal bleeds (UGIB).
H. Constipation related to phosphate binders, oral iron, limited fluid intake, decreased fiber intake, decreased activity/mobility, and/or defying the urge to defecate while undergoing dialysis.

VII. Transplant-related factors.

A. Chronic steroid use and/or intermittent high-dose steroids to combat rejection.
B. Use of low protein diets to control the course of rejection.
C. Gastrointestinal side effects of antirejection medications.

VIII. Miscellaneous factors.

A. Nonkidney comorbidities.
B. Multiple, complex diet restrictions with numerous caregivers providing information that can be conflicting.
C. Socioeconomic barriers/limited literacy skills.
D. Long-term use of low protein diets to slow the progression of CKD, which may also be insufficient in calories or maintained without appropriate monitoring of nutritional adequacy and status.
E. Depression.
F. Polypharmacy/nutrient-drug interactions.
G. Recurrent hospitalizations resulting in frequent — sometimes prolonged — NPO/clear liquid diet status.

Diabetes and Kidney Disease

I. Incidence.

A. Diabetes is a primary cause of CKD, and is the major cause of ESRD in the U.S. The prevalence of diabetes in the dialysis population is 36.2%, and the incidence of diabetes in patients new to dialysis is 44.8%, according to the 2005 USRDS.

II. Importance of glucose control.

A. Controlling blood glucose helps prevent the onset of diabetes. The Diabetes Prevention Program produced a 58% risk reduction in persons with prediabetes from progressing to diabetes. This study used lifestyle modification consisting of weight loss facilitated by diet and exercise.

B. Tight glucose control has been shown to benefit persons with type 1 diabetes. The Diabetes Control and Complications Trial (DCCT) demonstrated a 34% risk reduction of microalbuminuria and a 56% risk reduction in persons with microalbuminuria from progressing to proteinuria.

C. A similar decrease in the rate of complications in persons with type 2 diabetes was noted in the United Kingdom Prospective Diabetes Study (UKPDS).

D. In a smaller study of persons with diabetes on dialysis, intensive diabetes education and care management produced significant decreases in hemoglobin A1c (HbA1c), amputations, and diabetes-related or vascular-related hospital admissions, compared to the control group.

III. Making diabetic meal plans kidney friendly.

A. Modifying a traditional meal plan that had a focus on carbohydrate, protein, and fat to one with restrictions on sodium, potassium, phosphorus, and fluid can be challenging, and should be planned by an experienced renal dietitian.

B. Many foods considered "free" in the diabetic food lists, due to their low caloric content, are high in sodium, potassium, phosphorus, and/or fluid.
  1. High sodium "free" foods: bouillon, broth, many condiments such as soy sauce, dill pickles, commercial taco sauce, seasoned salt, and other salt and spice blends.
  2. High potassium "free" foods: low-sodium bouillon cubes or granules, mushrooms, spinach, and tomatoes.
  3. High phosphorus "free" foods: diet colas.
  4. High fluid "free" foods: broth, coffee, tea, sugar-free beverages, water, diet gelatin dessert, ice, and sugar-free popsicles.

C. The carbohydrate content of breads, cereals, fruit, and milk is similar per serving at 12–15 grams. However, the potassium content of fruit and milk is much higher. A higher percentage of carbohydrate needs to come from breads and cereals for persons on a potassium restriction.

D. Another issue in potassium control is seen in the starch/bread list itself. Potatoes, sweet potatoes, corn on the cob, winter squash, dried beans, lentils, lima beans, and wheat germ are technically in the diabetic starch/bread list, but are all high in potassium.

E. Traditionally, "diabetic snacks" have included a protein source, often from cheese, peanut butter, nuts, or milk. These foods are all high in potassium and/or phosphorus. Furthermore, protein does not prevent blood glucose from dropping and does not prevent subsequent hypoglycemia when used to treat a low blood sugar.

IV. Alcohol.

A. The effect of alcohol on blood glucose levels is related to the quantity of alcohol and its timing with other food consumed. Alcohol is a source of energy, but is not converted to glucose. Alcohol can suppress gluconeogenesis, especially in a fasting state. Therefore hypoglycemia may result if alcohol is taken while fasting by persons on insulin or oral insulin secretagogues (sulphonylureas).

B. For persons with diabetes choosing to drink, alcohol should be limited to one drink for women and two drinks for men. One drink contains 15 g of alcohol, equivalent to 12 oz of beer, 5 oz of wine, and 1½ oz of distilled spirits.

C. When diabetes is well-controlled, moderate use of alcohol should not affect blood glucose levels. Alcohol does not need insulin for its metabolism.

D. See Chapter 4. V. in this section for additional considerations.

V. Monitoring glucose and HbA1c.

A. Because the kidney is partially involved in the breakdown of insulin, the effect of insulin on blood glucose in CKD becomes more intense and prolonged as kidney disease progresses. Oral hypoglycemic medications and insulin should be adjusted accordingly. Patients and their caregivers should be more alert to the signs, symptoms, and possibility of hypoglycemia.

B. The American Diabetes Association's clinical practice recommendations include a fasting plasma glucose of < 120 mg/dL and HbA1c levels < 7%, with daily glucose goals 70–120 mg/dL before meals and 150–180 mg/dL 2 hours after meals.

C. The authors of *Handbook of Dialysis* state that tight glucose control in persons on dialysis is difficult to achieve, citing variations in food intake and absorption, and the dialysis treatment itself. Their recommendations state a fasting glucose of < 140 mg/dL, a postprandial of < 200 mg/dL, and a HbA1c of 100–120% of the normal range (which would essentially be < 7.0).

D. Only certain assays can be accurately used to test HbA1c when uremia is present, including affinity chromatography, colorimetric, or enzyme-linked immunoassays. In-house units commonly used in physician offices are acceptable.

E. The HbA1c reflects an average blood glucose of 3 months in non-CKD patients. This timeframe is reduced in uremia to 4 to 6 weeks, due to the reduced RBC survival rate.

F. Monitoring HbA1c levels on a quarterly basis is reasonable, considering the fragile medical condition and frequent history of uncontrolled blood sugars in many persons in this population.

VI. Treating hyperglycemia and hypoglycemia.

A. Because of the increased sensitivity to insulin in CKD, the treatment of hyperglycemia is usually modified compared to a patient's previous care. An altered sliding scale schedule may become necessary also.

B. Due to the reduction or absence of urine output in persons on dialysis, the "safety valve" effect of glucosuria is also reduced or absent. Severe hyperglycemia with glucose levels > 1000 mg/dL

may develop as a result. However, severe hyperosmolality is unusual since the kidney cannot compensate with osmotic diuresis. Therefore, the treatment does not include large amounts of fluid, but does involve insulin administration and potassium monitoring.

C. Treating low blood glucose with orange juice is contraindicated in patients on a potassium restriction.

D. Appropriate foods to treat low blood glucose are high in sugar and dissolve quickly in the stomach. They may need to be low in salt, potassium, phosphorus, and fluid, depending on the patient's dietary restrictions. "Safe" choices to provide 15 g of carbohydrate include:
   1. Plain table sugar: 4 teaspoons, 3 packets, or 3 sugar cubes.
   2. ½ cup regular nonphosphorus-containing soda pop, such as Sprite or 7-Up.
   3. ½ cup apple juice.
   4. 6 jelly beans.
   5. 5 lifesavers or gumdrops.
   6. 3 glucose tablets.

E. Foods usually NOT appropriate include:
   1. Milk or milk products.
   2. Chocolate.
   3. Salty crackers and salty snack foods.
   4. Peanuts, peanut butter, and other nuts.
   5. Many fruits and fruit juices.

F. The 15/15 rule is appropriate to treat hypoglycemia. Take 15 g of a safe carbohydrate, wait 15 minutes, and retest. Repeat until blood glucose normalizes.

G. Persons on peritoneal dialysis are exposed to a high glucose load, both on CAPD and CCPD, due to the peritoneal absorption of dextrose.

VII. Gastroparesis.

A. Gastroparesis, or delayed stomach emptying, is a common complication of diabetes during any stage of CKD.

B. Usual symptoms include early satiety, bloating, nausea, vomiting, heartburn, and constipation. These affect nutrient intake and absorption, and result in unpredictable blood glucose levels.

C. Dietary treatment includes frequent small meals

and snacks, four to six times daily, which are low in fat and fiber.

D. More frequent blood glucose monitoring with related adjustments in insulin or oral medications may be necessary to optimize glucose control.

E. Medications target the underlying problem of less frequent gastric contractions, or the symptoms, such as diarrhea or constipation.
    1. Metoclopramide (Reglan) is an antiemetic, gastroprokinetic agent.
    2. Domperidome (Motilin), another prokinetic, has not been available in the U.S. since January of 2001.
    3. Cisapride (Propulsid) is contraindicated in the kidney population due to potentially fatal dysrhythmias.
    4. Antidiarrheal medications include loperamide (Imodium), diphenoxylate and atropine (Lomotil), and cholestyramine resin (Questran).
    5. Treatment for constipation includes stool softeners and laxatives.

VIII. Medications for diabetes.

A. Safe oral hypoglycemic agents for persons with CKD are primarily metabolized in the liver rather than the kidney, and are short-acting.

B. Some sulfonylureas, such as acetohexamide (Dymelor), chlorpropamide (Diabinese), and tolazamide (Tolinase), are largely excreted in the urine, and should not be used in persons on dialysis.

C. The biguanide metformin (Glucophage) or the metformin combination (Glucovance and Avandamet) are contraindicated in the dialysis population due to the potential for lactic acidosis.

D. Acarbose (Precose) slows both the conversion of sucrose (table sugar) to glucose and the absorption of fructose and sucrose. Persons taking Precose should treat hypoglycemia with glucose rather than candy, etc.

E. Rapid, short, intermediate, and long-acting insulin may all be used in CKD, while considering the longer half-life of insulin.

F. Regular insulin may be used successfully in peritoneal dialysis solutions for blood glucose control when certain situations exist: use of an intraperitoneal insulin protocol, trained staff, and alert, compliant patients or their caregivers.

IX. Enteral and oral supplements.

A. Some kidney-specific enteral or oral supplements were designed for persons on hemodialysis, and are therefore restricted in potassium and phosphorus, but are higher in calories and sugar.

B. Predialysis formulations are lower in protein and higher in carbohydrate in comparison.

C. Most diabetes-specific enteral and oral supplements contain significant amounts of potassium and phosphorus, while controlling for carbohydrate type and amount.

D. Choosing an appropriate formula for a person with both diabetes and CKD requires the skills and assessment ability of an experienced renal dietitian. Formula content, cost, and availability should be matched with the prioritized medical and nutritional needs of the patient.

E. See Table 8.2. Comparisons of Renal and Diabetic Enteral and Oral Formulations.

F. For those dialysis patients who are on both insulin and a tube feeding formula, care must be taken to match the insulin timing with the formula administration. Continuous tube feeding formulas are usually stopped for dialysis treatments. This period might be approximately 6 hours, 4 for dialysis and 2 for transit time. In order to provide 100% of the formula volume in 18 hours rather than 24, the tube feeding pump speed must be increased accordingly. If a patient is on the morning shift, and the tube feeding is stopped at 6 a.m. in preparation for dialysis, the morning insulin needs to be moved to a later time when the patient has resumed the formula, to prevent hypoglycemia. To maintain consistency, using the same formula and insulin schedule 7 days a week instead of different ones on dialysis days may be less confusing for caregivers.

X. Diabetes self-management training (DSMT).

A. Many persons on dialysis were diagnosed with diabetes before the DSMT classes became popular.

B. Patients may or may not have been referred to these or to alternate comprehensive training programs, either at diagnosis, or at a subsequent time.

Table 8.2

Comparisons of Renal and Diabetic Enteral and Oral Formulations

Product	Manufacturer	Nutrients per 1000 Calories						
		Pro g	Carb g	Fat g	K+ mg	Na mg	Phos mg	Vit A iu
Diabetic								
Glucerna	Ross	41.8	95.6	54.4	1570	930	705	3520
ReSource Diabetic TF	Novartis Nutrition	59.4	93.4	44.3	1679	915	1038	2405
Diabetic Source AC	Novartis Nutrition	50	83	49	1433	883	667	3350
Glytrol	Nestle	45	100	47.5	1400	740	720	4000
Boost Diabetic	Novartis Nutrition	55	80	47	980	980	875	2388
Predialysis								
Amin-Aid	R & D Laboratories	9.7	183	23	NA	<173	NA	NA
Renalcal	Nestle	17.2	145.2	41.2	NA	NA	NA	NA
Suplena	Ross	15	127.6	47.8	560	395	365	530
Dialysis								
Nutren Renal	Nestle	35	102.4	52	628	370	350	832
NovaSource Renal	Novartis Nutrition	37	100	50	405	500	325	1650
Nepro	Ross	35	111.2	47.8	530	423	343	351
Med Pass No Sugar Added	Hormel HealthLabs	49	59	59	1519	956	613	3064

C. However, because many persons with diabetes have lived with their disease for many years, they are unaware of their lack of updated or even basic knowledge. As a result, many persons with diabetes initially arrive at dialysis facilities lacking adequate diabetes education, skill development, and glucose control, and may or may not have a close working relationship with an endocrinologist. Furthermore, they are often frustrated with the additional dietary restrictions imposed by their failing kidneys.

D. CMS (Centers for Medicare and Medicaid Services), on a one-time basis, will cover 80% of the cost of approved DSMT programs for all Medicare recipients who have diabetes, regardless of the diagnosis date. This includes 9 hours of group training and 1 hour of individual training or assessment. In addition, 2 hours of individual or group training are allowed annually. These resources, especially the annual retraining hours, are underused in the diabetic dialysis population.

XI. Supplies and reimbursement.

A. CMS covers blood glucose testing supplies for Medicare recipients who have Part B. This includes strips, lancets, and control solution. Glucose monitors are allowed every 5 years, although many suppliers will provide these free of charge to their clients. Batteries and lancet injectors may be provided every 6 months.

B. Therapeutic shoes and thermal foot gauntlets are allowed once every calendar year for certain diagnoses, including peripheral neuropathy and poor circulation, under Part B.

C. Part B will not cover insulin, syringes, skin care products, or therapeutic socks. Medicare Part D will cover insulin, and some Part D plans will cover syringes.

D. CMS will cover 80% of the cost of allowed supplies. Suppliers may or may not bill a patient separately for the 20% copay who has no secondary insurance.

E. The USRDS 2005 Data Report reveals that these resources are underused. More than 60% of persons with diabetes and ESRD have no test strip prescription. The number of patients prescribed at least 2 strips per day is 12% and 16% in urban and rural areas, respectively. *Complete monitoring*, defined as at least four annual HbA1c tests, two or more annual lipid tests, and two or more test strips per day, existed in only 3.4% of diabetic ESRD patients in 2004. Less than 25% of this population received "minimal care" consisting of one HbA1c and lipid test, and one or more testing strip.

Geriatric Patients with Kidney Disease

I. General considerations.

A. Inadequate energy and protein intakes in older hemodialysis patients have been associated with lower markers of nutrition and functional status, as well as higher comorbidities than with younger patients.

B. Malnutrition in elderly hemodialysis patients has been shown to influence overall survival despite adequate dialysis treatment.

II. Nutritional needs.

A. Energy: 30 kcal/kg ideal body weight (IBW) per day (> 60 years of age).

B. Protein.
1. CKD (without dialysis): 0.8 g/kg IBW per day.
2. Dialysis: at least 1.2 g/kg IBW/day (hemodialysis); 1.2–1.3 g/kg IBW/day (PD).

C. Vitamins/minerals.
1. General multivitamin until later stages of CKD, then change to renal vitamin. May need to use liquid renal vitamin if difficulty swallowing.
2. Calcium supplements and/or phosphorus binders if needed based on lab values. Determine best binder if difficulty swallowing or tube feeding required.
3. Potassium restriction may or may not be necessary, even in stage 5 CKD. Elderly patients who eat poorly or have diarrhea may not require strict dietary potassium or phosphorus limitation.

D. Fluid intake. Probably no need to restrict until stage 5 CKD, then work with patient and/or caretakers if difficulty eating due to limited fluid allowed.

III. Factors affecting nutritional status in the elderly.

A. Living situation.
1. Home. If living alone or with elderly spouse, obtaining food and meal preparation may be difficult or impossible; need to work with social worker to obtain delivered meals or assistance with grocery shopping and meal preparation. Nutritional supplements (if possible to obtain) may be an easy meal replacement.
2. Long-term care (LTC) facility. These issues need to be explored and addressed if nutrition status declines:
   a. Many elderly patients live in LTC facilities where they may dislike the food and, therefore, eat very little.
   b. Diet may be too restrictive.
   c. Patients needing to be fed may not always be helped or receive enough due to insufficient staffing.

B. Comorbid conditions.
1. Dentition. Consistency of food may need to be modified if dentition is poor or dentures do not fit.
2. Wounds.
   a. Pressure sores occur frequently with immobility. Protein, vitamin, and mineral needs are then increased to facilitate healing.
   b. Nutritional supplements often needed (see *Nutrition Care for the Patient Receiving Dialysis*: VI. F. Wound healing).

3. CVA.
   a. Residual loss of swallowing ability causing risk for aspiration and inability to consume adequate amounts of food and/or dislike of food consistency required.
   b. Work with caretaker or LTC facility staff to have patient evaluated periodically to upgrade food consistency if possible.
4. Depression.
   a. Can cause anorexia.
   b. Antidepressant therapy may be needed.
   c. Patient may need to be referred to primary care physician and/or geriatric psychiatry for treatment.
5. Dementia.
   a. May interfere with adequate nutrition if memory loss causes decreased food intake.
   b. Reminders to eat or help with eating (in later stages) may be needed.

C. Other issues.
1. Decreased sense of smell, taste, and saliva production in elderly patients.
   a. If sodium does not have to be strictly limited, intake of food may be better with a more liberal sodium intake.
   b. Use a variety of herbs, spices, and seasonings to enhance taste of food.
   c. Encourage allowed liquids with foods.
2. Constipation.
   a. Ensure that stool softeners are used regularly.
   b. Consider fiber supplements that do not require large amounts of liquid.
3. Diarrhea.
   a. Need to determine reason and treat if possible.
   b. During or after antibiotic therapy consider probiotics such as acidophilus or lactobacillus and/or check for *C-difficile*.
   c. If no treatable cause, consider soluble fiber added to oral diet or tube feeding (if receiving) and products containing glutamine.
4. Drug interactions or inappropriate medication use.
   a. Can lead to confusion, memory loss and anorexia in geriatric patients.
   b. Frequent medication review.
   c. Aid with organizing medications may be needed.

IV. Nutrition management.

A. Communication with caretakers.
1. Family.
   a. Need to ensure that family is aware of patient's nutritional needs and dietary modifications.
   b. Need to call or meet with family frequently if nutritional status is suboptimal or labs are abnormal.
2. LTC staff.
   a. Monthly review of labs necessary.
   b. Frequently the dialysis dietitian will send labs to the nursing home dietitian with a nutrition note on a monthly basis.
   c. Inservices to LTC facility staff, if possible, may be helpful regarding needs of the dialysis patient (including nutrition).

B. Obtaining nutritional supplements.
1. Patients at home.
   a. If feasible, have patients and/or family purchase supplements.
   b. If unable to afford, work with social worker to obtain financial assistance through medical insurance plans, monetary grants, kidney funds, or other agencies.
2. Patients in LTC facilities.
   a. Work with dietitian there to obtain available supplements suitable for the patient.
   b. Renal-specific supplements may not be necessary based on laboratory values.

C. Liberalization of diet restrictions.
1. Diet restrictions should not be imposed if not necessary, especially in LTC facilities.
2. Individualized needs must be encouraged based on labs, fluid retention, and nutrition status.

D. Use of appetite stimulants.
1. Megesterol acetate has been used to stimulate appetite for some elderly patients on dialysis, but caution must be taken with side effects, especially if the patient is immobile.
2. Other medications used for this purpose may be investigated as well.

Pediatric Patients with Kidney Disease

I. Causes of kidney failure in the pediatric patient.

A. Congenital – polycystic kidney disease, kidney dysplasia and hypoplasia, obstructive uropathy, reflux nephropathy, congenital nephrotic syndrome, cystinosis.

B. Acquired – glomerulonephritis, interstitial nephritis, hemolytic uremic syndrome (HUS), cortical and tubular necrosis, renal arterial or venous thrombosis, vasculitis, hypertension.

II. **Nutritional goals are to promote optimal** nutritional status, growth, and development while controlling the biochemical and metabolic consequences associated with the disease state.

III. **Barriers to achieving nutritional goals in pediatric patients.**

A. Anorexia and poor energy intake. Poor nutrient intake (< 80% of assessed needs) will impair linear growth and weight gain. This is often associated with changes in taste due to kidney failure and metabolic abnormalities. Multiple dietary restrictions can also contribute to poor energy intake.

B. CKD mineral and bone disorder. Calcium and phosphorus imbalance and hyperparathyroidism will interfere with bone growth.

C. Acidosis. Low CO_2 levels contribute to the poor appetite and intake associated with kidney failure. It also interferes with bone growth.

D. Hormonal/metabolic abnormalities. The anemia frequently seen in children with chronic kidney disease can negatively impact appetite and intake.

E. Corticosteroids. These may be used to treat several types of kidney disorders and as immunosuppressive therapy for transplant patients and can impair linear growth.

F. Cultural influences. It may be difficult to meet calorie and protein requirements due to food preferences and religious beliefs.

G. Psychosocial issues. Depression, family financial concerns, changes in family structure, increased fatigue, lethargy, changes in mental status, confusion, poor concentration, and forgetfulness can all contribute to poor appetite and intake.

H. Oral aversion. This is frequently associated with chronic kidney disease in infancy and may make it difficult to meet nutritional needs by mouth.

IV. **Nutritional assessment of the pediatric kidney patient.**

A. The nutritional assessment of the pediatric kidney patient is best performed by an experienced pediatric renal dietitian. This individual has received formal and informal education in renal nutrition and is skilled in managing patients with chronic kidney disease, including nutritional assessment, monitoring growth and weight gain, dietary counseling and education, and encouraging dietary adherence. Diet education should be provided to both the patient and family or other caregivers as appropriate.

B. Anthropometric measurements. Scheduled interval measurements of growth and nutrition parameters need to be obtained. Infants may require more frequent intervals to monitor adequacy of intake, feeding tolerance, and growth parameters. Ideally, measurements should be obtained by the same person each time.
   1. Length/height.
      a. Length measurements should be obtained in children up to 24 months of age or in older children who are unable to stand without assistance. This should be done on a measuring board by two people in order to get an accurate measurement. One person will hold the crown of the head against the headboard and the other person will move the footboard up to the heels of the infant's feet as the legs are straightened. Measurements are recorded to the nearest 0.1 cm.
      b. Height measurements are to be done on children older than 24 months who are able to stand unassisted using a wall-mounted stadiometer. The child should remove his or her shoes and stand on the floor, looking straight ahead. Measurements are recorded to the nearest 0.1 cm.
   2. Weight.
      a. Infants should be undressed to be weighed and the weight should be obtained on an infant scale. Weight should be recorded to the nearest 0.1 kg.
      b. Children should be weighed in light clothing without footwear standing up. Weight should be recorded to the nearest 0.1 kg.
      c. The fluid status of the patient should be considered when evaluating for weight gain since positive fluid balance may be misinterpreted as actual weight gain and increase in lean body mass.

3. Head circumference (OFC). Measured in children up to 36 months of age. The maximum head circumference is obtained and recorded to the nearest 0.1 cm.
4. Weight for height/body mass index (BMI). Important in assessing whether patient is the appropriate weight for stature.
5. Mid-arm circumference (MAC).
6. Tricep skinfold (TSF). May be falsely increased if patient is edematous.
7. Mid-arm muscle circumference (MAMC).

C. Medical and dietary history.
1. Concurrent disease (acute and chronic).
2. Usual dietary intake.
3. Food preferences and allergies.
4. Questions regarding consumption of unusual nonfood substances such as paper (pica).

D. Laboratory data.
1. Blood urea nitrogen (BUN).
2. Creatinine.
3. Sodium.
4. Potassium.
5. Calcium.
6. Phosphorus.
7. Albumin.
8. Hematocrit.
9. Iron studies (iron, % saturation, ferritin).
10. Parathyroid hormone or PTH (intact or bio-intact).
11. Bicarbonate (HCO_3 content).

E. Urine, stool, emesis, and ostomy output.
1. Urinary protein losses.
2. Diarrhea/constipation.
3. Nausea/vomiting.

F. Medications.
1. Phosphate binders (calcium and noncalcium based).
2. BP medications.
3. Erythropoietin (subcutaneous or intravenous).
4. Iron (oral and IV).
5. Bicarbonate.
6. Vitamins.
7. Herbals/supplements.

G. Psychosocial status.
1. Depression, anger, fear, denial.
2. Lethargy, increased fatigue.
3. Mental status changes, confusion, poor memory.
4. Psychomotor development.

H. Blood pressure.

I. Fluid balance.
1. Edema.
2. Dehydration.

J. Physical eating skills.
1. Chewing/swallowing skills.
2. Liquids/solids.
3. Developmental delays.

K. Appearance of hair, tongue, skin, and teeth; smell of breath.
1. Dental caries.
2. Oral lesions.
3. Dry skin.
4. Thinning hair.

V. Poor growth and chronic kidney disease.

A. Decreased rate of linear growth is common even if calorie intake is adequate.

B. Need to correct metabolic acidosis to help promote optimal growth and weight gain.

C. Need to achieve optimal calcium and phosphorus balance, PTH, calcium/phosphorus product to optimize linear growth.

D. Adequate nutrient intake may help to promote linear growth, but will not achieve catch-up growth. Use of recombinant growth hormone in children with documented poor linear growth can help achieve an improved rate of linear growth. Need to have good biochemical control for optimal effect. Growth hormone is given as an injection on a daily basis.

VI. Nutritional concerns for infants with kidney failure.

A. Inadequate nutrient intake is common in infants with chronic kidney disease. Decreased appetite and oral aversion are frequently present and the infant will refuse formula and/or solids orally. Enteral feedings (nasogastric, nasojejunal, gastrostomy tube) are often needed to meet 100% of nutritional requirements.

B. Gastrointestinal disturbances including gastroesophageal reflux, delayed gastric emptying, vomiting, early satiety, constipation, and diarrhea are frequently seen. These disorders may require medical intervention such as proton pump inhibitors, H-2 antagonists, motility agents, antidiarrheal agents, antimicrobial agents, and pro-biotic therapy. Dosages for these medications may need to be adjusted in kidney failure. Gastro-jejunostomy feedings may be helpful for children who vomit frequently.

C. Specialized infant formulas designed for children with chronic kidney disease may be necessary to maintain optimal biochemical control. These formulas are lower in sodium, potassium, and phosphorus with a lower renal solute load than standard infant formulas. They typically should not be concentrated, and modular components (protein, carbohydrate, fat) may be added to increase the caloric density without increasing the electrolyte and mineral content of the formula. Renal formulas designed for adults with chronic kidney disease are usually not recommended in children less than 2 years of age due to the increased osmolality and inappropriate vitamin and mineral content of these formulas.

D. Infants with nonoliguric chronic kidney disease (usually due to congenital kidney dysplasia) may be unable to concentrate their urine and will, there-fore, require increased fluid intake. They also may have increased urinary sodium losses necessitating sodium supplementation to achieve optimal linear growth and weight gain.

E. Introduction of solids should be done on a normal schedule when developmentally appropriate. The infant may benefit from occupational therapy and speech therapy involvement to promote oral intake and avoid or limit oral aversion.

F. "Powerpacking" using calorically dense foods such as simple carbohydrates and fats/oils may help to increase calorie intake and meet nutritional needs while staying within dietary limitations.

G. Fluid restriction for infants on dialysis may limit the ability to meet nutritional needs. May need to use modular components such as protein powders, carbohydrate powders, and fats to help meet calorie and protein needs and maintain good biochemical control within fluid restrictions.

H. Behavioral/control issues of the infant/toddler with chronic kidney disease may contribute to inadequate nutrient intake. Parents/caregivers are frequently extremely anxious in regards to

providing adequate nutrition to their child and this may be reflected in an increased focus on feedings. Emotional support should be provided to both the parents and the child related to feeding issues by the health care providers.

VII. Nutritional concerns for school-aged children with kidney failure.

A. Short stature related to chronic kidney disease may become problematic at this age since peers may tease the child and adults may treat the child younger than actual age.

B. School breakfast and lunch programs may need to be modified to accommodate the diet limitations of the child.

C. The child with chronic kidney disease should be included in discussions related to diet, nutrition, growth, laboratory data, and medications between medical staff and parents/caregivers (when devel-opmentally appropriate).

VIII. Nutritional concerns for adolescents with kidney failure.

A. Dietary adherence may be adversely affected by the patient's need to assert independence.

B. Irregular eating patterns and skipping meals may compromise the patient's ability to meet his or her nutritional needs.

C. Peer pressure may make dietary and medication adherence more difficult.

D. Onset of puberty will lead to closure of bone epiphysis and result in short stature as an adult if the child has short stature at the onset of puberty.

E. The adolescent with chronic kidney disease should be included in discussions related to diet, nutrition, growth, laboratory data, and medications between medical staff and parents/caregivers (when devel-opmentally appropriate).

IX. Nutritional recommendations for children with chronic kidney disease prior to dialysis or transplant (see Table 8.3: *Daily Nutrient Recommendations for Children with Chronic Kidney Disease*).

A. Dietary restrictions are only initiated when indicat-ed necessary by laboratory values, progression of kidney insufficiency, or presence of hypertension or edema.

Table 8.3

Daily Nutrient Recommendations for Children with Chronic Kidney Disease

Note: Restrictions should be implemented only where warranted and kept as liberal as possible to optimize energy intake and prevent malnutrition. Pediatric dietary restrictions usually take the form of a "low-nutrient X diet" with education about avoiding or limiting foods high in that nutrient. Depending on the response in the parameter relevant to that nutrient (e.g., blood pressure; biochemical value) the restriction can be liberalized or tightened. Prescriptions for specific amounts of a nutrient (e.g., 3 mEq nutrient X/kg) are rarely used in pediatrics. Amounts provided in the table can be used as references for assessment of daily intake obtained from food records.

Nutrient	Infant, birth to 1 y	Toddler, 1-2 y	Child, 3-8 y	Adolescent 9-13 y	Adolescent 14-18 y
Energy (kcal/kg/d)* Boys:	Birth to 6 mo: 95 7-12 mo: 82	87	87	63	52
Girls:	Birth to 6 mo: 87 7-12 mo: 75	82	82	60	44
Protein (g/kg/d)	Birth to 6 mo: 1.52† 7-12 mo: 1.1-1.5‡	0.88-1.10‡	0.76-0.95‡	0.76-0.95‡	Boys: 0.73-0.85‡ Girls: 0.71-0.85‡
Sodium (Recommendations for patients who are oliguric/anuric, edematous, or hypertensive	• No salt shaker and avoid salty foods (≥ 200 mg/serving). • Infants and toddlers: Restrict to 1-3 mEq/kg/d.§ • Children and adolescents: Restrict to 87-174 mEq/day§ (2-4 g/d).				
Potassium (Recommendations for patients with hyperkalemia)	• Avoid foods with high potassium levels, such as bananas, chocolate, and orange juice. Infants and toddlers restrict to 1-3 mEq/kg/day. • Children and adolescents: Restrict to 51-103 mEq/d§ (2-4 g/d).				
Calcium (mg/d)	• 100% of the DRI. • Monitor total calcium load, including calcium from phosphate binders.				
Phosphorus (mg/d) (recommendations for patients with hyperphosphatemia)	Restrict to low-phosphorus formula and foods	≤ 400–600		≤ 600	800
Vitamins	• If needed, supplement to 100% of the DRI. • Supplement with vitamin D metabolite to prevent hyperparathyroidism and renal osteodystrophy.				
Trace minerals	• If needed, supplement to 100% of the DRI. • Iron supplementation is usually needed with erythropoietin therapy.				
Fluids	• Unrestricted unless warranted for fluid management (indications would be decreased urine output, edema, or hypertension). • If restriction is needed: Total Fluid Intake (TFI) = Insensible losses + Urine output + Other losses.				

* Energy recommendations are the estimated energy requirements (EERs). They are based on active physical activity levels (PAL) as the level recommended tomaintain health and decrease risk of chronic disease and disability. EERs are presented in kcal/kg as determined by dividing the active PAL EER (total kcal/day) by the reference weight for each respective age.

† Protein recommendations are the adequate intake (AI) for ages birth to 6 months.

‡ Protein recommendations ar the range of estimated average requirement (EAR) to recommended dietary allowance (RDA) for ages 7 months to 18 years.

§ For sodium and potassium, mEq-mmol.

Data are from selected *Dietary Reference Intake* publications (34-42).

Source: Byham-Gray, L., & Wiesen, K. (Eds.) (2004). *A clinical guide to nutrition care in kidney disease.* Chicago: The American Dietetic Association.

B. Protein restriction below established adequate intake (AI) for infants 0–6 months of age is not recommended. Protein restriction below the range of estimated average requirement (EAR) to recommended dietary allowance (RDA) for ages 7 months to 18 years is not recommended. Protein restriction may impair linear growth and weight gain in children with chronic kidney disease.

C. Dietary calcium intake should meet 100% of the Dietary Reference Intake (DRI) for age. Total calcium intake should not exceed 2x DRI for age or 2500 mg elemental calcium/day including dietary calcium and elemental calcium from phosphate binders.

D. Dietary phosphorus should be decreased to the DRI for age when the serum PTH concentration is above the target range for the stage of chronic kidney disease (CKD) and serum phosphorus is within the target range for age. Dietary phosphorus intake should be decreased to 80% of the DRI for age when the serum PTH concentration is above the target range for the stage of CKD and serum phosphorus is above the target range for age. Infants, toddlers, and children may require restriction of ≤ 300–500 mg/day while adolescents may require limitation of phosphorus intake to ≤ 800–1000 mg/day. Foods high in phosphorus such as milk, cheese, yogurt, cola, and standard infant formulas may need to be limited. Good adherence to phosphate binders will facilitate allowance of more liberal phosphorus intake. Ideally, phosphate binders should be given 10–15 minutes before or during a meal or high phosphorus snack. Serum phosphorus should be monitored at least every 3 months.

E. Active vitamin D therapy is dependent on the stage of kidney disease the child is in and serum calcium, phosphorus, and PTH levels. Serum calcium, phosphorus and PTH levels should be measured regularly with changes in active vitamin D therapy made accordingly. Vitamin D2 (ergocalciferol) supplementation may also be necessary.

X. **Nutritional recommendations for children on hemodialysis** (see Table 8.4: *Daily Nutrient Recommendations for Children on Dialysis*).

A. Calorie needs are initially based on the RDA (Recommended Dietary Allowance) for chronologic age, but may be adjusted depending on nutritional status, growth, medical complications, intercurrent illnesses, activity level and other factors that could impact calorie needs.

B. Protein needs are increased above the RDA for chronologic age due to protein losses associated with the dialysis process.

C. Interdialytic weight gain should be between 3% and 5% of body weight. Fluid restriction is based on achieving this goal.

Total fluid intake = Insensible losses + Urine output + Ultrafiltration capacity + Other losses – Amount to deficit.

Insensible losses will vary depending on the size of the child. They will also increase with fever, phototherapy, open warmers (newborns), or tachypnea. They will decrease in patients who are ventilated with humidified air. Therefore, total fluid intake allowed may vary depending on the medical condition of the child.

D. Dietary restrictions of sodium, potassium, and phosphorus are only implemented when warranted based on laboratory values to optimize calorie and protein intake and avoid malnutrition.

E. Sodium restriction is necessary for patients who are oliguric/anuric, edematous, or hypertensive. Food should not be salted at the table and high sodium foods (≥ 200 mg sodium/serving) should be avoided. Infants and toddlers will typically require restriction of 1–3 mEq/kg/day (unless there are urinary sodium losses) and children and adolescents will require a restriction of 87–174 mEq/day (2–4 g/day).

F. Potassium restriction is necessary for patients with hyperkalemia. High potassium foods such as bananas, oranges, potatoes, tomatoes, chocolate, and milk should be limited. In infants and toddlers, restrict intake to 1–3 mEq/kg/day and in children and adolescents, restrict intake to 51–103 mEq/day (2-4 g/day).

G. Phosphorus restriction is necessary for patients with hyperphosphatemia and/or hyperparathyroidism. Dietary phosphorus should be decreased to the Dietary Reference Intake (DRI) for age when the serum PTH concentration is above the target range and serum phosphorus is within the target range for a dialysis patient. Dietary phosphorus should be decreased to 80% of the DRI for age when the serum PTH concentration is above the target range for a dialysis patient and serum phos-

Table 8.4

Daily Nutrient Recommendations for Children on Dialysis

Note: Restrictions should be implemented only where warranted and kept as liberal as possible to optimize energy intake and prevent malnutrition.

Pediatric dietary restrictions usually take the form of a "low-nutrient X diet" with education about avoiding or limiting foods high in that nutrient. Depending on the response in the parameter relevant to that nutrient (eg, blood pressure; biochemical value) the restriction can be liberalized or tightened.

Prescriptions for specific amounts of a nutrient (eg, 3 mEq nutrient X/kg) are rarely used in pediatrics. Amounts provided in the table can be used as references for assessment of daily intake obtained from food records.

Nutrient	Infant, birth to 1 y	Toddler, 1-3 y	Child, 4-10 y	Adolescent 11-14 y	Adolescent 15-18 y
Energy (kcal/kg/d)*	Birth to 6 mo: 108 7-12 mo: 98	102	4-6 y: 90 7-10 y: 70	Boys: 55 Girls: 47	Boys: 45 Girls: 40
Protein (g/kg/d)* For HD patients	Birth to 6 mo: 2.6 7-12 mo: 2.0	1.6	4-6 y: 1.6 7-10 y: 1.4	Boys: 1.4 Girls: 1.4	Boys: 1.3 Girls: 1.2
For PD patients	Birth to 6 mo: 2.9-3.0 7-12 mo: 2.3-2.4	1.9-2.0	4-6 y: 1.9-2.0 7-10 y: 1.7-1.8	Boys: 1.7-1.8 Girls: 1.7-1.8	Boys: 1.4-1.5[†] Girls: 1.4-1.5[†]
Sodium (Recommendations for patients who are oliguric/anuric, edematous, or hypertensive	• No salt shaker and avoid salty foods (> 200 mg Na/serving). • Infants and toddlers; restrict to 1-3 mEq/kg/d.[‡] • Children and adolescents: restrict to 87-174 mEq/day+ (2-4 g/d).				
Potassium (Recommendations for patients with hyperkalemia)	• Avoid foods with high potassium levels, such as bananas, chocolate, and orange juice. • Infants and toddlers: restrict to 1-3 mEq/kg/d.[‡] • Children and adolescents: restrict to 51-103 mEq/d[‡] (2-4 g/d).				
Calcium (mg/d)	• 100% of the DRI. • Monitor total calcium load, including calcium from phosphate binders.				
Phosphorus (mg/d) (recommendations for patients with hyperphosphatemia)	Restrict to low phosphorus formula and foods	≤ 400–600		≤ 600–800	
Vitamins*	If needed, supplement to 100% of the DRI for thiamin, riboflavin, pyridoxine, folic acid, and vitamin B-12, and 100% of the RDA for vitamins A, C, E and K. Supplement with vitamin D metabolite to prevent hyperparathyroidism and renal osteodystrophy.				
Trace minerals*	If needed supplement to 100% of the RDA for copper and zinc. Iron supplementation is usually needed with erythropoietin therapy.				
Fluids	Total fluid intake (TFI) = Insensible losses + Urine output + Ultrafiltration capacity + Other losses – Amount to deficit.				

* Future modification of K/DOQI guidelines will need to consider new recommendations for macronutrients, vitamins, minerals, and trace elements.

† Based on growth potential.

‡ For sodium and potassium: mEq = mmol.

Data are from K/DOQI guidelines (8) and selected *Dietary Reference Intakes* publications. (38, 40, 41, 43).

Source: Byham-Gray, L., & Wiesen, K. (Eds.) (2004). *A clinical guide to nutrition care in kidney disease*. Chicago: The American Dietetic Association.

phorus is above the target range for age. Infants, toddlers, and children may require restriction of ≤ 300–500 mg/day while adolescents may require limitation of phosphorus intake to ≤ 800–1000 mg/day. Foods high in phosphorus such as milk, cheese, yogurt, cola, and standard infant formulas should be limited. Good adherence to phosphate binders will facilitate allowance of more liberal phosphorus intake. Ideally, phosphate binders should be given 10–15 minutes before or during a meal or high phosphorus snack.

H. Sodium bicarbonate therapy may be necessary to maintain $HCO_3 > 22$ mEq/L. This will facilitate good growth and weight gain.

I. Total calcium intake should not exceed up to 2x DRI for calcium for age or 2500 mg elemental calcium/day including dietary calcium and elemental calcium from phosphate binders.

J. Vitamin D metabolites are used to prevent and treat hyperparathyroidism and renal osteodystrophy. Active vitamin D sterol (calcitriol) is given to patients with serum PTH >300 pg/mL to achieve a target range of 200–300 pg/mL. This is usually given IV to children on hemodialysis.

K. Vitamin intake may be supplemented to meet 100% of the DRI (Dietary Reference Intakes) for thiamin (B_1), riboflavin (B_2), pyridoxine (B_6), folic acid, and vitamin B_{12} and 100% of the RDA for vitamins A, C, E, and K. Copper and zinc, if needed, to be supplemented to 100% of the RDA. A renal multivitamin may be used.

L. Iron supplementation is typically given IV for patients on hemodialysis and is usually necessary for those patients on erythropoietin therapy. May also be given orally.

M. Calorically dense, renal supplements may be used to help meet nutritional needs.

N. Nutritionally-related medications, such as phosphate binders, iron, bicarbonate, vitamin D metabolites, and vitamins are usually available in both liquid and solid forms. The age, size, development, and preference of the child and parent will determine which type of preparation is used.

XI. **Nutritional recommendations for children on peritoneal dialysis** (see Table 8.4: *Daily Nutrient Recommendations for Children on Dialysis*).

A. Calorie needs are initially based on the RDA for chronologic age, but may be adjusted depending on nutritional status, growth, medical complications, intercurrent illnesses, activity level, and other factors that could impact calorie needs. Need to include calories absorbed from dialysate solution in total nutrient intake.

B. Protein needs are increased above the RDA for chronologic age due to increased protein losses associated with the peritoneal dialysis process.

C. Sodium restriction is usually not necessary unless the patient is edematous or hypertensive. Infants may require sodium supplementation.

D. Potassium restriction is usually not necessary if dialysis adequacy is adequate.

E. Phosphorus restriction is necessary for patients with hyperphosphatemia and/or hyperparathyroidism. Dietary phosphorus should be decreased to the Dietary Reference Intake (DRI) for age when the serum PTH concentration is above the target range and serum phosphorus is within the target range for a dialysis patient. Dietary phosphorus should be decreased to 80% of the DRI for age when the serum PTH concentration is above the target range for a dialysis patient and serum phosphorus is above the target range for age. Infants, toddlers, and children may require restriction of ≤ 300–500 mg/day while adolescents may require limitation of phosphorus intake to ≤ 800–1000 mg/day. Foods high in phosphorus such as milk, cheese, yogurt, cola, and standard infant formulas should be limited. Good adherence to phosphate binders will facilitate allowance of more liberal phosphorus intake. Ideally, phosphate binders should be given 10–15 minutes before or during a meal or high phosphorus snack.

F. Sodium bicarbonate therapy may be necessary to maintain $HCO_3 > 22$ mEq/L. This will facilitate good growth and weight gain.

G. Total calcium intake should not exceed 2x DRI for calcium for age or 2500 mg elemental calcium/day including dietary calcium and elemental calcium from phosphate binders.

H. Vitamin D metabolites are used to prevent and treat hyperparathyroidism and renal osteodystrophy. Active vitamin D sterol (calcitriol) is given to patients with serum PTH > 300 pg/mL to achieve a target range of 200–300 pg/mL. This is usually given orally to patients on peritoneal dialysis.

I. Vitamin intake may be supplemented to meet 100% of the DRI for thiamin(B_1), riboflavin (B_2), pyridoxine (B_6), folic acid, and vitamin B_{12} and 100% of the RDA for vitamins A, C, E, and K. Copper and zinc, if needed, to be supplemented to 100% of the RDA. A renal multivitamin may be used.

J. Iron supplementation is typically given orally for patients on peritoneal dialysis and is usually necessary for those patients on erythropoietin therapy. May also be given IV.

K. Standard and renal oral supplements (depending on laboratory values) may be used to help meet nutritional needs.

L. Nutritionally related medications, such as phosphate binders, iron, bicarbonate, vitamin D metabolites, and vitamins are usually available in both liquid and solid forms. The age, size, development, and preference of the child and parent will determine which type of preparation is used.

XII. Nutritional recommendations for children who have received a kidney transplant (see Table 8.5: *Daily Nutrient Recommendations for Children with Kidney Transplants*).

A. The nutritional goals following a kidney transplant are to promote wound healing and anabolism, prevent infection, promote optimal growth, minimize medication side effects, maintain electrolytes and minerals within normal limits, and maintain blood pressure within normal limits.

B. Need to continue to monitor nutritional status and growth closely. Acceleration in rate of linear growth may occur, particularly in younger children. The use of recombinant growth hormone following transplant is controversial due to the potential for deterioration in kidney function. Excess weight gain may occur due to increased appetite/intake, more liberal diet than in past, immunosuppressive medications, and decreased physical activity/inactive lifestyle.

C. Caloric needs are based on the estimated energy requirements (EERs) for age and are based on active physical activity levels as the level recommended to maintain health and decrease risk of chronic disease and disability. A low fat diet may

be necessary for those patients with hyperlipidemia or excess weight gain following transplantation. Hyperlipidemia in transplant patients is often related to immunosuppressive medications.

D. Protein needs are increased for the first 3 months after transplant (1.2–1.5 x DRI) and return to the DRI for age after 3 months.

E. Moderate sodium intake is recommended for patients with edema or hypertension. Food should not be salted at the table and high sodium foods (>200 mg sodium/serving) should be avoided. Infants and toddlers will typically require restriction of 1–3 mEq/kg/day and children and adolescents will require a restriction of 87–174 mEq/day (2–4 g/day) when needed.

F. Potassium is generally not restricted unless the patient has hyperkalemia (may be associated with immunosuppressive drug toxicity, use of ACE inhibitors, impaired kidney function in the allograft). If hyperkalemia is present, temporarily limit intake of high potassium foods such as bananas, oranges, tomatoes, potatoes, chocolate, and milk until potassium is within normal range.

G. Calcium intake should meet 100% of the DRI for age.

H. Phosphorus intake should meet 100% of the DRI for age. Supplementation may be necessary initially due to hyperparathyroidism and hypophosphatemia.

I. Vitamin supplementation is generally not necessary, except for the possible exception of vitamin D. 100% of DRI for age is acceptable.

J. Trace minerals may be supplemented up to 100% of DRI. Magnesium supplementation may be indicated initially due to hypomagnesemia.

K. High fluid intake should be encouraged to avoid dehydration and volume depletion.

L. Herbals and botanicals are currently contraindicated.

XIII. Nutritional support for the pediatric kidney patient.

A. Enteral nutrition.
1. If oral intake is inadequate to support growth and weight gain and achieve and maintain optimal nutritional status despite functioning GI tract, enteral nutrition may be necessary to avoid malnutrition.

Table 8.5

Daily Nutrient Recommendations for Children with Kidney Transplantation

Note: Restrictions should be implemented only where warranted and kept as liberal as possible to optimize energy intake and prevent malnutrition.

Pediatric dietary restrictions usually take the form of a "low-nutrient X diet" with education about avoiding or limiting foods high in that nutrient. Depending on the response in the parameter relevant to that nutrient (e.g., blood pressure; biochemical value) the restriction can be liberalized or tightened.

Prescriptions for specific amounts of a nutrient (e.g., 3 mEq nutrient X/kg) are rarely used in pediatrics. Amounts provided in the table can be used as references for assessment of daily intake obtained from food records.

Nutrient	Infant, birth to 1 y	Toddler, 1-2 y	Child, 3-8 y	Adolescent 9-13 y	Adolescent 14-18 y
Energy (kcal/kg/d)* Boys:	Birth to 6 mo: 95 7-12 mo: 82	87	87	63	52
Girls:	Birth to 6 mo: 87 7-12 mo: 75	82	82	60	44
Protein (g/kg/d)	• First 3 mo after transplant: 1.2-1.5 times the DRI. • After 3 mo posttransplant: DRI.				
Sodium (Recommendations for patients who are oliguric/anuric, edematous, or hypertensive	• No salt shaker and avoid salty foods (≥ 200 mg/serving). • Infants and toddlers: Restrict to 1-3 mEq/kg/d.[†] • Children and adolescents: Restrict to 87-174 mEq/day[†] (2-4 g/d).				
Potassium (Recommendations for patients with hyperkalemia)	• Restriction generally unnecessary. • Temporarily avoid foods with high potassium levels, such as bananas, chocolate, and orange juice, until serum levels are within normal range.				
Calcium (mg/d)	• 100% of the DRI.				
Phosphorus (mg/d) (recommendations for patients with hyperphosphatemia)	• 100% of the DRI. • Supplementation is usually indicated initially for hypophosphatemia.				
Vitamins	• 100% of the DRI. • Supplementation is generally unnecessary, with the possible exception of vitamin D.				
Trace minerals	• 100% of the DRI. • Magnesium supplementation is usually indicated initially for hypomagnesemia				
Fluids	High fluid intake is encouraged.				

* Energy recommendations are the estimated energy requirements (EERs). They are based on active physical activity levels (PAL) as the level recommended to maintain health and decrease risk of chronic disease and disability. EERs are presented in kcal/kg as determined by dividing the active PAL EER (total kcal/day) by the reference weight for each respective age.

[†] For sodium. mEq-mmol.

Data are from selected *Dietary Reference Intake* publications (34-42).

Source: Byham-Gray, L., & Wiesen, K. (Eds.) (2004). *A clinical guide to nutrition care in kidney disease.* Chicago: The American Dietetic Association.

2. Nasogastric or nasojejunal enteral feedings may be used. If enteral feedings will be needed long-term, gastrostomy tubes may be placed either surgically or nonsurgically. However, placement of a gastrostomy tube in a patient on peritoneal dialysis has been associated with an increased risk of infectious complications. Need to consider the risks/benefits of placing a gastrostomy tube on an individual basis.

3. Enteral feedings can be given as either a bolus feeding or as a continuous feeding using a feeding pump. Bolus feedings are frequently not well-tolerated in infants and toddlers with chronic kidney disease; therefore, continuous feedings may be necessary. Continuous enteral feedings may be given overnight to encourage oral intake during the day. Continuous feedings are usually started at 1–3 mL/kg/day and increased as tolerated. Feeding schedules may need to be adjusted for patients on dialysis.

4. Choice of formula is based on age, nutritional requirements, fluid requirements, laboratory values, and concurrent medical problems (pancreatitis, malabsorption, diabetes, etc.).

B. Parenteral nutrition.

1. Parenteral nutrition may be necessary if the gastrointestinal (GI) tract is nonfunctioning or nonaccessible or if enteral feedings are insufficient to meet nutritional needs.

2. Fluid limitations, dialysis modality, and route of infusion (peripheral or central) may impair the ability to fully meet nutritional needs using parenteral nutrition.

3. The most concentrated forms of dextrose, amino acid, and lipid solutions available should be used to limit fluid intake in dialysis patients if parenteral nutrition is necessary. There is no scientific evidence to support the use of essential amino acid solutions in the kidney patient. Electrolytes should be individualized to meet the patient's needs. Standard dosages of multivitamins for parenteral nutrition as established by the American Medical Association Nutrition Advisory Committee and amended in 2000 are recommended. Need to monitor for potential vitamin A toxicity in patients on long-term parenteral nutrition.

C. Interdialytic Parenteral Nutrition (IDPN). IDPN is the provision of macronutrients (carbohydrate, protein, and fat) through the venous drip chamber of the hemodialysis machine. It will not fully meet the patient's nutritional needs, but may be helpful in supplementing enteral intake. Strict criteria must be met in order to justify use of IDPN.

D. Intraperitoneal parenteral nutrition (IPN).

1. Increased protein losses associated with peritoneal dialysis may make it difficult to fully meet patient's protein requirements.

2. IPN substitutes an amino acid solution for one or two glucose exchanges per day when on peritoneal dialysis and may be indicated in patients with malnutrition who have inadequate calorie and protein intake and are unable to tolerate oral or enteral supplementation. KDOQI guidelines for use should be followed.

XIV. Monitoring nutritional status in pediatric kidney patients.

A. Multiple parameters should be used when assessing the nutritional status of children with chronic kidney disease.

1. Anthropometric measures. At least monthly assessment of linear growth (recumbent length or height), weight, head circumference (in children less than 3 years), standard deviation score (SDS) for length/height for chronologic age, body mass index (BMI). Appropriate childhood growth charts developed by the Centers for Disease Control and Prevention (CDC) should be used. At least quarterly assessment of mid-arm circumference, tricep skinfold, and mid-arm muscle circumference. Ideally, all measurements should be obtained by the same person each month.

2. Laboratory data: albumin, bicarbonate, other.

3. Dietary intake should be evaluated using diet recall and food records to assess adequacy of calorie and protein intake.

B. The nutrition plan should be adjusted frequently depending on response to dietary intervention, growth and weight gain, biochemical control, changes in medical status or dialysis modality, and changes in medications.

Pregnancy in Dialysis and Transplantation

I. Dialysis.

A. Energy/protein needs.
  1. Kilocalories.
     a. ~35/kg pregravida IBW + 300 kcal (2nd and 3rd trimesters).
     b. With PD kcal from absorption of glucose in dialysis solutions should be estimated and included.
     c. Intakes should be evaluated frequently by dietitian.
     d. May need nutritional supplements to meet needs.
  2. Protein needs.
     a. HD: 1.2 g/kg IBW + 10 g/day.
     b. PD: 1.3 g/kg + 10 g/day.
     c. Evaluated frequently by dietitian.
     d. May need protein supplements to meet needs.

B. Minerals.
  1. Sodium, potassium, and phosphorus.
     a. Content of diet often liberalized with more frequent dialysis (see below).
     b. Restrict according to fluid retention and lab values.
  2. Calcium.
     a. Calcium needs of the fetus are increased, thus calcium containing phosphate binders are usually given.
     b. If the phosphorus is below goal range, these medications are given apart from meals, primarily for calcium supplementation.
  3. Iron.
     a. IV iron has been used without complications; usually given as iron gluconate or iron sucrose.
     b. Dose given depends on iron studies used for nonpregnant dialysis patients.
     c. Although not as well absorbed, oral iron preparations have also been used instead of intravenous iron, either alone or in combination with a vitamin.
  4. Zinc.
     a. At least 15 mg/day given to prevent increased risks of fetal malformation, preterm delivery, low birth weight, and pregnancy-induced hypertension.
     b. May be given alone or included in the renal vitamin prescribed.

C. Vitamins.
  1. Water-soluble vitamins are usually preferred over prenatal vitamins due to the need to avoid excess vitamin A for all individuals with CKD undergoing dialysis. With increased requirements for water-soluble vitamins during pregnancy, as well as increased losses anticipated with more intensive dialysis, a standard renal vitamin containing 1 mg folic acid is often doubled to ensure at least 2 mg of folic acid per day.
  2. Vitamin D analogs have been given IV during dialysis to treat high PTH and to maintain normal serum levels of calcium. There does not seem to be definitive information available, however, about whether these forms of vitamin D cross the placental barrier and, if so, whether they are safe relative to fetal development.

D. Other medications.
  1. Antihypertensives. Agents considered safe during pregnancy include methyldopa, beta blockers, labetelol, and probably calcium channel blockers/clonidine. Angiotensin-converting enzyme inhibitors (ACEIs) and angiotensin-receptive blockers (ARBs) are contraindicated during pregnancy.
  2. Epogen™ has been used safely to treat anemia, and frequently needs to be increased as the pregnancy progresses.

E. Weight gain is difficult to determine due to fluid retention. It has been suggested that estimated dry weight (EDW) be increased by .5 kg/week in the 2nd and 3rd trimesters, but weight gain throughout the pregnancy needs regular, careful evaluation by the kidney team.

F. Dialysis modifications.
  1. Hemodialysis.
     a. Usually 4–6 x/week with ≥ 20 hr/week to assimilate more normal kidney function during fetal development.
     b. Dialysate may need to have a higher K+ content with more frequent dialysis, but calcium content usually ~2.5 mEq/L.
     c. Transfer to inpatient dialysis setting for fetal monitoring during treatment at approximately 24 weeks gestation.
  2. Peritoneal dialysis.
     a. Smaller volumes with more exchange needed.
     b. Tidal PD may be more efficient and comfortable.

II. Transplantation.

A. Energy/protein needs.
  1. Kilocalories: 25–35/kg pregravida IBW + 300 per day (2nd and 3rd trimesters).
  2. Protein: 0.8–1.0 g/kg pregravida IBW + 10 g/day.

B. Minerals (guidelines for normal pregnancy).
  1. Sodium: usually 2–4 g/day.
  2. Potassium: liberal intake unless serum levels increased.
  3. Calcium: at least 1000 mg/day (1300 mg/day < 19 years of age).
  4. Phosphorus: at least 700 mg (1250 mg/day < 19 years of age).
  5. Zinc: at least 11 mg/day (12 mg/day < 19 years of age).
  6. Iron: at least 27 mg/day.

C. Vitamins (guidelines for normal pregnancy).
  1. Vitamin A: ~ 800 ug/day.
  2. Folic Acid: at least 600 mcg/day.
  3. Thiamine: 1.4 mg/day.
  4. Riboflavin: 1.4 mg/day.
  5. B_6: 1.9 mg/day.
  6. B_{12}: 2.6 mg/day.
  7. Biotin: 30 ug/day.
  8. Vitamin C: 85 mg/day.
  9. Vitamin D: 5 ug/day.
  10. Vitamin E: 15 mg/day.

D. Weight gain (normal pregnancy).
  1. Underweight (BMI < 19.8): 28–40 lb.
  2. Normal weight (BMI 19.8–26): 25–35 lb.
  3. Overweight (BMI 26–29): 15–25 lb.
  4. Obese (BMI > 29): at least 15 lb.

Chapter 41

Nutrition Intervention

Nutrients Important in the Management of Kidney Disease

I. Protein and amino acids.

A. Protein is a structural component of all living cells, found in muscles, nerves, bone, teeth, skin, hair, nails, blood, and glands. Almost all body fluids contain protein with the exception of urine, sweat, and bile.

B. Protein is a regulator of blood pH, osmotic pressure, and water balance. It forms antibodies, aids in building resistance to infections, and transports other substances in the blood, such as drugs.

C. Protein is stored in all lean tissues, but acute-critical illness or inadequate intake can lead to deficiency.

D. As kidney function declines, nitrogenous wastes accumulate, plasma protein concentrations are altered, and protein catabolism is increased secondary to metabolic acidosis.

E. In catabolic states or with inadequate protein intake, protein stores are broken down and can contribute to the accumulation of nitrogenous wastes.

F. Amino acids and peptides are lost with each hemodialysis treatment. Protein losses that occur with peritoneal dialysis can double with peritonitis. The catabolic effect of high-dose steroids can increase protein requirements in kidney transplant patients.

G. Essential amino acids must be provided by the diet. Nonessential amino acids can be synthesized by the body. Tyrosine, histidine, and serine are conditionally essential amino acids in kidney failure.

H. As a source of energy, protein yields 4 calories per gram. This function should be spared by fat and carbohydrate so that protein is used for building and repairing tissues.

I. An adjusted body weight is needed to calculate protein needs with underweight or overweight conditions.

II. Carbohydrate.

A. Carbohydrate is the primary source of heat and energy. It has a protein sparing effect and serves as the carbon skeleton for the synthesis of nonessential amino acids.

B. Glucose is the major energy source of the brain and other nervous tissues. Carbohydrate occurs in the body chiefly as glucose, and is stored as glycogen in liver and muscle.

C. Carbohydrate metabolism is altered in chronic kidney disease. Two major defects frequently noted are peripheral resistance to the action of insulin and impaired insulin secretion by the pancreas.

D. Elevated parathyroid hormone (PTH) levels/ secondary hyperparathyroidism can also contribute to glucose intolerance by inhibiting insulin secretion.

E. Hypoglycemia may be noted in diabetic as well as nondiabetic patients when GFR falls below 40 mL/min. Insulin is metabolized and cleared by the kidney. Therefore, the half-life is increased as kidney disease progresses.

F. Carbohydrate yields 4 calories per gram and provides 45–50% of the calories in the typical American diet.

III. Fats.

A. Fat is a carrier of fat-soluble vitamins, is part of the essential structure of cells, adds palatability and satiety value to the diet, and has a protein-sparing effect.

B. Fat is stored as adipose tissue, found mainly in subcutaneous tissue and around visceral organs, and insulates the body against heat loss.

C. Fat provides the most concentrated source of calories, yielding 9 calories per gram. Fat stores are filled up or depleted depending on the balance between energy intake from food and energy expenditure.

D. Impaired kidney function and uremia are both associated with lipid abnormalities. These dyslipidemias are a contributing factor to the high incidence of atherosclerosis in CKD stage 5 patients.

E. In the nephrotic syndrome, increased cholesterol production and decreased clearance of lipids result in hypercholesterolemia and hypertriglyceridemia.

F. Hemodialysis patients frequently have elevated serum triglyderides and very low-density lipoprotein (VLDL) cholesterol, and low serum levels of high-density lipoprotein (HDL) cholesterol.

G. Peritoneal dialysis patients tend to have higher serum cholesterol, triglyceride, and low density lipoprotein (LDL) cholesterol levels than hemodialysis patients, possibly secondary to loss of proteins into the peritoneal dialysate and excessive absorption of glucose from the dialysate.

H. After kidney transplant, immunosuppressive therapy can lead to elevated serum cholesterol and triglycerides.

I. No Dietary Reference Intake (DRI) exists for fat, but guidelines suggest that 25–35% of daily caloric needs should be provided by fat, with less than 10% from saturated fat.

J. When Therapeutic Lifestyle Changes (TLC) are implemented to lower elevated lipid levels, total fat may be restricted to 25–30% of calories, and saturated fat to < 7% of calories.

IV. Energy.

A. Actual energy requirements vary, based on age, growth, medical condition, activity, and amount of lean body tissue compared to total edema-free weight. An adjusted body weight should be calculated to account for these variables, but the wide-spread acceptance of one formula which accounts for these multiple contributing factors is still elusive.

B. Persons on peritoneal dialysis are exposed to a high glucose load, both on CAPD and APD, due to the peritoneal absorption of dextrose (see Chapter 39, *Nutrition Care for the Patient Receiving Dialysis*, III. Peritoneal Dialysis, G, H, and I to estimate caloric load).

V. Alcohol.

A. Alcohol is metabolized primarily in the liver. Excessive consumption may lead to elevated levels of ketones, triglycerides, uric acid, lactic acid, acidosis, blood pressure, and stroke risk.

B. Alcohol should be avoided in pregnancy, pancreatitis, alcohol abuse, advanced neuropathy, and severely elevated triglyceride levels.

C. Light to moderate intake of alcohol may provide benefits. Alcohol use raises HDL cholesterol, lowers LDL cholesterol, decreases the oxidation of LDL, and exerts anticlotting actions, all which decrease the risk of coronary heart disease.

D. The consumption of alcohol along with certain medications is contraindicated due to the potential of alcohol as a stomach mucosal irritant, hepato-toxic agent, and as an agent that may produce additive toxicity during drug metabolism.

E. The fluid content of alcoholic beverages should be considered, along with other nutrients. The potassium content of wine ranges from 115 to 164 mg/5 oz serving. Mixed drinks may contain moderate to high potassium ingredients, such as tomato juice, orange juice, pineapple juice, and coconut cream.

F. See Chapter 40, *Diabetes and Kidney Disease*: IV. Alcohol, for considerations in diabetes.

VI. Fiber.

A. Dietary fiber is either soluble or insoluble. Soluble fiber, found in many vegetables and oatmeal, can moderately lower total and LDL cholesterol.

B. Many high fiber foods arc also high in potassium or phosphorus, such as prunes, dried beans and peas, bran, nuts, and certain fruits and vegetables, such as bananas, melon, and tomatoes. Safer choices within a potassium or phosphorus restriction include green beans, cabbage, carrots, cauliflower, corn, eggplant, onions, alfalfa sprouts, apple with skin, blueberries, raspberries, popcorn, brown rice, and oatmeal, among others.

C. Commercial fiber supplements, such as psyllium (Metamucil) and cellulose (Unifiber) contain 3 grams of fiber per tablespoon, and may be used when dietary fiber intake is insufficient. *Note*: Sugar-free, orange-flavored effervescent Metamucil is high in potassium.

D. Recommended intake is 20 to 25 g per day, with 20 to 30 grams recommended for Therapeutic Lifestyle Changes.

VII. Vitamins.

A. The recommended daily intake of vitamins varies depending on gender, age, and other conditions, such as pregnancy, lactation, and health status.

B. Chronic kidney disease alters vitamin status, and both deficiencies and abnormally high levels of vitamins have been reported with kidney disease.

C. Little data is available on vitamin requirements for acute kidney injury, but water-soluble vitamins should be supplemented to compensate for losses in HD and PD.

D. The Hemo Study demonstrated that mortality rates were improved in patients on dialysis who took vitamin supplements.

E. Water-soluble: Most water-soluble vitamins are not stored so daily intake is required, although vitamin B_{12} is the exception.
   1. Vitamin C.
      a. Vitamin C is necessary for the synthesis of collagen, for wound healing, and for the ability to withstand the stress of injury and infection. It also enhances the absorption of iron and influences cellular and humoral immune responses.
      b. Losses occur with HD (about 50 mg per HD treatment) and PD.
      c. Recommended supplementation is 60 to 100 mg per day.
   2. Vitamin B complex.
      a. B complex vitamins include eight vitamins: thiamine, riboflavin, niacin, B_6 or pyridoxine, pantothenic acid, biotin, B_{12} or cobalamin, and folic acid.
      b. Vitamins in this complex serve as coenzymes in a variety of biochemical reactions, including the production of energy; metabolism of proteins, lipids, and carbohydrates; and synthesis of body tissues.
      c. Primary sources are protein foods, whole grains, and fortified grains and cereals. Many B vitamins tend to be present in the same foods. Therefore, a deficiency of one may point to a deficiency in another, with some exceptions.
      d. Requirements increase when metabolism is accelerated by fever, stress, or injury.
      e. Recommended intake for CKD, HD, and PD:
         (1) Thiamin: 1.1–1.2 mg/day.
         (2) Riboflavin: 1.1–1.3 mg/day.

(3) B_6: 5–10 mg/day.
(4) B_{12}: 2.4–400 mcg/day.
(5) Niacin: 14–20 mg/day.
(6) Folic acid: 0.8–5.0 mg/day.
(7) Pantothenic acid: 5 mg/day.
(8) Biotin: 30–300 mcg/day.
f. AKI: Dietary Reference Intake; adjust to degree of catabolism.
g. Transplant: Dietary Reference Intake.

F. Fat soluble vitamins are stored in the body. Deficiencies can occur in fat malabsorption secondary to GI disorders, or with inadequate intake.
1. Vitamin A.
a. Vitamin A is necessary for photoreception in rod and cone cells of the retina, bone growth and development, epithelial tissue development and maintenance, and immunity.
b. Increased plasma levels occur in kidney failure. The vitamin A carrier, retinol-binding protein, is catabolized in the tubules, and this process decreases as kidney function drops. Vitamin A toxicity has been reported with supplementation.
c. No losses occur with HD. Very small losses have been reported in PD. Serum levels eventually return to normal after transplantation.
d. Supplementation is usually not necessary. Renal vitamins do not contain Vitamin A.
2. Vitamin D.
a. The functions of the active form include:
(1) Stimulating active GI absorption of calcium and phosphorus.
(2) Working in conjunction with PTH to mobilize calcium and phosphate from the bone to maintain serum calcium and phosphate levels.
b. The ability to synthesize 1,25-dihydroxyvitamin D_3 decreases as kidney function declines and supplementation with vitamin D analogs is needed in CKD, HD, and PD. Supplementation may also be needed in some transplant patients.
c. Besides issues related to bone metabolism, calcitriol is involved in metabolic processes affecting cardiovascular disease, such as congestive heart failure, hypertension, and left ventricular hypotrophy, and certain cancers, such as prostate.
d. The nonactive form of vitamin D is a required nutrient, even in persons with CKD. Uremic kidneys can lose vitamin D binding protein in the urine, potentially causing a

vitamin D deficiency. The elderly, housebound patients and people living in northern climates are also at risk.
e. In CKD stages 3 and 4, if PTH levels are > 70 or 110, respectively, the nonactive form of vitamin D should be measured (serum 25-hydroxyvitamin D). Supplement with ergocalciferol (OTC) if levels are < 30 ng/mL. Supplementation requirements for CKD stage 5 for the nonactive form have not been determined.
3. Vitamin E.
a. Functions of vitamin E.
(1) Antioxidant; used commercially to retard spoilage.
(2) Preserves intregrity of red blood cells.
(3) May protect structure and function of muscle tissues.
(4) Prevents oxidation of unsaturated fats and LDL.
b. Supplementation beyond the dietary intake is controversial. Vitamin E coated dialyzers may decrease oxidative stress, but their use is not widespread.
4. Vitamin K.
a. Vitamin K is essential for both prothrombin formation for blood coagulation, and for bone formation.
b. The main source is *E. coli* synthesis in the large intestine.
c. Generally, supplementation is not indicated, but hospitalized patients with poor intake and an extended course of antibiotics are at risk for developing a deficiency, and supplementation may be necessary, since body stores are small.
d. Patients who take warfarin (Coumadin) need to maintain a steady intake of vitamin K to prevent blood coagulation problems.

VIII. Minerals.

A. Sodium (23 mg = 1 mEq).
1. Sodium is the major cation in extracellular fluid.
2. Functions of sodium.
a. Regulation of extracellular fluid volume.
b. Conduction of nerve impulses.
c. Control of muscle contraction.
d. Acid-base regulation.
e. Cell membrane permeability.
3. Recommended intake.
a. AKI: 1000–2000 mg/day; adjust according to fluid status and blood pressure; replace in diuretic phase.

b. CKD: 1000–3000 mg/day.
c. HD: 1000–3000 mg/day.
d. PD: 2000–4000 mg/day.
e. Transplant: 2000–4000 mg/day.
f. Healthy adults: no Dietary Reference Intake (DRI) established.

B. Potassium (39 mg = 1 mEq).
1. Potassium is the major cation of intracellular fluid. Potassium makes up 5% of the total mineral content of the body.
2. Major functions of potassium.
   a. Aids in maintaining normal water balance, osmotic equilibrium, and acid-base balance.
   b. Aids in regulation of neuromuscular activity, particularly in transmission of electrical impulses in the heart.
   c. Participates in the conversion of glucose to glycogen.
3. Normally 80–90% of ingested potassium is excreted in the urine, and 10–20% is lost in the feces.
4. Potassium can shift from intracellular to extracellular fluid in conditions of acidosis and hyperglycemia.
5. Recommended intake.
   a. AKI: 2000 mg/day; maintain serum levels < 5 mEq/L; replace in diuretic phase.
   b. CKD: usually not restricted unless serum levels are elevated.
   c. HD: 2000–3000 mg/day.
   d. PD: 3000–4000 mg/day; adjust based on serum levels; may need a potassium supplement to maintain serum levels.
   e. Transplant: restrict if hyperkalemic.
   f. Healthy adults: no DRI established.

C. Calcium (20 mg = 1 mEq).
1. Calcium is the most abundant mineral found in the body, with 99% located in hard tissues, bone, and teeth.
2. Functions of calcium.
   a. Build and maintain bones and teeth.
   b. Activation of enzymes for metabolic functions.
   c. Blood coagulation.
   d. Permeability of cell membrane.
   e. Transmission of nerve impulses.
   f. Contraction of skeletal, cardiac, and smooth muscle fibers.
3. Only 10–30% of ingested calcium is absorbed.
   a. Absorption is increased by activated vitamin D, acidic medium, lactose, and increased body need.
   b. Absorption is decreased by vitamin D

deficiency, oxalic acid, phytic acid, fiber, alkaline medium, immobilizations, and trauma.
4. Recommended intake.
   a. Correct lab-reported serum calcium level for low serum albumin level, to prevent overadministration or underadministration of calcium supplements.

   Corrected serum calcium = Total calcium mg/dL + [0.8 x (4.0 – serum albumin (g/dL)].

   b. AKI: maintain serum levels within normal limits.
   c. CKD: 1000–1500 mg/day.
   d. HD and PD: < 2000 mg/day, including diet and binders; and a consideration of the dialysate used.
   e. Transplant: 800–1500 mg/day.
   f. Healthy adult: 1000–1300 mg/day, depending on age and gender.

D. Phosphorus (31 mg = 1 mEq).
1. Phosphorus is the second most abundant mineral in the body. Approximately 80% is located in the bones and teeth.
2. Functions of phosphorus.
   a. Building and maintaining bones and teeth.
   b. Transfer of energy within cells.
   c. Activation of vitamin D.
   d. Normal nerve and muscle function.
   e. Fat transportation as phospholipids.
   f. Acid-base regulation.
3. Phosphate binders are needed to decrease phosphate absorption in the GI tract in acute and chronic kidney failure to maintain acceptable serum levels.
4. Recommended intake.
   a. AKI: maintain serum values within normal limits.
   b. CKD, HD, and PD: 800 to 1000 mg/day (adjusted for protein requirements) when serum levels are > 4.6 mg/dL in stages 3 and 4, and > 5.5 mg/dL in stage 5, or if PTH levels are above target.
   c. Transplant: DRI; supplement as needed.
   d. Healthy adult: 800–1200 mg/day depending on age and gender.

E. Iron.
1. Iron is an essential component of hemoglobin and myoglobin. It is important in oxygen transport and cellular oxidation.
2. Between 60% and 70% of iron is in the

functional form as transferrin, while 30–40% is stored as ferritin.

3. Absorption is dependent on the amount of body stores, other medications, inflammation status, form of iron, and presence or absence of other meal components, such as vitamin C or phytic acid. Generally, 5–15% of iron intake is absorbed.

4. Recommended intake.
   a. AKI: not well-defined.
   b. CKD: 10–18 mg/day; individualize.
   c. HD: individualized; IV iron is usually required to maintain acceptable stores.
   d. PD: individualized; IV iron is sometimes needed to maintain acceptable stores.
   e. Transplant: DRI, but may need supplementation.
   f. Healthy adult: 8–18 mg/day depending on age and gender.

F. Zinc.
   1. The most important function of zinc is in the metabolic activity of cells. It is required for the activity of over 300 enzymes. Zinc is especially important in protein synthesis and taste and smell acuity.
   2. A zinc deficiency leads to extreme undernutrition and delayed wound healing.
   3. Zinc is primarily transported by albumin in plasma. Conditions which cause protein loss can also contribute to a loss of zinc.
   4. Zinc absorption is decreased with calcium-based binders and oral iron use.
   5. Recommended intake.
      a. AKI: not well defined.
      b. CKD: DRI; individualize.
      c. HD: DRI; individualize.
      d. PD: DRI; individualize.
      e. Transplant: DRI, but may require supplementation for wound healing.
      f. Healthy adult: 8–11 mg/day, depending on age and gender.

I. Fluid.

A. Water is an essential component of all living matter.
   1. Water is the largest single component of the body, making up 60% of body weight.
   2. The proportion of body water as a percentage of total body weight decreases with age.
   3. Intracellular water makes up 40% of body weight.
   4. Extracellular fluids, made up of interstitial fluid, plasma, lymph, spinal fluid, and secretions, make up 20% of body weight.

B. Functions.
   1. Water provides an aqueous environment necessary for all metabolism.
   2. It gives structure and form to the body.
   3. Water acts as a transport medium for nutrients and wastes.

C. Recommended daily intake.
   1. AKI: 500 cc plus urine output.
   2. CKD: no restriction.
   3. HD: 1000 cc plus amount equal to urine output; acceptable interdialytic weight gains are 2–5% of estimated dry weight.
   4. PD: maintain fluid balance.
   5. Transplant: no restriction unless fluid overloaded; liberal fluid intake.
   6. Healthy adults: intake to maintain fluid balance.

Education Strategies and Behavior Modification

I. **One in 5 American adults have reading skills below the 5th grade level.**

II. **Illiteracy is a problem found among all races and all socioeconomic levels** and does not correlate with the years of formal education.

III. **Evaluate the readability of written materials you** use for education. Materials should be written at the 4th or 5th grade level.

IV. **Assess the patient's ability to read and understand, even in his or her own native language.**

V. **Place emphasis on learning the patient's needs first.**

VI. **Assess the patient's readiness to learn and/or** determine which stage of behavior change the patient currently exhibits.

A. Precontemplation – patient is unaware, unwilling, or discouraged regarding the need to change.
B. Contemplation – patient is actively considering a change.
C. Preparation – patient has full intentions on changing in the very near term.
D. Action – patient is taking action to create change.
E. Maintenance – the stage where the change needs to be sustained, and the focus should be on lifestyle modifications to avoid a setback.

F. Relapse – the stage where a setback occurs.

VII. Focus on activities that can positively influence the interaction between the patient and clinician.

A. Ask nonjudgmental, open-ended questions.
B. Listen carefully and empathetically.
C. Use reflective listening.
D. Talk less than your patient does.
E. Offer reflections for every question asked.

VIII. Allow patients to choose the way they prefer to learn.

IX. Allow patients to set the agenda for learning.

X. Set diet and nutrition goals with the patient and not for the patient.

XI. Keep diet instruction simple. Teach the smallest amount possible to accomplish goals.

XII. Use simple language. Avoid technical or medical jargon. Illustrate whenever possible.

XIII. Have the patient restate or paraphrase the information in his or her own words.

XIV. Provide opportunities for the patient to demonstrate or practice their newly learned skill.

XV. Space the learning as appropriate, presenting the most important information first.

XVI. Involve the patient in problem solving. As adults, we are better able to remember instructions if we are involved in identifying obstacles and seeking realistic solutions.

XVII. Review often.

Considerations for Cultural Diversity

I. Cultural competence is an essential part of being a modern day healthcare professional. Committing to cultural awareness and education will improve communication and outcome in patients with kidney disease.

II. Factors that dictate food choices.

A. Geographic divisions.
B. Climate.
C. Religious beliefs.
D. Social and cultural beliefs.
E. Cultural influences.
F. Availability.
G. Food intolerances.
H. Age/generation.

III. Issues that interfere with treatment proposals.

A. Individual factors.
  1. Lack of understanding.
  2. Poor communication.
  3. Health beliefs.
  4. Dissatisfaction.
  5. Negative feedback.
  6. Failure to understand beliefs.

B. Disease related.
  1. Severity of conditions.
  2. Presence or absence of symptoms.
  3. Stability of symptoms.

C. Treatment related.
  1. Treatment setting.
  2. Lack of cohesiveness in treatment delivery.
  3. Lack of understanding cultural beliefs.
  4. Inconvenience.

D. Social.
  1. Social stigma.
  2. Peer pressure.

E. Generational differences.
  1. The struggle to balance native culture with new culture.
  2. Immigrants who came 40–50 years ago vs. 20 years ago.
  3. American born.

IV. Nutrition assessment requires information about specific food avoidance and health-related attitudes and practices.

A. Use of herbs and supplements.
B. Fasting and meditation practices.
C. Avoidance of certain foods at certain times.
D. Feasting and special occasions.
E. Acculturation; depends on gender, age, marital status, caste, years in the U.S.

V. General strategies and counseling tips for effective communication.

A. Nutrition education should involve significant others and family members.

B. Consider the client's learning style, literacy level, and preferred language.

C. Use translators to solve language barrier. Children act as translators.

D. Respect for elderly is a very important issue. A polite, unhurried conversation is appreciated.

E. Learn about your client's culture and cultural food habits.

F. Indicate benefits of following prescribed treatment.

G. Simplify educational material.

H. Learn about traditional medicine, herbal medications and food theories. Discuss side effects of herbal medications and limiting the use, if not appropriate.

I. Provide feedback, careful explanation to help overcome fears.

J. Expect gradual behavior modification (see previous subdivision: Education Strategies and Behavior Modification).

K. Interpersonal relationship and trust in providers is a significant issue.

L. Set clear limits as well as reasonable goals.

M. Extended families are very important. Women retain great influence in the family circle. Individual involvement is equally important.

VI. Considerations for planning renal diets.

A. Individualize meal pattern with consideration of the individual's cultural food habits, food preferences and beliefs.

B. Recommend fresh meat and meat substitutes for high sodium cured and canned dried beef, pork, fish, and eggs.

C. Encourage use of appropriate spices and condiments.
   1. Many cultures use liberal amounts of salt in their cooking. For example, Filipino people use a salt solution called "patis" which contains 500 mg of sodium in 1 tablespoon of solution.
   2. Soy sauce, oyster sauce, fish sauce, and MSG are condiments commonly used in Asian cooking methods.

D. May need to limit servings of high sodium, ready-to-eat snacks and savories.

E. Limit high potassium containing fruits and vegetables. Recommend appropriate substitutes and portion control.

F. Liberalize use of appropriate sweets and candies to increase caloric intake to prevent malnutrition and weight loss.

G. May need to limit intake of tea and sodas in these cultures for fluid control and to prevent fluid retention-related complications.

H. Discuss cultural and religious holidays and holiday foods. Help plan renal diets to allow appropriate holiday foods for better adherence.

VII. Vegetarian renal diets.

A. Reasons patients follow vegetarian diet are religious/spiritual, ethnic tradition, health reasons, and lack of taste for meat.

B. Vegetarian health practices, beliefs, and attitudes.
   1. Vegetarians more commonly take vitamins as well as mineral and other supplements.
      a. Brewer's yeast – related to belief that megavitamin therapy could cure certain diseases.
      b. Seaweed is believed to benefit thyroid and protect from radiation.
   2. Many vegetarians believe that disease is caused by an imbalance of nutrients.
   3. Common belief is that diseases can be cured by fasting and avoidance of certain foods.
   4. More commonly believe in alternative treatment for disease.
   5. Common belief is that mind, body, and soul are all interconnected.
   6. Ayurvedic therapy is used to achieve balance. Ayur means "longevity." Veda means "science or knowledge."
      a. Uses diet, herbal remedies, and meditation to reestablish equilibrium between the sick person and the universe.
      b. Diet is considered the most significant part of the therapy.
      c. Foods are classifies as "yin and yang" (hot and cold) depending on their effect on the body.
      d. Herbal infusions are prevalent.

C. Vegetarian renal diet concerns.
   1. Protein.
   2. Potassium.
   3. Phosphorus.

4. Use of meat analogs.
5. Sodium.
6. Herbs, fasting, and holiday foods.

D. Protein considerations.
1. Protein quality is determined by digestibility and amino acid content.
2. Dietary protein requirements.
   a. All essential and nonessential amino acids can be supplied by plant sources as long as a reasonable variety of foods is consumed daily and calorie intake is adequate to meet energy needs.
   b. Complementation is not necessary at each meal or at the same time.
3. Renal diet recommendation = 1.0–1.3 g Pro/kg, with 10% of calories from protein.
4. Benefits of vegetable proteins.
   a. Milder renal histologic damage.
   b. Reduced rate of progressive kidney failure.

c. Less proteinuria.
d. Improved lipid profile.
e. Maintenance of good nutritional status.

E. Minimizing uremic toxicity.
1. Phosphorus management is difficult since the lowest quantity of phosphorus (mg) per gram of protein comes from animal products. Consumption of a vegetarian diet will likely require an increase in the number of phosphate binders for patients on dialysis.
2. Potassium control requires selection of lower potassium-containing fruits and vegetables to allow the use of some dairy products, legumes, nuts and seeds, which are higher in potassium. Use of herbal supplements, roots, juices, and leaves will also contribute to potassium intake.
3. Sodium intake can be affected by salted nuts and seeds and use of meat analogs.

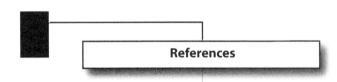

References

Alexander, J.W., Goodman, H.R., Gersin, K., Cardi, M., Austin, J., Goel, S., et al. (2004). Gastric bypass in morbidly obese patients with chronic renal failure and kidney transplant. *Transplantation, 78*(3), 469-474.

Aparicio, M., Chauveau, P., & Combe, C. (2001). Low protein diet and outcome of renal patients. *Journal of Nephrology 14,* 433-439.

Aparicio, M., Chauveau, P., Deprecigout, V., Bouchet, J.L., Lasseur, C., & Combe, C. (2000). Nutrition and outcome on renal replacement therapy of patients with chronic renal failure treated by a supplemented very low protein diet. *Journal of the American Society of Nephrology, 11,* 708-716.

Bergstrom, J. (1995). Why are dialysis patients malnourished? *American Journal of Kidney Diseases, 26*(1), 229-241.

Bistrian, B.R. (1998). Role of the systemic inflammatory response syndrome in the development of protein-calorie malnutrition in ESRD. *American Journal of Kidney Diseases, 32*(6), S113-S117.

Bistrian, B.R., McCowen, K.C., & Chan, S. (1999). Protein energy malnutrition in dialysis patients. *American Journal of Kidney Diseases, 33*(1), 172-175.

Brem, A.S., Lambert, C., Hill, C., Kitsen, J., & Shemin, D.G. (2002). Prevalence of protein malnutrition in children maintained on peritoneal dialysis. *Pediatric Nephrology, 17*(7), 527-530.

Burgess, E. (1999). Conservative treatment to slow deterioration of renal function: evidence-based recommendations. *Kidney International, 55,* S17-S25.

Burrowes, J.D., Cockram, D., Dwyer, J.T., Larive, B., Paranandi, L., Bergen, C., et al., and the Hemodialysis (HEMO) Study Group. (2002). Cross-sectional relationship between dietary protein and energy intake, nutritional status, functional statu-sand comorbidity in older verses younger hemodialysis patients. *Journal of Renal Nutrition, 12*(2), 87-95.

Byham-Gray, L., & Wiesen, K. (Eds.) (2004). *A clinical guide to nutrition care in kidney disease.* Chicago: The American Dietetic Association.

Chang, H., Miller, M.A., & Bruns, F.J. (2002). Tidal peritoneal dialysis during pregnancy improves clearance and abdominal symptoms. *Peritoneal Dialysis International, 22*(2), 272-274.

Chauveau, P., Combe, C., Laville, M., Fouque, D., Azar, R., Cano, N., et al., for the French Study Group for Nutrition In Dialysis. (2001). Factors influencing survival in hemodialysis patients aged older than 75 years: 2.5 year outcome study. *American Journal of Kidney Disease, 37*(5), 997-1003.

Combs, G.F. (1992). *The vitamins: Fundamental aspects in nutrition and health.* San Diego: Academic Press.

Cotton, A.B. (2005). Feeding the patient on dialysis with wounds to heal. *Nephrology Nursing Journal, 32*(4), 555-556.

DeGowin, R.L. (1994). *DeGowin and DeGowin's diagnostic examination* (6th ed.). New York: McGraw-Hill.

Diabetes Control and Complications Trial Research Group. (1993). The effect of intensive treatment of diabetes on the development and progression of long-term complications in insulin-dependent diabetes mellitus. *New England Journal of Medicine, 329,* 977-986.

Ducloux, D., Motte, G., Nguyen, N.U., Abdelfatah, A., Gibey, R., Chalopin, J., et al. (2002). Homocysteine, nutritional status and insulin in renal transplant recipients. *Nephrology Dialysis Transplantation, 17,* 1674-1677.

Escott-Stump, S. (2002). Geriatric nutrition. In *Nutrition and diagnosis-related care* (5th ed., pp. 35-40). Baltimore: Lippincott Williams & Wilkins.

Evans-Stoner, N. (1997). Nutrition assessment: A practical approach. *Nursing Clinics of North America, 32*(4), 637-650.

Foster, B.J., & Leonard, M.B. (2004). Measuring nutritional status in children with chronic kidney disease. *The American Journal of Clinical Nutrition, 80*(4), 801-814.

Franch, H.A., & Mitch, W.E. (1998). Catabolism in uremia: The impact of metabolic acidosis. *Journal of the American Society of Nephrology, 9*, S78-S81.

Furth, S.L. (2005). Growth and nutrition in children with chronic kidney disease. *Advances in Chronic Kidney Disease, 12*(4), 366-371.

Goldstein-Fuchs, J. (2006). Nutrition and chronic kidney disease. In A. Molzahn & E. Butera (Eds.), *Contemporary nephrology nursing: Principles and practice* (2nd ed., pp. 371-391). Pitman, NJ: American Nephrology Nurses' Association.

Gore, J.L., Pham, P.T., Danovitch, G.M., Wilkinson, A.H., Rosenthal, J.T., Lipshutz, G.S., et al. (2006). Obesity and outcome following renal transplantation. *American Journal of Transplantation, 6*, 357-363.

Grossman, S., & Hou, S. (2000). Obstetrics and gynecology. In J.T. Daugirdas, P.G. Blake, & T.S. Ing (Eds.), *Handbook of dialysis* (3rd ed., pp. 624-636). Baltimore: Lippincott Williams & Wilkins.

Haase, M., Morgera, S., Bamberg, C., Halle, H., Martini, S., Hocher, B., et al. (2005). A systematic approach to managing pregnant dialysis patients – The importance of an intensified haemodiafiltration protocol. *Nephrology, Dialysis & Transplantation, 20*(11), 2537-2542.

Hammond, K. (1997). Physical assessment: A nutritional perspective. *Nursing Clinics of North America, 32*(4), 779-790.

Hammond, K. (1999). The nutritional dimension of physical assessment. *Nutrition, 15*, 411-419.

Harvey, K.S. (2002). *A healthy food guide for people on dialysis* (2nd ed.). Chicago: American Dietetic Association.

Hasse, J.M., & Blue, L.S. (Eds.). (2002). *Comprehensive guide to transplant nutrition*. Chicago: American Dietetic Association.

Heimburger, O., Bergstrom, J., & Lindholm, B. (1994). Maintenance of optimal nutrition in CAPD. *Kidney International, 46*, S39-S46.

Hou, S. (2002). Modification of dialysis regimens for pregnancy. *Journal of Artificial Organs, 25*, 823-826.

Ikizler, T.A. (1997). Biochemical markers: Clincal aspects. *Journal of Renal Nutrition, 7*(2), 61-64.

Ikizler, T.A., Green, J.H., Wingard, R.L., Parker, R.A, & Haskim, R.M. (1995). Spontaneous dietary protein intake during progression of chronic renal failure. *Journal of the American Society of Nephrology, 6*, 1386-1391.

Ikizler, T.A., & Hakim, R.M. (1996). Nutrition in end-stage renal disease. *Kidney International, 50*, 343-357.

Klahr, S., Levey, A.S., Beck, G.J., Caggiula, A.W., Hunsicker, L., Kusek, J.W., et al. (1994). The effects of dietary protein restriction and blood-pressure control on the progression of chronic renal disease. *New England Journal of Medicine, 330*, 877-884.

Kleinman, R.E. (Ed.). (2004). *Pediatric nutrition handbook* (5th ed.). Elk Grove Village, IL: American Academy of Pediatrics.

Kopple, J.D. (1998). Dietary protein and energy requirements in ESRD patients. *American Journal of Kidney Diseases, 32*, S97-S104.

Kopple, J.D. (1999). Therapeutic approaches to malnutrition in chronic dialysis patients: The different modalities of nutritional support. *American Journal of Kidney Diseases, 33*(1), 180-185.

Kopple, J.D., & Massrey, S.G. (Eds.) (2004). *Nutritional management of renal disease* (2nd ed.). Philadelphia: Lippincott Williams & Wilkins.

Krause, I., Shamir, R., Davidovits, M., Frishman, S., Cleper, R., Gamzo, Z., et al. (2002). Intradialytic parenteral nutrition in malnourished children treated with hemodialysis. *The Journal of Renal Nutrition, 12*(1), 55-59.

Lacey, K., & Pritchett, E. (2003). Nutrition care process and model: ADA adopts road map to quality care and outcomes management. *Journal of the American Dietetic Association, 103*(8), 1061-1072.

Ledermann, S.E., Shaw, V., & Trompeter, R.S. (1999). Long-term enteral nutrition in infants and young children with chronic renal failure. *Pediatric Nephrology, 13*(9), 870-875.

Ledermann, S.E., Spitz, L., Moloney, J., Rees, L., & Trompeter, R.S. (2002). Gastrostomy feeding in infants and children on peritoneal dialysis. *Pediatric Nephrology, 17*(4), 246-250.

Leung, J., & Dwyer, J. (1998). Renal DETERMINE nutrition screening tools for the identification and treatment of malnutrition. *Journal of Renal Nutrition, 8*, 95-103.

Liano, F., & Pascual, J. (1999). Acute renal failure: Causes and prognosis. In T. Berl & J.V. Bonventure (Eds.), *Atlas of disease of the kidney* (pp. 8.3-8.4). Philadelphia: Current Medicine.

Lien, Y.H., & Ruffenach, S.J. (1996). Low dose megestrol increases serum albumin in malnourished dialysis patient. *The International Journal of Artificial Organs, 19*, 147-150.

Lowrie, E.G. (1990). Death risk in hemodialysis patients: The predictive value of commonly measured variables and an evaluation of death rate differences between facilities. *American Journal of Kidney Diseases, 15*(5), 458-482.

Lowrie, E.G. (1998). Acute phase inflammatory process contributes to malnutrition, anemia, and possibly other abnormalities in dialysis patients. *American Journal of Kidney Diseases, 32*(6), S105-S112.

Mahan, J.D., Warady, B.A., & Consensus Committee. (2006). Assessment and treatment of short stature in pediatric patients with chronic kidney disease: A consensus statement. *Pediatric Nephrology, 21*(7), 917-930.

Marconi, B.J. (1998). Protein restriction in the pre-end-stage renal disease (ESRD) patient: Who, when, how, and the effect on subsequent ESRD outcome. *Journal of the American Society of Nephrology, 9*, S100-S106.

McCann, L. (1998). *Pocket guide to nutritional assessment of the renal patient* (3rd ed.). New York: National Kidney Foundation Council on Renal Nutrition.

McMurray, S., Johnson, G., Davis, S., & McDougall, K. (2002). Diabetes education can care management significantly improve patient outcomes in the dialysis unit. *American Journal of Kidney Diseases, 40*(3), 566-575.

Miller, W.L., & Rollnick, S. (2002). *Motivational interviewing* (2nd ed.). New York: The Guilford Press.

Mitch, W.E., & Klahr, S. (1998). *Handbook of nutrition and the kidney* (3rd ed.). Philadelphia: Lippincott-Raven.

Mitch, W.E., & Marconi, B.J. (1999). Factors causing malnutrition in patients with chronic uremia. *American Journal of Kidney Diseases, 33*, 176-179.

Modification of Diet in Renal Disease Study Group. (2000). Relationship between nutritional status and the glomerular filtration rate: Results from the MDRD Study. *Kidney International, 57*, 1688-1703.

National Kidney Foundation (NKF). (2000). Kidney Disease Outcomes Quality Initiative (K/DOQI) clinical practice guidelines for nutrition in chronic renal failure. *American Journal of Kidney Disease, 35*(6)(Suppl. 2).

National Kidney Foundation (NKF). (2004). *Kidney Disease Outcomes Quality Initiative (K/DOQI) clinical practice guidelines for bone metabolism and disease in chronic kidney disease.* Retrieved June 19, 2006, from http://www.kidney.org/professionals/kdoqi/guidelines_bone/index.htm

National Kidney Foundation (NKF). (2005). *Kidney Disease Outcomes Quality Initiative (K/DOQI) clinical practice guidelines for bone metabolism and disease in children with chronic kidney disease.* Retrieved June 12, 2006, from http://www.kidney.org/professionals/kdoqi/guidelines_pedbone/index.htm

National Research Council, Food and Nutrition Board. (1989). *Recommended dietary allowances* (10th ed.). Washington, DC: National Academy of Sciences.

National Research Council, Food and Nutrition Board. (2004). *Dietary reference intakes: Recommended intakes for individuals, vitamins and dietary reference intakes: Recommended intakes for individuals, elements.* Washington, DC: National Academy of Sciences.

Nelson, E. (1991). Anthropometry in the nutrition assessment of adults with ESRD. *Journal of Renal Nutrition, 1*, 162-172.

Norman, L.J., Macdonald, I.A., & Watson, A.R. (2004). Optimising nutrition in chronic renal insufficiency – Growth. *Pediatric Nephrology, 19*(11), 1245-1252.

Parekh, R.S., Flynn, J.T., Smoyer, W.E., Milne, J.L., Kershaw, D.B., Bunchman, T.E., et al. (2001). Improved growth in young children with severe chronic renal insufficiency who use specified nutritional therapy. *Journal of the American Society of Nephrology, 12*, 2418-2426.

Partnership for Food Safety Education. (2006). *Safe food handling.* Retrieved June 21, 2006, from http://www.fightbac.org/content/view/6/11

Pupim, L.B., Cuppari, L., & Ikizler, T.A. (2006) Nutrition and metabolism in kidney disease. *Seminars in Nephrology, 26*(2), 134-157.

Rodriquex, D., & Lewis, S.L. (1997). Nutritional management of patients with acute renal failure. *Nephrology Nursing Journal, 24*, 232-241.

Savica, V., Santoro, D., Ciolino, F., Mallamace, A., Calvani, M., Savica, R., et al. (2005). Nutritional therapy in chronic kidney disease. *Nutrition in Clinical Care, 8*(2), 70-76.

Schulman, G. (2003). Nutrition in daily hemodialysis. American *Journal of Kidney Disease, 41*(3 Suppl 1), 2112-2115.

Schulman, G. (2004). The dose of dialysis in hemodialysis: impact on nutrition. *Seminars in Dialysis, 17*(6), 479-488.

Seidel, H.M., Ball, J.W., Dains, J.E., & Benedict, G.W. (1999). *Mosby's guide to physical assessment* (4th ed.). St. Louis: Mosby.

Shemin, D. (2003). Dialysis in pregnant women with chronic kidney disease. *Seminars in Dialysis, 16*(5), 379-383.

Teplan, V., Schuck, O., Stollova, M., & Vitko, S. (2003). Obesity and hyperhomocysteinaemia after kidney transplatation. *Nephrology Dialysis Transplantation, 18* (Suppl 5), 71-73.

Tzamaloukas, A.H., & Friedman, E.A. (2001). Diabetes. In J.T. Daugirdas, P.G. Blake, & T.S. Ing (Eds.), *Handbook of dialysis* (3rd ed.). Philadelphia: Lippincott Williams & Wilkins.

U.K. Prospective Diabetes Study Group. (1998). Intensive blood-glucose control with sulphonylureas or insulin complared with conventional treatment and risk of complications in patients with type 2 diabetes (UKPDS 33). *Lancet, 352*, 854-865.

U.S. Renal Data Systems (USRDS). (2006). *USRDS 2005 annual data report.* Bethesda, MD: The National Institutes of Health, National Institute of Diabetes and Digestive and Kidney Diseases.

Vidal, M.L., Ursu, M., Martinez, A., Roland, S.S., Wibmer, E., Pereira, D., et al. (1998). Nutritional control of pregnant women on chronic hemodialysis. *Journal of Renal Nutrition, 8*(3), 150-156.

Wiggins, K.L. (2002). Nutrition care of adult pregnant ESRD patients. In *Nutrition care of renal patients* (3rd ed., p. 105). Chicago: American Dietetic Association.

Wood, S. (1998). Practical procedures for nurses: Nutrition assessment. *Nursing Times, 94* (9), 1-2.

Yeun, J.Y., & Kaysen, G.A. (1998). Factors influencing serum albumin in dialysis patients. *American Journal of Kidney Diseases, 32*(6), S118-S1125.

Suggested Readings

Burrowes, J.D., & Van Houten, G. (2006). Herbs and dietary supplement use in patients with stage 5 chronic kidney disease. *Nephrology Nursing Journal, 33*(1), 85-88.

Charney, P. (2004). Enteral nutrition in kidney disease. In L. Byham-Gray & K. Wiesen (Eds.), *A clinical guide to nutrition care in kidney disease* (pp. 151-158). Chicago: American Dietetic Association.

Kopple, J.D., & Massry, S.G. (2003). *Kopple and Massry's nutritional management of renal disease.* Baltimore: Lippincott Williams & Wilkins.

Section 9

Pharmacologic Aspects of Chronic Kidney Disease

Editor

Elizabeth Cincotta, PharmD, BCPS

Authors

Kristine S. Schonder, PharmD

Elizabeth Cincotta, PharmD, BCPS

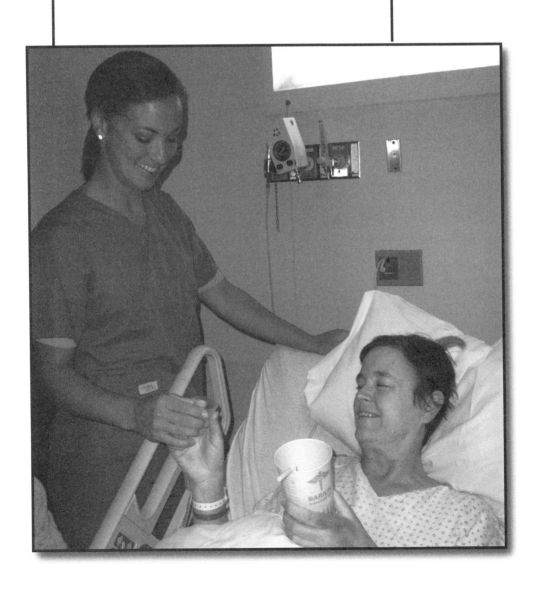

About the Authors

Kristine S. Schonder, PharmD, Section Editor and Author, is an Assistant Professor at the University of Pittsburgh School of Pharmacy in Pittsburgh, Pennsylvania.

Elizabeth Cincotta, PharmD, BCPS, is a Clinical Pharmacy Specialist in Nephrology and Solid Organ Transplant at Harper University Hospital/Detroit Medical Center in Detroit, Michigan.

Acknowledgment

Thanks to Charold L. Baer, PhD, RN, FCCM, CCRN, previous author of this material in the fourth edition of the *Core Curriculum*.

Section 9

Pharmacologic Aspects of Chronic Kidney Disease

Section

9

Pharmacologic Aspects of Chronic Kidney Disease

Purpose

The purpose of this section is to assist the clinician in meeting the challenges involved in the pharmacologic management of patients with chronic kidney disease (CKD). To provide such assistance, the following topics are included:

1. Drug characteristics including pharmacokinetics, pharmacodynamics, and pharmacotherapeutics.
2. The effects of patient adherence on drug therapy.
3. The effects of CKD on drug therapy.
4. Classifications of drugs commonly used with patients with CKD, including the purpose, an example, and major caveats.
5. The impact of dialysis on drug therapy.
6. The clinical significance for nursing, including monitoring and administering medications, educating the patient, and fostering adherence.

Objectives

Upon completion of this section, the learner will be able to:

1. Define the four processes involved in pharmacokinetics.
2. Identify the effects of the following factors on the rate of absorption: the physicochemical properties of the drug, the concentration of the drug, the dosage form, the route of administration, the perfusion rate at the site of absorption, and the surface area of the absorption site.
3. Identify the effects of the following factors on the distribution of a drug: protein binding, tissue binding, lipid solubility, polarity, the capillary permeability of various organs, the volume of body water, perfusion rates, and redistribution.
4. Identify seven influencing factors on the metabolism of a drug.
5. List the six body systems involved in excreting drugs.
6. Define the following as they relate to the pharmacokinetics of a drug: half-life, and steady state, protein binding and time course of action.
7. Define the following in terms of their influence on the pharmacodynamics of a drug: drug effects, mechanisms of action, and the dose-response.
8. Define the concepts of therapeutic index and drug interactions in relation to a drug.
9. Identify the effects of patient adherence on normal drug activity.
10. Describe the pharmacokinetic and pharmacodynamic changes that occur as a result of CKD.
11. Describe the effects of CKD on the drug characteristics and patient adherence in the process of normal drug activity.
12. List the purpose, at least one example, the major caveats or relevant facts, and the clinical significance of CKD related to the following classifications of drugs used to treat patients with CKD: analgesics, antacids (systemic),

Objectives, continued

antianemics, antidiarrheals, antiemetics, antihyperlipidemics, antihypertensives, antimicrobials,cardiotonics, cation-exchange resins, diuretics, glucocorticoids, heavy metal chelating agents, histamine H_1 and H_2 receptor antagonists, mineralocorticoids, phosphate binders, prokinetic agents, proton pump inhibitors, sedative-hypnotics, stool softeners, cathartics, and vitamins..
13. Define the concept of dialyzability in relation to drugs.
14. List six factors that determine the effect of dialysis on the half-life, or concentration, of a drug.
15. Describe the approach to determining dosing adjustments for patients with CKD.

Introduction

The urinary system, which includes the kidneys, ureters, bladder, and urethra, is the major excretory system for most drugs and their metabolites. It also regulates the internal environment of the body in which all other drug-related processes occur. Thus, normal kidney function is an important prerequisite for normal drug activity. When the urinary system is dysfunctional, major alterations occur in the processes associated with drug activity and the individual is confronted with three major problems.
1. A need for prolonged therapeutic drug intervention to cope with the systemic effects of CKD.
2. A more variable therapeutic response to the drug.
3. An increased potential for the drug to reach toxic levels due to retention and accumulation.

Chapter 42

Interactions between Drugs and the Body

The interactions between drugs and the body are described by two terms. *Pharmacokinetics* refers to the way the body handles the drug. *Pharmacodynamics* refers to the effects of the drug on the body.

I. **Pharmacokinetics is the study of drug absorption, distribution, metabolism, and excretion.** The pharmacokinetics of a drug will determine its plasma concentration levels at any given time. Other important concepts related to pharmacokinetics include bioavailablity, half-life, and steady state.

A. Absorption.
1. Definition. Absorption is the process by which drugs pass from the skin, lungs, or GI tract into in the systemic circulation.
2. Influencing factors. The rate of absorption is influenced by the factors listed below.
a. The physicochemical properties of the drug.
b. The concentration of the drug.
c. The dosage form.
d. The route of administration.
e. The perfusion rate at the site of absorption. (Table 9.1 summarizes these factors, their specific properties, and their effect on the rate of absorption.)

Table 9.1

Factors Affecting the Rate of Absorption

Factor	Specific Properties	Effect on Absorption Rate
Physicochemical properties	Molecular size 　Large 　Small Degree of ionization 　Ionized 　Nonionized Lipid solubility 　High 　Low	 Decreased Increased Decreased Increased Increased Decreased
Concentration	High Low	Increased Decreased
Dosage form	Liquid 　Aqueous solution 　Oily solution 　Suspension Solid	 Increased Increased over solid forms Increased over some solid forms Decreased in comparison to many 　liquids
Route of administration	Intravenous Intramuscular Subcutaneous Pulmonary (gases, vapors, and 　aerosols) Oral Sublingual/buccal Rectal Topical 　Mucous membranes 　Skin	Circumvented – may have 　immediate effects Rapid Rapid from aqueous solutions Rapid Variable – drug dependent Rapid Variable and often incomplete Semi-rapid Slow
Perfusion rate at absorption site	High flow rate Low flow rate	Increased Decreased
Surface area of absorption site	Large surface area Small surface area	Increased Decreased
pH at absorption site	Acidic pH Basic pH	Incresed for acidic compounds Decreased for acidic compounds
First-pass metabolism	High Low	Decreased Increased

3. Related term: bioavailability.
 a. Definition. Bioavailability is the extent or concentration of a drug that reaches the systemic circulation once it has been absorbed. The bioavailability relates the amount of drug that has been absorbed by a certain route of administration (e.g., oral, subcutaneous, intraperitoneal, etc.) to the intravenous route.

b. Clinical significance. The bioavailability is an important factor to determine the concentration of the drug at the site of action and the ultimate potential therapeutic or adverse effects. In addition to the factors that influence absorption of the drug, bioavailability is also influenced by the rate of absorption and first-pass metabolism, or the rate of hepatic extraction from the circulation for orally administered medications. For example, if a drug is 100% absorbed through the gastrointestinal tract, but then 75% is eliminated during first-pass metabolism, then the bioavailability is 0.25, or 25%.

B. Distribution.
 1. Definition. Distribution is the movement of an absorbed drug from the site of administration to other locations in the body. The distribution of a drug will continue until its concentration in the plasma and tissues reaches equilibrium.
 2. Influencing factors. The extent of distribution of a drug is dependent upon the factors listed below. Table 9.2 summarizes these factors, their specific properties, and their effects on drug distribution.
    a. Protein binding.
    b. Tissue binding.
    c. Lipid solubility.
    d. Polarity.
    e. The capillary permeability of various organs.
    f. The volume of body water.
    g. Perfusion rates.
    h. Redistribution.
 3. Related terms.
    a. Volume of distribution.
      (1) Definition. The volume of distribution is a term that relates the amount of drug distributed throughout the body to the amount of drug in the blood or intravascular space. It is an apparent volume that may exceed the physical amount of volume in a person.
      (2) Clinical significance. The volume of distribution is important to describe drug disposition and can give an indication of which compartment of the body (i.e., intravascular or extravascular) the drug has been distributed into. Drugs with a high volume of distribution generally have higher concentrations in the extravascular compartment. On the other hand, drugs with a volume of distribution similar to the volume of blood (i.e., 0.04

Table 9.2

Factors Affecting Drug Distribution

Factor	Specific Properties	Effect on Distribution
Protein binding	High percentage Low percentage	Decreased Increased
Tissue binding	High percentage Low percentage	Increased Decreased
Lipid solubility	High degree Low degree	Increased Decreased
Polarity	Polar Nonpolar	Decreased Increased
Capillary permeability	Increased Decreased	Increased Decreased
Volume of body water	Increased Decreased	Increased Decreased
Perfusion rates	Increased Decreased	Increased Decreased
Redistribution	Increased Decreased	Increased Decreased

l/kg of body weight) are found primarily in the intravascular compartment.
    b. Protein binding.
      (1) Definition. Drugs are often carried to the site of action by a carrier protein. Examples of carrier proteins.
        (a) Albumin.
        (b) Alpha1-acid glycoprotein.
        (c) Other blood cells, such as erythrocytes.
      (2) Clinical significance. Drugs that are bound to carrier proteins (protein-bound) are not active to exert the intended effect. The drug must be released from the protein (free drug) to exert its effect at the site of action. Only the free drug is considered to be active. Increases or decreases in plasma protein binding can have an effect on volume of distribution. As protein binding decreases, free drug increases and more drug is active and available to distribute throughout the body, resulting in an increase in volume

of distribution. The opposite is also true: as protein binding increases, there is less free drug to distribute and the volume of distribution is decreased. Dissolution from protein binding sites generally occurs passively, from areas of higher concentration to lower concentration.

(3) Principles of protein binding.

(a) Serum blood concentrations for many drugs are a measure of the total concentration of drug in the body, including free drug and protein-bound drug. These are often referred to as total serum concentration.

(b) The therapeutic effect of a drug that corresponds to a total serum blood concentration will vary depending on the amount of drug that is bound to protein. At the same total serum concentration, a drug that is bound to more protein in the bloodstream will have less effect than if more drug is in the free state.

(c) Metabolism and excretion are also dependent on protein binding. If more drug is bound to protein, less drug will be extracted by the liver for metabolism or by the kidney for excretion.

(d) A drug can be displaced from protein binding sites by other drugs with a greater affinity for the protein. This will increase the amount of free drug in the bloodstream and increase the therapeutic or adverse effects of the drug.

C. Metabolism.
1. Definition. Metabolism is the biochemical conversion of a drug to another chemical form via the processes of oxidation, reduction, hydrolysis, glucuronidation, or conjugation. Metabolism occurs primarily in the liver using the microsomal enzyme system, but it also takes place in the kidney, and to a lesser degree, in the lungs, plasma, and gastrointestinal tract. The result of metabolism is the production of drug metabolites that are usually more water soluble, less lipid soluble, more ionized at a normal pH, less protein bound, and less likely to be stored than the original drug. Drug metabolites are often excreted by the kidneys.
2. Influencing factors. The factors that influence the hepatic microsomal enzyme system include the following:
   a. The specific drugs.
   b. The maturational age of the person.
   c. The perfusion rate to the metabolic site.
   d. Nutritional state.
   e. System dysfunction (see Table 9.3).
   f. Environmental factors.
   g. Plasma protein binding.
3. The most important of these factors, however, is the individual drugs. The following specific relationships regarding these factors have been documented:
   a. Neonates have fewer metabolizing enzymes available and therefore are more sensitive to drugs.
   b. Starvation and diets deficient in ascorbic acid, calcium, or protein will impair the metabolic process.
   c. Hepatic disease, damage, or failure impedes metabolism.
   d. The elderly have decreased functioning hepatocytes.
   e. Exogenous chemicals produced by certain drugs and food constituents can alter the activity of the drug-metabolizing enzymes.

D. Excretion.
1. Definition. Excretion is the process of eliminating drugs from the body in either their unaltered states or as metabolites. The urinary system performs its excretory function through the processes of glomerular filtration, tubular secretion, and tubular reabsorption.
2. Influencing factors. The amount of drug that is filtered by the glomerulus and enters the tubular system is dependent upon the concentration of the drug, its degree of plasma protein binding, perfusion rates, and the glomerular filtration rate. The renal clearance of a drug is determined by dividing the amount of the drug that is excreted over time by the plasma concentration of the drug.
3. Other systems involved in excreting drugs and their metabolites include the biliary, intestinal, pulmonary, integumentary, and glandular secretory systems. Of these other systems, the biliary system is the most significant. The biliary system excretes drug metabolites into the intestines via bile.

E. Clearance.
1. Definition. Clearance, also referred to as elimination, is the removal of active drug from the

Table 9.3

A Summary of the Effects of Dysfunctional Organ Systems on Pharmacokinetics

Dysfunctional Organ/System	Absorption	Distribution	Metabolism	Excretion
Kidneys	• Minimal effect • Some decrease due to delayed gastric emptying	• Increased due to hypoalbuminemia and uremic competition for existing protein binding sites • Increased due to fluid volume expansion	• Normal or increased oxidation • Decreased reduction • Decreased hydrolysis • Normal or decreased synthesis	• Decreased and accompanied by prolonged half-lives for those drugs that are primarily excreted by the kidney
Liver	• Minimal effect	• Increased due to hypoalbuminemia • Increased due to fluid volume expansion and ascites	• Decreased due to impaired function of the microsomal drug metabolizing enzyme system	• Decreased due to decreased hepatic blood flow
Cardiovascular	• Decreased for some drugs for undocumented reasons	• Increased due to decreased protein binding resulting from hypoalbuminemia and the production of endogenous binding inhibitors • Increased due to fluid volume expansion	• Decreased due to decreased cardiac output and resulting decreases in hepatic and renal perfusion	• Decreased due to decreased cardiac output and resulting decreases in renal and hepatic perfusion
Gastrointestinal	• Decreased in episodes of hypermotility • Increased in episodes of hypomotility • Decreased due to decreased GI perfusion • Variable depending upon changes in gastric pH and bacterial flora • Decreased due to delayed gastric emptying • Decreased in jejunal disease due to decreased folic acid absorption • Decreased in ileal disease due to the impaired transport of bile salts	• No documented effect	• No documented effect	• No documented effect
Pulmonary	• Decreased due to decreased gastrointestinal blood flow resulting from pulmonary redistribution • Decreased due to tissue hypoxia, altered blood pH, and decreased tissue perfusion	• Minimal effect	• Minimal effect	• Increased for some drugs but no rationale is documented
Thyroid	• Decreased in hyperthyroidism due to increased gastric motility • Increased in hypothyroidism due to decreased gastric motility	• No documented effect	• Increased in hyperthyroidism due to increased hepatic microsomal drug metabolizing enzyme activity • Decreased in hypothyroidism due to decreased hepatic microsomal enzyme activity	• Increased in hyperthyroidism due to increased renal perfusion • Decreased in hypothyroidism due to decreased renal perfusion

bloodstream. Clearance involves one or two processes: metabolism and/or excretion. Metabolism transforms the active drug into a metabolite, which may be active or inactive. Excretion involves the removal of the active drug directly from the bloodstream, usually by the kidney.
2. Clinical significance. The clearance of a drug is critical in determining the duration of effect of a drug. The clearance is also used to determine the half-life of a drug.

F. Half-life.
1. Definition. The half-life is the amount of time that it takes the body to decrease the concentration of the drug in the blood by one-half. As time continues to elapse in increments equal to the half-life of the drug, exponential elimination of the drug will also continue.
2. Clinical significance. The half-life of a drug is a crucial element in determining the appropriate dosing intervals necessary for a drug to maintain therapeutic concentration levels in the body. Establishing time intervals for repeated dosages of a drug that are shorter than the amount of time required for elimination of the drug (approximately five half-lives) will result in accumulation of the drug. Such accumulation could lead to toxicity or significant adverse effects for the patient.

G. Steady state.
1. Definition. When a drug is administered repeatedly at a constant dosage and interval, it accumulates and the concentration in the blood reaches a plateau. The level of the concentration plateau is a function of the actual drug dosage and the dosage intervals. The time that is required for the concentration to reach the plateau is directly dependent upon the half-life of the drug. Once a plateau is reached, it will be maintained as long as the dosage and frequency of administration remain constant. Fluctuations in concentration will occur during the interim periods between dosage administrations; however, these fluctuations occur around the plateau mean at identical intervals. Once steady state is achieved, the rate of drug going into the body equals the rate of drug being cleared from the body.
2. Clinical significance. The steady state concept, or plateau principle, of a drug suggests the importance of maintaining constant dosages and dosage intervals in achieving the specific,

predictable pharmacologic action of a drug.
3. Principles of steady state.
a. A loading dose is a bolus dose that can be administered to reach the concentration plateau corresponding to the steady state of the drug faster. A maintenance dose is then administered to maintain the steady state concentration.
b. Often loading doses are administered intravenously, but can also be administered as a larger dose via other routes of administration.
c. If a loading dose is not administered, the time to reach steady state is generally equal to 4 to 5 half-lives of most drugs.

H. Time course of action.
1. Regardless of which route of administration is used to give a patient a drug, certain amounts of time must elapse as the drug is processed by the body. As depicted in Figure 9.1, there are five significant time designations in the time course of action of a drug:
a. Time of administration.
b. Time the threshold for action is reached.
c. Time of peak action.
d. Time at which a minimal clinical response ceases to be elicited.
e. Time of elimination of a drug.
2. Onset of action is the time that elapses between the time of administration and time to reach the threshold of action.

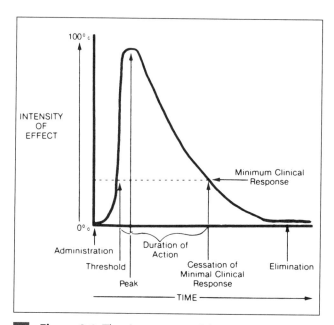

Figure 9.1. The time course of drug action.

3. Peak effect is length of time between drug administration and the time of maximal effect.
4. Duration of drug action is the time that elapses between administration and the time at which a minimal clinical response is elicited.
5. All of these time designations are specific for each drug and each individual and are dependent upon the pharmacokinetics of the drug.

II. Pharmacodynamics is the study of how a drug acts on the body. It refers to the biochemical effects and mechanisms of action of a drug in relation to specific dosages. The specific aspects of the drug that are important to pharmacodynamics are the effects, mechanisms of action, dosage-response curve of the drug, and therapeutic index.

A. Drug effects.
   1. Definition. Drug effects are those events that occur subsequent to the action of a drug. The action of a drug is the initial result of the interaction between a drug and a cell. During the interaction of a drug and a cell, cell function alters and begins a series of biochemical and physiologic changes that are characteristic of the drug. The initial result is the action of the drug, and all subsequent events constitute the effect of the drug.
   2. Example. The action of heparin is that it binds to a protein in the blood and inactivates clotting factors, while its effect is that it alters coagulation.

B. Mechanisms of action.
   1. Sites of action. In general, drugs act at one of three different sites within the body.
      a. Extracellularly.
      b. At the cellular membrane.
      c. Intracellularly.
   2. Mechanisms of action. Drugs act in one of three different ways.
      a. Altering the chemical properties of a body fluid. Examples of drugs that act by altering the chemical properties of body fluids include antacids, such as sodium bicarbonate, and acidifying agents, such as ammonium chloride.
      b. Nonspecifically interacting with cell membranes. General anesthetics, cathartics such as magnesium sulfate, and germicides, such as detergents, alcohol, hydrogen peroxide, and phenol derivatives are examples of drugs that interact nonspecifically with the cell membrane.

c. Selectively and specifically interacting with receptors.
   (1) Examples of drugs that interact via receptors encompass almost all of the other categories of pharmacologic agents.
   (2) The receptor theory.
      (a) Definition. The receptor theory of drug action implies that most drugs act in the body by associating with specific molecules on cells. The concepts of selectivity and specificity refer to the ability of a drug to act at these sites, or receptors, and produce a pharmacologic effect, while its presence at other sites produces no pharmacologic response. Selectivity and specificity are direct results of receptor activity, or the ability to recognize, bind, and interact with a drug to produce an effect. The chemical structure of the drug determines whether or not the drug can bind to a specific receptor. The traditional analogy used to describe the receptor theory is the lock and key fit. In other words, drugs with specific chemical structures can bind only to receptors with complementary or accepting structures.
      (b) Significance. Receptors are important in normal drug activity because they:
         [1] Determine the selectivity of drug action.
         [2] Determine the quantitative relationships between drug dosage or concentration and the pharmacologic effects.
         [3] Mediate the actions of pharmacologic antagonists, or those substances that bind to receptor sites and thus negate the binding of other drugs of similar chemical structure at that site.

C. Dose-response curve. The dose-response curve of a drug graphically displays the observed patient responses to a drug in terms of the drug doses required to elicit those responses. A dose-response curve illustrates the threshold and maximal efficacy levels of a drug. Figure 9.2 presents an example of a generic dose-response curve.

D. Therapeutic index. The therapeutic index of a drug is an approximate quantification of its

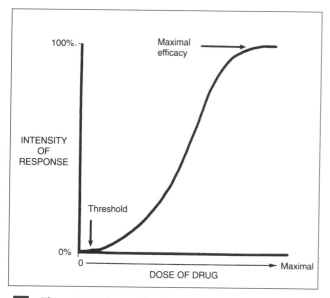

Figure 9.2. A generic dose-response curve.

relative safety as a clinical agent. It relates the minimum effective dose to the maximum tolerated dose.
1. The therapeutic index of a drug is expressed as a ratio of the median toxic or lethal dose to the median therapeutic dose.
2. As the therapeutic index of a drug becomes higher (expressed by increasingly wide ratios), the relative safety of the drug increases.
3. As the therapeutic index of a drug narrows, the margin of safety becomes smaller, and the chances of toxicity or other adverse reactions increase.

4. Because no drug produces only a single effect, a drug may have more than one therapeutic index.
5. Therapeutic indexes are computed for every desired effect of a drug.

E. Drug interactions.
1. Previously, concurrently, or subsequently administered drugs can modify the effects of another drug, often by altering the pharmacokinetics or pharmacodynamics of the drug.
2. Such drug interactions may enhance or detract from the original therapeutic intent of the drug.

III. **Patient adherence with a prescribed health care regimen is a primary component that directly influences drug activity.** Current research suggests that 30–50% of all patients are not adherent with their medication regimens. Seven of the most frequently cited reasons for not adhering to medication regimens are listed below.

A. Personal dissatisfaction with the regimen.
B. Noticeable improvement without having taken any medications.
C. Feeling better after completing only part of the drug regimen.
D. Forgetfulness in taking the medication.
E. Discontinued use of medications because of fear of side effects.
F. Lack of confidence that the medication will treat the condition.
G. Cost of the medication.

Chapter 43

Effects of Chronic Kidney Disease on Drug Activity

Chronic kidney disease (CKD) emphatically alters the pharmacokinetics and pharmacodynamics of drugs. The clinical significance of such alterations is that the patient is more vulnerable to the actions of pharmacologic agents and more likely to develop adverse reactions. In many instances, toxicity becomes the most common adverse reaction experienced by the patient with CKD.

I. **Pharmacokinetics.** The influence of CKD on the pharmacokinetics of drug activity is most obvious in the distribution and excretion processes.

However, absorption and metabolism are also somewhat altered by this pathophysiologic state.

A. Absorption. Existing information regarding the influence of CKD on absorption is minimal. In most cases, the primary effect discussed is related to mechanisms that delay gastric emptying. These mechanisms, however, are more a function of the pharmacologic agents used to treat the effects of CKD rather than a manifestation of renal impairment.

1. Factors affecting absorption.
   a. Increased gastric pH.
      (1) Urea in saliva increases gastric ammonia production.
      (2) Antacids.
   b. Altered GI transit time.
      (1) Diarrhea.
      (2) Vomiting.
      (3) Diabetic gastroparesis.
   c. Multiple medications and potential drug-drug interactions.
   d. Alterations in first-pass metabolism can vary.

B. Distribution. The effect of CKD on the distribution of a drug is primarily related to the increased fluid volume and decreased amount of protein binding that occurs in uremic patients.
   1. Alterations in fluid volume.
      a. Increased fluid volume increases the volume of distribution of water-soluble drugs because the drug distributes into the fluid, resulting in decreased plasma levels.
      b. Increased fluid volume increases the volume of distribution of protein-bound drugs because the proteins distribute into the fluid, resulting in decreased plasma levels.
      c. Dehydration and muscle wasting can decrease the volume of distribution, resulting in higher plasma levels.
      d. Hemodialysis will alter fluid status as fluid is removed.
   2. Alterations in protein binding.
      a. Decreased serum albumin.
         (1) Serum albumin levels may be decreased in CKD due to malnutrition or chronic disease.
         (2) Decreased albumin results in decreased protein binding for acidic drugs, increasing free drug concentrations.
      b. Uremia.
         (1) Uremia alters the structural orientation and decreases number of binding sites on plasma proteins, altering the binding affinity of drugs and results in higher free drug concentrations.
         (2) Endogenous substances accumulate in CKD and compete with binding sites on plasma proteins, increasing free drug concentrations.
      c. Increased alpha1-acid glycoprotein.
         (1) Serum levels of alpha1-acid glycoprotein are increased by hemodialysis and kidney transplantation.
         (2) Increased alpha1-acid glycoprotein results in increased protein binding for basic drugs, decreasing free drug concentrations.

C. Metabolism. The effects of CKD on nonrenal metabolism varies. These effects are specific for different drugs depending on whether the primary mechanism of metabolism is oxidation, reduction, hydrolysis, or synthesis. In general, CKD creates the following effects in those metabolic pathways.
   1. Oxidation is maintained at a normal or accelerated rate.
   2. Reduction is decreased.
   3. Hydrolysis is decreased.
   4. Hepatic microsomal enzyme system function may be decreased from accumulation of uremic toxins and oxidative stress.

D. Excretion. The extent to which CKD influences drug excretion is a function of the percent of drug that is cleared unchanged by the kidney and by the pharmacologic activity of its metabolites.
   1. Drugs that are dependent upon the kidneys for excretion will have a prolonged half-life in the presence of CKD.
   2. The half-life of a drug increases gradually as the creatinine clearance decreases until the creatinine clearance falls below approximately 30 mL per minute. From that point, the half-life increases rapidly as the creatinine clearance continues to decrease. Figure 9.3 illustrates this relationship.
   3. If the metabolites of a drug are also dependent upon the kidney for excretion, the effect of the CKD may be magnified. These metabolites may exhibit the desired effect of the parent drug (active metabolites) or they may exhibit toxic adverse reactions.

E. Time course of action, half-life, and steady state. The time course of action, half-life, and steady state of a drug will be altered by CKD.
   1. The time course of action of a drug may be delayed by CKD because of its effects on the pharmacokinetics of the drug.
   2. The half-life of a drug may be prolonged by CKD.
   3. The steady state is reflective of the half-life and dosing schedule of a drug. In patients with CKD, the steady state may be higher, more rapidly attained, and of longer duration than it is in healthy individuals. Meticulous monitoring and altering drug dosage schedules accordingly

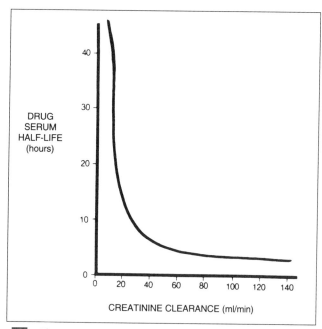

Figure 9.3. The relationship between drug half-life and creatinine clearance.

will assist in maintaining a steady state that more closely approximates the normal range for a given drug.

II. Pharmacodynamics.

A. The effects, mechanisms of action, and dose-response curve of a drug are all altered by CKD because of the impact on the pharmacokinetics of the drug.

B. To avoid toxic levels of drugs during repeated dosing in uremic patients, it may be necessary to:
1. Decrease the dose but maintain the normal dosage interval.
2. Maintain the dose but lengthen the dosage interval.
3. Decrease the dose and lengthen the dosage interval.

C. The decision to alter the dosing regimen by one of the above methods will depend upon the specific pharmacokinetics and pharmacodynamics of each drug.

D. It is important to note, however, that loading doses of medications are usually not altered in uremic patients because of the time required to reach therapeutic levels without them.

E. Therapeutic index. The effects of CKD on the therapeutic index of a drug are based on the interference of CKD with the pharmacokinetic parameters of the drug. Research indicates that CKD increases the frequency of adverse drug reactions in patients by about 2.5 times. There is an increased potential for more interactive drug effects because of the prolonged half-life of the various drugs. All of these factors functioning in concert create a significant threat for the patient with CKD who must rely on the therapeutic effects of many drugs to survive.

III. Patient adherence.

The systemic influences of CKD create a complex series of imbalances for patients that require several prolonged types of therapeutic interventions for effective management. As a consequence, the patient's life becomes restructured based on the interferences of externally imposed obligations. For example, not only is the patient required to take several types of medications at varying times throughout the day, but he or she must also ingest only the approved amounts and types of fluids and foods; adhere to a preset dialysis schedule either at home or in a specific facility; follow through with specifically established clinic appointments for continued monitoring; and assume responsibility for caring for surgically created vascular or abdominal access sites. Such activities require an inordinate amount of self-discipline and attention.

Chapter 44

Classifications of Drugs Frequently Used to Treat Patients with Chronic Kidney Disease

The systemic effects of CKD are so extensive that numerous pharmacologic agents are required to maintain the patient at an optimal level of well-being. Some of the more frequently prescribed medications are from the following classifications of drugs: analgesics, antacids, antianemics, antidiarrheals, antiemetics, antihyperlipidemics, antihypertensives, antimicrobials, cardiotonics, cation-exchange resins, diuretics, glucocorticoids, heavy metal chelating agents, histamine H_1 and H_2 receptor antagonists, mineralocorticoids, phosphate binders, prokinetic agents, proton pump inhibitors, sedative-hypnotics, stool softeners, cathartics, and vitamins.

I. Analgesics.

A. Purpose. Analgesics, both narcotic and nonnarcotic, are used to control pain in CKD patients when other types of interventions either do not work or are not appropriate.

B. Mechanism of action. Narcotic analgesics alter the perception of the painful experience, alter the pain threshold, or interfere with the conduction and response to pain in the central nervous system. Nonnarcotic analgesics decrease the sensitization of peripheral pain receptors and alter the response to pain by the central nervous system. Gabapentin and pregabalin have antinociceptive properties by inhibiting excitatory neurotransmitter release and are used specifically for neuropathic pain.

C. Examples.
1. Narcotic.
   a. Morphine.
   b. Codeine.
   c. Hydromorphone (Dilaudid®).
   c. Meperidine (Demerol®).
2. Nonnarcotic.
   a. Acetylsalicylic acid (aspirin).
   b. Acetaminophen (Tylenol®).
   c. Nonsteroidal antiinflammatory drugs (NSAIDs).
      (1) Ibuprofen (Advil®, Motrin®).
      (2) Indomethacini (Indocin®).
      (3) Naproxen (Aleve®, Naprosyn®).
      (4) Cyclooxygenase 2 (COX 2) inhibitors; celecoxib (Celebrex®).
   d. Miscellaneous.
      (1) Gabapentin (Neurontin®).
      (2) Pregabalin (Lyrica®).

D. Caveats and facts. Relevant facts related to administering analgesics to CKD patients.
1. All vital signs must be monitored before administration and after the peak effect has been reached.
2. The smallest effective doses for alleviating the pain should be administered.
3. Acetylsalicylic acid (aspirin) should be avoided in high doses in uremic patients because of the bleeding tendencies created by the effect of uremia on the platelets. However, low dosages (e.g., 81–325 mg/day) are often used for myocardial infarction prophylaxis.
4. Many narcotic analgesics are available in combination with nonnarcotic analgesics (e.g., hydrocodone/acetaminophen (Vicodin®, Norco®, Lortab®).
5. Meperidine metabolites can accumulate in patients with kidney insufficiency and may cause seizures. Use of this drug is not recommended in these patients.
6. Most narcotic analgesics require no dosage adjustments in patients with CKD and are not removed by dialysis. However, morphine and codeine have an active metabolite that is eliminated by the kidney and may accumulate in patients with kidney insufficiency. Repetitive doses should be avoided.
7. NSAIDs are used for both antiinflammatory and analgesic properties. The primary mechanism of action is the inhibition of prostaglandin synthesis. This action can compromise renal blood flow and result in CKD, particularly in individuals with preexisting extrarenal or renal disease that has already decreased renal perfusion. In addition, even though NSAIDs depend on hepatic biotransformation for their metabolism, they are excreted by the kidneys, so the potential for toxic effects when high doses are used is always present.

8. COX 2 inhibitors selectively inhibit COX 2, which is involved in the prostaglandin production at the site of inflammation, but not at other sites such as the GI tract. However, COX 2 inhibitors can also decrease renal blood flow, similar to the NSAIDs. Similar precautions should be taken in patients with CKD.
9. Gabapentin and pregabalin are primarily eliminated by the kidney and require dosage adjustment on patients with renal insufficiency.

II. Antacids (systemic).

A. Purpose. Systemic antacids are used in patients with CKD to assist in treating metabolic acidosis.

B. Mechanism of action. Oral systemic antacids neutralize gastric acid using exogenous bicarbonate. The excess amounts of bicarbonate are then absorbed into the extracellular fluid. Intravenous bicarbonate also neutralizes acids within the extrarenal fluid.

C. Examples.
1. Sodium bicarbonate.
2. Citrate and citric acid solutions (Shohl's solution, and Bicitra®).

D. Caveats and facts. The following are relevant facts to remember when administering antacids to patients with CKD.
1. Sodium bicarbonate can enhance fluid retention.
2. Oral antacids must be given 30 minutes to an hour after most other medications because the antacids delay absorption from the stomach.
3. Medications containing citrate must not be used with aluminum-containing agents because citrate significantly increases aluminum absorption. Aluminum accumulation can lead to encephalopathy and/or osteomalacia.

III. Antianemics.

A. Patients with CKD develop a normochromic, normocytic anemia due to the lack of erythropoietin production by the kidney. Anemia is a significant component of kidney disease that negatively affects the patient's quality of life. Thus, there has been much research conducted on all aspects of the anemia that accompanies CKD. The Anemia Work Group of the National Kidney Foundation's (NKF) Kidney Disease Outcomes Quality Initiative (KDOQI) Project developed Clinical Practice Guidelines to assist the clinician with the management of anemia associated with CKD.

B. Significant and general facts relevant to administering antianemics to patients with CKD.
1. Erythropoietin is a protein primarily produced by the kidney that is required to produce red blood cells. Normal erythropoiesis requires a complex interplay of erythropoietin in combination with various vitamins and minerals within erythroid tissues in the bone marrow to maintain red blood cell production.
2. Anemia can be the result of nutritional and metabolic disorders. These must be corrected before initiating antianemic therapy.
3. Iron and vitamin B deficiencies are common causes of anemia in patients with CKD. It is important to ensure adequate levels of iron and vitamin B when treating anemia associated with CKD.
4. As kidney function declines, the ability to produce erythropoietin also decreases, until adequate red cell production cannot be maintained.
5. The benefits of treating anemia include an increased sense of well being, more energy, increased appetite, normalization of cardiac output, regression of left ventricular hypertrophy and a general improvement in cognitive function.
6. The KDOQI Guidelines for Anemia in CKD recommend a target of hemoglobin 11–12 g/dL (dialysis and nondialysis patients).

C. Two basic categories of antianemic agents are used to treat anemia associated with CKD.
1. Erythropoiesis stimulating agents (ESAs).
2. Vitamins and minerals.
   a. Iron supplements.
   b. Vitamin B supplements.

D. Erythropoiesis-stimulating agents (ESAs).
1. Purpose. These agents replace the erythropoietin that is not being produced by the failing kidneys in sufficient quantity to maintain adequate red blood cell production.
2. Mechanism of action. Erythropoiesis-stimulating agents (ESAs) are glycoproteins that are biologically and immunologically similar to endogenous erythropoietin and function by acting on erythroid tissues within the bone marrow to stimulate differentiation of erythroid progenitor and early precursor cells.
3. Examples.
   a. Epoetin alfa (Epogen®, Procrit®).
   b. Darbepoetin alfa (Aranesp®).
4. Caveats and facts. Following are relevant facts

to remember when administering ESAs to patients with CKD:

a. Epoetin alfa is a recombinant human erythropoietin that is identical in structure and pharmacokinetics to endogenous erythropoietin.

b. Darbepoetin alfa is a novel erythropoietin stimulating protein. Two additional carbohydrate chains on the erythropoietin molecule result in a half-life that is two to three times longer than epoetin alfa.

c. Administration of ESAs can elevate blood pressure. Caution should be used when administering ESAs to patients with uncontrolled hypertension.

d. As the patient's hematocrit rises with ESA therapy, dialyzer clearance for substances such as creatinine, BUN, potassium, and phosphate may decrease, resulting in higher predialysis values for those substances. Thus, the adequacy of the patient's dialysis therapy should be assessed at least monthly and the prescription adjusted to meet the goal.

e. As the patient's appetite increases during ESA therapy, dietary intake also changes and may require alterations in diet or the dialysis prescription.

f. ESA therapy can result in increased activity levels, improved cognitive function, improved sexual function, and an overall perception of an increased quality of life for patients with CKD.

g. ESA therapy may also prevent possible long-term problems for the patient, including hypertensive cardiovascular disease, left ventricular hypertrophy, electrolyte abnormalities, and dialysis prescription adequacy.

E. Vitamin and minerals.
1. Iron supplements.
   a. Purpose. Iron is a necessary component in the erythropoiesis cascade of red blood cell production. Iron deficiency is a common cause of anemia in patients with CKD.
   b. Mechanism of action. Iron supplements replace iron stores to ensure adequate erythropoiesis. Iron deficiency results in a microcytic, hypochromic anemia. Iron is actively absorbed from all parts of the small intestine. After it is absorbed, it immediately combines with apotransferrin, a beta globulin, to form transferrin, which is transported in the plasma. The iron is loosely bound to the globulin and can easily be released to tissue

cells at any time. Excess iron is deposited in all tissue cells, but 60% of it is deposited in liver cells. In the liver, it combines with apoferritin to form ferritin, which is also called storage iron. When the iron level of the plasma decreases, iron is removed from ferritin and transported by transferrin to the sites where it is needed. Transferrin delivers iron to erythroblasts. Free iron that results from the destruction of RBCs is either stored as ferritin or reused to form additional hemoglobin.

   c. Examples.
      (1) Oral iron supplements.
         (a) Ferrous salts (ferrous sulfate, ferrous gluconate).
         (b) Polysaccharide iron complex (Niferex®).
      (2) Intravenous iron supplements.
         (a) Iron dextran (INFeD®, DexFerrum®).
         (b) Sodium ferric gluconate (Ferrlecit®).
         (c) Iron sucrose (Venofer®).
   d. Caveats and facts. Following are relevant facts to remember when administering iron supplements to patients with CKD.
      (1) Oral iron preparations are best absorbed in a fasting state.
      (2) Oral iron preparations can be given after meals to decrease gastric irritation and still provide adequate absorption.
      (3) Administering antacids or phosphate binders and iron preparations together significantly decreases iron absorption and bioavailability.
      (4) The excretion of iron preparations darkens the color of feces and may cause constipation.
      (5) The transferrin saturation (TSAT) is the ratio of the serum iron to the total iron binding capacity (TIBC). TIBC is the sum of the saturated and unsaturated transferrin. Transferrin saturation is calculated by the following formula: TSAT = (serum iron/TIBC) x 100. The normal value for TSAT is 20%–40%. TIBC can be calculated from the serum transferrin value by multiplying the serum transferrin value by 1.25. Transferrin can be calculated from the TIBC by multiplying the TIBC value by 0.7.
      (6) Iron stores must be adequate to support the bone marrow formation of new RBCs before initiating therapy with

ESAs and throughout their use. The KDOQI Clinical Practice Guidelines for Anemia in CKD recommend the TSAT to be at least 20%, and serum ferritin to be at least 200 ng/mL in hemodialysis patients and 100 ng/mL in peritoneal dialysis and nondialysis CKD patients.

(7) The preferred route of iron administration in hemodialysis patients is intravenous. Oral or intravenous iron may be used in peritoneal dialysis or nondialysis CKD patients.

(8) Intravenous iron preparations have been associated with hypersensitivity reactions. All patients receiving intravenous iron should be monitored closely. Iron dextran exhibits the highest risk, and a test dose must be administered prior to the dose.

(9) If the iron stores become depleted during therapy, replacement therapy should be initiated, and ESA therapy continued.

2. Vitamin B supplements.
   a. Purpose. Vitamin B is a necessary component in the erythropoiesis cascade of red blood cell production. Vitamin B deficiencies are often associated with distinct types of megaloblastic anemias.
   b. Mechanism of action. Vitamin B supplements replace lost or deficient stores in patients with CKD. Vitamin B is important in DNA synthesis and RBC proliferation.
   c. Examples.
      (1) Cyanocobalamin (vitamin B_{12}).
      (2) Folic acid (Folvite®).
      (3) Pyridoxine (vitamin B_6).
   d. Caveats and facts. Following are relevant facts to remember when administering vitamin B supplements to patients with CKD.
      (1) Vitamin B is removed by dialysis. Most dialysis patients are prescribed a vitamin containing cyanocobalamin, folic acid and pyridoxine to replace what is removed by dialysis.
      (2) Cyanocobalamin, folic acid, and pyridoxine must be present in sufficient quantities for a patient to respond appropriately to ESA therapy.

IV. Antidiarrheals.

A. Purpose. Antidiarrheals are used to treat persistent diarrhea resulting from intestinal irritation, medications, and other causative factors.

B. Mechanism of action. Loperamide and diphenoxylate are opioid derivatives. They act on the intestine through the opioid receptor inhibiting GI motility.

C. Examples.
   1. Loperamide (Immodium®).
   2. Diphenoxylate/atropine (Lomotil®).

D. Caveats and facts. Following are relevant facts to remember when administering antidiarrheals to patients with CKD.
   1. Both agents may cause drowsiness or dizziness.
   2. Diphenoxylate preparations contain atropine in order to discourage abuse. However, this may cause flushing, dry skin and mucous membranes, hyperthermia, tachycardia, and urinary retention.
   3. Diphenoxylate interacts with monoamine oxidase inhibitors and can precipitate a hypertensive crisis.

V. Antiemetics.

A. Purpose. Antiemetics are used to relieve persistent nausea and vomiting. Patients with CKD must be able to digest appropriate amounts of calories to maintain an anabolic state and not further enhance the uremic state due to catabolism. The use of these agents facilitates maintaining adequate nutrition.

B. Mechanism of action. The phenothiazines (prochlorperazine and promethazine) and butyrophenone (droperidol) antiemetic agents antagonize the D2 dopamine receptors in the chemoreceptor trigger zone (CTZ). The serotonin 5-HT3 receptor antagonists (ondansetron, dolasetron, and granisetron) antagonize the serotonin 5-HT3 receptors in the CTZ and possibly the periphery.

C. Examples.
   1. Phenothiazines.
      a. Prochlorperazine (Compazine®).
      b. Promethazine (Phenergan®).
   2. Droperidol (Inapsine®).
   3. Serotonin 5-HT3 receptor antagonists.
      a. Ondansetron (Zofran®).
      b. Dolasetron (Anzemet®).
      c. Granisetron (Kytril®).

D. Caveats and facts. Following are relevant facts to remember when administering antiemetics to patients with CKD.
   1. These agents depress the CNS and may cause drowsiness.

2. These agents have been reported to alter cardiac conduction and prolong QT interval.
3. The antiemetic effects of the phenothiazines increase with the dose; however, the side effects also increase with the dose. The more frequently observed side effects include hypotension, sedation, and extrapyramidal movement disorders. These side effects often limit the use of these agents.
4. Droperidol produces hypotension and sedation, and it also potentiates the action of other CNS depressants.
5. The effects of IV droperidol are usually noted within 3 to 10 minutes after administration, but peak effect is not seen for approximately 30 minutes.
6. Ondansetron, dolasetron, and granisetron require 30 to 60 minutes for peak effect and usually are well tolerated with only mild adverse effects, such as headache, constipation, and dizziness.

VI. Antilipemic agents.

A. Purpose. These agents are used to treat hyperlipidemia, which also decreases the incidence of atherosclerotic effects.

B. Significant general facts relevant to administering antilipemic agents to patients with CKD.
   1. Hyperlipidemia plays a significant role in the risk of cardiovascular disease in patients with CKD.
   2. Hyperlipidemia may be worse in patients with nephrotic syndrome.
   3. Most antilipemic agents are not removed by hemodialysis and do not require supplemental doses.

C. Five basic categories of antilipemic agents used to decrease cholesterol.
   1. Bile-sequestering agents.
   2. Fibric acid derivatives.
   3. Cholesterol synthesis inhibitors.
   4. Cholesterol absorption inhibitors.
   5. Nicotinic acid.

D. Bile-sequestering agents.
   1. Mechanism of action. These agents combine with the bile acids in the GI tract to form insoluble complexes. This decreases the bile acid level in the gallbladder and triggers the liver to synthesize more bile acids from their precursor, cholesterol. The overall effect is to decrease the serum cholesterol levels.

2. Examples.
   a. Cholestyramine (Questran®).
   b. Colestipol (Colestid®).
   c. Probucol (Lorelco®).
3. Caveats and facts. Following are relevant facts to remember when administering bile-sequestering agents to patients with CKD.
   a. Bile-sequestering agents bind to the drugs in the GI tract and decrease absorption. Thus, administration of these agents should be separated by at least 2 hours before or 4 hours after any other medications.
   b. The most common adverse effects associated with these agents are GI-related effects, including constipation, diarrhea, flatulence, abdominal pain, and bloating.

E. Fibric acid derivatives.
   1. Mechanism of action. These agents are thought to decrease cholesterol formation, mobilize cholesterol from the tissues, increase sterol excretion, decrease lipoprotein synthesis and secretion, and decrease triglyceride synthesis.
   2. Examples.
      a. Clofibrate (Atromid-S®).
      b. Gemfibrozil (Lopid®).
      c. Fenofibrate (Lofibra®, Tricor®).
   3. Caveats and facts. Following are relevant facts to remember when administering fibric acid derivatives to patients with CKD.
      a. These agents are useful in decreasing triglyceride levels.
      b. The most common adverse effect associated with fibric acid derivatives includes myopathies and rhabdomyolysis. Patients should be advised to contact their physician if they experience muscle pains.
      c. These agents can also increase liver enzymes. Liver function tests (LFTs) should be monitored routinely in patients receiving fibric acid derivatives.

F. Cholesterol synthesis inhibitors (HMG CoA reductase inhibitors).
   1. Mechanism of action. These agents inhibit the biochemical conversion of the precursor of cholesterol by inhibiting hydroxymethylglutaryl-coenzyme A (HMG CoA) reductase. This increases the expression of LDL receptors on the surface of various cells, which increases the clearance of LDL from the bloodstream, thus decreasing LDL concentrations.
   2. Examples.
      a. Atorvastatin (Lipitor®).
      b. Fluvastatin (Lescol®).

c. Lovastatin (Mevacor®).

d. Pravastatin (Pravachol®).

e. Rosuvastatin (Crestor®).

f. Simvastatin (Zocor®).

3. Caveats and facts. Following are relevant facts to remember when administering HMG CoA reductase inhibitors to patients with CKD.

a. These agents are commonly referred to as *statins*.

b. These agents are very useful in patients with CKD because they decrease cholesterol, triglycerides, and LDL cholesterol, and increase HDL cholesterol.

c. Side effects associated with these agents are myopathies and rhabdomyolysis. Patients should be advised to contact their physician if they experience muscle pains. Patients are especially at risk if taking with other drugs that inhibit the oxidative metabolism of these drugs.

d. These agents can also increase liver enzymes. LFTs should be monitored routinely in patients receiving HMG CoA reductase inhibitors.

G. Cholesterol absorption inhibitors.

1. Mechanism of action. These agents block the absorption of cholesterol from the intestines, reducing the uptake of cholesterol from the intestines into the liver. This decreases the amount of cholesterol stored in the liver and increases the clearance of cholesterol from the bloodstream.

2. Example: ezetimibe (Zetia®).

3. Caveats and facts. Following are relevant facts to remember when administering ezetimibe to patients with CKD.

a. Because it has a unique mechanism of action, ezetimibe is a very useful addition to HMG CoA reductase inhibitors to lower cholesterol levels even further than either agent alone.

b. The most common side effects associated with ezetimibe are GI related, including abdominal pain and diarrhea.

H. Nicotinic acid (niacin).

1. Mechanims of action. This agent inhibits lipolysis in adipose tissue, decreases esterification of triglycerides in the liver, and increases lipoprotein lipase activity.

2. Examples: nicotinic acid (niacin, Niaspan®).

3. Caveats and facts. Following are relevant facts to remember when administering nicotinic acid to patients with CKD.

a. Nicotinic acid is useful to reduce cholesterol, triglyceride, and LDL cholesterol levels, and increase HDL cholesterol levels.

b. The most common side effect of nicotinic acid is flushing that results from vasodilation of peripheral blood vessels. Aspirin can be administered 30 minutes before nicotinic acid to reduce the incidence of flushing.

c. Nicotinic acid can increase liver enzymes. LFTs should be monitored routinely in patients receiving nicotinic acid.

VII. Antihypertensives.

A. Hypertension is a major problem for most patients with CKD, and management of hypertension often requires the use of two or more concurrently administered antihypertensive agents.

B. Significant general facts relevant to administering antihypertensives to patients with CKD.

1. The blood pressure should be monitored before each administration and at the time of the peak effect of the dose of the drug.

2. The patient must be instructed about the possibilities of developing postural hypotension.

3. Alterations in dosages must be made in gradual increments or decrements.

4. Consistency in dosage amounts and intervals must be maintained whenever possible.

5. Most antihypertensive agents are not removed by dialysis. Decreases in blood pressure may occur during dialysis as fluid is removed. Therefore, consideration must be given to the appropriate time for administration on dialysis days. Many nephrology providers recommend evening administration for long acting medications and holding or decreasing the predialysis dose for short-acting medications.

C. Three basic categories of antihypertensive agents that directly decrease blood pressure.

1. Sympatholytics. There are four subcategories of sympatholytics that are used in patients with CKD.

a. Central acting agents.

b. Beta adrenergic agents.

c. Alpha-1 adrenergic blockers.

d. Mixed adrenergic blockers.

2. Vasodilators. There are two subcategories of vasodilators.

a. Direct.

b. Calcium channel blockers.

3. Renin-angiotensin-aldosterone system antagonists.

a. Angiotensin-converting enzyme (ACE) inhibitors.
b. Angiotensin II receptor blockers (ARBs).

D. Sympatholytics.
  1. Central acting agents.
    a. Mechanism of action. These agents decrease blood pressure by reducing sympathetic activity and subsequently decreasing arteriolar vasoconstriction. Clonidine stimulates inhibitory alpha-2 adrenergic receptors in the medulla to decrease sympathetic tone, peripheral resistance, heart rate, and cardiac output. Methyldopa forms a false neurotransmitter that stimulates the alpha adrenergic receptors and decreases sympathetic tone and renal vascular resistance; it may increase overall plasma volume. Both drugs decrease plasma renin activity.
    b. Examples.
      (1) Clonidine (Catapres®).
      (2) Methyldopa (Aldomet®).
    c. Caveats and facts. Following are relevant facts to remember when administering central-acting agents to patients with CKD.
      (1) Both drugs frequently produce a dry mouth, drowsiness, and sedation.
      (2) Impotency may result.
      (3) Both agents produce less orthostatic hypotension than the peripherally-acting agents.
      (4) Sudden withdrawal of these agents may result in a rebound hypertension.
  2. Beta adrenergic blockers.
    a. Mechanism of action. These drugs decrease blood pressure by competing with norepinephrine for beta receptor sites, antagonizing the membrane effect of norepinephrine and epinephrine and blocking sympathetic stimulation. Their pharmacologic effects produce the following: decreased heart rate and cardiac output; prolonged, decreased velocity of mechanical systole; inhibition of renin secretion; decreased sympathetic outflow from vasomotor centers in the brain; and gradual decreases in blood pressure. Because of the pharmacologic effects, they are also used to treat patients after an MI and those with chronic heart failure. In addition, they are useful in managing digitalis or catecholamine-induced dysrhythmias. In higher doses, they exert an anesthetic-like membrane effect that alters cardiac action potentials and depresses myocardial function. All

of these agents decrease cardiac output and heart rate and all, except pindolol, decrease plasma renin activity. Atenolol and propranolol also decrease renal blood flow and GFR, while metoprolol and pindolol decrease peripheral resistance.
    b. Examples.
      (1) B1 selective.
        (a) Atenolol (Tenormin®).
        (b) Metoprolol (Lopressor®).
      (2) B1 + B2 nonselective.
        (a) Nadolol (Corgard®).
        (b) Pindolol (Visken®).
        (c) Propranolol (Inderal®).
        (d) Timolol (Blocadren®).
    c. Caveats and facts. Following are relevant facts to remember when administering beta adrenergic blockers to patients with CKD.
      (1) All of these agents can produce sedation, bradycardia, hypotension, and heart failure.
      (2) All of these agents can mask the signs and symptoms of hypoglycemia in patients with diabetes.
      (3) All of these agents can precipitate or worsen depression.
      (4) All of these agents must have their dosages tapered before discontinuation to avoid rebound hypertension.
      (5) All require frequent monitoring of the apical pulse and blood pressure.
      (6) All have the potential of producing fluid retention and overload, particularly when sodium is not restricted.
      (7) All potentiate the hypoglycemic action of insulin.
      (8) Most require no dosage adjustment in patients with CKD.
      (9) Most are not removed by hemodialysis.
  3. Alpha-1 adrenergic blockers.
    a. Mechanism of action. These drugs decrease blood pressure by occupying the alpha-1 receptors of the sympathetic nervous system and blocking the effects of epinephrine and norepinephrine at those sites. The result is vasodilation due to relaxed smooth muscle, decreased peripheral resistance, and decreased plasma renin activity.
    b. Examples.
      (1) Prazosin (Minipres®).
      (2) Terazosin (Hytrin®).
      (3) Doxazosin (Cardura®).
    c. Caveats and facts. Following are relevant facts to remember when administering alpha-1

adrenergic blockers to patients with CKD.
   (1) All of these agents produce significant orthostatic hypotension and first-dose syncope.
   (2) They improve maximal urine flow in males with BPH.
   (3) They may maintain or improve sexual function in males.
4. Mixed alpha and beta adrenergic blockers.
   a. Mechanism of action. These agents decrease blood pressure by blocking alpha and beta adrenergic receptors. As a result, they decrease peripheral resistance, plasma renin levels, aldosterone levels, renal vascular resistance, and cardiac output. They also may increase plasma volume, renal blood flow, and GFR.
   b. Examples.
      (1) Labetalol (Normodyne®, Trandate®).
      (2) Carvedilol (Coreg®).
   c. Caveats and facts. The use of mixed alpha and beta adrenergic blockers can result in the following adverse effects in patients.
      (1) Bronchospasms.
      (2) Masking the signs and symptoms of hypoglycemia in patients with diabetes.
      (3) Significant orthostatic hypotension.

E. Vasodilators.
   1. Direct.
      a. Mechanism of action. These drugs decrease blood pressure by relaxing arteriolar smooth muscle and producing vasodilation. Hydralazine and minoxidil also alter cellular calcium metabolism and inhibit calcium movement within the vascular smooth muscle. All of these agents decrease peripheral resistance and increase plasma volume, plasma renin activity, and heart rate. They all increase cardiac output. In addition, hydralazine and diazoxide also increase renal blood flow and GFR.
      b. Examples.
         (1) Diazoxide (Hyperstat®).
         (2) Hydralazine (Apresoline®).
         (3) Minoxidil (Loniten®).
         (4) Nitroprusside (Nipride®).
      c. Caveats and facts. Following are relevant facts to remember when administering vasodilators to patients with CKD.
         (1) All of these agents may produce a reflex tachycardia, palpitations, S3 or S4 gallop, angina, peripheral edema, and headaches.
         (2) Sympathetic blocking agents are often given concurrently with these drugs to

decrease the reflex sympathetic stimulation due to baroreceptor response.
         (3) Diazoxide increases sodium and water retention, leads to hyperuricemia, and results in hyperglycemia.
         (4) Minoxidil may cause fluid retention and hypertrichosis as seen by thickening, elongation, and hyperpigmentation of fine body hair. The presence of excessive hair, particularly facial, may limit its use with women.
         (5) Diazoxide and nitroprusside are available only in intravenous form.
   2. Calcium channel blockers.
      a. Mechanism of action. These agents decrease blood pressure by preventing the entry of calcium into the cell and decreasing the contraction of vascular smooth muscle. They also decrease peripheral vascular resistance and myocardial contractility; increase cardiac output, coronary artery dilation, and myocardial perfusion; and inhibit renin activity. There are three categories of calcium channel blockers: phenylalkylamines, benzothiazepines, and dihydropyridines. The three categories are all similar in that they act on the slow calcium channel; however, they have different degrees of selectivity in their effects on vascular smooth muscle, myocardium, or specialized conduction and pacemaker tissues. The phenylalkylamines slow AV conduction and prolong the effective refractory period within the AV node, thus decreasing ventricular response secondary to atrial flutter or atrial fibrillation. They also can restore normal sinus rhythm in supraventricular tachycardia and can induce sinus arrest in patients with sick sinus syndrome. Overall, they depress the amplitude and velocity of depolarization and conduction in depressed atrial fibers and decrease myocardial contractility and peripheral vascular resistance. The benzothiazepines decrease SA and AV conduction, heart rate, myocardial contractility, and peripheral vascular resistance, and slightly increase cardiac output. They dihydropyridines exert their maximum effect on decreasing peripheral resistance. However, some of them also increase cardiac output and heart rate. Short-acting dihydropyridines produce significant vascular side effects, blood pressure swings, and concurrent increases in adrenergic responses such that they are not frequently used in treating hypertension in patients with

CKD. It has also been suggested that the short-acting agents not be used in high doses to treat hypertension in general.

  b. Examples.

(1) Phenylalkylamine: verapamil (Isoptin®, Calan®).

(2) Benzothiazepine: diltiazem (Cardizem®).

(3) Dihydropyridines.

(a) Amlodipine (Norvasc®).

(b) Felodipine (Plendil®).

(c) Isradipine (DynaCirc®).

(d) Nicardipine (Cardene®).

(e) Nifedipine (Procardia XL®, Adalat CC®).

(f) Nisoldipine (Sular®).

  c. Caveats and facts. Following are relevant facts to remember when administering calcium channel blockers to patients with CKD.

(1) Most of these drugs produce bradycardia, hypotension, headache, constipation, and edema.

(2) Nondihydropyridines, such as verapamil and diltiazem, have some negative cardiac inotropic effects and must be used with caution in patients who have left ventricular dysfunction.

(3) Nondihydropyridines have greater antiproteinuric effects than the dihydropyridines.

(4) Calcium channel blockers can inhibit platelet function.

(5) Long-acting dihydrophyridines are often used as first line agents in patients with angina because they may also decrease coronary vasospasm.

F. Renin-Angiotensin-Aldosterone system antagonists.

  1. Mechanism of action. These drugs decrease blood pressure by interrupting the renin-angiotensin-aldosterone system.

  a. Angiotensin converting enzyme (ACE) inhibitors. These agents block ACE, the enzyme that converts angiotensin I to angiotensin II. They also decrease sodium and water retention and peripheral resistance, and increase cardiac output and renal blood flow. They do not appear to significantly alter GFR in most individuals. However, they slow the progression of kidney disease in patients with proteinuria and decrease GFR in patients with renal artery stenosis.

  b. Angiotensin II receptor blockers (ARBs). These agents decrease blood pressure by blocking angiotensin II receptors on target tissues, thus relaxing smooth muscle and facilitating vasodilation. They also increase renal sodium and water excretion, decrease plasma volume, and decrease cellular hypertrophy.

  2. Examples.

  a. ACE inhibitors.

(1) Captopril (Capoten®).

(2) Benazepril (Lotensin®).

(3) Enalapril (Vasotec®).

(4) Fosinopril (Monopril®).

(5) Lisinopril (Prinivil®, Zestril®).

(6) Moexipril (Univasc®).

(7) Quinapril (Accupril®).

(8) Rampril (Altace®).

  b. ARBs.

(1) Candesartan (Atacand®).

(2) Irbesartan (Avapro®).

(3) Losartan (Cozaar®).

(4) Telmisartan (Micardis®).

(5) Valsartan (Diovan®).

  3. Caveats and facts. Following are relevant facts to remember when administering ACE inhibitors and ARBs to patients with CKD.

  a. Studies have shown that these agents can decrease protein excretion, which may be beneficial in slowing the progression of kidney disease.

  b. These agents are very useful in treating patients with diabetes because they slow the progression of diabetic glomerulopathy. They may also be useful in slowing the progression of glomerulosclerosis in patients with kidney dysfunction.

  c. These agents are useful for patients with left ventricular hypertrophy or ischemic heart disease with systolic dysfunction of the left ventricle.

  d. Adverse reactions that may accompany the use of ACE inhibitors include angioedema, proteinuria, agranulocytosis, significant orthostatic hypotension, hyperkalemia, impaired taste perception, and chronic cough.

  e. ARBs may produce less cough compared to ACE inhibitors.

  f. These agents may decrease kidney function, especially if renal artery stenosis is present, so frequent monitoring of BUN and serum creatinine levels are indicated.

  g. Many of the ACE inhibitors are removed by hemodialysis and the patient may require supplemental dosing after hemodialysis therapy.

h. The ARBs appear to need no dosage adjustments in patients with CKD, nor do they require supplemental dosing after hemodialysis.

VIII. Antimicrobials.

A. Purpose. CKD increases the susceptibility to infection. As a result, these patients frequently require antimicrobial agents to combat infections.

B. Mechanism of action. Most antimicrobial agents function in one of the following ways:
1. Inhibiting bacterial cell wall synthesis.
2. Altering the permeability of the cell membrane.
3. Altering nucleic acid metabolism.
4. Inhibiting protein synthesis by altering ribosomes.
5. Acting as antimetabolites.

C. Examples.
1. Antifungal agents.
    a. Amphotericin B (Abelcet®, Ambisome®, Fungizone®).
    b. Miconazole (Monistat®).
    c. Itraconazole (Sporanox®).
    d. Fluconazole (Diflucan®).
    e. Ketoconazole (Nizoral®).
    f. Voriconazole (Vfend®).
    g. Caspogungin (Cancidas®).
    h. Micafungin (Mycamine®).
2. Aminoglycosides.
    a. Gentamicin (Garamycin®).
    b. Kanamycin (Kentrex®).
    c. Tobramycin (Tobrex®).
    d. Amikacin (Amikin®).
3. Cephalosporins.
    a. Cefazolin (Ancef®).
    b. Cephalexin (Keflex®).
    c. Cefoxitin (Mefoxitin®).
    d. Cefotetan (Cefotan®).
    e. Cefotaxime (Claforan®).
    f. Ceftazidime (Fortaz®).
    g. Ceftriaxone (Rocephin®).
    h. Cefuroxime (Ceftin®).
    i. Cefepime (Maxipime®).
4. Penicillins.
    a. Ampicillin (Omnipen®).
    b. Amoxicillin (Amoxil®).
    c. Carbenicillin (Geocillin®).
    d. Nafcillin (Unipen®).
    e. Penicillin G, penicillin VK.
    f. Piperacillin (Pipracil®).
    g. Ticarcillin (Ticar®).

5. Tetracyclines.
    a. Doxycycline (Vibramycin®).
    b. Minocycline (Minocin®).
    c. Tetracycline (Acromycin®, Sumycin®).
6. Macrolides.
    a. Erythromycin (E-Mycin®).
    b. Clarithromycin (Biaxin®).
    c. Azithromycin (Zithromax®).
7. Carbapenams.
    a. Ertapenem (Invanz®).
    b. Imipenam (Primaxin®).
    c. Meropenem (Merrem®).
8. Beta lactam/Beta lactamase inhibitors.
    a. Amoxicillin/clavulanate (Augmentin®).
    b. Ampicillin/sulbactam (Unasyn®).
    c. Piperacillin/tazobactam (Zosyn®).
    d. Ticarcillin/clavulanate (Timentin®).
9. Fluoroquinolones.
    a. Ciprofloxacin (Cipro®).
    b. Levofloxacin (Levaquin®).
    c. Moxifloxacin (Avelox®).
    d. Norfloxacin (Noroxin®).
    e. Ofloxacin (Floxin®).
10. Others.
    a. Chloramphenicol (Chloromycetin®).
    b. Clindamycin (Cleocin®).
    c. Daptomycin (Cubicin®).
    d. Linezolid (Zyvox®).
    e. Metronidazole (Flagyl®).
    f. Vancomycin (Vancocin®).

D. Caveats and facts. Following are relevant facts to remember when administering antimicrobial agents to patients with CKD.
1. CKD must be continually monitored using the appropriate lab values during the course of antimicrobial therapy.
2. Serum electrolyte values may be increased by the electrolyte composition (particularly sodium and potassium) of the drug.
3. The patient needs to be closely monitored for signs of superinfection.
4. Drug plasma concentrations may be periodically assessed.
5. Many antimicrobial agents require dosage adjustments when being administered to patients with CKD. Table 9.4 lists selected antimicrobial agents that require varying levels of dosage adjustments for use in these patients.

| Table 9.4 |

Selected Antimicrobial Agents and the Type of Dosage or Interval Adjustment Required for CKD Patients

No Adjustment	Minor Adjustment	Significant Adjustment
Amphotericin B*	Amoxicillin	Amikacin*
Azithromycin	Ampicillin	Aztreonam
Caspofungin	Cephalothin	Carbenicillin
Chloramphenicol	Isoniazid	Cefazolin
Clindamycin		Ceftazidime
Doxycycline		Cefotetan
Erythromycin		Cefoxitin
Ketoconazole		Ciprofloxacin
Linezolid		Daptomycin
Metronidazole		Fluconazole
Micafungin		Gentamicin*
Moxifloxacin		Imipenem/Cilastin
Nafcillin		Kanamycin*
Rifampin		Levofloxacin
		Neomycin*
		Penicillin G
		Piperacillin/tazobactam
		Streptomycin*
		Sulfamethoxazole/Trimethoprim
		Ticarcilllin
		Tobramycin*
		Vancomycin

ˣ Can be nephrotoxic.

IX. Antivirals.

A. Purpose. Patients with CKD are susceptible to all types of organisms. Viruses present still another potential for infection.

B. Mechanism of action. Most antiviral agents act by inhibiting RNA and DNA synthesis and replication of the virus.

C. Examples.
  1. Acyclovir (Zovirax®).
  2. Famciclovir (Famvir®).
  3. Ganciclovir (Cytovene®).
  4. Amantadine (Symmetrel®).
  5. Valacyclovir (Valtrex®).
  6. Valganciclovir (Valcyte®).
  7. Foscarnet (Foscavir®).

D. Caveats and facts. Following are relevant facts to remember when administering antivirals to patients with CKD.
  1. Most of these agents are metabolized by the liver and other tissues and excreted in the urine.
  2. Kidney dysfunction is a possible result of using most of these agents, so frequent monitoring is mandatory.
  3. Ganciclovir and amantadine are not metabolized and are excreted unchanged by the kidney.
  4. Agents that inhibit DNA synthesis can result in bone marrow suppression. The CBC should be monitored during therapy with acyclovir, famciclovir, ganciclovir, valacyclovir, and valganciclovir.
  5. Acyclovir, famciclovir, foscarnet, ganciclovir, valacyclovir, and valganciclovir require a dosage adjustment when used with patients who have a creatinine clearance less than 60 mL/min.

X. Calcimimetics.

A. Purpose. This agent is used to treat hypercalcemia and secondary hyperparathyroidism that can result from excessively elevated phosphorus levels.

B. Mechanism of action. This agent acts by increasing the sensitivity of the calcium receptors on the parathyroid gland to reduce the production and secretion of PTH, thereby reducing GI absorption and bone resorption of calcium.

C. Example: Cinacalcet (Sensipar®).

D. Caveats and facts. Following are relevant facts to remember when administering cinacalcet to patients with CKD.
  1. Cinacalcet has minimal effects on serum calcium levels. Therefore, it is very useful in patients with CKD who have secondary hyper-parathyroidism in conjunction with hypercal-cemia.
  2. The adverse effects that have been reported for cinacalcet include nausea, vomiting, and hypocalcemia.

XI. Cardiotonics.

A. Purpose. Cardiotonic agents are used to manage the congestive heart failure that often occurs as one of the systemic manifestations of CKD.

B. Mechanism of action. Cardiotonics function by:
  1. Increasing cardiac contractility and the cardiac output without increasing cardiac oxygen consumption.
  2. Decreasing venous pressure.
  3. Increasing stroke volume and circulatory velocity.
  4. Prolonging diastole.
  5. Decreasing the volume of blood toward a more normal level.

C. Example: Digoxin (Lanoxin®).

D. Caveats and facts. Following are relevant facts to remember when administering cardiotonics to patients with CKD.
  1. Digoxin is primarily excreted by the kidney.
  2. Apical pulses must be monitored before the administration of the drug.
  3. Serum electrolyte levels, especially potassium and calcium, must be periodically assessed.
  4. Digoxin has a narrow therapeutic index.

Therefore serum drug levels should be assessed in order to avoid potential toxicity.
  5. Constant dosage intervals must be maintained to promote appropriate concentrations of the drug.
  6. Dosage adjustments are usually required in patients with diminished CKD.
  7. Digoxin is not removed by dialysis.

XII. Cation-exchange resins.

A. Purpose. Cation-exchange resins are used in patients with CKD to treat hyperkalemia.

B. Mechanism of action. Cation-exchange resins function primarily in the large intestine where they exchange sodium ions for potassium ions. The potassium ions are then excreted in the feces.

C. Example: Sodium polystyrene sulfonate (Kayexalate®) is the most frequently use cation-exchange resin.

D. Caveats and facts. Following are relevant facts to remember when administering cation-exchange resins to patients with CKD.
  1. When given by enema, the drug must be retained in the intestine 30–45 minutes to be effective.
  2. When given orally, the concurrent administra-tion of an osmotic laxative, such as sorbitol, facilitates the exchange process by promoting the movement of extracellular fluid into the lumen of the gut and also helps to prevent fecal impaction.
  3. Hours are required for the drug to significantly alter potassium levels, so it is not appropriate as the only treatment for acute hyperkalemia.
  4. The patient must be closely monitored for hypokalemia, hypocalcemia, hypomagnesemia, and hypernatremia.
  5. The digitalized patient must be frequently monitored for digoxin toxicity that can be exacerbated by hypokalemia.

XIII. Diuretics.

A. Purpose. Diuretics are used in patients with CKD to increase the formation of urine and enhance the excretion of fluids and solutes. In many cases, the major contribution lies in the ability to potentiate the effect of the antihypertensive agents.

B. Mechanism of action. Diuretics exert their effects according to the pharmacologic mechanisms of action inherent in each classification.
   1. Promoting osmosis by altering concentration of increased amounts of pharmacologically inert substances.
   2. Inhibiting the tubular generation of carbonic acid.
   3. Selectively and nonselectively inhibiting the renal tubular reabsorption of sodium and water.
   4. Altering sodium and water reabsorption from the ascending limb of the loop of Henle.
   5. Promoting sodium excretion through the increased reabsorption of potassium.
   6. Dilating the renal vessels.

C. Examples.
   1. Osmotics.
      a. Mannitol (Osmitrol®).
      b. Urea (Ureaphil®, Urevert®).
   2. Carbonic anyhdrase inhibitors.
      a. Acetazolamide (Diamox®).
      b. Ethoxzolamide (Cardrase®, Ethamide®).
   3. Thiazides.
      a. Chlorothiazide (Diuril®).
      b. Hydrochlorothiazide (Esidrix®, HydroDiuril®).
      c. Chlorthalidone (Thalitone®).
   4. Loop-acting.
      a. Furosemide (Lasix®).
      b. Bumetanide (Bumex®).
      c. Torsemide (Demadex®).
      d. Ethacrynic acid (Edecrin®).
   5. Potassium sparing.
      a. Spironolactone (Aldactone®).
      b. Triamterene (Dyrenium®).
   6. Thiazide-like.
      a. Metolazone (Zaroxolyn®).
      b. Indapamide (Lozol®).

D. Caveats and facts. Following are relevant facts to remember when administering diuretics to patients with CKD.
   1. Patients should be frequently monitored for fluid and electrolyte imbalances.
   2. Daily weights and intake and output records can help validate the effects of diuretics.
   3. Diuretics can promote the nephrotoxicity of other pharmacologic agents, such as aminoglycosides, primarily by altering the hydration state.
   4. Kidney function must be frequently monitored using the appropriate serum lab values for the duration of diuretic therapy.

   5. The little information that is available suggests that diuretics are not removed by dialysis.
   6. Furosemide and metolazone are the diuretics that are most commonly useful in advanced CKD.
   7. Carbonic anhydrase inhibitors are primarily used to treat glaucoma and some forms of edema, such as drug-induced, or to prevent altitude sickness. They are not usually used to treat patients with CKD because of their major side effect, metabolic acidosis.
   8. Potassium-sparing diuretics are not usually used to treat patients with advanced kidney dysfunction because of their potential to produce hyperkalemia, which would only add to the already existing potassium excess created by the diminished kidney function.

XIV. Glucocorticoids.

A. Purpose. Systemic glucocorticoids are used in patients with CKD primarily for their antiinflammatory properties. They may be used to treat underlying kidney disease, such as glomerulonephritis, or a specific complication. They are also used in conjunction with other immunosuppressive agents after tissue or organ transplantation.

B. Mechanism of action. The mechanism of action of systemic glucocorticoids is not well understood, but they appear to suppress hypersensitivity and immune response by preventing cell mediated immune reactions; decrease the binding of antibodies to cell surface receptors; and inhibit interleukin synthesis. In addition, they stabilize lysosomal membranes, prevent plasma exudation, inhibit phagocytosis, decrease antibody formation in injured or infected tissues, and interfere with wound healing. They also influence lipid, protein, and carbohydrate metabolism and enhance sodium retention.

C. Examples.
   1. Prednisone (Deltasone®).
   2. Methylprednisolone sodium succinate (Solu-Medrol®).

D. Caveats and facts. Following are relevant facts to remember when administering systemic glucocorticoids to patients with CKD.
   1. Long-term administration may result in Cushing's syndrome characterized by acne, moon face, hirsutism and masculinization,

cervicodorsal fate, protruding abdomen, central obesity, amenorrhea, purplish abdominal striae, edema, atrophy of extremities, muscle weakness, hypertension, hyperglycemia, immunosuppression, and mental status changes.
2. These agents will increase catabolism, serum glucose, potassium excretion, sodium retention, and water retention, and decrease wound healing.
3. These agents can create GI ulcerations.
4. Administer these agents with milk or food.

XV. Heavy metal chelating agents.

A. Purpose. Heavy metal chelating agents are used to treat aluminum and iron toxicity in patients with CKD.

B. Mechanism of action. These agents function by forming complexes with the heavy metals, thus preventing the metallic cations from entering into further chemical reactions in the body. Chelating agents have the following characteristics:
1. Water solubility.
2. Resistance to metabolic degradation.
3. Ability to penetrate metal storage sites.
4. Easy excretion by the kidney.
5. Ability to retain chelating activity at the pH of the body fluids.
6. The property of forming metal complexes that are less toxic than the free metal ion.

C. Example: Deferoxamine mesylate (Desferal®) is the best example of a heavy metal chelating agent that is used in patients with CKD. This drug is used most frequently to treat iron overdose or aluminum intoxication in dialysis patients.
It is administered intravenously near the end of a dialysis treatment and forms dialyzable metal-drug complexes that are removed by subsequent dialysis treatments. For maximal effectiveness, it should be administered through the venous blood line.

D. Caveats and facts. Following are relevant facts to remember when administering deferoxamine to patients with CKD.
1. It gives the urine a reddish coloration.
2. If given parenterally, it must be administered slowly.
3. Patients must be frequently monitored for allergic-type reactions following administration.
4. Patients must be frequently monitored for adverse reactions because the drug is primarily excreted by the kidneys.

XVI. Histamine H1 receptor antagonists.

A. Purpose. These agents are used to block the effects of histamine and perhaps decrease pruritus that is associated with CKD.

B. Mechanism of action. These agents function by inhibiting the H1 receptors in the effector cells in the gastrointestinal tract, blood vessels and respiratory tract.

C. Examples.
1. Sedating H1 receptor antagonists.
   a. Diphenhydramine (Benadryl®).
   b. Hydroxyzine (Atarax®).
2. Nonsedating H1 receptor antagonists.
   a. Cetirizine (Zyrtec®).
   b. Fexofenadrine (Allegra®).
   c. Loratadine (Claritin®).

D. Caveats and facts. Following are relevant facts to remember when administering antihistamines to patients with CKD.
1. The sedating H1 antagonists cause CNS depression.
2. Higher doses of the non-sedating H1 receptor antagonists may cause CNS depression and sedation.
3. The sedating H1 receptor antagonists may have anticholinergic effects.

XVII. Histamine H2 receptor antagonists.

A. Purpose. Histamine H2 receptor antagonists are used to decrease the potential gastric irritation, ulceration, and bleeding occurring secondary to CKD.

B. Mechanism of action. These agents function by competitively inhibiting the action of histamine at the histamine H2 receptor sites of the gastric parietal cells. As a result, the volume and hydrogen ion concentration of gastric acid secretions is decreased.

C. Examples.
1. Cimetidine (Tagamet®).
2. Ranitidine (Zantac®).
3. Famotidine (Pepcid®).
4. Nizatidine (Axid®).

D. Caveats and facts. Following are relevant facts to remember when administering H2 receptor antagonists to patients with CKD.

1. When given orally, antacids may interfere with their absorption.
2. Dosage adjustment is recommended for patients with hepatic and renal insufficiency.
3. Smoking decreases the effectiveness of the drug.
4. The levels of these drugs are decreased by dialysis.

XVIII. Mineralocorticoids.

A. Purpose. Mineralocorticoids may be used in patients with CKD to treat hyperkalemia.

B. Mechanism of action. Mineralocorticoids mimic aldosterone to increase sodium retention in the kidney and increase potassium excretion by the kidney. They also mimic the effects of aldosterone on the colonic excretion of potassium, which is the primary effect these agents have in patients with CKD.

C. Example: fludrocortisone (Florinef®).

D. Caveats and facts. Following are relevant facts to remember when administering mineralocorticoids to patients with CKD.
1. Sodium retention can lead to fluid retention, which can worsen hypertension, edema and chronic heart failure and can limit the use of these agents in patients with CKD.
2. These agents should not be discontinued abruptly, but slowly tapered to minimize adrenal suppression.

XIX. Phosphate binders.

A. Purpose. Calcium products, aluminum-based products, phosphate binding polymers, and lanthanum are administered to assist in managing the hyperphosphatemia that is associated with CKD.

B. Mechanism of action. These agents act by binding phosphate in the GI tract and facilitate the excretion of phosphate in the feces.

C. Examples.
1. Calcium-based phosphate binders.
   a. Calcium acetate (PhosLo®).
   b. Calcium carbonate (Os-Cal®, Tums®).
2. Aluminum-based phosphate binders.
   a. Aluminum hydroxide gel (Amphojel®, Alternagel®, Aludrox®, Dialume®).
   b. Basic aluminum carbonate (Basaljel®).

3. Phosphate binding polymers: sevelamer hydrochloride (Renagel®).
4. Lanthanum carbonate (Fosrenol®).

D. Caveats and facts. Following are relevant facts to remember when administering phosphate binding agents to patients with CKD.
1. Serum calcium and phosphate levels must be monitored frequently during the therapy.
2. Dietary phosphate should be restricted during the therapy.
3. All of these agents should be administered with meals to bind to phosphate in the GI tract.
4. The dose of the phosphate binders should be adjusted to maintain a calcium-phosphate product less than 55 mg/dL.
5. Aluminum-based phosphate binders are rarely used in patients with chronic CKD because they can result in increased systemic aluminum levels. They should only be used for short durations when serum phosphorus levels are > 7 mg/dL to avoid aluminum toxicity. The potential for aluminum toxicity is increased if the dialysis water contains aluminum.
6. Calcium-based phosphate binders can result in hypercalcemia. It is important to monitor serum calcium levels closely.
7. Calcium acetate binds approximately twice the amount of phosphate as an equivalent amount of calcium carbonate.
8. Phosphate binders should maintain a serum phosphate level of approximately 3.5–5.5 mg/dl in patients with Stage 5 CKD and 2.7–3.6 mg/dl in patients with Stage 3 or 4 CKD.
9. Sevelamer is not absorbed into the bloodstream.
10. Sevelamer and lanthanum do not contain aluminum or calcium.
11. The phosphate binding agents should not be used in patients with hypophosphatemia or who have a bowel obstruction. They should be used with caution in patients with swallowing disorders of severe GI motility disorders.
12. Other drugs should be administered 2 hours before or 4 hours after sevelamer to prevent possible concomitant binding that could affect blood levels of the other drug.
13. Lanthanum is a chewable phosphate binder and cannot be swallowed whole.

XX. Prokinetic agents.

A. Purpose. These agents are used to treat patients who experience hypomotility of the GI tract, or gastroparesis, and thus have a delayed emptying of the stomach resulting in clinical signs and symptoms, such as nausea, vomiting, indigestion, or gastroesophageal reflux.

B. Mechanism of action. These agents act as dopamine antagonists, resulting in inhibition of relaxation, enhanced coordinated antral-duodenal motility, and accelerated gastric emptying and transit in the small intestine.

C. Example: metoclopramide (Reglan®).

D. Caveats and facts. Following are relevant facts to remember when administering metoclopramide to patients with CKD:
1. Metoclopramide can result in restlessness, drowsiness, fatigue, depression, extrapyramidal symptoms, and tardive dyskinesia.
2. Metoclopramide should not be used with patients in whom an increased GI motility might be hazardous, such as those with GI bleeding or obstructions.

XXI. Proton pump inhibitors.

A. Purpose. These agents produce a dose related inhibition of gastric acid secretion and are useful in treating and preventing ulcers within the GI tract and for gastroesophageal reflux disease (GERD).

B. Mechanism of action. These agents inhibit the H+-K+-ATPase and the proton pump in the gastric parietal cells. They produce only small changes in the volume of gastric juice, pepsin secretion, and intrinsic factor secretion, and do not affect gastric motility.

C. Examples.
1. Omeprazole (Prilosec®).
2. Lansoprazole (Prevacid®).
3. Rabeprazole (Aciphex®).
4. Pantoprazole (Protonix®).
5. Esomeprazole (Nexium®).

D. Caveats and facts. Following are relevant facts to remember when administering proton pump inhibitors to patients with CKD.
1. These agents are metabolized in the liver and do not require dosage adjustments.
2. These drugs may produce the following adverse effects: nausea, vomiting, diarrhea, abdominal pain, headache, dizziness, somnolence and rash.
3. All of these agents increase the gastric pH and can decrease the effect of the ferrous salts, indomethacin, ketoconazole, tetracyclines, digoxin, and fluconazole.

XXII. Sedative-hypnotics.

A. Purpose. Sedative-hypnotic agents are used primarily to induce sleep, if necessary, in patients with CKD.

B. Mechanism of action. In general, these agents depress the activity of excitable tissues and produce drowsiness.

C. Examples.
1. Temazepam (Restoril®).
2. Zolpidem (Ambien®).
3. Zaleplon (Sonata®).
4. Eszopiclone (Lunesta®).

D. Caveats and facts. Following are relevant facts to remember when administering sedative-hypnotic agents to patients with CKD.
1. These drugs are primarily excreted by nonrenal mechanisms, so dosage adjustments are not necessary.
2. Patients should be monitored for excessive drowsiness.
3. Most of these drugs are not removed by dialysis.

XXIII. Stool softeners and cathartics.

A. Purpose. Emollient laxatives (stool softeners) and other cathartics are frequently prescribed for patients with CKD because they are prone to constipation for a variety of physiologic, therapeutic, and pharamcologic reasons. In most cases, bulk-forming or stimulant cathartics are preferable to saline cathartics that contain magnesium, sodium, phosphate, and/or potassium.

B. Mechanism of action. Stool softeners and cathartics exert their effects by one of the following mechanisms:
1. Increasing the penetration of water into the stool.
2. Increasing bulk of stool to stimulate peristalsis in the GI tract.
3. Increase peristalsis in the GI tract.

C. Examples.
1. Emollient laxatives.
   a. Docusate sodium (Colace®).
   b. Docusate calcium (Surfak®).
2. Cathartics.
   a. Bulk-forming.
      (1) Methylcellulose (Citrucel®).

(2) Psyllium (Metamucil®).
b. Stimulant.
(1) Castor oil (Neoloid®).
(2) Bisacodyl (Dulcolax®).
(3) Senna (Senakot®).
c. Osmotic: lactulose (Chronulac®, Cephulac®).

D. Caveats and facts. Following are relevant facts to remember when administering stool softeners and laxatives to patients with CKD.
1. These drugs are excreted by nonrenal mechanisms and are not removed by dialysis.
2. These agents should be avoided in patients with bowel obstruction.
3. Avoid the use of magnesium-based and phosphate-based cathartics.

XXIV. Vitamins.

A. Purpose. Vitamin supplements are frequently prescribed for patients with CKD because of their dietary restrictions, dialysis therapy, and metabolic disturbances.

B. Examples.
1. All B and C.
2. Vitamin B complex and C.
3. Nephrocaps®.
4. Nephro-Vite®.

C. Caveats and facts. Following are relevant facts to remember when administering vitamins to patients with CKD.
1. In most patients, water-soluble vitamins are administered daily, and on dialysis days, they are usually administered after dialytic therapy.
2. Administration of vitamin A, a fat soluble vitamin, can lead to vitamin A toxicity in patients with CKD.

XXV. Vitamin D.

A. Purpose. Vitamin D and vitamin analogs are used to treat vitamin D deficiency, hypocalcemia, and secondary hyperparathyroidism.

B. Mechanism of action. These agents function by either directly replacing vitamin D or by acting like vitamin D to enhance calcium absorption and provide negative feedback to the parathyroid gland to reduce PTH secretion.

C. Examples: vitamin D and analogs.
a. Calcitriol (Calcijex®, Rocaltrol®).

b. Doxercalciferol (Hectorol®).
c. Paricalcitol (Zemplar®).

D. Caveats and facts. Following are relevant facts to remember when administering vitamin D therapy to patients with CKD.
1. Calcitriol and doxercalciferol can increase serum calcium and phosphate levels by increasing the absorption from the GI tract and resorption from the bones. It is important that phosphorus levels are controlled before initiating therapy with these agents to minimize further elevations in phosphate levels or increases in the calcium-phosphate product.
2. Paricalcitol suppresses PTH secretion in patients with CKD with minimal effect on GI absorption or bone resorption of calcium and phosphorus.
3. Oral vitamin D can be administered daily or three times weekly.
4. Intravenous vitamin D is generally administered three times weekly with dialysis therapy.
5. Serum calcium and phosphorus levels and the calcium-phosphorus product must be monitored frequently in patients receiving vitamin D therapy.
6. The dosage of vitamin D can be adjusted based on serum calcium or PTH levels.

Chapter 45

Dialysis and Drug Therapy

Dialysis therapy significantly influences the pharmacologic management of patients with CKD. In general, if a drug is normally primarily excreted by the kidney, then it is usually also dialyzable through hemodialysis. Because of the selectivity of the peritoneal clearances for many drugs, this general statement does not necessarily apply to peritoneal dialysis. Thus, the concentrations of many drugs may be decreased by hemodialysis and not by peritoneal dialysis.

I. **The dialyzability of drugs.**

A. Definition. A drug is considered to be dialyzable if the serum concentration levels can be depleted through the interaction with a dialysis process.

B. Influencing factors. The effect of hemodialysis on the half-life, or concentration of a drug, is a function of the following factors:
   1. Hemodialysis.
      a. Dialysis dependent factors.
         (1) Dialysate flow rate.
         (2) The dialysis membrane.
            (a) Permeability.
            (b) Surface area.
            (c) Pore size.
         (3) Length of dialysis.
         (4) Type of dialysis.
         (5) Blood flow rates.
      b. Drug dependent factors.
         (1) Molecular weight and particle size. Drugs with a high molecular weight or a large particle size are not able to pass through dialysis membrane.
         (2) Percent of protein binding. Drugs that are largely protein bound are not removed by dialysis because the protein cannot pass through the dialysis membrane.
         (3) Lipid affinity. Drugs with high lipid affinity are not able to diffuse into the dialysate fluid to be removed.
         (4) Volume of distribution. Drugs with a low volume of distribution are contained primarily in the vascular space and are more likely to be removed by dialysis.

   2. Peritoneal dialysis.
      a. Dialysis dependent factors.
         (1) Surface area of peritoneum.
         (2) Blood flow rates to the peritoneum.
         (3) Type of dialysis.
      b. Drug dependent factors.
         (1) Molecular weight and particle size. Drugs with a high molecular weight or a large particle size are not able to pass through dialysis membrane.
         (2) Percent of protein binding. Drugs that are largely protein bound are not removed by dialysis because the protein cannot pass through the dialysis membrane.
         (3) Volume of distribution. Drugs with a low volume of distribution are contained primarily in the vascular space and are more likely to be removed by dialysis.
         (4) Drug ionization at physiologic pH. Drugs that are ionized at physiologic pH are not able to be removed by peritoneal dialysis.

II. **Alterations in dosage and frequency.**

A. General approach to determining the appropriate dosing adjustment for patients with CKD.
   1. Obtain the history and relevant clinical information from the patient.
   2. Estimate the creatinine clearance to determine kidney function.
   3. Identify medications requiring dosage adjustments.
   4. Determine treatment goals.
   5. Calculate the dose.
   6. Monitor for drug response and toxicity.
   7. Adjust the drug regimen based on drug response or change in patient status.

B. Specific considerations to determine dosage adjustments in patients with CKD.
   1. Treatment goals.
      a. Maintain similar peak levels for drugs whose effect or toxicity is correlated with the peak level.
         (1) Example: aminoglycosides.

(2) Dosing adjustment strategy: increasing the dosing interval will maintain similar peak levels.

b. Maintain similar trough levels for most drugs whose effect is dependent on a minimum concentration.
   (1) Examples.
      (a) Phenytoin.
      (b) Phenobarbital.
   (2) Dosing adjustment strategies.
      (a) Decreasing the dose will maintain similar trough levels for drugs with a short half-life.
      (b) Monitoring free drug concentrations for the drug whenever possible will allow a more accurate determination of the necessary dosing adjustment.

c. Maintain average steady state drug levels for drugs that have no specific target peak or tough levels.
   (1) Examples.
      (a) Antihypertensives.
      (b) Benzodiazepines.
      (c) Most antibiotics.
   (2) Dosing adjustment strategies.
      (a) Decreasing the dose will maintain adequate drug levels for most drugs.
      (b) A combination of decreasing the dose and increasing the dosing interval may be required for some drugs, particularly as kidney function worsens and for patients receiving dialysis.

C. Supplemental dosing.
   1. Principles of supplemental dosing in patients receiving hemodialysis.
      a. As the concentration of a drug decreases because of dialysis, consideration must be given to providing supplemental doses to reestablish or maintain therapeutic levels.
      b. Supplemental dosing after hemodialysis is based on the half-life of the drug, the dosage interval in relation to the hemodialysis schedule, and the amount of drug rebound or redistribution that occurs after dialysis.
      c. The key to supplemental dosing is to replace the amount of the drug that was actually removed during hemodialysis.
      d. This extra dosing does not replace the maintenance dose, but is given in addition to it.
   2. Determining efficacy. The efficacy of supplemental dosing can be determined by monitoring the plasma concentration of the drug at peak and trough intervals.
   3. Examples. Table 9.5 summarizes the dialyzability of selected drugs that are frequently used in treating patients with CKD.

Chapter 46

The Clinical Significance for Nursing

From a nursing perspective, the clinical significance of this discussion on the pharmacologic aspects of CKD is related to three essential areas of patient care: monitoring and administering medications, educating the patient, and fostering patient adherence.

I. **Monitoring and administering medications.** Many beneficial effects can be enhanced and many adverse effects can be avoided when the nurse attends closely to the details of appropriately monitoring and administering pharmacologic agents. Monitoring medications includes the following activities:

A. Be aware of all of the medications a patient may be taking. A nurse can easily become aware of all the medications that are prescribed for a patient by checking the physician's orders and the medication record.

B. Understand the pharmacokinetic and pharmacodynamic parameters of medications can be accomplished by considering the following questions in relation to each medication:
   1. Is the drug readily absorbed?
   2. Will the absorption be altered by CKD?
   3. Will the distribution be altered by CKD?
   4. Is the drug excreted unchanged or does it undergo significant metabolism?
   5. What is the primary route of excretion?
   6. Does CKD influence the excretion of the drug or its metabolites?

Table 9.5

The Dialyzability of Selected Pharmacologic Agents

Drug	Removed by hemodialysis (Differences noted for high permeability dialysis when applicable)	Removed by peritoneal dialysis	Supplemental dose required (H = hemodialysis)	Drug	Removed by hemodialysis (Differences noted for high permeability dialysis when applicable)	Removed by peritoneal dialysis	Supplemental dose required (H = hemodialysis)
Analgesics				**Antihyperlipidemics**			
Acetaminophen	Yes	No	Yes H	Fibric acid derivatives	No	No	No
Aspirin	Yes	Yes	Yes	Niacin	No	No	No
Codeine	No	?	No H	Statins	No	?	No
Fentanyl	?	?	?				
Meperidine	No	No	No	**Antihypertensives**			
Methadone	No	No	No	Acebutolol	Yes	No	Yes H
Morphine	No (Yes)	?	No H	Amlodipine	No	No	No
Pentazocine	Yes	?	Yes H	Atenolol	Yes	No	Yes H
Propoxyphene	No	No	No	Benzapril	No	?	No
Salsalate	Yes	No	Yes H	Candesartan	No	?	No
				Captopril	Yes	No	Yes H
Antiarrhythmics				Clonidine	No	No	No
Amiodarone	No	No	No	Diltiazem	No	No	No
Bretylium	Yes	?	Yes H	Doxazosin	No	No	No
Disopyramide	No	?	No	Enalapril	Yes	Yes	Yes
Flecanide	No	?	No H	Esmolol	Yes	Yes	Yes
Lidocaine	No	?	No H	Felodipine	No	?	No H
Mexiletine	Yes	No	Yes II	Hydralazine	No	No	No
N-Acetylprocainamide	Yes	No	Yes H	Irbesartan	No	?	No
Procainamide	Yes	No	Yes H	Labetalol	No	No	No
Propafenone	No	No	No	Lisinopril	Yes	?	Yes H
Sotalol	Yes	?	Yes H	Losartan	No	No	No
Tocainide	Yes	?	Yes H	Methyldopa	Yes	Yes	Yes
				Metoprolol	Yes	?	Yes H
Anticoagulants				Minoxidil	Yes	Yes	Yes
Dalteparin	No	No	No	Nadolol	Yes	?	Yes H
Enoxaparin	No	No	No	Nicardipine	No	?	No H
Fondaparinux	No	No	No	Nifedipine	No	No	No
Heparin	No	No	No	Nimodipine	No	No	No
Tinzaparin	No	No	No	Nitrendipine	No	?	No H
Warfarin	No	No	No	Nitroprusside	Yes	Yes	Yes
				Quinapril	No	No	No
Anticonvulsants				Penbutolol	No	No	No
Carbamazepine	No	No	No	Prazosin	No	No	No
Ethosuximide	Yes	?	Yes H	Propranolol	No	No	No
Lamotrigine	No	No	No	Ramipril	Yes	?	Yes H
Phenobarbital	Yes	Yes	Yes	Reserpine	No	No	No
Phenytoin	No (Yes)	No	No	Terazosin	No	No	No
Primidone	Yes	?	Yes H	Timolol	No	No	No
Topiramate	Yes	?	Yes	Valsartan	No	No	No
Valproic acid	No	No	No	Verapamil	No	No	No
Antidepressants							
Amitriptyline	No	No	No	**Antiinflammatories**			
Buproprion	No	No	No	Celecoxib	?	?	?
Citalopram	No	No	No	Cortisone	No	No	No
Desipramine	No	No	No	Dexamethasone	No	No	No
Doxepin	No	No	No	Fenoprofen	No	?	No
Escitalopram	?	?	?	Ibuprofen	No	?	No
Fluoxetine	No	No	No	Indomethacin	No	?	No
Imipramine	No	No	No	Mefenamic acid	No	?	No
Nortriptyline	No	No	No	Methylprednisolone	Yes	?	Yes H
Paroxetine	No	No	No	Naproxen	No	?	No H
Sertraline	No	No	No	Prednisolone	No	No	No
				Prednisone	No	No	No
Antihistamines							
Cetirizine	No	No	No				
Chlorpheniramine	Yes	No	Yes				
Fexofenadine	No	No	No				
Hydroxyzine	No	No	No				
Loratidine	No	No	No				

Table continues on next page

Table 9.5 (continued)

The Dialyzability of Selected Pharmacologic Agents

Drug	Removed by hemodialysis (Differences noted for high permeability dialysis when applicable)	Removed by peritoneal dialysis	Supplemental dose required (H = hemodialysis)	Drug	Removed by hemodialysis (Differences noted for high permeability dialysis when applicable)	Removed by peritoneal dialysis	Supplemental dose required (H = hemodialysis)
Antimicrobials				**Antineoplastics**			
Amikacin	Yes	Yes	Yes	Bleomycin	No	No	No
Amoxicillin	Yes	No	Yes H	Carboplatin	Yes	?	Yes H
Ampicillin	Yes	No	Yes	Carmustine	No	?	No H
Azithromycin	No	No	No	Chlorabucil	No	No	No
Aztreonam	Yes	?	Yes H	Cyclophosphamide	Yes	?	Yes H
Carbenicillin	Yes	No	Yes H	Doxorubicin	No	?	No H
Cefaclor	Yes	Yes	Yes	Etoposide	No	No	No
Cefadroxil	Yes	No	Yes H	Fluorouracil	Yes	?	Yes H
Cefamandole	Yes	?	Yes H	Hydroxyurea	No	?	No H
Cefazolin	Yes	Yes	Yes	Lomustine	No	?	No H
Cefepime	No	No	No	Mercaptopurine	Yes	?	Yes H
Cefixime	No	No	No	Methotrexate	Yes	No	Yes H
Cefoperazone	No	No	No				
Cefotaxime	Yes	No	Yes H	**Antipsychotics**			
Cefotetan	Yes	Yes	Yes	Buspirone	Yes	?	Yes H
Cefoxitin	Yes	No	Yes H	Chlorpromazine	No	No	No
Ceftazidime	Yes	Yes	Yes	Haloperidol	No	No	No
Ceftriaxone	No	No	No	Mirtazapine	No	No	No
Cephalexin	Yes	No	Yes H	Olanzapine	No	No	No
Cephalothin	Yes	No	Yes H	Trifluoperazine	No	No	No
Cephadrine	Yes	Yes	Yes				
Chloramphenicol	Yes	No	Yes	**Antituberculosis**			
Cilastatin	Yes	?	Yes H	Aminosalicylic acid	Yes	?	Yes H
Ciprofloxacin	No	No	No	Ethambutol	No	?	No
Clarithromycin	?	?	?	Isoniazid	No	No	No
Clindamycin	No	No	No	Pyrazinamide	Yes	No	Yes H
Cloxacillin	No	No	No				
Dicloxacillin	No	No	No	**Antivirals**			
Doxycycline	No	No	No	Acyclovir	Yes	No	Yes H
Erythromycin	No	No	No	Adefovir	No	No	No
Gentamicin	Yes	Yes	Yes	Amantadine	No	No	No
Imipenem	Yes	Yes	Yes	Foscarnet	Yes	?	Yes H
Kanamycin	Yes	Yes	Yes	Ganciclovir	Yes	?	Yes H
Lincomycin	No	No	No	Lamivudine	No	No	No
Methicilin	No	No	No	Valacyclovir	Yes	?	Yes H
Nafcillin	Yes	Yes	Yes	Valganciclovir	Yes	?	Yes H
Norfloxacin	No	?	No H				
Oxacillin	No	No	Yes H	**Cardiotonics**			
Penicillin G	Yes	No	Yes H	Digitoxin	No	No	No
Pentamidine	No	No	No	Digoxin	No	No	No
Piperacillin	Yes	No	Yes H				
Rifampin	No	No	No	**Diuretics**			
Streptomycin	Yes	Yes	Yes	Bumetanide	No	?	No H
Sulbactam	Yes	No	Yes H	Chlorthalidone	No	?	No H
Sulfamethoxazole	Yes	No	Yes H	Ethacrynic acid	No	No	No
Sulfisoxazole	Yes	Yes	Yes	Furosemide	No	?	No H
Tetracycline	No	No	No	Hydrochlorothiazide	No	?	No H
Ticarcillin	Yes	No	Yes H	Indapamide	No	?	No H
Tobramycin	Yes	Yes	Yes	Metolazone	No	?	No H
Trimethoprim	Yes	?	Yes H	Spironolactone	No	No	No
Vancomycin	No (Yes)	No	No	Torsemide	No	No	No
Antimycotics							
Amphotericin B	No	No	No				
Caspofungin	No	No	No				
Fluconazole	Yes	No	Yes H				
Flucytosine	Yes	Yes	Yes				
Ketoconazole	No	No	No				
Miconazole	No	No	No	*Table continues on next page*			
Voriconazole	No	No	No				

Table 9.5 (continued)

The Dialyzability of Selected Pharmacologic Agents

Drug	Removed by hemodialysis (Differences noted for high permeability dialysis when applicable)	Removed by peritoneal dialysis	Supplemental dose required (H = hemodialysis)	Drug	Removed by hemodialysis (Differences noted for high permeability dialysis when applicable)	Removed by peritoneal dialysis	Supplemental dose required (H = hemodialysis)
Gastrointestinal agents				Filgrastim	No	No	No
Cimetidine	Yes	No	Yes H	Fludrocortisone	?	?	?
Famotidine	No	No	No	Gabapentin	Yes	?	Yes H
Granisetron	?	?	?	Gold Na Thiomalate	No	?	No H
Lansoprazole	No	No	No	Interferon	No	?	No H
Metoclopramide	No	No	No	Iron dextran	No	No	No
Nizatidine	No	No	No	Iron sucrose	No	No	No
Omeprazole	?	?	?	Penicillamine	Yes	?	Yes H
Ondansetron	?	?	?	Quinidine	No	No	No
Raniditine	No	No	No	Theophylline	Yes	?	Yes H
Sucralfate	No	No	No	Tolbutamide	No	?	No H
Hypoglycemic agents				**Sedatives-Hypnotics**			
Glipizide	No	No	No	Alprazolam	No	?	No H
Glyburide	No	?	No H	Chloral hydrate	Yes	Yes	Yes
Insulin (all types)	No	No	No	Chlordiazepoxide	No	?	No H
Metformin	Yes	?	Yes H	Clonazepam	No	?	No H
Nateglinide	No	No	No	Clorazepate	No	?	No H
Pioglitazone	No	No	No	Diazepam	No	?	No H
Rosiglitazone	No	No	No	Flurazepam	No	?	No H
				Meprobamate	Yes	Yes	Yes
Immunosuppressants				Midazolam	No	?	No H
Azathioprine	Yes	?	Yes H	Oxazepam	No	?	No H
Cyclosporine	No	No	No	Pentobarbital	No	?	No H
Mycophenolate	No	No	No	Secobarbital	No	No	No
Sirolimus	?	?	?	Temazepam	No	?	No H
Tacrolimus	No	?	No	Triazolam	No	?	No H
				Zaleplon	?	?	?
Miscellaneous agents				Zolpidem	No	No	No
Allopurinol	Yes	?	Yes H				
Calcitriol	No	No	No	**Vasodilators**			
Darbepoetin	?	?	?	Isosorbide dinitrate	No	No	No
Doxercalciferol	No	No	No	Isosorbide mononitrate	Yes	No	Yes H
Epoetin (EPO)	No	No	No	Nitroglycerin	No	No	No
Ferric gluconate	No	No	No				
Ferrous salts	No	No	No				

7. What are the major characteristics of its metabolites?
8. Is the drug nephrotoxic, and, if so, at what levels?
9. What is the onset and duration of the pharmacologic effect?
10. What is the influence of CKD on the half-life of the drug?
11. Are dosage and frequency interval adjustments required in patients with CKD?
12. Is the drug dialyzable?
13. Will alterations in the normal administration schedule be necessary on dialysis days?

14. Is supplemental dosing necessary after dialysis?
15. What are the potential side effects of the drug?
16. How is the drug likely to interact with other medications that the patient is taking?

C. Evaluate the serum levels of medications and electrolytes daily or as appropriate. Assessing serum drug and electrolyte levels daily is almost second nature to nurses caring for nephrology patients. However, it should not become such a routine task that its importance is slighted. All of these values are significant in the pharmacologic management of the patient with CKD.

D. Assess kidney function periodically. In most cases, kidney function is assessed using serum creatinine and BUN levels. Because these values do not give a clear indication of kidney function, particularly when patterns or trends in value levels are used, they may not be sufficient.

1. Cockcroft and Gault equation. Cockcroft and Gault developed a formula for estimating creatinine clearance that provides additional data for assessing kidney function. This formula is based on the fact that creatinine clearance is proportional to body mass and inversely proportional to age. The formula is:

$$\text{Creatinine clearance} = \frac{(140 - \text{age}) \times (\text{body weight in kg})}{(72) \times (\text{serum creatinine in mg/dl})}$$

This formula appears to be an accurate method for estimating creatinine clearance. When it is used with female patients, however, the result should be decreased by about 10–15% to account for inaccuracies that tend to overestimate creatinine clearance in that gender. The Cockcroft Gault equation is often used when calculating creatinine clearance for medications that require dosage adjustments in CKD.

2. MDRD equation. The Modification of Diet in Renal Disease (MDRD) Study data was used to develop an equation to estimate GFR in patients with CKD. The original formula included six parameters: age, sex, ethnicity, serum creatinine, BUN, and serum albumin level. An abbreviated version provides similar accuracy in estimating GFR utilizing four of those parameters: age, gender, ethnicity, and serum creatinine concentration. The formula is:

$$\text{GFR (ml/min/1.73m}^2) = 186 \times (\text{SCr})^{-1.154} \times (\text{Age})^{-0.203} \times (0.742 \text{ if female}) \times (1.21 \text{ if African American})$$

The NKF has developed guidelines for evaluating, classifying and stratifying CKD. The guidelines recommend using the MDRD abbreviated equation to evaluate and classify CKD.

3. Timed urine collection. A timed urine collection is the most accurate method to determine actual kidney function. A 24-hour urine collection is more accurate compared to a fixed time interval because it accounts for diurnal variations in the production and excretion of creatinine throughout the day. However, patient error in the collection technique may compromise the results of the study. The patient should be carefully instructed in the following key elements of a timed urine collection to obtain the most accurate result:

a. Completely void before starting the timed urine collection. Discard the urine from this void.

b. Accurately record the time of the complete void as the start time of the urine collection.

c. Collect the urine from each void over the entire time course of the timed collection.

d. Ensure proper storage of the urine collection during and after the time collection.

e. At the end of the time collection period, completely void and collect the final urine void.

f. Accurately record the time of the final urine void as the end time of the urine collection.

E. Medication administration and patient safety.

1. Medication Errors. According to the FDA, medication errors cause at least one death every day and injure approximately 1.3 million people annually in the United States. Common causes of errors include similar product names/packaging, poor communication, and misinterpreting abbreviations or handwriting. Medication errors can occur at any time during medication ordering, transcribing, dispensing and/or preparing, or administration.

2. Five "rights" of medication administration. Prior to the administration of any medication, the five "rights" should be verified: *right patient, right medication, right dose, right time,* and *right route.*

a. Right patient. Before administering any medication, it should be verified that the medication is being given to the correct patient. Using at least two patient identifiers such as name, birthdate, social security number or medical record number, will help to avoid this error. Many hospitals have implemented bar coding systems on patient wristbands to prevent a medication being administered to the wrong patient during hospitalization.

b. Right medication. Factors that may contribute to administering the wrong medication include similar color or writing of medications, or medication packaging, sound-alike medications (example Zantac®/Zyrtec®, dopamine/dobutamine), and transcribing orders. If it's necessary to take a verbal order from a prescriber, write down the order immediately and read it back to the prescriber out loud to verify. It is also important to always clarify orders if they are incomplete or illegible. Do not assume any part of an order.

c. Right dose. Administering the correct dose of medication is very important. Always use leading zeros and avoid using trailing zeros (see "Error-Prone Abbreviations" below) when transcribing to avoid ten-fold errors in dosing. Any unfamiliar doses should be verified by a reference and/or with the prescriber and dosing calculations should always be double checked before administration.

d. Right time. Timing of medication administration is sometimes important. Some drugs need to be separated by a given amount of time to avoid drug-drug interactions. For example, certain antibiotics must be separated from calcium, magnesium and iron to ensure proper absorption. Drug-food interactions can also be significant and some medications should be given on an empty stomach or full stomach depending on their pharmacokinetic properties. Timing of medications is also especially important in patients who are on dialysis. Some medications should be held until after dialysis or supplemented after dialysis because a significant proportion is removed during the hemodialysis procedure.

e. Right route. Many drugs can be given by multiple routes of administration such as intravenous, oral, intramuscular, subcutaneous, rectal, transdermal, and/or intraperitoneal. The dosage prescribed often depends on the bioavailability of the drug for the specific route of administration (see Chapter 42, I. Pharmacokinetics, for definition and discussion of bioavailability). For example, many medications require higher oral dosages than intravenous dosages and an oral dosage given intravenously could result in toxic adverse effects.

3. Error-prone abbreviations. Many health care organizations such as the Institute for Safe Medication Practices (ISMP) and the Joint Commission on Accreditation of Healthcare Organizations (JCAHO) support avoiding error-prone abbreviations when ordering medications. There are many abbreviations that have routinely resulted in harmful errors. A few examples of abbreviations to avoid include:

a. q.d or QD. Although the usual intended meaning of this abbreviation is once daily, it has been mistaken as q.i.d (4 times daily) or q.o.d. (every other day). It is recommended to use the word "daily" instead.

b. q.o.d. or QOD. This may be interpreted as q.d. or QD. Use "every other day" instead.

c. U or u. This abbreviation commonly used for "unit" has resulted in insulin errors because U may be read as 0 or 4. For example 2U may be read as 20. Using the word "unit" instead of U or u will help to avoid these errors.

d. Leading and trailing zeros. Avoiding trailing zeros will help to prevent dosing errors. 2.0 mg may be seen as 20 mg if the decimal point is not seen. In addition, using a leading zero is recommended when ordering dosages less than 1mg. Avoid potential errors by using 0.1 mg rather than .1 mg.

II. Educating the patient.

When educating the patient about medications, the following information must be included:

A. The prescribed drug.

B. The purpose and actions of the drug.

C. The frequency, dosage and route of administration of the drug.

D. The major side effects of the drug.

III. Fostering adherence.

Nurses can be particularly influential in promoting patient adherence because of their prolonged and involved contact with the patient. Some of the mechanisms that have been documented by research to be helpful in fostering patient adherence include:

A. Helping the patient understand the rationale for treatment.

B. Encouraging the patient to become an active participant in the therapy.

C. Simplifying the medication regimen to fit the patient's daily routine.

D. Providing consistent continuity of care and supervision for the patient when he or she is assuming responsibility for the medication regimen.

E. Providing adequate, liberal amounts of feedback and positive reinforcement.

F. Encouraging the family to become involved in the therapy so they can act as a support system for the patient.

G. Providing written as well as verbal instructions and information regarding the medications.

H. Establishing contacts with the patient to help in modifying behavior.

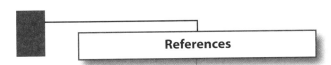

References

Aiello, J. (2002). Anemia management protocols and epoetin alfa administration: An algorithm approach. Case study of the anemic patient. *Nephrology Nursing Journal, 29*(3), 297-300.

Arnoff, G.R., Berns, J.S., Brier, M.E., Golper, T.A., Morrison, G., Singer, I., et al. (1999). *Drug prescribing in renal failure* (4th ed.). Philadelphia: American College of Physicians.

Brommage, D., & Gallgano, C. (2005). The role of cinacalcet in treating secondary hyperparathyroidism. *Nephrology Nursing Journal, 32*(2), 229-231.

Brunton, L.L., Lazo, J.S., Buxton, I.L.O., & Blumenthal, D.K. (2006). *Goodman & Gilman's the pharmacologic basis of therapeutics* (11th ed.). New York: McGraw-Hill.

Chmielewski, C. (2002). Aranesp (darbepoetin alfa): A new erythropoiesis-stimulating protein. *Nephrology Nursing Journal 29*(1), 67-68.

Curtin, R.B., Svarstad, B.L., & Keller, T.H. (1999). Hemodialysis patients' noncompliance with oral medications. *ANNA Journal, 26*(3), 307-316.

DiPiro, J.T., Talbert, R.L., Yee, G.C., Matzke, G.R., Wells, B.G., & Posey, L.M. (2005). *Pharmacotherapy: A pathophysiologic approach* (6th ed.). New York: McGraw-Hill.

Drug facts and comparisons. (2006). St. Louis: Wolters Kluwer Company.

Food and Drug Administration (FDA). (1998). *Medication errors.* Retrieved October 24, 2006, from http://www.fda.gov/cder/handbook/mederror.htm

Foret, J.P. (2002). Diagnosing and treating anemia and iron deficiency in hemodialysis patients. *Nephrology Nursing Journal 2*(3), 292-296.

Katzung, B.G. (2004). *Basic and clinical pharmacology* (9th ed.). New York: McGraw-Hill.

Michael, M., & Garcia, D. (2004). Secondary hyperparathyroidism in chronic kidney disease: Clinical consequences and challenges. *Nephrology Nursing Journal 31*(2),185-194.

Minneman, K.P. (2004). *Brody's human pharmacology: Molecular to clinical* (4th ed.). St. Louis: Mosby.

National Kidney Foundation (NKF). (2002). K/DOQI clinical practice guidelines for chronic kidney disease: Evaluation, classification and stratification. *American Journal of Kidney Diseases, 39*(Suppl. 1), S1-S246.

National Kidney Foundation (NKF). (2003a). K/DOQI clinical practice guidelines for bone metabolism and disease in chronic kidney disease. *American Journal of Kidney Diseases, 42*(Suppl. 3), S1-S202.

National Kidney Foundation (NKF). (2003b). K/DOQI clinical practice guidelines for managing dyslipidemias in chronic kidney disease. *American Journal of Kidney Diseases, 41*(Suppl. 3), S1-S92.

National Kidney Foundation (NKF). (2004). K/DOQI clinical practice guidelines on hypertension and antihypertensive agents in chronic kidney disease. *American Journal of Kidney Diseases, 43*(Suppl. 1), S1-S290.

National Kidney Foundation (NKF). (2005). K/DOQI clinical practice guidelines for cardiovascular disease in dialysis patients. *American Journal of Kidney Diseases, 45*(Suppl. 3), S1-S154.

National Kidney Foundation (NKF). (2006). K/DOQI clinical practice guidelines and clinical practice recommendations for anemia in chronic kidney disease. *American Journal of Kidney Diseases, 47*(Suppl. 3), S1-S85.

Vogel, S., Schweitzer, S., & Seiler, S. (1999). Iron management: Innovative solutions to persistent challenges – Focus on Ferrlecit. *ANNA Journal 26*(5), 515-521.

Wish, J.B., & Weigel, K.A. (2001). Management of anemia in chronic kidney disease (predialysis) patients: Nephrology nursing implications. *Nephrology Nursing Journal, 28*(3), 341-345.

Section 10

Transplantation

Section Editor

Kim Alleman, MS, RN, FNP-C, APRN, CNN

Authors

Kim Alleman, MS, RN, FNP-C, APRN, CNN

Sharon Longton, BSN, RN, CNN, CCTC

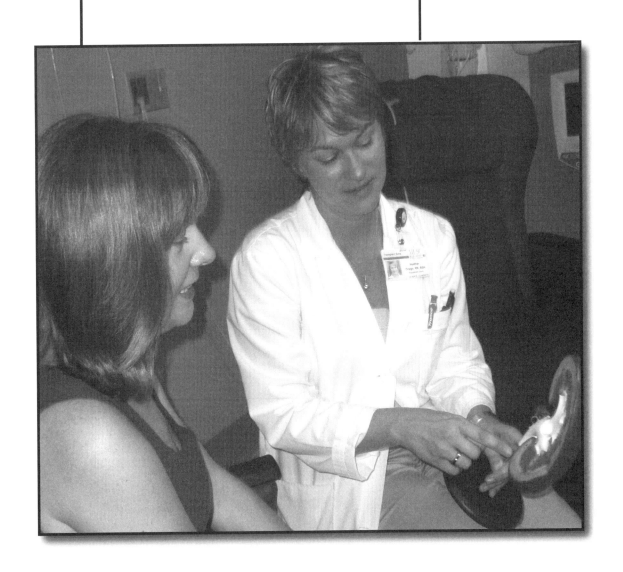

About the Authors

Kim Alleman, MS, RN, FNP-C, APRN, CNN, Section Editor and Author, is a Nurse Practitioner at the Hartford Hospital Transplant Program in Hartford, Connecticut.

Sharon Longton, BSN, RN, CNN, CCTC, is a Kidney/Pancreas Transplant Coordinator at Harper University Hospital in Detroit, Michigan.

Acknowledgment

Thanks to Roberta Billman, MSN, RN, CNN, CCTC, for her contribution to the chapter on kidney transplantation in this section. Her helpfulness and assistance in preparing the introduction are greatly appreciated.

Thanks also to the previous authors of this material:

Nancy M. Albert
Marilyn Rossman Bartucci
Mandy Bass
Jerita Payne
Barbara Schanbacher

Section 10

Transplantation

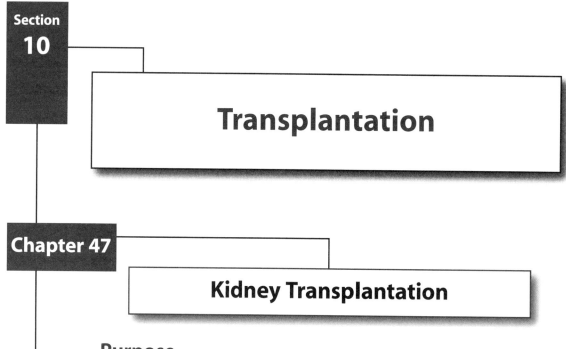

Section 10

Transplantation

Chapter 47

Kidney Transplantation

Purpose

The purpose of this chapter is to discuss concepts of kidney transplantation.

Objectives

Upon completion of this chapter, the learner will be able to:
1. Discuss important historical events related to organ transplantation.
2. Discuss patient acceptance criteria for kidney transplantation.
3. Define transplant rejection.
4. Describe the pathophysiology of an acute rejection episode.
5. Discuss the signs and symptoms of the different types of rejection.
6. Explain methods for modification of the immune system as related to organ transplantation.
7. List major side effects of selected immunosuppressive agents.
8. Discuss criteria for living and deceased donors.
9. Outline the preoperative care of the kidney transplant recipient.
10. Describe the operative procedure for the kidney transplant recipient and living donor.
11. Develop a collaborative care plan for the transplant recipient during the postoperative period.
12. Discuss long-term complications of kidney transplantation.

Introduction

A. Kidney transplantation has evolved from an experimental procedure to an accepted modality for kidney replacement therapy. The 1950s offered the first long-term successful transplant. Since that period of time, advances in immunosuppression, understanding of the immune system, and refinement of surgical techniques have served to improve the morbidity and mortality of patients with chronic kidney disease.

B. Overview of statistics.
1. Kidney transplantation is the preferred treatment modality for patients with CKD stage 4–5 end-stage renal disease (ESRD). It is not a cure.
2. Pre-emptive kidney transplantation (transplant prior to dialysis) is the best option, but this only happens in about 2% of the ESRD population and usually with an available living donor.
3. A patient must have a glomerular filtration rate (GFR) less than or equal to 20 cc per minute in order to gain waiting time points on the United Network for Organ Sharing (UNOS) List.
4. Overall graft survival is 89% at 1 year and 66% at 5 years. The actual half-life is less than 10 years for deceased (formerly referred to as "cadaveric") donor kidney transplants.
5. Survival statistics.
   a. Patient survival at 1 year with a deceased donor transplant is 94.2%.
   b. Patient survival at 5 years with a deceased donor transplant is 80.2%.
   c. Graft survival at 1 year with a deceased donor transplant is 88.7%.
   d. Graft survival at 5 years with a deceased donor transplant is 65.7%.
   e. Patient survival at 1 year with a living donor transplant is 97.5%.
   f. Patient survival at 5 years with a living donor is 90.1%.
   g. Graft survival at 1 year with a living donor is 94.3%.
   h. Graft survival at 5 years with a living donor is 78.6%.
6. The transplant process can be viewed in four phases.
   a. Pretransplant.
   b. Maintenance on the list.
   c. Transplant.
   d. Posttransplant.

C. Brief history of transplantation.
1. Surgical techniques for vascular suturing were first developed in the early 20th century by Drs. Alexis Carrel and Charles Guthrie.
2. The first successful kidney transplant was performed by Dr. Joseph Murray and Dr. Hartwell Harrison in 1954, at Peter Bent Brigham Hospital in Boston. The kidney was donated by an identical twin.
3. The importance of the immune system and immunology began to be recognized and understood, first during World War II, then even more so during the 1950s.
4. The development and refinement of immunosuppressive medications and regimens have continued to advance the field.
5. Tissue typing became the accepted procedure to match donor and recipient in 1962.
6. Later in the 1960s, the relationship between a positive crossmatch and hyperacute rejection was recognized.
7. In the 1970s, the use of deceased organ donors became accepted practice, and the concept of brain death was established.
8. In 1972, a landmark contribution to end-stage renal disease treatment was the passage of Public Law 92-603 (HR-1), which legislated Medicare coverage for dialysis and kidney transplantation.
9. In 1978, cyclosporine was first used in clinical trials as an immunosuppressant.
10. In 1978, the use of HLA-DR matching became accepted practice.
11. In 1987, the United Network for Organ Sharing was awarded the federal government contract to govern organ sharing distribution and establish scientific registries.
12. Development of newer immunosuppressants, antibody reduction protocols, clearer understanding of immunology, and other research continue to advance the field.

Organ Donation and Preservation

I. **Living donor.**

A. Related or biologically related: parent, sibling, child, aunt, uncle, cousin, and grandparent.

B. Unrelated or biologically unrelated: spouse, in-laws, adoptive parent, friend, significant other, and anonymous or altruistic.

C. Evaluation.
  1. Information/explanation of process.
    a. Information on donation process.
      (1) Orientation conference.
      (2) Review benefits and risks to recipient.
        (a) Explain an additional treatment option for CKD.
        (b) Procedure is elective, not life-saving.
      (3) Risks to donor.
      (4) Donor evaluation process.
      (5) Postoperative recovery.
      (6) Long-term risks and benefits.
    b. Discuss with someone who has donated a kidney.
    c. Psychosocial assessment may include social worker, psychiatric nurse, psychologist, and/or psychiatrist.
    d. Assessment of willingness to donate.
      (1) Assess family dynamics.
      (2) Relationship between donor and recipient.
      (3) Consideration of other family members opinion on donation.
    e. Financial considerations.
      (1) Potential future health insurance implications.
      (2) Personal/family expenses while off work for evaluation and postoperative recovery.
      (3) Travel to transplant center for donation.
    f. Implications of recipient graft loss or death.
  2. Medical assessment.
    a. ABO typing.
    b. Histocompatibility testing.
    c. Age – generally between 18 and 65.
    d. Thorough health history and physical assessment.
      (1) Rule out hypertension, diabetes mellitus, cardiovascular disease, chronic obstructive pulmonary disease, kidney disease, malignancies, infections, substance abuse, obesity, current pregnancy, and other systemic diseases with implications for renal involvement.
      (2) Review family and social history.
      (3) Review current medications, non-prescription medications, and herbal preparations.
    e. Chest x-ray.
    f. EKG.
    g. Hematology, chemistries, serologies, and cultures.
    h. Urine studies to assess kidney function.
    i. Spiral CT scan or MRI/MRA to document anatomy of kidneys, ureter, bladder.

D. Living donor procedures.
  1. Pretransplant cytotoxic crossmatch with recipient sera.
  2. Surgical procedure.
    a. Open nephrectomy.
      (1) Flank incision.
      (2) Left side preferred but dependent on anatomy.
      (3) The procedure usually takes 4 to 6 hours.
    b. Laparoscopic donor nephrectomy.
      (1) Minimally invasive.
      (2) Three small incisions.
      (3) Less postoperative morbidity, less pain, shorter hospital stay and earlier return to work.
    c. Hand-assisted laparascopic donor nephrectomy.
      (1) Similar to laparoscopic donor nephrectomy.
      (2) A small abdominal incision is created for the surgeon to place his/her hand through a pneumosleeve to remove the kidney.
      (3) This decreases the operative time and warm ischemic time for the kidney.
  3. Postoperative nursing care.
    a. Frequent monitoring of vital signs.
    b. Meticulous pulmonary toilet.
    c. Early ambulation.
    d. Maintenance of fluid and electrolyte balance.
    e. Record intake and output.
    f. Monitor for signs of bleeding.
    g. Daily weights.
    h. Prevent infection.
      (1) Frequent coughing and deep breathing.
      (2) Aseptic wound care.
      (3) Aseptic intravenous line care.
      (4) Urinary catheter care.
    i. Pain control.
      (1) Analgesia (preferably patient controlled) as needed.
      (2) Monitor bowel function because of constipation from narcotic use.
    j. Emotional support.
    k. Patient education.

II. Deceased donor.

A. Criteria.
  1. Heart beating donor must have irreversible cessation of spontaneous brain function (brain death).
    a. No seizures or posturing.
    b. No response to pain in cranial nerve distribution; spinal reflexes may be present.

c. Apnea in response to acidosis or hypercarbia.
d. No pupillary or corneal reflexes.
e. No oculocephalic or vestibular reflexes.
f. No tracheobronchial reflexes.
g. Absent brain stem function.
2. Expanded criteria donors.
    a. Non-heart-beating.
        (1) Controlled situation.
        (2) Irreversible brain injury, but does not meet criteria for brain death.
        (3) Discontinuation of ventilatory support in a controlled environment. Cardiopulmonary arrest occurs within one hour of discontinuation of ventilatory support.
        (4) Family gives informed consent prior to discontinuation of ventilatory support.
    b. Uncontrolled situation.
        (1) Cardiopulmonary arrest occurs.
        (2) No response to cardiopulmonary resuscitation and death is declared.
        (3) Family gives informed consent.
        (4) Organs are recovered immediately to minimize warm ischemic time.
    c. Older donors (60 years or greater).
    d. Donors aged 50–59 with history of cerebral vascular accident (CVA), hypertension, and/or creatinine > 1.5 mg/dL.
    e. Medical conditions associated with decreased graft survival.
        (1) Diabetes.
        (2) Hypertension.
        (3) Certain infections.
            (a) Hepatitis B.
            (b) Hepatitis C.
            (c) Other infections when cleared by infectious disease specialist.
        (4) High risk social behavior.
        (5) Hemodynamic instability.
        (6) Chemical imbalances.
        (7) Increased organ preservation time.
    f. The kidneys are usually biopsied prior to transplantation.
3. Medical criteria for deceased donors.
    a. Absence of malignancy except for some primary brain tumors or skin cancers.
    b. Absence of active systemic infections or transmissible disease.
    c. Absence of significant kidney disease or uncontrolled hypertension.
    d. Generally less than 70 years of age.
    e. Evaluation of organ function.
    f. No high risk behaviors for transmissible diseases.

4. Deceased donor care.
    a. Maintenance of adequate blood pressure and urine output with intravenous solution, such as crystalloid, colloid, and inotropic medications.
    b. Support for the donor family throughout the process.
5. Other considerations.
    a. Mandatory request protocols for every hospital require the designated trained hospital representative (physician, nurse, chaplain, social worker) to offer the option of organ and tissue donation to families of patients who meet the criteria for donation.
    b. Permission is obtained from next of kin.
    c. Impact of multiorgan procurement.
        (1) The retrieval process for multiple organs and tissues may result in multiple teams congregating at once.
        (2) May cause delays in the organ recovery process.
        (3) Occasionally is an obstacle to achieving an efficient organ donation process.
    d. Education of health care professionals, especially those that work in the critical care units and emergency departments, about the need for organs and tissues is an important part of organ donor care.
    e. Organ recovery.
        (1) Minimize warm ischemia time using in situ flush of cold intracellular solution. The acceptable limit of warm ischemia time is 0 to 5 minutes.
        (2) Preserving vasculature requires careful techniques to prevent intimal tears in the renal veins and arteries, which may result in thrombosis or partial occlusion and loss of graft.
        (3) Coordination of multiorgan retrieval.
    f. Organ preservation.
        (1) Cold storage. Kidneys are flushed with cold intracellular solution, packed in sterile containers, and packed in ice (most common method of storage).
        (2) Pulsatile perfusion. The perfusion machine pumps cool solutions through the renal vasculature to continuously cool, oxygenate, and allow for longer storage times than the simple cold storage provides.
        (3) The viability of the organs remain intact for as long as 72 hours regardless of preservation method used. The goal is to transplant the kidney in less than 24 hours to reduce the possibility of delayed graft function.

g. Histocompatibility testing is done as soon as possible after donor identification. Crossmatching is done with potential recipients.

III. Organ sharing and distribution.

A. Organ Procurement and Transplant Network (OPTN). Its purpose is to assure that each person on the waiting list has equitable access to organs. It also serves to maintain a scientific registry for organ donations and transplant procedures as legislated by the National Transplant Act of 1984.

B. United Network for Organ Sharing (UNOS).
   1. Awarded the OPTN contract in 1986.
   2. Established membership standards for transplant centers and organ procurement organizations (OPO).
   3. Established an equitable organ allocation system. Allocation based on an objective point system consisting of:
      a. ABO matching.
      b. Histocompatibility matching.
      c. Pediatric status.
      d. Waiting time on the list.
      e. Level of preformed antibodies.
      f. Medical urgency.
      g. Standardized listing criteria (i.e., creatinine clearance < 20 mL/min).
      h. Previous kidney donor.
   4. Organs distributed locally, regionally, and nationally. Mandatory sharing of six antigen, or phenotypically identically matched kidney, must be offered to the patient (transplant center) no matter where located. UNOS data and data from the Renal Transplant Registry support the superior success rates in these patients.
   5. Monitors distribution of all organs in the United States.
   6. Maintains scientific registries for all organs to facilitate data acquisition and management.
   7. Facilitates organ placement throughout the country.

Organ Transplantation

I. Definition of terminology.

A. Autograft. Transplantation of a person's own tissue from one body site to another (e.g., skin or a vein

for a coronary artery bypass graft). Because no foreign antigens are introduced, there is no problem with rejection of an autograft.

B. Isograft. Transplantation of tissues between monozygotic identical (same genetic make-up) twins.

C. Allograft or homograft. Transplantation of tissues between of the same species (from one person to another with different genetic make-up). Because foreign antigens are introduced into the recipient, rejection of an allograft is a possibility.

D. Xenograft. Transplantation of tissues between members of different species. Because of the extreme antigenic differences between the donor and recipient of a xenograft, the incidence of rejection is very high.

II. Evaluation of the kidney transplant candidate.

A. All Medicare ESRD patients are entitled to be referred for transplant.

B. The patient is referred to a transplant center by the nephrologist, nurse, or social worker at the dialysis unit. Some patients are self-referred.

C. Early referral, prior to initiation of dialysis, is encouraged.

D. The purpose of the pretransplant evaluation is to determine the patient's suitability for transplant by identifying and, where possible, correcting those medical and psychosocial factors that would affect a successful outcome in the short and long term.

E. A patient's candidacy is considered on an individual basis. Broad groups of patients are no longer automatically excluded.

F. Transplant centers vary in the way that they accomplish the evaluation, but the transplant team members in this initial phase usually include:
   1. Transplant Coordinator.
   2. Transplant Surgeon.
   3. Transplant Nephrologist.
   4. Transplant Social Worker.
   5. Financial Coordinator.
   6. Dietitian.

III. Pretransplant patient education.

A. An informational session allows the patient to consider if transplantation is the right choice for him/her.

B. Patient education about transplant includes:
1. Transplant as one of the options for CKD stage 5, but not a "cure."
2. Patient and graft survival statistics.
3. The risks and benefits of transplantation.
4. Potential complications of surgery and immunosuppression.
5. Potential long-term complications including, but not limited to rejection, infection, malignancy, and diabetes.
6. Sources of donors.
    a. Living.
        (1) Living related.
        (2) Living unrelated.
        (3) Good samaritan (also known as altruistic).
    b. Deceased.
        (1) Standard.
        (2) Expanded.
        (3) Donation after cardiac death.
7. Advantages and disadvantages of both.
8. Small but possible risk of disease transmission (infection, cancer) despite donor testing.
9. Discussion regarding the illegality of buying and selling of organs.
10. UNOS policy and the center's policy regarding nontraditional donors; solicitation of donors, including the Internet.
11. UNOS Waiting List and organ allocation policies.
12. Options of multiple listing and wait time transfer.
13. Discussion of special programs throughout the country.
    a. Living donor paired exchange ("Swap").
    b. ABO incompatible recipient and donor.
    c. Crossmatch positive recipient and donor.
    d. HIV positive patients.
    e. Older patients (> age 70).
14. Rights and responsibilities of patients and transplant staff.
15. Other educational resources.
    a. UNOS (United Network for Organ Sharing).
    b. NKF (National Kidney Foundation).
    c. AKF (American Kidney Fund).
    d. AST (American Society of Transplant).
    e. ANNA (American Nephrology Nurses' Association).
    f. ITNS (International Transplant Nurses Society).

IV. Workup and selection of potential recipient.

A. Every transplant center has its own acceptance criteria for candidacy, protocol for evaluation, and absolute and relative contraindications. However, most centers are in agreement regarding major indications and contraindications for transplant.

B. Contraindications.
1. Current or recent malignancy (excluding noninvasive skin cancers).
2. Active or chronic untreated infection.
3. Severe irreversible extrarenal disease (e.g., inoperable cardiac disease, chronic lung disease, severe peripheral vascular disease).
4. Active autoimmune disease.
5. Morbid obesity (BMI > 35).
6. Current substance abuse.
7. Psychiatric illness that would prevent informed consent or adherence to treatment regimen.
8. Significant history of nonadherence to treatment regimens.

C. History and physical examination.
1. Age.
    a. Physiologic age is more important than chronologic age.
    b. Patients over age 70 are accepted at some centers.
    c. Older patients are at increased risk of death related to cardiovascular disease.
    d. Rejection episodes may be less due to a less reactive immune system in older adults.
    e. For pediatric patients transplant is the treatment of choice, and when possible, pre-emptive with a living donor.
2. Etiology of renal disease.
    a. Determine native kidney disease.
        (1) Obtain renal biopsy results, if done.
        (2) Important to know the cause since some diseases can recur in the transplanted kidney and some have comorbidities that could influence outcome.
        (3) It can also affect the type of donor chosen, especially when living donation is being considered.
    b. Type of dialysis, how long, response to treatment.
    c. Determine if patient has had a previous transplant. It is important to know transplant course, treatment, and complications to assess risk in next transplant.
    d. Diabetes mellitus is associated with cerebro-vascular disease, peripheral vascular disease, infections, gastroparesis, and neuropathy

(neurogenic bladder). All can increase the risk for perioperative and postoperative complications.

e. Autoimmune diseases need to be quiescent prior to transplant.

f. Polycystic kidney disease may require nephrectomy prior to or after transplant if very enlarged or excessive bleeding from cysts or recurrent infections. May need cerebral imaging to rule out associated aneurysm. PKD can be inherited in families and must be taken into consideration if considering living related donor.

g. Alport's syndrome is also familial.

h. Chronic pyelonephritis may also require nephrectomy to prevent infection post-transplant.

i. Many diseases may recur in the transplanted kidney including focal and segmental glomerulosclerosis (FSGS), MPGN I and II, IgA nephropathy, membranous nephropathy, diabetic nephropathy, certain types of oxalosis, Wegener's disease, Fabry disease, systemic lupus erythematosis, and thrombotic thrombocytopenic purpura (TTP).

3. Urinary tract.

a. Patients with a history of recurrent infection, reflux, kidney or bladder stones, chronic urinary diversion, bladder dysfunction, neurogenic bladder, benign prostatic hypertrophy, or obstructive uropathy will require evaluation to ensure bladder function after transplant.

b. The patient must be free of active urinary tract infections.

c. Urine output is important to assess before transplant as it may be important to assess early function of the allograft.

d. Assessment of bladder function.

(1) The potential recipient must have a functional bladder, or successful renal transplantation may be performed in patients with ileal conduits or other methods of urinary diversion.

(2) Patients with neurogenic bladders or atonicity may be required to perform periodic self-catheterization.

(3) Voiding cystourethrogram with postvoid films, if indicated.

(4) Urodynamic studies, if indicated.

(5) Routine urinalysis and culture, if indicated.

(6) Catheterization for postvoid residual, if indicated.

(7) Evaluation by a urologist, if indicated.

4. Cardiovascular system.

a. Cardiac disease is the leading cause of death with functioning graft in transplant recipients.

b. Risk of surgery is increased by ischemic heart disease, therefore pre-emptive treatment, medically or surgically, is recommended.

c. Patients with peripheral vascular disease and/or aortoiliac disease may have compromised blood flow to the transplanted kidney or lower extremities.

d. Patients with a history of claudication, lower-extremity amputations, history of cardiovascular or cerebrovascular disease warrant further investigation.

e. The patient must have:

(1) Adequate cardiac function.

(2) Patent iliac vasculature.

(3) Absence of severe atherosclerosis.

(4) A thorough assessment of prior cardiac and vascular events.

(5) Corrective interventions prior to transplantation: coronary artery bypass surgery, stent placement, valve replacement, peripheral bypass surgery.

f. Screening of asymptomatic patients with risk factors for coronary artery disease is recommended.

g. Assessment.

(1) History and physical examination.

(2) EKG.

(3) Echocardiogram, if indicated.

(4) If there are any positive findings in the history, the patient may also need stress testing, cardiac catheterization, evaluation by a cardiologist, and Doppler studies.

(5) CT or MRA of abdominal and pelvic vessels, if indicated.

(6) Noninvasive lower extremity arterial studies with measurement of ABI (ankle brachial index), if indicated.

(7) Angiography, if indicated.

(8) Evaluation by vascular surgeon, if indicated.

5. Pulmonary system.

a. The potential for posttransplant pulmonary complications in the immunosuppressed host must be evaluated prior to transplantation.

b. Lung disease can increase the risk of anesthesia and surgery. Fluid overload, ventilator dependency, and pneumonia are all potential complications.

c. Patients with a history of chronic obstructive lung disease or restrictive lung disease may need further evaluation.

d. Patients who smoke tobacco should be encouraged to stop. Some programs do not transplant patients who are currently smoking.

e. Patients with a positive PPD should be treated prophylactically with INH for 6 months.

f. Assessment.
   (1) History and physical examination.
   (2) Chest x-ray, PA and lateral views.
   (3) Pulmonary function studies, if indicated.
   (4) PPD testing, if indicated.
   (5) Pneumococcal pneumonia immunization.
   (6) Evaluation by a pulmonologist, if indicated.

6. Neurologic system.
   a. Patients with a history of CVA, TIA, seizure disorder, or other neurologic event are at risk for increased complications in perioperative and postoperative periods.
   b. Anti-seizure medications may need to be changed because of potential interaction with immunosuppressives. This should be done in collaboration with the patient's neurologist.
   c. Assessment.
      (1) History and physical.
      (2) Carotid duplex.
      (3) Brain imaging for PKD patients with history of headaches or sudden death in family to rule out cerebral aneurysm.
      (4) Evaluation by a neurologist, if indicated.

7. Gastrointestinal system.
   a. Active peptic ulcer disease, pancreatitis, cholecystitis, and diverticulitis must be medically or surgically treated to prevent complications associated with the use of immunosuppressive medications after transplant.
   b. Active or chronic liver disease must be evaluated.
   c. Liver enzyme elevations must be investigated.
   d. The patient with severe gastroparesis must have a thorough evaluation of his or her gastric emptying ability.
   e. Esophageal infections must be completely treated prior to transplantation.
   f. Assessment.
      (1) History and physical examination.
      (2) Stool examination for occult blood.
      (3) Radiologic studies as indicated.
      (4) Depending on age, colonoscopy and/or barium enema.
      (5) Hepatitis B immunization.
      (6) Liver function tests and hepatitis B and C screening.
      (7) Evaluation by a gastroenterologist and/or hepatologist.

8. Endocrine system.
   a. Evaluation and treatment of hyperparathyroidism is completed prior to transplantation.
   b. Evaluation of patient with diabetes.
   c. Females must have recent (within 12 months) gynecologic examination, PAP smear (if sexually active or > 18 years of age), and mammogram (if 40 or older, or at high risk for breast cancer).
   d. Assessment.
      (1) History and physical examination.
      (2) Parathyroid hormone level, serum calcium, and phosphorus.
      (3) Pap smear.
      (4) Mammogram.

9. Dental system.
   a. Teeth or gum disease must be resolved prior to transplantation.
   b. Presence of infected teeth or gums may threaten the life of the postoperative immunosuppressed patient.
   c. Assessment.
      (1) History and physical examination.
      (2) Statement from dentist regarding status of teeth and gums.

10. Cancer screening.
    a. Patients with ESRD have a higher risk of cancer than the general population.
    b. Patients who underwent immunosuppression for treatment of their original kidney disease or for a prior transplant are at increased risk for cancer.
    c. Prior history of cancer that was treated does not preclude transplant.
       (1) Each patient should be individually evaluated regarding risk of recurrence and time frame for transplantation.
       (2) A waiting period of 2–5 years, depending on the malignancy is recommended.
       (3) No waiting period may be necessary for malignancies with a low chance of metastasis such as basal cell carcinomas, encapsulated renal cell carcinoma, primary CNS tumors, and in-situ tumors.
    d. All patients should have routine cancer screenings according to American Cancer Society guidelines.

11. Infection.
    a. Infections are a major cause of morbidity and mortality after transplantation.
    b. An active infection is a contraindication to transplant.
    c. Patients with hepatitis B or C may be

considered for kidney transplantation after evaluation including viral load and liver biopsy. Antiviral therapy prior to transplant may be done.

   d. Assessment.

     (1) History and physical examination.

     (2) Viral and fungal screening (CMV, EBV, and varicella in children).

     (3) Hepatitis B and C screening.

12. Immunologic system.

   a. A thorough assessment of immunologic status will aid in predicting the graft outcome.

   b. Previous transplants, blood transfusions, and pregnancy may alter the host response to additional foreign antigens.

   c. Autoimmune diseases must be quiescent before transplantation is undertaken.

   d. Pretransplant modification of the immune system.

     (1) Splenectomy, total body irradiation, and thoracic lymph duct drainage were once used to decrease the number of circulating lymphocytes. These procedures are rarely used presently.

     (2) Plasmapheresis is sometimes used to decrease the presence of cytotoxic antibodies. This is usually done in the form of an antibody reduction protocol in conjunction with intravenous immunoglobulin and immunosuppression.

   e. Assessment.

     (1) ABO testing identifies the blood type of the donor and recipient. The following shows acceptable donor to recipient combinations.

Donor Blood Type	Compatible Recipient Blood Type
O	O, A, B, AB
A	A, AB
B	B, AB
AB	AB only

     (2) Histocompatibility testing is the detection of antigens on cell membranes or in cell walls that determines the genetic composition and defines whether foreign tissue is accepted or rejected by the host.

     (3) Cytotoxic screening or panel reactive antibodies (PRA) is a blood test using lymphocytotoxic antibodies obtained from multiparous females or from recipients of multiple blood transfusions to determine the presence of preformed antibodies to human leukocyte antigens (HLA). The results range from 0% to 100% and reflect the percentage of antigens on the test panel against which the potential recipient has preformed antibodies.

     (4) Review of transfusion history since last serum sample submitted for cytotoxic screening.

     (5) Review of status of autoimmune disease (titers). Transplantation cannot be performed in the presence of active autoimmune disease processes, which may adversely affect the transplanted kidney (e.g., if the patient has lupus, it is important to wait until quiescent).

     (6) Review of pregnancy history. Challenges to the immune system (multiple pregnancies) may result in the development of significant cytotoxic antibodies.

     (7) Review of HLA antigens of previous transplants. Exposure to foreign HLA antigens from prior transplants may result in development of specific antibody.

     (8) A current, positive cytotoxic T cell crossmatch between donor and recipient lymphocytes, indicating the presence of preformed antibodies, is an absolute contraindication to transplantation. Most centers have adopted protocols relating to the T cell and B cell crossmatches with respect to length of negativity.

     (9) Some centers use flow cytometry crossmatches to detect very low levels of circulating antibodies, especially in high-risk patients (e.g., retransplants). False positives may be a limitation of this crossmatch.

13. Other medical conditions.

   a. Hypercoagulable state.

     (1) Prevalence of thrombophilia in the CKD population increases the risk of graft loss due to renal vein or artery thrombosis.

     (2) History of thrombosis, multiple clotting of AV fistulas or grafts, requires more in-depth coagulation screening and possible referral to a hematologist.

     (3) Assessment.

       (a) Prior history of deep vein thrombosis (DVT).

       (b) Further laboratory tests as indicated.

         [1] Antiphospholipid antibodies.

         [2] Lupus anticoagulant.

         [3] Anticardiolipin antibody.

[4] Protein C.
[5] Protein S.
[6] Homocysteine.
[7] Factor V Leiden.
[8] Prothrombin gene mutation (G20210A).
[9] Antithrombin III.
[10] Activated Protein C.
(c) Evaluation by a hematologist, as indicated.
b. Obesity.
(1) Obese patients are at greater risk for delayed graft function, surgical/wound complications, posttransplant diabetes mellitus, and cardiovascular disease.
(2) A BMI (Body Mass Index) of > 30 kg/m² is considered a contraindication to transplant at some centers, although many centers consider it up to 35, or look at the patient on a case by case basis.
(3) Weight loss is recommended.
(4) Bariatric surgery for those morbidly obese may be considered.
c. Diabetes.
(1) Transplantation is preferred renal replacement therapy because of a greater potential for rehabilitation and decreased incidence of cardiac disease and stroke, as compared to remaining on dialysis.
(2) Consider simultaneous kidney/pancreas transplantation for type I diabetics to prevent recurrence of diabetic complications in the renal graft and prevent or delay other secondary complications of diabetes.
(3) Assessment.
(a) Meticulous assessment of cardiac function.
[1] Stress testing.
[2] Cardiac catheterization, some centers do even if stress test is normal.
[3] Cardiology evaluation.
(b) Ophthalmologic examination (protocols vary).
(c) Neurologic evaluation.
(d) Gastrointestinal evaluation.
(e) Urologic evaluation.
14. Psychosocial system.
a. Social work interview with patient and family provides information about the patient's illness history, coping ability, and support system, all of which can impact transplant outcome.

b. Should determine patient's ability to provide informed consent.
c. Patient and staff should use the pretransplant period to plan for transplant surgery and posttransplant needs.
(1) Getting to the hospital for transplant.
(2) Assistance at home after surgery.
(3) Transportation to follow-up clinic visits.
(4) Adequate medical and medication coverage.
d. Assessment.
(1) Adjustment and understanding of present illness and therapy options.
(2) Living situation.
(3) Educational background.
(4) Employment history.
(5) Lifestyle prior to illness.
(6) Adherence to treatment regimen.
(a) Dialyzes as scheduled or misses treatments, doctors' appointments?
(b) Takes medications as prescribed?
(c) Follows diet?
(7) History of substance abuse.
(8) History of psychiatric illness.
(9) Medical insurance and drug coverage for transplant medications.
(10) Financial resources.
(11) The financial coordinator gives financial clearance for the transplant and frequently works in tandem with the social worker regarding the last two issues.

V. Role of the referring physician.

A. May perform the candidate evaluation using local consultants and resources in collaboration with the transplant center.

B. Communication between referring physician and transplant center is essential.

C. Transplant center must provide written and verbal reports of hospitalizations and transplant clinic visits.

VI. Immediate preoperative care of the kidney transplant recipient.

A. Preparation for surgery.
1. Communication with referring physician regarding patient's candidacy.
a. Any current illnesses that may preclude transplantation.
b. Determine when patient was last dialyzed.

2. NPO for 6 to 8 hours before surgery to prevent perioperative aspiration and postoperative nausea and vomiting.
3. History and physical are performed to determine that there are no current medical contraindications to transplantation.
4. Laboratory testing. Pretransplant hematology, chemistries, viral titers, and urine culture are performed to detect any abnormalities and provide baseline data for postoperative comparisons.
5. Chest x-ray to assess for fluid overload, pneumonia, or new lesions.
6. EKG obtained to document cardiac function.
7. Vital signs and baseline weight.
8. Shower and skin preparation.
9. Vascular access or peritoneal dialysis catheter assessment to assure the absence of infection.
10. Insertion of intravenous lines, peripheral and or/central lines.
11. Immunosuppression may be ordered to be given prior to the operation.
12. Antibiotics are ordered perioperatively.
13. Patient and family education.
14. A final cytotoxic crossmatch performed.

15. Pretransplant dialysis may be done if there has been significant weight gain, hyperkalemia, or fluid overload to permit safe induction of general anesthesia.

VII. The kidney transplant surgical procedure.

A. The kidney is usually placed in the anterior iliac fossa, extraperitoneally (see Figure 10.1).
　1. Adult kidneys into infants or small children may require intraperitoneal placement.
　2. Renal artery is anastomosed to external iliac artery.
　3. Renal vein is anastomosed to iliac vein.
　4. Ureter is tunneled into the bladder or anastomosed end-to-side to recipient's native ureter or anastomosed to previously created ileal conduit.

B. The anatomic placement of the graft assists in the ease of patient assessment.
　1. Ease of vascular and ureteral placement.
　2. Facilitates diagnosis of rejection.
　　a. Graft tenderness is easily assessed.
　　b. Easy access for percutaneous needle biopsy to diagnose renal allograft dysfunction.
　3. Obviates need for pretransplant native nephrectomy.

VIII. Postoperative management of the kidney transplant recipient.

A. Maintain circulatory function.
　1. Frequent monitoring of vital signs (blood pressure, temperature, pulse, respirations, central venous pressure).
　2. Monitor femoral, popliteal, and pedal pulses.
　3. Monitor cardiac status.

B. Maintain pulmonary function.
　1. Turn, cough, and deep breathe frequently.
　2. Encourage use of respiratory inspiratory devices.
　3. Early ambulation.

C. Monitor fluid and electrolyte balance.
　1. Monitor fluid intake and urine output.
　2. Daily weight.
　3. Monitor vital signs frequently, per center protocol.
　4. Replace fluids according to protocol.
　5. Daily laboratory testing to evaluate potassium, creatinine, phosphorus, etc.
　6. Physical assessment of fluid imbalance, observe for hypotension, dry mucous membranes, poor

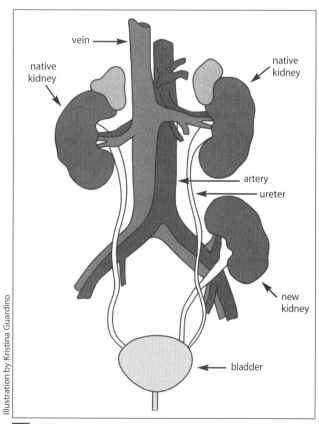

Figure 10.1. Kidney transplant placement.

Illustration by Kristina Guardino

skin turgor, concentrated urine, shortness of breath, presence of edema.
7. Administer diuretics as prescribed and monitor response.
8. Avoid hypotension due to risk of arterial or venous thrombosis and graft loss.

D. Prevention of infection.
1. Pulmonary toilet.
2. Careful hand washing techniques.
3. Promote adequate nutrition for wound healing.
4. Aseptic care of intravenous lines, wound, and urinary catheter.
5. Isolate infected patients.
6. Facilitate oral and skin hygiene.
7. Isolate recipient with leukopenia.
8. Assess patients for signs and symptoms of infection.
9. Administer prophylactic antiviral agents and antibiotics as prescribed.

E. Provide and monitor immunosuppressive regimen.

F. Assess and assist with treatment for complications.
1. Short-term complications.
   a. Rejection.
   b. Renal artery thrombosis.
      (1) Uncommon, usually occurs in early transplant period.
      (2) Requires early detection for treatment (surgical removal) to be effective.
      (3) Signs and symptoms: sudden anuria, graft tenderness.
   c. Renal vein thrombosis.
      (1) Symptoms include decreased urine output, proteinuria, hematuria, and swelling of graft, thigh, and leg.
      (2) Treated with anticoagulation therapy or attempt at surgical removal.
      (3) May require nephrectomy.
   d. Graft rupture.
      (1) Signs and symptoms: swollen painful graft and hematuria.
      (2) Usually caused by swelling of the graft during a rejection episode.
      (3) Surgical repair or graft nephrectomy is always required.
   e. Urologic complications.
      (1) Urine leak results from ureteral leakage, ureteral disruption, or leak from the bladder.
      (2) Usually a result of poor tissue healing, ureteral stenosis, or poor vascularity with tissue necrosis.

f. Delayed graft function (DGF).
   (1) Etiology.
      (a) Prolonged organ storage time before transplantation.
      (b) Prolonged warm ischemia time.
      (c) Severe rejection episode.
   (2) Symptoms.
      (a) Decreased urine volume.
      (b) Elevated BUN and creatinine.
   (3) Treatment.
      (a) Alteration of diet; decrease potassium intake.
      (b) Manage hyperkalemia.
      (c) Dialysis may be indicated.
      (d) Avoid nephrotoxic medications.
g. Acute tubular necrosis (ATN).
   (1) Etiology.
      (a) Usually an ischemic injury.
      (b) Can be volume depletion in the recipient.
      (c) Similar to DGF.
   (2) Symptoms are similar to DGF.
      (a) Decreased urine output.
      (b) Elevated BUN and creatinine.
      (c) Nonoliguric ATN (high urine volume with low clearance).
   (3) Treatment.
      (a) Alteration in diet, decrease potassium intake.
      (b) Manage hyperkalemia.
      (c) Dialysis if indicated.
g. Wound complications.
   (1) Perinephric hematomas, urinomas, lymphoceles, and abesses can mechanically compress the kidney or ureters and result in deterioration of kidney function.
   (2) Wound infection.
   (3) Signs and symptoms.
      (a) Swollen, tender allograft.
      (b) Fever.
      (c) Wound drainage.
      (d) Elevated WBC.
      (e) Lower extremity edema on same side as the transplant.
h. Metabolic. Hypertension, immuno-suppression-induced diabetes mellitus, disorders of calcium and phosphorus metabolism, Cushingoid effects.
i. Psychosocial. Depression, sexual dysfunction, adjustment to wellness, coping with body changes.
2. Long-term complications.
   a. Chronic allograft nephropathy (CAN), also known as chronic rejection.

(1) The most common cause of kidney transplant failure in the first 10 years following transplant.

(2) Slow, variable rate of decline.

(3) Proteinuria and hypertension.

(4) Other causes of graft dysfunction need to be ruled out first.

(5) Biopsy findings nonspecific.
    (a) Atherosclerosis.
    (b) Glomerular lesions.
    (c) Glomerular sclerosis.
    (d) Intersititial fibrosis.
    (e) Tubular atrophy.

(6) Risk factors.
    (a) Donor age.
    (b) Prolonged ischemic time.
    (c) Delayed graft function.
    (d) Acute rejection episodes.
    (e) Calcineurin inhibitor toxicity.
    (f) Infection.
    (g) Medication nonadherence.
    (h) Hyperlipidemia.
    (i) Cigarette smoking.
    (j) Suboptimal immunosuppression.

(7) Currently no treatment, but control of blood pressure, treatment of hyperlipidemia, and avoidance of acute rejection are thought to be most helpful. Some centers use ACE inhibitors and nonnephrotoxic immunosuppressive regimens, but more studies need to be done.

b. Gastrointestinal. Ulcers, liver disease, cholecystitis, pancreatitis.

c. Ophthalmic. Cataracts, visual disturbances.

d. Metabolic. Hypertension, immunosupression induced diabetes mellitus, disorders of calcium and phosphorus metabolism, Cushingoid effects.

e. Renal artery stenosis.
(1) Usually occurs 6–12 months after transplant, but can occur later.
(2) Uncontrolled hypertension with multiple medications, new bruit over graft.
(3) Sometimes occurs with renal dysfunction, particularly after addition of an ACE inhibitor.
(4) Can be diagnosed with ultrasound, but arteriography is definitive.
(5) Treatment includes antihypertensive therapy, surgical repair, or balloon angioplasty.

f. Cardiovascular. Hypertension, coronary artery disease, cerebral vascular disease, peripheral vascular disease.

g. Malignancy. Squamous cell skin cancer (most common), solid organ tumors, lymphomas.

h. Recurrence of original disease in the transplant.

i. Osteoporosis.
(1) Risk of osteoporosis quite high with use of glucocorticosteroids and pre-existing bone disease.
(2) Screen with bone density scan (DEXA) every 1 to 2 years.
(3) Use calcium with vitamin D supplements (in patients with normal calcium levels).
(4) Use biphosphonates or calcitonin depending on kidney function.
(5) Encourage weight-bearing exercise.

j. Posttransplant chronic kidney disease.
(1) Almost all patients have stage 2 or greater kidney disease.
(2) Use the same guidelines as for non-transplant patients with CKD.

k. Pregnancy after transplantation.
(1) Patients can have a successful pregnancy after transplantation.
(2) Usually encourage patient to wait at least one to two years after transplant and when kidney function is stable.
(3) Counsel patients on contraception as fertility usually returns after transplant.
(4) Pre-pregnancy planning includes evaluation of immunosuppression and other medications to avoid teratogenic medications, if possible.
(5) Close monitoring is required during pregnancy and at the time of delivery.

l. Obesity.
(1) Very common due to medications, liberalization of dietary restrictions, and sedentary lifestyle.
(2) Work in collaboration with patient and dietitian to help maintain a healthy weight.

G. Administer pain medication as needed.

H. Discharge planning.
1. Patient/family education begins in the early posttransplant period and consists of:
a. General postoperative care.
b. Medications: name, dose, action, frequency, and side effects.
c. Signs and symptoms of rejection: how and when to report.
d. Follow-up tests and visits to clinic: frequency and purpose.
e. Record keeping: intake and output, daily weight, temperature and blood pressure

monitoring, home-glucose monitoring.
f. Diet.
g. Posttransplant activity: when to drive, resuming sexual activity, birth control, and exercise.
h. Prevention of infection.
i. Arranging for administration of outpatient medications and treatments.
2. Scheduling for posttransplant patient follow-up.
a. Local laboratory testing and clinic visits.
b. Monitor for short and long term complications.
3. Communicate with referring physician.
4. Rehabilitation.
a. Facilitate return to pre-illness level of activity.
b. Vocational rehabilitation.
c. Financial considerations.
d. Disincentives to rehabilitation.
(1) Hiring practices of employers: fear of increased time off for illness and follow-up care.
(2) Added insurance burden to employer.
(3) Local community resources.
(4) Provision of accurate information to agencies.
(5) Potential lack of disability income.

I. Miscellaneous considerations.
1. Changes in family relationships.
a. Role reversal. Dependency to independence.
b. Recovery from illness.
c. Effective body image changes.
d. Sexual concerns.
2. Economic concerns.
a. Cost of medications and follow-up.
b. Return to employment.
c. State and local financial assistance.
d. Difficulties obtaining insurance.
e. Post-Medicare reimbursement expenses.
3. Concerns about graft failure/death.
a. First 12 months require close monitoring.
b. Potential for chronic allograft nephropathy.
c. Education and counseling regarding lifetime commitment to health care and necessity of lifetime immunosuppressive medications.
d. Importance of meticulous adherence with prescribed therapy.
e. Preparation for possible return to dialysis or retransplantation.

Pathophysiology of Organ Transplant Rejection

Rejection is the process by which the recipient's immune system recognizes and mounts an immune response to eliminate foreign antigens on transplanted tissue. The transplanted tissue or organ is destroyed in the process.

I. **Terminology – components of the immune response.**

A. Major histocompatibility complex (MHC) – a cluster of genes that controls the molecules expressed on the surface of cells (HLA molecules).

B. Human leukocyte antigen (HLA) – the primary antigens that help the body recognize "self from nonself."

C. T lymphocytes – killer cells that contain microbes or foreign cells.

D. Antigen presenting cells (APCs) – activates antigen specific T–cells.

E. Dendritic cells – initiate immune response by presenting foreign antigens to T cells.

F. Macrophage – a phagocytic cell, engulfs and destroys infectious organisms and other particles.

G. B lymphocytes – component of the humoral response, present foreign antigens to T–cells, generate antibody formation.

H. Antigen – any molecule that can be recognized by the immune system and elicit an immune response.

I. Antibody – a protein produced by lymphocytes in response to an antigen.

J. Crossmatch – recipient cells are combined with donor cells to determine the presence of antibody from the recipient toward the donor. A positive crossmatch indicates that the patient could have early graft rejection.

II. **Immune response to the transplanted kidney.**

A. The main function of the immune system is to defend against infections.

B. Direct recognition (see Figure 10.2).
1. Donor tissue is first recognized by circulating T–cells.

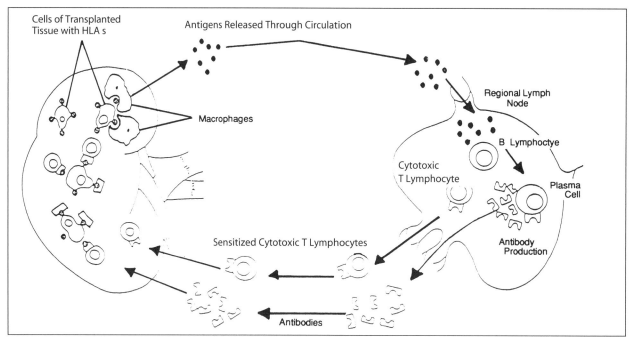

Figure 10.2. Mechanisms of transplanted tissue rejection. Macrophages recognize and process foreign HLAs, and antigenic material is released into the circulation. Lymphocytes in lymph nodes produce activated cytotoxic T lymphocytes and antibodies, which then destroy the transplanted tissue. (See text for details.)

2. Helper T lymphocytes release cytokines such as interleukin 2 and interferon-gamma to activate cytotoxic T cells.
3. The T lymphocytes then regulate the gene expression for IL-1 and IL-2 receptors.
4. IL-2 stimulates T lymphocyte proliferation and activation of other lymphocytes.
5. Other cytokines are involved in B lymphocyte activation.
6. The activated T cells release other inflammatory cytokines that result in cell damage and allograft injury.
7. Important in acute rejection.

C. Indirect recognition.
1. APCs of the recipient take up MHCs shed from the donor cells. This then activates recipient lymphocytes.
2. More important in the process of chronic rejection.

III. Types of rejection.

A. Hyperacute rejection.
1. Onset is minutes to hours.
2. As a result of preformed antidonor antibodies and complement.
3. This process usually involves memory B lymphocytes.

4. Irreversible and untreatable.
5. Circulating preformed antibodies recognize and bind with the transplanted tissue. The complement and coagulation systems are activated by antigen-antibody binding. As a result of this process, ischemia, hypoxia, and acidosis occur in the transplanted tissue.
6. Can be prevented by performing crossmatch prior to transplant.
7. Transplant nephrectomy is necessary for treatment.

B. Accelerated rejection.
1. Onset is days.
2. Caused by reactivation of sensitized T lymphocytes, similar to hyperacute rejection.
3. At the time of the transplant, the number of circulating preformed antibodies is insufficient to mount a rejection episode. Over a few days they proliferate rapidly and cause rejection.
4. Clinical signs and symptoms.
   a. Profound oliguria.
   b. Fever.
   c. Rapid loss of transplanted kidney function.
   d. Systemic toxicity.
5. Can be prevented by performing crossmatch prior to transplant.
6. Transplant nephrectomy is usually necessary for

treatment, although plasmapheresis is sometimes attempted.

C. Acute rejection.
1. Onset is days to weeks.
2. Caused by activation of T lymphocytes.
3. Signs and symptoms: fever, elevated leukocyte count, malaise, increased creatinine, increased BUN, decreased urine output, electrolyte imbalances, edema, graft tenderness.
4. Mononuclear leukocytes accumulate inside the capillaries of the transplanted organ, lymphocytes migrate into the interstitial spaces. Lymphokines are released and attract and cause multiplication of other inflammatory-immune cells. Pronounced edema, perivascular hemorrhages, and cellular necrosis result from the immune attack on the transplanted organ. Later, thrombosis of blood vessels and organ necrosis occur.
5. Acute rejection can usually be treated with increased immunosuppression.

D. Chronic rejection (also known as chronic allograft nephropathy).
1. Onset is months to years.
2. Cause is unclear, but is likely a combination of T lymphocyte and B lymphocyte mediated rejection.
3. Events of the inflammatory immune response cause internal damage to blood vessels and glomeruli. Gradual ischemia causes chronic tissue necrosis and attempts at repair by fibroblast proliferation and collagen deposition. This causes scarring, the interstitium is filled with collagen, and blood vessels are blocked by proliferation of intima.
4. There is no successful treatment.

Modifications of Immune Responsiveness

The goal of immunosuppression is to modify the immune system enough to prevent rejection, but not so much as to allow infection, malignancies, and other side effects.

I. Glucocorticoids.

A. Most commonly used forms are prednisone and methylprednisolone.

B. Dosage and schedule of administration vary widely based on concurrent use of other immunosuppressive therapies.

C. Many centers use very briefly, if at all.

D. Peak blood concentration is reached in 1 to 2 hours. Biologic effects persist 12 to 24 hours.

E. Action.
1. Exact action of corticosteroids in altering the immune response has not been clearly delineated.
2. Corticosteroids prevent release of interleukin-1 from macrophages, thus decreasing the activity of T lymphocytes.
3. Corticosteroids decrease the antigenicity of transplanted tissue.
4. Corticosteroids exert anti-inflammatory effects that result in a decreased inflammatory reaction at the transplanted site (e.g., decreased edema, capillary permeability, leukocyte migration, deposition of a fibrin mesh, and phagocytosis).

F. Nursing implications.
1. Administer as prescribed.
2. Observe for side effects (see Table 10.1).
3. Administer antacids, H2 antagonists, or proton pump inhibitors as ordered to prevent gastrointestinal ulcers.
4. Administer antifungal medications (either systemic or mouthwashes) as prescribed.
5. Encourage early and frequent ambulation to minimize muscle weakness.
6. Monitor blood glucose levels.
7. Provide emotional support in adaptation to changing body image.

II. Mycophenolate mofetil, mycophenolic acid (Cellcept®, MMF®, Myfortic®, MPA®).

A. Action.
1. Mycophenolate mofetil is an antimetabolite that selectively inhibits the proliferation of T and B lymphocytes by interfering with purine nucleotide synthesis.
2. This drug has replaced azathioprine at most transplant centers as a maintenance agent because it has significantly decreased the incidence of acute rejection.
3. The drug is largely metabolized in the liver and eliminated through the kidney. The elimination half-life is approximately 18 hours.
B. Nursing implications.
1. Administer as prescribed.

2. Monitor WBC.
3. Observe for side effects (see Table 10.1).

III. Sirolimus (Rapamune®).

A. Action.
1. Sirolimus inhibits T lymphocyte activation and proliferation that occurs in response to antigenic and cytokine stimulation by a mechanism that is distinct from that of other immunosuppressants.
2. This drug also inhibits antibody production.
3. Nonnephrotoxic agent.
4. Sometimes used with chronic allograft nephropathy.

B. Nursing implications.
1. Administer as prescribed.
2. Observe for side effects (see Table 10.1).

IV. Azathioprine (Imuran®).

A. Action.
1. Azathioprine is an antimetabolite that interferes with deoxyribonucleic acid (DNA) synthesis, thus decreasing the division of rapidly reproducing cells, including leukocytes.
2. The number of killer cells is reduced, antigen receptor sites on T lymphocytes are inhibited, and B lymphocyte activity is inhibited.
3. Azathioprine is almost always used in conjunction with other immunosuppressive medications.
4. The drug is detoxified by the kidney. Therefore, good renal function is essential to prevent toxicity.

B. Nursing implications.
1. Administer as prescribed.
2. Monitor WBC and liver function tests.
3. Observe for side effects (see Table 10.1).

V. Cyclosporine (Sandimmune®, Neoral®, Gengraf®).

A. Action.
1. Cyclosporine acts by interfering with the production of interleukin-1 (T lymphocyte activation factor) by macrophages and the production of interleukin-2 (T lymphocyte growth factor) from T lymphocytes. It has no direct effect on macrophage production.
2. As a result, even though macrophages and T lymphocytes can recognize the transplanted tissue as foreign, the lymphocytes cannot mount an immune response.

3. Two different formulations modified and non-modified (see Table 10.1)

B. Nursing implications.
1. Administer as prescribed.
2. Observe for side effects (see Table 10.1).

VI. Tacrolimus (FK506®, Prograf®).

A. Action.
1. Tacrolimus inhibits T cell activation and proliferation in vitro primarily by impairing the activation or induction of gene coding for interleukin-2 (IL-2), IL-3, IL-4, and tumor necrosis factor and gamma interferon.
2. Tacrolimus also inhibits B cell activation and causes a significant, but transient, decrease in the number of B cells secreting immunoglobulins.

B. Nursing implications.
1. Administer as prescribed.
2. Observe for side effects (see Table 10.1).

VII. Polyclonal preparations (e.g., antilymphocyte globulin, thymoglobulin (Atgam®).

A. Method of preparation.
1. An animal (e.g., horse, goat, rabbit) is injected with human lymphocytes.
2. The animal then produces antibodies to the foreign human cells.
3. The globulin, which is the part of the serum containing the antibodies, is separated from the plasma, purified, and stored.
4. The ALG (antilymphocyte globulin) containing the antibodies is then administered to the organ transplant recipient.

B. Action.
1. It is known to act specifically against T lymphocytes and decreases their activity and number by coating T lymphocytes and rendering them ineffective. In addition, ALG forms blocking antibodies and destroys T lymphocytes by direct antigen-antibody complex formation.

C. Nursing implications.
1. Administer as prescribed through a central line to prevent sclerosis of peripheral veins.
2. Observe for side effects (see Table 10.1).
3. May be used for induction or rejection therapy.

Text continues on page 629

Table 10.1 ———— Immunosuppressive Medications

Name of Agent	Purpose	Dose	Method of Administration	Side Effects
Azathioprine (Imuran®) Generic available	Maintenance immunosuppression	1.5–2 mg/kg Tablet size: 50 mg	Intravenous initially, then orally once a day.	Bone marrow suppression: anemia thrombocytopenia bleeding leukopenia Hair thinning and loss Infections Gastrointestinal problems Mouth ulcers Hepatic dysfunction; hepatitis Malignancies
Cyclosporine Two formulations that are not bioequivalent and cannot be used interchangeably Modified: Neoral®, Gengraf® cyclosporine modified – microemulsion allowing for more consistent absorption Nonmodified: Sandimmune® cyclosporine nonmodified – variable rate of absorption	Maintenance immunosuppression	Adjusted to serum drug levels or per protocol; usually 3-4 mg/kg as maintenance dose. Solution: 100 mg/mL 100 mg capsules 25 mg capsules	Intravenous initially, then orally; mixed in milk or citrus juice for solution. Usually twice a day dose unless pharmacokinetics dictate otherwise (protocols vary).	Nephrotoxicity Hepatotoxicity Hand tremors Hypertrichosis Gingival hyperplasia Seizures Flushing Hyperesthesia Gastrointestinal distress: nausea/vomiting anorexia diarrhea feeling of fullness Headaches Mild anemia Hyperkalemia Hypertension Malignancies Hirsutism Hyperlipidemia
Cyclophosphamide (Cytoxan®) (Rarely used)	Maintenance immunosuppression if unable to tolerate Imuran® or Cellcept®	50–75 mg/day for adults	Orally once a day in the morning to prevent hemorraghic cystitis.	Leukopenia Thrombocytopenia Bladder fibrosis GI disturbances Hemorraghic cystitis

Table 10.1 continues on next page

Table 10.1 ———— Immunosuppressive Medications (continued)

Name of Agent	Purpose	Dose	Method of Administration	Side Effects
Tacrolimus (FK-506, Prograf®)	Maintenance immunosuppression	Adjusted to serum drug levels or per protocol. 5 mg capsules 1 mg capsules 0.5 mg capsules IV preparation: 5 mg/mL	Intravenous until able to take orally. Orally twice a day.	Nephrotoxicity Hypertension Infections Neurotoxicity: tremors or tingling sensations in palms of hands or soles of feet Paresthesias Insomnia Headache Tinnitus Increased visual sensitivity to light Nightmares/sleep disturbances Mood changes Diabetes Malignancies

Prednisone	Maintenance immunosuppression	Usual maintenance dose 0.2 mg/kg
		Tablet size:
		  50 mg
		  20 mg
		  10 mg
		  5 mg
		  2.5 mg
			Intravenous initially, then orally in divided doses until maintenance dose achieved, then once a day.	*Common*
				Cushingoid appearance
				Increased appetite
				Na+/water retention
				GI disturbances
				Peptic ulcers with bleeding
				Easy bruising
				Impaired wound healing
				Acne
				Diaphoresis
				Infections (especially opportunistic)
				Hyperlipidemia
				Osteoporosis
				Less Common
				Avascular joint necrosis
				Steroid induced diabetes
				Cataracts
				Growth retardation
				Pancreatitis
				Anemia
				Thrombocytopenia
				Leukopenia
				Hypertension
				Emotional disturbances
				Malignancies

Table 10.1 continues on next page

Table 10.1 — Immunosuppressive Medications (continued)

Name of Agent	Purpose	Dose	Method of Administration	Side Effects
Solu-Medrol®	Rejection therapy	15 mg/kg for no more than 3 days	Intravenous as a bolus through peripheral IV site.	See Prednisone
Monoclonal Antibody (OKT3®)	Rejection or induction therapy	5 mg daily for 5–14 days	Intravenous push through peripheral vein. Premedicate with hydrocortisone, Tylenol®, Benadryl® for first 1-3 doses until side effects abate.	*First Dose* Flu-like syndrome: fever chills tremors nausea/vomiting dyspnea wheezing chest pain and tightness pulmonary edema (rare) *Long-term Complications* Viral infections Lymphoma
Polyclonal preparations (ATG, ALG, ALS, ATS) Thymoglobulin, Atgam®	Rejection or induction therapy	10–15 mg/kg daily for 5–10 days	Intravenous infusion over 6 hours through high flow vein (central line, fistula). Premedicate with Benadryl® and Tylenol®.	Hypersensitivity response: generalized rash tachycardia dyspnea chills fever chest pain back pain hypotension anaphylaxis Leukopenia Thrombocytopenia Arthralgia and myalgia Fluid retention (if diluted with normal saline) Opportunistic infections, especially: Cytomegalic virus (CMV) Herpes viruses *Pneumocystis carinii* *Cryptococcus neoformans*

Table 10.1 continues on next page

Table 10.1 ——————**Immunosuppressive Medications (continued)**

Name of Agent	Purpose	Dose	Method of Administration	Side Effects
Mycophenolate mofetil Mycophenolic acid, Myfortic® Cellcept®	Maintenance immunosuppression	1000 mg–1500 mg Tablet size: 250 mg 500 mg Liquid available for pediatrics. 180 mg, 360 mg, 720 mg	Orally q 12 hours.	Bone marrow suppression: anemia leukopenia thrombocytopenia bleeding Gastrointestinal distress nausea/vomiting anorexia diarrhea Malignancies
Sirolimus (Rapamune®)	Maintenance immunosuppression	2 mg–5 mg: adjust to serum drug levels Available in multidose bottle or laminated aluminum pouches of 1 mg, 2 mg, or 5 mg doses 1 mg tablet	Orally; mixed in orange juice or water; once a day.	Hyperlipidemia Hypercholesterolemia Diarrhea Anemia Arthralgia Acne Thrombocytopenia Hypokalemia Delayed wound healing Rash Mouth sores
Basiliximab (Simulect®)	Induction therapy	20 mg	Intravenously in 50 mL normal saline over 15-20 minutes through a peripheral vein. Doses are administered on the day of transplant and on postoperative day 4.	Does not add to the background of adverse events seen in organ transplant patients.
Daclizumab (Zenapax®)	Induction therapy	1 mg/kg per dose	Intravenously in 50 mL normal saline over 15 minutes through a peripheral vein. Five doses are administered beginning the day of transplant and then every 2 weeks. Alternative dosing is one dose with repeat in dose in 10 days.	Does not add to the background of adverse events seen in organ transplant patients.

Continued from page 624

VIII. Monoclonal preparations: muromonab CD3 (Orthoclone OKT3®).

A. Action.
1. Developed to react to one specific marker on the surface of T lymphocytes. These markers are composed of 3 polypeptide chains (the CD3 complex) that signal the T lymphocyte to respond to a foreign antigen.
2. OKT3 combines with the CD3 complex, and as a result, inhibits T lymphocyte proliferation and lysis of transplanted cells by T lymphocyte activity.

B. Nursing implications.
1. Administer as prescribed.
2. Observe for side effects (see Table 10.1).

IX. Interleukin-2 receptor antagonists: basiliximab (Simulect®), daclizumab (Zenapax®).

A. Action.
1. Basiliximab (chimeric) and daclizumab (humanized) are monoclonal antibodies that bind to the CD25 or Tac subunit of the IL-2 receptor expressed on activated T lymphocytes, thereby inhibiting IL-2 mediated activation and proliferation.
2. Both drugs have long half-lives secondary to decreased inactivation of human antibodies.

B. Nursing implications.
1. Administer as prescribed through a peripheral or central line.
2. Observe for side effects (see Table 10.1).

Chapter 48

Pancreas Transplantation

Purpose

The purpose of this chapter is to discuss concepts related to pancreas transplantation.

Objectives

Upon completion of this chapter, the learner will be able to:
1. Outline important historical events related to pancreas transplantation.
2. Outline the rationale for pancreas transplantation.
3. Identify the steps of the evaluative process for pancreas transplantation.
4. Discuss acceptance criteria for pancreas transplantation.
5. Describe the organ procurement process for pancreas transplantation.
6. Discuss various options of transplantation.
   a. Solitary pancreas transplant.
   b. Pancreas transplant alone (PTA).
   c. Pancreas after kidney transplant (PAK).
   d. Simultaneous pancreas-kidney transplant (SPK).
7. Differentiate various techniques for handling the exocrine drainage and the advantages of each: enteric drainage and bladder drainage.
8. Describe the operative procedure for pancreas transplantation.
9. Explain methods for modification of the immune system after transplantation.
10. List major side effects of selected immunosuppression.
11. Define pancreas transplant rejection.
12. Identify complications of pancreas transplantation.
13. Discuss the long-term effects of pancreas transplantation on diabetes.
14. Describe quality of life issues that have been identified for pancreas transplant recipients.
15. Develop a collaborative care plan for a pancreas transplant recipient during the postoperative period.

I. Historical perspectives of pancreas transplantation.

A. First human whole pancreas transplant performed by Kelly and Lillehei at the University of Minnesota in 1966. The recipient survived 2 months, and then died of sepsis and rejection.

B. From 1966 to 1977, 64 pancreas transplants were performed. Two patients had a 1-year graft survival (3%). There was a 40% 1-year patient survival rate. Failures were attributed to technical difficulties and postoperative complications, including graft thrombosis, fistula formation, necrosis from poor preservation, and difficulties in balancing immunosuppression therapy to control rejection and prevent infection.

C. Graft survival has continued to increase and is attributed to advancements in immunosuppressive therapy.

D. Several surgical techniques have been used to manage pancreas graft exocrine secretions.
   1. Enteric drainage was used in the earliest transplants.
   2. Dubernard originated duct injection in the mid-1970s.
   3. Sollinger introduced a technique to connect the pancreas to the bladder in the early 1980s.
   4. In the mid-1980s, Nghiem and Corry modified this technique to suture a duodenal cuff from the donor with the pancreas to the recipient bladder. This allows the exocrine drainage from the pancreas to drain into the bladder.
   5. From 1987 to 1997, over 90% of the pancreas transplants done in the United States were bladder-drained (Auchincloss & Shaffer, 1999).

E. Since October 1987, all U.S. pancreas transplants must be reported to the Scientific Registry of the United Network of Organ Sharing (UNOS).

F. There are currently 143 centers that perform pancreas transplants in the United States.

G. In 2004, the number of pancreas transplant performed totaled 1,484 (185 PTAs, 419 PAKs, and 880 SPKs) (UNOS, 2005).

H. As of June 7, 2006, there were 2,481 candidates on the UNOS waiting list for a simultaneous pancreas-kidney transplant and 1,740 listed for a pancreas transplant. This total of 4,221 patients waiting for a simultaneous pancreas-kidney or solitary pancreas transplant is an increase of 74% from the 3,133 candidates who were waiting in April 2000.

I. UNOS reports national graft and patient survival statistics.
   1. From 1998 to 2003, the graft survival at 1 year, 3 years, and 5 years for SPK was 86%, 79%, and 71%, respectively.
   2. At 1 year, 3 years, and 5 years, graft survival for PAK was 78%, 66%, and 57%, respectively, and for PTA was 77%, 62%, and 56%, respectively (UNOS, 2005).

J. For SPK, patient survival rates at 1 year for transplants performed between 2002 and 2003, at 3 years for transplants done between 2000 and 2003, and at 5 years for SPKs done in 1998-2003 were 95%, 91%, and 86%, respectively. PAK transplant recipient survival rates at 1 year, 3 years, and 5 years was 96%, 90%, and 84%, respectively and for PTA was 96%, 94%, and 91%, respectively (UNOS, 2005).

K. By the end of 2004, over 23,000 pancreas transplantations have been performed nationally.

II. Basic concepts and goals of pancreas transplantation.

A. American Diabetes Association (ADA) reports that diabetes mellitus is an endocrine disease that has been diagnosed in 14.8 million Americans. However, 6.2 million are unaware they have diabetes. In 2005 there were 1.5 million new cases of diabetes diagnosed in adults 20 years of age or older (ADA, 2006). Diabetes is the most prevalent chronic disease encountered in health care (Semb, 2000).

B. The ADA reports that the total yearly economic cost of diabetes was $132 billion in 2002. The per capita health care spending rose from an annual cost of $10,071 per person in 1997 to $13,243 in 2002 (greater than 30% increase).

C. The ADA has classified two types of diabetes. Type 1 diabetes accounts for 5-10% of those diagnosed with diabetes. Type 2, the most frequent type of diabetes, accounts for 90-95% of diabetes.

D. Those with type 1 diabetes secrete little or no insulin from the beta cells of the pancreas. People with type 1 diabetes depend on exogenous insulin for the control of carbohydrate metabolism and prevention of ketoacidosis and wide fluctuations in plasma glucose levels. High glucose levels can result in hypotonic fluid loss, dehydration, and electrolyte depletion.

E. Type 1 diabetes is associated with other diseases, such as retinopathy, neuropathy, nephropathy, and cardiovascular diseases (angina, myocardial infarction, cerebral vascular accident; often grouped together as macrovascular disease).

F. In adults, diabetic retinopathy causes 12,000-24,000 new cases of blindness every year. As the leading cause of chronic kidney disease, diabetes accounted for 44% of the new diagnoses in 2002. Heart disease death rates and the risk of stroke are 2 to 4 times higher in adults with diabetes. About 60-70% have mild to severe neuropathy and more than 60% of nontraumatic lower-limb amputations occur in diabetic people.

G. The Diabetes Control and Complications Trial (DCCT) Research Group reported, in 1993, that intensive therapy effectively delays the onset and slows the progression of diabetic retinopathy, nephropathy, and neuropathy in patients with type 1 diabetes. A total of 1,441 patients were involved in this study. Study conclusions recommended that patients "be treated with the goal to maintain their glycemic state as close to the normal range as safely possible."

H. Pancreas transplantation is performed to treat Type 1 diabetes and to restore a euglycemic state for the transplant recipient. Patient survival following SPK transplantation is excellent and has increased incrementally since 1995 (UNOS, 2005). However, the transplant community remains uncertain as to whether PTA or PAK transplantation has a survival advantage. As with any treatment option, risk vs. benefit of transplantation/immunosuppression or insulin independence must be carefully evaluated to determine the best choice available for each patient.

I. The ADA position on pancreas transplantation (1998) states that pancreas transplantation "should be considered an acceptable therapeutic alternative to continued insulin therapy in diabetic patients with end-stage renal disease who have had or plan to have a kidney transplant." The ADA also supports pancreas transplant alone in cases where

there is "frequent severe metabolic complications requiring medical attention" and "failure of other therapeutic approaches."

J. Questions to consider when evaluating a patient as a potential pancreas transplant candidate.
1. Is a pancreas transplant the optimal choice for replacement of pancreas endocrine function?
2. What is the best timing for pancreas transplantation related to progression of nephropathy and the other diseases associated with diabetes?
3. Do the benefits of a pancreas transplant alone and immunosuppression outweigh the risks of the long-term complications of diabetes and insulin management?
4. What is the likelihood that pancreas transplantation will prevent and/or stop the progression of retinopathy, neuropathy, nephropathy, cardiac, and vascular diseases associated with type 1 diabetes?

K. Research documents that patients who receive a pancreas transplant report a better quality of life after transplantation. Because of the increasing success rates, more research pointing toward the decrease in complications of diabetes after pancreas transplantation, and reports of better quality of life, pancreas transplantation is a viable and worthwhile treatment of type 1 diabetes.

L. Research indicates that patients who receive a pancreas transplant report a better quality of life and improved physical and psychological well-being after transplantation. The benefits of having a normal blood sugar, no insulin shots or reactions, and no diabetic diet have contributed to pancreas transplant recipients reporting feeling more positive and hopeful about the future. Because of the success rates, the decrease in diabetic complications after pancreas transplantation, and reports of improved quality of life, pancreas transplantation is a viable and worthwhile treatment of type 1 diabetes.

III. **Evaluative process and options for potential pancreas transplant recipients.**

A. Simultaneous pancreas-kidney transplant offers the patient with diabetes and kidney failure the option of correcting uremia and becoming euglycemic, thereby preventing or ameliorating the secondary complications of diabetes. The goal is to perform the procedure in the early stages of kidney failure, and before the other associated diseases of diabetes have occurred. Auchincloss and Shaffer (1999) suggest that simultaneous pancreas-kidney transplantation should occur before the serum creatinine is above 2 mg/dL. Patients do not accumulate wait time points from UNOS until their glomerular filtration rate (GFR) is ≤ 20 mL/min.

B. Pancreas transplant after kidney transplantation is another option to control the effects of diabetes, because kidney transplant alone does not control the effects of diabetes at the microvascular or macrovascular level.

C. Pancreas transplant alone in nonuremic patients is also performed in some institutions. The belief is that with lower rejection rates of organs and better technical ability to perform the surgery this option is a viable one for patients with type 1 diabetes.

D. Living transplantation may also be done with a segmental pancreas transplant. This option remains in the research phase and has not yet had the positive outcomes hoped for.

E. Refer to the section on kidney transplantation for general guidelines for candidate criteria. This section includes the specific assessment of the patient with diabetes who is being evaluated for pancreas transplantation.

F. Candidate criteria and assessment for pancreas transplantation.
   1. Age.
      a. Emphasis on complications of type 1 diabetes rather than chronologic age.
      b. Some programs require recipients to be at least 18 years of age and not older than 60 years of age.
      c. Research has shown that the most significant risks were in recipients older than 45 years of age (Gruessner et al., 1994).
   2. Laboratory assessment of potential recipients may include:
      a. Metabolic studies.
         (1) Glucose tolerance test.
         (2) Serum C-peptide levels.
         (3) Glycosylated hemoglobin.
         (4) Antibodies to islet cells.
      b. Kidney function studies.
      c. Thyroid function studies.
      d. Complete electrolyte and chemistry profile.
      e. Serum amylase.

f. Lipoprotein profile.
g. Hematology studies.
h. Serology for infectious diseases.
   (1) Cytomegalovirus (CMV).
   (2) Epstein-Barr virus (EBV).
   (3) Herpes virus.
   (4) Hepatitis.
   (5) Human immunodeficiency virus (HIV).
   (6) Bacterial and fungal cultures, as indicated.
   (7) Syphyllis (VDRL).
   3. Cardiovascular system assessment.
      a. Most attention is given to this system in preoperative evaluation owing to the incidence and risks of macrovascular and microvascular disease in persons with type 1 diabetes. Persons with diabetic neuropathy can have significant coronary artery disease without angina.
      b. The more advanced the cardiovascular or peripheral vascular disease in the potential recipient, the more likely the candidate is to have a higher morbidity and mortality rate following pancreas transplantation (Cosimi & Conti, 1989).
      c. Some centers will transplant recipients with previous myocardial infarction or cardiovascular disease once the potential candidate undergoes coronary artery bypass grafting or angioplasty.
      d. Work-up for the cardiovascular system includes:
         1. Electrocardiogram (EKG).
         2. Stress EKG.
         3. Thallium stress test with follow-up coronary angiogram if the stress eletrocardiogram is positive or there is a history of angina or myocardial infarction.
         4. Peripheral vascular studies, including Doppler examination of the lower extremities, and, if needed, carotid plethysmography.
   4. Neurologic system work-up.
      a. Neurologic evaluation includes the evaluation of the motor, sensory, and autonomic nervous systems.
      b. Work-up of the neurologic system includes:
         (1) History and physical examination for evidence of sensory and autonomic neuropathy, such as gastroparesis, diarrhea, impotence, and neurologic ulcerations. Injury related to loss of sensation of pain, temperature, and position are also assessed.

(2) Peripheral nerve conduction velocity studies to assess motor nerve conduction. Gross motor disease is also detected by observing for muscle atrophy, weakness, and foot drop.

5. Urinary tract and bladder function assessment. Because one of the methods of exocrine drainage in the transplanted pancreas is through the bladder, the function of the urinary system and bladder is important.
    a. Urinalysis and culture.
    b. Urine protein studies.
    c. Voiding cystourethrography with postvoid films.
6. Ophthalmologic studies.
    a. Retinopathy and blindness are major complications of type 1 diabetes and indicative of microvascular disease.
    b. Assessment.
        (1) Fundus examination including the retina, optic disc, and blood vessels.
        (2) Refraction index. Measurement of ability to see an object at an specific distance.
        (3) Retinal photography. Uses a fluorescein dye to take pictures with a special camera to analyze the circulation of the retina and choroid.
        (4) Slit-lamp examination. Uses low power microscope combined with a high intensity light to evaluate the structures at the front of the eye.
7. Psychosocial assessment (social worker, psychologist, and/or psychiatrist).
    a. Current adjustment to illness.
        (1) Onset, adjustment to therapy.
        (2) Emotional impact of illness.
        (3) Understanding of diagnosis and disease process.
        (4) Adherence to current medical treatment.
        (5) Lifestyle changes, including work, activity, sexual, self-esteem.
    b. Family and social history.
        (1) Social support system, impact of illness on family.
        (2) Educational level.
    c. Work and financial history.
        (1) Employment status.
        (2) Financial resources.
        (3) Status with insurance resources.
    d. Transplantation history.
        (1) Understanding of preoperative and postoperative regimen.
        (2) Expectations of process and outcome.
        (3) Why transplantation is being chosen by patient.

(4) Understanding of donor process and recipient transplant selection criteria.
    e. Assessment conclusions.
        (1) Coping skills.
        (2) Adaptation response and anticipated adaptation response after transplantation.
        (3) Willingness and ability to adhere to treatment regimen.
        (4) Understanding of process and potential effects of immunosuppression.
8. Gastrointestinal, endocrine, pulmonary, dental, and immunologic systems assessment is similar to what is discussed in the kidney transplantation section.
9. Pancreas transplantation is contraindicated in any of the following:
    a. Inoperable cardiovascular or peripheral vascular disease.
    b. Incapacitating neuropathies.
    c. Active peptic ulcer disease.
    d. Active malignancy.
    e. Acute infectious process.
    f. Active alcohol or drug addiction.
    g. Psychosis.
    h. Body mass index (BMI) greater than 35.
10. The majority of transplant programs currently do not offer pancreas transplantation to individuals who are HIV positive.
11. SPK and PAK ideal candidate.
    a. 18–50 years of age.
    b. BMI 25–30, depending on transplant center.
    c. Nonsmoker.
    d. No history of heart disease.
    e. Functional vision.
    f. No peripheral vascular disease.
12. SPK and PAK higher-risk candidate.
    a. 50-60 years of age.
    b. BMI > 30.
    c. Previous myocardial infarction.
    d. Previous stroke.
    e. Significant peripheral vascular disease.
13. Once accepted for pancreas transplantation, the potential recipient's name is placed on the national waiting list, unless a partial segmental donation from a living donor is to be done.

IV. Organ procurement process for pancreas transplantation.

A. Pancreas or kidney-pancreas organs for transplantation are largely obtained from deceased donors. The need for donors greatly exceeds the number of donors annually. Therefore, strategies to expand the donor pool are constantly being researched. Donor selection in some transplant centers has been expanded to include donors older than 45 years, and as young as 5 years, and donors who have been on vasopressors. Kapur et al. (1999) report that in their series of expanded criteria donor use, organs with calcification, extensive fatty infiltration, or fibrosis were not procured. Despite the use of what previously was considered expanded criteria donors for pancreas transplantation, recipients of expanded criteria donor grafts did not have higher complication rates than other recipients. This group also had an overall graft survival rate of 83%, with a mean follow-up of 23 months. This a 1% greater graft survival rate than the national 1-year statistics.

B. Many pancreas transplant centers still believe that donors over 45 years of age are thought of as high-risk donors for pancreas transplantation.

C. Kapur et al. (1999) report that donor amylase, lipase, and glucose values range greatly in marginal donors. Amylase levels ranged from 5 to 1411 IU/dL, with a mean of 136 IU/dL. Lipase ranged from 9 to 1373 IU/dL, with a mean of 116 IU/dL, and glucose ranged from 100 to 648 mg/dL, with a mean of 285 mg/dL.

D. The donor's history must be negative for cancer (excluding skin or primary brain), diabetes, tuberculosis, chronic hypertension, alcoholism, hepatitis, syphilis, and HIV. Positive CMV status does not preclude donation.

E. Organ procurement process.
1. During procurement, amphotericin B solution may be given through a nasogastric tube inserted into the duodenum to decrease the risk of fungal infection.
2. The spleen is mobilized to use as a handle to decrease manipulation and potential trauma of the pancreas during procurement. The pancreas and its respective vessels are mobilized. A portion of the duodenum is transected with the pancreas.
3. The pancreas is flushed with preservation solution to prevent ion flux across the cell membranes. The duodenal section may be flushed again with amphotericin B or preservation solution, depending on center protocols.
4. Variation of this procedure may include removal of several abdominal organs with dissection and preservation ex vivo.

5. Pancreas cold ischemic time may be up to 24 hours, if necessary. The goal is to transplant the graft in less than 24 hours.

V. Organ options of pancreas transplantation.

A. Pancreas transplant alone (PTA).
1. Is no longer considered experimental due to the good success rates.
   a. Candidates' qualifications.
      (1) Must be diabetic without chronic kidney disease and have good kidney function.
      (2) Are typically labile with frequent episodes of ketoacidosis and hypoglycemia.
      (3) May have hypoglycemia unawareness.
      (4) May require multiple daily blood sugar checks to maintain control.
      (5) May have poor control despite multiple insulin injections or pump use.
      (6) May not be able to live independently or hold a job.
   b. May be required to have a referral or evaluation by an endocrinologist and an evaluation by a transplant clinical psychologist before being considered as an eligible pancreas transplant alone candidate.
2. PTA transplants performed in the United States in 2004 totaled 185, a 14% increase from 2003 with a 1-year graft survival increasing to 77% (UNOS, 2005) as compared to 74% in 1997 (Sutherland et al., 1999). Improved results reflect more advanced immunosuppression resulting in a decrease in rejection rates and a decrease in technical failure.

B. Pancreas after kidney transplant (PAK).
1. PAK transplant is usually performed from a deceased donor after successful kidney transplant to control the medical complications of diabetes. May potentially also be done from a living donor.
   a. Transplant performed on a person with diabetes with a well-functioning prior kidney transplant.
   b. Pancreas comes from a donor different from the kidney donor.
   c. Creatinine clearance must be > 40 mL/min.
   d. PAK ameliorates recurrence of diabetic nephropathy in the transplanted kidney.
   e. Long-term kidney graft function is likely to be improved.
2. PAK transplants performed in the United States in 2004 totaled 419, an 18% increase from 2003

with a 1-year graft survival of 78% (UNOS, 2005) as compared to 72% in 1997 (Sutherland et al., 1999).

C. Simultaneous pancreas-kidney transplant (SPK).
1. Candidates must meet the medical indications and criteria for kidney transplantation and have significant clinical problems with insulin therapy.
2. Kidney and pancreas from the same deceased donor are transplanted into a person with diabetes and CKD during one surgical procedure.
   a. Addition of the pancreas does not jeopardize the transplanted kidney's long-term survival or function.
   b. New pancreas may improve the recipient's long-term survival since many of the medical complications related to diabetes may be eliminated or significantly improved.
3. SPK transplantation outcome is improved if the dual transplant is done early in the course of kidney failure. This does not often happen due to the long waiting times for organ donation patients usually encounter. Some regions require that patients be on dialysis before being listed for a transplant, and then list candidates together with those waiting for a kidney only. These patients can wait several years before getting a simultaneous pancreas-kidney donor.
4. The rationale for performing a simultaneous pancreas-kidney transplant is that one is not adding the risk of immunosuppression. Also, the immunology is the same for both organs, so rejection can be detected by well-established methods of detecting kidney transplant rejection, compared to the difficulty of diagnosing rejection in the transplanted pancreas.
5. SPK transplants performed in the United States in 2004 totaled 880 which was a slight increase from the 870 transplants performed in 2003. The 1-year graft survival of 86% (UNOS, 2005) as compared to 82% in 1997.
6. Based on the above statistics, simultaneous pancreas-kidney transplant offers the greatest 1-year graft survival as compared with pancreas transplant alone or pancreas after kidney transplant.
7. Patients listed for a simultaneous pancreas kidney transplant remain eligible to receive a kidney transplant alone should an acceptable kidney become available without the pancreas. If a kidney transplant alone occurs, patients may still be eligible for re-evaluation for a pancreas after kidney transplant.

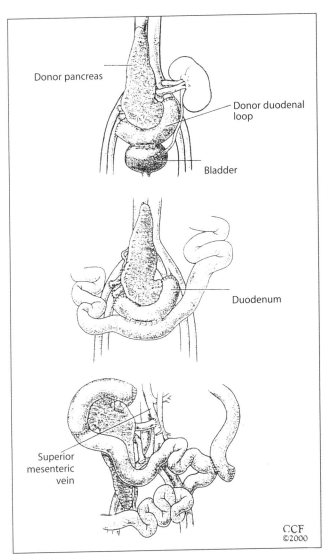

Figure 10.3. Three surgical options for pancreas transplantation. **Top**: procedure developed by Ngheim and others, in which the exocrine secretions of the pancreas are drained into the bladder. **Middle**: enteric drainage into the recipient jejunum. **Bottom**: enteric drainage into the jejunum and venous drainage into the superior mesenteric vein.

Source: Mayes, J.T., Dennis, V.W., & Hoogwerf, B.J. (2000). Pancreas transplantation in type 1 diabetes: Hope vs reality. *Cleveland Clinic Journal of Medicine, 67*(4), 283. Used with permission.

VI. Surgical options for pancreas transplantation (see Figure 10.3).

A. The exocrine function of the native pancreas is not affected by diabetes so the recipient's pancreas is left in to continue its exocrine function.

B. The transplanted pancreas also maintains its exocrine function, leading to the high risk of fluid and bicarbonate losses, fistula formation, and related infection. Exocrine drainage management is the most difficult technical aspect of pancreas transplantation. Currently, in the United States there are two surgical options for pancreas transplantation. Duct occlusion, once an option for handling exocrine drainage, is currently not reported in the United States.

1. Bladder drainage.
   a. Was the standard approach in the United States.
   b. Exocrine secretions are drained through the bladder via a small segment of the donor duodenum.
   c. The pancreas is transplanted with a duodenal cuff from the donor, which is sutured to the recipient's bladder in a side-to-side anastomosis, or duodenocystostomy.
   d. Pancreatic enzymes are secreted in a largely inactive form, so they do not damage the bladder.
   e. Measurement of urinary amylase can then assist with detection of pancreas function and rejection after this procedure.
   f. There is a reduced chance of infection and fistula formation related to other methods of anastomoses because the urinary tract is free from bacteria.
   g. Complications.
      (1) Metabolic acidosis due to normal losses of bicarbonate via the transplanted pancreas and the bladder's inability to reabsorb the bicarbonate.
      (2) Cystitis related to irritation of the bladder with exocrine enzymes.
      (3) Bleeding of the duodenal cuff.
      (4) Fluid losses through the pancreas with dehydration and hypotension.
2. Enteric drainage.
   a. Because of the complications of bladder drainage, along with the decreased rejection rate, pancreas biopsy techniques, and better radiologic studies, the majority of institutions in the U.S. are using enteric drainage.
   b. Exocrine function is managed by anastomosis of the graft to the jejunum with or without a Roux-en-Y loop.
   c. This is the most physiologic method of handling exocrine function.
   d. Exocrine secretions can be absorbed and metabolic imbalances are theoretically reduced.
   e. Complications leading to repeat laparotomy include graft thrombosis, infection, and duodenal leak.

   f. Some centers use the superior mesenteric vein for venous drainage.

C. Segmental versus whole pancreas transplantation.
   1. Segmental pancreas procurement occurs in living donation and can be done for deceased donation also.
      a. The tail of the pancreas is taken for transplantation.
      b. When the donor is a live donor, there has been a 13% complication rate reported by Sutherland et al. (1999) Complications include need for splenectomy; abscess formation, successfully treated by drainage; sterile fluid collections; and two patients who needed repeat laparotomy. All donors were normoglycemic after donation.
   2. Exocrine drainage for segmental pancreas transplantation is controlled by a Roux-en-Y pancreaticojejunostomy.
   3. There seems to be no clinical significance between whole versus segmental pancreas transplantation in the long term (Tajra et al., 1994).

D. Operative procedure for SPK transplant differs from a kidney transplant alone.
   1. For a kidney transplant alone, the incision is along the groin area with the kidney being placed outside the abdominal cavity.
   2. For a SPK transplant, the incision is down the middle of the abdomen with the pancreas and kidney being placed within the iliac fossa of the abdominal cavity.
   3. The kidney is first transplanted to protect the pancreas from unnecessary trauma. It is placed in the left iliac fossa to save the right fossa for the pancreas. Refer to the section on kidney transplantation for further information on the operative procedure for kidney transplantation.
   4. The pancreas is placed in the right iliac fossa because there is less chance of portal vein kinking after venous anastomosis when it is placed on the right side (Auchincloss & Shaffer, 1999).
   5. The pancreas can be placed intraperitoneally to prevent deep wound infections, although it is easier to place the pancreas extraperitoneally.
   6. The donor spleen may be removed either before transplantation, during the transplant procedure, or just before closing the abdomen. Leaving the spleen with the pancreas transplant can cause graft-versus-host disease (Deierhoi et al., 1986).

7. Exocrine management occurs as previously described.

VII. Complications of pancreas transplantation (see Table 10.2).

A. Arterial or venous thrombosis related to poor preservation, long preservation time, or decreased blood flow after ligation of the splenic artery may occur postoperatively. It is usual practice to anticoagulate pancreas recipients in the immediate postoperative period. Systemic heparinization may result in bleeding, so other methods of anti-coagulation are often used. This may be done with:
   1. Low molecular weight dextran IV or subcutaneous heparin for up to 5 days postoperatively, as long as there is no postoperative bleeding, and low dose acetylsalicylic acid (aspirin) from day 1 to 4 months posttransplantation.
   2. Postoperative bed rest may be necessary for 1–3 days to prevent hip flexion and secondary shifting to protect the vascular anastomoses.
   3. Arterial thrombosis occurs with a sudden rise in serum glucose levels and stable amylase.
   4. Venous thrombosis occurs with sudden abdominal pain and hyperamylasemia. Upon surgical reentry, the pancreas appears large, engorged, and dark-blue in color.
   5. Diagnosis is made with Doppler ultrasound or computed tomography (CT) angiogram or magnetic resonance (MR) angiogram.
   6. Prompt surgical intervention is required to prevent serious infection; usually the graft is lost.

B. Bleeding related to anastomosis complications or anticoagulation therapy.
   1. Hematuria occurs in up to 15.7% of cases (Sollinger et al., 1993) and can be handled with aggressive bladder irrigation using sterile normal saline to prevent bladder outlet obstruction or cystoscopy for clot evacuation.
   2. Anticoagulation therapy may need to be discontinued if that is the cause of the bleeding.
   3. Postoperative bleeding that is significant may require re-exploration surgically to prevent severe hemorrhage.

C. Local infection as either a urinary tract infection, wound infection, or CMV infection occurs in 37–60% of patients. As technique improves, wound infection rates have decreased dramatically (Auchincloss & Shaffer, 1999).

Table 10.2

Surgical Complications of Pancreas Transplantation

- Thrombosis of vessels supplying pancreas
- Bleeding from vessel
- Hematuria
- Local infection
- Anastomotic leak
- Pancreatitis

D. Anastomotic leaks are one of the most common complications within the first 3 months after transplantation (Cupples & Ohler, 2003).
   1. Foley catheter is used to keep the bladder decompressed and prevent tension on sutures.
   2. Symptoms include lower abdominal pain, fever, leukocytosis, and hyperamylasemia.
   3. Diagnosis is made by cystogram.
   4. Leaks can cause fistula or abscess formation. Surgical re-exploration may be required to prevent these secondary complications. Some smaller anastomotic leaks may be treated with stent placement.
   5. Leaks that occur late after transplantation in bladder drained pancreas transplants may need to be converted to enteric drainage.

E. Early allograft pancreatitis can occur secondary to preservation injury, ischemia, surgical handling, or other technical complications. Signs and symptoms include "hyperamylasemia, perigraft fluid collections, graft tenderness, and glycemic discontrol" (Cheng & Munn, 1994). Peak serum amylase levels are reached within 72 hours of the pancreas transplant and usually decrease by postoperative day 5. A consistent rise in serum amylase and/or graft site tenderness may be indicative of rejection which needs to be ruled out. Pancreatitis may also occur later after transplantation due to anastomotic strictures (Cupples & Ohler, 2003).

F. Sepsis occurs more frequently in pancreas transplantation than in any other transplant and is the most common cause of patient death.
   1. Acidic enzymes cause septic pancreatitis.
   2. Symptoms include fever, abdominal tenderness, and increased blood glucose levels.
   3. Requires aggressive intravenous antibiotics and monitoring of blood glucose levels.
   4. Frequently requires surgical re-exploration.

Table 10.3

Signs and Symptoms of Pancreas Rejection

- Fever > 100° F
- Tenderness at graft site
- Decreased urinary amylase (in patients with bladder drainage)
- Urine pH < 7.5 (in patients with bladder drainage)
- Hyperglycemia (late)
- Increased amylase and lipase

VIII. Immunosuppression and rejection after pancreas transplantation.

A. See Chapter 47 for immunogenetic basis of tissue transplantation, rejection, and immune modification. Same principles apply for pancreas transplantation.

B. Immunosuppression protocols for pancreas transplantation have a similar combination as in kidney transplantation.

C. Induction therapy for PAK and SPK were similar in 2004 with 80% receiving some type of induction (UNOS, 2005).
   1. In SPK transplantation, the most common induction therapies used were antithymocyte globulin (ATG [44%]), alemtuzumab (Cam-Path® [19%]), and either basiliximab (Simulect®) or daclizumab (Zenepax® [18% for both]).
   2. In PAK transplantation, 58% received ATG, 20% received alemtuzumab, and 12% received basiliximab or daclizumab.
   3. In PTA transplantation, 51% received ATG, 43% received alemtuzumab, and 9% received daclizumab.

D. The majority of recipients currently receive tacrolimus (Prograf®), mycophenolate mofetil (MMF®), and steroids as their initial maintenance immunosuppression. Cyclosporine (CsA) and sirolimus (Rapamune®) are also used.
   1. Steroids, CsA, and Prograf may all contribute to hyperglycemia.
   2. The number of recipients on steroid-free immunosuppression has continued to increase with 50% of PTA recipients being steroid free in 2004 (UNOS, 2005).

3. Drug dosing varies by each institution's specific protocol and is based on desired trough levels.

E. Potential common side effects of immunosuppressive therapy.
   1. MMF. GI distress (diarrhea, nausea, vomiting) and bone marrow suppression (leukopenia, thrombocytopenia).
   2. Prograf. Diabetes, nephrotoxicity, hypertension, and infections.
   3. Rapamune. Delayed wound healing, diarrhea, thrombocytopenia, hyperlipidemia, and hypercholesterolemia.
   4. CsA. Nephrotoxicity, GI distress (diarrhea, nausea, vomiting), hyperkalemia, hypertension, and hyperlipidemia.
   5. Prednisone. Increased appetite, GI disturbances, impaired wound healing, infection, hyperlipidemia, and easy bruising.

F. The goal of immunosuppression is to prevent rejection in the transplanted organ, and not over-immunosuppress so that infection occurs. Therefore, the least amount of immunosuppression that can be given to prevent rejection is used. Continual monitoring for rejection is done. The patient is taught the signs and symptoms of rejection to continue as much of that observation as possible after discharge from the hospital.

G. Signs and symptoms of pancreas rejection (see Table 10.3), although they lack real specificity, include:
   1. Low amylase levels in the urine when bladder drainage procedure is done. Amylase levels in the urine usually exceed 30,000 units/24 hours (Cosimi & Conti, 1989).
   2. Urine pH less than 7.5.
   3. Graft tenderness.
   4. Fever greater than 100 degrees F.
   5. Hyperglycemia, which is a very late sign of rejection.
      a. Occurs after about 90% of the pancreas is damaged. At this point, significant vascular and islet cell infiltration with lymphocytes, as well as fibrosis, has occurred (Bartucci et al., 1992).
      b. This damage is often irreversible and requires removal of the pancreas.

H. When simultaneous pancreas-kidney transplant is done, the kidney may become the sentinel organ to monitor for rejection. Signs and symptoms include:

1. Decreased urine output.
2. Increased serum creatinine and blood urea nitrogen.
3. Tenderness over graft site.
4. Weight gain, greater than 2 pounds over 24 hours.
5. Hypertension.
6. Fever.

I. The kidney allows for an earlier diagnosis and treatment of rejection, thereby accounting for the improved graft survival of simultaneous pancreas-kidney transplant.

J. Detecting rejection after pancreas transplantation is still considered one of the major problems of pancreas transplantation because of its difficulty. Various institutions use various methods, and continued research is being conducted to create a gold standard for detecting pancreas rejection (see Table 10.4).
   1. With simultaneous pancreas-kidney transplants, rejection may be detected by kidney rejection and by frank signs and symptoms of pancreas rejection listed above.
   2. Cytoscopic transduodenal pancreas-transplant biopsy is another option for bladder-drained transplants (Jones et al., 1994).
      a. Done under ultrasound guidance for best visualization of the pancreatic vessels and iliac vessels and to prevent biopsy of the bowel or vascular structures.
      b. Nephroscope is used for the cystoscopy.
      c. Biopsy forceps are used for the duodenal biopsy through the cystoscope.
      d. Core-cutting biopsy needles are used with the aid of a biopsy gun for the transcystoscopic biopsy of the pancreas to allow for adequate tissue samples.
      e. Adequate pancreas tissue was obtained in 80% of the sample as compared to 57% in other biopsy protocols, which led to better ability to diagnose rejection of the pancreas (Jones et al., 1994).
      f. Complications include hematuria after biopsy, treated with bladder irrigation until clear. No patients required transfusion, and no grafts were lost because of biopsy complications.
      g. Other postbiopsy complications reported include clot retention and transient hyperamylasemia.
   3. Percutaneous pancreas biopsy also is an option to diagnose rejection.
      a. 18-gauge biopsy needle is used with Doppler ultrasound localization.

Table 10.4

Detection of Rejection in Pancreas Transplantation

Noninvasive Methods
- Assessment for signs and symptoms of rejection in either the kidney or pancreas
- Experimental techniques
  - Serum anodal trypsinogen
  - Pancreas specific protein
  - Urine cytology

Invasive Methods
- Percutaneous pancreas biopsy
- Cystoscopic transduodenal pancreas biopsy

      b. Adequate tissue for examination was obtained in 88% of cases in one study reported. Two (2.2%) cases resulted in intraabdominal bleeding. There were no reported cases of graft pancreatitis, pancreatic fistula, or pseudocyst formation.
   4. Reliable techniques or laboratory studies for noninvasive diagnosis of rejection is being sought by other institutions.
      a. Serologic markers for pancreatic exocrine function currently being considered include serum anodal trypsinogen and pancreas specific protein (Auchincloss & Shaffer, 1999; Nyberg et al., 1991; Perkal et al., 1992).
      b. Urine cytology and glucose disappearance rates have also been reported as helpful in diagnosing rejection (Auchincloss & Shaffer, 1999; Elmer et al., 1995; Radio et al., 1993).
      c. Serum amylase remains a poor indicator of rejection because it may also rise in pancreatitis after pancreas transplantation.

IX. **Other postoperative management of the pancreas transplant recipient.**

In general, pancreas transplant recipients no longer require intensive care monitoring in the postoperative period. Depending upon each individual transplant program protocol, once extubated, patients may be moved from the recovery room to a specialized transplant/surgery nursing unit. If an arterial line was placed during surgery and the patient does not go to the intensive care unit, it is removed in the recovery room to decrease risk of infection. A regular insulin infusion is administered intraoperatively and is frequently discontinued in the recovery room due to the immediate function of the newly transplanted pancreas.

A. Acute postoperative nursing care.
1. Hemodynamic and fluid status monitoring.
   a. Vital signs.
      (1) Blood pressure monitoring; a decrease in systolic blood pressure of 20 mmHg may signify dehydration (Trusler, 1992).
      (2) Cardiac monitoring; an increase of 25 beats per minute may indicate dehydration (Trusler, 1992).
      (3) Central venous pressure monitored by central line.
   b. Observe for bleeding.
      (1) Urine may be bloody. Monitor for clots and irrigate bladder as ordered.
      (2) Jackson Pratt (JP) drain(s) may be in place. Monitor output if present. Assess amount and color of drainage.
      (3) Observe for drainage on bandages. Circle, date, and time drainage and monitor rate of increase (if any) in drainage.
      (4) Monitor hematocrit as ordered for sudden decrease or downward trend.
   c. Monitor fluid and electrolyte status. Osmotic diuresis may occur posttransplantation.
      (1) Assess for signs of dehydration.
      (2) Monitor for hypokalemia related to diuresis.
      (3) Hyponatremia may occur with osmotic shift.
      (4) Monitor for hypotension. Hypotension may increase the risk of vessel thrombosis.
2. Monitor for potential thrombosis.
   a. Unilateral lower extremity edema on side of pancreas transplant (usually the right side).
   b. Maintain bed rest for 1 to 3 days posttransplantation with no hip flexion to preserve integrity of the vessel anastomoses and prevent thrombosis.
   c. Maintain subcutaneous heparin or enteric-coated aspirin for thrombosis prophylaxis.
3. Monitor for anastomosis leakage. Maintain integrity of urinary catheter for up to 5 days posttransplantation for bladder decompression and decreased tension on sutures.
4. Maintain integrity of nasogastric tube. Because pancreas is often placed intraperitoneally, there will be decreased bowel motility. Assess patient for bowel sounds and effects of potential gastroparesis secondary to diabetes.

5. Monitor metabolic function related to pancreas function.
   a. If bladder drainage of pancreas is the operative procedure done, check urine pH and urine amylase every 4 hours. Urine pH should be > 7.5 secondary to bicarbonate excreted from transplanted pancreas into the bladder. Urine amylase should be 10,000–200,000 IU/L.
   b. If arterial line present, monitor arterial blood gases for metabolic acidosis secondary to bicarbonate losses through the pancreas. If arterial line is not present, monitor venous CO_2 or pulse oximetry.
   c. Monitor blood glucose levels every 1 to 2 hours.
   d. Regular insulin infusion may be used in the early postoperative period. Maintain blood glucose levels less than 150 mg/dL since chronic hyperglycemia is detrimental to beta cells.
   e. If not on insulin and the newly transplanted pancreas is functioning well, the patient may require high-concentration dextrose infusions to compensate for an initial outpouring of insulin.
   f. Monitor serum amylase for signs of pancreatitis immediately postoperatively and every 12 hours.
   g. Monitor immunologic function via white blood cell counts and body temperature.
6. Infection prophylaxis.
   a. Intravenous antibiotics and antifungals are generally continued for 48 hours or longer.
   b. Pneumocystis carinii (PCP) and cytomegalovirus (CMV) prophylaxis is started.

B. Intermediate care.
1. There is a decreased need for hemodynamic monitoring 24 hours after surgery as long as the patient remains stable. Therefore, the arterial and central lines can be discontinued as soon as possible because of the risk of infection and sepsis in the immunosuppressed patient. Noninvasive blood pressure monitoring continues until the patient is more mobile and has stable fluid balance.
2. Metabolic monitoring is still important, but need not be done as often as in the first 24 hours as long as the patient is stable.
   a. Blood glucose levels can be drawn when the patient is fasting, and then every 4 to 6 hours, depending on the results.
   b. Urine and serum amylase levels are done once daily.

c. Urine pH continues to be monitored every 4 to 8 hours, then daily as the patient progresses.
3. Drains and tubes are discontinued as soon as possible because of the risk of contamination and subsequent sepsis. However:
   a. The urinary catheter is left in up to 5 days to decompress the bladder and drain exocrine secretions from the pancreas.
   b. The JP drains are left in for several days until there is a negative ultrasound, about day 5 postoperatively. Specifically there should be no fluid collections around the pancreas or the kidney, if a kidney transplant was also done.
   c. The nasogastric tube is taken out when there are bowel sounds present, usually about day 2 to 3 postoperatively. The patient gradually is allowed clear liquids and progresses slowly to a regular diet. Continue monitoring for:
      (1) Pancreatitis secondary to preservation injury, handling of the pancreas during the time of transplantation, or inflammation postoperatively.
      (2) Gastroparesis secondary to diabetes.
   d. The patient may get out of bed day 1 to 3 after surgery. Assessment for orthostatic hypotension is done the first several times that the patient gets out of bed. Orthostatic hypotension can either be caused by fluid depletion or be secondary to peripheral neuropathy related to diabetes.
   e. Infection and immunologic assessments are done through monitoring of:
      (1) Temperature every 4 hours.
      (2) Wound site every 8 hours.
      (3) White blood cell count monitoring.
      (4) Cultures weekly of JP fluid and urine, if indicated.
      (5) Chest x-ray weekly, if indicated.
      (6) CMV antigenemia, if indicated.
      (7) With temperatures greater than 100° F, urine, blood, and sputum cultures may be done.

C. Rehabilitation to discharge.
   1. Metabolic effects of the pancreas transplant continue to be monitored.
      a. Glycosylated hemoglobin (hemoglobin A1c) can be monitored. Normal value is between 3.5% and 5% and may vary slightly with lab variation.
      b. C peptide can be monitored which reflects secretory function of the beta cells in the transplanted pancreas.
      c. Blood glucose levels continue to be monitored because of the effects of steroids on glucose metabolism. Rising glucose is not a good indicator for rejection.
      d. Urine amylase continues to be monitored to assist with the diagnosis of pancreatitis or rejection.
   2. Discharge preparation is done through patient teaching (see Tables 10.5 and 10.6), which includes:
      a. Medications, including names, indications, doses, times taken, and side effects.
         (1) A teaching booklet is a good reference for the patient because there is so much to learn in the postoperative period.
         (2) A teaching card with medications, doses, and times to take the medications is helpful for the patient to initially learn and then to review medications.
         (3) Medications at the bedside for the patient to prepare and have checked by the nurse reinforces learning.
      b. Signs and symptoms of rejection and infection.
      c. Immunization history and immunizations allowed.
      d. Hygiene and self-care are stressed, with emphasis on emptying bladder.
      e. Good foot care.
      f. Follow-up clinic appointments are made before discharge.
      g. Other issues are also discussed (see Tables 10.5 and 10.6).
      h. Average length of stay has decreased to 5–10 days.

X. Long-term benefits of pancreas transplantation.

A. Nephropathy.
   1. Various studies have shown that pancreas transplantation prevents progression of diabetic nephropathy in the transplanted kidney.

B. Polyneuropathy.
   1. Improvements in polyneuropathy have been seen in pancreas transplant recipients.
   2. It is difficult to determine if this is secondary to improvement in uremia or euglycemia.

C. Diabetic retinopathy.
   1. No reversal of retinopathy is seen with pancreas transplantation but data suggests that stabilization occurs.

Table 10.5

Patient Outcomes – Combined Kidney/Pancreas Transplant

☐ 1. Can state rationale for taking daily temperatures.

☐ 2. Can recognize fever (temperature greater than 38.5° C or 101° F).

☐ 3. Can take and record oral temperature (has thermometer).

☐ 4. Can explain susceptibility to infection.

☐ 5. Can describe signs and symptoms of infection and appropriate action to take.

☐ 6. Can explain need to take and record weight daily (has scale).

☐ 7. Can recognize weight gain (greater than 2 lb/day or 4 lb/week).

☐ 8. Can explain rationale for measuring and recording intake and output, if needed.

☐ 9. Can measure and record intake and output, if needed.

☐ 10. Can correctly perform and record blood glucose (has blood glucose monitoring machine).

☐ 11. Can state blood glucose parameters that require physician notification.

☐ 12. Can measure and record urine pH (has urine test strips), if bladder drainage.

☐ 13. Can state urine pH parameters that require physician notification, if bladder drainage.

☐ 14. Can state precautions to avoid trauma to transplanted kidney/pancreas.

☐ 15. Can describe typical changes in sexual functioning following transplant.

☐ 16. Can explain importance of avoiding pregnancy for 1 year after transplant.

☐ 17. Can describe signs and symptoms of rejection and appropriate action to take.

☐ 18. Can state actions, dosages, and side effects of medications.

☐ 19. Can explain routine for immunosuppressive blood test monitoring.

☐ 20. Can state how to ensure medication supply.

☐ 21. Can describe identification patient will carry as a transplant recipient.

☐ 22. Can describe dietary and fluid prescriptions.

☐ 23. Has Kidney/Pancreas Transplant Book.

☐ 24. Has written medication instructions that have been reviewed with nurse (including medication cards).

☐ 25. Has rejection and infection cards.

☐ 26. Has written dietary and fluid instructions.

☐ 27. Has arranged for physical therapy consult, if needed.

☐ 28. Has arranged for social service consult.

☐ 29. Has all appropriate telephone numbers for emergencies (physician, clinical nurse specialist, transplant office, transplant unit).

☐ 30. Has follow-up appointment.

Primary Nurse Signature _____

Discharging Nurse Signature _____

Date of Discharge _____

Source: Bartucci, M.R., Loughman, K.A., & Moir, E.J. (1992). Kidney-pancreas transplantation: A treatment option for ESRD and type 1 diabetes. *ANNA Journal, 19*(5), 471. Used with permission.

D. Gastroenteropathy. Some improvement is seen after pancreas transplantation.

E. Vascular disease.
1. Cardiac function was shown to improve after transplantation.
2. Peripheral vascular disease does not seem to be affected by pancreas transplantation.

F. Lipid metabolism. Several studies have shown improvement in lipid profiles posttransplantation.

G. Pregnancy. Pregnancy outcomes are followed through the National Transplant Pregnancy Registry database for kidney–pancreas recipients.

H. Quality of life after pancreas transplantation.
1. Quality of life is important in terms of pancreas transplantation because pancreas transplantation is not meant to be life saving, but done to improve the life of a diabetic.
2. Although important to analyze, quality of life is rather difficult to assess. It makes up the physical, social, and psychic well being of an individual, based on his or her own perception of these domains.
3. Quality of life has been studied in pancreas transplant recipients by various groups of practitioners, but there are no standardized tools used to look at quality of life, and no conclusive data. There does seem to be a trend that shows pancreas transplant recipients experience improved quality of life after transplantation.

Table 10.6

What Patients Need to Know about Their Medications Before Leaving the Hospital

- Names of all medications (brand, generic, and common nicknames)
- The rationale for the medication
- Frequency, times, and whether the medication can be taken with food or with other medications
- Instructions for taking medications when blood is to be drawn
- How long the patient can expect to be on the medication
- Common side effects
- What to do if a dose is missed
- What to do in the event the patient cannot take the medication
- Where to store the medication
- How to get a refill
- How much it costs and what insurance will/will not cover

Source: Conway, P., Davis, C., Hartel, T., & Russell, G. (1998). Simultaneous kidney pancreas transplantation: Patient issues and nursing interventions. *ANNA Journal, 25*(5), 459. Used with permission.

Chapter 49

Islet Cell Transplantation

Purpose

The purpose of this chapter is to discuss concepts related to islet cell transplantation.

Objectives

Upon completion of this chapter, the learner will be able to:
1. Outline important historical events related to islet cell transplantation.
2. Discuss concepts of islet cell transplantation.
3. Discuss recipient selection for islet cell transplantation.
4. Describe the different sites for islet cell infusion.
5. Explain methods for modification of the immune system after islet cell transplantation.
6. Discuss future directions and challenges related to islet cell transplantation.

I. **Historical perspectives of pancreas transplantation.**

A. The first known report of transplanting portions of the pancreas in diabetic patients was in 1894. This involved using pieces of sheep pancreas in humans and was not successful.

B. The first successful effort was reported in 1972 by Ballinger and Lacy in a rat model.

C. The 1980s brought the first successful islet transplantation in patients with type 1 diabetes, although the rates of sustained success were quite low.

D. More recently, the rates of successful transplant are higher, although on only small numbers of patients.

II. **Basic concepts of islet cell transplantation.**

A. The islets of Langerhans are clusters of endocrine cells scattered throughout the pancreas that are responsible for glucose metabolism in the body.

B. Beta cells, which are located in the islets, secrete insulin in response to hyperglycemia.

C. The pancreas contains approximately 1 million islets that make up approximately 2–3% of the total pancreatic volume.

D. Islets are isolated from procured pancreata from deceased donors close to the same way that pancreata are procured for whole organ transplantation.
   1. The pancreatic duct is then cannulated, and collagenase is infused to separate islets from exocrine and ductal tissue.
   2. The cells are purified by centrifugation to remove cellular debris.
   3. The purified cells are infused via catheter through the portal vein where they travel to the liver sinusoids.
   4. It may take up from one to four donors to yield enough islet cells for one patient.

E. Islet cell transplantation is minimally invasive. It is therefore without the risks of the major surgery of pancreatic transplantation and its ensuing complications.

F. Currently still investigational, it is still not routine care for diabetics.

III. Recipient selection.

A. Persons with type 1 diabetes with kidney failure after kidney transplant (who also meet other criteria, see section on pancreas transplantation – recipient selection).

B. Nonuremic patients with hypoglycemic unawareness or metabolic instability despite intensive work to attempt to control glucose.

IV. Sites for islet cell infusion.

A. The hepatic circulation via the portal vein is the most common site.
   1. Most sustained results are via this site of infusion.
   2. Potential complications include bleeding, portal venous thrombosis, and portal hypertension.
   3. There are also risks that the islets may be exposed to environmental toxins as well as medications.
   4. Intrahepatic islet cells are unable to release glucagon during periods of hypoglycemia.

B. Research is being conducted regarding other sites including the peritoneal cavity and omentum.

V. Immunosuppression in islet cell transplantation.

A. The most promising results have been from Edmonton, Canada, using low-dose tacrolimus,

sirolimus, and daclizumab. This protocol is steroid-free.

B. Other protocols have been used, using other combinations of immunosuppression (see Chapter 47 on kidney transplantation).

VI. Challenges and future directions in pancreatic islet cell transplantation.

A. Several donor pancreatic organs are needed to procure enough islets for one patient.

B. Most patients require more than one islet cell infusion.

C. Detection of rejection is currently very difficult. As with whole organ transplantation, hyperglycemia occurs late in the process, when it is likely too late to salvage the cells.

D. Patients must be carefully monitored for insulin requirements following islet infusion. It may take days, weeks, or even months to achieve insulin independence.

E. Because immunosuppression is required to prevent rejection, patients still have all of the risks associated with immunosuppression.

F. Currently, research is being conducted to culture islet cells in vitro, cryopreservation, minimization of immunosuppression, induction of tolerance, and encapsulation of the islets with some type of device is being investigated.

Chapter 50

Chronic Kidney Disease in the Transplant Recipient

Purpose

Part 1. The purpose of this chapter, Part 1, is to provide an understanding of factors that affect kidney function in advanced heart failure, to discuss concepts related to acute and chronic kidney disease after cardiac transplantation, and to describe clinical implications before and after cardiac transplantation related to renal function.

Part 2. The purpose of this chapter, Part 2, is to provide an understanding of factors that affect kidney function in advanced liver disease, to discuss concepts related to acute and chronic kidney failure after liver transplantation, and to describe clinical implications before and after liver transplantation related to kidney function.

Objectives

Upon completion of this chapter, the learner will be able to:

Part 1.

1. Discuss mechanisms that could worsen kidney function prior to cardiac transplantation.
2. Discuss the significance and nursing implications of worsening kidney dysfunction in advanced chronic systolic heart failure.
3. Describe kidney injury characteristics that are frequent, common, and uncommon after cardiac transplant.
4. Describe ways to minimize the toxic effects of posttransplant medications.
5. List treatment strategies that may reduce the incidence or severity of medication nephrotoxicity.
6. Describe the implications and considerations of dialysis in the cardiac transplant recipient.

Part 2.

1. Discuss the underfill and overfill theories of renal sodium and water retention in liver disease.
2. Discuss causes of reabsorption of sodium during end-stage liver disease.
3. Describe mechanisms of ascites in liver disease.
4. Identify causes and treatments of hyponatremia and hypernatremia in liver disease.
5. Discuss the four types of acid-base imbalances in liver disease and their pathophysiologic mechanisms.
6. Define hepatorenal syndrome and discuss how it differs from other types of kidney failure.
7. Discuss the management of patients with liver disease associated kidney failure.
8. Discuss chronic kidney disease and the liver transplant recipient.

Part 1

Chronic Kidney Disease in Cardiac Transplant Recipients

I. Chronic kidney disease with left ventricular dysfunction.

A. Abnormalities in kidney function frequently occur in patients with chronic left ventricular systolic dysfunction.

B. Intrinsic kidney disease may be caused most often by advanced age, atherosclerosis (renovascular disease), hypertension (causes lower effective renal plasma flow and higher mean renovascular resistance), and diabetes mellitus (diabetic nephropathy).

C. Hemodynamic abnormalities that diminish kidney function are decreased cardiac output and renal blood flow and an elevation in renal vein pressure secondary to an elevated right atrial pressure and tricuspid regurgitation.
   1. Hypotension may result in poor renal perfusion.
   2. Atrial fibrillation leads to atrial structure changes (electrical and mechanical remodeling) and atrial natriuretic peptide release, which influences renal volume. Loss of atrial kick may decrease cardiac output and affect renal perfusion.

D. Neurohormonal abnormalities lead to vasoconstriction from increased concentrations or enhanced responsiveness to norepinephrine, endothelin, and angiotensin II. Neurohormonal abnormalities prevent the release of endogenous vasodilators or diminish their responsiveness (natriuretic peptides and nitric oxide).
   1. Initially, angiotensin II causes an increase in efferent glomerular arterial resistance, leading to maintenance of glomerular filtration rate when renal blood flow is reduced. Over time, glomerular filtration rate may fall.
   2. Markedly elevated plasma renin levels and hyponatremia are signs of great risk for worsening renal function during ACE inhibitor therapy since maintenance of glomerular filtration rate is dependent on angiotensin II.

E. Therapies for heart failure may influence kidney function.
   1. ACE inhibitors and angiotensin II receptor blockers decrease the glomerular filtration rate by inhibiting efferent renal arteriolar resistance, thus, reducing glomerular blood flow. Serum creatinine rises, leading to renal dysfunction.
      a. The effect of ACE inhibitors and angiotensin II receptor blockers on kidney function is unpredictable. It is influenced by volume status, serum sodium level, and concurrent medications. A rise in serum creatinine and blood urea nitrogen of 10–20% is not unlikely.
      b. Rises in serum creatinine to 3 mg/dL or higher do not preclude the continuation of therapy as long as the serum creatinine is stabilized and hyperkalemia does not occur.
   2. Diuretic therapy (all classes) depletes sodium and volume, leading to decreased renal blood flow.
      a. Loop diuretics directly activate neuro-endocrine systems (sympathetic nervous system, renin-angiotensin system, and antidiuretic hormone), leading to an imbalance between renal sympathetic activation, angiotensin II, and natriuretic peptides.
      b. During aggressive diuresis with loop diuretics and in the presence of angiotensin-converting enzyme inhibitors, natriuretic peptide levels are reduced, and angiotensin II is diminished. In addition, sympathetic activation and increased vasopressin levels alter the glomerular filtration rate, resulting in kidney function deterioration.
   3. Beta-blocker therapy appears to be renoprotective and may decrease the risk for developing worsening kidney function by 30%. Beta-blocker therapy lowers plasma renin level activity, which will decrease dependence on angiotensin II for maintaining glomerrular filtration rate.

F. Concurrent therapies for comorbid conditions may influence kidney function. Nonsteroidal anti-inflammatory drugs (NSAIDs) and aspirin may inhibit renal vasodilatory prostaglandins and afferent arteriole vasodilatation.

G. A moderate degree of chronic kidney disease stage 3, or GFR < 60 mL/min, is associated with an increase in all-cause mortality in patients with mild to moderate left ventricular systolic dysfunction. Risk for pump failure death and the combined endpoint of death or hospitalization for heart failure increases in patients with moderate CKD. Since CKD leads to heart failure progression, data suggest that adequacy of kidney function may influence disease progression and compensation.

II. Collaborative management of chronic kidney disease prior to cardiac transplantation.

A. Permanent discontinuation of ACE inhibitors is rarely necessary when creatinine is moderately elevated. Decreases in kidney function that lead to interruption in therapy might prevent optimization of afterload and preload, potentially leading to further compromise of left ventricular function and perpetuation of symptoms.

B. Patients who develop an elevated serum creatinine from ACE inhibitor or angiotensin II receptor blocking therapies may derive the greatest benefit from the therapies, especially when left ventricular systolic dysfunction is advanced.

C. Beta-blocker therapy is initiated and maintained whenever possible.

D. If atrial fibrillation develops, attempts to restore normal sinus rhythm are a priority.

E. Renal insufficiency serves as a marker for more advanced heart failure. Measurement of GFR (not baseline serum creatinine level) should be monitored, especially when there is an increase in the blood urea nitrogen/serum creatinine ratio, suggesting prerenal failure.

F. Since comorbid conditions influence the prevalence of renal insufficiency, treatment should reflect current consensus recommendations.

G. Kidney replacement therapies improve prognosis when kidney dysfunction occurs as a result of heart failure and/or the therapies used to treat the condition while awaiting cardiac transplantation.
1. Therapies allow for controlled removal of excess sodium and volume, even when diuretic resistance occurs.
2. Therapies replace kidney function when conventional fluid removal with diuretics leads to prerenal depletion and impaired kidney function.
3. Continuous kidney replacement therapies are the first choice during periods of hemodynamic instability.

III. Chronic kidney disease after cardiac transplantation: incidence, definition, outcomes.

A. Early acute kidney failure refers to the immediate postoperative period of 0–30 days. The incidence is approximately 50%.
1. Predisposing factors.
   a. Use of calcineurin inhibitors (cyclosporine or tacrolimus) in the early postoperative period. Increased incidence with intravenous dosing or higher drug trough levels.
   b. Preoperative kidney dysfunction.
   c. Preoperative cardiovascular compromise (presence of hypotension), requiring continuous intravenous vasopressor support.
   d. Any hospitalization before transplantation.
   e. Perioperative hemodynamic compromise.
   f. Sepsis.
2. Signs that suggest severe kidney hypoperfusion with intact tubular function.
   a. Oliguria or anuria.
   b. High serum creatinine and BUN, which peak 4–5 days postoperatively (BUN not reliable indicator as steroids can significantly increase BUN postoperatively); elevated BUN/creatinine ratio.
   c. Low urine sodium (less than 10 mEq/L) — however, this may be inaccurate if the patient is receiving diuretics; hyponatremia; low fractional excretion of sodium (less than 1%); and metabolic acidosis.
   d. Hyperkalemia disproportionate to elevated serum creatinine.
   e. Normal urine sediment.
3. Outcome.
   a. If calcineurin inhibitor use was the only factor that produced the decrease in kidney function, and the dosage was reduced, the outcome is favorable with a spontaneous recovery in 7–10 days. (In general, mortality is lower following open heart surgery for cardiac transplantation than when acute renal failure [ARF] occurs after other open heart surgery procedures.)
   b. If graft function was poor and when multifactorial causes were present, mortality rates range from a low of 20–29% to approximately 50%. Deaths were unrelated to renal causes.
   c. If kidney failure lasts beyond 7–10 days and is complicated by septicemia or surgery or calcineurin inhibitor dose cannot be reduced, irreversible kidney failure may ensue.

B. Late acute kidney injury occurs after 30 days and has a low incidence of 1–2%. The first 6 to 8 weeks after transplantation are when the greatest risk of nephrotoxic effects occur.
   1. Predisposing factors.
      a. Use of nephrotoxic drugs together with calcineurin inhibitor, causing a synergistic toxic effect, i.e., amphotericin, ganciclovir, and NSAIDs.
      b. Use of drugs that interact with and increase the blood levels of calcineurin inhibitors, causing kidney dysfunction and severe infection.
      c. Multisystem organ failure syndrome.
      d. Hypertension and hyperlipidemia have been suggested as potential factors that may lead to accelerated atherosclerosis.
   2. Signs.
      a. Elevation of serum creatinine with or without oliguria. Significant deterioration noted after the third month posttransplant.
      b. Low fractional excretion of sodium in the absence of heart failure.
      c. No relation has been found between calcineurin inhibitor dose and trough levels and the incidence of acute kidney dysfunction.
   3. Outcome is favorable if there is no heart failure.

IV. Chronic kidney disease after cardiac transplantation: Injury characteristics.

A. Kidney biopsy findings in patients with calcineurin inhibitor toxicity.
   1. Tubulointerstitial damage: interstitial fibrosis with tubular atrophy (most frequent finding).
   2. Microvascular changes from vasoconstriction of the afferent artioles causes obliterative vasculopathy, endothelial swelling, and microthrombi from deposition of protein material in necrotic arterial walls (second most common finding). In later stages, fibrous endarteritis occurs.
   3. Arterial changes lead to an occlusive disorder of the afferent arterioles and ischemic damage to nephrons, causing obliteration and retraction of the affected glomerulus (not common).

B. Electron microscopy.
   1. Vacuolization of the proximal tubular cells with destruction of apical microvilli.
   2. Giant mitochondria.
   3. Dilation of the ergastoplasmic cisternae.
   4. Numerous lysosomes.

C. Physiologic findings.
   1. Increased renal vascular resistance from persistent renal vasoconstriction, cortical renal artery spasm, and ischemia. These findings are related to loss of vasodilatory effects of prostanoids, altered levels of circulating catecholamines, alteration in efferent sympathetic signals to the kidney and possibly by the stimulation of endothelin-1 (a potent vasoconstricting peptide that is derived from the endothelium).
   2. Decreased glomerular filtration rate and renal plasma flow.

V. Chronic kidney disease after cardiac transplantation: Minimizing nephrotoxic effects of calcineurin inhibitors.

A. Dosage should be tailored to individual patient.

B. Routine monitoring of the trough level is integral to maintaining adequate immunosuppression, yet it may be inadequate in minimizing nephrotoxic effects.

C. Avoidance of intravenous calcineurin inhibitors, if possible.

D. Strict monitoring of hemodynamic status postoperatively and maintenance of euvolemia are essential to prevent compromise that would require aggressive use of vasopressor or diuretic medications, since their use enhances the renal toxicity associated with calcineurin inhibitors.

E. Reduction in the dose with early, mild kidney function impairment, whenever possible.

F. Specific drug therapies when calcineurin nephrotoxicity occurs.
   1. Minimize vasoconstriction effects by administration of calcium channel blockers. Careful monitoring for hemodynamic compromise is necessary since these agents have negative inotropic properties.
   2. Other drugs that minimize calcineurin inhibitor effects are atrial natriuretic peptide, cilastatin, dopamine (at low dopaminergic dose), pentoxifylline, and dietary antioxidant supplementation.
   3. Consider change in immunosuppressive regimen using sirolimus instead of calcineurin inhibitor (currently FDA approved for kidney transplant only).

Table 10.7

Drug Interactions Affecting Calcineurin Inhibitors (Cyclosporine and Tacrolimus)

Increased Blood Levels	Decreased Blood Levels	Increased Nephrotoxicity
acetazolamide	carbamazepine	acyclovir
azithromycin	cholestyramine	aminoglycosides
cimetidine	glutethimide	amphotericin B
clarithromycin	isoniazid	cimetidine
corticosteroids	phenobarbital	ciprofloxacin
• methylprednisolone	phenytoin	cephalosporins
• prednisolone	primidone	diclofenac
diltiazem	rifampin	lovastatin
erythromycin	IV sulfatrimethoprim	melphalan
fluconazole	IV trimethoprim/sulfamethoxazole	NSAIDs
imipenem-cilastatin	warfarin	pravastatin
itraconazole		ranitidine
ketoconazole		simvastatin
nicardipine		trimethoprim/sulfamethoxazole
verapamil		
grapefruit juice		

IV = intravenous; NSAIDs = nonsteroidal antiinflammatory drugs

VI. Chronic kidney disease after cardiac transplantation: Other treatment strategies.

A. Conservative measures.
1. Correct disorders of electrolyte imbalance (sodium and potassium), acid-base balance, and hypovolemia.
2. Careful calculation of intake and urinary output.
3. Detect and correct graft dysfunction and infection immediately. Optimal wound care in the early postoperative period.
4. Avoid over-immunosuppression (which can lead to infection and sepsis).
5. If antibiotics are needed, facilitate the use of non-nephrotoxic agents.
6. Use care in administering agents that increase the blood level of cyclosporine or tacrolimus (see Table 10.7). Educate patients to avoid these agents.
7. Use the same recommendations as for any patient with CKD (e.g., control of blood pressure, diabetes, treatment of anemia, hyperlipidemia, etc.).

B. Kidney replacement therapy.
1. Initiate kidney replacement therapy as for any patient with CKD stage 5.
2. Careful monitoring for infection with early intervention because of immunosuppressed state.
3. Very little data on dialysis outcomes for cardiac transplant recipients, but hemodialysis appears to be preferable to peritoneal dialysis.
4. Consider kidney transplantation, if possible.

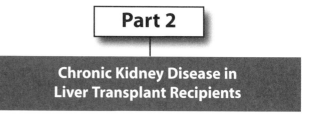

Part 2

Chronic Kidney Disease in Liver Transplant Recipients

I. Chronic kidney disease prior to liver transplantation.

A. Renal sodium and water retention in liver disease. Renal sodium and water retention is a frequent complication of end-stage liver disease (ESLD).

The mechanisms involved in these processes are not completely understood, but they eventually lead to sequelae such as ascites, spontaneous bacterial peritonitis, portal hypertension, varices and variceal bleeding, and hepatorenal syndrome (HRS). These sequelae are major causes of morbidity and mortality before transplantation and also complicate the care of patients after transplantation. The cause(s) of renal sodium and water retention in ESLD are not due to an intrinsic abnormality of the kidneys, but rather to extrarenal mechanisms that control the handling of water and sodium. Several theories about these control mechanisms will be discussed.

1. Afferent factors.
    a. Underfilling. Circulating blood volume and distribution are important factors in the pathology of liver disease associated kidney failure. In patients with ESLD, the amount of blood volume available to the kidneys is decreased because of an increase in vascular capacity. Vasodilatation is the initial cause of the decreased blood volume, leading to an imbalance between the increased vascular capacity and the amount of available blood. This imbalance causes a decrease in the volume of blood that can be used effectively by the kidneys. Vasodilatation causes hemodynamic alterations, including an increased cardiac output and decreased systemic resistance, and low arterial blood pressure. Often, these changes are similar to arteriovenous shunts. Even though the total extracellular volume is increasing, fluid is shifted to other compartments, which does not allow a normal blood volume to reach the kidneys. Correction is aimed at redistribution of the blood to allow the available blood volume to return to normal. (see Figure 10.4) According to this theory, ascites is the main event that leads to underfilled circulation and associated renal salt retention. In summary, this theory postulates that there is an increase in hepatic resistance to blood flow in addition to low serum oncotic pressure, which causes the extravasation of fluid into the peritoneal cavity. The kidneys then recognize a decrease in blood volume and respond by retaining sodium and water.
    b. Overfilling. The overfill theory proposes that retention of excess sodium by the kidneys leads to fluid retention and eventually the development of ascites. It is believed that, in

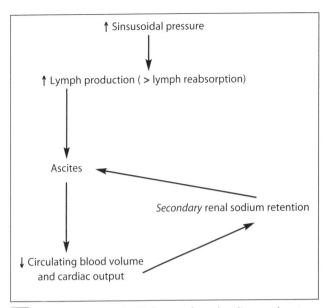

Figure 10.4. Underfill theory of renal sodium and water retention in liver disease.

liver disease, with the reduction of plasma colloid osmotic (oncotic) pressure and portal venous hypertension, the expanded plasma volume moves to the peritoneal spaces and causes ascites formation. Therefore, the retention of renal sodium and the expansion of the plasma volume are causes of, rather than results of, ascites. Normal splanchnic perfusion is unable to increase sinusoidal pressure to the degree necessary to cause ascites formation. However, venous outflow obstruction causes the retention of renal sodium independent of a decrease in intravascular volume. Sodium retention then leads to an increase in plasma volume, cardiac output, and splanchnic perfusion, which causes an increase in portal and sinusoidal pressures to the point that fluid moves from the interstitial space into the peritoneum and causes overflow/overfill ascites (see Figure 10.5). In summary, this theory proposes that the kidneys inappropriately retain sodium as the initial event, leading to an increase in the plasma volume, which causes the formation of ascites.

2. Efferent factors. While blood volume and distribution, and therefore, a decrease in the GFR, play a role in the kidney's ability to absorb or excrete sodium, often sodium is retained with a normal GFR. Renal sodium retention in

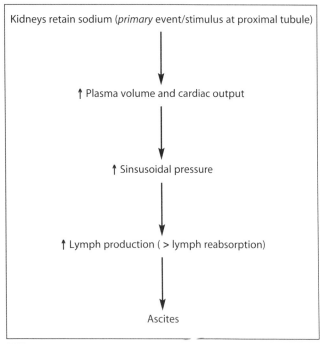

Figure 10.5. Overfill theory of renal sodium and water retention in liver disease.

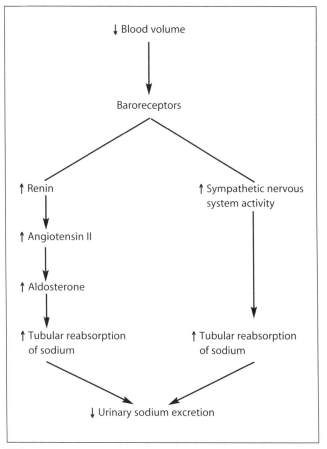

Figure 10.6. Efferent theory of renal sodium and water retention in liver disease with normal glomerular filtration rate.

patients with ESLD is due to enhanced tubular reabsorption as opposed to changes in the filtered sodium load. The majority of sodium reabsorption occurs along the proximal tubule. The causes of this reabsorption are not completely understood, but include the renin-angiotensin-aldosterone system, changes in distribution of intrarenal blood flow, and an increase in activity of the sympathetic nervous system (see Figure 10.6). An increase in renal sympathetic activity directly stimulates the release of renin from the juxtaglomerular complex of the kidney. Renin is released due to impaired renal perfusion from increased afferent arterial tone and decreased renal perfusion. Additionally, impaired hepatic metabolism and inactivation of renin are possible alternative factors.

B. Ascites.
1. Collection of free fluid in the peritoneal space.
2. The ascitic fluid comes from the vascular space of the hepatic circulation and is derived from the liver and intestines.
3. The constant formation of ascites is due to salt and water retention, which shows there is a relationship between the formation ascites and the onset of urinary sodium retention.
4. Once portal hypertension develops and the

patient's albumin decreases, fluid moves from the sinusoids and hepatic circulation to the peritoneal cavity. This causes a decrease in the amount of useful blood volume, causing a decrease in the vascular space, which then stimulates the renal tubule to reabsorb sodium and water.

C. Electrolyte imbalances.
1. Hyponatremia.
    a. Usually due to dilution by large amounts of body water.
    b. ADH levels are increased due to nonosmotic stimulation brought on by a decrease in blood volume to the kidneys.
    c. The best therapy is prevention.
        (1) Serial monitoring of electrolytes and response to diuretics.
        (2) Restriction of water intake.
        (3) Hypertonic saline is not a recommended therapy since most patients have

decreased intravascular oncotic pressure and are not responsive to diuretic therapy.
   (4) Complications include confusion, delirium, seizures, lethargy, weakness, and cerebral edema.
2. Hypernatremia.
   a. Usually due to dehydration or decrease in total body water.
   b. Usually caused by lactulose (the hallmark treatment for hepatic encephalopathy) due to the osmotic effect in which water moves from the plasma to the bowel, causing diarrhea. More water than sodium is excreted since sodium is absorbed by the colon.
   c. Also occurs in hospitalized patients due to insensible water losses from sepsis, fever, tachypnea, and dehydration associated with diuresis.
   d. The best therapy is prevention.
      (1) Monitor fluid balance.
      (2) Monitor electrolytes.
      (3) Decrease lactulose as appropriate.

D. Acid-base imbalances.
   1. Respiratory alkalosis. The cause of respiratory alkalosis in ESLD is not well defined. It may be caused by hypoxemia associated with ascites and ventilation-perfusion imbalances, increased ammonia levels, and hyponatremia. Another cause may be intracellular acidosis, which can cause hyperventilation.
   2. Metabolic alkalosis. Usually due to iatrogenic or extrarenal causes. Diuretics may cause a secondary aldosteronism, which can cause alkalosis. The amount of sodium that actually arrives at the collecting tubule is limited by the sodium reabsorption at the proximal tubule. Therefore, the amount of sodium increases the potassium and hydrogen secretion that results from the sodium reabsorption. If diuretics are administered, more sodium arrives at the distal most nephron and hypokalemia and alkalosis result.
   3. Metabolic acidosis. Lactic acidosis usually occurs in combination with factors such as bleeding or sepsis that decrease the hepatic blood flow, thereby diminishing the use of lactate by the liver and kidneys or causing an increase in the formation of lactate. Other causative factors include alcohol use, medications, hypotension, and hyperventilation.
   4. Respiratory acidosis. Respiratory acidosis is very common in liver disease. It usually occurs in association with severe restrictive lung disease

due to massive ascites and pleural effusion. Additionally, respiratory failure may ensue with the associated respiratory muscle weakness that is due to hypokalemia or respiratory depression from the drugs that the liver usually detoxifies.

E. Hepatorenal syndrome (HRS).
   1. Characterized by a decrease in renal blood flow and GFR in which there is no abnormality of the kidney and no other identified causes of kidney failure.
   2. Other causes of kidney failure must first be ruled out, including nephritis, obstruction, acute tubular necrosis, or dehydration.
   3. Defined by BUN > 50 mg/dL and/or serum creatinine > 2 mg/dL, urine sodium concentration < 10 mEq/L, urine-to-plasma osmolality ratio > 1, no urinary sediment, negative proteinuria, no kidney improvement after albumin or saline administration, and no other cause of kidney failure.
   4. Potential causes.
      a. Severe renal vasoconstriction due to portal hypertension, peripheral arteriolar vasodilatation, increased plasma volume, arterial hypotension, activation of the sympathetic nervous system, activation of the renin-angiotensin system, and oversecretion of ADH.
      b. Impaired liver metabolism, with or without adequate volume may also lead to HRS. Since the mechanisms are independent of volume status, they are not triggered by volume stimuli and may decrease peripheral vascular resistance. This causes vasodilatation, a decrease in systemic blood pressure and effective blood volume, which may then cause efferent stimulation and renal vasoconstriction.
      c. Mechanisms to protect glomerular capillary pressures and decrease renal vasoconstriction are lost or reduced in patients with HRS even though they typically have a decreased blood volume. This may also lead to a further decrease in the GFR.
      d. Decrease in "effective" blood volume is another cause of HRS. Ascites is formed when the splanchnic vessels and hepatic sinusoids create an overabundance of lymph to such an extent that it cannot be returned to circulation. The lymph then accumulates in the peritoneal space, which leads to a decrease in the blood volume. As ascites continues to develop plasma volume is constantly redistributed. Patients who retain water and sodium have a decreased total

peripheral resistance. Even though there is an increase in total plasma volume, the amount of available blood is decreased. Hence, the total extracellular fluid volume is moved to other fluid compartments, leading to a decrease in effective blood volume.

e. Other factors that play a role include changes in the renin-angiotensin system and increased sympathetic nervous system (SNS) stimulation. The renin-angiotensin system helps to maintain the vasoconstriction associated with HRS. Patients with ESLD have elevated plasma renin levels that may be due to the inability of the liver to inactivate renin or more likely, due to the kidney's continued secretion of renin. This may occur due to decreased perfusion of the kidney leading to stimulation of the renin-angiotensin system or a secondary response to a decrease in blood volume. Additionally, the secretion of the angiotensin II causes a more profound decrease in perfusion and GFR.

f. An increase in the SNS stimulation may also contribute to the cause of HRS. A decrease in blood volume is recognized as a decrease in arterial pressure. Through a chain of events, the sympathetic nervous system is activated, which produces renal vasconstriction and a decreased GFR.

5. Management of hepatorenal syndrome.
   a. No specific treatment except liver transplantation.
   b. Focus should be on prevention and support of the kidneys.

F. Hepatitis C associated kidney disease.
   1. Membranous nephropathy.
      a. Usually presents as nephrotic syndrome.
      b. May also have microscopic hematuria.
      c. Diagnosis by kidney biopsy.
      d. Management – control of nephrotic syndrome.
         (1) ACE inhibitors and/or ARBs.
         (2) Control of hypertension.
         (3) Treatment of hyperlipidemia.
         (4) In some cases, prednisone and cyclophosphamide are used.
         (5) Some patients may be considered for combined liver and kidney transplant.
   2. Membranoproliferative glomerulonephritis – Type I.
      a. Usually associated with mild nephrotic syndrome.

b. May also have hypertension and microhematuria with preserved kidney function.
c. Also associated with circulating cryoglobulins, weakness, arthralgias, and palpable purpura.
d. Diagnosis is made by measuring serum complement levels (decreased) and hepatitis serologies. Kidney biopsy is most definitive way to diagnose.
e. Management – control of nephrotic syndrome.
   (1) ACE inhibitors and/or ARBs.
   (2) Control of hypertension.
   (3) Antiviral therapy for HCV. Pegylated interferon with or without ribavirin (depending on degree of renal insufficiency).
   (4) Some patients may be considered for combined liver and kidney transplant, though recurrence of disease is common.

II. Chronic kidney disease after liver transplantation.

Patients who had some degree of renal insufficiency before transplantation are at a greater risk for morbidity and mortality than those who had normal function. Determination of cause and treatment can be difficult in these patients. Therefore, it is best to follow a general approach and then move to possible specific causes of renal impairment such as drug toxicities.

A. Intraoperative and postoperative events may contribute to renal insufficiency. These events include hemorrhage, hypotension, hypovolemia, infection, graft failure, and antibiotic and immunosupppressant use. Usually there are multiple causative factors. In most patients, these factors lead to acute tubular necrosis (ATN) for a short time that usually resolves in less than a month if there is adequate liver function. Routine assessment of serum creatinine, creatinine clearance, and drug levels is necessary.

B. As with other patients on calcineurin inhibitors, careful monitoring of drug levels is required with adjustment of dosage as needed.
   1. Dosage should be tailored to individual patient.
   2. Routine monitoring of the trough level is integral to maintaining adequate immunosuppression, yet it may be inadequate in minimizing nephrotoxic effects.
   3. Avoidance of intravenous calcineurin inhibitors, if possible.

Processing

4. Strict monitoring of hemodynamic status postoperatively and maintenance of euvolemia are essential to prevent compromise that would require aggressive use of vasopressor or diuretic medications, since their use enhances the renal toxicity associated with calcineurin inhibitors.

5. Reduction in the dose with early, mild renal function impairment, whenever possible.

6. Specific drug therapies when calcineurin nephrotoxicity occurs.

7. Consider change in immunosuppressive regimen using sirolimus instead of calcineurin inhibitor (currently FDA approved for kidney transplant only).

C. In patients with hepatitis C as cause of liver disease, concerns regarding membraneous nephritis.

III. Chronic kidney disease after liver transplantation: Other treatment strategies.

A. Conservative measures.
1. Correct disorders of electrolyte imbalance (sodium and potassium), acid-base balance, and hypovolemia.
2. Careful calculation of intake and urinary output.
3. Detect and correct graft dysfunction and infection immediately.
4. Meticulous wound care.
5. Avoid over immunosuppression which can lead to infection and sepsis.
6. If antibiotics are needed, facilitate the use of non-nephrotoxic agents.
7. Use care in administering agents that increase the blood level of cyclosporine or tacrolimus (Table 10.7). Educate patients to avoid these agents.
8. Use the same recommendations as for any patient with CKD (e.g., control of blood pressure, diabetes, treatment of anemia, hyperlipidemia, etc.).

B. Kidney replacement therapy.
1. Initiate kidney replacement therapy as for any patient with CKD stage 5.
2. Careful monitoring for infection with early intervention because of immunosuppressed state.
3. Very little data on dialysis outcomes for liver transplant recipients, but mortality increased in transplant recipient compared to the nontransplant patient.
4. Consider kidney transplantation, if possible.

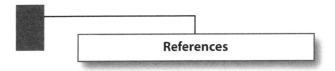

References

Ader, J., & Rostaing, L. (1998). Cyclosporin nephrotoxicity: Pathophysiology and comparison with FK-506. *Current Opinion in Nephrology and Hypertension, 7*(5), 539-545.

American Diabetes Association (ADA). (2006). *Web site.* Retrieved June 7, 2006, from http://www.diabetes.org

Auchincloss, H., & Shaffer, D. (1999). Pancreas transplantation. In L.C. Ginns, A.B. Cosimi, & P.J. Morris (Eds.), *Transplantation.* Malden, MA: Blackwell Science.

Barone, C., Martin-Watson, A., & Barone, G. (2004). The postoperative care of the adult renal transplant recipient. *MEDSURG Nursing, 13*(5), 296-302.

Bartucci, M.R., Loughman, K.A., & Moir, E.J. (1992). Kidney-pancreas transplantation: A treatment option for ESRD and type 1 diabetes. *ANNA Journal, 19*(5), 467-474.

Bloom, R.D., & Doyle, A.M. (2006). Kidney disease after heart and lung transplantation. *American Journal of Transplantation, 6,* 671-679.

Burrows-Hudson, S., & Prowant, B.F. (Eds.). (2005). *Nephrology nursing standards of practice and guidelines for care.* Pitman, NJ: American Nephrology Nurses' Association.

Cheng, S.S., & Munn, S.R. (1994). Posttransplant hyper-amylasemia is associated with decreased patient and graft survival in pancreas allograft recipients. *Transplantation Proceedings, 26*(2), 428-429.

Conway, P., Davis, C., Hartel, T., & Russell, G. (1998). Simultaneous kidney pancreas transplantation: Patient issues and nursing interventions. *American Nephrology Nursing Journal, 25*(3), 455-478.

Corsini, J.M., White-Williams, C., & Cupples, S.A. (2003). Evaluation of patients for solid organ transplantation. In S.A. Cupples & L. Ohler (Eds.), *Transplantation nursing secrets* (pp. 27-44). Philadelphia: Hanley & Belfus, Inc.

Cosimi, A.B., & Conti, D.J. (1989). Pancreas transplantation. *Comprehensive Therapy, 15*(5), 56-61.

Cupples, S.A., & Ohler, L. (Eds.). (2003). *Transplantation nursing secrets.* Philadelphia: Hanley & Belfus, Inc.

Danovitch, G.M. (Ed.). (2005). *Handbook of kidney transplantation* (4th ed.). Philadelphia: Lippincott Williams & Wilkins.

Davis, C.L. (2004). Transplant: Immunology and treatment of rejection. *American Journal of Kidney Diseases, 43*(6), 1116-1134.

Deierhoi, M.H., Sollinger, H.W., Bozdech, M.J., & Belter, F.O. (1986). Lethal graft-versus-host disease in a recipient of a pancreas-spleen transplant. *Transplantation, 41,* 544-545.

Elmer, D.S., Hughes, T.A., Hathaway, D.K., Shokouh-Amiri, M.H., Gaber, L.W., Nymann, T., et al. (1995). Use of glucose disappearance rates to monitor B-cell function of pancreas allografts. *Transplantation Proceedings, 27*(6), 2985-2986.

Fishman, J.A., & Rubin, R.H. (1998). Infection in organ-transplant recipients. *The New England Journal of Medicine, 338*(24), 1741-1751.

Friedman, A., Miskulin, D., Rosenberg, I., & Levey, A. (2003). Demographics and trends in overweight and obesity in patients at time of kidney transplantation. *American Journal of Kidney Diseases, 41*(2), 480-487.

Ghobrial, R.M., Rosen, H.R., & Martin, P. (2001). Long-term issues in liver transplantation. In D. Norman & L. Turka (Eds.), *Primer on transplantation* (2nd ed., pp. 581-590). Mt. Laurel, NJ: American Society of Transplantation.

Gruessner, A.C., & Sutherland, D.E.R. (2005). Pancreas transplant outcomes for United States (U.S.) and non-U.S. cases as reported to the United Network for Organ Sharing (UNOS) and the International Pancreas Transplant Registry (IPTR) as of June 2004. *Clinical Tranplantation, 19*, 433-455.

Gruessner, R.W.G., Troppmann, C., Barroui, B., Dunn, D.L., Moudry-Munns, K.C., Najarian, J.S., et al. (1994). Assessment of donor and recipient risk factors on pancreas transplant outcome. *Transplantation Proceedings, 26*(2), 437-438.

Hoffman, F.M., Nelson, B.J., Drangstveit, M.B., Flynn, B.M., Watercott, E.A., & Zirbes, J.M. (2006). Caring for transplant recipients in a nontransplant setting. *Critical Care Nurse, 26*(2), 53-73.

Jindal, R., & Zawada, E. (2004). Obesity and kidney transplantation. *American Journal of Kidney Diseases, 43*(6), 943-952.

Jones, J.W., Nakhleh, R.E., Casanova, D., Sutherland, D.E.R., & Gruessner, R.W.G. (1994). Cystoscopic transduodenal pancreas transplant biopsy: A new needle. *Transplantation Proceedings, 26*(2), 527-528.

Kapur, S., Bonham, C.A., Dodson, S.F., Dvochik, I., & Corry, R.J. (1999). Strategies to expand the donor pool for pancreas transplantation. *Transplantation, 67*(2), 284-290.

Kasiske, B.L., Heim-Duthoy, K.L., Tortorice, K.L., & Rao, K.V. (1991). The variable nature of chronic declines in renal allograft function. *Transplantation, 51*(2), 330-334.

Miller, B., & Brennan, D. (2006). Maintenance immunosuppressive therapy in renal transplantation in adults [Electronic version]. *UpToDate Online.*

Mize, J.B. (2003). Pancreas and simultaneous pancreas-kidney transplantation. In S.A. Cupples & L. Ohler (Eds.), *Transplantation nursing secrets* (pp. 143-149). Philadelphia: Hanley & Belfus, Inc.

Molzahn, A.E., & Butera, E. (Eds.). (2006). *Contemporary nephrology nursing: Principles and practice* (2nd ed.). Pitman, NJ: American Nephrology Nurses' Association.

Mylonakis, E., Goes, N., Rubin, R., Cosimi, A.B., Colvin, R.B., & Fishman, J.A. (2001). BK virus in solid organ transplant recipients: An emerging syndrome. *Transplantation, 72*(10), 1587-1592.

Nyberg, G., Olausson, M., Norden, G., Mjornstedt, L., Blohme, I., & Hedman, L. (1991). Pancreas specific protein (PASP) monitoring in pancreas transplantation. *Transplantation Proceedings, 23*(1), 1604-1605.

Ojo, A.O., Held, P.J., Port, F.K., Wolfe, R.A., Leichtman, A.B., Young, E.W., et al. (2003). Chronic renal failure after transplantation of a nonrenal organ. *The New England Journal of Medicine, 349*(10), 931-940.

Organ Procurement and Transplantation Network (OPTN). (2003). *Organ datasource.* Retrieved June 7, 2006, from http://www.optn.org/organDatasource

Organ Procurement and Transplantation Network (OPTN). (2006). *Web site.* Retrieved February 15, 2008, from http://www.optn.org

Pascual, M., Theruvath, T., Kawai, T., Tolkoff-Rubin, N., & Cosimi, A.B. (2002). Stategies to improve long-term outcomes after renal transplantation. *The New England Journal of Medicine, 346*(8), 580-590.

Paul, L.C. (1999). Chronic allograft nephropathy: An update. *Kidney International, 56*, 783-793.

Penn, I. (1993). Incidence and treatment of neoplasia after transplantation. *The Journal of Heart and Lung Transplantation, 12*(6), S328-S336.

Perkal, M., Marks, C., Lorber, M., & Marks, W.H. (1992). A three-year experience with serum anoidal trypsinogen as a biochemical marker for rejection in pancreatic allografts. *Transplantation, 53*(2), 415-419.

Pirsch, J.D., & Stratta, R.J. (1998). Pancreas and simultaneous kidney-pancreas transplantation. In D.J. Norman & W.N. Suki (Eds.), *Primer on transplantation* (pp. 501-511). Thorofare, NJ: American Society of Transplant Physicians.

Radio, S.J., Stratta, R.J., Taylor, R.J., & Linder, J. (1993). The utility of urine cytology in the diagnosis of allograft rejection after combined pancreas-kidney transplantation. *Transplantation, 55*(3), 509-516.

Robertson, R.P. (2004). Islet transplantation as a treatment for diabetes – A work in progress. *The New England Journal of Medicine, 350*(7), 694-705.

Roche Pharmaceuticals. (2004). *PDR 2004 transplant disease management guide* (1st ed). Montvale, NJ: Thompson PDR.

Schrier, R.W. (Ed.). (1995). *Manual of nephrology* (4th ed.). Boston: Little, Brown and Company.

Semb, S. (2000). *Diabetes care: Competencies for patient teaching.* Sacramento, CA: Continuing Medical Education Resource.

Sollinger, H.M., Messing, E.M., Eckhoff, D.E., Pirsch, J.D., D'Alessandro, A.M., Kalayoglu, M., et al. (1993). Urological complications in 210 consecutive simultaneous pancreas-kidney transplants with bladder drainage. *Annals of Surgery, 218*(4), 561-568.

Steen, D.C. (1999). The current state of pancreas transplantation. *AACN Clinical Issues, 10*(2), 164-175.

Stuart, F.P., Abecassis, M.M., & Kaufman, D.B. (2003). *Organ transplantation* (2nd ed.). Georgetown: Landes Bioscience.

Sutherland, D.E.R., Cecka, M., & Gruessner, A.C. (1999). Report from the international Pancreas transplant registry – 1998. *Transplantation Proceedings, 31*, 597-601.

Tajra, L.C., Molina, G., Albalate, P., Lefrancois, M., Brunet, M., Martin, X., et al. (1994). Early post-operative period: Study of metabolic profiles after segmental or total pancreas transplantation. *Transplantation Proceedings, 26*(2), 478-479.

Trusler, L.A. (1992). Management of the patient receiving simultaneous kidney-pancreas transplantation. *Critical Care Nursing Clinics of North America, 41*(1), 89-95.

United Network for Organ Sharing (UNOS). (2005). *Organ donation and transplantation.* Retrieved June 7, 2006, from http://www.unos.org

Vella, J., & Brennan, D. (2006). Induction immunosupressive therapy in renal transplantation [Electronic version]. *UpToDate Online.*

Wallace, M. (2003). What is new with renal transplantation? *AORN Journal, 77*(5), 945-970.

Wilcox, C.S., & Tisher, C.C. (Eds.). (2005). *Handbook of nephrology & hypertension* (5th ed.). Philadelphia: Lippincott Williams & Wilkins.

Zand, M.S. (Ed.). (2001). Care of the well transplant patient. *Graft, 4*(4).

Section 11

Hemodialysis

Section Editor

Karen C. Robbins, MS, RN, CNN

Authors

Rebecca L. Amato, BSN, RN

Diana Hlebovy, BSN, RN, CHN, CNN

Betsy King, MSN, RN, CNN

Patricia Baltz Salai, MSN, RN, CRNP, CNN

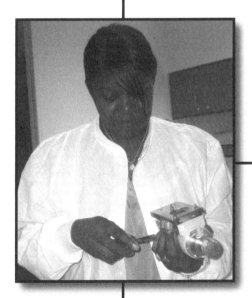

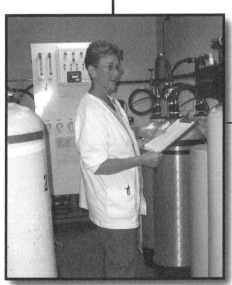

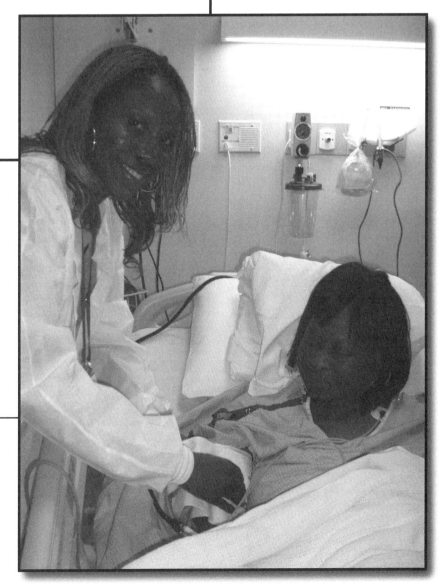

About the Authors

Karen C. Robbins, MS, RN, CNN, Section Editor, is the Nurse Educator for Dialysis Services and Transplant at Hartford Hospital in Hartford, Connecticut. She is the Associate Editor of the *Nephrology Nursing Journal*, Journal of the American Nephrology Nurses' Association.

Rebecca L. Amato, BSN, RN, is a Staff Nurse at Highline Medical Center in Seattle, Washington.

Diana Hlebovy, BSN, RN, CHN, CNN, is Director of Clinical Affairs at Hema Metrics in Kaysville, Utah.

Betsy King, MSN, RN, CNN, is a Clinical Services Specialist at DaVita, Inc., in White Plains, New York.

Patricia Baltz Salai, MSN, RN, CRNP, CNN, is a Nephrology Nurse Practitioner at Veterans Affairs Pittsburgh Healthcare System in Pittsburgh, Pennsylvania.

Acknowledgment

The authors thank Marcia L. Keen, Larrry E. Lancaster, Lowanna S. Binkley, Marguerite F. Hartigan, and Randee Breiterman White, authors of the fourth edition of the *Core Curriculum*, upon which some of this content is based.

Section 11

Hemodialysis

Section

11

Hemodialysis

Purpose

The purpose of this section is to describe the principles of hemodialysis and current technologies available. It focuses on providing hemodialysis treatments that are not only safe and accurate, but are also appropriate for the individual patient. Strategies that can be used to reach desired patient outcomes while avoiding adverse events are addressed. Complications associated with the dialysis procedure are explained. Additionally, it discusses how to establish and reach the dry weight of the patient on hemodialysis while minimizing untoward effects. This section will provide an overview of hematocrit-based blood volume monitoring, descriptions of the most common profiles displayed, and suggested interventions for more effective strategies for fluid volume management to enhance patient outcomes.

Objectives

Upon completion of this section, the learner will be able to:
1. Describe the process of diffusion as it relates to hemodialysis.
2. List factors affecting the rate of diffusion.
3. List factors affecting net flux of solute during hemodialysis.
4. Describe how hydrostatic pressures are used during hemodialysis.
5. Describe how to calculate the transmembrane pressure to obtain desired ultrafiltration rate during hemodialysis.
6. Discuss the function and operation of the blood pump.
7. Describe dialyzer design.
8. List the composition of a typical dialysate solution.
9. List the conditions causing blood and dialysate compartment alarms.
10. Describe the use of urea kinetic modeling in patients on hemodialysis.
11. Define Kt/V and current target values for hemodialysis adequacy.
12. Outline the causes, signs and symptoms, prevention, and treatment of complications of the hemodialysis procedure.
13. Summarize how hematocrit-based blood volume monitoring improves fluid management during hemodialysis.
14. Identify the various categories of blood volume profiles observed during hematocrit-based blood volume monitoring.
15. Describe general guidelines for interventions with observed blood volume monitoring profiles.

Significant Dates in the History of Dialysis

1861 – Thomas Graham is considered to be the father of modern dialysis. This colloid chemist from London coined the term "dialysis."

1890 – Bicarbonate peritoneal lavage was used in Europe to treat cholera.

1913 – The term *artificial kidney* was coined by John J. Abel, Leonard Rowntree, and B.B. Turner at Johns Hopkins University in Baltimore. They devised a "kidney" using celloidin tubing for membranes and crushed leech heads (hirudin) for anticoagulation. The "kidney" was not efficient enough for humans, and hirudin was toxic to humans.

1923 – In Germany, Nicheles used the peritoneal membrane from an ox to make an "artificial kidney."

1924 – In Giessen, Germany, Georg Haas performed the first human dialysis.

1935 – Heparin was purified and replaced the toxic and expensive hirudin; regenerated cellulose tubing was developed.

1940 – Willem Johan Kolff in Gronigen, was unable to save a young patient dying from uremia. Kolff began simple experiments studying the dialyzability of urea using cellophane.

1942-43 – Kolff designed the rotating drum artificial kidney, which was used in Holland for successful treatment of patients with acute renal failure.

1945 – Kolff performed the first successful dialysis treatments on a 67-year-old female with acute renal failure who recovered kidney function and lived another 7 years.

1946 – Kolff wrote that the artificial kidney should be used for acute renal failure but was not indicated for chronic therapy.

1946 – Gordon Murray performed the first hemodialysis in North America. The patient eventually recovered complete renal function and survived.

1946-47 – The events of World War II prevented communication among physicians working around the world on treatment of uremia.

1947 – Kolff found effectiveness of hemodialysis superior to peritoneal and intestinal lavage for urea removal. His artificial kidney was shipped to Canada, New York and London. Kolff came to the United States where he assisted in the initiation of the first dialysis at Mount Sinai Hospital in New York City. Drs. John Merrill and George Thorne were present and made the decision to launch a program in Boston to support a transplant unit they were planning to start.

1947 – Van Garretts, in Copenhagen, made a hand-wound coil kidney and used it successfully to treat humans.

Early 1950s – Kolff went to Boston and worked with Edward Olsen, a machinist, and Dr. Carl Walters to modify Kolff's design. The Kolff-Brigham artificial kidney evolved and was the machine used by military physicians of the United States Army.

1950-53 – Teschan, Schreiner, and colleagues used artificial kidneys to treat acute renal failure from battle injuries in Korean War MASH units. The survival rate of acute renal failure patients improved.

1956 – Kolff developed a disposable coil dialyzer and gave it to Travenol; no other company thought it had any practical application. Repeated vascular access remained a significant challenge to chronic therapy.

1957 – Kiil developed the first flat plate parallel flow dialyzer that was widely used.

1959 – After development of the Quinton-Scribner external shunt, the first two patients on chronic maintenance dialysis were started using the Kiil dialyzer.

1960 – David Dillard, a pediatric heart surgeon, implanted the first Scribner shunt developed by Belding Scribner, to dialyze Clyde Shields in Seattle, Washington, the first person on chronic dialysis. He survived lived 11 years and succumbed to a heart attack.

1964 – Home dialysis was started by Curtis and Scribner in Seattle; Shaldon in London; and Merrill, Schupak, and Hampers in Boston.

1965 – The internal arteriovenous fistula was developed by Brescia and Cimino.

1967 – The first hollow fiber kidney was developed and clinically tested.

1973 – Federal support for treatment of end-stage renal disease (ESRD) became available in the United States.

1974 – Large surface-area dialyzers that allowed a decrease in treatment time became available.

1978 – Polytetrafluorethylene (PTFE) was configured into graft material for arteriovenous vascular access.

Late 1970s – Reprocessing of dialyzers implemented for cost containment.

1980s – Volumetric hemodialysis machines allowed for more highly permeable membranes to be safely used.

1980s – Automated peritoneal dialysis and continuous ambulatory peritoneal dialysis were widely accepted as maintenance dialysis modalities.

1980s – Hepatitis outbreak occurred as it set the stage for personal protective equipment (PPE).

1989 – Recombinant human erythropoietin was commercially available for use in patients with ESRD on dialysis.

Early 1990s – Intravenous forms of vitamin D analogs commercially available for management of bone and parathyroid disease.

1990s – Noninvasive blood volume monitoring becomes available for monitoring intravascular volume during hemodialysis.

1997 – National Kidney Foundation published Dialysis Outcomes Quality Initiative (DOQI) Clinical Practice Guidelines for Adequacy of Hemodialysis, Adequacy of Peritoneal Dialysis, Treatment of Anemia of Chronic Renal Failure, and Vascular Access.

Late 1990s into 2000s – Resurgence of interest in return to home hemodialysis with daily or nightly therapy.

2002 – National Kidney Foundation publishes The Kidney Disease Outcomes Quality Initiative (KDOQI) Clinical Practice Guidelines for Chronic Kidney Disease. Subsequent revisions and expansions serve as guidelines for the care of patients with all stages of chronic kidney disease including patients on hemodialysis.

2005-2006 – Additional KDOQI Guidelines released and earlier Guidelines revised.

Chapter 51

Principles of Hemodialysis

I. Solute removal (mass transfer).

A. Diffusion is the movement of a molecule from a region of higher solute concentration to a region of lower solute concentration and is the result of random movement of molecules driven by thermal energy.

1. Diffusion in hemodialysis occurs across the semipermeable membrane that separates the blood compartment from the dialysate compartment. A semipermeable membrane allows passage of some molecules while restricting or preventing the transit of others.

2. Factors affecting the rate of diffusion in hemodialysis.

a. Molecule size. Molecules that are too large to pass through the pores in a semipermeable membrane are nondiffusable. Depending on certain characteristics, they may exert an effect that causes water to move into the compartment that contains the nondiffusable molecule.

b. Size and number of pores in a semipermeable membrane. The greater the number of pores, the faster the diffusion; larger pores allow diffusion of larger molecules.

c. Surface area of semipermeable membrane. Generally the larger the surface area, the more rapid diffusion occurs.

d. Temperature of the solutions on either side of the semipermeable membrane: the higher the temperature of the solutions, the more rapid diffusion occurs.

e. Concentration of solutes in the blood as compared to concentration of solutes in the dialysate.
   (1) The greater the concentration gradient for a given solute, the more rapidly diffusion occurs, given the above constraints.
   (2) When equilibrium of a solute on the two sides of the membrane is reached, diffusion ceases.
   (3) Diffusion can occur in either direction, depending on the solute concentration in the respective compartments.

f. Thickness of the semipermeable membrane may exert an influence on diffusion rate; thick membranes may decrease the rate of diffusion but diffusion is not always proportional to membrane thickness.

g. Resistance to diffusion retards the rate at which solutes move to the membrane edge in the blood compartment, across the membrane, and away from the membrane edge into the flowing dialysate stream. A film layer develops on both the blood and dialysate sides of the membrane which can slow the rate of diffusion.

h. Solute drag or convective removal. Solutes move across the semipermeable membrane in conjunction with water movement.

3. The rate at which solutes diffuse through the triple laminated solution of blood, membrane and dialysate is termed *overall permeability*. It is expressed as the overall transport coefficient of Ko in cm^2/min.

a. The Ko is a unique value for each solute; it measures the efficiency of a dialyzer design.

b. The Ko is the summed value of the reciprocals for each of the resistances in the triple laminate of blood, membrane, and dialysate.

4. The product of Ko and membrane surface area (A) gives the overall mass transport coefficient (KoA) of a given dialyzer expressed as mL/min or L/min. In a perfect dialyzer, this value would be stable and independent of blood or dialysate flow rates.

B. Net flux.
1. Net flux is the amount of solute leaving the blood and entering the dialysate (or opposite, depending on the concentration gradient) per unit of time.

2. The equation for net flux from either blood side or dialysate side.
Equation 1
J = (QbiCbi – QboCbo) = (QbiCbi) – (Qbi – Qf)Cbo = [(Qdi + Qf)Cdo] – [(Qdi) – (Cdi)]
where:
J = solute flux in mg/min
Qbi = blood flow rate into the dialyzer in mL/min
Qbo = blood flow rate leaving the dialyzer in mL/min
Cbi = solute concentration of blood entering the dialyzer in mg/mL
Cbo = solute concentration of blood leaving the dialyzer in mg/mL
Qf = ultrafiltration rate in mL/min
Qdi = dialysate flow rate into the dialyzer in mL/min
Qdo = dialysate flow rate leaving the dialyzer in mL/min
Cdi = solute concentration of dialysate entering the dialyzer in mL/min
Cdo = solute concentration of dialysate leaving the dialyzer in mL/min
Example:
Cbi BUN = 80 mg/dL or 0.8 mg/mL
Cbo BUN = 20 mg/dL or 0.2 mg/mL
Qbi = 300 mL/min
Qf = 10 mL/min
Qbo = 290 mL/min
Qdi = 500 mL/hr
Cdi BUN = 0
Cdo BUN = 35.6 mg/dL or 0.356 mg/mL
J = [(300 x 0.8) – (290 x 0.2)] = [(300 x 0.8) – (300 – 10)0.2] = [(500 + 10) 0.356] – (500 x 0) = 182 mg/min

3. Mechanism is defined by the product of KoA and log mean concentration gradient. It is proportional to the concentration gradient and can increase only by increasing Ko or A.

4. Mass balance is when the amount of solute recovered on the dialysate side is equal to the amount of solute lost from the blood side.
5. Factors affecting net flux.
   a. Membrane surface area: generally net flux increases as surface area increases.
   b. Permeability of membrane for a specific solute (molecular size or weight) or Ko. Net flux is generally higher for small molecules and lower for large molecules.
   c. Mean concentration gradient between blood and dialysate. Net flux is more rapid with large concentration gradients.
   d. Blood-dialysate flow configuration.
      (1) Cocurrent or concurrent: blood and dialysate flow in the same direction from dialyzer inlet to outlet. Concentration gradient and net flux decrease as blood and dialysate approach the outlet.
      (2) Countercurrent flow: blood and dialysate flow in opposite direction; maintains an optimal blood-dialysate concentration gradient (high net flux) throughout the dialyzer until blood and dialysate flows approach similar concentrations; usually requires 2–2.5 times higher dialysate flow rate relative to blood flow rate to achieve maximum efficiency.

C. Clearance.
   1. Clearance expresses the performance of the dialyzer for solute removal. The amount of blood completely cleared of a solute per unit time, usually expressed as mL/min or L/min.
   2. Formula for clearance.
      Equation 2
      K = Qb[(Cbi-Cbo)/Cbi] + Qf(Cbo/Cbi)
      where:
      K = clearance of solute in mL/min Cbi, Cbi, Qbi, Qf: see above under Equation 1.
      Example:
      Cbi BUN = 80 mg/dL or 0.8 mg/mL
      Cbo BUN = 20 mg/dL or 0.2 mg/mL
      Qf = 10 mL/min
      Qbi = 300 mL/min
      K = 300[(0.8 – 0.2) / 0.8] + 10(0.2/0.8) = 227.5 mL/min
   3. Factors affecting clearance.
      a. Membrane permeability for a given solute and surface area, KoA.
      b. Blood flow rate. Clearance is equal to blood flow rate up to some level at which clearance will be limited by KoA (see Figure 11.1).
      c. Dialysate flow rate and flow configuration.

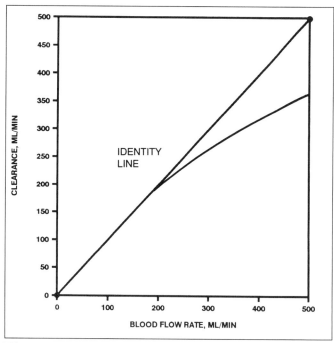

Figure 11.1. The relationship between blood flow (Ob) in mL/min and clearance in mL/min in a typical dialyzer. Clearance increases with blood flow; at some point it diverges from the identity line with Qb as a function of membrane permeability (Ko) and area (A).

4. Clearance is not dependent on the incoming blood solute concentration because this is the volume-cleared parameter (constant regardless of incoming blood concentration) while net flux is the mass of solute removed per unit time and is dependent on the clearance-concentration product.

D. Dialysance.
   1. Dialysance expresses dialyzer efficiency when solute concentration in the dialysate is not zero (such as recirculating dialysate systems)(see III.D.2 for information on regenerative dialysis delivery systems). The volume of blood cleared of that solute per minute if the dialysate concentration was zero.
   2. Formula for dialysance.
      Equation 3
      D = Qbi[(Cbi - Cbo)/(Cbi – Cdi)] + Qf(Cbo/Cbi)
      where:
      D = dialysance in mL/min
      Cbi, Cbo, Qf, etc.: see above under Equation 1.
   3. Factors affecting dialysance are similar to those affecting clearance.
   4. Does not represent actual effective clearance in recirculating systems since effective clearance is

decreased because of the diminished blood-to-dialysate concentration gradient.

5. In single-pass dialysate systems, where dialysate concentration for many solutes is zero, clearance and dialysance are the same.

II. Water removal.

A. Ultrafiltration is the process by which plasma water is removed (expressed in mL/min, mL/hour, or L/hour) because of a pressure gradient between the blood and dialysate compartments. There are two types of pressure that may influence ultrafiltration.

1. Osmosis: the movement of water across a membrane permeable only to water; water moves from an area of lesser solute concentration to an area of greater solute concentration to equalize the concentration between the components.
   a. Osmotic pressure: the amount of pressure required to exactly oppose this water movement across the semipermeable membrane separating these two compartments with unequal solute concentrations.
   b. During dialysis, plasma proteins exert osmotic pressure in the blood compartment and oppose water movement out of that compartment. This is termed oncotic pressure; expressed as mm Hg; usually exerts a relatively small effect during dialysis.
2. Hydraulic pressure, the actual pressure that forces water out of one compartment into another compartment; expressed as mm Hg.

B. Ultrafiltration during dialysis is the result of net transmembrane pressure (TMP) in the dialyzer that moves plasma water from the blood compartment to the dialysate compartment because of the net pressure gradient.

1. Equation for mean TMP, which is the net pressure difference across the membrane:
   Equation 4
   $$TMP = [Pbi + Pbo)/2] - [Pdi + Pdo)/2]$$
   where:
   TMP = transmembrane pressure in mm Hg
   Pbi = inlet blood compartment pressure in mm Hg
   Pbo = outlet blood compartment pressure in mm Hg
   Pdi = inlet dialysate compartment pressure in mm Hg
   Pdo = outlet dialysate compartment pressure in mm Hg

   a. Blood compartment pressure decreases from the inlet to the outlet side of the dialyzer with the typical blood circuit configuration.
   b. Dialysate compartment pressure decreases from the inlet side to the outlet side of the dialyzer. With negative pressure in the compartment, absolute pressure is lower (more negative at Pdo than Pdi). The same relationship holds with positive pressure on the dialysate.
2. Can be accomplished with either positive pressure on the blood compartment, negative pressure on the dialysate compartment, or some combination of both; the rate per mm Hg is the same in a given dialyzer, independent of the approach used.
3. Factors affecting ultrafiltration.
   a. Transmembrane pressure.
   b. Membrane water permeability.
   c. Dialyzer surface area may be decreased with thrombus formation or dialyzer clotting.

C. The ultrafiltration coefficient (KUF in mL/hr/mm Hg) is a dialyzer characteristic that expresses relative efficiency of water removal; reflects membrane water permeability and surface area.

1. TMP is calculated for the length of time ultrafiltration will be done using the known or estimated KUF of the dialyzer.
2. If using volumetric ultrafiltration control delivery systems, the operator calculates the ultrafiltration rate per hour and does not need to calculate TMP.
   Example:
   Total fluid removal = 3 kg or 3000 mL
   Treatment time = 3 hours
   Ultrafiltration rate = 3000/3 = 1000 mL/hour
3. Programmable ultrafiltration is available on some delivery systems. Rather than the ultrafiltration rate remaining the same throughout the treatment, the rate can be set higher during the beginning of the treatment, and lower toward the end of the treatment to stabilize the patient and allow for maximum fluid removal.

III. Components of a hemodialysis system (see Figure 11.2).

A. Blood pump.
1. The blood pump is responsible for pumping blood through the tubing and dialyzer (extracorporeal circuit). Resistance in vascular access (needles, arteriovenous fistulae or grafts

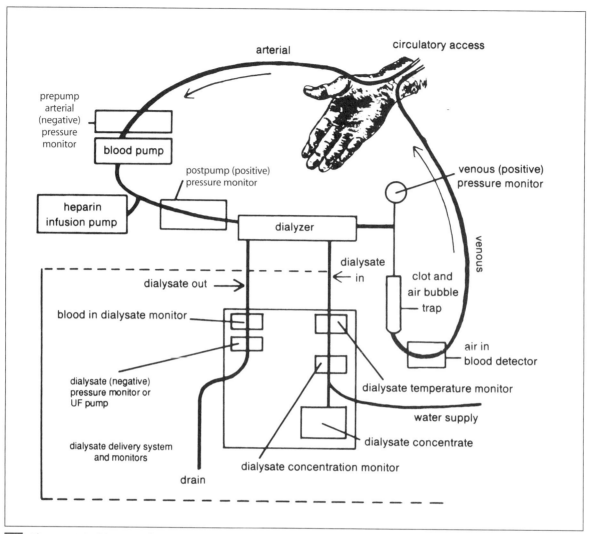

Figure 11.2. Diagram of components of a typical hemodialysis system.

Source: Wick, G.S., & Parker, J. (1984). *Protecting the future of quality care through an understanding of hemodialysis principles.* Pitman, NJ: The American Nephrology Nurses' Association. Used with permission.

or central vein catheters) and the extracorporeal circuit is high and prevents passive flow.

2. Two or more rollers rotate in a closed compartment and compress the blood tubing against a semicircular pump housing wall.
   a. Rollers are self-occluding in most equipment to provide the appropriate compression against the housing to deliver an accurate blood flow rate through the dialyzer.
   b. Pump calibration is checked periodically to assure stable and accurate blood flow rates.
   c. Calibration for the blood tubing is critical to ensure accurate measurement and delivery of blood flow.
3. Factors affecting blood pump functioning.
   a. There must be no extraneous high resistance to flow of blood through blood tubing and dialyzer.

b. If obstruction exists inside the dialyzer or between the blood outlet of the dialyzer and patient (e.g., dialyzer clotting, venous drip chamber clotting, kinked lines), pressure will increase inside the dialyzer and increase blood compartment pressure. If the pressure exceeds roller occlusion tolerance (+300 to +400 mm Hg), retrograde flow across the rollers may occur and decrease effective stroke volume per revolution and therefore, blood flow rate.

c. If obstruction exists between the circulatory access site and the pump (e.g., kinked line, clotted access needle or catheter), the arterial blood compartment pressure (up to the blood pump) will decrease (become more negative) and exceed maximum specified pressure value.

(1) High negative pressure may cause a pressure alarm or arterial bloodline collapse or cavitation as a consequence of insufficient flow into the blood pump, decrease stroke volume per roller revolution, and thus diminish effective blood flow rate through the dialyzer.

(2) If negative pressure is high enough (equal to or greater than -250 mm Hg at the needle), subclinical hemolysis may result.

(3) Blood pump should be stopped until problem(s) is/are corrected.

B. Dialyzers.
 1. Description.
  a. Blood and dialysate compartments are discrete areas of the dialyzer and are completely separated by the semipermeable membrane.
  b. The blood contains excess quantities of specific solutes (e.g., metabolic waste products and some electrolytes) and inadequate concentrations of other physiologic solutes (e.g., bicarbonate and calcium).
  c. The dialysate is free of metabolic waste products and generally has a lesser concentration of some electrolytes (e.g., K^+, Mg^{++}) than the blood, although Na^+, $HCO3^-$ (or acetate), and Ca^{++} content may be higher.
  d. Solutes, electrolytes, and water will cross the semipermeable membrane as a consequence of diffusion and convection according to concentration and hydraulic pressure gradients.
 2. Types of membrane composition.
  a. Cellulose treated by cuprammonium process (Cuprophane®) with or without various agents (e.g., cellulose acetate [CA]; saponified cellulose ester [SCE]) are considered symmetric membranes because inside and outside of the membrane looks the same. Material induces leucopenia and complement activation (i.e., inflammatory response to membrane material) during dialysis when membrane is new; described as not biocompatible.
  b. Modified cellulosic membranes (e.g., cellulose triacetate) are generally produced in hollow fiber configuration; induces milder inflammatory response and considered more biocompatible than cellulose.
  c. Synthetic membranes include polyacrylonitrile (PAN), polysulfone (PSF),

polymethylmethacrylate (PMMA), polycarbonate, polyamide.
  (1) Some can be made in flat sheets, but primarily used in hollow fiber devices.
  (2) An asymmetric membrane with the thin permeable skin on the blood contacting surface with a thick supporting structure around its skin.
  (3) Described as biocompatible because they induce less leukopenia and/or complement activation even when the membrane is new.
 3. Factors affecting dialyzer performance.
  a. Dialyzing membrane surface area: the larger the surface area of a given membrane, generally the greater the clearance and ultrafiltration.
  b. Pore size or permeability. Pores in the membrane must be large enough to permit uremic toxins, electrolytes, and water to pass through with ease, but small enough to prevent passage of blood cells, proteins, bacteria, endotoxin, and viruses.
  c. Pore size distribution. Large population of larger pores gives higher clearance of larger solutes; water permeability is less affected by pore size and distribution.
  d. Ultrafiltration coefficient and ultrafiltration predictability; ideally predictable and consistent with each treatment.
  e. Compliance. The volume of the dialyzer should remain small and relatively constant with changes in TMP as found in fixed geometry dialyzers such as hollow fibers; more compliance is seen in flat plate dialyzers.
  f. Blood leak rate/blood recovery. The blood leak rate should be negligible and the dialyzer should allow for almost complete return of blood to the patient at the end of dialysis.
  g. Resistance to clotting. Dialyzer should allow for minimal anticoagulation without resulting in thrombus formation and loss of dialyzer efficiency.
  h. Biocompatibility. Membrane should be biocompatible (i.e., elicits only mild inflammatory response).
 4. Types of dialyzer configurations.
  a. Parallel-flow or flat plate dialyzer is no longer used in the United States (see Figure 11.3).
  b. Hollow fiber dialyzer is most commonly used dialyzer in the United States (see Figure 11.4).
   (1) Design. Thousands of hollow fibers of cellulosic or synthetic membrane are

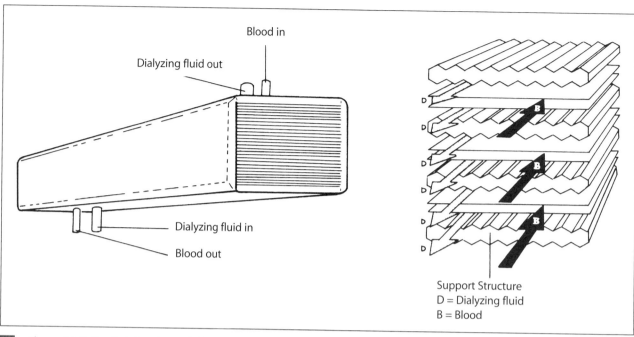

Figure 11.3. Parallel plate hemodialyzer.

Source: Wick, G.S., & Parker, J. (1984). *Protecting the future of quality care through an understanding of hemodialysis principles*. Pitman, NJ: The American Nephrology Nurses' Association. Used with permission.

embedded at each end in potting material; the entire bundle with potting material is encased in hard clear plastic jacket.

(2) Flow geometry is counter current; blood flows through the hollow fibers while dialysate flows counter current along the outside of the fibers.

(3) Compliance is very small; does not increase with increasing blood flow rate or dialysate pressure.

(4) Ultrafiltration is achieved by applying negative pressure to dialysate compartment, positive pressure to the blood compartment, or some combination of both.

5. Categories of dialyzers.

  a. Conventional dialyzers:

    (1) Smallest surface area.

    (2) Low KUF.

    (3) Efficient low-molecular-weight clearance up to 5000 daltons.

    (4) Longer treatment time may be needed to achieve adequate dialysis.

    (5) Membrane material is usually cellulose.

  b. High-efficiency dialyzers.

    (1) Larger surface area.

    (2) Medium KUF.

    (3) Efficient low-molecular-weight clearance up to 5000 daltons.

    (4) Membrane material can be modified cellulose or synthetic.

  c. High-flux dialyzers.

    (1) Medium to large surface area.

    (2) High KUF.

    (3) High molecular weight cutoffs up to 15,000 daltons.

    (4) Membrane material is synthetic and more biocompatible than other types of membranes.

    (5) Requires use of volumetric ultrafiltration control systems.

    (6) Dialysate flow rates range from 500 to 1000 mL/min.

D. Dialysate delivery system.

  1. Proportioning system (see Figure 11.5).

    a. Definition: a system that mechanically mixes an appropriate amount of water and concentrate to achieve physiologic dialysate composition.

    b. Can be accomplished through a fixed proportioning ratio of water to concentrate or with a feedback control system that automatically proportions an amount of concentrate relative to water to achieve the desired dialysate composition and conductivity.

    c. With bicarbonate dialysate, two concentrate

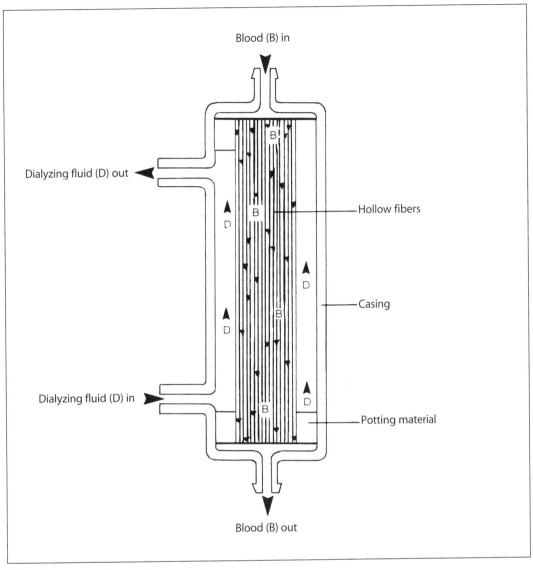

Blood (B) in

Dialyzing fluid (D) out

Hollow fibers

Casing

Dialyzing fluid (D) in

Potting material

Blood (B) out

Figure 11.4. Hollow fiber hemodialyzer.

Source: Wick, G.S., & Parker, J. (1984). *Protecting the future of quality care through an understanding of hemodialysis principles.* Pitman, NJ: The American Nephrology Nurses' Association. Used with permission.

streams are proportioned to achieve the desired buffer concentration.

d. Central proportioning unit is a larger stationary unit that mixes, heats, monitors, and delivers dialysate for multiple stations or dialyzers at the desired individual flow rates. This type of delivery system is not commonly used in the United States.
   (1) Each station or dialyzer has a unit that may control dialysate flow rate, independently monitor the blood compartment parameters, and provide ultrafiltration capability.
   (2) Advantages: efficient for dialysate preparation and monitoring dialysate parameters for multiple patients.
   (3) Disadvantages: equipment failure may disable treatment for all patients; malfunction may deliver unsuitable dialysate to a number of patients; no flexibility in electrolyte composition in dialysate.

e. Individual proportioning unit is a relatively small device that mixes, heats, monitors, and delivers dialysate for a single dialyzer at 500–1000 mL/min. This is the most commonly used dialysate delivery system in the United States.

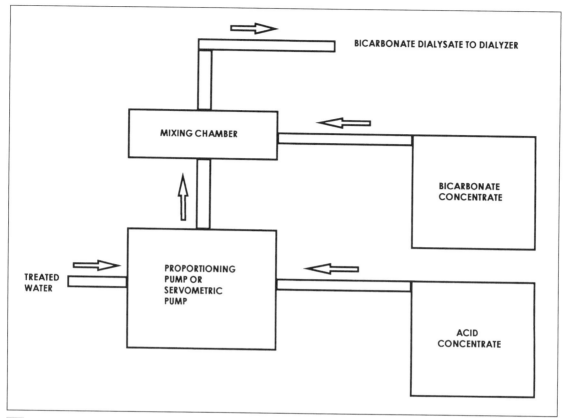

Figure 11.5. Single proportioning system.

(1) Requires electrical and water source with adequate pressure and appropriate drain for spent dialysate.
(2) In addition to dialysate monitoring functions, the unit also monitors blood compartment parameters and may incorporate a blood pump and heparin pump.
(3) Advantages: can individualize dialysate composition; rapid setup and production of suitable dialysate; easy to replace if equipment fails.
(4) Disadvantage: more equipment to maintain.
2. Regenerative system.
a. Definition: the use of sorbents packed in a multilayer cartridge to purify and regenerate a constant recirculating volume of dialysate.
b. The binding capacity and specificity of the sorbents used will determine the type and amount of uremic solutes and electrolytes removed from the patient and adsorbed by the cartridge.
(1) Urease, an enzyme, is used to adsorb and

degrade urea to ammonium for absorption by zirconium; produces bicarbonate as a result of the process.
(2) Activated carbon layer that protects the urease from trace metal contamination and chlorine, chloramines, bleach, or solutions used to disinfect the system.
(3) Zirconium phosphate acts as a cation exchanger, while zirconium oxide functions as an anion exchanger and removes phosphate.
(4) Activated charcoal adsorbs nonionic organic solutes, such as creatinine, uric acid, phenols, and other large molecules.
c. Advantages: small water requirement for dialysate preparation; does not require water pretreatment; small and portable.
d. Disadvantages: low efficiency because of the dialysate flow rate of 250–300 mL/min; may have an initial drop in dialysate pH; because calcium, magnesium, and potassium are removed, must reinfuse at least calcium and magnesium into the dialysate reservoir using an infusion pump.

E. Dialysate composition.
 1. Sodium.
  a. Major cation of dialysate and the extracellular compartment of total body water.
  b. Physiologic dialysate concentration may range from 125 to155 mEq/L. The frequent concentrations used in dialysate range from 135 to145 mEq/L.
  c. Dialysate sodium concentration lower than plasma sodium concentration may induce intracellular movement of water and plasma volume depletion.
  d. Dialysate sodium concentration higher than plasma sodium concentration may induce extracellular movement of water, intracellular dehydration, and stimulation of thirst.
  e. The objective in dialysis is to achieve euvolemic status and normal body sodium content at the end of the treatment. The sodium concentration required to accomplish this objective may vary depending on salt and water intake or loss during dialysis.
  f. Sodium modeling during dialysis.
   (1) Using various profiles (e.g., step, linear, exponential) have been used to reduce the incidence of intradialytic hypotension in some patients.
   (2) Higher dialysate sodium or sodium profiles should be avoided due to the increase in extracellular osmolality stimulating thirst, increasing water intake and increasing interdialytic weight gains, especially in patients with poor residual kidney function (RKF).
   (3) The NKF-KDOQI Clinical Practice Guidelines for Adequacy recommend that high dialysate sodium concentrations and sodium profiling be avoided. Dietary restriction of sodium and adequate management of ultrafiltration during treatment should be employed to facilitate achieving the patient's true dry weight.
 2. Potassium.
  a. Major intracellular cation in the body.
  b. Dialysate concentration varies from 0 to 4 mEq/L, depending on the need to decrease serum potassium level.
  c. Low dialysate potassium concentration has been associated with cardiac dysrhythmias, especially in patients receiving digitalis preparations.
  d. Rapid potassium removal during dialysis is

more likely to produce dysrhythmias than total amount removed.
  e. Clinical consequence of low postdialysis serum potassium is not certain, but it may contribute to postdialysis fatigue and muscle cramps.
 3. Magnesium.
  a. An abundant intracellular cation.
  b. Dialysate concentration may vary from 0 to 3 mEq/L.
 4. Calcium.
  a. Calcium flux from dialysate to blood may be desired to increase serum calcium levels; this is accomplished by increasing the dialysate calcium concentration above the average ionized serum fraction.
  b. Normal values for serum calcium is 8.4 to 10.2 mg/dL. Use of calcium-containing phosphate binders and active vitamin D sterols has led some clinicians to lower dialysate calcium concentration to decrease the calcium load. As an alternative, non-calcium containing phosphate binders and/or a calcimimetic agent such as cinacalcet hydrochloride may be prescribed to a blood volume maintain a serum calcium level within target range.
 5. Chloride.
  a. Dialysate contains combinations of sodium chloride, potassium chloride, and calcium chloride, and the actual concentration of the various combinations will vary depending on the specific concentration formulations and anion concentrations. Total dialysate concentration will be in the range of 95–105 mEq/L.
 6. Glucose.
  a. Glucose is usually added to prevent loss of sizable amounts of glucose. This may be particularly problematic in the patient with diabetes and/or the patient who is fasting.
  b. When present, dialysate glucose concentration ranges from 100 to 250 mg/dL.
 7. Buffer.
  a. The most frequent buffer used for acid-base correction in chronic hemodialysis patients is bicarbonate; concentrations range from 25 to 40 mEq/L. If acetate is used as the buffer, concentrations range from 29 to 39 mEq/L.
  b. Acetate requires metabolic activities (the citric acid cycle) to take up a hydrogen ion, thereby repleting body buffer stores.
  c. Bicarbonate is a more physiologic buffer, thought to be associated with fewer

symptoms and better tolerance than acetate to ultrafiltration during dialysis.

d. Bicarbonate is available in liquid or powder form that is reconstituted before use.

e. High dialysate bicarbonate concentrations increase the likelihood of precipitate formation and delivery system malfunction.

f. Dilute acetic acid or sodium hypochlorite may be used to remove precipitates from the flow path during dialysis equipment cleaning.

g. Bicarbonate is more susceptible to bacterial growth because, unlike acetate, the concentrate is not bacteriostatic or bacteriocidal.

h. Bicarbonate is not stable; reconstituted bicarbonate in an open container loses carbon dioxide and solution buffer becomes carbonate.

IV. Monitoring systems of the hemodialysis machines.

A. Blood compartment of the extracorporeal circuit.
1. Prepump arterial pressure.
   a. Arterial pressure is measured in the blood circuit between the patient and the blood pump (prepump). The pressure reading will be negative, or below zero.
   b. Pressure (mm Hg) is read on a gauge, meter, light emitting diode (LED), or video screen.
   c. Upper and lower limits may be manually set or set automatically by the equipment or user.
   d. Excursions above or below limits will activate an audible and visual alarm, stop the blood pump and require user intervention, there will be a temporary cessation of ultrafiltration until the alarm is corrected.
   e. Lower limit of pressure monitor should not exceed -250 mm Hg because of possible hemolysis from high vacuum.
   f. Pressure will generally decrease (become more negative) during dialysis with ultrafiltration because of increasing blood viscosity (increasing hematocrit) and/or decreasing cardiac output with plasma volume reduction. Given the same needle gauge, pressure will be lower (more negative) with higher hematocrit and higher blood flow rates.
   g. Conditions causing alarm.
      (1) Low alarm (more negative).
         (a) Hypotension or vasoconstriction.
         (b) Occlusion or insufficiency in arterial supply from the vascular access.
         (c) Compression or kinking of the bloodline between the patient and

the arterial monitoring site.
         (d) Malposition or infiltration of the arterial fistula needle.
         (e) Blood pump set at a rate exceeding that which the vascular access can supply, i.e., the pump speed is greater than the access flow rate.
         (f) "Flooding" the transducer monitor or monitoring line so that pressures are not accurately measured.
         (g) Failure to unclamp the monitoring line.
      (2) High alarm (less negative).
         (a) If upper limit is set at some point below zero, separation of the bloodline will cause the pressure to return to zero and activate the high limit alarm.
         (b) Any air leak between the patient and the monitoring site, such as with the saline infusion line; because pressure is generally negative in this segment, air will be pulled into the circuit and pressure will move toward zero.
         (c) Decrease in blood pump speed.
2. Postpump or predialyzer arterial pressure.
   a. Pressure is measured between the blood pump and the dialyzer. The pressure reading is positive, or above zero.
   b. Readout is in the form of gauge, meter, LED, or video screen in mm Hg.
   c. Upper and lower limits may be manually or automatically set by the equipment or user.
   d. Excursions above or below the set limits will activate an audible and visual alarm, stop the blood pump, and require user intervention. In some equipment there will be a temporary cessation of ultrafiltration until alarm is corrected.
   e. Primary utility is in monitoring clotting in the dialyzer.
   f. Pressure will generally increase during dialysis with ultrafiltration, because of increasing blood viscosity. Under some clinical circumstances such as high hematocrit and/or high blood flow rates, high pressures may be observed (> 400 mm Hg).
   g. Conditions causing alarm.
      (1) Low alarm.
         (a) Line separation between monitoring point and downstream circuit to the patient; any leak in this segment of the extracorporeal circuit; because pressure is positive in this segment,

blood will leak from this site; lower limit should be set above zero.
(b) Occlusion in the bloodline between the blood pump and the monitoring site.
(c) Decrease in blood pump speed.
(2) High alarm.
(a) Kink in bloodline between the monitoring site and patient.
(b) Malposition or infiltration of the venous fistula needle.
(c) Increase in blood pump speed.
(d) Clotting in the dialyzer.
3. Venous pressure in the extracorporeal circuit.
a. Measures pressure and integrity of the extracorporeal circuit from the monitoring site to the venous return to the patient (access).
b. Readout is in the form of a gauge, meter, LED, or video screen, in mm Hg.
c. Upper and lower limits are manually set or automatically set by the equipment or user.
d. Excursions above or below the set limits will activate an audible and visual alarm, stop the blood pump, and require user intervention. In some equipment, there will be a temporary cessation of ultrafiltration until the alarm condition is corrected.
e. Pressure will generally be greater than zero or positive.
f. Pressure will generally increase during dialysis with ultrafiltration because of increasing blood viscosity.
g. Given the same needle gauge, higher pressure will be seen with higher hematocrit or higher blood flow rate.
h. Initial high pressures may be associated with early access failure due to venous stenosis.
i. Conditions causing an alarm.
(1) Low alarm.
(a) Separation of bloodline from venous fistula needle; leak in this segment of the extracorporeal circuit; because pressure is generally positive in this segment, blood will leak from the site.
(b) Decrease in blood pump speed.
(c) Occlusion in bloodline between dialyzer and monitoring site.
(d) A severely clotted dialyzer may decrease pressure sufficient to trigger low alarm.
(e) "Flooding" the transducer monitor or monitoring line so that pressures are

not accurately measured; failure to unclamp the monitoring line.
(2) High alarm.
(a) Occlusion or obstruction in bloodline between the monitoring site and the patient.
(b) Malposition or infiltration of the venous needle.
(c) Embolus (sufficient in size to completely or partially occlude the bloodline or fistula needle) from dialyzer or venous drip chamber into downstream bloodline.
4. Air detector.
a. Detects air bubbles and foam in the venous bloodline by change in light transmission to a photoelectric cell or ultrasonic detection device located on or below the venous drip chamber.
b. Manually armed or automatically set by the equipment when sensor head is in place.
c. When alarm is activated, blood pump is automatically stopped and venous bloodline clamp activated below the sensing site; requires user intervention to correct or override.
d. Condition causing alarm: air, foam, or microbubbles at sensing site.

B. Dialysate circuit electronic monitors.
1. Dialysate composition (conductivity).
a. Continuously measures electrical conductance or conductivity of dialysate, which is dependent on the concentration and mobility of the contained ions; expressed in milliohms; reflects the concentration of sodium salts, the major electrolyte in the dialysate.
b. Upper and lower limits on the physiologic range of conductivity are usually preset by the manufacturer; upper and lower limits within the physiologic range may be manually set or automatically set as a function of the base conductivity for proportioned dialysate.
c. When conductivity exceeds the upper or lower limits, system should immediately go into bypass to divert dialysate to drain; should be accompanied by audible and visual alarms.
d. Conditions causing alarm: incorrect composition of dialysate.
(1) Low conductivity: too much water, too little concentrate, or only one of the acid

or bicarbonate concentrates required for bicarbonate dialysate is available.

(2) High conductivity: too little water or too much concentrate.

2. Dialysate flow rate.
   a. Measures and displays the dialysate flow rate on the front panel of the delivery system.
   b. Flow rate may be preset by manufacturer. In newer equipment, operator may be able to change flow rate to several settings or to completely turn off dialysate.
   c. Divergence from desired rate may decrease dialyzer efficiency or consume more concentrate. Poses no lethal threat to patient.
   d. Conditions causing an alarm.
      (1) Dialysate pump failure.
      (2) Power failure.
      (3) Inadequate water pressure.
      (4) Obstruction in outflow.
      (5) Inadequate availability of concentrate.

3. Dialysate temperature.
   a. Thermostat controls electric heater or hot and cold mixing valve; heat exchanger may be incorporated in dialysate circuit to conserve energy required to heat cold water to normal dialysate temperature setting; thermostat or monitor in dialysate circuit before the dialyzer monitors dialysate temperature.
   b. Range is usually preset by manufacturer.
   c. Dialysate temperature.
      (1) High limit of 42° C as protein denaturation and hemolysis can occur at greater than 45° C.
      (2) Low dialysate temperature may induce chilling in patients.
   d. Excursion above the high temperature limit activates an audible and visual alarm, and opens the bypass valve to divert dialysate to drain until alarm condition is rectified; low temperature may activate an alarm, but may or may not activate the bypass valve.
   e. Conditions causing alarm.
      (1) Mechanical malfunction of heater.
      (2) Power supply failure.

4. Blood leak detector.
   a. Photoelectric cell in the dialysate circuit after the dialyzer which detects light transmission changes in effluent dialysate.
   b. Sensitivity may be preset by manufacturer or may be modified by user; may have several sensitivity settings that can be manually selected.
   c. When blood in effluent dialysate is detected, audible and visual alarms are activated and the blood pump stops; in some equipment,

there will be cessation of ultrafiltration.
   d. Validation of blood in effluent may be done with blood leak testing strips.
   e. Generally requires replacement of the dialyzer.
   f. Conditions causing alarm.
      (1) Membrane leak or rupture.
      (2) Fouling of photoelectric cell from dialysate residue or bicarbonate precipitate.
      (3) Excessive air in dialysate stream.
   g. Do not reinfuse the patient's blood as there is the potential for direct mixing of the dialysate with the patient's blood.

5. Dialysate pressure or transmembrane pressure (TMP).
   a. Measures negative pressure or, in some equipment, the TMP (transmembrane pressure); may be a passive monitor in some equipment; in other delivery systems, it may incorporate the actual mechanism for generating pressure for ultrafiltration.
   b. May have upper and lower limits that can be manually set.
   c. If limits are in place, will activate an audible and visual alarm; in some equipment, it will stop the blood pump and ultrafiltration, while in other systems, it will stop dialysate flow and ultrafiltration.
   d. Conditions causing an alarm.
      (1) Mechanical malfunction of the negative pressure pump.
      (2) Failure of the pump in a volumetric ultrafiltration control system.
      (3) Obstructed blood side transducer; leads to incorrect venous pressure reading and a drift in TMP (usually to the positive side) sufficient to cause alarm.
      (4) Power supply failure.
      (5) Excursions beyond limits.
   e. It is important to maintain a minimum UFR, especially when using a high flux dialyzer, to avoid the risk of reverse ultrafiltration of dialysate with a zero, or near zero UFR. Refer to the dialyzer manufacturer's recommendations for the given configurations of that dialyzer.

V. Urea kinetic modeling.

A. Background and rationale.
   1. Urea kinetic modeling (UKM) is the formal mathematical analysis of predialysis and postdialysis blood urea nitrogen (BUN) concentrations, and selected treatment and patient information to develop an appropriate

dialysis prescription. It is used to assess the consistency of delivery of that prescription. It reflects the changes in the patient's BUN level during a single dialysis treatment.

2. Increased protein catabolism has been associated with the severity of clinical manifestations of uremia; urea is the bulk catabolite of protein.

3. BUN can serve as a marker for small molecular weight solutes in patients on dialysis.
   a. Can be used to determine the net amount of protein catabolized/day in patients on dialysis.
      (1) Urea generation is linearly related to protein catabolism.
      (2) With accurate measurement of BUN concentrations and formal mathematical analyses, a reliable estimate of dietary protein intake can be made in stable patients in nitrogen balance.
   b. From the calculation of dietary protein intake, phosphate ingestion and hydrogen ion liberation can be calculated (see Figure 11.6).
      (1) Each gram of dietary protein catabolized

in a whole-food North American diet contains approximately 15 mg of phosphate. Dairy protein contains approximately 28 mg of phosphate/gram of protein catabolized; most hemodialysis patients require phosphate binders to manage phosphate concentrations.
      (2) Each gram of protein catabolized liberates 0.75 mEq of hydrogen. Large protein intakes are associated with large acid loads which must be buffered from available body base stores including bone; buffer must be repleted during dialysis by dialysate bicarbonate.
   c. Can be used as a marker solute to quantify dialysis therapy and individualize the dialysis dose prescription based on unique patient and treatment parameters; can serve as quality assurance tool to determine the dose of dialysis delivered relative to the dose prescribed.

B. Application of the urea kinetic model.
   1. Requires determination of specific patient

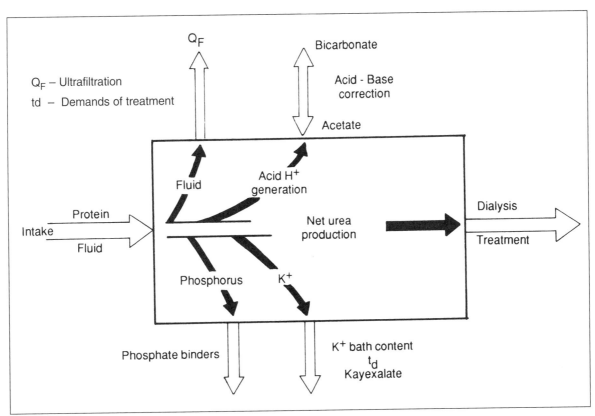

Figure 11.6. Protein catabolism yields urea, other nitrogenous waste products, phosphate, and hydrogen.

parameters and an understanding of the interaction between patient and treatment variables.

2. Most frequently used model is the variable volume, single pool urea model.
   a. The NKF-KDOQI Clinical Practice Guidelines for Hemodialysis Adequacy recommends that the dose of dialysis should be measured and monitored routinely; that the delivered dose of hemodialysis in adult and pediatric patients should be measured using formal urea kinetic modeling, a single-pool, variable-volume model.
   b. Assumes urea is distributed in a single, well-mixed volume or pool.
3. Patient parameters of the model are those parameters associated with unique characteristics of each patient.
   a. Urea volume (V) is the body water volume of distribution for urea; considered to be total body water (TBW), expressed in mL or L.
      (1) With normal body composition, it is approximately 58% of body weight; fat tissue contains less water and muscle tissue relatively more water.
      (2) In obese individuals, TBW may be less than 58%, and may range from 40 to 50% of body weight.
      (3) In lean, muscular males, TBW may be greater than 58%, and range from 60 to 70% of body weight.
      (4) Lean, elderly males with relatively little body fat may also have higher TBW, in the range of 60 to 70% of body weight.
   b. V (urea volume) in the kinetic model can be calculated in several ways:
      (1) From the drop in during dialysis with a known dialyzer urea clearance, operated for a known length of time; calculation is complicated and requires computational assistance.
      (2) From surface area as a function of height, weight, and gender; and anthropometric measures.
      (3) As some fixed percentage of body weight; this is the least accurate method to estimate V.
   c. TBW can accurately be determined with radioisotope dilution methods; bioelectrical impedance has been proposed as a suitable method to determine TBW.
4. As protein is catabolized, urea is generated and distributed in body water in mg/min.
   a. The breakdown of ingested protein produces

urea, which is normally excreted by the kidneys.
   b. Other products of protein catabolism include creatinine in small amounts, uric acid, phosphate, sulfur, and fecal nitrogen.
   c. In the absence of renal excretion of urea, the concentration of BUN increases; rate of increase reflects the net generation of BUN or Gu.
   d. Gu can be calculated from the change in body urea content from the end of one dialysis to the beginning of the next dialysis.
   e. Computer solution of both V and Gu equations can now be done with a single set of predialysis/postdialysis BUN values and suitable treatment information.
      (1) To express concentration in SI units, the BUN multiplied by 0.357 can be used to convert BUN values to urea concentration in mmol/L.
      (2) To convert BUN to urea nitrogen values, the BUN multiplied by 0.1667 will give urea nitrogen values in mmol/L.
   f. From Gu, the clinician can calculate the net amount of protein catabolized; if the patient is stable or in zero nitrogen balance, this is equal to dietary protein intake.
      (1) The equation to calculate net grams of protein catabolized/24 hours (PCR, g/24 hours) from Gu in the adult patient is as follows: PCR, g/24 hr = 9.35(Gu)+11.04.
      (2) If patient is catabolic or anabolic, PCR will not equal dietary protein intake. If patient is catabolic, PCR will overestimate dietary intake. If patient is anabolic, PCR will underestimate protein intake.
      (3) If residual renal urea clearance is present but not measured, PCR will be underestimated.
5. Normalized protein catabolic rate (NPCR) is the net amount of protein catabolized or ingested per kilogram of normalized body weight per 24 hours; is expressed as NPCR in g/kg/day.
   a. NPCR is expressed per unit of normalized or ideal body weight; PCR is the total grams of protein catabolized per 24 hours. Protein is prescribed as g/kg of normalized body weight/24 hours.
Example:
Patient #1 is obese with a body weight of 75 kg or V=30 L. The prescribed dietary protein intake would be V/.58 or 30/.58 = ideal body weight of 51 kg. The diet prescription would be 50–55 g of protein/24 hours or 1.0 g/kg/24 hours for ideal

body weight rather than 75 g/24 hours using actual body weight.

b. The frequent dietary prescription for hemodialysis patients is 1.0 to 1.2 g/kg/24 hours.

(1) Assures adequate protein nutrition if 2/3 of the protein is high-biologic-value protein (i.e., meat, milk, fish, eggs).

(2) Is considered adequate for nutritional needs, but avoids generating excessive amounts of urea, phosphate, and hydrogen ions, as discussed above.

6. KrU is the residual renal urea clearance in mL/min.

a. Will be a lower value than residual creatinine clearance and is generally about 0.55 to 0.60 of residual renal creatinine clearance.

b. Residual renal urea clearance represents one of the urea removal mechanisms, since it operates 24 hr/day compared to the intermittent removal by hemodialysis.

c. KrU in mL/min is calculated from urine volume (Uv in mL), urine urea concentration (Uu in mg/dL), mean BUN in mg/dL, and time of collection (t in min). The calculation is as follows: KrU = (Uu/Mean BUN)(Uv/t).

d. In the patient with chronic kidney disease who does not require dialysis (steady state conditions), Gu can be calculated from the measured KrU and BUN concentrations which bracket the urine collection. Gu in mg/min = (Kru in mL/min)(Mean BUN in mg/dL). PCR can be calculated as shown above from Gu.

7. In the patient on hemodialysis, where BUN concentration oscillates as a function of the removal during treatment and accumulation between treatments, the BUN concentration in the body is equal to the following: C = (Urea input – Urea output)/V and is a function of V, PCR, KrU, and dialysis dose.

a. V will influence BUN if input is constant. *Example*: the same amount of protein ingested by a patient with a large V will result in a lower BUN concentration than the same protein load ingested by a patient with a small V.

b. Input will be represented by PCR or NPCR. Rate of rise in BUN will be dependent on the net amount of protein catabolized between treatments and the V into which urea nitrogen is generated. Higher protein intake will increase the rate of BUN rise relative to a low protein intake in the same patient.

c. Output will be primarily controlled by urea removal during dialysis.

C. Treatment parameters related to the urea kinetic model are those aspects that constitute the primarily urea removal mechanisms. They generally can be controlled or manipulated.

1. K or dialyzer urea clearance is the rate at which available blood through the dialyzer is completely cleared urea (see dialyzer section).

a. K is a function of membrane permeability, size and membrane area (KoA in mL/min), blood flow rate (Qb in mL/min or L/min), and dialysate flow rate (Qd in mL/min); it can be influenced by a change in membrane, Qb, KoA, and Qd.

b. K is manipulated to achieve a drop in BUN concentration during dialysis; the desired K will be achieved by manipulation of Qb during dialysis or by selection of a dialyzer (KoA) that will provide the desired clearance.

c. The curvilinear drop in BUN concentration that occurs during dialysis follows first order phenomenon. The bulk amount of urea removed (flux) is a function of BUN concentration (although dialyzer urea clearance is constant). As concentration falls, the flux decreases and BUN concentration decays at a slower rate.

2. A major parameter that influences the drop in BUN concentration during dialysis is the length of dialysis or t in min.

a. A dialyzer with a known urea clearance operated for a specified time will produce a predictable drop in BUN concentration.

b. The length of time required to achieve that drop in BUN will be a function of dialyzer urea clearance, and patient V or volume to be cleared.

c. These three parameters, K, t, and V, are integrally related and control the rate at which BUN concentration drops during dialysis as well as the total decrease in BUN concentration that occurs over the hemodialysis treatment.

D. Kt/V is a tool to prescribe the dose of dialysis.

1. A treatment prescription can be defined as the use of a specified dialyzer for a prescribed treatment time with prescribed blood and dialysate flow rates.

2. A dialysis prescription can be written using Kt/V.

a. Kt/V is a dialyzer urea clearance (K in mL or

L/min) times the length of dialysis (t in min) and the product divided by patient V (V in mL or L).

Example:
Dialyzer K is 220 mL/min or .220 L/min;
Treatment time is 3.5 hours or 210 minutes;
Patient V is 35 L
Kt/V = [(.220)(210)]/35 = 1.32.

  b. NKF-KDOQI Clinical Practice Guidelines for Hemodialysis Adequacy recommend that the prescribed dose of dialysis be at least 1.43 to maximize the chance that a minimum dose of 1.2 per treatment will be attained when a patient dialyzes three times a week; the respective URR would be 70%.

E. Urea kinetic modeling can be used to assess treatment delivery relative to the prescription.
  1. Knowledge of the model and application in the development of an appropriate dialysis prescription allows the caregiver to assess adequacy of a given therapy by accepted criteria, and manipulate treatment variables to obtain the desired dialysis prescription.
  2. Actual treatment delivery can be assessed from predialysis and postdialysis BUN concentrations and patient weights, and treatment information from the specific dialysis.
    a. With BUN concentrations, weights, dialyzer type, blood and dialysate flow rates, and treatment time, the delivered Kt/V and NPCR can be calculated using rigorous mathematical analysis.
    b. The NKF-KDOQI Clinical Practice Guidelines for Hemodialysis Adequacy state that all patients on hemodialysis within a facility should have a delivered dose of dialysis measured using the same method.
    c. NKF-KDOQI Clinical Practice Guidelines for Hemodialysis Adequacy state that the delivered dose of dialysis should be monitored at least once a month in adult and pediatric patients.
  3. The total drop in BUN concentration during dialysis will be a function of patient size, as represented by the volume of distribution for urea (total body water) or V, the dialyzer urea clearance (K), and the length of dialysis or t; the drop in BUN concentration will be inversely related to the V (e.g., given the same treatment conditions, a smaller drop in BUN concentration represents a larger V) (see Figure 11.7).
    a. If the drop in BUN concentration during dialysis is less than expected, the prescribed

therapy was underdelivered or less therapy was given than expected.
    b. If the drop in BUN concentration during dialysis is more than expected, the delivered therapy appears to be higher than the prescription.
      (1) May be the result of drawing the postdialysis BUN sample from the venous bloodline rather than the arterial line at the end of dialysis.
      (2) May be related to urea rebound. During dialysis, BUN concentration disequilibrium exists between two compartments. At the end of dialysis, there is rapid equilibrium between the two compartments and BUN concentration rises rapidly; this represents the two pool distribution of urea.
      (3) Disequilibrium may be between the intracellular BUN concentration and the extracellular compartment of which the vascular compartment is one component. This is the result of relatively slow transport of urea from one compartment to the other.
    c. The disequilibrium may reflect the relatively low blood flow to the large urea-containing compartment or volume (skin, bone, and muscle) compared to the high blood flow to the smaller urea-containing compartment. This is the flow-volume disequilibrium concept.
    d. Equilibration occurs usually within 30–60 minutes after the end of dialysis.
    e. The magnitude of urea rebound seems to be associated with the rate of urea clearance relative to urea volume (K/V). The magnitude of urea rebound may be as high as 50% of the postdialysis BUN concentration. For example, if the postdialysis concentration is 20 mg/dL and there is 50% urea rebound, the equilibrated BUN will be 30 mg/dL.
      (1) NKF-KDOQI Clinical Practice Recommendations suggest that women, smaller patients, and patients who are malnourished may need more dialysis to reach target prescription due to possible differences in urea distribution and/or postdialysis rebound.
      (2) Delivered Kt/V may be further complicated by cardiopulmonary recirculation, where well-dialyzed blood is returned to the venous circulation and heart, where this blood reduces the effective systemic BUN concentration coming back to the dialyzer; reduces the

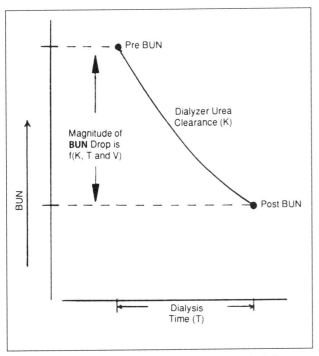

Figure 11.7. Drop in BUN concentration with dialyzer urea clearance (K) and treatment time (T).

effective concentration gradient in the dialyzer; it is usually dissipated within 2 minutes after dialysis.

(3) NKF-KDOQI Clinical Practice Guidelines for Hemodialysis Adequacy state that predialysis and postdialysis samples should be drawn on the same hemodialysis treatment.

(4) NKF-KDOQI Clinical Practice Guidelines for Hemodialysis Adequacy state that the predialysis BUN sample should be drawn just prior to the dialysis treatment, avoiding the dilution of the blood sample by saline or heparin; the postdialysis BUN sample should be drawn using the slow flow/stop pump technique.

(a) At the end of dialysis, the ultrafiltration is stopped, dialysate flow is reduced or discontinued, the blood pump is reduced to 50–100 mL/min. After 15 seconds, the postdialysis BUN sample is drawn from the arterial sample port closest to the patient.

(b) This avoids spurisously low BUN concentration from access recirculation.

4. The dialyzer clearance (K), treatment time (t) information, and predialysis/postdialysis BUN concentrations and weights allow the calculation of effective V (urea volume) to uniquely fit these data. Obviously errors occur in K and t, but calculation of effective V provides useful information.

a. Identifies persistent technical problems.

(1) Errors in dialyzer clearance (K).
(a) Fistula recirculation.
(b) Inaccurate estimate of dialyzer performance.
(c) Errors in blood pump setting.
(d) Blood pump calibration errors.
(e) Variability in cross-sectional area of the blood pump tubing segment which affects stroke volume per revolution of the blood pump.
(f) Inadequate dialyzer reprocessing.
(g) Dialysate flow errors.

(2) Treatment time (t) errors.
(a) Treatment time measured by wall clock or personal wristwatch.
(b) Blood pump is gradually increased over the first 15–30 minutes of dialysis.
(c) Blood pump speed is reduced for hypotension or muscle cramps.
(d) Frequent extracorporeal blood compartment pressure alarms or dialysate compartment alarms.
(e) Needle manipulation/infiltration.
(f) Dialyzer blood leak.
(g) Treatment time electively changed by patient or care provider.

(3) BUN measurement errors.
(a) Predialysis BUN sample diluted by saline in the fistula needle.
(b) Predialysis BUN sample drawn after the start of dialysis.
(c) Postdialysis BUN sample drwn from the venous port.
(d) Laboratory error.
(e) Laboratory calibration error.
(f) Analysis of the two samples on different laboratory equipment or different analysis runs.

b. Allows comparison of kinetic V with the anthropometric V (height, weight, gender, and age) as a check on accuracy.
c. Allows calculation of NPCR.
d. Allows quantification of the prescription changes necessary to achieve desired Kt/V.

F. All parameters of the model are integrally related and change or modification in any one of these components may have an effect on the entire model system.

1. Modification in protein intake (input) in a patient will change the rate of urea production and the predialysis BUN value.

2. A reduction in treatment time or clearance (output) will remove less urea during dialysis which will be reflected in a higher postdialysis BUN value; if protein during the interdialystic interval is the same, the next predialysis BUN value will be higher.

3. The parameters that can be manipulated more easily are those associated with dialysis. Protein intake may or may not be amenable to modification.

4. The three variable, BUN, NPCR, and Kt/V are predictably related.
    a. A specific Kt/V with a known NPCR will produce a unique predialysis BUN.
    b. As shown in Figure 11.8, on a three-variable plot, if two variables are known, the remaining variable can be determined.
        Example:
        If measured midweek predialysis BUN is 73 mg/dL; the delivered Kt/V is 1.1; the NPCR that intersects these two points is 0.96 g/kg/24 hours.
    c. The three-variable plot for eKt/V is shown in Figure 11.9.

5. As shown in Figure 11.8, with the same Kt/V of 1.1, midweek predialysis BUN concentration may range from 29 mg/dL (at NPCR 0.5 g/kg/day) to 81 mg/dL with NPCR 1.1 g/kg/day; demonstrates the difficulty of assessing adequacy of dialysis prescription or dialysis delivered dose from a single predialysis BUN concentration.
    a. A predialysis and postdialysis BUN value measured on a single dialysis each month, with appropriate treatment information, allows one to determine the actual treatment delivered to the patient compared to that prescribed.
        (1) If NPCR varies, but the actual delivered dialysis dose remains constant, the predialysis BUN concentration will move along one of the diagonal Kt/V treatment lines.
        (2) If NPCR is constant, but therapy delivery varies, the measured predialysis BUN concentration will move vertically and cross different Kt/V lines.
    b. This type of graphic display of treatment information will facilitate evaluation of the consistency of treatment delivery as well as provide information about the patient's NPCR.

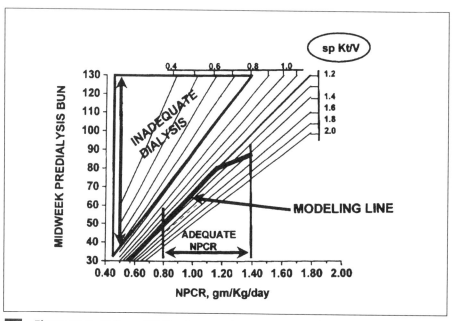

Figure 11.8. Delivered Kt/Vsp therapy plot – correlation of 3 variables, Kt/V, NPCR, and BUN concentration.

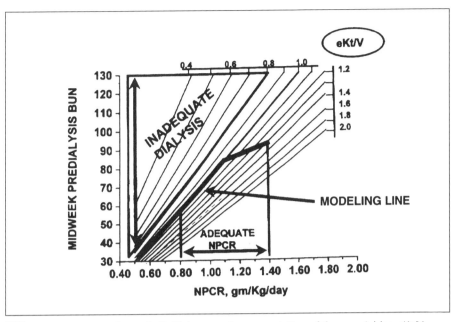

Figure 11.9. Delivered eKt/V therapy plot – correlation of three variables, eKt/V, NPCR, and BUN concentration.

G. There are several disadvantages to formal urea kinetic modeling.
  1. The assumption that urea is distributed in a single, well-mixed volume is not correct. Urea is distributed in two pools.
  2. Formal urea kinetic modeling requires the effort and personnel time to process data. User must be able to understand the patient-dialyzer system to use information; requires comprehensive knowledge of dialysis and clinical events to interpret results of kinetic modeling.

H. Urea reduction ratio (URR) calculation is a simplified approximation of formal urea kinetic modeling that can be used to assess treatment delivery.

  1. URR uses predialysis and postdialysis BUN concentrations to calculate the following: URR = (Predialysis BUN – Postdialysis BUN/Predialysis BUN in mg/dL)(100).
  Example:
  Predialysis BUN = 100 mg/dL
  Postdialysis BUN = 30 mg/dL [(100-30](100) x 100 = 70%
  2. Clinical data and NKF-KDOQI Guidelines state a URR of 70% or greater is needed.
  3. There is a correlation with Kt/V.
  4. Is a simple calculation, requiring only a calculator and two BUN values.
  5. Cannot derive NPCR.
  6. Ignores volume changes during the dialytic interval and may lead to some error in actual delivered dose.

Chapter 52

Water Treatment

I. The purposes of water treatment.

A. To prepare safe water for all facets of HD including preprocessing and reprocessing of hemodialyzers, concentrate mixing, dialysate proportioning, and machine cleaning and disinfection, that is sufficiently pure and free of contaminants to meet the minimum recommended standards for water quality set by the Association for the Advancement of Medical Instrumentation (AAMI) and enforced by the Centers for Medicare and Medicaid Services (CMS).

B. To prevent the consequences of inadequately purified water including anemia, hemolysis, bone disease, neurologic deterioration, methemoglobinemia, metabolic acidosis, sepsis, pyrogenic reactions, and death in patients receiving HD.

C. To protect the patient from developing potential complications related to long-term exposure to low levels of endotoxins that eminate from dead gram-negative bacteria, and other bacterial-derived products that may cause chronic inflammatory disease in patients.
   1. Patients do not have an overt pyrogenic reaction, but exhibit other symptoms over time.
   2. Symptoms may include resistence to epogen, albumin reduction, malnutrition, decreased transferrin levels, beta-2 microglobulin amyloidosis (e.g., carpal tunnel syndrome) and accelerated atherosclerosis leading to enhanced cardiovascular risk and mortality.

II. Quality.

A. Bacteria levels in water for hemodialysis purposes shall not exceed 200 CFU/mL (colony forming units) with an action level of 50 CFU/mL.

B. Endotoxin levels in water for hemodialysis applications shall not exceed 2 EU (endotoxin units) with an action level of 1 EU.

C. AAMI analysis of the product water should not exceed recommended safe levels (see Table 11.1) at all times.

III. Testing.

A. Water samples for bacteria shall be collected minimally from the first and last outlets of the water distribution loop, entrance to reprocessing equipment and concentrate mixing, exiting the deionizer (DI), ultraviolet (UV), ultrafiltration (UF) and storage tank systems and anywhere water is dispensed.
   1. Do not disinfect sampling ports, simply flush with water for 60 seconds.
   2. Bacteria samples should be tested at least once per month.
   3. Microbial samples should be assayed within 1–2 hours, or refrigerated at 4–6° C up to 24 hours of collection. Total viable counts shall be obtained using membrane filtration technique or spread plate technique and grown on trypticase soy agar or equivalent.
   4. The calibrated loop method should not be used, nor blood or chocolate agar.
   5. Samples shall be incubated at 35° C for 48 hours and counted with a magnifying device.

B. The above testing method only tests for free-floating (planktonic) bacteria and not for attached (sessile) bacteria and may underestimate the bioburden of a water treatment system, especially if there is biofilm present.

C. Endotoxin testing shall be done with the Limulus amoebocyte lysate (LAL) assay using either a kinetic assay (more accurate) or gel-clot assay.
   1. When drawing the water samples for endotoxin testing, the same technique applies as for bacteria testing.
   2. Endotoxin testing must be done if reprocessing is used, and after DI, UV, and UF.

D. AAMI analysis on the water for hemodialysis should be performed at least annually at the most distal portion of the loop (some states require more frequent testing). It should be performed more often if the percent rejection of the reverse osmosis (RO) falls below 90% or the water quality degrades below a predetermined set point.

IV. Water supply.

A. Water contaminants can be classified into inorganic and organic chemicals: ionic compounds such as dissolved salts, minerals and metals, gases; and organics such as bacteria, viruses, and algae.

1. To make the water potable, the water supplier may add chemicals such as chlorine/chloramines for disinfection, aluminum for clarity, fluoride to prevent dental caries, and phosphates and other pH adjusters to preclude pipe corrosion.

2. If not reduced to safe levels, such chemicals can cause serious injury and death to patients on HD due to the high water permeability of the dialyzer.

3. All drinking water should meet EPA standards (Environmental Protection Agency).

B. An emergency contingency plan for loss of water should be in place.

V. Water treatment system.

A. Water treatment for hemodialysis consists of four segments: pretreatment, purification, posttreatment, and distribution.

B. Pretreatment or conditioning of the feed water is to diminish damage to the RO membrane, help the RO to perform optimally, and prevent harm to the patients.

1. Temperature blending valve increases incoming water temperature to around 77° F. The colder the water, the less purified water the RO will produce.

   a. For every one degree F drop, 1.5% purified water production is lost.

   b. Monitor posttemperature with a thermometer and record daily.

2. Chemical injection systems are used to decrease the pH of the incoming feed water to between 5 and 8 units so the RO membrane and carbon tanks can perform optimally.

   a. May use hydrochloric or sulfuric acid for pH alteration, or sodium metabisulfite for chloramine reduction.

   b. If using for chloramine reduction, the appropriate amount of carbon tanks must accompany the chemical

injection. This is not to replace the appropriate carbon setup.

   c. Should be followed by a depth filter to remove the solidified particles.

   d. Monitor the pH after the acid injection system and record daily.

   e. Need to demonstrate safe reduction of chemical byproducts.

Table 11.1

AAMI and EPA Maximum Allowable Levels of Contaminants in Water

Contaminant	Drinking water (mg/L) (condensed list) July 2002	Concentration for Hemodialysis Water (mg/L)	Associated with Hemodialysis Toxicity (mg/L)
Calcium	Not regulated	2 (0.1 mEq/L)	88
Magnesium	Not regulated	4 (0.3 mEq/L)	
Potassium	Not regulated	8 (0.2 mEq/L)	
Sodium	Not regulated	70 (3.0 mEq/L)	300
Antimony	0.006	0.006	
Arsenic	0.005 (0.010 on 1/23/06)	0.05	
Barium	2	0.10	
Beryllium	0.004	0.0004	
Cadmium	0.005	0.001	
Chromium	0.10	0.014	
Lead	0.015**	0.005	
Mercury	0.002	0.0002	
Selenium	0.05	0.09	
Silver	0.10	0.005	
Aluminum	0.05-0.2*	0.01	0.06
Chloramines	4.0*	0.10	0.25
Free Chlorine	4.0*	0.50	
Copper	1.3**	0.10	0.49
Fluoride	2.0*-4.0	0.20	1.0
Nitrate (as Nitrogen)	10	2.0	21
Sulfate	250*	100	200
Thallium	0.002	0.002	
Zinc	5*	0.10	0.2
Bacteria	HPC Bacteria: 500 cfu/mL Coliform bacteria: 0-5%***	200 cfu/mL (action level 50 cfu/mL)	>200 cfu/mL
Endotoxin	Not regulated	2 EU/mL (action level 1 EU/mL)	5 EU/kg/ body weight

* Unenforceable maximum contaminant level goal (secondary standard)
** Action level at 90th percentile
*** 95% of the samples (all positive results must be resolved)
HPC = heterotrophic plate count; EU = endotoxin unit

Source: Association for the Advancement of Medical Instrumentation (AAMI). (2001). *AAMI Standards. Vol. 3: Dialysis*. WQD. Richmond, VA: AAMI. Table previously printed in Amato, R.L. (2005). Water treatment for hemodialysis – Updated to include the latest AAMI Standards for Dialysate (RD52: 2004). *Nephrology Nursing Journal, 32*(2), 151-167.

3. Depth filtration (multimedia filter).
   a. Removes particulates and colloidal matter greater than 10 microns from the incoming water supply.
   b. These foulants can clog the pretreatment devices and RO membrane that follow.
   c. Monitor and record the prepressure and postpressure and backwash (cleans the tank of debris) routinely or when delta pressure equal to or greater than 10 is reached (meaning the filter is clogging).
4. Softener removes scaling factors from the feed water that would otherwise deposit on the RO membrane surface and foul it off.
   a. Calcium and magnesium cause the feed water to be "hard."
   b. Works on a cation exchange process, exchanges two sodiums (monovalent bond) for one calcium or magnesium ion (divalent bond), and to a lesser degree, iron. Sodium does not cause scale on the RO membrane and is highly rejected.
   c. Must have a regeneration lockout device so the softener cannot regenerate during patient treatments.
   d. Test hardness daily after softener at end of operation. May test the softener preoperation to demonstrate it regenerated properly before use.
   e. Monitor prepressure and postpressure and record daily.
   f. Regenerate with clean pelletized salt routinely or with hardness breakthrough (greater than 1 grain or 17.5 mg/L hardness).
5. Carbon adsorption, a chemical process, removes chlorine, chloramines, and other low-molecular-weight synthetic and organic compounds such as herbicides, pesticides, and industrial solvents from the feed water.
   a. Chloramine and chlorine can cause severe hemolytic anemia, met-hemoglobinemia, and death in patients if exceeds the AAMI limits of 0.1 and 0.5 respectively.
   b. The setup shall have two tanks in series configuration.
      (1) The first is the "worker" that is the primary source of chloramine and chlorine removal.
      (2) The second is the "polisher" for any residual chloramine/chlorine.
      (3) There should be a total of 10 minutes EBCT (empty bed contact time) with 5 minutes in each tank at the maximum flow rate.
   c. GAC (granular activated carbon) shall have a

minimum iodine rating of 900 or equivalent, be virgin carbon (nonregenerated) and have a mesh size of 12 x 40 or smaller.
   d. Test after first tank for total chlorine level and free chlorine. The difference between the two is assumed to be the chloramine level. If using a single total chlorine indicator, the limit shall be 0.1 mg/L (assume all total chlorine is chloramine since no differentiation is made). Test before every patient shift, or every 4 hours if no shift.
   e. If breakthrough occurs, test after the second tank. Assuming there is no breakthrough of chlorine/chloramines, HD may continue if testing is done more frequently (e.g., every 1–2 hours) and arrangements for a new tank made. Whenever possible, the second tank should be rotated into the first position, or all carbon changed out.
   f. Backwashing does not regenerate carbon. Backwash on a regular basis. Exchange carbon for new on a routine schedule as it can grow bacteria and bioburden the RO membrane.
   g. Monitor prepressure and postpressure and record daily.

C. Purification.
   1. Reverse osmosis (RO) systems have a prefilter to remove particulates emanating from the pretreatment, a pump to increase water pressure, and RO membranes to purify the pretreated water.
      a. Produces purified water through the use of a semipermeable membrane with pressurized water that is forced through the membrane, leaving most of its contaminants behind (overcoming natural osmosis using hydraulic pressure, creating "reverse osmosis"). The incoming stream is split into two, one as the purified product stream and one as the waste stream (see Figure 11.10).
      b. RO membranes will reject charged particles in an approximate range from 95 to 99%. Contaminants with no charge (bacteria, viruses, endotoxin) will be sieved at a greater than 200 molecular weight cut-off. pH, temperature, and damage to the RO membrane will change rejection characteristics.
      c. RO membranes are made of a spiral wound polyamide material that is damaged by oxidants such as total chlorine and high levels of peracetic acid.
      d. RO membrane performance is measured by percent rejection, which is the percent of charged contaminants that are removed to waste drain (e.g., 95% rejected).

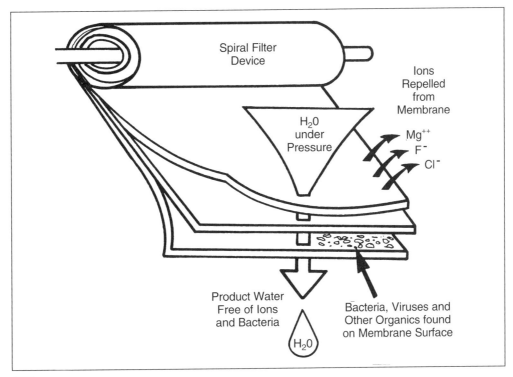

Figure 11.10. Reverse osmosis.

Source: Wick, G.S., & Parker, J. (1984). *Protecting the future of quality care through an understanding of hemodialysis principles*. Pitman, NJ: The American Nephrology Nurses' Association. Used with permission.

e. Final water quality is measured by either conductivity in microsiemens/cm or total dissolved solids (TDS) displayed as mg/L or parts per million (PPM) and shows what ions remain in the RO product water.

f. The percent rejection and conductivity/TDS display will vary depending on how well the RO membrane is functioning and the amount of dissolved solids in the feed water.

g. Both percent rejection and a water quality monitor shall be used and continuously displayed with a visual and audible alarm that can be heard in the patient care area. An AAMI analysis must be done on the product water to validate if the readings meet the criteria.

h. If a predetermined set point for water quality is violated, the system should have a divert-to-drain so inadequately purified water is not sent to patient use.

i. Record all water quality, flow meters and pressure gauges daily.

D. Posttreatment components.
1. Deionization (DI) contains resin beads that remove both positively and negatively charged ions from the water in exchange for hydroxyl (OH-) and hydrogen (H+) which combine to form H2O. It is usually used as a polisher for RO product water that does not meet the AAMI standards, or as an emergency backup in case of breakdown.
   a. Types of deionizers.
      (1) Mixed bed deionizers contain both cationic and anionic resin beads.
      (2) Dual bed deionizers have either all cationic or anionic resins in one tank that need to be used together to remove ions and should be followed by a mixed bed deionizer.
   b. DI has a finite capacity. Once exhausted, it will dump mass quantities of retained ions, especially the weakly attracted ones such as aluminum and fluoride. This has caused serious injury and death in patients.
   c. Water quality is measured using resistivity (inverse of conductivity).
   d. Resistivity shall be continuously monitored with an audible and visual, temperature compensated alarm. The staff must be able to hear the alarm in the patient care area.
   e. The DI shall divert-to-drain for a resistivity less than 1 meg-ohm/cm and shall not be used until the tanks are replaced.
   f. Bacteria and endotoxin will not be removed as

they do not contain a charge. DI tanks tend to grow microbes and should be exchanged regularly.

g. The DI shall be followed by ultrafiltration (UF) to remove both endotoxin and bacteria.

h. DI is not intended to be used for primary purification without the RO. DI coupled with UF is unable to remove low-molecular-weight bacterial byproducts such as microcystins (toxins from blue-green algae), which have caused liver failure and death in patients.

i. Must use designated medical or potable water grade resins that are regenerated at the supplier separately from other more contaminated resins. The tanks should also be disinfected at the supplier.

j. Carbon filtration shall precede DI to prevent formation of carcinogenic nitrosamines.

k. Two tanks should be used in a series configuration, one as the worker, one as a backup.

l. Record resistivity twice daily, and before and after tank pressures once a day.

2. Ultraviolet irradiation (UV) is a low pressure mercury vapor lamp enclosed in a transparent quartz sleeve that emits a germicidal 254 nm wavelength that delivers a dose of radiant energy to inhibit microbial growth.

a. UV is able to penetrate the cell wall of bacteria to destroy it or render it unable to replicate.

b. UV resistant strains may develop if the equipment is not maintained properly.

c. UV shall be equipped with an intensity meter that delivers 16 milliwatt-sec/cm^2 or, if no meter, delivers a radiant dose of at least 30 milli-watt-sec/cm^2.

d. Endotoxin levels may increase as a result of destruction of microbes.

e. UV shall be followed by ultrafiltration (UF).

f. Replace the UV bulb every 8000 hours, or annually and clean quartz sleeve routinely. Daily record radiant output and prepressure and postpressure.

3. Ultrafiltration is a membrane filter that is either a cross-flow design (with a feed stream, a product stream and a waste stream) or a dead-ended design (with one stream that flows in then out).

a. UF removes bacteria and endotoxin (submicron filtration only removes bacteria).

b. UF shall be post DI and UV.

c. UF should be validated for medical use (absolute rating).

d. UF will grow bacteria if not routinely disinfected or replaced.

e. May be used at points of use (e.g., reprocessing equipment, on dialysate line, etc.).

f. Pressure differential should be monitored and recorded at least daily.
   (1) A differential reading of zero might indicate that water is flowing around and not through the filter.
   (2) A high delta pressure reading would indicate the filter is clogged.

E. Distribution system.
1. There are two types of distribution systems, direct and indirect. Direct systems deliver water from the RO directly to the loop for use. Indirect distribution systems deliver the water to a storage tank first.

a. Direct feed systems should have a minimum velocity at peak demand (all equipment operating) measured in the distal portion of the loop of 1.5 ft/sec to impede microbial attachment (biofilm) and proliferation.

b. Biofilms are communities of microorganisms attached to surfaces that secrete a gelatinous substance (extracellular polymer, glycocalyx) to protect themselves and create an endless supply of food.

c. Unused product water should loop back to the RO.

2. Water storage tank accumulates the product water and delivers it to the distribution loop. Unused product water is recirculated back into the tank.

a. The large surface area is conducive for microbial growth.

b. To reduce microbial growth, the tank should be designed with a cone shaped bottom, a tight fitting lid that is vented with a microbial air filter, an internal spray mechanism, and all parts made of inert materials that do not leach contaminants.

c. The tank should be just large enough to meet peak water demands without exceeding it.

d. Minimum velocity at peak demand (all equipment that draws running water) measured at the distal portion of the loop should be 3 ft/sec to impede microbial attachment and growth (biofilm).

e. An aggressive and frequent disinfection program should be employed.

f. Monitor and record before and after recirculation pump pressures and velocity daily.

3. Water distribution piping systems should be a continuous loop design where water is returned to the RO or storage tank and designed to minimize biofilm formation.
   a. Made of inert materials only. No copper, brass, aluminum, lead, zinc or other toxic materials shall be used.
   b. No dead-ends or multiple branches should exist.
   c. Rough joints must be avoided.
   d. Low flow velocity and large pipes will lead to biofilm formation.
   e. To minimize biofilm formation, there should always be flow in the piping and storage tank.
   f. Frequent disinfection and vigilant monitoring of the velocity where it returns to the RO or storage tank will impede biofilm formation.

VI. Records.

A. All monitoring sheets for record keeping should have parameters where appropriate so users know when a limit has been violated.

B. A record of maintenance of the water treatment system will be maintained.

C. Proper training of personnel who monitor and maintain the system will be recorded.

D. Flow diagrams of the water treatment system should be posted and each device labeled with its individual operation.

E. The medical director should be notified when any water quality parameter is exceeded or component limit is violated.

Chapter 53

Patient Management – The Dialysis Procedure

I. Predialysis equipment preparation. The dialysis equipment is prepared and tested to assure a safe and effective dialysis treatment.

A. The dialyzer is prepared as follows:
   1. Using aseptic technique, bloodlines are attached to appropriate dialyzer ports.
   2. Normal saline is used to rinse extracorporeal circuit to remove air, glycerin, sterilants and/or disinfectants, and any other manufacturing residue, according to manufacturer's recommendations.
   3. Dialysate compartment of dialyzer is rinsed with dialysate of physiologic concentration, the procedure should follow manufacturer's recommendations.
   4. Dialyzer must be tested for any residual disinfectant or sterilant after rinsing procedure but before use on patient. It must adhere to manufacturer's instructions for testing.
   5. If preparing a reused dialyzer, verify and document that this is the correct dialyzer for this patient and that the dialyzer has tested positive for the presence of sterilant before priming.

6. Minimize the length of time supplies and extracorporeal system are prepared in advance and recirculated per unit policy. *Editor's note*: At the time of this publication, no documented evidence could be found regarding the appropriate time that the extracorporeal system could be safely prepared in advance.

2. Delivery system preparation will depend on the particular system used and may depend on the type of buffer used.
   1. Any disinfectant/sterilant present in the system must first be rinsed and the system tested to assure that no residual remains.
   2. Temperature and conductivity must be within acceptable and safe limits.
   3. All alarms must be tested and functioning correctly.
   4. Hydraulic pressure testing may be performed with volumetric ultrafiltration machines.
   5. Many, if not all steps, should be documented.
   6. The primed dialyzer should be placed in recirculation mode until patient begins dialysis; for reused dialyzers, the recirculation mode is important to prevent sterilant rebound from

dialyzer potting compound into the extracorporeal circuit. It is common practice for facilities to dispose of unused bloodlines and discard or reprocess the hemodialyzer after recirculating for the unit specified number of hours, per unit policy.

II. Predialysis patient assessment and preparation.

Also see Fluid Assessment parameters under Chapter 54: *Fluid Removal: Obtaining Estimated Dry Weight During Hemodialysis.*

A. The patient is assessed predialysis to ensure a safe and appropriate dialysis treatment.
   1. Assessment should include but not be limited to:
      a. Predialysis weight. Compare to weight from end of previous dialysis and patient's estimated dry body weight.
      b. Thorough evaluation of fluid status including assessment of edema (facial, periorbital, sacral and lower extremity), skin turgor, and evaluation for jugular venous distention in supine and Fowler's or semi-Fowler's position.
      c. Blood pressure (sitting and standing, if appropriate and possible for patient's condition), comparing to those from previous dialysis (normotension is desired).
      d. Heart rate and rhythm, presence of pericardial rub, gallop, or other abnormalities.
      e. Respiratory rate, rhythm, and quality, presence of wheezes, rales, diminished breath sounds.
      f. Temperature (average 96.8° F).
      g. Peripheral pulses.
      h. Mental status (orientation, confusion, restlessness, mood, speech, and thought processes).
      i. Ability to ambulate and gait changes, if appropriate.
      j. Skin (turgor, color, temperature).
      k. Condition and patency of vascular access. (Also see Section 12, Vascular Access.)
      l. Residual kidney function (RKF)/urine output.
      m. Level of functioning.
      n. General sense of well-being.
      o. Current complaints of or interdialytic history of headache, dizziness, blurred vision, nausea, vomiting, diarrhea, constipation, tarry stool, change in appetite, muscle cramps, shortness of breath, dyspnea, chest pain or palpitations, weakness, fatigue, insomnia, pain, fever/chills, bleeding, urgency or frequency of urination, or other problems patient has experienced since last dialysis.
      p. Review of any pertinent laboratory data, such as electrolytes, blood glucose, hemoglobin or hematocrit, etc.
      q. Fluid losses related to draining wounds, nasogastric tube.
   2. Adjust and plan to administer the prescribed hemodialysis treatment based on the predialysis assessment findings. Components of the hemodialysis prescription include:
      a. Hemodialysis treatment time.
      b. Blood flow rate.
      c. Dialysate flow rate.
      d. Dialysate composition.
      e. Anticoagulation approach.
      f. Fluid removal plan.
         (1) Ultrafiltration as appropriate for the type of equipment being used. Either calculate the TMP or the ultrafiltration rate in mL/hr or L/hr. Calculations will determine the total amount of fluid to be removed during dialysis should include any projected intake or fluid losses during the treatment.
         (2) Blood or blood products, fluid intake, ice, saline expected to be given, or drugs that are given in some volume of diluent should be included in projected intake during the treatment.
         (3) Projected intake should also include the saline volume that the patient receives from priming the extracorporeal circuit and when blood is returned to the patient at the end of dialysis.
         (4) Urine or emesis should be considered outputs for the purpose of calculating the total amount of fluid removal during the treatment.

III. Initiation of hemodialysis.

A. This section outlines the basic steps necessary to initiate a dialysis treatment.
   1. Vascular access is prepared and cannulated according to unit procedure.
   2. Any blood sampling for biochemical or hematologic analyses is done following vascular access cannulation; must ensure that sample is not diluted with saline from fistula needle (if used for needle preparation).
   3. Administer heparin loading dose as indicated by unit policy and wait until patient is systemically heparinized (approximately

3 minutes). This reduces the potential for thrombus formation in the dialyzer.

4. Arterial bloodline is attached and secured to the arterial access, preferably with secure Luer-Lok connections, and all clamps released on dynamic bloodlines. (*Note: Some facilities may apply tape over the Luer-lok connections.*)

5. Blood pump is started at less than 200 mL/min and extracorporeal monitor lines are opened. This allows visual inspection of pressures to assure adequate arterial supply and the absence of clamps on the bloodlines.

6. If patient is to receive the equivalent of the normal saline prime, flush circuit with fresh normal saline before connecting the arterial and venous bloodlines to patient.

7. On rare occasions, such as overt pulmonary edema or other medical reasons, the normal saline prime is discarded as to not add extra volume to the patient. In this case, allow blood to fill the circuit to beyond the venous drip chamber, then connect the venous bloodline to the venous access. (*Note: This procedure requires great caution because of the risk of accidental exsanguination. Because of the potential for this lethal complication, this practice has been restricted to special circumstances or eliminated in most dialysis facilities.*)

8. Initiate extracorporeal circuit pressure monitoring, if it has not already been done.

9. Establish desired blood flow rate and note time. This is the start of dialysis time.

10. Manually set limits on all monitors if necessary, or check to see that they are set appropriately.

11. Set dialysate flow rate.

12. Initiate anticoagulation infusion per unit protocol.

13. Ultrafiltration is set for patient-desired fluid loss.

14. Bloodlines are adequately secured to patient per unit protocol.

IV. Intradialytic patient assessment and management.

A. The patient is monitored during dialysis to assure a safe and effective treatment and to determine the patient's response to the delivery of the hemodialysis prescription. Also see *Intradialytic Complications, Blood Volume Monitoring,* and *Fluid Removal: Obtaining Estimated Dry Weight During Hemodialysis.*

1. Patient assessment includes:
   a. Blood pressure and pulse, comparing to predialysis values and to established acceptable parameters.
   b. Weight or amount of fluid removed.
   c. Respiratory rate and quality.
   d. Temperature, if indicated.
   e. Hemodialysis access (see Section 12, Vascular Access).
   f. Any new complaint reported by the patient (could be early signs of complications or an adverse response to dialysis).
      (1) Headache, dizziness, or blurred vision.
      (2) Nausea, vomiting.
      (3) Fever, chills.
      (4) Chest pain or palpitations.
      (5) Shortness of breath, dyspnea.
      (6) Change in mental status, e.g., agitation, confusion, restlessness.
      (7) Tachycardia.
   g. Response to anticoagulation approach.

2. Once dialysis is initiated, assess integrity of extracorporeal circuit, including connections, and delivery system alarms.
   a. Bleeding at access site.
   b. Signs of clotting in the extracorporeal system.

3. Patient and equipment monitoring are performed and documented immediately upon the initiation of dialysis, and at some regular interval during dialysis, depending on patient condition and unit policy.

4. The patient is taught and encouraged to recognize and report early signs of adverse responses to dialysis so that preventive measures can be taken.

5. Monitor the patient throughout treatment for the onset of signs and symptoms of treatment and equipment-related complications (see Chapter 55: *Complications of Hemodialysis: Prevention and Management*).
   a. Pyrogenic reaction.
   b. Dialyzer reaction.
      (1) Hypersensitivity reaction (most severe).
      (2) Complement activation by dialyzer.
   c. Hemolysis.
   d. Air embolism.
   e. Exsanguination.

6. Based on patient assessment, modify the treatment plan as necessary to prevent complications (see Chapter 55).

7. Treat complications, as appropriate, if they occur (see Chapter 55).

8. Administer medications as prescribed.

V. Discontinuation of hemodialysis.

A. This part outlines the steps required to terminate the dialysis treatment in a safe and efficient manner.

1. The heparin infusion or bolus dosing may be discontinued before the termination of dialysis, depending on unit procedure. This may shorten postdialysis bleeding from needle sites.
2. All patient and machine parameters are documented.
   a. If a postdialysis blood sample is to be drawn the blood pump is reduced to a slow speed (100 mL/min).
   b. The NKF-DOQI Clinical Practice Guidelines for Hemodialysis Adequacy recommend that the postdialysis blood sample for determining Kt/V be drawn from the arterial bloodline injection site approximately 15 seconds after the blood pump speed has been reduced to 50–100 mL/min at the end of the dialysis treatment (see Chapter 51, V. Urea kinetic modeling).
3. The blood pump is stopped, sample obtained, and blood is returned to the patient as per routine practice with normal saline.
4. It may be useful to continue blood compartment monitoring until a patent circuit is terminated. The air detector should remain armed until the venous bloodline is disconnected from the patient.
5. Please see Section 12 for management of the vascular access postdialysis.

VI. Postdialysis patient assessment.

A. The patient is assessed after dialysis to determine the patient's response to the delivered hemodialysis prescription.
   1. The assessment should include, but not be limited to:
      a. Blood pressure and pulse, comparing to predialysis values and to established acceptable parameters.
      b. Temperature, comparing to predialysis value.
      c. Condition of access and any difficulty achieving homeostasis after needle removal is noted.
      d. Patient condition and method of departure from the unit.
   2. All predialysis, intradialysis, and postdialysis assessment information should be compared and interpreted. Additional treatments and interventions and teaching should be initiated as appropriate.
   3. Adequacy of dialysis may be determined by one or more of the following:
      a. Blood chemistries.

   b. Absence or amelioration of uremic signs and symptoms.
   c. Patient self-report of well-being.
   d. Fluid status.
   e. Morbidity during or between dialysis treatments.
   f. Quantification of the delivered dose of dialysis (see Chapter 51, V. Urea kinetic modeling).
4. Delivery system is rinsed and/or sterilized according to manufacturer's recommendations.

VII. Anticoagulation during hemodialysis.

A. Rationale for anticoagulation during hemodialysis.
   1. When blood comes into contact with foreign surfaces, such as the bloodlines and the dialyzer membrane or with air, such as in the drip chambers, the clotting mechanism is activated beginning with a coating of the surfaces by plasma proteins followed by platelet adherence and aggregation, thromboxane A2 generation, and activation of the intrinsic coagulation cascade.
   2. The clotting cascade may then continue on to significant thrombus formation, fibrin deposition and clotting in the extracorporeal circuit.
   3. Other factors such as blood flow through the dialyzer, the extent of recirculation in the extracorporeal circuit, the amount of ultrafiltration, and the length, diameter, and composition of the bloodlines affect intradialytic clotting.
   4. Anticoagulation agents and methods are part of the hemodialysis prescription.
   5. Anticoagulation with heparin is the most common method of preventing clotting in the extracorporeal system.

B. Pharmacology of heparin.
   1. Derived from porcine intestinal mucosa (mucosal heparin) or beef lung (beef heparin). (*Note*: Beef lung heparin may not be available.)
   2. Acts by accelerating the activity of antithrombin binding to thrombin. It is most effective in thrombosis prophylaxis, and more heparin is required if thrombosis has developed. Heparin has little inhibitory effect on platelet-surface interaction.
   3. In commercial preparation, heparin is a heterogenous material of active and inactive species with varying molecular size. A more homogenous heparin preparation has been

developed and used for anticoagulation in this patient population (low-molecular-weight heparin).

4. Removed from the circulation through the reticuloendothelial system at a low but constant rate; metabolized in the liver and excreted in the urine.

C. Methods of heparin administration.
   1. Continuous: heparin is continuously infused into the extracorporeal circuit during dialysis with a calibrated infusion pump. It is usually infused into the arterial limb of the extracorporeal circuit after the blood pump to avoid accidental excessive infusion due to the negative pressure in the prepump arterial circuit. This may be combined with a bolus loading dose before initiation of dialysis.
   2. Intermittent: a bolus loading dose of heparin is administered to the patient 3 to 5 minutes before the start of the dialysis treatment; additional bolus doses of heparin may be administered during dialysis.

D. Anticoagulation approaches.
   1. Systemic routine heparinization.
      a. Used for patients at normal risk for bleeding, not for those considered to be at an unusually high risk for bleeding.
      b. The objective is to achieve some designated prolongation of a patient's clotting time (usually 1.5 to 2.0 times normal value) to prevent thrombus formation in the extracorporeal circuit.
      c. Anticoagulation is initially achieved with a bolus dose before start of the dialysis treatment; heparin is continuously infused as described above.
      d. The heparin may be a standard dosing regimen for all patients or given as individualized doses.
   2. Fractional, tight, or minimal heparinization.
      a. This is prescribed for patients who are at slight risk for bleeding.
      b. The objective is to only slightly prolong the patient's clotting time, without inducing thrombus formation in the extracorporeal circuit, through the judicious administration of heparin.
      c. Small doses of heparin are given. Clotting times may be measured frequently.
      d. Usually given with an initial bolus of heparin followed by a constant infusion.
      e. The target activated clotting time, ACT, is

25% (fractional) or 15% (tight fractional) above baseline.
   3. Regional heparinization.
      a. The objective is to prolong the clotting time in the extracorporeal circuit without significant prolongation of the patient's innate clotting time.
      b. Indications for use are any pathologic state in which prolongation of the patient's clotting time puts the patient at risk of hemorrhage.
      c. It is achieved with an infusion of heparin into the arterial bloodline and an infusion of protamine into the venous bloodline.
         (1) Pharmacology of protamine.
            (a) Highly alkaline and neutralizes the highly acidic heparin. This is a reversible bond.
            (b) Neutralizes heparin by weight not by anticoagulant activity; 1–1.5 mg of protamine neutralizes approximately 100 units of heparin.
            (c) Protamine has an anticoagulant action in large doses.
            (d) Heparin rebound caused by a breakdown of the heparin-protamine complex in the reticuloendothelial system and the liberation of heparin into the circulation; may occur 2 to 4 hours after the cessation of dialysis and may persist for up to 10 hours.
         (2) This method is rarely used today because of new anticoagulation techniques and associated difficulties of rational control of dual drug infusions and the potential for heparin rebound.
   4. Alternative methods for anticoagulation with patients at risk for bleeding.
      a. Regional citrate anticoagulation: infuses sodium citrate into the arterial bloodline to form a complex with calcium to prevent activation of the clotting cascade. Calcium is infused into the venous bloodline to restore serum calcium to normal value.
         (1) Must use calcium-free dialysate.
         (2) Complications may be hypocalcemia and citrate toxicity, which may be expressed as nausea, paresthesias, muscle cramps, and tetany.
      b. Heparin-free dialysis: using high blood flow rates (at least equal to or greater than 300 mL/min) and intermittent saline flush through the dialyzer (50–100 mL every 15 minutes) to prevent and observe for clotting. Dialysis has been successfully performed with no heparin

or anticoagulant. The equivalent of the administered saline volume must be removed by ultrafiltration during the dialysis treatment.

E. Assessing outcomes of anticoagulation therapy.
1. Assess the patient predialysis for any interdialytic changes in condition or events, signs of bleeding, or risk of bleeding.
   a. Open or closed injuries.
   b. Falls.
   c. Bruising or contusions.
   d. Hemorrhage, including the eye.
   e. Surgical, dental or biopsy procedures that have been performed or to be performed.
   f. Signs and symptoms of pericarditis.
2. Intradialytic inspection of the dialyzer and extracorporeal circuit for visual signs of clotting.
   a. Extremely dark blood or black streaks in the dialyzer.
   b. Clot formation in drip chambers and headers of the dialyzer.
   c. Rapid filling of venous chamber and/or transducer filters with blood.
   d. Changes in arterial or venous pressures, depending on where the clot is occurring.
3. Postdialysis inspection of the dialyzer and extra-corporeal circuit for visual signs of clotting.
   a. Large amounts of clotting indicate need for increase in anticoagulation.
   b. Decrease in total cell volume (in dialyzer

reuse) can indicate dialyzer clotting.
4. Activated clotting time (ACT).
5. Whole blood activated partial thromboplastin time (WBPTT).
6. Plasma partial thromboplastin time (PTT).
7. Platelets.
   a. Heparin-induced thrombocytopenia, type II, is a complication of heparin therapy occurring in 5–10% of patients treated with heparin.
   b. Related to the presence of heparin-induced antiplatelet antibodies.
   c. Presents initially as thrombocytopenia (a reduction in platelet count to 30–50% of baseline value).
   d. Associated with venous and/or arterial thrombosis in 20–50% of cases.

F. Federal regulations have constrained the ability to perform anticoagulation monitoring in the dialysis unit by staff.
1. Dialysis staff can perform anticoagulation monitoring only by using laboratory certified methods which are subjected to regular laboratory quality control.
2. In the absence of in-unit heparin monitoring, less quantitative methods of anticoagulation monitoring are used (e.g., visual inspection of the extracorporeal circuit for thrombus formation).

Chapter 54

Fluid Removal: Obtaining Estimated Dry Weight during Hemodialysis

I. Definition of true dry weight.

A. The weight when fluid volume is optimal.

B. The ultrafiltration component of the hemodialysis prescription should be optimized with a goal to render the patient euvolemic and normotensive.

II. Significance of obtaining dry weight.

A. Extra fluid that accumulates in the various body compartments must be safely removed during hemodialysis (HD) with ultrafiltration (UF).
1. Hypervolemia, is the most common cause of

hypertension, left ventricular hypertrophy, and cardiovascular disease effecting the mortality rate of patients on HD.
2. Inaccurate overestimation of dry weight has significant consequences.
3. Hypovolemia can cause intradialytic morbidities (IDMs), ischemia, and damage to vital organs (e.g., brain, heart), loss of residual kidney function (RKF) and increases mortality rate (see Hypotension in Chapter 55).

B. The most common admitting diagnoses for patients with stage 3 chronic kidney disease (CKD) are pulmonary edema and acute coronary syndrome.

C. The goal is to obtain normovolemia without IDMs. This combined with solute clearances equals adequacy of dialysis.

III. Patient outcome: The patient will maintain optimal fluid volume status.

A. Nursing management.
   1. Fluid assessment parameters.
     a. Weight: predialysis and postdialysis.
     b. Blood pressure (sitting and standing, if appropriate and possible for patient's condition), comparing those to previous HD (normotension is desired), predialysis, intradialysis and postdialysis.
     c. Apical and peripheral pulses: quality, rate, rhythm.
     d. Respiratory rate and quality; O_2 saturation if available.
     e. Temperature: predialysis and postdialysis with the goal of isothermia.
     f. Neck vein distention, jugular venous pressure.
     g. Capillary refill.
     h. Heart sounds.
     i. Breath sounds.
     j. Dependent and peripheral edema. (*Note:* A patient can have fluid excess in the absence of gross clinical evidence of volume expansion, a phenomenon termed "silent overhydration" or "silent volume.")
     k. Skin turgor and mucous membranes.
     l. Residual kidney function(RKF). Assess at least every 2 months if urinary output is greater than 100 mL/day.
     m. Fluid intake (oral, parenteral and intradialytic).
     n. Sodium intake (include water source).
     o. Medication regimen and types. Ingestion of some medications may stimulate thirst and/or fluid retention, i.e., calcium channel blockers, clonidine, and other vasodilator meds such as narcotics, analgesics, beta blockers. Physicians instruct most patients to hold antihypertensive medications until after HD. As patient nears "ideal" dry weight, adjustment of BP medications is paramount. Diuretic therapy is effective only when RKF is high enough to provide daily urine output of at least 100 mL.
     p. Measure abdominal girth. Assess abdominal distention caused by extravasation of fluids related to bowel dysfunction, ascites, and lymphocele posttransplant.
     q. Assess for comorbities that may affect fluid removal during hemodialysis, e.g., diabetes, autonomic neuropathy, sepsis, high output renal failure, ileostomy, cardiac disease, carnitine deficiency.
     r. Assess previous and/or current adherence to prescribed plan of care in consultation with the multidisciplinary team and/or family.
     s. Review previous treatment record, paying special attention to pre/post treatment BPs.
      (1) Note any interventions for hypotension or other intradialytic morbidities.
      (2) National Kidney Foundation Kidney Disease Outcomes Quality Inititiative (NKF-KDOQI) Clinical Practice Guidelines suggest that a dialysis log summarizing the relevant information such as body weights, blood pressures, and IDMs is essential to provide a longitudinal dynamic view of ECF volume and blood pressure changes.
     t. Assess patient's knowledge of fluid ingestion quantification, e.g., liquids, "wet" foods, ice; individual fluid allowance, generally urinary output plus 1000 mL per day (four 8-ounce glasses).
     u. Assess patient's knowledge of recommended weight gains (not to exceed 1 kg between dialyses during the week; 1.5– 2 kg during the weekend).
     v. Assess patient's knowledge of sodium restriction (no more than 2.0 grams with a more stringent limitation of 1 to 1.5 g sodium for dialysis patients who are hypertensive).
     w. Assess amount of daily exercise.
     x. Consider recent hospitalizations, current stressors and holidays as indications for possible weight adjustments.
   2. Laboratory test results.
     a. Hemoglobin/hematocrit.
     b. BUN, serum creatinine.
     c. Sodium.
     d. Blood glucose.
     e. Serum albumin.
     f. Atrial natriuretic peptide and brain natriuretic peptide (ANP/BNP) (acute treatments only).
     g. CO_2 (serum bicarbonate) levels.
     h. Carnitine levels if indicated.
     i. Angiotension levels (elevated levels increase thirst).
   3. Interdialytic concerns.
     a. Complaints such as weakness, fatigue, dizziness, gastrointestinal (GI) symptoms (e.g. appetite changes, nausea, vomiting, diarrhea, constipation), respiratory difficulties (e.g., shortness of breath at rest,

dyspnea on exertion, orthopnea, orthostatic hypotension).
b. How/when patient resumes BP medications posttreatment.
c. Fluid losses related to draining wounds, nasogastric tube, fever, diarrhea (greater than 5–6 loose stools a day), diaphoresis, hyperventilation, and dialysis ultrafiltrate.
d. Changes in amount of residual urine output.
4. Intradialytic complaints or symptoms, e.g., cramping, hypotension, tachycardia, nausea, vomiting, dizziness.
5. Intervention (see Hypotension in Chapter 55).
a. Determine degree of ultrafiltration (UF) for each dialysis treatment and feasibility of reaching UF goal safely, without inducing hypotension.
b. Monitor and adjust UF based on patient's response.
   (1) Achieving true dry weight through ultrafiltration should be accomplished gradually over a number of dialysis treatments.
   (2) While decreasing the patient's fluid volume, net fluid loss ideally should not exceed 1–2 kg/wk.
   (3) More fluid may be removed during hematocrit-based blood volume monitoring (Hct-based BVM) since the patient's plasma refill rate relative to the current UFR can be observed via the display (see Chapter 56: *Obtaining Ideal Dry Weight through Hematocrit-Based Blood Volume Monitoring*).
c. Administer fluids according to treatment plan and prescription. Avoid hypertonic injections the last 1/2 hour of treatment and prevent the need for administration of extra fluids/volume expanders during the the last 1/2 hour other than the amount for reinfusion.
d. Use sodium modeling cautiously and with discretion for patients with reduced plasma osmolality.
   (1) Ensure return to baseline sodium level for the last 1/2 hour as the patient's postdialysis serum sodium is a function of the time-averaged dialysate level, not the terminal level of sodium in the dialysate (see sodium profiling in Chapter 55).
   (2) The NKF-KDOQI Clinical Practice Guidelines do not support the use of sodium profiling or high dialysate sodium levels.
      (a) Avoid their use to avoid thirst, fluid gains, and hypertension.
      (b) Uncertain benefits and possible risk of hypotension have been reported.
      (c) Satisfactory experiences have been reported with a dialysate sodium of 138 mmol/L.
e. Recommend changes in estimated dry weight as indicated. *Note: True dry weight is subject to change related to conditions that cause a loss or gain of nonfluid body tissue.*
f. Collaborate with physician and renal dietitian in planning appropriate fluid and sodium intake and medication prescription.
g. Encourage fluid and dietary management according to prescription.
h. Identify resources to assist patient to achieve goals of fluid management.
i. Initiate consultations as needed.
j. Prolonging treatments (adjusting for longer, or shorter more frequent HD time) may be necessary.
k. Obtaining ideal dry weight through Hct-Based BVM (see Chapter 56).
l. Use thermal control, modified Trendelenburg, reassess medication list, treat hypoxemia.
6. Patient/family education on fluid management. Instruct patient/family regarding:
a. Renal function and relationship to fluid balance.
b. Diet and fluid management.
   (1) Thirst.
      (a) Relationships between fluid and sodium intake, blood sugar, elevated angiotension levels, and medications.
      (b) Use of antithirst sprays.
      (c) Avoid drinking water purified by a water softener which exchanges calcium for sodium. *Note: attempts at water restriction are futile if sodium limitation is not taught and observed simultaneously.*
   (2) Review sodium restrictions, preferred low-sodium foods.
   (3) Individual fluid allowance: generally urinary output plus 1000 mL per day (four 8-ounce glasses).
   (4) Weight changes: 1 kg between treatments during the week; 1.5–2 kg during the weekend.
   (5) Rationale for not eating during HD; small meal before and for 1 hour after HD.
c. Signs, symptoms, and management of hypervolemia and hypovolemia.

d. Importance of preventing IDMs to avoid long-term complications.

e. Differentiation between solid weight gain (body mass) and fluid weight gain.

f. Frequent causes of intradialytic morbidities (IDM) unrelated to fluid removal (e.g., eating, UFR, medications, increasing core temperature, posture, hypoxemia).

g. Patients can experience an IDM even though they are not at their dry weight due to intravascular hypovolemia, even though the tissues may still have fluid.

h. Three compartmental fluid shifts occurring during dialysis (extracellular, intracellular, and intravascular).

i. The meaning of plasma refill.

j. The causes, effects, and treatment of hypoxemia.

k. Positive effects of exercise in between treatments to prevent fluid gain, and during the last hour of dialysis to prevent IDMs.

l. Self-monitoring of blood pressure and weight measurements.

m. Blood pressure parameters: normotensive pretreatment without antihypertensive medications.

n. Parameters for when to take or hold BP medications predialysis and postdialysis.

o. Effects of posture change.

p. Report changes in prescribed and over-the-counter medications; interdialytic symptoms.

IV. Principles of fluid removal.

A. Water removal (see Chapter 51).

B. The Guyton curve (see Figure 11.11).
Note: Guyton's curve is an approximation of fluid dynamics and is patient specific.

1. The Guyton curve.
   a. Illustrates the approximate relationship between extracellular fluid volume and blood volume.
   b. Demonstrates a limit to blood volume as fluid levels continue to increase past a normal range.
   c. As fluid volume is added or removed, the body will distribute its fluid load according to this curve.

2. At ideal dry weight, the average 70 kg adult has approximately 5 liters of blood volume in the intravascular space.
   a. This corresponds to a normal extracellular (tissue) fluid level of approximately 17 liters on Guyton's curve.
   b. Approximately 23 liters of fluid are in the intracellular space.

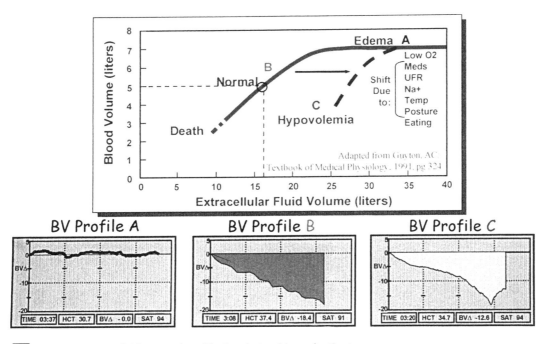

Figure 11.11. Fluid removal profiles in relationship to the Guyton curve.
Used with permission from Hema Metrics.

3. "Silent volume" phenomenon.
   a. A person can have fluid excess in the absence of gross clinical evidence of volume expansion.
   b. An excess of even 3–5 liters does not cause clinical signs or complaints in some patients.
4. When fluid is added and not removed (as between HD treatments):
   a. When the intravascular capacity of approximately 7 liters is reached, the extracellular tissue space will have expanded from 17 liters to approximately 22 liters.
   b. The presence of edema can then be assessed when this expansion has occurred as PRR is at a lesser rate than the UFR.
   c. All additional fluid thereafter expands into the extracellular tissue space.
   d. This area of edema is noted as "A" on the Guyton curve.
5. The extracellular tissue spaces can hold as much as 20–40 liters, sometimes referred to as "third spacing."
6. The goal of fluid removal is to gently reduce the patient's blood volume down the knee of the Guyton's curve to "normal."
   a. The blood volume is normovolemic and the tissues are at the patient's true dry state (ideal dry weight).
   b. This area is noted as "B" on the Guyton curve.
7. Symptoms occurring below "normal" are considered a "dry" crash (both the tissue and intravascular spaces area below "normal").
8. Symptoms occurring on the edema section of Guyton's curve, when the patient is still over-loaded, are considered a "wet" crash. This is noted as "C" on the Guyton curve.
9. Causes of a "wet" crash include, but are not limited to:
   a. Hypoxemia.
   b. Medications.
   c. Incorrect ultrafiltration rate (UFR).
   d. Sudden change in position.
   e. Temperature elevation.
   f. Decreased plasma osmolality.
   g. Eating.
   h. Anemia.
   i. Unstable cardiac status.
   j. Arrhythmia.
   k. Electrolyte/acid-base imbalance.
10. The areas noted as "A," "B," and "C" on the Guyton curve correspond to the "A," "B," and "C" profiles described with "Hct-based blood volume monitoring."

C. Plasma refill rate.
   1. During the dialysis process, fluid is removed directly from the intravascular space through ultrafiltration.
      a. Refer to the Three Compartment Model in Figure 11.12.
      b. Volumes listed under each compartment are for the average 70 kg adult at ideal dry weight.
      c. Volumes increase with fluid gains as described with the Guyton curve above.
   2. Fluid removal from the plasma decreases hydrostatic pressure and increases plasma oncotic pressure. This combination enables fluid to move from the extracellular (tissue) space into the intravascular space.
   3. The rate of this process is known as the plasma refill rate (PRR).
      a. Plasma refill continues for 30 to 60 minutes after ultrafiltration has been set to minimum or postdialysis.
      b. The majority takes place within 10 minutes.
   4. Maintenance of blood volume depends upon rapid refilling of the intravascular space.
      a. Hypotension eventually occurs when the ultrafiltration rate (UFR) exceeds PRR and plasma volume falls (hypovolemia).
      b. A change in blood volume greater than -8% an hour ("C profile") is an indication of impending hypovolemia as PRR is at a significantly lesser rate than the UFR, depleting the intravascular space.
   5. In the absence of preexisting complications, e.g., serious cardiovascular disease, autonomic dysfunction and acetate intolerance, the average adult patient can tolerate 500–1000 mL of ultrafiltration/hour.
      a. The PRR is capable of replacing the blood volume removed to prevent hypovolemia.
      b. A change in blood volume of -3% to -8% per hour up to a total of approximately -10% to -15% ("B profile)" is generally well tolerated in the average overloaded patient on HD (see Chapter 56).
   6. The PRR may be be impaired in patients with:
      a. Reduced plasma osmolality.
      b. Low serum albumin.
      c. Hypoxemia.
      d. Ischemia.
      e. Cardiac dysfunction.
      f. Arrhythmias.
      g. Low predialytic diastolic blood pressure.
      h. Increased temperature.
      i. Septicemia.
      j. The use of antihypertensive medications or steroids.
      k. Other patient variables.

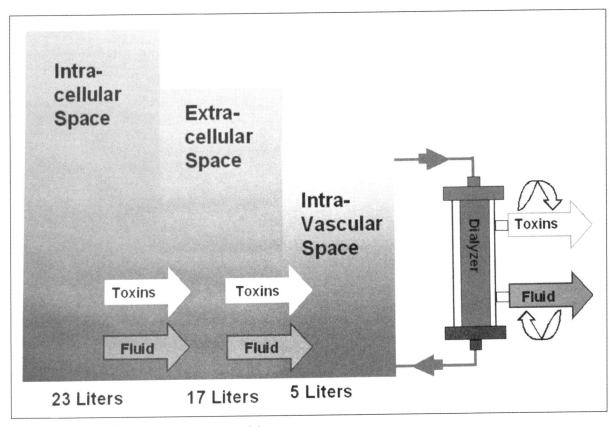

Figure 11.12. Three compartment model.
Used with permission from Hema Metrics.

7. PRR diminishes as the patient approaches dry weight.
   a. Frequency of IDMs increase toward the end of HD.
   b. With linear (constant) UFR, frequency can be up to 10 times higher than at the start of treatment.
8. During the first hour, plasma osmolality is highest related to initial concentratrions of plasma proteins, urea, atrial natremic protein (ANP), and middle molecules.
   a. Blood sugar is generally higher and core body temperature lower in the first hour.
   b. All of these conditions during the first hour promote plasma refill.
   c. Optimal time to remove excess fluid.
9. Ultrafiltration may be less tolerated and the patient may have symptoms of decreased plasma volume despite still being fluid overloaded (a "wet" crash).
   a. The patient could still be on the edema ("A") section of Guyton's curve.
   b. A change in blood volume of less than -3% per hour, no change in blood volume (a flat line), or a positive change with the UFR greater than minimum is an indication of fluid overload. This is referred to as an "A" profile (see Chapter 56).
10. For the above reasons, using the occurrence of signs and symptoms of hypovolemia may result in inappropriate high dry weight estimation.
11. Based on the average refill rate noted above, the minimum UFR for an adult is equal to or less than 400 mL/hour.
12. Putting the patient in minimum UFR for 10–15 minutes and watching for refill on a BVM can assist in determining true or "ideal" dry weight (IDW) (see Chapter 56).

D. Starling's curve (see Figure 11.14).
   1. The most common causes of IDM: a rapid decrease in blood volume or reduced peripheral vascular resistance (PVR).
   2. Measurements/data.
      a. BP = cardiac output (CO) x peripheral vascular resistance (PVR)
      b. Cardiac output = stroke volume (SV) x heart rate (HR)
      c. BP = SV x HR x PVR

3. Hypotension is a consequence of reduction in CO and/or PVR. Any minor decrease in PVR can precipitate a drop in BP as the CO cannot increase to compensate during blood volume depletion.

4. Loss of the ability to vasoconstrict the resistance vessels (decreasing PVR) is a significant cause of UF-induced hypotension, more so than hypovolemia.

5. PVR is affected by:
   a. Antihypertensive and other medications.
   b. Hypoxemia (see G. Hypoxemia).
   c. Dialysate temperature at or above 36° C (see section V.F. Thermal Control).
   d. Dialysate pH/acidotic blood pH, pO_2, pCO_2.
   e. Neural tone/sympathetic nerve activity.
   f. Neuropathies from diabetes or other causes.
   g. Cardiovascular disease (CVD).
   h. Other comorbidities.
   i. Viscosity of blood/anemia.
   j. Vessel radius.
   k. Eating prior to/during dialysis (splanchic vasodilatation).

6. Splanchic vasodilatation results from ingestion of food immediately prior to, during or after HD.
   a. This can cause increase in these blood vessels' capacity, resulting in a decrease in systemic BP.
   b. The food effect lasts at least 2 hours.
   c. A change of greater than -8% an hour, with accompanying hypoxemia is generally noted during blood volume monitoring (see Figure 11.13).

7. Effects from blood volume loss (see Figure 11.14 and Table 11.2).
   a. Aproximately 10% of the total blood volume can be removed with no significant effect on arterial pressure or cardiac output.
   b. CO begins to fall slighty starting at approximately 15% decrease of blood volume loss.
   c. CO begins to plummet at approximately 20% decrease of blood volume.
   d. BP can stay up for 10–20–40 or more minutes (sometimes referred to the "Golden Hour") related to compensatory mechanisms (increased heart

rate, PVR) before it begins to plummet. The time depends on the individual patient's ability to compensate.
   e. Both CO and BP start falling to zero when about 35% to 45% of the total blood volume has been removed.
   f. Death occurs with 50% loss of blood volume (see Figure 11.14 and Table 11.2).

8. BP is a late indicator or post facto measurement for ensuing IDMs (see Figure 11.14).
   a. The KDOQI Guidelines do not support BP or symptoms of hypotension as an indicator of EDW.
   b. The KDOQI Guidelines address concern about the clinical practice of routinely and deliberately provoking hypotension to operationally define a patient's EDW.

E. The inverse relationship between blood volume and blood pressure (see Figure 11.15).
   1. Increased intravascular volume may increase the tension in the myocardium to such a degree that it cannot pump effectively.

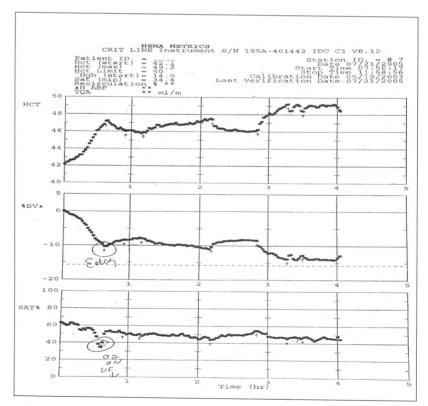

Figure 11.13. The effects of eating. A change of greater than -8% an hour, with accompanying hypoxemia.

Used with permission from Hema Metrics.

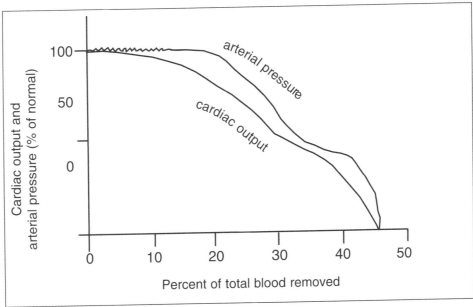

Figure 11.14. The Starling curve effects of blood loss on cardiac output and arterial pressure. BP is a post facto measurement.

Adapted from Guyton, A.C. (1987). *Textbook of Medical Physiology* (4th ed.), p. 63. Used with permission from Hema Metrics.

2. Frank Starling mechanism.
   a. Cardiac output can be decreased when the muscle itself becomes overstretched as occurs with hypervolemia.
   b. The heart cannot contract effectively and stroke volume decreases resulting in heart failure.
   c. Hypotension follows.
3. Laplace's theorem.
   a. Tension in the wall of the myocardium increases as the radius in the chamber increases with hypervolemia.
   b. Wall tension is directly related to the myocardium's demand for oxygen.
   c. When the radius is dilated to such an extent that the demand for oxygen to the heart can no longer be met, CO declines and the pump begins to fail.
   d. Hypotension follows.
4. When hypotension develops in this scenario, the tendency is to decrease UF and replace volume while the opposite may be indicated, i.e., contraction of the volume and decreasing left ventricular dilation to increase CO.

F. Blood pressure lag time phenomenon.
   1. 90% of patients on HD could be normotensive by lowering dry weight. However, the blood pressure response to

Table 11.2

Clinical Result of Hemorrhage

Loss of BV	Likely Result
5–10%	Little change in BP Spontaneous recovery
12–20%	Moderate hypotension Spontaneous recovery
20–30%	Early shock Rapid drop in CO Usually reversible
30–40%	Serious shock May be irreversible

Source: Smith, J.J. (1990). *Textbook of circulatory physiology: The essentials* (3rd ed., p. 267). Baltimore: Lippincott Williams & Wilkins. Used with permission from Hema Metrics.

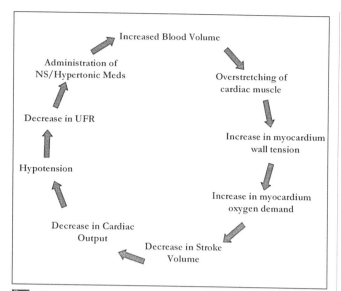

Figure 11.15. Inverse relationship between blood volume and blood pressure.

Used with permission from Hema Metrics.

extracellular volume (ECV) reduction is delayed by some weeks.
2. Days to weeks are required to reach a new steady state in which blood pressure will rise. It will eventually decrease after fluid volume excess (FVE) has been corrected and dry weight is achieved.
3. With gradual removal of FVE, blood pressure begins to decreases in 3–4 weeks after lowering dry weight, but it eventually reaches a plateau only after 6–12 months (may be sooner with Hct-based BVM).
4. BP will not increase with increasing body mass.
5. As patients lose excess fluid and their hypertension improves, antihypertensive medications will need to be systematically tapered or discontinued in order to continue removing fluid to obtain dry weight without IDM.
6. The exact mechanism responsible for this lag time is not fully understood. Several explanations for this time lag are offered.
   a. Autoregulation of vascular resistances including functional and structural (remodeling) changes.
   b. Reduced formation or inhibition of vasoactive substances leading to decrease in vascular tone such as increases in:
      (1) Asymmetric dimethylarginine (ADMA) leading to nitric oxide production.
      (2) Sodium-potassium-adenosine triphosphatase.

c. Sodium restriction can cause vascular relaxation.
7. Health care providers and patients should be aware of the lag time phenomenon and not become discouraged if it takes weeks or months of dry weight adjustments to achieve a lower blood pressure (when antihypertensive medications are not administered at the same time).

G. Hypoxemia (also see Chapter 55, II.).
1. Significant complication of hemodialysis causing periods of ischemia and ensuing intradialytic morbid (IDM) events related to the release of adenosine and subsequent decrease of peripheral vascular resistence (PVR).
2. Adenosine has intrinsic vasodilatory properties and blocks the release of norepinephrine from sympathetic nerve terminals.
3. Symptoms exhibited resemble symptoms of hypovolemia, e.g., nausea, vomiting, restlessness, low blood pressure, cramps, etc.
4. Measurement/data sources.
   a. If available, arterial blood gas analysis for SaO_2, PaO_2; SvO_2 from central venous catheter (CVC), or hemoglobin/hematocrit laboratory result.
   b. Noninvasive: pulse oximetry SpO_2; Crit-Line Monitor® (Hema-Metrics, UT).
   c. SaO_2 from fistula or graft.
   d. Venous saturation (SvO_2) from CVC; hemoglobin/hematocrit (Hct).
5. Data.
   a. Oxygen saturation: the percent to which the hemoglobin is filled with oxygen. Circulation of blood volume and hemoglobin from the lungs to tissues must be adequate to prevent tissue hypoxia.
   b. 97% means that 97% of the total amount of hemoglobin in the blood volume is filled with oxygen molecules.
   c. Fewer total hemoglobin molecules causes the total amount of oxygen available to the tissues to be low even though the hemoglobin present is full of oxygen.
   d. The normal range of overall oxygen-carrying capacity is 19 to 20 mL/dL. This is calculated by multiplying 1.39 mL (the amount of oxygen each gram of hemoglobin carries) x hemoglobin x SaO_2 (or SpO_2).
   e. The target predialysis hemoglobin is a minimum of 11 g/dL (Hct 33%).
6. Arterial blood saturation provides information on how well the lungs are oxygenating the blood.
   a. 90–100% is considered normal for arterial saturations (SaO_2).

b. Mechanisms for intradialytic hypoxemia include:
   (1) Pulmonary edema.
   (2) Chronic obstructive pulmonary disease (COPD).
   (3) Congestive heart failure (CHF).
   (4) Sleep apnea (see Figure 11.16).
   (5) Rebound of reuse agent.
   (6) Bioincompatibility/first use syndrome.
   (7) Pulmonary leukostasis.
   (8) Pulmonary microembolizaton.
   (9) Dialysate composition.
   (10) Alveolar hypoventilation due to CO_2 loss through the dialyzer.
   (11) Warm dialysate temperature > 36° C.
   (12) Anemia: Hgb ≤ 10 g/dL.
   (13) Hemolysis.

7. SvO_2 is considered a mixed venous sat. Mixture of blood from the upper and lower vena cava caused by rotation of the blood pump.
   a. Mixed venous blood saturation (SvO_2) provides information regarding the adequacy of tissue oxygenation.
   b. Tissue oxygen need is met when the amount of oxygen being delivered to the tissues is sufficient to meet the amount of oxygen being consumed. When the oxygen delivery falls below oxygen consumption needs, lactic acidosis develops(SvO_2 less than 30%).
   c. SvO_2 is the measurement of the amount of O₂ returning to the right side of the heart that is left over after tissue needs.
   d. If SvO_2 is normal, both ventilation and circulation are adequate.
   e. 60–80% is considered normal for mixed venous sats; less than 60% indicates cardiac dysfunction; less than 50% indicates severe cardiac dysfunction; less than 30% anaerobic metabolism with lactic acidosis begins.
   f. SvO_2 assists in determining if the CO is adequate to meet tissue O₂ needs. Hence SvO_2 in determining if the CO is providing adequate perfusion.
   g. The continuous monitoring of SvO_2 is a sensitive parameter of continuous CO.
   h. A decreasing CO causes a compensatory rise in oxygen extraction at the tissue level.
      (1) Increased O₂ extraction is the fastest and often the single compensation of the organism following inadequate CO (i.e., a decreased SvO_2 indicates that the CO is not high enough to meet tissue oxygen needs).
      (2) SvO_2 can indicate whether the CO is high enough to meet the need.
   i. A rise in SvO_2 demonstrates a decrease in oxygen extraction, and usually indicates that the cardiac output is meeting the tissue oxygen need.
   j. A return of the SvO_2 to normal, in the presence of a normal or improving lactate,

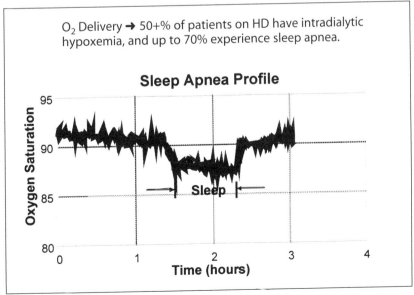

O₂ Delivery ➜ 50+% of patients on HD have intradialytic hypoxemia, and up to 70% experience sleep apnea.

Sleep Apnea Profile

Figure 11.16. Oxygen delivery issues.

Used with permission from Hema Metrics.

suggests patient improvement.

k. A rise in SvO_2 (greater than 80%) in the presence of a rising lactate is an inappropriate and ominous finding, suggesting that the tissues are unable to extract oxygen. It can be seen in burns, late septic shock, or in cell poisoning such as cyanide.

l. SvO_2 can be very helpful when attempting to determine whether a change in therapy is beneficial. Measuring SvO_2 before and after a change can assist in determining whether the therapy made the patient better or worse.

m. Four causes for a drop in SvO_2.
(1) The CO is not high enough (CO = heart rate x stroke volume); i.e., heart rate is too fast, too slow, irregular; hypo/hypervolemia; poor ejection fraction.
(2) The Hgb is too low, i.e., ≤ 10 g/dL (see Figure 11.17).
(3) The SaO_2 is too low.
(4) The oxygen consumption has increased without an increase in oxygen delivery (not common in HD).

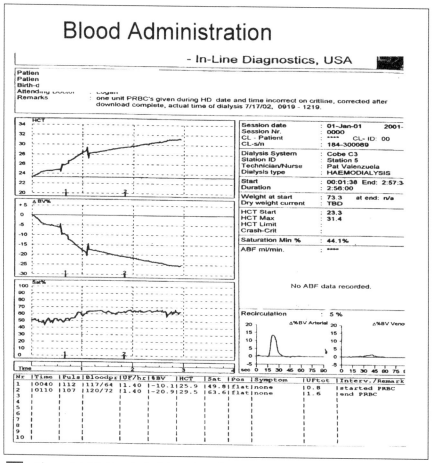

Figure 11.17. Blood administration: Changes in SvO_2 with Hct increase. Blood transfusion started at approximately 50 minutes into the treatment as noted by marker. Note SvO_2 improvements with blood transfusion.

Used with permission from Hema Metrics.

V. Technologies used to obtain dry weight.

A. Volumetric or ultrafiltration-controlled dialysis equipment provides more precise management of fluid removal to reach the ultrafiltration goal set for the patient.

B. Bioimpedence spectroscopy.
1. Noninvasive indicator of total body weight measuring distribution in the intracellular fluid (ICF) and extracellular fluid (ECF) spaces.
2. Measurements are taken before and after varying periods of UF.

C. Sodium profiling used to enhance PRR by increasing ECF osmolarity through various higher dialysate sodium concentrations.
1. This technique increases dialysate sodium concentrations early in HD (e.g., 145–155 mmol/L) followed by a progressive decrease to a lower value (e.g., 135–140 mmol/L) at the end of the HD session.
2. Various profiles exist (linear, step, or logarithmic) and offer different changes in the delivered dialysate sodium.
3. Hypertonic saline has been used in the absence of sodium profiling. A large portion is retained even when given 2 hours before the end of the HD; 78% of hypertonic saline is retained when given even 1 hour prior to the end of therapy.

4. Both strategies have been shown to lead to the vicious cycle of increased thirst, increased inter-dialytic weight gains, hypertension, and the need for excessive UF with the risk for hypotension or muscle cramp (see also Patient Outcomes, Interventions).

D. UF profiling facilitates movement of fluid from the intravascular space into the dialysate by varying the rate of fluid removal to permit periods of plasma refill.
   1. Goal is to individualize UF rate according to the patient's individual response to HD to avoid hypotension.
   2. An individual profile may seem to emerge but caution must be used as this may need to vary from one HD to the next.
   3. Factors influencing this profile include, but are not limited to:
      a. ECF osmolarity from albumin.
      b. Sodium level.
      c. Glucose levels.
      d. Tissue hydration.
      e. Medication.
      f. Changes in lean body mass.

E. Isolated ultrafiltration (IU) is also referred to as sequential ultrafiltration.
   1. Removes iso-osmolar fluid from the systemic circulation via convection; removes excess fluid without changing blood solute concentrations.
   2. Involves bypassing the dialysate solution to drain allowing UF only.
   3. Temperature of the blood returning to the patient is lower with IU than HD.
   4. The effects of increasing osmolality, lowering core body temperature, and increase in PVR allow for large amounts of fluid to be removed. The rate is dependent on cardiovascular stability, amount of overhydration and PRR.
   5. Typical prescription is for 1 hour prior to regularly prescribed dialysis time to avoid poor dialysis solute removal adequacy. Clearance via diffusion does not take place as there is no circulating dialysate through the dialyzer.
   6. Hyperkalemia and other fatal complications have occurred. Performing HD immediately following IU significantly reduces this risk.

F. Thermal control (cooler dialysate). A cool dialysate temperature may improve hemodynamic stability by increasing venous tone, oxygenation, PVR, and cardiac contractility. The goal is to keep the patient's pre-, intra- and post-temperature the same (isothermia).
   1. Dialysate temperature of 37° C is warmer than the temperature of most patients on HD. The lower body temperature is related to anemia, uremia, immunosuppression, and lowered metabolism. The average patient temperature is 36° C.
   2. Dialysate temperature greater then 36° C adds to the warming of the patient's core and decreasing PVR. Core heating is a powerful vasodilatory stimulus resulting in both venous and arteriolar dilatation.
   3. Cooler dialysate (34–36° C) appears to dissipate some of heat generated from UF that contributes to vasodilitation.
   4. More extracorporeal cooling is necessary with more ultrafiltration to keep patients at a constant temperature (isothermic).
   5. Dialysate temperatures may need to be decreased for patients with a high ultrafiltration to maintain stability.
   6. Cooler dialysate prevents hypoxemia by decreasing oxygen diffusion through the dialyzer; patients report feeling more energetic after HD.
   7. Cooler dialysate can decrease complement activation and the inflammatory process that occurs during hemodialysis.

G. HCT-based BVM: monitoring of blood volume changes that occur over the course of the HD treatment observed using an optical technique to monitor absolute Hct changes, or protein density changes through ultrasound (see Chapter 56).
   1. Current monitors require a disposable blood chamber or dedicated bloodline to obtain arterial measurements during HD.
   2. Oxygen saturation can also be observed through the select BV monitors.
   3. The clinician can observe the maximum Hct and BV achieved without symptoms and guide the following treatments accordingly.
   4. With monitors that display an absolute Hct, the value can be used to diagnose and treat anemia and its trend.
   5. The displayed blood volume profile enables the clinician to determine the patient's rate of plasma refill into the intravascular space relative to the current ultrafiltration rate of the dialysis machine.
   6. Proper adjustment of the UFR by the clinician proactively allows reduction in intradialytic hypervolemia and optimizes fluid removal

while avoiding intradialytic morbidities. This is based on:
a. Feedback from the blood volume profile.
b. The patient's maximum hematocrit.
7. A customized UF profile can be followed based upon the patient's actual PRR during each *individual* treatment to:
a. Promote optimization of extracellular fluid status.

b. Reduce intradialysis *and* postdialysis morbid complications.
c. Increase improvements in patient well-being.
d. Provide an objective way of assigning ideal, true dry weight through plasma refill or "dry weight check" near treatment end (see Chapter 56, VII: Dry Weight Check in Hct-Based BVM).

Chapter 55

Complications of Hemodialysis – Prevention and Management

Complications: adverse events requiring intervention are estimated to occur in 20–30% of hemodialysis treatments.

Note: Also see Chapter 54: Fluid Removal: Obtaining Estimated Dry Weight During Hemodialysis.

I. Hypotension.

A. Background.
1. It is estimated that hypotension occurs in 20–50% of hemodialysis (HD) treatments.
2. Hypotension during HD has many adverse effects and potential life-threatening consequences.
3. By impairing tissue perfusion, low blood pressure can compromise dialysis adequacy, contribute to loss of residual kidney function, and predispose patients to coronary and/or cerebral ischemia.
4. Post BP less than 110 correlates with a 2.5x increase risk of death. Two or more hypotensive episodes per week increases the mortality rate to 70%.

B. Etiology. BP = cardiac output (CO) x peripheral vascular resistance (PVR). Cardiac output = stroke volume x heart rate. Hypotension is a consequence of reduction in CO and/or PVR. Any minor decrease in PVR can precipitate a drop in BP as the CO cannot increase to compensate during

blood volume depletion. The inability to vasoconstrict the resistance vessels is a significant cause of ultrafiltration (UF) induced hypotension-more so than hypovolemia. Causes include:
1. Posture changes. Autonomic neuropathy from diabetes or uremia blunts the normal PVR response to postural/orthostatic hypotension.
2. Hypoxemia and tissue ischemia cause a release of adenosine, a potent vasodilator.
3. Medications: antihypertensives, or other vasodilator medications (narcotics, analgesics); beta-blockers decrease cardiac contractility and rate.
4. Decrease in PVR related to vasoactive substances that are administered or released by cells during dialysis. Chemical inflammatory mediators from cells may induce potent vasodilatory effects.
5. Inaccurate ultrafiltration rate (UFR) or amount causes inaccurate volume depletion or overload. Decreased cardiac filling pressure and stroke volume can occur with either hypervolemia or hypovolemia.
a. The rate of plasma volume change will be the difference between UF from the vascular compartment and the plasma refilling rate (PRR) from the interstitial compartment.
b. The mismatch in these rates, and the precipitous fall in PRR supports the activation of the cardiodepressor (Bezold-Jarisch) reflex leading to sudden loss of sympathetic tone and increased vascular bed capacitance (the ability to hold or contain).

c. This reflex is initiated by cardiac stretch receptors that are maladaptively triggered by the hyperdynamic left ventricle becoming hypovolemic with UF.
   d. Autonomic neuropathy from diabetes or uremia may blunt the normal compensatory responses to a decrease in CO, attenuating the UF-induced contraction of the capacitance vessels and shift of volume from periphery to central circulation (DeJager-Krogh Phenomenon).
6. Incorrect goal or target end dialysis body weight.
7. Reduced plasma osmolality. Low serum albumin, or low dialysate sodium relative to plasma sodium, can lead to movement of water into the intracellular compartment and reduces the extracellular compartment.
8. Core body heating stimulates vasodilatation.
   a. Dialysate greater than 36° C: average temperature for patients on HD is 36° C (96.8° F).
   b. High UF rates generate heat and lead to heat accumulation, and eventual vasodilatation.
9. Eating immediately prior to or during dialysis causes splanchnic vasodilatation. Effects can last up to 2 hours.
10. Electrolyte imbalance can affect cardiac contractility and heart rate.
11. Acid-base imbalance can cause vasodilatation. Acetate bath may contribute to hypotension from vasodilatation if high blood concentrations are achieved during dialysis.
12. Anemia (Hct less than 30%/Hgb less than 10 g/dL). Viscosity of blood affects PVR; anemia leads to hypoxemia and tissue ischemia; anemia can lead to decreased cardiac reserve related to chronic high output state.
13. Unstable cardiovascular status, arrhythmias, pericardial tamponade, myocardial infarction, stiff hypertrophied heart. These compromise the heart's ability to maintain or increase CO in response to volume depletion.
14. Septicemia causes vasodilatation.
15. Dialyzer reaction, pulmonary leukostasis, hemolysis, air embolism causes hypoxemia with resultant vasodilatation.
16. Carnitine deficiency alters cardiac and skeletal muscle function.
17. Hypotension perpetuates hypotension.
    a. Tissue ischemia causes the release of adenosine.
    b. Abrupt episodes support the activation of a cardiodepressor (Bezold-Jarisch reflex), which causes a loss of sympathetic tone and PVR.

B. Signs and symptoms.
   1. Low blood pressure may be associated with pallor, nausea and vomiting, perspiration or cold, clammy skin, visual complaints, cramping.
   2. A complaint of feeling warm and fanning himself or herself or subtle complaints of "not feeling well" may be early signs.
   3. Dizziness on standing.
   4. Tachycardia.
   5. Decreased mental status, loss of consciousness.
   6. Posttreatment malaise and fatigue.
   7. Serious vascular complications include cerebral ischemia, atrophy, infarct; vision loss, vascular access thrombosis, nonocclusive mesenteric ischemia, cardiac ischemia, arrhythmias, infarct, decrease in residual renal function, increased mortality.

C. Treatment.
   1. Place patient in modified Trendelenburg position. Elevate legs 30 to 45 degrees, flexing at the hip, with the trunk remaining horizontal, head level with trunk.
   2. Reduce ultrafiltration rate to minimum (a minimum UFR prevents backflow of dialysate across the membrane).
   3. Administer oxygen to prevent or treat tissue ischemia and improve myocardial function.
   4. If necessary to reverse hypotension, administer suitable agents. If volume replacement is needed, the severity of symptoms will influence the volume.
      a. Normal saline (NS) replacement, if severe, can be used in bolus doses of 100–200 mL. *Note: There are disadvantages to giving NS.*
         (1) Fluid removal during HD will be less.
         (2) If given late in or after HD, the patient may experience postdialysis thirst resulting in increased interdialytic weight gain.
         (3) Rapid infusion of a large bolus may cause dysrhythmia or CHF.
      b. Osmotic agents, such as mannitol, albumin, hypertonic saline, or hypertonic glucose solutions will facilitate movement of water from the interstitial and intracellular compartments into the vascular compartment. See limitations below.
         (1) Unless cramps are also present, use of hypertonic solutions appears to offer no benefit over normal saline.
         (2) Use above agents with caution. Disadvantages:
            (a) Hyperosmolality of hypertonic sodium chloride.

[1] Increases postdialysis thirst.

[2] A large portion is retained even when given 2 hours before the end of the HD.

[3] 78% is retained when given 1 hour prior to the end of the HD.

(b) Mannitol has a long half-life.

[1] Tends to accumulate in the extracellular fluid.

[2] The continued hyperoncotic effects fluid shifts between HD.

[3] Its administration depresses serum sodium potentially exacerbating cramping.

[4] A 6- hour HD removes only 14% of circulating mannitol.

[5] Not recommended for patients with diabetes.

(c) Hypertonic glucose solutions are better tolerated in patients without diabetes; there is no evidence to support this practice.

c. Administer oral fluids if less severe: water; black coffee, if allowed, will increase sympathetic tone.

D. Prevention.

1. Accurate predialysis and postdialysis weights.

2. As accurate an estimate of dry body weight as possible. See Chapters 53 and 54.

3. Dry weight should be systematically reevaluated after each dialysis treatment as it may change under various conditions (e.g., intercurrent illness leading to loss of muscle mass and tissue weight, a patient newly dialyzed becoming less uremic and regains appetite, muscle and nonfluid weight changes).

4. BP and pulse before, during and after HD; rapid pulse may indicate compensation.

5. NKF-KDOQI Clinical Practice Guidelines suggest use of a dialysis log to summarize relevant information, e.g., body weights, blood pressures and intradialytic incidents, to provide a longitudinal dynamic view of extracellular fluid volume and blood pressure changes.

6. Start HD with patient's feet one notch off the floor, elevate prophylactically. Instruct patient to sit up and stand up slowly after HD.

7. Assess for and treat hypoxemia prior to symptoms.

8. Withhold antihypertensive medications immediately before and during dialysis per order.

a. Reassess medication list frequently to look for possible side effects, interactions, and current need.

b. Reductions in antihypertensive medication(s) may occur with fluid removal and achieving/maintaining ideal dry weight.

9. Dialyze with volumetrically controlled HD ultrafiltration systems, especially if using mid-flux or high-flux dialyzer.

10. Adjust UFR to avoid intravascular volume depletion, hypotension, and other intradialytic morbidities. Net fluid loss ideally should not exceed 1–2 kg/week unless guided by hematocrit based blood volume monitoring (BVM) to observe PRR. See Hct-based BVM (see Chapter 56).

a. UF profiling: varies the rate of fluid removal permitting the vascular space to refill.

b. Isolated ultrafiltration (IU – no dialysate flow) also referred to as sequential ultrafiltration.

(1) Bypasses the dialysate solution to drain allowing UF only.

(2) Removes iso-osmolar fluid from the systemic circulation via convection.

(3) Removes excess fluid without changing blood solute concentrations.

(4) Typical prescription is for 1 hour of IU prior to regularly prescribed HD time to avoid poor dialysis solute removal adequacy.

(5) To avoid rebound hyperkalemia, it is suggested that IU be immediately followed by HD.

(a) Intensive IU may lead to rebound hyperkalemia, perhaps from the exit of intracellular potassium into the extracellular fluid.

(b) Although this complication is controversial, possible hyperkalemia can be avoided by immediate HD following IU.

(6) The IU time is in addition to the prescribed HD treatment as it provides UF only, not dialysis.

c. Hct-based blood volume monitoring noninvasively provides a measure of blood volume changes, Hct and oxygen saturation (see Chapter 56).

(1) Allows for the calculation of plasma volume changes, UFR, and PRR mismatch to proactively prevent intravascular volume depletion.

(2) Promotes optimization of extracellular fluid status.

(3) Reduces intra and post HD morbid complications.

(4) Increases improvements in patient well-being.

(5) Provides an objective way of assigning ideal, true dry weight through plasma refill or "dry weight check" near treatment end.

(6) Provides numerical values for Hct and oxygen saturation for assessment of anemia/hypoxemia as potential causes of hypotension.

11. Sodium profiling if needed due to reduced plasma osmolality.
   a. This technique increases dialysate sodium concentrations early in HD (e.g., 145–155 mmol/L) followed by a progressive decrease (linear, step, or logarithmic) to a lower value (e.g., 135–140 mmol/L) at the end of HD.
   b. NKF-KDOQI Clinical Practice Guidelines state that increasing positive sodium balance by "sodium profiling" or using a high dialysate sodium concentration should be avoided to decrease thirst, fluid gains, and hypertension. Reviews showed uncertain benefit.
   c. The risk of intradialytic hypotension increases 13% for each 1 mEq fall in dialysate to serum sodium.
   d. The time-weighted average concentration determines the post serum sodium (e.g., using 150 mmol/L to 140 mmol/L linear is equivalent to a 145 mmol/L fixed sodium dialysate).
12. Cool dialysate.
   a. Thermal control (dialysate temperatures between 34–36° C to improve hemodynamic stability).
   b. Goal is for isothermic dialyis. More extra-corporeal cooling is necessary with more ultrafiltration to keep patients at a constant temperature.
   c. Dialysate temperatures may need to be decreased for patients with a high UF rate to maintain stability.
13. Encourage patients to eat a small high quality protein meal an hour before and after HD. Discourage eating immediately prior to or during HD.
14. Assess labs to identify and correct electrolyte/acid-base imbalances. The use of bicarbonate versus acetate dialysate is recommended as the buffer of choice.
15. Maintain adequate hemoglobin/hematocrit. Transfuse blood products as needed.
16. Assess for and treat cardiovascular problems.
17. Correct identified carnitine deficiency.
18. Assess for and treat septicemia.
19. Follow procedures to avoid dialyzer reaction, hemolysis, air embolism.
20. Administer an alpha-adrenergic agonist such as midodrine 15–30 minutes prior to HD. It may be repeated midway if needed to avoid hypotension in patients with autonomic neuropathy leading to impaired PVR, or those with a tendency for hypotension.
21. Teach the patient to recognize and report early signs and symptoms.
22. Instruct patients on taking BP at home and prior to taking BP medications post HD.
23. Encourage fluid restriction between HD to 1 liter (L) plus urinary output.
   a. Ideal fluid gain is limited to 1 kg between treatments during the week.
   b. Ideal fluid gain is limited to 1.5–2 kg during the weekend, or less than or equal to 3% of body weight.
24. Daily dietary sodium intake should be restricted to no more than 2.0 g of sodium; a more stringent daily sodium limit of 1–1.5 g is recommended for patients on HD who have hypertension.

II. Hypoxemia occurs in 50% of patient treatments.

A. Etiology (see Hypoxemia in Chapter 54).
   1. HD itself can provoke significant tissue hypoxemia.
   2. Pulmonary leukostasis.
   3. Pulmonary microembolization.
   4. Alveolar hypoventilation due to CO_2 loss through dialyzer.
   5. Alkalosis.
   6. Diffusion of oxygen through the dialyzer.
   7. Dialysate composition.
   8. Warm dialysate (greater than 36° C).
   9. Bioincompatibility.
   10. First use syndrome.
   11. Sleep apnea occurs in as many as 70% of patients on HD related to uremic effects on sleep center and throat mechanics.
   12. Congestive heart failure (CHF)/cardiovascular disease (CVD).
   13. Pulmonary edema.
   14. Chronic obstructive pulmonary disease (COPD).
   15. Rebound of reuse agent.
   16. Anemia (HCT equal to or less than 30%/Hgb equal to or less than 10 g/dL).
   17. Eating during HD (see Figure 11.13).

B. Signs and symptoms (related to ensuing ischemia and/or vasodilation).
   1. Shortness of breath.
   2. Tachycardia.
   3. Hypotension.

4. Cramping.
5. Tachypnea.
6. Cyanosis.
7. Dizziness.
8. Nausea and vomiting.
9. Blurred vision.
10. Confusion.
11. Restlessness.
12. Seizure.
13. Chest pain.

C. Treatment.
   1. Supplemental oxygen.
   2. Nasal oxygen is usually sufficient.
   3. Support BP.

D. Prevention.
   1. Consider supplemental oxygen proactively in the following situations (see Hypoxemia in Chapter 54).
      a. Arterial saturation less than 90%.
      b. Oxygen-carrying capacity below 19–20 mL/dL.
         (1) The normal range of overall oxygen-carrying capacity is 19 to 20 mL/dL.
         (2) This is calculated by multiplying 1.39 mL (the amount of oxygen each gram of hemoglobin carries) x hemoglobin x SaO_2 or SpO_2.
      c. Venous saturation less than 60%.
      d. Anemia (Hct less than 30%, hemoglobin less than 10 g/dL).
      e. Respiratory rate is greater than 24.
      f. Pulse less than 60 or greater than 100 bpm.
      g. Systolic BP less than 100 mm Hg.
      h. Unresolved edema.
      i. Patients who frequently exhibit symptoms.
      j. Patients with a history of cardiac or respiratory disease.
      k. Sleep apnea.
   2. Refrain from weaning patient/or decreasing oxygen during HD; if applied during HD, continue until patient is discharged to promote plasma refill.
   3. Have patient evaluated if sleep apnea is suspected.
   4. Bicarbonate dialysate.
   5. Use thermal control for isothemic dialysis.
      a. Dialysate temperature significantly affects diffusion of oxygen, decreasing PaO_2.
      b. Most patients benefit from cool dialysate for prevention of hypoxia and report increased energy post HD.
   6. Use a dialyzer made of biocompatible materials to reduce complement activation, especially in high-risk patients.

7. If dialyzers are being reprocessed, follow facility policies for removing and assessing for residual reuse agent and prevent rebound (see Chapter 57).
8. Maintain Hct within target range.
9. Discourage eating immediately prior to and during HD.
10. Use Hct-based BVM to attain and maintain ideal dry weight to avoid CHF/pulmonary edema.

III. Muscle cramps occur in 5–20% of HD treatments.

A. Etiology.
   1. Excessive or rapid fluid removal.
   2. Hypo-osmolality.
   3. Tissue hypoxemia/ischemia.
   4. Electrolyte disorders or imbalances: low sodium, calcium, potassium, magnesium.
   5. Any local irritating factor or metabolic abnormality of a muscle, e.g., severe cold, lack of blood flow, over-exercise.
   6. Skeletal muscle structural changes.
   7. Neuromuscular (motor system) diseases.
   8. Polyneuropathy.
   9. Postdialytic alkalemia.
   10. Carnitine deficiency.

B. Signs and symptoms.
   1. Painful cramps generally occurring in, but not limited to, the extremities or abdomen.
   2. Muscle cramps usually occur late in dialysis.

C. Treatment.
   1. Suitable dialysate potassium and sodium concentrations.
   2. Thermal control (dialysate 34–36° C).
   3. Correction of anemia (Hct less than 30%, hemoglobin less than 10 g/dL).
   4. Treatment of hypoxemia (PaO_2 less than 90%; SvO_2 less than 60%; oxygen-carrying capacity below 19–20 mL/dL).
   5. Reducing UFR to minimum.
   6. Stretching of affected muscle, e.g., dorsiflexion of foot.
   7. Bolus dose of osmotic agents such as hypertonic saline, mannitol, or 50% dextrose should be used with extreme caution. See caution statement under "Hypotension" regarding the use of osmotic agents.
   8. Volume expansion with saline.
   9. Application of heat.
   10. Treatment of identified carnitine deficiency with carnitine replacement.

D. Prevention.
1. Appropriate dietary control of fluid and electrolytes.
2. Adjust UFR to avoid intravascular volume depletion. Net fluid loss ideally should not exceed 1–2 kg/week unless guided by Hct-based BVM to observe PRR (see Chapter 56).
3. Frequent assessment of correct target end dialysis body weight.
4. Evaluate appropriate dialysate sodium concentration.
5. Refrain from eating on dialysis.
6. Proactively identify and treat hypoxemia.
7. Correct anemia.
8. Use Hct-based BVM to attain and maintain ideal dry weight.

IV. **Angina/chest pain occurs in 2–5% of HD.**

A. Etiology.
1. Anemia.
2. Hypoxemia.
3. Arteriosclerotic cardiovascular disease (ASCVD).
4. Coronary artery spasm.
5. Severe vascular volume depletion in susceptible individuals.
6. Hemolysis.
7. Type B dialyzer reaction (see XIV: Membrane biocompatibility).

B. Signs and symptoms: pain or tightness in the chest, back, arm, or jaw.

C. Treatment and prevention.
1. Prevent hypovolemia.
2. Decrease ultrafiltration rate to minimum.
3. Administer oxygen.
4. Maintain oxygen carrying capacity greater than 19–20 mL/dL.
5. Maintain hemoglobin at asymptomatic level.
6. Place in reclining position.
7. Volume replacement if needed.
8. Give nitroglycerin per order if blood pressure is acceptable.
9. Cardiac monitoring for EKG changes.
10. Notify physician.
11. Discontinue dialysis if chest pain is severe or unresolved.
12. Assess EDW and UF goal.

V. **Fever and chills/pyrogenic reaction occurs in less than 1% of HD.**

A. Etiology.
1. Infection (suspect with even small increases in temperature (98–99° F) as average temperature for patients on HD is 96.8° F.
2. Introduction of pyrogens or endotoxins via dialysate, water or reprocessed dialyzers. Low-molecular-weight endotoxin fragments may be able to cross any dialyzer membrane.
3. Dialysate temperature higher than patient's pretemperature can contribute to core body heating.

B. Signs and symptoms.
1. Patient feels cold after initiation of dialysis, often followed by involuntary shaking and sometimes fever.
2. Increase in temperature.
3. Fever caused by pyrogenic or endotoxin reaction, most likely will occur within the first 45–75 minutes of treatment, especially when the patient is afebrile prior to treatment.
4. Hemodynamic instability.
5. Myalgia.
6. Headache.
7. Nausea and vomiting.

C. Treatment.
1. Assess for sources and signs of infection such as vascular access, foot ulcers, respiratory or urinary tract infections.
2. Obtain vital signs including temperature.
3. Notify physician.
4. Obtain blood, inlet and outlet dialysate and water cultures.
5. Perform Limulus amoebocyte lysate (LAL) assay to determine the presence of endotoxin in the water and/or dialysate.
6. Discontinue HD without returning the blood if a pyrogen or endotoxin reaction is suspected.
7. Administer antipyretics and antibiotics as ordered.
8. Assess for and maintain proper dialysate temperature (34–36° C).

D. Prevention.
1. Proper water treatment.
2. Appropriate reuse procedures for dialyzers (see Chapter 57).
3. Careful preparation of equipment and supplies, and aseptic treatment initiation to prevent contamination.
4. Minimize the length of time supplies and

extracorporeal system are prepared before treatment initiation (no longer than 2 hours prior to initiation).

5. Protect the patient from known infectious agents.
6. Careful handling of bicarbonate concentrate to avoid contamination.
7. Prevent backflow of dialysate by maintaining a minimum UFR.
8. Regular cleaning and disinfection of water treatment and distribution system, and dialysate delivery system.
9. Regular cleaning and disinfection of concentrate containers, particularly those used with bicarbonate concentrate.

VI. Dialysis disequilibrium syndrome (DDS).

A. Etiology.
1. During HD, the BUN concentration in the blood is often reduced more rapidly than the concentration in the cerebrospinal fluid (CSF) and brain tissue due to the relatively slow transport of urea across the blood-brain barrier in the CSF.
2. Osmolality in the CSF falls more slowly than in the blood, leading to water movement into the brain. Pressure increases during dialysis and cerebral edema occurs.
3. DDS occurs more often in acute renal failure when BUN concentrations are very high. It is less likely to occur in patients on chronic hemodialysis unless they are underdialyzed for a variety of reasons, e.g., poor access flows, skipping treatments.
4. DDS is more common in elderly and pediatric populations, patients recently started on HD, patients with severe metabolic acidosis and pre-existing neurologic disorders, e.g., recent stroke, head trauma, subdural hematoma, malignant hypertension.
5. Other factors: rapid pH changes and electrolyte shifts.

B. Signs and symptoms usually occur toward the end of the HD, but may be delayed for up to 24 hours.
1. Headache.
2. Nausea and vomiting.
3. Restlessness.
4. Hypertension.
5. Increased pulse pressure.
6. Blurred vision.
7. Cardiac arrhythmias.
8. Decreased sensorium, seizures, coma, and death can occur as the DDS progresses.

C. Treatment and prevention for susceptible patients.
1. Early recognition of mild symptoms.
2. Reduce the efficiency of dialysis by one or all of the following.
   a. Use a less efficient dialyzer, i.e,. a dialyzer with lower clearances/solute removal.
   b. Decrease treatment time.
   c. Decrease blood and dialysate flows.
   d. Use cocurrent dialysate flow.
3. Short, more frequent dialysis treatments.
4. Bicarbonate dialysis.
5. Administer osmotic agents such as mannitol, glucose or hypertonic sodium chloride to counteract the rapid fall in plasma osmolality (see cautionary note for use of hypertonic solutions under "Hypotension").
6. Use a higher dialysate sodium concentration (greater than 140 mEq/L) to blunt the fall in plasma osmolality.
7. Terminate the dialysis treatment if severe or progressive signs and symptoms occur.

VII. Acute hemolysis.

A. Etiology. Rupture of red blood cells due to problems with the dialysate solution, overheated dialysate, or malfunctioning equipment.
1. Hypotonic or hypertonic dialysate.
   a. Inappropriate dialysate composition outside of physiologic limits caused by obstruction of dialysate concentrate source, malfunction of concentration pump, or faulty concentrate.
   b. Failure of conductivity meter caused by significant calibration error, malfunction/fouling of the probe or meter, or failure to set correct limits.
   c. Bypass mechanical failure caused by equipment malfunction or a retrograde leak across the bypass valve.
2. Hypotonic/hypertonic IV solutions.
   a. Administration of rapid bolus doses of hypertonic saline (23.4%) for muscle cramps or hypotension. The osmotic effect is sizable and can cause local hemolysis. Administration using limited doses should not induce severe hemolysis.
   b. Iatrogenic bolus administration of distilled water as diluent for medications.
3. Overheated dialysate (greater than 42° C).
   a. Dialysate heater malfunction caused by significant calibration error for high temperature limit, calibration error in dialysate temperature range, or major malfunction in the heater cycle.

b. Dialysate temperature monitor failure.

c. Bypass valve failure caused by mechanical failure or retrograde leak across the valve.

4. High negative pressure in the extracorporeal circuit.

   a. Prepump arterial pressure more negative than minus 250 mm Hg.

   b. Access blood flow (QA) is less than blood pump (QB).

   c. Kinks in the bloodline immediately before the blood pump.

   d. Improperly occluded roller blood pump.

   e. *Note*: Red blood cells can tolerate more extreme positive pressure (greater than 1500 mm Hg) but are susceptible to more modest negative pressure/vacuum.

5. Trauma to the RBC as it passes over a defective area in the extracorporeal circuit, narrowed tubing, needle trauma, or catheter malfunction.

6. Blood flow rate rate is high and dialysis needle or catheter holes are relatively small.

7. Oxidant hemolysis.

   a. Copper piping in dialysate machines leached as a consequence of low water/dialysate pH.

   b. Chloramine used as a bactericidal agent in city water supplies.

   c. Nitrates in well water used for dialysate preparation.

8. Causes of sterilant presence in dialysate (formaldehyde, bleach, peracetic acid): inadequate rinsing of dialyzer, dialysate delivery system, water treatment system, or distribution system.

B. Signs and symptoms.

1. Chest, back, and/or abdominal pain with possible crescendo of that pain, especially back pain.

2. Dyspnea.

3. Hypotension.

4. Translucent deep burgundy or cherry-red color to the blood in the venous bloodline.

5. Localized burning and pain in the vascular access return site.

6. If hyperthermic dialysate, patient will complain of feeling hot.

7. Dysrhythmias.

8. Acute decrease in Hgb/Hct (see caution statement under Hypotension).

9. Hyperkalemia.

10. Hypoxemia.

11. Increased LDH, unconjugated bilirubin, decrease in serum haptoglobin.

12. Pancreatitis can follow an acute episode.

C. Treatment.

1. Discontinue dialysis.

2. Immediately clamp the venous line and do not reinfuse hemolyzed blood.

3. Administer oxygen.

4. Notify physician.

5. Monitor vital signs and cardiac rhythm. Watch for dysrhythmias, hypotension, and shortness of breath.

6. Check hemoglobin, haptoglobin, and electrolytes, LDH. Hyperkalemia may occur due to the release of potassium from ruptured red blood cells. Acute anemia may develop if significant hemolysis occurs.

7. If necessary, replace volume and/or blood if symptoms are severe.

8. Collect dialysate samples for analysis as indicated.

9. Save extracorporeal circuit for analysis.

D. Prevention.

1. Verify dialysate conductivity and temperature immediately before dialysis is initiated.

2. Assure conductivity and temperature monitors are working properly and they trigger the bypass mechanism to stop dialysate flow to the dialyzer.

3. Clean concentrate containers, lines, and filters per manufacturers recommended process and frequency.

4. Shield all electrical components from corrosive effects of dialysate and concentrate.

5. Assure regular preventive maintenance of monitors, alarms, and bypass mechanism.

6. Monitor preblood pump arterial pressures to ensure that it does not become more negative than -250 mm Hg.

7. Use appropriate blood flow rates for type and size of access.

8. Removal of copper pipe in water treatment, distribution, and dialysate preparation system.

9. Charcoal filtration of water supply to remove chloramines and chlorine (see Chapter 52).

10. Verification and documentation of results of testing procedure for presence of sterilant in water system, dialyzer, and dialysate preparation system.

11. Administer hypertonic saline, 23.4%, in limited, divided doses, e.g., 10 mL over 30 seconds and given through the venous chamber to enhance dilution to minimize hemolysis and sclerosing of the vessels. Use caution with hyperosmolar solutions (see Chapter 55 for more information).

12. Assess extracorporeal system to ensure absence of kinks and other manufacturer defects.

13. Monitor the patient throughout treatment for the onset of signs and symptoms of treatment and equipment-related complications.
14. The patient should not be left unattended during the HD treatment.

VIII. Air embolism.

A. Etiology. Introduction of a large quantity of air into the venous circulation can be caused by:
   1. Defective or disarmed extracorporeal air detector.
   2. Loose connections at the arterial needle, small leak in the extracorporeal circuit before the blood pump, or an open end of a central venous catheter.
   3. Empty air-vented IV bottles/bags attached to the extracorporeal circuit.
   4. Air dissolved in very cold water may exceed the deaeration capacity of the delivery system; air may pass from the dialysate to blood in the dialyzer.
   5. Microemboli created by blood passing over a defective area in the extracorporeal circuit.

B. Signs and symptoms.
   1. Signs and symptoms depend on the position of the patient at the time of the air introduction.
      a. If the patient is upright, air will travel to the cerebral venous system.
      b. If the patient is lying flat, air may enter the pulmonary circulation or significantly impair cardiac performance.
      c. If the patient is in Trendelenburg position, air may pass to the lower extremities causing patchy cyanosis.
   2. Visualization of air pockets or foam in the venous bloodline.
   3. Feeling of air rushing into the circulation, the patient complains of hearing the "sound of a train" or hear "rushing air."
   4. Chest pain, dyspnea, coughing, cyanosis.
   5. Visual disturbances.
   6. Churning sound on auscultation of the heart.
   7. Neurologic deficits: confusion, coma, hemiparesis.
   8. Death.

C. Treatment.
   1. Stop infusion of air immediately.
   2. Place patient on the left side in Trendelenburg position to trap the air in the apex of the right ventricle, away from the pulmonary valve.
   3. Administer oxygen. 100% oxygen by mask is preferred. Hyperbaric oxygen therapy may be beneficial.
   4. Monitor vital signs. Cardiac massage should not be attempted until air is removed from right ventricle via needle aspiration. Performing chest compressions could cause the distribution of air to other organs/parts of the body.
   5. Notify physician.

D. Prevention.
   1. Correct use of a calibrated air foam detector at all times when the patient is on dialysis.
   2. Visual inspection of the venous bloodline before connecting to access.
   3. Secure Luer-Lok connections throughout the extracorporeal circuit.
   4. Return patient's blood with saline and with air foam detector armed.
   5. During dialysis, administer saline as a bolus dose rather than as a constant slow infusion unless via an infusion pump. Observe infusions into the extracorporeal circuit carefully.
   6. Use solutions in collapsible bags rather than glass air-vented bottles.
   7. Heparin infusion site should be after the blood pump.
   8. Double clamp saline administration line and all stagnant lines.
   9. Monitor the patient throughout treatment for the onset of signs and symptoms of treatment and equipment-related complications.
   10. The patient should not be left unattended during the HD treatment.

IX. Dysrhythmias occur in 50% of patients on HD.

A. Etiology.
   1. Electrolyte and pH changes induced by dialysis.
   2. Hyperkalemia/hypokalemia.
   3. Underlying heart disease.
   4. Hypoxemia.
   5. Hypovolemia/hypervolemia.
   6. Rapid infusion of large bolus of IV solution.
   7. Removal of antiarrhythmic drugs during dialysis.
   8. Use of incorrect dialysate for patient.

B. Signs and symptoms.
   1. Irregular, slow, or fast pulse.
   2. Patient complaints of palpitations.
   3. Patient complaints of anxiety.
   4. Often asymptomatic.

C. Treatment.
1. Administer oxygen.
2. Antiarrythmic drugs as ordered.
3. Dialysate potassium concentration as deemed appropriate.
4. Discontinue dialysis for severe, symptomatic dysrhythmias.
5. Cardiac monitoring for EKG changes.
6. Use of AED (automated external defribrillator) if available) to diagnose and treat ventricular arrhythmias.
7. Refer to cardiologist for possible pacemaker and/or internal defibrillator.

D. Prevention.
1. Use higher dialysate potassium concentration never less than 2 meq/L, if the patient is on digoxin.
2. Administer antiarrhythmic drugs as ordered.
3. Monitor heart rate and rhythm, report changes.
4. Limit amount of IV solution given as bolus.
5. Reinfuse blood at lower blood pump speed at treatment termination.
6. Adjust UFR to avoid intravascular volume depletion, hypotension; net fluid loss ideally should not exceed 1–2 kg/week. unless guided by Hct based BVM to observe PRR (see Chapter 56).

X. **Cardiac arrest occurs in 7 per 100,000 HD treatments.**

A. Etiology.
1. Electrolyte/acid-base imbalance.
2. Dysrhythmias.
3. Myocardial infarction.
4. Hypoxemia.
5. Hypovolemia.
6. Cardiac tamponade.
7. Large air embolism.
8. Hemolysis.
9. Anemia.
10. Too rapid transfusion of cold blood.
11. Exsanguination.
12. Hyperthermia/overheated dialysate.
13. Profound shock.
14. Unsafe dialysate composition.
15. Exposure to dialyzer sterilant.

B. Signs and symptoms.
1. Absence of apical or carotid pulse.
2. Lack of spontaneous respiratory effort.
3. Unresponsive.
4. Asystole or ventricular fibrillation on cardiac monitor.

C. Treatment.
1. Assess for signs noted above.
2. Begin cardiopulmonary resuscitation and activate the emergency resources used for cardiac arrest.
3. Discontinue dialysis and return blood to patient if appropriate. Leave access line in place for fluid and medication administration.
4. Use of AED (automated external defibrillator) if available) to diagnose and treat ventricular arrhythmias.

D. Prevention.
1. Prevent conditions that could lead to cardiac arrest, such as profound shock and rapid potassium shifts in susceptible patients.
2. Ensure dialysate concentration is appropriate for patient.
3. Adjust UFR to avoid intravascular volume depletion, hypotension; net fluid loss ideally should not exceed 1–2 kg/week. unless guided by Hct based BVM to observe PRR (see Chapter 56).
4. Ongoing careful assessment during HD.
5. Refer patients with dysrhythmias to cardiologist for possible pacemaker and/or internal defibrillator.
6. EKG/BVM monitoring during dialysis for patients considered to be at risk.
7. Monitor the patient throughout treatment for the onset of signs and symptoms of treatment and equipment-related complications.
8. The patient should not be left unattended during the HD treatment.

XI. **Seizures occur in less than 10% of HD transplants.**

A. Etiology.
1. Dialysis fisequilibrium syndrome (DDS).
2. Electrolyte/acid-base imbalances.
3. Hypotension.
4. Hypovolemia.
5. Hypoglycemia.
6. Hypoxemia.
7. Intracranial bleeding hastened by heparin.
8. Removal of anticonvulsants by HD.
9. Hemodynamic instability including rapid changes in BP.
10. Severe hypertension.
11. Too rapid transfusion.
12. Dialysate composition errors.

B. Signs and symptoms.
1. Change in level of consciousness.

2. Twitching and jerking movements of the extremities.

C. Treatment.
1. Protect the patient and access arm from harm.
2. Treat hypotension and hypoglycemia if indicated.
3. Administer oxygen.
4. Treat DDS if indicated.
5. Terminate treatment for severe seizures.
6. Provide airway support.
7. Obtain laboratory studies for glucose, calcium, other electrolytes.

D. Prevention.
1. Predialysis assessment of risk factors.
2. Avoid large drops in BUN concentration during dialysis.
3. Monitor blood pressure during HD.
4. Minimize osmotic changes during HD.
5. Administer anticonvulsant medication as ordered.
6. Administer oxygen for patients with underlying cardiac or respiratory disease.
7. Adjust UFR to avoid intravascular volume depletion, hypotension; net fluid loss ideally should not exceed 1–2 kg/week. unless guided by Hct based BVM to observe PRR (see Chapter 56).
8. Monitor the patient throughout treatment for the onset of signs and symptoms of treatment and equipment-related complications.
9. The patient should not be left unattended during the HD treatment.

XII. Exsanguination.

A. Etiology.
1. Accidental or traumatic separation of bloodlines.
2. Accidental dislodgement of needles from vascular access site.
3. Rupture of vascular access aneurysm or anastomosis.
4. Open central venous catheter limb or dislodgement of catheter.
5. Dialyzer membrane rupture with failure of dialysate blood leak detector.
6. Failure to connect the venous bloodline to the patient when dumping the prime.
7. Undetected internal bleeding after heparinization (e.g., cardiac tamponade, GI, intracranial bleed) or inaccurate CVC placement.

B. Signs and symptoms.
1. Visualization of source of bleeding.
2. Hypotension, increased heart rate.
3. Decrease in Hct/hemoglobin.
4. Shock, seizures, cardiovascuar collapse.

C. Treatment.
1. Immediately turn off the blood pump, and place a clamp on both sides of the separated bloodlines or catheter.
2. Apply pressure to any bleeding site. Apply tourniquet to site if unable to control bleeding.
3. Evaluate suitability of returning blood to the patient from a ruptured dialyzer.
4. Administer oxygen if the blood loss is significant.
5. Administer volume expander if patient is hypotensive.
6. Obtain laboratory studies: Hgb/Hct.
7. Blood replacement in timely manner as indicated.

D. Prevention.
1. Securely locking luer connections on all bloodlines and access lines.
2. Tape needles to avoid significant movement of needles in any direction.
3. Allow for visualization of the entire extra-corporeal circuit throughout the treatment, including the patient's vascular access.
4. Assure arterial and venous pressure monitors, and the dialysate blood leak detector are functioning properly.
5. Appropriately cap and secure central venous catheters.
6. Connect both arterial and venous bloodlines to access lines at initiation of HD.
7. Monitor the patient throughout treatment for the onset of signs and symptoms of treatment and equipment-related complications.
8. The patient should not be left unattended during the HD treatment.
9. Ensure complete stasis of access site prior to leaving or discharging patient.

XIII. Dialysis encephalopathy.

A. Etiology.
1. Neurologic disorder caused by accumulation of aluminum in the body.
2. Aluminum toxicity.
   a. Results from water not properly treated for HD.
   b. The administration of large quantities or long-term use of aluminum-containing phosphate binders.

3. Incidence has declined greatly because of water treatment and the use of non-aluminum-containing phosphate binders.

B. Signs and symptoms.
   1. Neurologic signs: speech disturbances including apraxia, dysarthria, aphasia, stuttering; personality changes; gait changes; myoclonus; seizures; EEG changes; dementia.
   2. Other signs: aluminum-related osteomalacia and anemia.

C. Treatment.
   1. Discontinue oral aluminum-based medications.
   2. Chelation of aluminum with desferoxamine.
   3. Renal transplant.

D. Prevention.
   1. Properly treated water.
   2. Use of non-aluminum-based phosphorous binders.

XIV. Membrane biocompatibility.

A. Etiology.
   1. Two types of reactions can occur: anaphylactic reactions (Type A) and a nonspecific reaction (Type B). Type A reactions can be severe while Type B reactions are milder and occur much less frequently than in the past.
   2. Type A reactions.
      a. Sensitivity to ethylene oxide (EO), a gas dialyzer sterilant.
      b. Allergy to the dialyzer membrane material. Reaction may be amplified in patients taking ACE inhibitors.
      c. Allergy to drugs such as heparin and iron dextran.
      d. Bacterial or endotoxin contamination of water for reprocessing or used to mix the bicarbonate.
   3. Type B reactions are nonspecific and less severe.
      a. May result from sensitivity to membrane material.
      b. Complement activation has been implicated.

B. Signs and symptoms.
   1. Type A reaction.
      a. Occur during the first 5 to 10 minutes (maximum 20) and progress in severity.
      b. Initial feeling of uneasiness, warmth, a sense of impending doom; followed by agitation, tightness in the chest, back pain, and nausea.
      c. Can progress to shortness of breath, coughing, wheezing, urticaria, facial, edema, flushing, anaphylaxis, cardiac arrest, and death.
      d. Milder case presents with itching, uticaria, cough, sneezing, watery eyes, or GI symptoms.
      e. BP can be high or low.
   2. Type B reaction.
      a. Occur later in dialysis, 20–40 minutes after initiation; generally resolves after the first hour.
      b. Associated with back or chest pain.
      c. Hypotension in some cases.

C. Treatment.
   1. Type A reaction.
      a. Immediate termination of dialysis. Do not return the patient's blood.
      b. Administer oxygen.
      c. Administer intravenous antihistamines, steroids, or epinephrine depending on the severity of the reaction.
      d. In an anaphylactic reaction, cardiopulmonary support may be required.
   2. Type B reaction.
      a. Treatment is supportive in nature. Oxygen for respiratory complaints, antihistamines or analgesics for pain; treat angina promptly.
      b. Symptoms often resolve, and the treatment does not usually need to be terminated.

D. Prevention.
   1. Type A reaction.
      a. Proper rinsing of dialyzers prior to treatment to remove ethylene oxide (ETO) sterilant, other sterilants, or other allergens.
      b. Use of dialyzer sterilized with electron beam, Gamma-radiation or steam to avoid such exposure and reactions.
      c. Administration of antihistamines prior to treatment.
      d. Place patient on reuse program or change to an alternate membrane or sterilant.
      e. Reprocess reuse dialyzers prior to first use.
      f. Follow AAMI standards for water treatment (see Chapter 52).
   2. Type B reactions may result from sensitivity to membrane material.
      a. Possible benefit from reuse program.
      b. Changing patient to a dialyzer with a more compatible membrane such as substituted cellulose, cellulosynthetic, or synthetic membranes may be helpful.
   3. Monitor the patient throughout treatment for the onset of signs and symptoms of treatment and equipment-related complications.

4. The patient should not be left unattended during the HD treatment.

XV. Nausea and vomiting occurs in 5–15% of treatments.

A. Etiology.
1. Most cases are related to hypotension.
2. Hypoxemia.
3. Nausea can also be an early manifestation of DDS.
4. Metabolic disturbance secondary to chronic kidney disease.
5. Medications.
6. GI: peptic ulcer, gallbladder, pancreas disease, pancreatitis, gastroparesis.
7. Pregnancy.

B. Signs and symptoms: nausea and vomiting.

C. Treatment.
1. Identify and treat appropriate cause.
2. Antiemetics if needed.
3. Consider alternate medications if related to medication administration.

D. Prevention.
1. Prevent hypotension and hypoxemia.
2. Antiemetics if needed.
3. Medications such as metoclopramide can control nausea and enhance gastric emptying.
4. Encourage a small meal 1 hour before and after HD. Discourage eating during HD.
5. Refer recurring nausea and vomiting to provider for further evaluation of underlying cause.

XVI. Dizziness.

A. Etiology.
1. Associated with volume depletion.
2. Hypoxemia.
3. Medications.
4. Orthostatic/postural hypotension.
5. Anemia.
6. Autonomic neuropathy.

B. Signs and symptoms.
1. Complaints of dizziness during HD.
2. Complaints of dizziness upon standing.
3. Complaints of interdialytic dizziness.

C. Treatment.
1. Assess BP. If needed, volume replacement will depend on severity of symptoms and BP.

a. NS replacement if severe.
b. Oral fluids: water, black coffee if allowed to increase sympathetic tone.
2. Sitting for 10–15 minutes to allow for plasma refill.
3. Administer oxygen if needed.
4. Maintain anemia management goals.
5. Blood transfusion if needed.

D. Prevention.
1. Frequent reassessment of dry weight.
2. Reduce UFR to minimum for last 10–15 minutes of HD to allow for refill and time to begin to re-equilibrate.
3. Change position slowly at end of treatment.
4. If oxygen was administered during treatment, leave it on until the patient is ready to leave the facility to facilitate plasma refill.
5. Have patient move legs/feet prior to standing to stimulate circulation.
6. Reassess antihypertensive medications as dry weight reductions occur.
7. Add approximately 0.2 to 0.5 kilogram to estimated dry weight.
8. Maintain anemia management goals.
9. Hct-based BVM to prevent intravascular volume depletion, assess refill at end of treatment, and assign ideal dry weight.
10. Instruct patient on BP parameters to resume BP medications at home after treatment.

Chapter 56

Obtaining Ideal Dry Weight through Hematocrit-Based Blood Volume Monitoring

Editor's note: Descriptions, labeling of profiles, terms, and generalized guidelines were obtained from information available at the time of writing. Refer to manufacturer for specific information.

I. Hct-based blood volume monitoring (BVM).

Blood volume monitoring must always be used in conjunction with the clinical assessment and existing medical history before altering a dialysis treatment.

A. Definition.
1. Monitoring of blood volume changes that occur over the course of the HD treatment using an optical technique to measure absolute Hct, or protein density changes through ultrasound to measure relative Hct.
2. Current monitors require a disposable blood chamber or dedicated bloodline to obtain arterial measurements.

B. Technology.
1. As fluid is removed from the intravascular compartment at a greater rate than plasma refill rate (PRR), the red blood cells (RBCs) becomes more concentrated increasing the Hct.
2. A noninvasive, continuous, hematocrit monitor, opens a "window" into the patient's intravascular compartment.
3. Monitor graphically displays the percent change in blood volume by continuously measuring the patient's absolute hematocrit, or is calculated as a relative hematocrit (RBVcrit) from protein density changes occurring during HD.
4. The Hct and BV profiles will be inversely proportionate: mirrors of each other (see Figure 11.18).
5. Oxygen saturation can also be observed through select BV monitors allowing proactive identification and treatment of hypoxemia and ensuing intradialytic morbidities (IDMs).
6. With monitors that display an absolute Hct, the value can be used to diagnose, treat and trend anemia.

C. Basic principles.
1. With a Hct reading, the clinician can observe the maximum Hct achieved without symptoms and guide subsequent treatments accordingly.
2. By observing the Hct changes the clinician can avoid the patient's Hct threshold, also known as the "crash crit."
   a. Referred to as "RBV crit" with relative measurements.
   b. The critical blood volume level identified by the Hct at which the patient experiences an IDM symptom (see Figure 11.18).
   c. The patient may or may not be at estimated dry weight (EDW) if the Hct threshold has been reached. Intravascular hypovolemia to the Hct threshold may have been caused by the rate, versus the amount of fluid removed (see Chapter 54).
3. The Hct threshold is specific for each patient and can be used to guide future treatments.
   a. UF will be adjusted so that in subsequent treatments the BV change results in maximum Hct being reached without reaching the Hct threshold or IDMs. This will allow for continued fluid removal without reaching hypovolemia and the Hct threshold.
   b. The Hct threshold is the gold standard outcome predictor repeatable for numerous treatments.
   c. The Hct threshold will change over time as the RBC mass changes, e.g., blood loss, blood transfusions, infection, intravenous iron therapy, erythropoietic stimulating agent (ESA) titration, e.g., epoetin alfa, darbapoetin alfa.
4. The average patient on HD with fluid overload will tolerate a change in Hct by approximately 10% to 15% as the blood volume changes with fluid removal. BV changes are inversely proportional (-10% to -15%) (see section IV. D. on Starling's curve for rationale for approximate total BV change in Chapter 54).
5. Tolerance to blood volume reductions differs among patients, and may change for the individual patient each treatment depending on numerous variables such as:

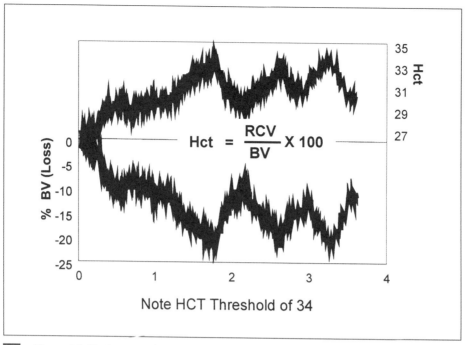

$$Hct = \frac{RCV}{BV} \times 100$$

Note HCT Threshold of 34

Figure 11.18. Inverse relationship of hematocrit and blood volume.

Used with permission from Hema Metrics.

a. Age.
b. Gender.
c. Comorbid conditions.
d. Neuropathies.
e. Cardiac dysfunction (i.e., myocardial insufficiency, cardiac arrhythmia, low predialytic diastolic blood pressure).
f. Patient temperature.
g. Electrolyte and acid-base balance.
h. Serum sodium.
i. Serum albumin.
j. Blood glucose levels.
k. Anemia status.
l. Hypoxemia.
m. Medications taken, etc.
n. Ultrafiltration rate.
o. Posture changes.
6. This explains why some patients have IDM to relatively small decreases in BV change, while others can have large changes without symptoms until much later.
7. The displayed blood volume profile enables the clinician to determine the patient's plasma refill rate (PRR) into the intravascular space relative to:
   a. The current ultrafiltration rate of the dialysis machine.
   b. The dialysis prescription.

c. The patient's comorbid conditions and other variables.
8. Proper adjustment of the ultrafiltration rate (UFR) by the clinician allows reduction in intradialytic hypervolemia and optimizes fluid removal while avoiding IDMs. This is based on:
   a. Feedback from the blood volume profile.
   b. The patient's maximum hematocrit.
   c. Hct threshold, proactively.
9. A customized UF profile can be followed based upon the patient's actual PRR during each individual treatment to:
   a. Promote optimization of extracellular fluid status.
   b. Reduce intradialysis and postdialysis morbid complications.
   c. Improve patient well-being.
   d. Provide an objective way of assigning true "ideal" dry weight through plasma refill or "dry weight check" near treatment end.
10. By adjusting the UFR to minimum (for adults, equal to or less than 400 mL/hour) for 10–15 minutes and watching the profile changes for PRR, the clinician can assess and assign true "ideal" dry weight (see Figure 11.19 for dry weight check example).
11. PRR continues for 30–60 minutes with UFR in minimum (or postdialysis) with the majority

taking place within the first 10 minutes.

II. **General profile descriptions:** Profiles and principles for intervention are based on Guyton and Starling curves as well as general fluid removal principles (see Fluid Removal in Chapter 54).

A. Profile A. Profile "A" represents fluid overload. The plasma refill rate (PRR) is equal to, greater than, or near the ultrafiltration rate (UFR). The profile appears as a flat, positive, or a slope slower than -3% BV change per hour (with the UFR above minimum). This profile may present an opportunity to increase the UFR until a decrease in BV is reflected by an increased Hct.

   1. Profile "A" flat: The patient is refilling at or near the same UFR. This can occur in spite of considerable amounts of fluid removal (see Figure 11.20).
      a. BV is slightly positive at end of treatment.
      b. The Hct is slightly more dilute.
      c. The patient is at risk of developing pulmonary edema/CHF after treatment.

   2. Exceptions. Profile "A" flat: A flat BV curve is acceptable if at any time during fluid removal challenge, a dry weight check is conducted by reducing the UFR to minimum (equal to or less than 400 mL/hr for an adult) for 10–15 minutes and the curve becomes flat.
      a. These patients are already near their HCT threshold ("crash crit") or dry weight.
      b. Conditions that place patients near their HCT threshold include:
         (1) Small weight gain.
         (2) High residual urine output (greater than 800 to 1000 mL/day).
         (3) High output renal failure.
         (4) High residual kidney function (RKF).

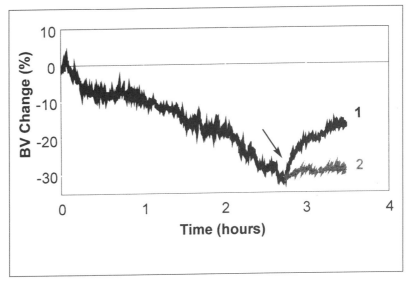

Figure 11.19. Dry weight check: assessing for refill an indicator of overhydration. The arrow denotes minimum UFR applied. Patient #1 still has fluid to remove as refill is evident by plasma refilling. Patient #2 is near ideal dry weight as there is little evidence of plasma refilling.

Used with permission from Hema Metrics.

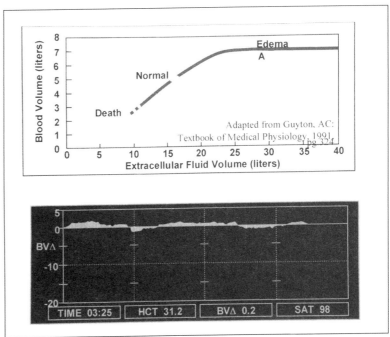

Figure 11.20. Typical "A" profile compared to the Guyton curve.

Used with permission from Hema Metrics.

(5) Dehydration.
(6) Ileostomy.
(7) Pregnancy.
(8) Leg/limb amputation.
3. Profile "A" positive slope. The PRR is greater than UFR: the blood volume in the intravascular space is increasing for the majority of treatment. In Figure 11.21, there is very little change in BV or Hct by end of treatment.
   a. A positive slope can be caused by massive fluid overload, infusion of NS, osmotic agents such as albumin, administration of hypertonic injections, use of sodium modeling, inaccurate goal or UFR.
   b. Depending on the condition of the heart, hypertension or hypotension may ensue (see the inverse relationship of BV and BP in Chapter 54).
   c. This patient is at high risk of developing pulmonary edema/CHF during and after the treatment.

B. "B" profile: recommended fluid removal profile for the patient on HD who is not at dry weight related to extra fluid volume.
   1. The "B" profile suggests treatments with consistent fluid removal without intervention or complications.
   2. "B" profiles can be obtained through "Linear" or "Fly the Curve" methodologies (see Figures 11.22 and 11.23).
3. The Linear "B" profile (see Figure 11.22).
   a. UF progresses faster than the body's ability to refill (the ultra-filtration rate is greater than the PRR), but at a rate that is generally well tolerated. Reduced volume of the intravascular space is displayed as a reduction in blood volume.
   b. Profile resembles a 45-degree angle, obtaining a gradual BV slope of -3% to -8% per hour (average -5% per hour) to a total BV change of approximately -10% to -15% for the average patient presenting with fluid volume excess (FVE).
   c. Well tolerated in the patient on HD who is not at his dry weight related to extra fluid volume. Symptoms generally will not occur until the intravascular space nears the Hct threshold.
   d. Patients with exceptions may include cardiac dysfunction (myocardial insufficiency, cardiac arrhythmia, low predialytic diastolic blood pressure), septicemia, high output renal failures, high RKF, pregnancy, amputations, ileostomy, dehydration, ischemia, hypoxemia, etc. These patients may only tolerate smaller maximum BV changes of approximately -5% to -10%, total.
   e. The maximum percent change in BV is still a

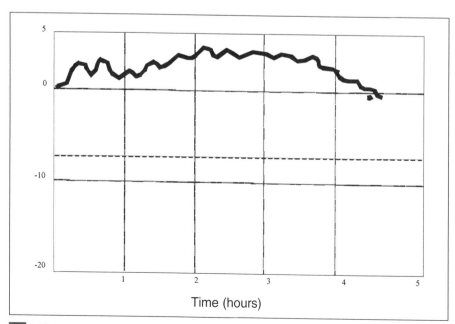

Figure 11.21. "A" profile: Positive slope.

Used with permission from Hema Metrics.

relative measure with limited predictive value.

   (1) Treatment to treatment profiles may be clearly different in shape and BV endpoint.

   (2) Continuous absolute Hct is the control parameter.

   (3) *Example*: If the starting Hct is 29, and the Hct threshold is 37, the % BV changes is -21.6%. However, if the patient comes in next treatment with a starting Hct of 34, and his Hct threshold is 37, he may experience an IDM at a % BV change of only -8.1%.

4. The Flying the Curve "B" profile (Figure 11.23).

  a. The Fly the Curve profile is not recommended to be used without blood volume monitoring. A high UFR is set for the first hour of treatment and monitoring of the percent blood volume change is required.

  b. UFR is adjusted to obtain up to 1/2 of the goal for the first hour to create a profile that appears as a rapid BV slope during that hour (no greater than -8% BV change). This is followed by a more gradual profile slope (of approximately -3% to -4% BV change per hour) to obtain the total goal over the remainder of the HD (to maximum of -15% total BV change). (See manufacturer's guidelines for more specific steps.)

  c. Rationale.

   (1) PRR diminishes as the patient approaches dry weight. Frequency of IDMs increase toward the end of HD. With linear (constant) UFR this can be up to 10 times higher than at the start of the treatment.

   (2) Related to the high UFR during the first hour, the plasma osmolality increases secondary to increases in plasma proteins, urea, atrial natremic protein (ANP), and middle molecules as fluid is rapidly removed. Blood sugar is generally higher

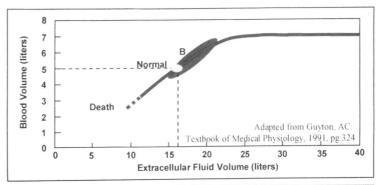

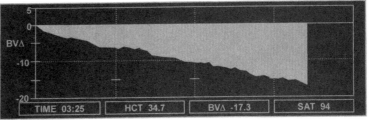

Figure 11.22. Typical linear "B" profile in comparison to the Guyton curve.

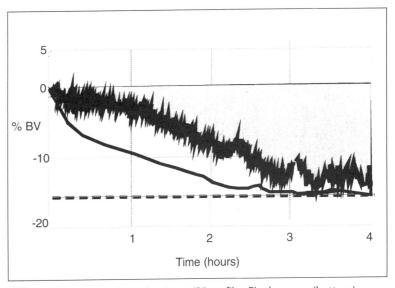

Figure 11.23. Flying the Curve "B" profile: Fly the curve (bottom) profile as compared to Linear (top) profile.

Used with permission from Hema Metrics.

and core body temperature lower in the first hour. All of these conditions promote plasma refill.

   (3) Since as much as half of the UF goal may be obtained early in the treatment, this profile creates the highest mobilization of tissue fluid by increasing albumin/oncotic pressure.

d. Improved URR occurs related to the creation of a diffusion gradient for urea and by preventing ischemia and shunting (80% urea is in the skin, muscle, bone).

e. The Fly the Curve profile may eliminate the need for isolated UF (IU) as it maximizes fluid removal using the same principles without sacrificing clearance of solutes and risk of rebound hyperkalemia.

C. The "C" profile: represents an impending "crash." The UFR is significantly greater than the patient's PRR. Proactive interventions are needed to prevent IDM from intravascular hypovolemia. The three profiles in Figure 11.24 show "C" profiles at different stages during a treatment.

1. Appears as a steep slope of greater than -8% BV change per hour, and can occur at any time during the treatment.

2. The PRR is not able to keep up with the UFR. Hypovolemia will ensue if there is no intervention.
   Note: -8% is only permissible in the first hour of a calculated "Fly the Curve" profile.

3. "C" profile can begin anywhere along the Guyton curve. It describes a dialysis session in which the patient will ultimately experience some type of intradialytic morbidity such as lightheadedness, nausea, vomiting, cramping, or hypotension, a condition often called "crashing."

III. General guidelines: Adjust UFR to obtain a "B" profile through "Linear" or "Fly the Curve" methodologies. (Refer to monitor's manufacturer for specific recommended protocols.)

A. Observe the Hct and avoid the Hct threshold (crash crit).

1. Assess RKF. Reassess every 2 months if RKF is greater than 100 mL per day.

2. Review clinical assessment, patient's medical history, medication list, last dialysis treatment data, and profile to determine initial UF goal and past tolerance to fluid removal.

3. Dry weight will be decreased initially by 1/2 kg if postdialysis blood pressure was greater than 135/85 mm Hg and/or current predialysis blood pressure exceeds 150/85 mm Hg, regardless of the presence or absence of postdialysis edema unless otherwise directed by physician.

4. No UF modeling will be used during BVM as individual profiles will be made each treatment.

5. Per NKF-KDOQI Practice Guidelines, sodium modeling is not generally recommended.

6. Thermal control (dialysate temperatures between 34° and 36° C).

7. Patients will be instructed to hold their antihypertensive medications until after dialysis unless otherwise directed by physician.

8. Patients will be instructed not to eat on hemodialysis.

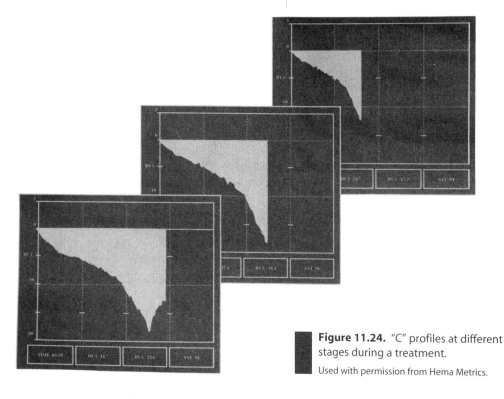

Figure 11.24. "C" profiles at different stages during a treatment.

Used with permission from Hema Metrics.

9. Verify accuracy of monitor per manufacturer's recommendations.
10. Each patient's blood volume will be monitored during the entire treatment.
11. When attempting to decrease dry weight from treatment to treatment, do not remove more than 1–2 kg less than the previous postweight.
12. The amount of increase or decrease in the UF rate is patient-specific.
    a. Adjusting the UF rate by 100 to 500 mL every 20–30 minutes until the slope is at least -3% per hour is appropriate.
    b. Adjustments up to a total increase of 1–2 liters are appropriate unless otherwise directed by physician.
13. Monitor for patient symptoms/IDMs/"crashes" that require interventions.
14. Treat patient per facility protocol.
    a. Interventions.
       (1) Follow facility resuscitation protocol.
       (2) Change position to modified Trendelenburg.
       (3) Assessing for and treating hypoxemia (see below).
       (4) Thermal control to maintain isothermia.
       (5) Reassess dry weight. Reduce UFR to minimum, assess for the presence or absence of plasma refill.
       (6) Record Hct threshold/modify alarm line.
       (7) Record new dry weight if established.
    b. Follow up interventions for intradialytic morbidities with assessment and treatment of possible causes of the crash other than reaching or going below dry weight.
       (1) Hypoxemia.
       (2) Medications that cause vasodilatation.
       (3) Medications that decrease plasma refill, e.g., angiotension-converting enzyme (ACE) inhibitors, calcium channel blockers.
       (4) UF rate too rapid compared to patient refill rate.
       (5) Hypotonic vascular space.
       (6) Hypoalbuminemia.
       (7) Increased patient temperature.
       (8) Posture.
       (9) Eating during HD.
       (10) Severe anemia: Hgb $\leq$ 10 g/dL.
       (11) Occult hemorrhage.
       (12) Cardiac dysfunction.
       (13) Arrhythmia.
       (14) Septicemia.
       (15) Electrolyte/acid base imbalances.
       (16) Neuropathy.
       (17) Other comorbidities.

IV. **Identify and report the Hct threshold (crash crit).** The critical blood volume level in a patient, identified by the hematocrit at which the patient experiences an IDM. *Note*: The patient may or may not be at dry weight if the Hct threshold has been reached. Intravascular hypovolemia to the Hct threshold may have been caused by the rate, versus the amount of fluid removed.

A. The Hct threshold will remain unchanged if the patient's RBC mass remains stable. It is reassessed at least every 2–3 weeks through a dry weight (plasma refill) check.

B. Maximum Hct will be recorded following each treatment.

   1. UF will be adjusted so that in subsequent treatments the BV change results in maximum Hct being reached without reaching the Hct threshold or IDMs.
   2. This will allow for continued fluid removal without reaching hypovolemia and the Hct threshold.

V. **Set alarm limit: The alarm limit will be set at 1–2 Hct points below the identified Hct threshold in subsequent treatments.**

A. If the Hct threshold is unknown, the limit will be set at approximately 10% to15% above the starting Hct (-10 % to -15% BV change) for the patients on chronic HD with FVE.

B. Initially at 5% to 10% above the starting Hct (-5% to -10% BV change) for patients with exceptions as described under B.3.d.: Linear "B" profile (see page 720).

VI. **Identify and treat hypoxemia prior to symptomology.**

A. Hypoxemia may begin with an arterial saturation (SaO_2) from a fistula or graft below 90% or a venous saturation (SvO_2) from a central venous catheter (CVC) line below 60%.

B. Hypoxemia may occur with an acceptable arterial saturation in the presence of a low Hct/Hgb as oxygen carrying capacity may be low.
   1. The normal range of overall oxygen-carrying capacity is 19 to 20 mL/dL.
   2. This is calculated by multiplying 1.39 mL (the amount of oxygen each gram of hemoglobin carries) x hemoglobin x SaO_2 (or SpO_2) (see Chapter 54).

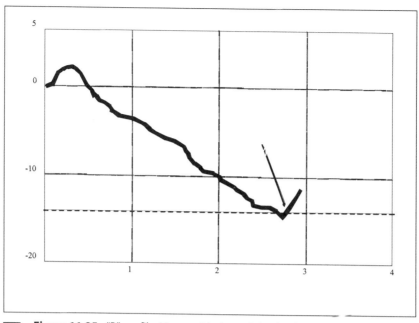

Figure 11.25. "B" profile: Linear with dry weight check. Plasma refill is observed (BV does not "level off" when UFR is in minimum and continues to rise by equal to or greater than +1.5%; Hct decreases by equal to or greater than 0.5%). True "ideal" dry weight has not yet been achieved.

Used with permission from Hema Metrics.

VII. Assess for plasma refill by conducting a dry weight check.

A. Set the UFR to minimum (equal to or less than 400 mL/hour for an adult) and wait 10–15 minutes. (Refer to manufacturer for recommended minimum rate on specific dialysis machines.)

B. In the last 10–15 minutes of each treatment in which the patient has been converted to a "B" profile slope, or at any point in the treatment if assessment is desired, a "dry weight" check will be done by reducing the UFR to minimum, and observe for plasma refill.

C. If plasma refill is observed (BV does not "level off" and continues to rise, i.e., becomes less negative by equal to or greater than 1.5%, Hct decreases by equal to or greater than 0.5%), true "ideal" dry weight has not yet been achieved. If plasma refill is noted at the end of the treatment, .25 kg (250 mL) will be added to the patient's goal the next treatment (see Figure 11.25).

VIII. Prescribed dry weight will be adjusted for next treatment based on assessment of patient profiles, maximum Hct achieved, if Hct threshold was identified, plasma refill, previous post and current pre blood pressures, and patient symptoms.

IX. Education on fluid removal (see Chapter 54).

Chapter 57

Hemodialyzer Reprocessing

I. Purpose.

A. The purpose of the dialyzer reprocessing procedure is to clean and sterilize or achieve a high level of disinfection of the blood and dialysate compartments of a hemodialyzer to render the device fully suitable, safe and effective for further use on the same patient.

B. Participating in reprocessing is voluntary. All benefits and risks must be explained to the patient and the patient must consent before being placed on reuse and annually thereafter.

C. Reasons for preprocessing and reprocessing of dialyzers vary but the main ones are:
   1. Preprocessing of the unused dialyzer decreases the hypersensitivity reaction in patients due to ethylene oxide (ETO) exposure.
      a. ETO is frequently used as a gas sterilant for new dialyzers in the United States.
      b. Patients with ETO sensitivity (often called "first use syndrome") can exhibit symptoms within the first 15 minutes of hemodialysis (HD) and include anxiety, pruritis, dyspnea, lower back pain, chest tightness, palpitations, hypotension, nausea, and vomiting. In rare cases, a patient can have an anaphylactic reaction which can include hives and respiratory arrest (see Chapter 55).
   2. Reprocessing of hemodialyzers allows the patient's blood to coat the fibers with the patient's own protein, making it more biocompatible, or more like the patient's own tissue.
   3. The most common nonmedical reason for reuse is cost. Reuse of hemodialyzers may reduce the cost per dialysis treatment.
   4. The environmental impact of reusing means there is less medical waste and is a cost benefit for the facility as disposal of biohazardous waste is costly.

D. Diaylzers should be reprocessed using the standards set forth by the Association for the Advancement of Medical Instrumentation (AAMI) and enforced by the Center for Medicare and Medicaid Services (CMS). The CMS has adopted the AAMI Guidelines as a condition of coverage.

II. Risks to patients.

A. The greatest risk to patients who participate in reuse is the possibility of infusion of germicide during HD.

B. Using proper procedure and double checks, reduces this risk of exposure significantly.

C. Possible signs and symptoms of an exposure to germicide.
   1. Burning at the access, the taste of gasoline in the mouth, along with shortness of breath, chest pain or tightness, nausea and vomiting, hypotension, palpitations, pruritis.
   2. Hemolysis (rupture of red blood cells [RBCs]– blood turns bright red).
   3. Crenation (shriveling of RBCs, blood turns black) is visualized within the blood tubing.

D. The potential for sepsis and/or pyrogenic reactions.

E. Inadequate levels of germicide or shortened germicide contact time.
   1. Some strains of gram positive mycobacteria may survive within an inadequately reprocessed hemodialyzer and form a protective biofilm.
   2. The gram positive mycobacteria do not produce endotoxin so will not induce a pyrogenic reaction. However, they can get into the bloodstream and cause sepsis.
   3. With sepsis, the patient may have a fever and general malaise and a positive blood culture result. The infection has the potential to be fatal.

F. Endotoxins from dead or dying gram-negative bacteria (endotoxin-producing bacteria) can absorb into the potting material of the hemodialyzer and other plastics of the dialyzer and leach out during HD with blood contact (the endotoxin needs protein to draw it out).

1. If the endotoxin exposure is high enough (5 EU[endotoxin unit]/kg/body weight), the exposure can cause a pyrogenic reaction in patients during the treatment.
2. Chills, rigors, fever spike, nausea, vomiting, body aches, and hypotension are some of the main symptoms a patient may exhibit when exposed to enough levels of endotoxin.

G. Patient's temperature should be taken pre and post HD. A temperature over 37.8° C (100° F) or chills with or without a fever should be reported to the physician.
   1. Initiate an investigation into the etiology.
   2. Possible causes of fever may include vascular access infection, poor reuse, inadequately purified water, contaminated dialysate, etc.
   3. Patients on HD typically have subnormal temperatures, averaging 96.8 ° F (36° C).

H. Other unusual symptoms such as access pain should also be reported.

III. Issues that decrease the number of reuses.

A. Inadequate heparinization of the extracorporeal unit and the patient will cause clotting in the fibers and decrease the number of times the dialyzer may be suitable for use.

B. Inadequate blood flow in a large surface dialyzer may lead to clotting because the velocity is sluggish or multiple alarms intermittently stop the blood pump during HD.

C. Allowing air in the extracorporeal circuit during priming (e.g., empty saline bag) will enhance clotting of the dialyzer.

D. Clotting leads to poor diffusion of molecules compromising the adequacy/clearances for the patient (see also Chapter 53, VII: Anticoagulation during hemodialysis).

IV. Records.

A. All records shall meet the requirements for medical records including completeness, legibility, and security.
   1. Complaint investigation and quality control and improvement should be part of the ongoing documentation.
   2. Maintenance of the records should be overseen by the medical director.

B. Records shall be kept that identify:
   1. The dialyzer.
   2. The date of each reprocessing step.
   3. The person performing the reprocessing.
   4. The results of the tests should be maintained in a log and/or in the patient's medical record.

V. Training.

A. All personnel reprocessing hemodialyzers must be trained in the procedure and that training will be overseen by the medical director.

B. The curriculum should include the policy and procedures with rationale, basic documentation requirements, the principles of hemodialysis, the operation of equipment, microbiology, risks and hazards to patients with consequences of not performing each task correctly, OSHA training for chemicals and emergency guidelines.

VI. Preprocessing should be done whenever possible.

A. It is performed to decrease the first-use syndrome in patients and to determine the baseline total cell volume (TCV) of the hemodialyzer.

B. Preprocessing and reprocessing can only be performed on dialyzers labeled for multiple use. Single use dialyzers must be disposed of after each use.

C. The stated volume of the dialyzer may be inaccurate from the manufacturer, so it is important to establish the actual volume of a dialyzer before use on a patient. If preprocessing is not possible, other methods such as volume averaging of the lot should be used.

D. Preprocessed dialyzers can be ready on the shelf with all of the necessary information except the patient's name. Before the dialyzer is used on a patient, it must be labeled with the patient's name and identifying number(s).

E. The preprocessing steps are the same as reprocessing given below.

VII. Reprocessing.

A. Reprocessing of hemodialyzers (often referred to as "reuse") requires a physician's order and can be done automatically or manually.
   1. The automated machine has the advantage of higher quality control, better efficiency, more

consistency, a better patient safety record and accurate documentation.
2. Maintenance records shall be maintained of all equipment used for reprocessing.
3. The multiple use of a hemodialyzer is repeated until the dialyzer does not meet the performance criteria, reaches the clinic-specific maximum allowable reuses, or is not aesthetically acceptable to staff or patient.

B. Hemodialyzer labeling.
1. Reprocessed dialyzers must be used on the same patient. Labeling must include the patient's first and last name, the patient's identifying number(s), the number of times it has been reprocessed and preprocessed, the date and time of both, the TCV, that it passed all tests, and the person performing the reprocessing.
2. Patients with similar last names shall have a distinctive same name alert on the dialyzer to notify the staff to use extra precautions when handling (e.g., red-edged label).
3. The label must be updated with each reuse.
4. The reuse label must not obscure any important manufacturer's information, must be small enough to visualize the blood path, and should have a transparent cover that can withstand normal reprocessing and dialysis procedures to keep it protected.
5. All information should be legible. If the name is not readable, the dialyzer shall not be used and discarded. A new label may be printed up for all but an illegible name.

C. Dialyzer transporting and handling.
1. All staff shall observe standard precautions when handling dirty, used dialyzers.
2. The Centers for Disease Control (CDC) recommendations should be followed for all patients and staff who participate in reuse. Hepatitis B surface antigen positive patients should not participate in reuse.
3. Visual inspection of the dialyzer should reveal no cracks, intact label, no chips or defects of the dialyzer.
4. At termination of the hemodialysis procedure, the dialyzer shall be handled in a clean and sanitary way (e.g., all ports should be capped and the dialyzer enclosed in a plastic disposable bag).
5. The dialyzer should be refrigerated in a temperature range of 2–10° C (should not freeze) to inhibit bacterial growth if it is not reprocessed within 2 hours.

6. The amount of time delay shall be validated by the facility and allow for safe reprocessing (e.g., 24–36 hours).

D. Rinsing and cleaning.
1. Many facilities will preclean the dialyzer to remove debris before the rinsing and cleaning process on the reprocessing device.
   a. One approach to precleaning is with reverse ultrafiltration.
   b. A cap is placed on the dialysate port and a controlled supply of water is locked onto the other dialysate port.
   c. The water pressure blows gross clots and blood products out of the fibers.
2. Some dialyzers have removable headers (end caps).
   a. Some dialysis facilities will remove the header to better preclean the dialyzer.
   b. If the headers are removed, they must be labeled appropriately and the O-ring and header must stay with their respective dialyzer.
   c. If instruments or materials are used to clean the headers (e.g., 4 x 4 gauze) it shall not cause damage to the end of the dialyzer and shall be new or disinfected between uses.
   d. The headers and O-rings shall be disinfected and not rinsed after returning to the dialyzer.
   e. Overtightening of the header may cause cracks and undertightening may cause blood leaks.
3. The rinsing water must meet the contaminant requirements set forth by AAMI (refer to Table 11.1 in Chapter 52) and shall have a bacterial colony count of less than 200 colony forming units/mL (CFU/mL), with an action level of 50 CFU/mL. Endotoxin levels shall be less than 2 EU/mL with an action level of 1 EU/mL (see Chapter 52, water section for testing criteria).
4. Dilute solutions of hydrogen peroxide, sodium hypochlorite, peracetic acid, or other chemicals may be used as cleaning agents.
   a. Any cleaning agent must be able to be reduced to safe levels after flushing.
   b. The integrity and performance of the dialyzer cannot be affected by the cleaning agent.
5. One disinfectant must be rinsed before another is introduced unless mixing is shown to be safe and effective. For example, mixing formaldehyde and bleach or peracetic acid and bleach create noxious vapors that are dangerous.
6. Both the blood and dialysate compartments of the dialyzer are flushed with the cleaning

solution until the effluent is clear and the dialyzer fibers are generally free of visible blood.

7. Ventilation of the reprocessing area must meet Occupational Safety and Health Adminstration (OSHA) Standards.

E. Performance measurements.

1. Performance measurements are done on the automated reuse system after precleaning and rinsing of the dialyzer. On a manual system, the performance tests are done by the reprocessing technician.

2. The TCV of the dialyzer is measured each time and compared with the baseline TCV (or averaged TCV). Once the volume falls below 80% of the new TCV, the dialyzer has failed the criteria and should not be used again.

3. A direct or indirect measurement of small molecule clearance shall be less than 10%.
   a. Data shows that a loss of less than 20% TCV corresponds to a less than 10% reduction in small molecule clearance (the "20/10" rule).
   b. The manufacturer of the dialyzer supplies information on removal of in-vitro small-molecule clearance such as sodium and urea, along with middle-molecule clearance. Since it is impractical to duplicate such clearances in the clinical setting, it can be assumed that if the TCV is above 80%, the clearance is above 90%.

4. A membrane integrity or air pressure leak test should be performed each time.
   a. Generally, the dialyzer is tested against a high TMP (e.g., 500 mm/Hg) and held there for a set amount of time.
   b. If the pressure decays too quickly, the dialyzer has failed the leak test and should not be used.
   c. This can also be done just before use on the dialysis machine.

5. Each individual dialyzer must be performance tested prior to use, batch testing is not acceptable.

6. Dialyzer failures must be documented correctly. It is part of the quality assurance permanent record and shows if the clinic (or manufacturer) is having a problem.

F. Germicide instillation.

1. Germicide instillation takes place once the dialyzer is cleaned and has passed all tests.

2. The blood compartment and dialysate compartment must be filled with a high level disinfectant (e.g., formaldehyde, gluteraldehye) or a sterilant (e.g., peracetic acid).

   a. All OSHA guidelines must be adhered to when handling any hazardous chemicals. Follow the Material Data Safety Sheets (MSDS) supplied by the manufacturer.

   b. When performing manual reprocessing, each batch of germicide must be tested prior to use to verify proper concentration (potency test). Automated systems will dilute the germicide from concentrate on line and should be checked once per month.

   c. The hemodialyzers shall be filled with the germicide solution until the concentration in the dialyzer is at least 90% of the prescribed concentration.
      (1) Only USP grade germicides, free of particulates, should be used.
      (2) Users must follow manufacturer guidelines for the concentration of peracetic acid since different types exist (e.g, Renalin® at 4%). A minimum of 11 hours contact time in the dialyzer is required.
      (3) Concentration for formaldehyde must be 4% with a minimum contact time of 24 hours at a temperature > 20° C.
      (4) If heat pasteurization is used along with formaldehyde, lower concentrations or shorter contact times may be appropriate if equivalent results can be demonstrated (e.g., 1% at 40° C for 24 hours).
      (5) If other options are used such as citric acid, the user must consult the literature. 1.5% citric acid at 95° C heat pasteurization for 20 hours has been shown to be effective.
      (6) Gluteraldehyde is another high level disinfectant option.
      (7) The germicide should not damage the integrity of the dialyzer and must be able to be rinsed from the dialyzer to safe levels before use.

   d. The water to dilute the germicide must be "RO" treated water that meets the AAMI chemical standards (refer to Table 11.1 in Chapter 52) and has a bacterial count less than 200 CFU/mL (action must be taken if the count reaches 50 CFUs) and an endotoxin level less than 2 EU (and an action level of 1 EU).

   e. The dialyzer must be completely filled with the germicide, both blood and dialysate compartments and the germicide should not degrade more than 10% original fill concentration after the dwell time is complete.

f. Disinfected ports should be placed on the blood ports and the dialysate ports.

g. The exterior of the dialyzer must be cleaned with a low level disinfectant such as 1:100 dilution of household strength bleach (sodium hypochlorite) or a 1% peracetic acid solution.

G. Storage of dialyzers.

1. Storage of dialyzers is important so that the conditions should keep deterioration of the germicide, contamination and breakage to a minimum.

2. Do not store reproecessed dialyzers with new ones. A system for separating clean dialyzers from dirty dialyzers must be in place.

3. The temperature of the storage and reprocessing areas should be appropriate for the germicide in use (e.g., less than 70° F for peracetic acid) and monitored and recorded routinely.

4. The shelf life of reprocessed and preprocessed dialyzers is 1 month. The dialyzer needs to be reprocessed before this time is exceeded.

H. Dialyzer inspection.

1. Dialyzer inspection should be repeated after the reprocessing step when it is placed in storage, and prior to use.

a. Check that the label is intact, complete, and legible.

b. No structural damage to the dialyzer exists.

c. All ports are capped and there is no leakage from ports and the volume of germicide is appropriate within the dialyzer (this will vary depending upon the germicide used).

d. The contact time has been sufficient for the germicide to work but not so long as to exceed acceptable shelf life (greater than 1 month).

e. The cosmetic appearance is acceptable to both the patient and the staff. There is minimal header clots and few clotted fibers. The overall appearance looks clean and sanitary.

f. At least two people verify and document with initials that the dialyzer is used on the correct patient. If possible, one of these people should be the patient.

g. The gross presence of germicide in the blood and dialysate compartments, including headers is confirmed.

I. Germicide rinsing.

1. Germicide rinsing of the dialyzer should be performed prior to the patient's hemodialysis.

2. Test the dialyzer for the gross presence of germicide prior to rinsing with normal saline.

3. With peracetic acid, the blood side of the dialyzer must be rinsed first (peracetic acid will react with the dialysate and cause much bubbling in the fibers).

4. Care must be taken to prevent the introduction of germicide into the:

a. Saline line or bag.

b. The heparin line.

c. The arterial and venous lines and respective chambers.

d. Clamp these lines before rinsing begins.

5. Once the dialyzer and bloodlines are rinsed and primed according to facility policy, the normal saline (NS) exiting the dialyzer must be tested for the reduction to safe level (the absence) of detectable germicide. This must be verified and documented by two staff members.

6. It is important that the absence test is performed just before the patient treatment is initiated. Rebound (where the disinfectant level increases) of disinfectant can occur with no flow through the dialyzer on either the dialysate side or blood side prior to treatment initiation.

7. Assure that the appropriate test is used for residual germicide levels; some tests are more accurate than others.

a. Formaldehyde levels must be less than 3 PPM.

b. Follow manufacturers' recommendations for the safe reduction of germicides, e.g., peracetic acid less than 3 PPM.

VIII. Quality monitoring.

A. Quality improvement and assurance must be an ongoing program with the reuse of hemodialyzers.

B. A complaint file must be kept for any problems with the dialyzers (e.g., cracked header, clotted dialyzer, inadequately filled with germicide, blood leaks, etc.).

C. Event (incident) reports should be completed for any significant event during dialysis such as a pyrogenic reaction.

D. Adequacy of dialysis must be monitored with any reprocessing program (e.g. Kt/V, URR) as part of the quality oversight.

E. Follow-up investigation of any discrepancies must be documented. Adjustments should be made to the reprocessing program whenever indicated and must involve the medical director.

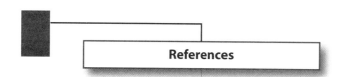

Chapter 51

Ahmad, S., Misra, M., Hoenich, N., & Daugirdas, J.T. (2007). Hemodialysis apparatus. In J.T. Daugirdas, P.G. Blake, & T.S. Ing (Eds.), *Handbook of dialysis* (4th ed., pp. 59-78). Philadelphia: Lippincott Williams & Wilkins.

Burrows-Hudson, S., & Prowant, B. (2005). *Nephrology nursing standards of practice and guidelines for care.* Pitman, NJ: American Nephrology Nurses' Association.

Daugirdas, J.T. (2007). Chronic hemodialysis prescription: A urea kinetic approach. In J.T. Daugirdas, P.G. Blake, & T.S. Ing (Eds.), *Handbook of dialysis* (4th ed., pp.146-169). Philadelphia: Lippincott Williams & Wilkins.

Fresenius Medical Care. (n.d.). *History of hemodialysis.* Retrieved October 6, 2007, from http://www.fmc-ag.com/internet/fmc/fmcag/agintpub.nsf/Content/History+of+Dialysisfmcag/agintpub.nsf/Content/History+of+Dialysis

Gotch, F., & Keen, M. (2005). Kinetic modeling in hemodialysis. In A.R. Nissenson & R.N. Finc (Eds.), *Clinical dialysis* (4th ed., pp. 153-202). New York: McGraw Hill.

Latham, C.E. (2006). Hemodialysis technology. In A.E. Molzahn & E. Butera (Eds.), *Contemporary nephrology nursing: Principles and practice* (2nd ed., pp. 529-558). Pitman, NJ: American Nephrology Nurses' Association.

Levin, N.W., & Ronco, C. (2002). Complications during hemodialysis: Common clinical problems during hemodialysis. In A.R. Nissenson & R.N. Fine (Eds.), *Dialysis therapy* (pp. 171-179). Philadelphia: Hanley & Belfus, Inc.

National Kidney Foundation Kidney (NKF). (2006). *Clinical practice guidelines for hemodialysis adequacy: Update 2006.* Retrieved January 1, 2008, from http://www.kidney.org/professionals/KDOQI/guideline_upHD_PD_VA/index.htm

Pittard, J. (2002). Safety monitors in hemodialysis. In A.R. Nissenson & R.N. Fine (Eds.), *Dialysis therapy* (pp. 68-82). Philadelphia: Hanley & Belfus, Inc.

Robbins, K.C. (2006). Hemodialysis: Prevention and management of treatment complications. In A.E. Molzahn & E. Butera (Eds.), *Contemporary nephrology nursing: Principles and practice* (2nd ed.). Pitman, NJ: American Nephrology Nurses' Association.

Chapter 52

Amato, R.L. (2005). Water treatment for hemodialysis – Updated to include the latest AAMI Standards for Dialysate (RD52: 2004). *Nephrology Nursing Journal, 32*(2), 151-167.

Association for the Advancement of Medical Instrumentation (AAMI). (2002). *Hemodialysis systems. ANSI/AAMI, RD62-2001* (Volume 3). Arlington, VA: Author.

Burrows-Hudson, S., & Prowant, B. (2005). *Nephrology nursing standards of practice and guidelines for care.* Pitman, NJ: American Nephrology Nurses' Association.

Canaud, B., Bosc, J.Y., Leray, H., Morena, M., & Stec, F. (2000). Microbiologic purity of dialysate: Rationale and technical aspects. In J. Botella, H. Klinkmann, G. La Greca, & P.

Zuccheli (Eds.), *Chronic inflammation in hemodialysis* (pp. 34-47). Switzerland: S. Karger AG.

Food and Drug Administration (FDA). (1988). *FDA safety alert: Chloramine contamination of hemodialysis water supplies.* Rockville, MD: Author.

Jochimsen, E.M., Carmichael W.W., An, J.S., Cardo, D.M., Cookson, S.T., Holmes, C.E., et al. (1998). Liver failure and death after exposure to microcystins at a hemodialysis center in Brazil. *New England Journal of Medicine, 338*, 873-888.

Kirkwood, R.G., Dunn, S., Thomasson, L., & Simmonhoff, M.L. (1981). Generation of the precarcinogen dimethylnitrosamine (DMNA) in dialysate water. *Transactions of the American Society for Artificial Internal Organs, 27*, 168-171.

Latham, C.E. (2006). Hemodialysis technology. In A.E. Molzahn & E. Butera (Eds.), *Contemporary nephrology nursing: Principles and practice* (2nd ed.). Pitman, NJ: American Nephrology Nurses' Association.

Luehmann, D., Keshaviah, P., Ward, R., Klein, E., & Thomas, A. (1989). *A manual on water treatment for hemodialysis.* Rockville, MD: Food and Drug Administration.

Panichi, V., Migliori, M., De Pietro, S., Taccola, D., Bianchi, A.M., Norpoth, M., et al. (2000). C-reactive protein as a marker of chronic inflammation in uremic patients. *Blood Purification, 18*(3), 183-190.

Ward, R.A., & Ing, T.S. (2007). Product water and hemodialysis solution preparation. In J.T. Daugirdas, P.G. Blake, & T.S. Ing (Eds.), *Handbook of dialysis* (4th ed.). Philadelphia: Lippincott Williams & Wilkins.

Chapter 53

Burrows-Hudson, S., & Prowant, B. (Eds.). (2005). *Nephrology nursing standards of practice and guidelines for care.* Pitman, NJ: American Nephrology Nurses' Association.

De La Vega, L.P., Miller, R.S., Benda, M.M., Grill, D.E., Johnson, M.G., McCarty, J.T., et al. (2005). Association of heparin-induced antibodies and adverse outcomes in hemodialysis patients: A population-based study. *Mayo Clinical Proceedings, 80*(8), 995-1000.

Latham, C.E. (2006). *Hemodialysis technology.* In A. Molzhan & E. Butera (Eds.), *Contemporary nephrology nursing: Principles and practice* (2nd ed., pp. 529-558). Pitman, NJ: American Nephrology Nurses' Association.

Mureebe, L., Coats, R.D., Silliman, W.R., Shuster, T.A., Nichols, W.K., & Silver, D. (2004). Heparin-associated antiplatelet antibodies increase morbidity and mortality in hemodialysis patients. *Surgery, 136*(4), 848-853.

National Kidney Foundation (NKF). (2001). Kidney Disease Outcomes Quality Initiative (K/DOQI) clinical practice guidelines for hemodialysis adequacy: Update 2000. *American Journal of Kidney Diseases, 37*(1)(Suppl. 1), S7-S64.

Palomo, I., Pereira, J., Alarcón, M., Díaz, G., Hidalgo, P., Pizarro, I., et al. (2005). Prevalence of heparin-induced antibodies in patients with chronic renal failure undergoing hemodialysis. *Journal of Clinical Laboratory Analysis 19*, 189-195.

Chapter 54

Burrows-Hudson, S., & Prowant, B. (2005). *Nephrology nursing standards of practice and guidelines for care.* Pitman, NJ: American Nephrology Nurses' Association.

Carey, S. (2002, October). *Optimizing dry weight: Assessing, achieving, maintaining.* Paper presented at the American Nephrology Nurses Association Fall Meeting, Phoenix, AZ.

Charra, B. (1998). Dry weight in dialysis: The history of a concept. *Nephrology Dialysis Transplantation, 77*(13), 1882-1885.

Charra, B., Bergstrom, J., & Scribner, B.H. (1998). Blood pressure control in dialysis patients: The importance of the lag phenomenon. *American Journal of Kidney Diseases, 32,* 720.

Daugirdas, J.T., Blake, P.G., & Ing, T.S. (Eds.). (2007). *Handbook of dialysis* (4th ed.). Philadelphia: Lippincott Williams & Wilkins.

Diroll, A., & Hlebovy, D. (2003). Inverse relationship between blood volume and blood pressure. *Nephrology Nursing Journal, 30*(4), 460-461.

Eknoyan, G., Beck, G.J., Cheung, A.K., Daugirdas, J.T., Greene, T., & Kusek, J.W. (2002). Effect of dialysis dose and membrane flux in maintenance hemodialysis. *New England Journal of Medicine, 347,* 2010-2019.

Goldstein, S.L., Michael, M., & Brewer, E. (2004). Blood volume monitoring to achieve target weight in pediatric hemodialysis patients. *Pediatric Nephrology, 19,* 432-437.

Kallenbach, J.Z., Gutch, C.F., Stoner, M.G., & Corea, A.L. (Eds.). (2005). *Review of hemodialysis for nurses and dialysis technicians* (7th ed.). St Louis: Elsevier Mosby.

Guyton, A.C., & Hall, J.E. (2000). *Textbook of medical physiology.* (10th ed.). Philadelphia: W.B. Saunders.

Hardnett, J., Foley, R., Foley, R., Kent, G., Barre, P., Murray, D., et al. (1995). Congestive heart failure in dialysis patients: Prevalence, incidence, prognosis and risk factors. *International Society of Nephrology, 47,* 884-890.

Hegbrant, J., Sternby, J., Larsson, A., Martennson, L., Nielsen, A., & Thysell, H. (1997). Beneficial effect of cold dialysate for the prevention of hemodialysis induced hypoxemia. *Blood Purification, 15*(1), 15-24.

Hema Metrics. (2004). *Crit-Line III reference manual and training materials.* Kaysville, UT: Author.

Hlebovy, D. (2003). Inverse relationship between blood volume and blood pressure. *Nephrology Nursing Journal, 30*(4), 460.

Hlebovy, D. (2006). Fluid management: Moving and removing fluid during hemodialysis. *Nephrology Nursing Journal, 33*(4), 441-446.

Holechek, M.J. (2003). Renal hemodynamics: An overview. *Nephrology Nursing Journal, 30*(4), 441-448.

Hossli, S.M. (2005). Clinical management of intradialytic hypotension: Survey results. *Nephrology Nursing Journal, 32*(3), 287-292.

Jaeger, J.Q., & Mehta, R.L. (1999). Assessment of dry weight in hemodialysis: An overview. *Journal of the American Society of Nephrology, 10,* 392-403.

Kinnel, K. (2005). Should patients eat during hemodialysis treatments? *Nephrology Nursing Journal, 32*(5), 513-515.

Kutner, N. (2007, April). *Geriatric considerations in nephrology.* Presentation at the National Kidney Foundation Spring Clinical Meeting, Orlando, FL.

LePain, N., & Hlebovy, D. (2004). *Hematocrit-based blood volume monitoring and the hemodialysis patient.* Kaysville, UT: Hema Metrics.

Levin, N.W., & Ronco, C. (2002). Common clinical problems during hemodialysis. In A.R. Nissensen & R.N. Fine (Eds.), *Dialysis therapy* (3rd ed.). Philadelphia: Hanely & Belfus, Inc.

McLaren, P., & Hunter, C. (2007). Sodium profiling: The key to reducing symptoms of dialysis? *Nephrology Nursing Journal, 34*(4), 403-414.

Mees, E. (2004). Adequacy of dialysis: An inadequately applied concept. *Dialysis & Transplant, 33*(22), 738-748.

National Kidney Foundation (NKF). (1997). *Kidney Disease Outcomes Quality Initiative (K/DOQI) clinical practice guidelines for hemodialysis adequacy.* New York: Author.

National Kidney Foundation (NKF). (2006). Kidney Disease Outcomes Quality Initiative (K/DOQI) clinical practice guidelines for hemodialysis adequacy: Update 2006. *American Journal of Kidney Diseases, 48*(Suppl. 1), S2-S75.

Palma, J., & Pittard, J. (2001). Body water – Body weight (Part II). *Dialysis & Transplant, 792.*

Purcell, W., Manias, E., Williams, A., & Walker, R. (2004). Accurate dry weight assessment: Reducing the incidence hypertension and cardiac disease in patients on hemodialysis. *Nephrology Nursing Journal, 31*(6), 631-638.

Robbins, K.C. (2006). Hemodialysis: Prevention and management of treatment complications. In A.E. Molzahn & E. Butera (Eds.), *Contemporary nephrology nursing: Principles and practice* (2nd ed.). Pitman, NJ: American Nephrology Nurses' Association.

Rodriguez, H.J., Domenici, R., Diroll, A., & Goykhman, I. (2005). Assessment of dry weight by monitoring changes in blood volume using Crit-Line. *Kidney International, 68,* 854-861.

Schreiber, M.J. (2003, May). *Intradialytic complications.* Paper presented at the RCG Sixth Annual Medical Conference, Tucson, AZ.

Schroeder, K.L., Sallustio, J.E., & Ross, E.A. (2004). Continuous haematocrit monitoring during intradialytic hypotension: Precipitous decline in plasma refill rates. *Nephrology Dialysis Transplant, 19*(3), 652-656.

Sherman, R. (2007, April). *Managing intradialytic hypotension.* Paper presented at the National Kidney Foundation Spring Clinical Meeting, Orlando, FL.

Shoji, T., Tsubakihara, Y., Fujii, M., & Imai, E. (2004). Hemodialysis-associated hypotension as an independent factor for two-year mortality in hemodialysis patients. *Kidney International, 66,* 1212-1220.

Smith, K.J., & Kampine, J.P. (1990). *Circulatory physiology: The essentials* (3rd ed.). Baltimore: Lippincott Williams & Wilkins.

Sodemann, K., & Polascheggm, H.D. (2001). *Monitoring of mixed venous oxygen saturation by Critline III as a parameter of continuous cardiac output.* ASN/ISN World Congress of Nephrology: Abstract #553720.

Spiegal, P., Michelis, M., Panagopoulos, G., DeVita, M.V., & Schwimmer, J.A. (2005). Reducing hospital utilization by hemodialysis patients. *Dialysis and Transplantation, 34*(3), 131-136.

Chapter 55

Burrows-Hudson, S., & Prowant, B. (2005). *Nephrology nursing standards of practice and guidelines for care.* Pitman, NJ: American Nephrology Nurses' Association.

Carey, S. (2002, October). *Optimizing dry weight: Assessing, achieving, maintaining.* Paper presented at the American Nephrology Nurses' Association Fall Meeting, Phoenix, AZ.

Charra, B. (1998). Dry weight in dialysis: The history of a concept. *Nephrology Dialysis Transplantation, 77*(13), 1882-1885.

Charra, B., Bergstrom, J., & Scribner, B.H. (1998). Blood pressure control in dialysis patients: The importance of the lag phenomenon. *American Journal of Kidney Diseases, 32,* 720-724.

Daugirdas, J.T., Blake, P.G., & Ing, T.S. (Eds). (2007). *Handbook of dialysis* (4th ed.). Philadelphia: Lippincott Williams & Wilkins.

Diroll, A., & Hlebovy, D. (2003). Inverse relationship between blood volume and blood pressure. *Nephrology Nursing Journal, 30*(4), 460-461.

Eknoyan, G., Beck, G.J., Cheung, A.K., Daugirdas, J.T., Greene, T., & Kusek, J.W. (2002). Effect of dialysis dose and membrane flux in maintenance hemodialysis. *New England Journal of Medicine, 347,* 2010-2019.

Goldstein, S.L., Michael, M., & Brewer, E. (2004). Blood volume monitoring to achieve target weight in pediatric hemodialysis patients. *Pediatric Nephrology 19, 432-437.*

Guyton, A.C., & Hall, J.E. (2000). *Textbook of medical physiology* (10th ed.). Philadelphia: W.B. Saunders.

Hardnett, J., Foley, R., Foley, R., Kent, G., Barre, P., Murray, D., et al. (1995). Congestive heart failure in dialysis patients: Prevalence, incidence, prognosis and risk factors. *International Society of Nephrology, 47,* 884-890.

Hegbrant, J., Sternby, J., Larsson, A., Martennson, L., Nielsen, A., & Thysell, H. (1997). Beneficial effect of cold dialysate for the prevention of hemodialysis induced hypoxemia. *Blood Purification, 15*(1), 15-24.

Hema Metrics. (2004). *Crit-Line III reference manual and training materials.* Kaysville, UT: Author.

Hlebovy, D. (2006). Fluid management: Moving and removing fluid during hemodialysis. *Nephrology Nursing Journal, 33*(4), 441-446.

Holechek, M.J. (2003). Renal hemodynamics: An overview. *Nephrology Nursing Journal, 30*(4), 441-448.

Hossli, S.M. (2005). Clinical management of intradialytic hypotension: Survey results. *Nephrology Nursing Journal, 32*(3), 287-292.

Jaeger, J.Q., & Mehta, R.L. (1999) Assessment of dry weight in hemodialysis: An overview. *Journal of the American Society of Nephrology, 10,* 392-403.

Kallenbach, J.Z., Gutch, C.F., Stoner, M.G., & Corea, A.L. (Eds.). (2005). *Review of hemodialysis for nurses and dialysis technicians* (7th ed.). St Louis: Elsevier Mosby.

Kinnel, K. (2005). Should patients eat during hemodialysis treatments? *Nephrology Nursing Journal, 32*(5), 513-515.

Kutner, N. (2007, April). *Geriatric considerations in nephrology.* Presentation at the National Kidney Foundation Spring Clinical Meeting, Orlando, FL.

LePain, N., & Hlebovy, D. (2004). *Hematocrit-based blood volume monitoring and the hemodialysis patient.* Kaysville, UT: HemaMetrics.

Levin, N.W., & Ronco, C. (2002). Common clinical problems during hemodialysis. In A.R. Nissensen & R.N. Fine (Eds.), *Dialysis therapy* (3rd ed.). Philadelphia: Hanely & Belfus, Inc.

McLaren, P., & Hunter, C. (2007). Sodium profiling: The key to reducing symptoms of dialysis? *Nephrology Nursing Journal, 34*(4), 403-414.

Mees, E. (2004). Adequacy of dialysis: An inadequately applied concept. *Dialysis & Transplant, 33*(22), 738-748.

National Kidney Foundation (NKF). (1997). *Kidney Disease Outcomes Quality Initiative (K/DOQI) clinical practice guidelines for hemodialysis adequacy.* New York: Author.

National Kidney Foundation (NKF). (2006). Kidney Disease Outcomes Quality Initiative (K/DOQI) clinical practice guidelines for hemodialysis adequacy: Update 2006. *American Journal of Kidney Diseases, 48*(Suppl. 1), S2-S75.

Palma, J., & Pittard, J. (2001). Body water – Body weight (Part II). *Dialysis & Transplant,* 792.

Purcell, W., Manias, E., Williams, A., & Walker, R. (2004). Accurate dry weight assessment: Reducing the incidence hypertension and cardiac disease in patients on hemodialysis. *Nephrology Nursing Journal, 31*(6), 631-638.

Robbins, K.C. (2006). Hemodialysis: Prevention and management of treatment complications. In A.E. Molzahn & E. Butera (Eds.), *Contemporary nephrology nursing: Principles and practice* (2nd ed). Pitman, NJ: American Nephrology Nurses' Association.

Rodriguez, H.J., Domenici, R., Diroll, A., & Goykhman, I. (2005). Assessment of dry weight by monitoring changes in blood volume using Crit-Line. *Kidney International, 68,* 854-861.

Schreiber, M.J. (2003, May). *Intradialytic complications.* Paper presented at the RCG Sixth Annual Medical Conference, Tucson, AZ.

Schroeder, K.L., Sallustio, J.E., & Ross, E.A. (2004). Continuous haematocrit monitoring during intradialytic hypotension: Precipitous decline in plasma refill rates. *Nephrology Dialysis Transplant, 19*(3), 652-656.

Sherman, R. (2007, April). *Managing intradialytic hypotension.* Paper presented at the National Kidney Foundation Spring Clinical Meeting, Orlando, FL.

Shoji, T., Tsubakihara, Y., Fujii, M., & Imai, E. (2004). Hemodialysis-associated hypotension as an independent factor for two-year mortality in hemodialysis patients. *Kidney International, 66,* 1212-1220.

Sodemann, K., & Polaschegg, H.D. (2001). *Monitoring of mixed venous oxygen saturation by Critline III as a parameter of continuous cardiac output.* ASN/ISN World Congress of Nephrology: Abstract #553720.

Spiegal, P., Michelis, M., Panagopoulos, G., DeVita, M.V., & Schwimmer, J.A. (2005). Reducing hospital utilization by hemodialysis patients. *Dialysis and Transplantation, 34*(3), 131-136.

Chapter 56

Burrows-Hudson, S., & Prowant, B. (2005). *Nephrology nursing standards of practice and guidelines for care.* Pitman, NJ: American Nephrology Nurses' Association.

Carey, S. (2002, October). *Optimizing dry weight: Assessing, achieving, maintaining.* Paper presented at the American Nephrology Nurses' Association Fall Meeting, Phoenix, AZ.

Charra, B. (1998). Dry weight in dialysis: The history of a concept. *Nephrology Dialysis Transplantation, 77*(13), 1882-1885.

Charra, B., Bergstrom, J., & Scribner, B.H. (1998). Blood pressure control in dialysis patients: The importance of the lag phenomenon. *American Journal of Kidney Diseases, 32,* 720-724.

Daugirdas, J.T., Blake, P.G., & Ing, T.S. (Eds). (2007). *Handbook of dialysis* (4th ed.). Philadelphia: Lippincott Williams & Wilkins.

Diroll, A., & Hlebovy, D. (2003). Inverse relationship between blood volume and blood pressure. *Nephrology Nursing Journal, 30*(4), 460-461.

Eknoyan, G., Beck, G.J., Cheung, A.K., Daugirdas, J.T., Greene, T., & Kusek J.W. (2002). Effect of dialysis dose and membrane flux in maintenance hemodialysis. *New England Journal of Medicine, 347,* 2010-2019.

Goldstein, S.L., Michael, M., & Brewer, E. (2004). Blood volume monitoring to achieve target weight in pediatric hemodialysis patients. *Pediatric Nephrology, 19,* 432-437.

Guyton, A.C., & Hall, J.E. (2000). *Textbook of medical physiology* (10th ed.). Philadelphia: W.B. Saunders.

Hardnett, J., Foley, R., Foley, R., Kent, G., Barre, P., Murray, D., et al. (1995). Congestive heart failure in dialysis patients: Prevalence, incidence, prognosis and risk factors. *International Society of Nephrology, 47,* 884-890.

Hegbrant, J., Sternby, J., Larsson, A., Martennson, L., Nielsen, A., & Thysell, H. (1997). Beneficial effect of cold dialysate for the prevention of hemodialysis induced hypoxemia. *Blood Purification, 15*(1),15-24.

Hema Metrics. (2004). *Crit-Line III reference manual and training materials.* Kaysville, UT: Author.

Hlebovy, D. (2003). Inverse relationship between blood volume and blood pressure. *Nephrology Nursing Journal, 30*(4), 460.

Hlebovy, D. (2006). Fluid management: Moving and removing fluid during hemodialysis. *Nephrology Nursing Journal, 33*(4), 441-446.

Holechek, M.J. (2003). Renal hemodynamics: An overview. *Nephrology Nursing Journal, 30*(4), 441-448.

Hossli, S.M. (2005). Clinical management of intradialytic hypotension: Survey results. *Nephrology Nursing Journal, 32*(3), 287-292.

Jaeger, J.Q., & Mehta, R.L. (1999). Assessment of dry weight in hemodialysis: An overview. *Journal of the American Society of Nephrology, 10,* 392-403.

Kallenbach, J.Z., Gutch, C.F., Stoner, M.G., & Corea, A.L. (Eds.). (2005). *Review of hemodialysis for nurses and dialysis technicians* (7th ed.). St Louis: Elsevier Mosby.

Kinnel, K. (2005). Should patients eat during hemodialysis treatments? *Nephrology Nursing Journal, 32*(5), 513-515.

Kutner, N. (2007, April). *Geriatric considerations in nephrology.* Presentation at the National Kidney Foundation Spring Clinical Meeting, Orlando, FL.

LePain, N., & Hlebovy, D. (2004). *Hematocrit-based blood volume monitoring and the emodialysis patient.* Kayseville, UT: Hema Metrics.

Levin, N.W., & Ronco, C. (2002). Common clinical problems during hemodialysis. In A.R. Nissensen & R.N. Fine (Eds.), *Dialysis therapy* (3rd ed.). Philadelphia: Hanely & Belfus, Inc.

McLaren, P., & Hunter, C. (2007). Sodium profiling: The key to reducing symptoms of dialysis? *Nephrology Nursing Journal, 34*(4), 403-414.

Mees, E. (2004). Adequacy of dialysis: An inadequately applied concept. *Dialysis & Transplant, 33*(22), 738-748.

National Kidney Foundation (NKF). (1997). *Kidney Disease Outcomes Quality Initiative (K/DOQI) clinical practice guidelines for hemodialysis adequacy.* New York: Author.

National Kidney Foundation (NKF). (2006). Kidney Disease Outcomes Quality Initiative (K/DOQI) clinical practice guidelines for hemodialysis adequacy: Update 2006. *American Journal of Kidney Diseases, 48*(Suppl. 1), S2-S75.

Palma, J., & Pittard, J. (2001). Body water – Body weight (Part II). *Dialysis & Transplant, 792.*

Purcell, W., Manias, E., Williams, A., & Walker, R. (2004). Accurate dry weight assessment: Reducing the incidence hypertension and cardiac disease in patients on hemodialysis. *Nephrology Nursing Journal, 31*(6), 631-638.

Robbins, K.C. (2006). Hemodialysis: Prevention and management of treatment complications. In A.E. Molzahn & E. Butera (Eds.), *Contemporary nephrology nursing: Principles and practice* (2nd ed.). Pitman, NJ: American Nephrology Nurses' Association.

Rodriguez, H.J., Domenici, R., Diroll, A., & Goykhman I. (2005). Assessment of dry weight by monitoring changes in blood volume using Crit-Line. *Kidney International, 68,* 854-861.

Schreiber, M.J. (2003, May). *Intradialytic complications.* Paper presented at the RCG Sixth Annual Medical Conference. Tucson, AZ.

Schroeder, K.L., Sallustio, J.E., & Ross, E.A. (2004). Continuous haematocrit monitoring during intradialytic hypotension: precipitous decline in plasma refill rates. *Nephrology Dialysis Transplant, 19*(3), 652-656.

Sherman, R. (2007, April). *Managing intradialytic hypotension.* Paper presented at the National Kidney Foundation Spring Clinical, Meeting. Orlando, FL.

Shoji, T., Tsubakihara, Y., Fujii, M., & Imai, E. (2004). Hemodialysis-associated hypotension as an independent factor for two-year mortality in hemodialysis patients. *Kidney International, 66,* 1212-1220.

Sodemann, K., & Polaschegg, H.D. (2001). *Monitoring of mixed venous oxygen saturation by Critline III as a parameter of continuous cardiac output.* ASN/ISN World Congress of Nephrology: Abstract #553720.

Spiegal, P., Michelis, M., Panagopoulos, G., DeVita M.V., & Schwimmer, J.A., (2005). Reducing hospital utilization by hemodialysis patients. *Dialysis and Transplantation, 34*(3), 131-136.

Chapter 57

Association for the Advancement of Medical Instrumentation (AAMI). (2002). *Hemodialysis systems. ANSI/AAMI RD47-2002* (Volume 3). Arlington, VA: Author.

Burrows-Hudson, S., & Prowant, B. (2005). *Nephrology nursing standards of practice and guidelines for care.* Pitman, NJ: American Nephrology Nurses' Association.

Kaufman, A.M., Levin, R., Jayakaran R., & Levin, N.W. (2007). Dialyzer reuse. In J.T. Daugirdas, P.G. Blake, & T.S. Ing (Eds.), *Handbook of dialysis* (4th ed.) Philadelphia: Lippincott Williams & Wilkins.

Latham, C.E. (2006). Hemodialysis technology. In A.E. Molzahn & E. Butera (Eds.), *Contemporary nephrology nursing: Principles and practice* (2nd ed., pp. 529-558) Pitman, NJ: American Nephrology Nurses' Association.

Section 12

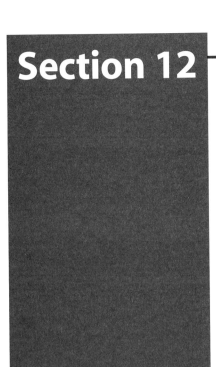

Vascular Access for Hemodialysis

Lesley C. Dinwiddie, MSN, RN, FNP, CNN

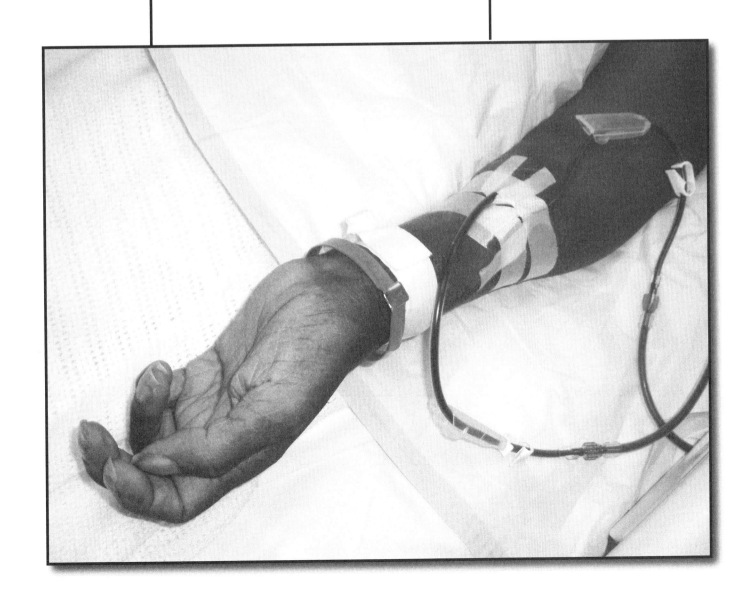

About the Author

Lesley C. Dinwiddie, MSN, RN, FNP, CNN, Section Editor and Author, is a Nephrology Nurse Consultant at Vascular Access Education and Research in Cary, North Carolina, and the Executive Director for the Institute of Excellence, Education and Research (ICEER).

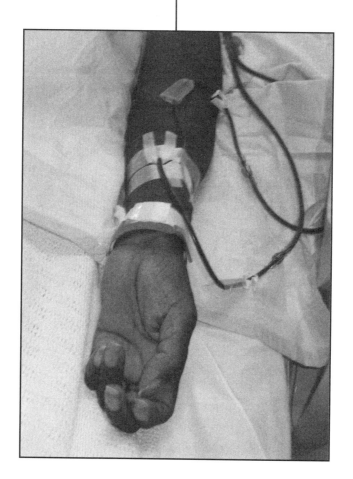

Section 12

Vascular Access for Hemodialysis

Vascular Access for Hemodialysis

Purpose

The purpose of this section is to provide an overview of the commonly used types of vascular access for hemodialysis as well as the nursing process necessary to assure the following patient outcomes (Burrows-Hudson & Prowant, 2005):

1. The patient's vascular access will provide a blood flow rate adequate to achieve the dialysis prescription.
2. The patient's vascular access will have a long use-life and be free of complications.
3. The patient will demonstrate knowledge regarding his/her vascular access.

Objectives

Upon completion of this section, the learner will be able to:

1. List the preferential order for vascular access according to the 2006 KDOQI guidelines and compare the indications, locations, advantages, and disadvantages of the arteriovenous fistula (AVF); the arteriovenous graft (AVG); and the central venous catheter (CVC) and catheter/port devices.
2. State the steps for assessment for each type of access.
3. List the possible causes and diagnoses of complications.
4. Describe routine planning for management of the vascular access, implementation (including cannulation), and interventions for complications.
5. Define the ongoing evaluation by the vascular access team through continuous quality improvement (CQI) and:
   a. Patient education.
   b. Staff education.
   c. Data collection and analyses.

Introduction

Vascular access is essential to hemodialysis (HD) therapy. Positive patient outcomes for hemodialysis are highly dependent on complication-free vascular access. The type of vascular access needed to achieve such outcomes depends upon the diagnosis and prognosis as well as the anatomic and physiologic potential and limitations of the patient. The ideal blood flow through a patient's fistula or graft is a flow sufficient to achieve prescribed blood flow rates through the dialyzer without compromising cardiac output or flow to the extremity distal to the access. While creation/placement of vascular access is primarily the purview of physicians, the routine maintenance, preservation, and patient education is the responsibility of the nephrology nurse.

Historical Perspectives

1960 Scribner and Quinton developed the first permanent access for chronic hemodialytic therapy. It consisted of Teflon tubes, one placed in an artery and one in a vein, which exited through the skin and were joined by a Teflon loop by means of swedge locks. (The detailed information on external AV shunts that has appeared in previous editions of the *Core Curriculum* has been archived to Historical Documents on the ANNA Web site, www.annanurse.org.)

1961 Shaldon described a technique for cannulation of femoral veins.

1962 Siliconized rubber used for external shunt loop and Teflon used for vessel tips. A curved loop connected the two cannulas forming the shunt, which was specifically made for each patient. Siliconized rubber segments had steps and bends formed in them to make them more comfortable for patients, and to extend the life of the shunt by bringing it back up to the limb and away from the joint (reverse-winged shunt).

1966 Brescia and Cimino developed the internal arteriovenous (AV) fistula for repeated venipunctures for maintenance hemodialysis.

1966 Ramirez developed the straight-winged shunt for better stabilization and easier declotting.

1966 Buselmeier shunt developed.

1972 Allen-Brown shunt developed.

1974 Bovine carotid artery graft used for circulatory access.

1975 Gore-tex® graft became commercially available for use as AV access for hemodialysis.

1977 Umbilical cord vein used for AV graft.

1977 Expanded polytetrafluoroethylene (ePTFE) used as AV conduit for hemodialysis.

1979 Uldall developed a catheter that allowed repeated cannulation of subclavian vein for temporary access for hemodialysis; introduced the concept of subclavian vein as temporary access to avoid destruction of peripheral vessels that later may be needed for creation of permanent vascular access. This led to the development of subclavian and jugular vein catheters that could be used as permanent circulatory access for hemodialysis when peripheral vasculature was inadequate to support creation and patency of either an AV fistula or an AV graft.

1980 Button needle-free vascular access for hemodialysis developed.

1980 Interventional radiology procedures for the (circa) treatment of underlying anatomic stenotic lesions emerged.

1980 Urokinase used for thrombolysis of AV access, (circa) especially catheters.

1983 The tunneled, cuffed catheter for long-term hemodialysis access introduced.

1997 National Kidney Foundation/Dialysis Outcome Quality Initiative (NKF-DOQI) Clinical Practice Guidelines published.

1998 Trials began for subcutaneous port/catheter devices for hemodialysis.

1999 Clinical Performance Measures (CPMs) based on the NKF-DOQI guidelines were introduced.

1999 Centers dedicated to vascular access were established with many using interventional nephrologists.

1999 Urokinase was removed from the market. Other lytics came to the forefront, most notably tissue plasminogen activator (tPA), to fill the need to lyse clot in thrombosed accesses.

2001 The DOQI guidelines were revised and renamed the Kidney Disease Outcomes Quality Initiative (KDOQI). The most significant change in these Vascular Access guidelines was in the section on Monitoring and Surveillance.

2003 The National Vascular Access Improvement Initiative (NVAII) began because the AVF growth and the catheter reduction goals in the KDOQI guidelines were not being realized. It soon came to be known as the Fistula First Program and in March 2005, this program was elevated by CMS to breakthrough initiative status and is now known as the Fistula First Breakthrough Initiative (FFBI).

2006 The KDOQI guidelines for Vascular Access were revised with major format changes. There are now eight clinical practice guidelines (CPG) and a section for clinical practice recommendations (CPR) with specific recommendations for pediatrics. The CPGs are evidence-based. The CPRs are supported by a combination of weaker evidence and expert opinion. Four topics were intensively reviewed and revised for this iteration and all others updated. While the goal for long-term catheter reduction (< 10%) is unchanged, the goal for AVFs, incident and prevalent, is now 65% (NKF KDOQI, 2006, CPG 8). It is to be noted that the KDOQI guidelines are not standards of care.

Chapter 58

Patient Evaluation for Long-term Access Selection

This chapter is based on NKF KDOQI, 2006, CPG 1.

I. **Patient history.** To optimize the choice of access type and placement, the following factors must be assessed.

A. Dominant arm.

B. Exercise capacity and current arm strength training (Leaf et al., 2003; Oder et al., 2003).

C. History of:
1. Previous vascular catheters, peripheral or central.
2. Previous vascular surgery for access.
3. Needle phobia.
4. Pacemaker or internal defibrillator.
5. Other arm, neck, breast, chest surgery, or trauma.
6. Any cardiovascular disease including stroke.
7. Diabetes mellitus.
8. Coagulopathies.
9. Other life-threatening comorbidities (e.g., malignancies).

D. Current anticoagulation therapy.

E. Kidney replacement therapy (KRT) modality plan.
1. Scheduled transplant from a living donor.
2. Potential candidate for peritoneal dialysis.
3. Undergoing a trial of hemodialysis to help decide between KRT or palliative care option.

II. **Physical examination.**

A. Examine skin for scarring.

B. Check arterial blood supply in all extremities, noting:
1. Character of peripheral pulses.
2. Color of digits.
3. Temperature of hands and feet.
4. Presence of lesions.
5. Deficits in function.

C. Perform Allen test (see Table 12.1).

D. Listen to apical pulse for rate and rhythm.

E. Measure bilateral upper arm blood pressures to detect differences in arterial flow.

F. Examine venous drainage in all extremities.
1. Compare both arms for:
   a. Presence and degree of edema.
   b. Differences in size (evidence of venous and/or lymphatic obstruction).
   c. Patency of veins noting compressibility and mobility of superficial veins in arms.
   d. Note degree of change in superficial vessels with application of tourniquet.
2. Compare both legs for:
   a. Presence and degree of edema.

Standards of Nursing Care for Vascular Access

The nephrology nurse:
A. Assesses the patient and collects comprehensive data pertinent to the maturation or routine management of the access for HD therapy.
B. Analyzes the assessment findings and/or data to determine normalcy of the access or the presence of pathology.
C. Identifies expected individual patient outcomes.
D. Develops a plan of care to attain the patient outcomes.
E. Implements the plan by:
1. Coordinating the delivery of care and assuring appropriate documentation.
2. Providing patient education including self-management.
F. Evaluates the status of the patient's progress in attaining the stated outcomes individually and as part of the vascular access team using the CQI process.

Table 12.1 ——— Allen Test

1. Patient clenches the fist of one hand to produce pallor in the hand.
2. Clinician occludes arterial flow by compressing both radial and ulnar arteries.
3. Patient opens clenched fist.
4. Clinician releases pressure on the ulnar artery and counts the seconds required for color to return to the hand. More than 3 seconds indicates decreased ulnar arterial supply to the hand if the radial artery is used for the vascular access.
5. Repeat the procedure, but release pressure on radial artery this time to assess radial arterial flow to hand.
6. Repeat procedure with opposite hand.

  b. Difference in size (evidence of lymphatic and/or venous obstruction).
  c. Presence of varicosities.
3. Look for swelling and presence of collateral veins in chest wall and neck indicating central venous obstruction.

III. Diagnostic evaluation.

A. Duplex ultrasound mapping of the upper extremity arteries and veins for all patients.

B. Central vein evaluation in the patient known to have:
  1. Previous catheter, pacemaker, and/or internal defibrillator.
  2. Edema or unilateral enlargement in the extremity of choice.
  3. Collateral veins above the planned access site.
  4. Evidence of any surgery or trauma to the neck, chest, breast, or arm involving the planned access vessels.

C. Central venography can be accomplished with dilute contrast, CO_2, magnetic resonance imaging (MRI), duplex ultrasound to avoid nephrotoxicity and preserve residual kidney function. However, gadolinium-based contrast agents for MRI should not be used in patients with CKD stage 4 or 5 due to risk of nephrogenic systemic fibrosis (NSF) (FDA, 2007).

Chapter 59

Vascular Access Type and Site of Placement

This chapter is based on NKF KDOQI, 2006, CPG 2.
Vascular access should be placed distally and in the upper extremities whenever possible. Because AVF provides the access with the longest patency rates and need for fewest interventions (Huber et al., 2003; NKF, 2006; Pisoni et al, 2002) options for AVF creation should be considered first, followed by prosthetic grafts, if AVF creation is not possible. Catheters should be avoided for HD and used only when the previous options are not possible, are contraindicated by the patient's condition, or the access for hemodialysis is short-term.

I. Arteriovenous fistulae (AVF).

A. Definition. A surgically created opening between an artery anastomosed to a juxtapositional

(nearby) vein allowing the high pressure arterial blood to flow into the vein causing engorgement, enlargement, and wall thickening. This process is known as arterialization or maturation of the vein and is necessary to provide a vessel with adequate flow for hemodialysis and sufficiently strong to effectively cannulate. The outflow vessel should be naturally superficial or surgically superficialized. The artery and the anastomosis site should never be cannulated. A variety of surgical anasomotic techniques are used to create the fistula and are illustrated in Figure 12.1.

B. Anatomic locations. The sites for creation of an AVF are limited only by the patient's suitable vasculature and the skill and creativity of the clinicians creating and caring for it.

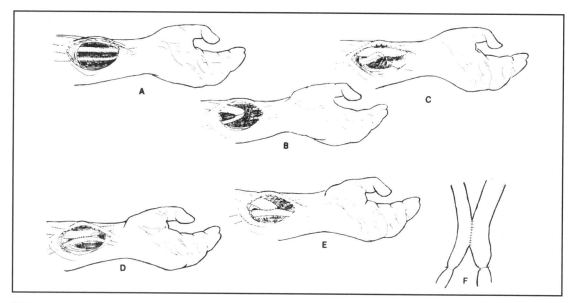

Figure 12.1. Examples of various configurations for AV fistula anastomoses: (a) normal artery-vein relationship, (b) end-to-end anastomosis, (c) end-vein to side-artery anastomosis, (d) side-to-side anastomosis, (e) side-vein to end-artery anastomosis, (f) side-to-side converted to end-to-end anastomosis.

C. Placement in order of priority.
  1. A wrist (radial-cephalic) primary fistula (see Figure 12.2).
  2. An elbow (brachial-cephalic) primary fistula.
  3. An upper arm (brachial-basilic) fistula with vein transposition.

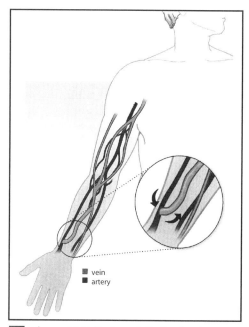

Figure 12.2. Preferred site for fistula. Actual site may vary depending on patient.

Used with permission from Arrow International Inc.

D. Classification of AVFs. The traditional AVF (such as the radial-cephalic or brachial-cephalic) is created with just the construction of the AV anastomosis — a one-step procedure, sometimes known as a primary fistula. With the increased impetus to give priority to AVF creation, more innovative surgical techniques are being used to superficialize the outflow vein such as transposition (surgically dissecting out and tunneling in a superficial, accessible area of limb) of the vein or surgical removal of the tissue between the skin and the vein (Roberts, 2005). AVFs with vein transposition are frequently created with two separate procedures to allow for arterialization of the vein prior to superficialization.

E. Indication for AVF creation. A fistula should be placed at least 6 months prior to the anticipated start of hemodialysis treatments. This timing allows for access evaluation and additional time for revision to ensure a working, fully functional fistula is available at initiation of dialysis (NKF KDOQI, 2006, CPG 1). Patients should be considered for construction of a fistula after failure of every dialysis AV access. In the patient performing PD, who is manifesting signs of modality failure, the decision to create a backup fistula should be individualized by periodically reassessing need (NKF KDOQI, 2006, CPG 2).

F. Advantages of AVF accesses.
1. Have the lowest rate of thrombosis and require the fewest interventions, providing longer survival of the access (Huber et al., 2003; Pisoni et al., 2002).
2. Have lower rates of infection than grafts (which, in turn, are less prone to infection than percutaneous catheters and subcutaneous port catheter systems).
3. Cost of implantation and access maintenance are the lowest long-term.
4. Are associated with increased survival (Dhingra et al., 2001) and lower hospitalization rates.
5. Avoid the complications associated with the venous anastomosis in AVGs.
6. Avoid potential for allergic response to synthetic materials.
7. Outflow veins are autogenous tissue which seals and heals after cannulation. Synthetic grafts only seal by means of a fibrin plug.
8. Can utilize the buttonhole cannulation technique.

G. Disadvantages of AVF accesses.
1. The vein may fail to enlarge or increase wall thickness (i.e., fail to mature). This may be caused by inadequate inflow or the presence of collateral or accessory veins that divert both volume and pressure from the intended outflow vein.
2. AVFs have comparatively long maturation times. Weeks to months must elapse following creation of these fistulae before they can be used. If the access has not been created several weeks in advance of the anticipated need for dialysis, an alternative method of vascular access must be used while the fistula matures.
3. In some individuals, the vein may be more difficult to cannulate than an AVG.
4. AVF creation and cannulation require different skill sets than for AVGs. Proficiency in one type of access does not assure proficiency in the other.
5. Thrombosed AVF may be more difficult in which to restore flow.
6. The enlarged vein may be visible, especially in the forearm and perceived as cosmetically unattractive by some individuals.
7. A hypertrophied outflow vein may significantly increase cardiac output (in turn increasing cardiopulmonary recirculation), and myocardial load and may cause steal syndrome in patients with compromised peripheral vasculature.

H. Complications of AVFs (KDOQI, 2006, CPG 5).
1. Nonmaturing outflow vein and early failure. Primary nondevelopment of the outflow vein may be secondary to:
   a. Insufficient vasculature caused by poor arterial flow and/or small vein size. Signs and symptoms.
      (1) Minimal increase in vein size and bruit limited to anastomosis area.
      (2) Absence of palpable thrill and bruit by auscultation along the outflow vein.
   b. Treatment is surgical revision if possible.
2. Disturbances in flow dynamics that are usually caused by venous stenosis (abnormal narrowing of the lumen of the vessel as a result of injury to the wall causing intimal hyperplasia). Related problems include:
   a. Venous hypertension: engorgement of vessels distal to anastomosis when resistance to flow is greater in proximal veins due to venous stenosis (Schanzer, 2002).
   b. Sore thumb syndrome: engorgement of thumb veins with sometimes painful throbbing or pulsating of distal veins and edema of thumb that may extend to entire hand; cyanotic nail bed with potential for serous oozing if obstruction of venous capillary drainage continues (White, 2006).
   c. Increased venous return can cause arm, breast, neck, chest, and face swelling if stenosis develops in the central vessels.
3. Accessory veins: arterial flow through multiple outflow veins prevents the arterialization of a single outflow vein and therefore the development of a functional fistula; thrill and bruit are present but appropriate vein development is absent. To detect the presence of an accessory vein, occlude the main outflow vein with finger pressure sequentially along the vein. Note the character of the flow with the occlusion. If there is no accessory, the flow will become an augmented pulse. If an accessory vein is present between the anastomosis and the occlusion point, the thrill will continue.
4. Medical diagnostics and treatment.
   a. Doppler ultrasound or fistulogram/venogram to measure flow and detect stenosis. Treatment for hemodynamically significant stenosis is balloon angioplasty.
   b. Treatment for venous hypertension is arm elevation above the level of the heart.
   c. Treatment for accessory veins is surgical ligation or percutaneous coil ablation (coils

are injected into the veins and expand to block and clot the veins) if no stenosis is detected in main outflow vein.

  d. Infection occurring within 3 weeks of surgery is generally considered perioperative infection and is usually prevented by prophylactic antibiotics at the time of surgery.

5. Late failure.

  a. Thrombosis.

    (1) Causes. *Items (a) through (d) are applicable for AVG also.*

      (a) Stenosis of main outflow vein without collateral circulation and/or

      (b) Significant hypotension due to volume depletion.

      (c) Hypercoagulable states.

      (d) Prolonged occlusive compression of access vessel vein from a pressure dressing, tight clothing or jewelry (anything that leaves an impression is too tight), supporting heavy objects such as a basket handle or a sleeping head. (Lifting heavy objects with the hands once the suture line is well healed [> 10 days postoperatively] will not damage the AVF.)

    (2) Signs and symptoms of impending thrombosis. *Items (b) through (h) are applicable for AVG as well.*

      (a) The vein is distended and does not soften when the arm is elevated overhead.

      (b) Significantly decreased intra-access blood flow (400–500 mL/min for AVF and < 600 mL/min for AVG) (NKF KDOQI, 2006, CPG 4).

      (c) Increased static venous pressures and standardized dynamic venous pressures with a ratio:

        [1] >0.5 for AVG venous segment and for AVG arterial segment ratio > 0.75.

        [2] >0.35 for AVF venous segment and > 0.43 for AVF arterial segment (NKF KDOQI, 2006, CPG 4).

      (d) Changes in the quality of the bruit.

      (e) Pulsation rather than thrill.

      (f) Difficulty cannulating or pain with cannulation.

      (g) Evacuation of clots even with needle properly inserted into the center of the vessel.

      (h) Increased viscosity of intra-access flow as evidenced by:

      [1] Difficulty maintaining extracorporeal blood flow at prescribed rate without increase in venous pressure and decrease in arterial pressure.

      [2] Access recirculation causing unexplained decrease in Kt/V and URR – this is a late sign.

      [3] Black blood syndrome that occurs when the same blood is being recirculated through the dialyzer and becomes deoxygenated as well as hemoconcentrated. Lightening of blood color in the arterial line when saline is introduced into the venous line confirms recirculation. This is a very late sign and constitutes an emergency requiring same day intervention.

    (3) Predominant signs of thrombosis in AVF and AVG are the absence of thrill and bruit along the access vessel. There may be a strong pulse in the artery at the inflow anastomosis. Do not cannulate vessel to confirm. Needle holes in a thrombosed access complicate or prevent lytic administration.

    (4) Treatment for AVF and AVG.

      (a) Urgent referral to an interventionalist or surgeon to:

      [1] Prevent thrombosis by detecting and treating stenosis or

      [2] Perform thrombectomy by lysing with a thrombolytic such as tPA (tissue plasminogen activator) to soften or resolve clot. This is frequently used before mechanical thrombectomy and can be followed by correction of causative stenoses if indicated with angioplasty or surgical revision.

      (b) Access monitoring and surveillance postprocedure to assure normal flow and pressure parameters.

      (c) Anticoagulation for proven hypercoagulable states.

      (d) Targeted ultrafiltration to patient tolerance.

      (e) Patient and staff education about prevention of:

      [1] Prolonged occlusive pressure.

      [2] Hypovolemic hypotension.

b. Infection (for both AVF and AVG).
   (1) Causes.
      (a) Poor patient hygiene (Kaplowitz et al., 1988).
      (b) Inadequate skin cleansing for cannulation.
      (c) Not using aseptic technique for cannulation (Schanzer, 2002).
      (d) Seeding from another infected site in the body.
   (2) Signs and symptoms.
      (a) Inflammation.
      (b) Pain.
      (c) Skin break with drainage along the course of the vessel.
      (d) Fever.
   (3) Intervention and treatment.
      (a) Culture of any exudates.
      (b) IV broad spectrum or organism sensitive antibiotics.
      (c) Surgical takedown of AVF if evidence of septic emboli. Surgical resection and removal of affected portion or all of graft.
   (4) Nursing management note: Cannulation of an access with an infected segment should be done *only* with a physician order if dialysis is extremely urgent. The infected area must be avoided.
c. High output cardiac failure (seen in AVF and progresses with AVF maturation).
   (1) Cause. Creation or development of an AVF that shunts more blood through the fistula to the detriment of the peripheral circulation causing tissue hypoxemia and a compensatory increase in cardiac output (Guyton & Hall, 2006). This condition can include the development of left ventricular hypertrophy, high-output cardiac failure, exacerbation of coronary ischemia, and the possible contribution to the development of central vein stenosis (MacRae et al., 2006) and is aggravated by a preexisting anemia and/or cardiovascular disease.
   (2) Signs and symptoms that occur at or near dry weight:
      (a) Tachycardia.
      (b) Shortness of breath.
      (c) Pulmonary crackles.
      (d) Cyanosis of lips and nail beds.
      (e) Pulmonary edema.
      (f) Peripheral edema.
      (g) Jugular vein distension (if patent).
      (h) Confusion.
   (3) Potential complications.
      (a) Pulmonary edema.
      (b) Angina.
      (c) Cardiac dysrhythmias.
   (4) Diagnosis is by:
      (a) Branham's sign: a decreasing pulse rate when the vein is compressed.
      (b) Echocardiography with and without AVF compression.
   (5) Treatment.
      (a) Surgical reduction of flow with a banding procedure or surgical ligation.
      (b) Correct anemia.
      (c) Review cardiac pharmacotherapy.
      (d) To reduce interdialytic symptoms, the AVF and outflow vein can be wrapped with an elastic bandage to reduce cardiac output. This requires a physician's or APN's order. The nurse or patient must be able to comfortably slide an index finger under the bandage to be sure the AVF is not occluded.

II. Arteriovenous grafts (AVG).

A. Definition. A synthetic or, less frequently, biologic conduit implanted subcutaneously and interposed between an artery and a vein. Needles are inserted into the graft (never into the anastomoses) to remove and return blood during hemodialysis. The average graft diameter is 6 mm.

B. Types. Synthetic grafts are usually made of expanded polytetrafluoroethylene (ePTFE/Teflon) and may be tapered for the arterial anastomosis or contain ringed segments to prevent kinking at the apex of the loop. Tapering and external reinforcement have not been shown to significantly improve AVG outcomes (NKF KDOQI, 2006, CPG 2). The composite/polyurethane graft has a temporary advantage over ePTFE. Because of its self-sealing property, it can be cannulated within hours of placement. Biologic grafts are sometimes autogenous vein or cryopreserved human vein but most frequently are from treated bovine vessels. The latter have been shown to provide functional access for patients who have failed PTFE.

C. Indications. Patients who do not have vasculature suitable for AVF or who have a failed AVF in the location of the planned AVG.

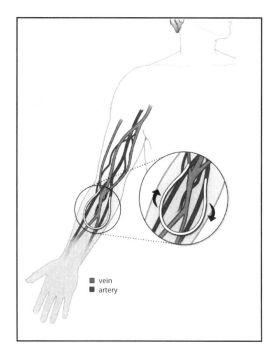

Figure 12.3. Forearm loop graft. Actual site may vary depending on patient.

Used with permission from Arrow International Inc.

D. Anatomic locations, configurations, and placement priority (NKF KDOQI, 2006 CPG 2) (see Figure 12.3).
   1. A forearm loop graft is preferable to a straight configuration.
   2. Upper arm graft – either an arc (preferred) or a loop.
   3. Chest wall or "necklace" prosthetic graft or lower-extremity fistula (rare) or graft; (all arm sites should be exhausted). "Femoral placement of access has been associated with proximal venous stenosis, which may be problematic later in patients receiving kidney transplantation" (NKF, 2006).

E. Advantages of AVGs.
   1. Have a large surface area available for cannulation.
   2. Are technically easier to cannulate than new AVFs.
   3. Lag time from insertion to maturation is short. For ePTFE grafts, it is recommended that not less than 14 days should elapse prior to cannulation to allow healing and incorporation of the surrounding tissue into the graft. Ideally 3–6 weeks are recommended to allow healing of incision and resolution of pain and swelling.

   4. Can be placed in many areas of the body including the upper surface of the thighs and the anterior chest wall.
   5. Can be placed in a variety of shapes to facilitate cannulation.
   6. Are easier for the surgeon to handle, implant, and construct the vascular anastomoses.
   7. Are comparatively easier to repair either surgically or endovascularly (gaining entry through the vascular system rather than through an incision).

F. Disadvantages of AVGs.
   1. Are associated with an increased incidence of thrombosis and infection over an AVF.
   2. Patients have a higher mortality risk than patients dialyzed with fistulae. Those without diabetes have a relative risk (RR) = 1.47, and those with diabetes have a RR = 2.47 (Dhingra et al., 2001).
   3. Have shorter patency rates than AVF (a primary patency in grafts at 18 months of 33% compared with fistulae at 51% and a secondary patency rate of 55% as compared with 77% in fistulae) (Huber et al., 2003).
   4. Cannulation sites seal but do not heal.
   5. Have the potential for an allergic response to nonautogenous material, especially PTFE.
   6. May cause steal syndrome in patients with compromised peripheral vasculature.

G. Complications of AVGs (NKF KDOQI, 2006, CPG 6).
   1. Extremity edema.
      a. Causes. Venous hypertension secondary to increased cardiac output and exacerbated by presence of one or more stenotic lesions in the proximal and central vessels.
      b. Treatment. If newly postoperative, arm should be elevated above the level of the heart whenever the patient is sitting or lying down. If swelling persists beyond 2–3 weeks, imaging to detect pathologic stenosis is indicated and corrected with angioplasty and maybe even stenting for a long, recoiling (returns after angioplasty) stenosis.
   2. Steal syndrome, usually early post-AVG placement, is ischemia of the extremity distal to the arterial anastomosis (may be seen late in AVF with hypertrophied upper arm with flows > 1.5 L/min).
      a. Caused by diverting significant volume of blood away from the peripheral circulation.

b. Complicated by patients, usually elderly, with:
(1) Peripheral vascular disease.
(2) Diabetes.
(3) History of multiple access surgeries in same extremity.

c. Signs and symptoms (that may increase intradialytically).
(1) Pain distal to anastomosis.
(2) Cold, pale hand.
(3) Impaired hand movement and strength.
(4) Paresthesias: numbness, tingling (pins and needles) which increases intradialytically.
(5) Poor capillary refill of affected nail beds (> 2 secs).
(6) May progress to ulcerated, necrotic fingertips.

d. Diagnosis, based on physical examination, can be confirmed with ultrasound to measure arterial flow to fingertips (plethysmyography/PPGs).

e. Treatment.
(1) Surgical reperfusion of the hand using the DRIL (distal revascularization-interval ligation) procedure (Diehl et al., 2003; Knox et al., 2002) while maintaining flow through AVG.
(2) Banding of inflow to AVF to reduce flow.
(3) Severe ischemia not amenable to surgical revision may require urgent ligation of the access.
(4) Symptoms of mild ischemia may be improved with the wearing of a glove, keeping the hand dependent as much as possible, exercise, and massage.

3. Graft degeneration and pseudoaneurysms in AVG and aneurysms in AVF outflow vein.
a. Causes.
(1) AVG. Repeated cannulation in same area of graft leading to extravasation (bleeding) into the incorporating tissue and creating a pseudoaneurysm. The expansion of the pseudoaneurysm can cause stretching of the overlying subcutaneous tissue and combined with the scar tissue of multiple cannulations can lead to compromise of the microcirculation. This causes tissue breakdown and puts the patient at risk for graft rupture.
(2) AVF. Repeated cannulation in same area of vein leading to weakening and subsequent ballooning of the vein wall.

What is the difference between an aneurysm and a pseudoaneurysm?

■ An aneurysm is an abnormal blood-filled dilation of a blood vessel wall (most commonly in arteries) resulting from disease or repeated injury of the vessel wall.

■ A pseudoaneurysm is a vascular abnormality that resembles an aneurysm, but the outpouching is not limited by a true vessel wall, but rather by external fibrous tissue.

Adapted from the glossary (NKF, 2006).

---

b. Signs (2–4 apply to both AVF and AVG).
(1) Sudden appearance of an irregular, pulsatile mass on the surface of the AVG.
(2) Increase in size of the pseudoaneurysm or aneurysm from increased pressure in vessel.
(3) Thinning of the overlying skin over the vessel giving a shiny appearance.
(4) Poor healing of needle sites.

c. Treatment.
(1) Never cannulate into a pseudoaneurysm or a large aneurysm. It causes further vessel degeneration and can be difficult to locate the center of the underlying vessel flow.
(2) A rapidly, progressing pseudoaneurysm or aneurysm is one that is more than twice the diameter of the vessel and must be surgically repaired or a covered stent placed. Those with skin degeneration should be surgically repaired as they put the patient at risk for infection and access rupture that is a life-threatening emergency. Cannulation through a stent is an off-label use of the device and should never be done without a physician's order.

4. Traumatic AVF.
a. Caused by needle passing through the vessel during cannulation and creating an abnormal fistula track between the vessel and an underlying artery. Blood from the artery shunts into the vessel, thereby disturbing the existing flow pattern (White, 2006).
b. Signs.
(1) Abnormal presence of a strong pulsation in area of vessel not previously observed. May be more pronounced than at the arterial anastomosis.

---

(2) Sudden increase in venous pressure not present during previous dialysis session is possible.
   c. Treatment is referral to an interventionalist for evaluation and/or to a surgeon for possible repair.
5. Thrombosis, impending and actual.
   a. Causes.
     (1) Stenosis at the anastomoses, intragraft, the outflow vein or the central veins. Though the venous anastomosis is the most common site of stenosis, inflow stenosis at the arterial anastomosis can be as high as 20 to 25%. Stenosis is the cause of 90% of thrombosed grafts (NKF KDOQI, 2006, CPG 6).
     (2) In the absence of stenosis, causes as for AVF.
   b. Signs of impending thrombosis (same as for AVF), plus:
     (1) Increasing static pressures proximal to the stenosis; can lead to extended time to hemostasis postdialysis and appearance of new pseudoaneurysms.
     (2) Decreasing flow through the graft to < than 600 mL/min.
     (3) Abnormal coagulation studies indicating a hypercoagulable state (LeSar et al., 1999; O'Shea et al., 2003).
   c. Treatment for preventing impending thrombosis.
     (1) Angiography with selective angioplasty of those stenoses that cause > 50% decrease in vessel lumen diameter and reduction in access flow with increased intra-access pressure.
     (2) Anticoagulation or antiplatelet therapy for hypercoagulable state.
     (3) Signs and treatment of thrombosis is as for AVF.
6. Infection (see complications of AVF).

III. Central venous catheters (CVC)/port catheter systems.

Catheters and ports are essential tools for providing urgent and, in some cases, long-term vascular access. Prevention and early treatment of complications should greatly reduce associated morbidity and mortality (NKF KDOQI, 2006, CPG 7).

A. Definition. A synthetic, relatively large (10–22 Fr. outer diameter in adults) tube placed into a high-flowing central vein. Because hemodialysis removes and returns blood at the same time, the catheter either has two side-by-side chambers or lumens (called a dual lumen catheter) or two single lumen catheters (called twin catheters). The end of the catheter that enters the patient's bloodstream is the "tip" and has holes for blood entry or exit. The other end, the "tail," is outside the body with the two lumens separated (see Figure 12.4). Each lumen has a threaded hub on the tail for attaching to the bloodlines. The exit site is where the catheter comes out through the skin. The port catheter system has one or two metal ports under the skin that are attached to single lumen catheters. These are accessed each treatment by cannulas.

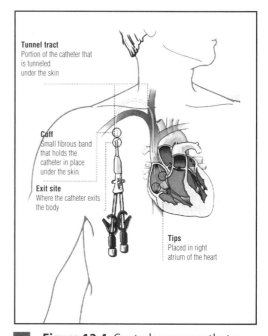

Figure 12.4. Central venous catheter.

Used with permission from Arrow International Inc.

B. Types. Catheters need to be made of rigid, semi-rigid material, or be structurally reinforced to prevent collapse of the lumen. Catheter lengths vary with the size of the patient and the site of placement.
   1. Nontunneled, noncuffed acute catheters for short-term use (see Figure 12.5). These should stay in no longer than a week, and the patient should not be discharged from hospital with this type of catheter. The tips should be in the superior vena cava (NKF KDOQI, 2006, CPG 2.)
   2. Tunneled, cuffed catheters (see Figure 12.6) and port catheter systems are for long-term use only in the patient who:

   a. Is not suitable for an AVF or AVG access.
   b. Has an AVF or AVG planned.
   c. Has an AVF or AVG waiting to mature.
   d. Is waiting for a scheduled live donor transplant.

   3. The tips of the catheter should be in the right mid-atrium with the arterial port medial (for neck and chest placements) (NKF KDOQI, 2006, CPG 2) (see Figure 12.4). The fibrous cuff, positioned about 1 cm from exit site inside the tunnel, is designed to incorporate the tunnel tissue thereby creating a barrier to organism entry as well preventing catheter dislodgment. In chest and neck placements, the exit site is usually a few centimeters below the clavicle. To determine whether the catheter is inserted into the internal jugular (IJ) or the subclavian vein, see Table 12.2.

C. Anatomic locations. Catheters or port/catheter devices should not be placed on the same side as a slowly maturing long-term access (NKF KDOQI, 2006, CPG 2). Catheters are always inserted into veins.
   1. Right internal (or external) jugular vein is the preferred site because this site offers a more direct route to the right atrium than the left-sided great veins (see Figure 12.4). Catheter insertion and maintenance in the right internal jugular vein are associated with a lower risk of complications compared to other potential catheter insertion sites.

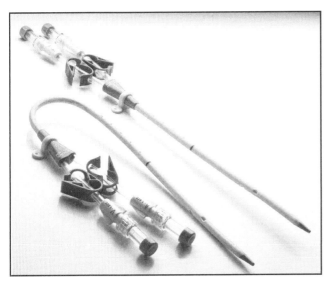

Figure 12.5. Nontunneled, noncuffed acute catheters for short-term use.

Used with permission from Arrow International Inc.

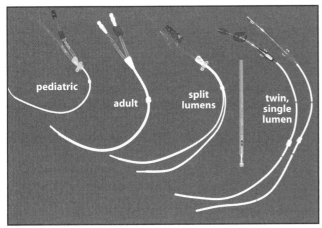

Figure 12.6. Cuffed catheters. The pencil is shown as a size comparison.

Table 12.2

How to Differentiate Between an IJ and a Subclavian Catheter Placement

Inspection
- Where is the exit site — above or below the clavicle?
- Can you see the outline of the catheter in a tunnel?
- Can you see the tunneled catheter crossing the clavicle?

Palpation
- With a gloved hand, feel the skin above the exit site. Can you feel the catheter in a tunnel?
- Trace the tunnel till you can no longer feel the catheter. If it crosses the clavicle, it's jugular. If not, it's probably subclavian.

2. Left internal jugular vein catheter placement potentially puts the left arm's vasculature in jeopardy for a long-term access on the same side. It may also be associated with poorer blood flow rates and higher rates of stenosis and thrombosis than the RIJ due to the increased length.
3. Femoral placement is associated with the highest infection rates and the catheter tip must be in the inferior vena cava to avoid regional recirculation (see Figure 12.7). Placement of a femoral catheter in a transplant candidate should be avoided because of potential damage to blood vessels needed for the transplant.
4. Subclavian veins on either side must be strictly avoided due to risk of stenosis, which can permanently exclude the possibility of upper extremity long-term AVF or AVG (NKF KDOQI, 2006, CPG 2). They should be used only when all access sites are exhausted in the ipsilateral (same side) arm. Subclavian placement puts patient at greater risk for pneumothorax and/or hemothorax during insertion.
5. When all the above sites are exhausted, catheters may be inserted into the inferior vena cava using the translumbar or transhepatic approach.

D. Advantages of catheters/ports.
   1. Are universally applicable – anyone can have one.
   2. Can be inserted into multiple sites relatively easily.
   3. Require no maturation time. They can be used immediately (after tip position is confirmed by fluoroscopy or chest x-ray).
   4. Cause no changes in cardiac output or myocardial load.
   5. Can provide access over a period of months, permitting AVF maturation in patients who require immediate hemodialysis.
   6. Percutaneous catheters only.
      a. Skin puncture not required for repeated vascular access for hemodialysis.
      b. Lower initial cost and replacement costs.

E. Disadvantages.
   1. High morbidity due to thrombosis and infection (Oliver et al., 2004; Pastan et al., 2003). Patients receiving catheters have a relative risk (RR) of death (RR = 2.3 for patients with diabetes and 1.83 for those without) greater than those with an AVF (Dhingra et al., 2001).
   2. Risk of permanent central venous stenosis or occlusion.
   3. Percutaneous catheters only.
      a. Discomfort and cosmetic disadvantage of an external appliance.
      b. Safety concern with inadvertent dislodgment of external appliance as well as need for protection of exit site.
      c. Shorter expected use-life than other access types.
      d. Overall lower blood flow rates, requiring longer dialysis times.
   4. Frequent episodes of occluded catheters due to thrombosis or fibrin sheaths may require use of a lytic agent or an interventional procedure to replace the catheter and possibly disrupt a sheath. These episodes may lead to reduced dialysis adequacy (lower BFRs and shortened or missed treatments) that is associated with increased morbidity and mortality.

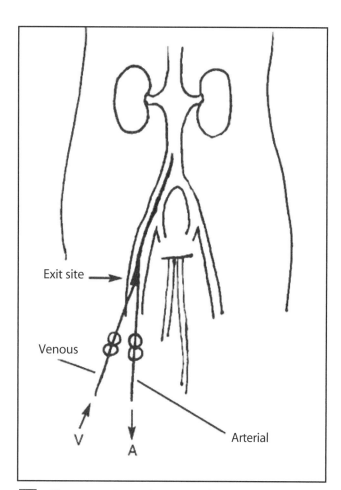

Figure 12.7. Femoral vein central venous catheter.

F. Complications.
  1. Immediate/early.
     a. All catheters should be placed using imaging such fluoroscopy or ultrasound (NKF KDOQI, 2006, CPG 2) to assure correct tip placement and minimize complications such as:
        (1) Carotid or femoral artery puncture.
        (2) Pneumothorax.
        (3) Hemothorax.
        (4) Cardiac dysrhythmias.
        (5) Tissue perforation (e.g., brachial plexus, trachea, superior vena cava, myocardium).
        (6) Poor flow from malpositioned tip.
     b. Operating room conditions and practice must be used for placement to prevent infection.
  2. Late complications.
     a. Infection. Local and systemic.
        (1) Causes.
           (a) Not using aseptic technique and appropriate cleansing for accessing catheter.
           (b) Poor patient hygiene.
           (c) Inadequate skin cleansing at dressing change.
        (2) Signs and symptoms.
           (a) Inflammation and pain around exit site and in tunnel.
           (b) Drainage at exit site or from tunnel.
           (c) Erosion of skin over catheter.
           (d) Fever and/or chills.
        (3) Treatment (NKF KDOQI, 2006, CPG 7).
           (a) IV broad spectrum or organism sensitive antibiotics for all infections except localized exit site where topical and/or oral antibiotics may be used.
           (b) Catheter exchange within 72 hours of initiating antibiotic therapy with follow-up cultures 1 week after antibiotic therapy.
           (c) Antibiotic lock therapy may be used instead of catheter exchange in cases where the patient is clinically stable and/or the catheter is reinfected with the same organism and catheter sites are limited (NKF KDOQI, 2006, CPR 7) (see Section 5, Table 5.6, for sample protocol).
           (d) Port pocket infections are treated with systemic antibiotics and pocket irrigation.

  b. Catheter dysfunction (BFR < 300 mL/min). Exceptions are for pediatric patients and small adults. Dysfunction for these categories is defined by a significant reduction in baseline flows.
     (1) Causes.
        (a) Mechanical. Line and catheter kinking, holes or cracks in catheter, drug precipitation.
        (b) Patient position.
        (c) Partial or complete occlusion due to intraluminal or mural thrombus or fibrin sheath.
     (2) Signs.
        (a) Inability to withdraw anticoagulant lock or blood.
        (b) Inability to maintain consistent BFR > 300 mL/min at an arterial < -250 mm/Hg. Arterial prepump pressure monitoring is mandatory.
        (c) Presence of leak from catheter.
     (3) Treatment. See algorithm in Nursing Process interventions (see Figure 12.8).
  c. Superior vena cava syndrome. Catheter insertion and long-term placement can cause endothelial injury, inflammation, stenosis, and occlusion of any vein. When this occurs in the superior vena cava, it has life-threatening implications and constitutes an emergency to be reported to the physician. It can have slow or rapid onset.
     (1) Signs and symptoms.
        (a) Swelling of the chest/breast, arms, neck, and face with periorbital edema.
        (b) Visible collateral veins on chest wall and jugular vein distension (if patent).
        (c) CNS disturbances such as vision changes, dizziness, confusion, pain.
        (d) Dyspnea (difficulty breathing) and/or dysphagia (difficulty swallowing).
     (2) Treatment.
        (a) Removal of any obstruction including an indwelling catheter.
        (b) Lysing of thrombus with a thrombolytic infusion.
        (c) Angioplasty of identified stenoses. Stents could be placed for recoiling stenoses.

     (Figure 12.8 on next page)

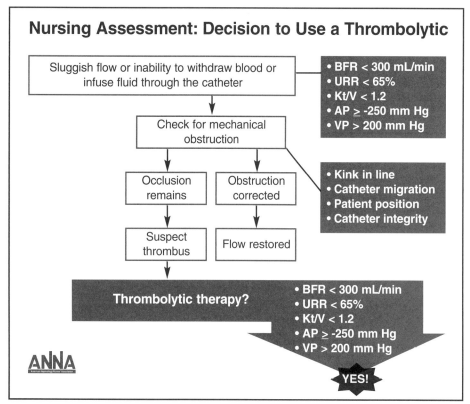

Nursing Assessment: Decision to Use a Thrombolytic

Sluggish flow or inability to withdraw blood or infuse fluid through the catheter

- BFR < 300 mL/min
- URR < 65%
- Kt/V < 1.2
- AP ≥ -250 mm Hg
- VP > 200 mm Hg

Check for mechanical obstruction

Occlusion remains | Obstruction corrected

- Kink in line
- Catheter migration
- Patient position
- Catheter integrity

Suspect thrombus | Flow restored

Thrombolytic therapy?

- BFR < 300 mL/min
- URR < 65%
- Kt/V < 1.2
- AP ≥ -250 mm Hg
- VP > 200 mm Hg

YES!

ANNA

Figure 12.8. Algorithm for catheter dysfunction.

Source: Dinwiddie, L.C. (2004). Managing catheter dysfunction for better patient outcomes: A team approach. *Nephrology Nursing Journal, 31*(6), 653-660.

Needle phobia

Needle phobia has been defined as a formal medical condition and is included in the American Psychiatric Association's Diagnostic and Statistical Manual of Mental Disorders, 4th edition (DSM-IV) within the diagnostic category of Blood-Injection-Injury. Needle phobia is evidenced by a vasovagal reflex (frequently inherited) that causes shock with needle puncture. With repeated needle exposure, those with vasovagal shock reflex tend to develop a fear of needles. According to the DSM-IV, a phobia is defined by the presence of fear and by avoidance behavior. While a dislike or mild fear of needles is very common, needle phobia can be more rigorously defined by objective clinical findings in addition to subjective symptoms.

Source: Hamilton, J.G. (1995). Needle phobia: A neglected diagnosis. *Journal of Family Practice, 41*(5), 437, 512.

Chapter 60

Nursing Process in the Routine Care of Vascular Access

I. Assessment of all accesses, mature or maturing.

A. Assess patient's subjective response to the vascular access, e.g. function, body image, self-concept, fears, need for local anesthesia. Many patients who suffer from needlephobia will require some form of local anesthetic. A cream containing lidocaine 2.5%/prilocaine 2.5% is the best choice. The patient self-administers the cream prior to coming to dialysis. He/she will need to be instructed on needle sites at the previous treatment time. This cream is expensive and can have systemic effects if

too much is absorbed (AstraZeneca, 2005). Therefore it should not be applied all over the vessel. If the patient does not have cream, lidocaine injection or ethyl chloride spray can be used. Lidocaine injections put the cannulator at twice the risk of needle accident and are thought to facilitate scarring as is ethyl chloride. Patients should be assessed frequently to determine if the local anesthetic can be discontinued.

B. Solicit access complaints from patient and evaluate prior to initiation of treatment.

1. Access problems during or since the last treatment.
2. Pain or tenderness at the access or exit site or incisions.
3. Sensations of coldness, numbness, tingling, or pain in access extremity.
4. Impairment of movement or function in access limb.
5. Bleeding or drainage from cannulation site or exit site.
6. Fever or chills.

C. Assessment related to arteriovenous fistula (AVF) or arteriovenous graft (AVG).
   1. Assess the patient's access extremity for:
      a. Character of pulses.
      b. Swelling.
      c. Change in color or temperature.
      d. Numbness or decreased sensation.
      e. Limitations of movement.
      f. Change in function.
      g. Capillary refill > 2 seconds in the nail beds.
      h. Comparison to contralateral (opposite) extremity.
   2. Assess the access vessel area for absence of:
      a. Redness.
      b. Bruising.
      c. Hematoma.
      d. Rash or break in skin.
      e. Bleeding or other exudate.
      f. Atypical warmth.
      g. Tenderness or pain.
      h. Aneurysm or pseudoaneurysm.
   3. Assess the vessel for:
      a. Maturation (see Table 12.3) defined as "the process by which a fistula becomes suitable for cannulation by developing adequate flow and wall thickness" (NKF, 2006).
      b. Direction of flow.
      c. Flow characteristics (thrill vs. pulse) by palpating arterial, mid, and venous sections.
      d. Auscultating for bruit all along the vein or graft noting changes in pitch (the quality of sound: high, medium, or low) and amplitude (the volume or abundance: full, moderate, or low).
      e. Identify cannulation pattern.
         (1) Rotation of sites.
         (2) Presence of buttonholes.

D. Assessment related to the percutaneous catheter and port/catheter device.
   1. Absence of:
      a. Facial or neck edema.
      b. Respiratory distress.

Table 12.3

Rule of 6's for AVF Maturation

- The AVF should be expertly assessed within 6 weeks of creation for maturation.

- Flow through the vessel should exceed 600 mL per min.

- The vessel should be greater than 6 mm in diameter.

- The vessel should be less than 6 mm from the skin surface.

(NKF KDOQI, 2006, CPG 3)

---

   c. Cardiac arrhythmia.
   d. Catheter occlusion as evidenced by inability to withdraw anticoagulant and blood.
   e. Thrombus in the catheter lumens or the vessel wall as evidenced by ease of anticoagulant removal and saline flushing.
   f. Fibrin sheath with tail blocking the tip holes as evidenced by ability to push saline but inability to pull.
   2. Further assessment for percutaneous catheter only.
      a. Integrity of catheter (no cracks, holes) and dressing.
      b. Well-healed exit site, with an absence of:
         (1) Redness.
         (2) Induration or swelling.
         (3) Discoloration or bruising.
         (4) Drainage or bleeding.
         (5) Evidence of catheter migration such as visible cuff.
   3. Further assessment for port/catheter device only.
      (a) Well-healed buttonhole.
      (b) Palpable port directly beneath buttonhole in an even plane, with an absence of:
         (1) Redness.
         (2) Bruising.
         (3) Edema.
         (4) Hematoma.
         (5) Rash or break in skin.
         (6) Drainage or bleeding.
         (7) Atypical warmth.
         (8) Tenderness or pain.

E. Assess the patient during the treatment (keeping catheter site, cannulated areas and connections in clear view at all times) for the following:
1. Complications of cannulation.
2. Degree of pain during cannulation and effectiveness of preventive measures.
3. Securely taped needles.
4. Infiltration or hematoma.
5. Secure connections or disconnected bloodlines.
6. Difficulty achieving or maintaining prescribed blood flow rate.
7. Arterial or venous pressure outside the established parameters.
8. Bleeding or oozing from cannulation site(s) or catheter exit site.
9. Pain.
10. Body temperature greater than established parameter.
11. Air or foam in lines.

F. In conjunction with routine monthly physical assessment, assess AVF or AVG for hemodynamically significant stenoses using one of the following surveillance methods (NKF KDOQI, 2006, CPR 4).
1. Intra-access flow measured at least monthly using one of the several methods outlined in Table 12.4 (NKF KDOQI, 2006, CPR 4).
2. Static venous dialysis pressure every 2 weeks using:
   a. A hydrophobic filter where the pressure is transmitted from the newly placed needle to a sphygmomanometer.
      Or
   b. The protocol in Table 12.5 (NKF KDOQI, 2006, CPR 4).
3. Dynamic venous pressure monitoring every treatment but not an acceptable method if a static pressure cannot be derived.
4. Measure for recirculation (in AVF only) (see Table 12.6).

II. Diagnosis/evaluation.

A. Notify the physician or advanced practice nurse of any predialysis assessment findings that require alteration in the hemodialysis treatment plan. If catheter occlusion or dysfunction is diagnosed proceed with standing orders for thrombolytics or notify physician or nurse practitioner.

B. Evaluate findings indicative of stenosis and report to vascular access team.
1. Decreased flows.

2. Increased pressures.
3. Arm edema.
4. Appearance of collateral veins.
5. Outflow vein of AVF not partially collapsed with arm elevation (predialysis).
6. Increase in postdialysis bleeding time.
7. Difficulty with cannulation.
8. Pain.
9. Altered characteristic of thrill or bruit
10. Recent pseudoaneurysm formation in AVG.

III. Intervention for dialysis treatment.

A. Cannulate AVG or AVF following established KDOQI guidelines (NKF KDOQI, 2006, CPG 3) using strict aseptic technique (see Figure 12.9. for cannulation illustration). For all rotation of sites/rope ladder technique cannulation:
1. Assure that patient has washed his/her hands and access site. For all health care facilities, the CDC recommends 15 seconds of vigorous hand washing with an antibacterial soap, rinsing, and then patting dry with a clean, disposable towel.
2. Wash your hands, wear gloves and personal protective equipment (PPE).
3. Take your time. A prepared, calm, confident cannulator will inspire patient confidence.
4. Confirm direction of flow.
5. Select sites away from recent entries.
6. Choose both sites prior to cannulation – 50% of the discernible vessel should be reserved for the arterial site and the remainder for the

---

Table 12.4

Intra-access Flow Measurement Methods

Duplex Doppler Ultrasound (quantitative color velocity imaging) (DDU)

Magnetic Resonance Angiography (MRA)

Variable Flow Doppler Ultrasound (VFDU)

Ultrasound Dilution (UDT)

Crit-Line III (optodilution by ultrafiltration) (OABF)

Crit-Line III (direct transcutaneous) (TQA)

Glucose Pump Infusion Technique (GPT)

Urea Dilution (UreaD)

Differential Conductivity (HDM)

In Line Dialysance (DD)

Table 12.5

Intra-access Static Pressure Measurement
(Adapted from NKF KDOQI, CPR 4)

1. Establish a baseline when the access has matured and shortly after the access is first used. Trend analysis is more useful than any single measurement.

2. Assure that the zero setting on the pressure transducers of the dialysis delivery system being used has been calibrated to be accurate within ± 5 mm Hg.

3. Measure the mean arterial blood pressure (MAP) in the arm contralateral to the access (MAP = systolic BP + 2 [diastolic BP]/3).

4. Enter the appropriate output or display screen where venous and arterial pressures can be visualized (this varies for each dialysis delivery system). If a gauge is used to display pressures, the pressure can be read from the gauge.

5. Stop the blood pump and cross clamp the venous line just proximal to the venous drip chamber with a hemostat. (This avoids having to stop ultrafiltration for the brief period needed for the measurement.) On the arterial line, no hemostat is needed since the occlusive roller pump serves as a clamp.

6. Wait 30 seconds until the venous pressure is stable. Then record the arterial and venous intra-access pressure (IAP) values. The arterial segment pressure can only be obtained if a pre-pump drip chamber is available and the dialysis system is capable of measuring absolute pressures greater than 40 mm Hg.

7. Unclamp the venous return line and restore the blood pump to its previous value.

8. Determine the height correction, $\triangle$h between the access and the drip chamber(s) either by direct measurement (A) or using a formula (B) based on the difference in height between the top of the drip chamber and the top of the arm rest of the dialysis chair ($\triangle$) . Both measurements need to be in cm. Height corrections are not needed if the measurements in step 6 are done with access level with the drip chamber.

   • Measure the height from the venous or arterial needle to the top of the blood in the venous drip chamber. The offset in Hg = height (cm) x 0.76.

   • Use the formula, offset in mm Hg = 3.6 + 0.35 x $\triangle$.

9. The same correction values can be used for both if the two drip chambers are at the same height. If the drip chambers are not at equal heights, the arterial and venous height offsets must be determined individually. In a given patient with a given access the height offsets need to be measured only once and then used until the access location is altered by construction of a new access.

10. Calculate the normalized arterial and venous segment static IAP ratio(s), P_{IA}/MAP

   Arterial ratio = (arterial IAP + arterial height correction)/MAP

   Venous ratio = (venous IAP + venous height correction)/MAP

Table 12.6

Procedure for Drawing Noninvasive, Two Needles, Stop Flow Percent Recirculation

1. Measure within the first 30 minutes after prescribed blood flow is established.

2. BUN samples are drawn simultaneously from the arterial and venous lines into syringes labeled "arterial" and "venous," then placed in tubes labeled "arterial sample" and "venous sample."

3. Ultrafiltration is reduced to minimum.

4. The blood pump is stopped.

5. Clamp arterial needle and blood lines.

6. Separate the arterial needle and blood line.

7. Withdraw 10 mL from the arterial needle line, keep sterile, and set aside.

8. Within 30 seconds of stopping blood flow, withdraw 5 mL from arterial needle line and place in tube. Label "Systemic Sample."

9. Return the 10 mL of sterile blood that was set aside.

10. Reconnect arterial needle and blood lines.

11. Reestablish blood flow.
Formula for percent recirculation of vascular access:

$$\frac{S - A}{S - V} \times 100 = \% \text{ recirculation}$$

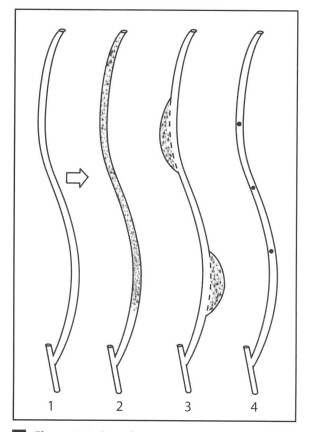

Figure 12.9. Cannulation types.
1. Uncannulated
2. Rope-ladder with site rotation
3. Pseudoaneurysms/one-site-it is
4. Buttonhole/constant site

Source: Twardowski, Z., & Kubara, H. (1979). Different sites vs. constant sites of needle insertion into arteriovenous fistulas for treatment by repeated dialysis. *Dialysis and Transplantation, 8*(10), 978-980. Reprinted with permission of John Wiley & Sons, Inc.

venous needle. Room should be left distal to the venous needle for recannulation if necessary.

7. Choose not only the entry site but the location of the tip once fully inserted. Steel needles do not bend, vessels do.

8. Choose needle length based on vessel depth and available vessel length.

9. Arterial (pull) needle is inserted closest to the arterial anastomosis and can be against the flow (retrograde) or with the flow (antegrade).

10. Venous (return) needle is always antegrade, (i.e., points away from the arterial anastomosis) which helps decrease resistance, and is downstream (closer to the heart in the vascular system) from the arterial needle (to prevent recirculation between the needles) (see Figure 12.10).

11. Never cannulate into anastomoses, aneurysms, or pseudoaneurysms.

12. Needle tip separation is dependent on rate of intra-access flow. Accesses with high flow can tolerate close approximation. Caution should be taken in smaller vessel AVFs with lower flows as

close tip approximation could result in recirculation of blood from the venous needle back to the arterial needle.

13. Prepare skin.
    a. Have patient wash his/her hands and access site with antibacterial soap upon entry to dialysis unit.
    b. Apply 2% chlorhexidine gluconate/70% isopropyl alcohol, 10% povidone-iodine, or 70% isopropyl alcohol to insertion site as per manufacturer's instructions.

    2% chlorhexidine gluconate/70% isopropyl alcohol antiseptic has a rapid (30 seconds) and persistent (up to 48 hours) antimicrobial activity on the skin. Apply solution using back and forth friction scrub for 30 seconds. Allow area to dry. Do not blot the solution.

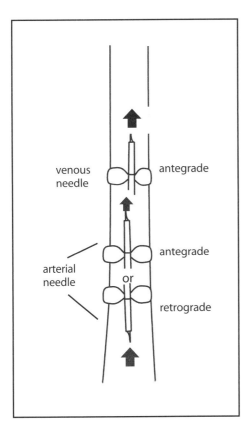

venous needle

arterial needle

antegrade

antegrade

or

retrograde

Figure 12.10. Direction of needles. Venous needle always points toward the venous return, while the arterial needle may point in either direction.

Source: Brouwer, D. (1995). Cannulation camp: Basic needle cannulation training for dialysis staff. *Dialysis and Transplantation, 24*(11), 606-612. Used with permission of John Wiley & Sons, Inc.

Alcohol has a short bacteriostatic action time and should be applied in a rubbing motion for 1 minute immediately prior to needle cannulation.

Povidone-iodine needs to be applied for 2–3 minutes for its full bacteriostatic action to take effect and must be allowed to dry prior to needle cannulation (NKF KDOQI, 2006, CPG 3).

  c. Do not palpate insertion site once area has been cleaned.

14. If intradermal lidocaine 1% is to be used, one syringe with a 25-gauge needle must be used for each site. Intradermal means that the needle is inserted just under the surface of the skin and lidocaine injected to form a bleb about 5 mm in diameter. Lidocaine must not be injected deeper as it may puncture the vessel and cause a hematoma over the vessel.

15. Determine direction of flow. In AVG compress midsection, the end that has the pulse is arterial.

16. Pull skin taut in opposite direction of needle insertion. (This compresses peripheral nerve endings between dermis and epidermis, providing some anesthetic effect and facilitates smoother incision of skin with less surface area contacting the cutting edge and enables better stabilization of vessel. When skin is released, it pushes the needle in direction of insertion rather than away.)

17. Insert needle through skin at angle appropriate to depth of vessel. A flashback of blood signals entry into the vessel.

18. Pause.

19. Hold vessel between nondominant thumb and index finger to stabilize vessel and reorient the needle in the direction of the vessel.

20. Thread the needle all the way to the hub in the center of the flow. Never probe blindly in a poorly defined vessel — get expert help. Such probing can puncture the backwall of the vessel causing bleeding internally (infiltration) and is very painful for the patient. If this occurs, remove the needle, hold pressure, and get help. Never force the needle against resistance. If resistance is encountered, pull the shaft back 1–2 mm, reorient away from resistance and advance to hub.

21. Do not "flip" (rotating axis 180°) needles routinely. Rotating the needle while in the vessel risks cutting or coring the endothelium. Back-eye needles are used for the arterial pull so that flow is maximized. Should rotating the needle be necessary, the needle should be withdrawn at angle of threading, re-angled to angle of entry, rotated, and rethreaded.

22. Tape needles securely using 1-inch tape across the wings to stabilize laterally, and 1/2-inch tape chevroned around wings to place traction in the direction of needle insertion (see Figure 12.11).

23. Flush the needles with saline to assure ease of flow and remove blood from the needle before connecting the extracorporeal circuit.

24. To prevent accidental dislodging of the needles, secure the bloodlines to the patient's limb or clothing (Brouwer, 1995).

B. For AVG cannulation only.
  1. Angle of insertion is approximately 45°. Less steep angles increase risk of dragging the tip along the top surface of the graft material. Steeper angles risk perforating the underside (backwall) of the graft.

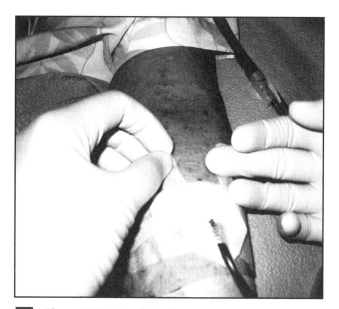

Figure 12.11. Needle taping.
Courtesy of Janet Holland and the FFBI.

2. The first cannulation of the AVG can occur after 2 weeks postoperative with most grafts. Both arterial and venous needles of the standard size should be inserted at the first cannulation. A PTFE graft has optimal flow and size when new and does not require the stepwise process commonly employed for patients with catheters and new AVFs. Assure that heparin administration is stopped one hour prior to termination of dialysis to prevent prolongation of partial thromboplastin time (PTT) and therefore bleeding from needle sites (Hertel, Keep, & Caruana, 2001).

C. For AVF cannulation only.
  1. Always use a tourniquet (firm enough to engorge vessel but not to occlude flow) to increase the surface tension of the skin allowing for a cleaner needle entry.
  2. Angle of insertion is approximately 25 degrees, depending on depth of vessel.
  3. Use rope ladder or constant site, buttonhole technique, with AVF. If the patient has established buttonhole sites but the cannulator does not feel confident doing the buttonhole cannulation, he/she may rotate sites being careful to stay at least 3/4-inch from buttonhole to avoid damaging tunnel wall (Ball, 2006).
  4. The first cannulation of newly matured AVF, if the patient has a functioning catheter in place, is to use one 17-gauge needle for the arterial or

"pull" segment with return to the venous circulation through the catheter. (This is sometimes referred to as the "one and one" method.) Using the needle for the outflow to the dialyzer both assures maturity of the vessel as well as lessens the risk of a severe and painful infiltration if blood is being pumped into the tissues at the rate of 300 mL/min. Attention needs to be directed to the use of heparin in the "one and one" circumstance. A lesser quantity for the loading bolus should be considered as well as making sure that no heparin is given in the last hour of dialysis. The lumen of the catheter not used for dialysis should be flushed and locked at the beginning of treatment so the amount of freshly circulating concentrated heparin is minimized at the end of dialysis. Though it is generally accepted that one needle should be used for three treatments before progressing to using two needles, the nurse should use her judgment to determine when to progress based on the individual patient need (Dinwiddie, 2007).

D. Buttonhole cannulation is the "repeated cannulation into the exact same puncture site and a scar tissue tunnel tract develops. The scar tissue tunnel tract allows the needle to pass through to the (outflow) vessel of the fistula following the same path each time" (Petersen, 2002). The buttonholes should be created by an expert cannulator who has assessed and chosen the most superficial, straight, and problem-free sites on the outflow vein. It takes at least 6 and as many as 12 sharp entries to establish each buttonhole (Ball, 2006; Petersen, 2002). Then the cannulator can switch to "dull" needles for all future cannulations. For cannulation of buttonholes:
  1. Wash your hands, wear gloves and personal protective equipment (PPE).
  2. Take your time. A prepared, calm, confident cannulator will inspire patient confidence.
  3. Prepare skin.
    a. Assure patient washes his/her hands and access site with bacterial soap upon entry to dialysis unit.
    b. Apply 2% chlorhexidine gluconate/70% isopropyl alcohol, 10% povidone-iodine, or 70% isopropyl alcohol to insertion site as per manufacturer's instructions. (See additional notes above in routine cannulation.)
    c. The skin around the buttonhole is then stretched away from the buttonhole and/or soaked with a bactericidal solution to loosen the scab.

d. The scab over the entry site is removed with a sterile piece of gauze or a sterile instrument. Never use the tip of the cannulating needle (Ball, 2006).

e. Perform a second skin cleaning as above after changing gloves.

f. The technique needed to find the vein through the tunnel with a dull needle requires needle insertion into the buttonhole, using a twisting motion if necessary to approach the vein. It may feel like the tip is bouncing on the vein wall as the venotomy can shift in relation to the track, perhaps due to fluid overload. The cannulator should go 20 degrees forward or back till the needle "drops" into the vein. "When the cannulator goes by feel (not sight) you know they've 'got it'" (Petersen, 2002). Think of the track like the hole of a pierced ear. Sharp needles should not be needed once the track is established.

g. Thread the needle all the way to the hub in the center of the flow.

h. Secure the needles as for the rope ladder technique.

E. Catheter accession.
1. Wash your hands. Wear gloves, mask, and appropriate PPE.
2. Patient wears a mask.
3. Clean catheter hub or connection with 10% povidone-iodine or 70% alcohol if the catheter material is suitable (CDC, 2002). Holding the connection site with one swab, clean the catheter away from the hub for 10 cm (4 inches). Discard. Then clean the cap and hub vigorously with the first swab. Allow to dry if using povidone-iodine.
4. Using strict aseptic technique, open catheter. Minimize the time that the catheter lumens are open to air. (There are now catheter caps that can be cleaned and accessed without removal. They are changed weekly, reducing the time that the lumen is exposed significantly.)
5. Withdraw locking solution, discard, and flush lumens with saline assessing for ease of flow.
6. Change dressing during or following each treatment using strict aseptic technique and with patient and clinician wearing masks. Clean the exit site using 2% chlorhexidine gluconate and 70% isopropyl alcohol, 10% povidone-iodine, or 70% alcohol if the catheter material is suitable. Clean twice, starting at the exit site and working outward in a circle, diameter of 10 cm. Chlorhexidine requires a scrubbing motion.

Allow to dry before applying the dressing which can be either gauze and tape or a transparent, breathable, plastic dressing. The dressing should be changed at each dialysis treatment and the patient should be taught to keep it clean and dry (NKF KDOQI, 2006, CPG 3). However, there are some chlorhexidine impregnated patches that are changed weekly.

F. Connect patient per facility procedure, turn flow to 200 mL/min, check vital signs, flow pressures, and patient comfort prior to setting prescribed flow.

G. Maintain visibility of the access and connections at all times.

H. Postdialysis, using appropriate PPE for staff/patient and strict aseptic technique.
1. Remove needles from AVG, AVF, or port at the same angle as entry using the needle safety device and discarding needles into sharps container immediately.
2. Compress the peripheral sites with two fingers following complete removal of the needle. (Pressure on the needle bevel is painful for the patient and can damage the vessel.) A new transparent sealing device that is taped over the needle at the insertion site at the time of insertion allows visualization of the insertion site during treatment and requires only one fingertip for hemostasis posttreatment.
3. Do not occlude the blood flow in peripheral access (check thrill distal to the site of pressure).
4. It is optimal to remove one needle at a time and have the patient hold pressure to hemostasis.

The Purpose of Locking Solutions for Catheters

Because there is no flow through the catheter between treatments, the blood must be flushed from both lumens and an anticoagulant locking solution must be instilled to prevent clot formation to maintain patency. Traditionally heparin in varying strengths has been used, but with the awareness of the contribution of bacteria-proliferating biofilm to the patient's risk of bacteremia, it has become apparent that the ideal locking solution should be both antimicrobial and anticoagulant. Such a solution is citrate 4% that is now FDA allowed (2007). Other prophylactic locking solutions are being investigated.

Many patients cannot "hold their sites," and clamps must sometimes be used. It is noteworthy, though, that some facilities have successfully "outlawed" clamps. Staff must be vigilant in leaving the clamps for the minimum time only if there is no alternative.

5. Sites can be dressed with an adhesive bandage, gauze, and tape that should neither be circumferential nor tight. Patients should be taught to remove any pressure dressing on arriving home and the adhesive bandage the next day.

6. For catheter (both percutaneous and port) disconnect.
   a. Clean the connections.
   b. Flush both lumens with 10 mL saline.
   c. Firmly infuse anticoagulant lock (usually 5000 units heparin per mL — to the volume of the lumen), displacing saline, and quickly reclamp lumen to prevent negative pressure in catheter pulling blood in the side holes.

7. Percutaneous catheter only: cap per facility protocol.

8. Remove port needles and apply light pressure for 1 minute. Gently massage the pockets to evacuate any old blood.

IV. Interventions to treat dialysis-related complications.

A. AVG or AVF complications.
   1. Poor flow.
      a. Reposition needle.
      b. If recannulation is required, use nursing judgment on whether to remove the initial, failed needle. Consider the amount of systemic heparin and the ability to hold pressure without compromising blood flow.
      c. Treat hypotension, if present.
   2. Infiltration.
      a. Do not recannulate if patient has a catheter access till the swelling has receded.
      b. Apply ice intermittently for the first 24 hours, then heat.
      c. If unable to clearly feel and see vessel and the patient has no catheter and needs dialysis, the Vascular Access Team (VAT) should consider the use of a short-term catheter.
   3. Bleeding. Attempt hemostasis, if bleeding persists, report to nephrologist or advanced practice nurse.
   4. Infection. Do not cannulate without medical caregiver's order. Obtain cultures, report findings and initiate antibiotic therapy as ordered.
   5. Thrombosis. Report immediately to vascular access team.
   6. Ischemia in limb. Report immediately to vascular access team.
   7. Skin breaks on shiny aneurysms or pseudoaneurysms or other risk of rupture. Report immediately to vascular access team.

B. Catheter and port/catheter complications.
   1. Algorithm for poor flow (less than 300 mL/min) (Dinwiddie, 2004; NKF KDOQI 2006, CPG 7) (see Figure 12.11).
      a. Check for and correct mechanical obstruction such as kinking of catheter or lines or clamp indentation.
      b. Check for dislodgement of catheter as evidenced by cuff extrusion from exit site. Do not push the catheter back in. Tape in place and report to vascular access team.
      c. Reposition patient. Putting the patient supine returns them to the position in which they were when the catheter was inserted and may reposition the tip of the catheter in the right atrium. Also when the patient is supine or in the Trendelenburg position, the central veins are maximally engorged. Changing the position of the head or having the patient cough can also increase flow.
      d. Flush each lumen with 10 mL of saline.
      e. Reverse lines (using aseptic technique and cleaning connections) to determine if arterial lumen port is malpositioned. If flow improves significantly without increase in arterial or venous pressure, continue treatment but report to vascular access team for further study.
      f. If flow problem persists the cause is likely to be thrombus in the lumens or on the wall of the vessel or a fibrin sheath. If the catheter flushes with ease but cannot pull, a fibrin sheath may be present. Use a thrombolytic agent per standing orders.
      g. Report flow problem to vascular access team if flow is not corrected to prescribed levels.
   2. Exit site infection as evidenced by purulent drainage.
      a. Obtain culture.
      b. Initiate antibiotic therapy as ordered.
      c. Report findings.
   3. Exit site bleeding.
      a. Aseptically attempt hemostasis.
      b. If bleeding persists, report to vascular access team.
   4. Fever and/or chills.
      a. Notify medical caregiver.
      b. Obtain blood cultures.
      c. Initiate antibiotic therapy as ordered.

d. Report findings.
e. Obtain surveillance cultures 1 week after antibiotics.

V. Interventions/evaluations for CQI.

A. Each center should establish a database and CQI process to track the types of accesses created and the complication rates for these accesses (NKF KDOQI, 2006, CPG 8).
1. The goals for permanent HD access placement should include:
a. Prevalent functional AVF placement rate of greater than 65% of patients.
b. Cuffed catheter for permanent dialysis access (e.g., not as a bridge) in less than 10% of patients. Chronic catheter access is defined as the use of a dialysis catheter for more than 3 months in the absence of a maturing permanent access — graft or fistula.
2. The primary access failure rates of HD accesses in the following locations and configurations should not be more than the following:
a. Forearm straight grafts: 15% (for each 100 AVGs placed, less than 15 should fail within 30 days).
b. Forearm loop grafts: 10%.
c. Upper arm grafts: 5%.
d. Tunneled catheters with a blood flow < 300 mL/min: 5%.
3. Access complications and performance.
a. Fistula complications/performance should be as follows:
(1) Fistula thrombosis: < 0.25 episodes per patient year at risk.
(2) Fistula infection: < 1% over the use-life of the access.
(3) Fistula patency of > 3.0 years (by life table analysis).
b. Graft complications/performance should be as follows:
(1) Graft thrombosis: < 0.5 thrombotic episodes per patient year at risk.
(2) Graft infection: < 10% over the use-life of the access.
(3) Graft patency >2 years (by life table analysis).
(4) Graft patency following PTA: > 4 months.
c. Catheter complications/performance should be as follows:
(1) Tunneled catheter-related infection < 10% at 3 months, and < than 50% at 1 year.
(2) The cumulative incidence of the following insertion complications should not exceed 1% of all catheter placements:
(a) Pneumothorax requiring a chest tube.
(b) Symptomatic air embolism.
(c) Hemothorax.
(d) Hemomediastinum.
(e) Hematoma requiring evacuation.
(3) Cumulative patency rate of tunneled cuffed catheters (TCCs): not specified.
(4) Efficacy of corrective intervention. The rate of certain milestones after correction of thrombosis or stenosis should be as follows:
(a) AVF patency following PTA: > 50% unassisted patency at 6 months (and < 30% residual stenosis post-procedure or lack of resolution of physical findings postprocedure).
(b) AVF patency following surgery: > 50% unassisted patency at 1 year.
(c) AVG patency following PTA: > 50% unassisted patency at 3 months and < 30% postprocedure residual stenosis or lack of postprocedure resolution of physical findings.
(d) AVG patency following surgery: > 50% unassisted patency at 6 months and > 40% at 1 year.
(e) AVG after either PTA or surgery: > 90% with postprocedure restoration of blood flow and > 85% postprocedure ability to complete one dialysis treatment.
(f) Surgical correction is set to a higher standard because of the use of venous vasculature, reducing the options for future sites.
4. Document vascular access data and findings appropriately. Maintain database to reflect:
a. Number of each type of functional access. Functional access is the access that is being used for dialysis. An AVF should not be recorded as the functional access until it can support extracorporeal flow independent of a catheter (i.e., two needles).
b. Surveillance data.
c. Incidence of infection.
d. Incidence of thrombosis.
5. Participate in CQI process/care planning with the vascular access team.
6. Initiate consultations or request referrals, as appropriate.
7. Do patient teaching.

a. Purpose and type of access.
b. Vein preservation.
    (1) Peripheral (both arms).
    (2) Blood draws and IV placement from/in the dorsum (back) of hands, never from the access arm.
    (3) Central. Avoid subclavian catheters.
c. Preferred access.
d. Exercises for maturation of AVF once surgical incisions are healed.
    (1) Squeezing a rubber ball with a light tourniquet on upper arm twice daily for forearm vein and muscle development.
    (2) Biceps curls with weight to tolerance for upper arm vein and muscle development.
e. Care and protection of access including:
    (1) Identifying activity and clothing appropriate for vascular access type and site.
    (2) Not allowing BP cuffs on access arm.
    (3) Not allowing catheter to be used for any purpose other than hemodialysis (CDC, 2000).
    (4) How to assess for patency in AVG or AVF.
    (5) Signs and symptoms of infection.
    (6) Signs and symptoms of complications, management strategies, and information to report to nurse.
    (7) Hand washing and access cleansing/disinfection prior to hemodialysis for AVF/AVGs.
    (8) Purpose of rotation of cannulation sites.
    (9) Purpose and care of the buttonholes.
    (10) Proper cannulation techniques.
    (11) Proper compression of access for hemostasis.
    (12) The appropriate site dressing and when to remove it.
    (13) Proper catheter connection techniques.
    (14) How to prevent catheter dislodgment.
f. Emergency care: prolonged bleeding from needle sites. Instruct how to hold pressure with clean fabric. If bleeding continues, contact medical provider (physician/NP/PA) on call or go to emergency room.
g. Absence of thrill or bruit. Go to dialysis unit to have staff check. If dialysis unit is closed patient should contact medical provider (physician/NP/PA) on call.
h. Emergency care: grafts or fistula rupture. Teach patient and family to place a tourniquet (such as a belt) above the point of rupture, and call 911.
i. Partial catheter dislodgment. Patient should tape catheter in place to prevent further movement and contact dialysis unit as soon as possible for instructions for access repair.
j. Accidental catheter removal. Patient should lie down and have pressure held on site for at least 10 minutes. Site should be covered with a clean dressing. If bleeding continues contact medical provider (physician/NP/PA) on call or go to emergency room. Otherwise, patient should contact dialysis unit as soon as possible to arrange for new access.
8. Self-management of access to the extent possible and the benefits of self-cannulation if appropriate.

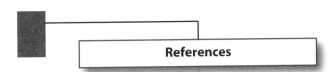

Allon, M. (2004). Dialysis catheter-related bacteremia: Treatment and prophylaxis. *American Journal of Kidney Disease, 44*(5), 779-791.

AstraZeneca. (2005). *EMLA cream.* Retrieved August 1, 2006, from http://www.astrazeneca-us.com/pi/EMLA.pdf

Ball, L. (2006). The buttonhole technique for arteriovenous fistula cannulation. *Nephrology Nursing Journal, 33*(3), 299-304.

Beathard, G. (2003). Catheter management protocol for catheter-related bacteremia prophylaxis. *Seminars in Dialysis, 16*(5), 403-405.

Brouwer, D.J. (1995). Cannulation camp: Basic needle cannulation training for dialysis staff. *Dialysis and Transplantation, 24*(11), 606-612.

Burrows-Hudson, S., & Prowant, B. (2005). *Nephrology nursing standards of practice and guidelines for care.* Pitman, NJ: American Nephrology Nurses' Association.

Centers for Disease Control and Prevention (CDC). (2002). Guidelines for the prevention of intravascular catheter-related infections. *Morbidity and Mortality Weekly Report, Recommendations and Reports, 51*(RR-10A), 1-29.

Dhingra, R.K., Young, E.W., Hulbert-Shearon, T.E., Leavey, S.F., & Port, F.K. (2001). Type of vascular access and mortality in U.S. hemodialysis patients. *Kidney International, 60,* 1443-1451.

Diehl, L., Johansen, K., & Watson, J. (2003). Operative management of distal ischemic complications of upper extremity dialysis access. *American Journal of Surgery, 186*(1), 17-19.

Dinwiddie, L.C. (2000). Identifying the insertion site of a central vein catheter. *Nephrology Nursing Journal, 27*(3), 326.

Dinwiddie, L.C. (2004). Managing catheter dysfunction for better patient outcomes: A team approach. *Nephrology Nursing Journal, 31*(6), 653-660.

Dinwiddie, L.C. (2007). Cannulation of hemodialysis vascular access: Science and art. In A.R. Nissenson & R.N. Fine (Eds.), *Handbook of dialysis therapy* (4th ed., pp. 383-392). Philadelphia: Saunders.

Food and Drug Administration (FDA). (n.d.). *FDA alert.* Retrieved May 31, 2007, from http://www.fda.gov/medwatch/safety/2007/safety07.htm#

Hertel, J., Keep, D., & Caruana, R. (2001). Anticoagulation. In J. Daugirdas, P. Blake, & T. Ing (Eds.), *Handbook of dialysis* (3rd ed., pp. 182-198). Philadelphia: Lippincott Williams & Wilkins.

Huber, T.S., Carter, J.S., Carter, R.L., & Seeger, J.M. (2003). Patency of autogenous and polytetrafluoroethylene upper extremity arteriovenous hemodialysis accesses: A systematic review. *Journal of Vascular Surgery, 38*(5), 1005-1011.

Kaplowitz, L.G., Comstock, J.A., Landwehr, D.M., Dalton, H.P., & Mayhall, C.G. (1988). A prospective study of infections in hemodialysis patients: Patients hygiene and other risk factors for infections. *Infection Control Hospital Epidemiology, 9*(12), 534-541.

Katzman, H.E., Glickman, M.H., Schild, A.F., Fujitani, R.M., & Lawson, J.H. (2005). Multicenter evaluation of the bovine mesenteric vein bioprostheses for hemodialysis access in patients with an earlier failed prosthetic graft. *Journal of the American College of Surgeons, 201*(2), 223-230.

Knox, R.C., Berman, S.S., Hughes, J.D., Gentile, A.T., & Mills, J.L. (2002). Distal revascularization-interval ligation. *Journal of Vascular Surgery, 36*(2), 250-255.

Leaf, D.A., MacRae, H.S., Grant, E., & Kraut, J. (2003). Isometric exercise increases the size of forearm veins in patients with chronic renal failure. *American Journal of Medical Science, 325,* 115-119.

LeSar, C.J., Merrick, H.W., & Smith, M.R. (1999). Thrombotic complications resulting from hypercoagulable states in chronic hemodialysis vascular access. *Journal of the American College of Surgeons, 189*(1), 73-79.

MacRae, J.M., Levin, A., & Belenkie, I. (2006).The cardiovascular effects of arteriovenous fistulas in chronic kidney disease: A cause for concern? *Seminars in Dialysis 19*(5), 349-352.

National Kidney Foundation (NKF). (2006). KDOQI clinical practice guidelines for vascular access: Update 2006. *American Journal of Kidney Diseases, 48*(1), S176-S307.

Oder, T.F., Teodorescu, V., & Uribarri, J. (2003). Effect of exercise on the diameter of arteriovenous fistulae in hemodialysis patients. *ASAIO Journal, 49,* 554-555.

Oliver, M.J., Rothwell, D.M., Fung, K., Hux, J.E., & Lok, C.E. (2004). Late creation of vascular access for hemodialysis and increased risk of sepsis. *Journal of the American Society of Nephrology, 15,* 1936-1942.

O'Shea, S.I., Lawson, J.H. Redden, D., Murphy, M., & Ortel, T.L. (2003). Hypercoagulable states and antithrombotic strategies in recurrent vascular access site thrombosis. *Journal of Vascular Surgery, 38*(3), 541-548.

Paston, S., Soucie, J.M., & McClellan, W.M. (2002). Vascular access and increased risk of death among hemodialysis patients. *Kidney International, 62*(2), 620-626.

Peterson, P. (2002). Fistula cannulation: The buttonhole technique. *Nephrology Nursing Journal, 29*(2), 195.

Pisoni, R.L., Young, E.W., Dykstra, D.M., Greenwood, R.N., Hecking, E., Gillespie, B., et al. (2002). Vascular access use in Europe and the United States: Results from the DOPPS. *Kidney International, 61,* 305-316.

Roberts, C. (2005). Saving a brachiocephalic fistula using lipectomy. *Nephrology Nursing Journal, 32*(3), 331.

Schanzer, H. (2002). Overview of complications and after vascular access creation. In R.J. Gray & J.J. Sands (Eds.), *Dialysis access: A multidisciplinary approach* (pp. 93-97). Philadelphia: Lippincott Williams & Wilkins.

Twardowski, Z., & Kubara, H. (1979). Different sites vs. constant sites of needle insertion into arteriovenous fistulas for treatment by repeated dialysis. *Dialysis and Transplantation, 8*(10), 978-980.

White, R.B. (2006). Vascular access for hemodialysis. In A. Molzahn & E. Butera (Eds.), *Contemporary nephrology nursing: Principles and practice* (2nd ed., pp. 561-578). Pitman, NJ: American Nephrology Nurses' Association.

Section 13

Peritoneal Dialysis

Section Editor

Barbara F. Prowant, MS, RN, CNN

Authors

Leonor P. Ponferrada, BSN, BSHSM, RN, CNN

Barbara F. Prowant, MS, RN, CNN

Roberta J. Satalowich, BS, RN, CNN

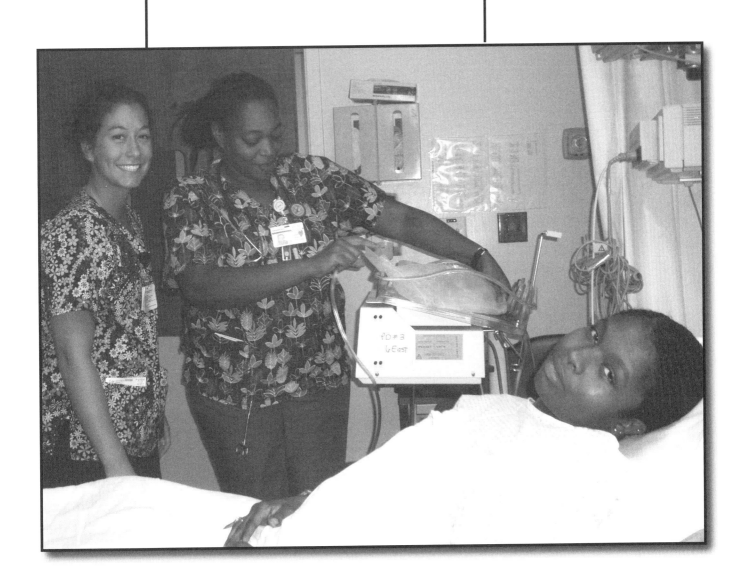

About the Authors

Barbara F. Prowant, MS, RN, CNN, Section Editor and Author, is a Research Associate in the Division of Nephrology, Department of Internal Medicine, at the University of Missouri in Columbia, Missouri.

Leonor P. Ponferrada, BSN, BSHSM, RN, CNN, is the Quality Management Coordinator at Dialysis Clinic, Inc., in Columbia, Missouri.

Roberta J. Satalowich, BS, RN, CNN, is a Staff Nurse in the Home Dialysis Department at Dialysis Clinic, Inc., in Columbia, Missouri.

Section 13

Peritoneal Dialysis

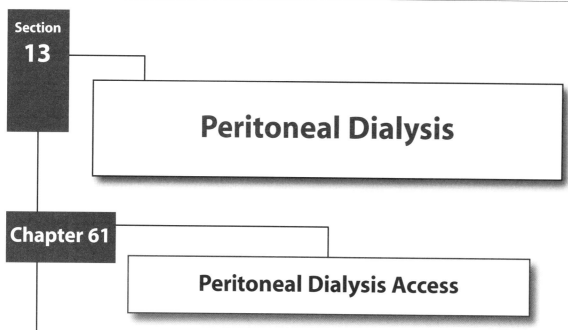

Section

13

Peritoneal Dialysis

Chapter 61

Peritoneal Dialysis Access

Purposes

The purposes of this chapter are to provide:
1. A brief history of peritoneal dialysis (PD) catheters.
2. A description of the catheters currently used for peritoneal dialysis.
3. An overview of catheter implantation and exit site healing.
4. A review of principles of nursing care for the PD access.
5. A cognitive understanding of etiology, assessment, and management of catheter-related complications.

Objectives

Upon completion of this chapter, the learner will be able to:
1. Differentiate between catheters used for acute and chronic peritoneal dialysis.
2. Discuss key characteristics of at least three different catheters used for chronic peritoneal dialysis.
3. State two functions of the cuffs used on chronic peritoneal dialysis catheters.
4. Describe four components of nursing care prior to peritoneal dialysis catheter insertion.
5. Cite two goals of peritoneal catheter break-in procedures.
6. State two ways intraabdominal pressure can be minimized after catheter insertion.
7. Differentiate between characteristics of normal healing of the catheter exit site after catheter insertion and early infection.
8. Differentiate between immediate postoperative and long-term care of the peritoneal dialysis catheter exit site.
9. Discuss basic principles of chronic peritoneal dialysis exit site care.
10. List at least six exit site features that are evaluated during a catheter exit site assessment.
11. List at least five activities or conditions that are detrimental to the peritoneal catheter exit site.
12. Discuss the risk factors, pathophysiology, nursing assessment, and collaborative management of the following complications related to the peritoneal dialysis access:
    a. Exit site infection.
    b. Catheter cuff or tunnel infection.
    c. Catheter malfunction.
13. List five indications for catheter removal and discuss under what circumstances simultaneous removal and reimplantation might be appropriate.

Where Level I or Level II evidence exists, treatment recommendations are identified as evidenced-based. Level I evidence is based on results from multiple well-designed, randomized, prospective, controlled studies. Level II evidence is based on at least one well-designed randomized, prospective, controlled study.

History

I. Earliest devices for PD access.

A. In the early years of PD, devices used for other medical procedures were used for PD access. These included needles, cannulas, sump drains, and Foley catheters. Many of the early procedures used two catheters: one for infusion, placed higher in the peritoneal cavity, and the other in the pelvis for drainage.

B. 1923 – Ganter used a needle for access in the first reported use of PD in a human.

C. 1927 – Heusser and Werder reported use of a needle for infusion and a rubber drain with multiple side perforations for drainage.

D. 1934 – Balázs and Rosenak performed continuous flow PD with two cannulas made of glass or fine wire with a bulbous tip and multiple holes.

E. 1937 – Wear, Sisk, and Trikle used two gall bladder trocars for acute PD. The drainage trocar had multiple side holes in the distal third.

F. 1946 – Fine, Frank, and Seligman reported continuous flow dialysis for acute renal failure using combinations of stainless steel tubes, whistle tip, and mushroom-type catheters for inflow and outflow devices. This was the first report of rubber catheters inserted through a trocar. They also reported the use of heparin to minimize fibrin formation and adhesions.

G. 1946 – Weiss and Mills reported use of a sump drain for outflow.

II. Development of access specifically for peritoneal dialysis.

A. 1948 – Rosenak and Oppenheimer develop the first "drain" specifically for PD. The intra-peritoneal segment was a spiral, stainless steel wire with a rounded tip and a plate for fixation to the abdominal wall. This was the first commercially available PD catheter.

B. 1948 – Frank, Seligman, Fine, and colleagues first reported use of a longer subcutaneous tunnel.

C. 1948 – Odel, Ferris, and Power first used polyvinyl for the drain catheter. The tubing had multiple perforations to drain the dialysate. Both inflow and outflow tubes were weighted to keep the tips in the true pelvis. They argued against the use of inline bacterial filters, because they reduce flow rates and provide a potential site for multiplication of microorganisms.

D. 1949 – Dérot and colleagues described a polyvinyl catheter inserted through a trocar.

E. 1951 – Grollman and colleagues reported a polyethylene plastic catheter, inserted through a trocar.

F. 1959 – Maxwell and colleagues used a "nonirritating," semi-rigid, nylon catheter with a rounded tip and numerous tiny side holes.

G. 1959 – Doolan et al. used a polyvinyl chloride catheter with grooves (20 per inch) designed to prevent omental wrapping.

H. 1962   Merrill and colleagues credit the availability of plastic catheters and commercial dialysis solution as instrumental in the wide acceptance of PD for treatment of renal failure in humans.

I. 1962 – Boen and colleagues implanted Teflon or rubber tubes in the abdominal wall for re-insertion of the catheter in intermittent peritoneal dialysis. This was known as "Boen's button."

J. 1962 – Gutch and colleagues reported on the successful use of a less rigid, more comfortable polyvinyl catheter left in place for 110 days in a patient with chronic renal failure.

K. 1963 – Barry and colleagues from Walter Reed Hospital reported a new catheter with a balloon at the distal end. After placement in the peritoneal cavity, the balloon was filled with saline to extend it.

L. 1963 – McDonald developed a smaller trocar specifically for PD. This significantly reduced leaks and bleeding.

M. 1963 – Palmer and Quinton developed a silicone rubber PD catheter with a coiled intraperitoneal segment: the prototype for current coiled catheters. The catheters were used for chronic renal failure and remained in place up to 2 years, but had problems associated with a tri-flange step located in the tunnel segment.

N. 1964 – Mallette and colleagues developed a conical shaped "button" implanted subcutaneously. The skin was punctured and a catheter inserted through the button for each treatment.

O. 1965 – Weston and Roberts invented a sharp, 3-sided, steel stylet that fit inside the PD catheter for insertion, eliminating the need for general anesthesia, and creating a snug fit around the catheter, further reducing the incidence of leaks.

P. 1968 – Tenckhoff and Schechter published results with a silicone elastomer (Silastic®) catheter for chronic dialysis with two Dacron® polyester felt cuffs, one preperitoneal and one below the skin. The relatively short subcutaneous tunnel and straight intraperitoneal segment allowed implantation at the bedside. Tenckhoff and colleagues also developed a trocar for catheter insertion and described in detail a bedside insertion technique. The "Tenckhoff catheter" was commercially produced, was widely used, and remains the most common catheter for PD access. It became the "gold standard" of peritoneal access, and is the prototype for most modern catheters.

Q. 1968 – McDonald and co-workers developed a Silastic catheter with a Dacron sleeve extending to the peritoneum and a velour "skirt" located just beneath the skin exit. This was the first of several attempts to locate the barrier just beneath the skin or at the skin surface, based on the premise that the sinus was the major cause of exit and tunnel infections.

R. 1968 – A dual lumen catheter was developed for continuous flow peritoneal dialysis.

S. 1969 – Deane's prosthesis, a short Teflon rod the same diameter as the catheter with a plastic head, was inserted into the sinus tract after catheter removal, keeping the established track open. The rod was removed for catheter placement for the next treatment. This was produced commercially and used through the early 1970s.

T. 1973 – The Goldberg catheter had larger side holes and a balloon located 3 inches from the tip. After insertion, the balloon was inflated with saline. The purpose of this "cuff" was to prevent obstruction of the catheter side holes by omentum.

U. 1976 – The Toronto Western Hospital (TWH) catheter had three silicone discs placed on the intraperitoneal segment to reduce the incidence of catheter migration.

V. 1980 – Ash and colleagues developed the "column disc" catheter implanted in the left lower quadrant.

W. 1981- Ash and colleagues successfully placed Tenckhoff catheters using peritoneoscopy.

X. 1982 – TWH-2 catheter was shorter than the original Toronto catheter and had only two silicone discs. This catheter had a Dacron disc or flange and silicone bead at the deep cuff to create a better seal and prevent leaks. It is still used, primarily in Canada.

Y. 1982 – Reports of successful placement of peritoneal dialysis catheters using laparoscopic technique.

Z. 1983 – The relatively short intraperitoneal segment of the Valli catheter is within a balloon reinforced with a longitudinal Silastic ring and two Silastic cords to keep it distended.

AA. 1983 – Lateral placement with deep cuff fixed in the rectus muscle was reported to decrease leakage and prolong catheter life.

BB. 1984 – The Gore-Tex® catheter was made of Silastic with a polytetrafluoroethylene (PTFE) flange and cuff. The flange was located subdermally with a collar protruding through the skin.

CC. 1985 – A short catheter was implanted very low, just above the symphysis pubis, based on the theory that a very short catheter could not migrate out of the true pelvis. This catheter was later named the Vicenza catheter and is still used, primarily in Europe.

DD. 1985 – Twardowski and colleagues developed a swan-neck catheter with a bent or curved subcutaneous segment. The goal was to overcome the problems associated with catheter shape memory, when a straight Silastic catheter is placed in a curved or arched tunnel (cuff extrusion and catheter malposition).

EE. 1987 – Antibiotics were bonded to PD catheters and tested in animals.

FF. 1988 – Cruz reported development of a polyurethane "pail-handle" catheter. This is currently manufactured and used in the United States.

GG. 1988 – Ash reported that a catheter with an intraperitoneal silver disc implanted in dogs was biocompatible and suggested that coating a PD catheter with silver, which has antimicrobial properties, would reduce infections at the catheter surface.

HH. 1990 – Antibiotic bonding to catheters prior to insertion did not decrease infections in humans.

II. 1990 – Japanese researchers used an alumina ceramic connector for the sinus portion of a PD catheter.

JJ. Early 1990s – many reports of successful laparoscopic surgery for malfunctioning or malpositioned catheters.

KK. 1991 – Moncrief and Popovich reported a technique for catheter implantation leaving the external segment buried subcutaneously for 4 weeks to allow healing and tissue ingrowth into cuffs in a sterile environment. Then the external segment is "exteriorized." This technique continues to be used with a variety of catheters.

LL. 1992 – Moncrief and colleagues reported a modified Silastic, swan-neck, coiled catheter with the subcutaneous cuff lengthened to 2.5 cm. Both ends of the cuff were tapered. This catheter was implanted with the external segment buried as described above. This catheter, manufactured in North America, is distributed and used in many countries.

MM. 1992 – A swan-neck catheter with a long tunnel, third cuff, and presternal exit site on the chest was developed by Twardowski and colleagues in an effort to reduce exit site complications and contamination. This presternal catheter is currently used in both adults and children.

NN. 1992 – A German group patented a silver ring that fits over the external segment of the catheter

just external to the exit site so the antimicrobial properties of silver would reduce bacterial colonization at the exit site.

OO. 1993 – A "T-fluted catheter" was developed with flutes or grooves along the surface to channel fluid. The intraperitoneal segment of this T-shaped catheter lies against the parietal peritoneum. Thus, the catheter cannot migrate. This catheter is manufactured in North America.

PP. 1996 – A "self-locating" catheter with a tungsten weight at the catheter tip was manufactured in Italy. This catheter remains in use in Europe.

QQ. Table 13.1 summarizes key developments leading to current PD catheter designs.

RR. Table 13.2 summarizes key developments leading to current catheter implantation techniques.

Peritoneal Dialysis Catheters

I. Acute catheters.

A. The rigid, nylon stylet catheter is designed for one acute use only (see Figure 13.1). These catheters and the bedside insertion technique are rarely used for patients with chronic kidney disease (CKD), so they are mostly of historic interest.
1. It is recommended that acute stylet catheters be used for no more than 48–72 hours.
2. Advantages.
   a. May be inserted by physician at the bedside.
   b. Dialysis may be initiated immediately.
   c. Less expensive than a cuffed, silicone catheter.
   d. Catheter is easily removed.
3. Disadvantages.
   a. Catheter rigidity.
      (1) Increased risk of organ perforation.
      (2) Causes discomfort to patient.
   b. Flow is not as reliable as with flexible Silastic catheters.
   c. Increased incidence of dialysate leak, which then increases the risk of infection.
   d. Risk of intraperitoneal catheter loss.
   e. Risk of peritonitis increases with length of use.
   f. Must be reinserted for each acute peritoneal dialysis treatment.

B. Single-cuff Silastic catheters.
1. Used almost exclusively for acute dialysis in North America.

Table 13.1

Key Developments in the Evolution of Current PD Catheters

1927 – Drain with multiple side holes used for PD
1948 – First commercially available PD catheter
1948 – Longer subcutaneous tunnel
1963 – Silicone rubber catheter material
1963 – Coiled intraperitoneal segment
1968 – Dacron polyester cuffs; double-cuffed catheter
1968 – Double-lumen catheter for continuous flow peritoneal dialysis
1982 – Flange and bead at deep cuff (TWH; later Missouri swan-neck)
1985 – Bent or curved tunnel segment (swan-neck catheter)
1988 – Polyurethane catheter material (Cruz catheter)
1992 – Longer, tapered cuff on Moncrief catheter
1992 – Presternal catheter exit site

Table 13.2

Key Developments in the Evolution of Current PD Catheter Implantation Techniques

1937 – Gall bladder trocars used for catheter insertion
1963 – Smaller trocar designed for PD catheters
1965 – Stylet designed for catheter insertion; anesthesia not required for this technique
1981 – Peritoneoscopic technique for catheter placement
1982 – Laparoscopic technique for catheter insertion
1983 – Lateral placement with deep cuff fixed in the rectus muscle
1991 – Technique to leave the external segment buried subcutaneously during healing (Moncrief-Popovich technique)

2. Require surgical insertion.
3. May continue to be used as chronic access, if necessary.
4. More comfortable than rigid nylon catheter.
5. Less risk of leak or perforation.
6. Procedures and care similar to chronic catheters.

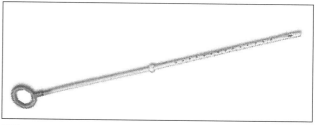

Figure 13.1. Polyvinyl catheter for acute peritoneal dialysis, threaded on stylet used for catheter insertion.

II. Features of chronic catheters.

A. Catheter materials.
   1. Most are made of silicone with a 5 mm outer diameter and 2.6 mm inner diameter. Silicone catheters typically have a radiopaque stripe to allow visualization on x-ray.
   2. The Cruz® catheter is made of polyurethane and has a 3.1 mm inner diameter. The catheter material is radiopaque.
   3. The Flex-Neck® and Advantage™ catheters are made of a special silicone rubber material. These catheters have an inner diameter of 3.5 mm.

B. Catheter segments.
   1. The intraperitoneal segment is approximately 11–15 cm in length and contains numerous 0.5–1 mm side holes as well as an open tip for solution flow.
   2. The subcutaneous segment is approximately 5–7 cm in length and passes from the peritoneal membrane through the muscle and subcutaneous fat to the external cuff or skin.
   3. The external segment is external to the subcutaneous cuff or skin exit.

C. Standard commercially available catheters come in a variety of sizes.
   1. Short and long intraperitoneal segments for very short or tall patients, or for surgical insertion very high or low in the abdomen.
   2. Longer subcutaneous segment for obese patients. Very short subcutaneous segment for very thin patients.
   3. Pediatric and neonatal sizes have shorter lengths and smaller diameters.

D. Catheter cuffs.
   1. Cuff material is usually polyester (Dacron).
   2. The purpose of the cuffs is to provide material for fibrous tissue ingrowth to:

a. Fix the catheter position and prevent piston-like movement with respiration and activity.
   b. Prevent migration of bacteria.
   c. Prevent dialysate leaks.

E. Placement of the cuffs.
   1. A double-cuff catheter typically has one cuff placed in the muscle just anterior to the posterior rectus sheath and the other cuff placed ~ 2 cm from the skin exit (subcutaneously).
   2. A single-cuff catheter may have the cuff placed either in the preperitoneal or subcutaneous position.
      a. Subcutaneous cuff position is recommended for acute dialysis catheters, due to ease of removal.
      b. Cuff positioned preperitoneally is recommended for chronic single-cuff catheters.

F. Double-cuff catheters have been shown to have higher survival rates in chronic PD patients.

G. Historically, single-cuff catheters have been associated with more exit infections, shorter time to first peritonitis, and shorter survival. However, a prospective study found that catheters with a single-cuff placed in the preperitoneal position had similar outcomes to double-cuff catheters (Eklund, Honkanen, Kyllonen, Salmela, & Kala, 1997).

H. Catheter adapters.
   1. The catheter adapter fits into the open end of the chronic PD catheter and provides a means of joining the catheter and solution administration set.
   2. Adapters are made of titanium, other lightweight metals, or plastic polymers.
   3. Adapters are inserted at the time of catheter placement.
   4. Each catheter adapter is made to fit the inner lumen of a specific size catheter.
      a. If the catheter lumen is larger than is appropriate for the adapter, the adapter may be loose or fall out.
      b. If the catheter lumen is smaller than is appropriate for the adapter, the adapter may damage the catheter.

I. A specific catheter adapter may only fit administration tubings from the same manufacturer. However, devices are available to make adapters compatible with other PD systems.

III. Chronic catheter function.

A. Features of an ideal PD catheter include reliable inflow and outflow, rapid flow rates, no leaks, and few infectious complications.

B. With standard silicone catheters, a 2-liter exchange volume infuses in less than 10 minutes and drains in 15–20 minutes.

C. The longer and more curved a catheter is, the longer it will take to infuse and drain. However, differences are not clinically significant.

D. Catheters made from materials with thinner walls and larger interior lumens have significantly faster flow rates.

E. The outflow rate decreases when about 75% of the volume has been drained. Toward the end of the drain, the outflow is very slow, almost imperceptible.

F. Even with a well-functioning catheter, there is typically 300–500 mL residual volume remaining in the peritoneal cavity at the end of the drain.

IV. Chronic catheters.

A. Chronic catheters most frequently used in North America are shown in Figure 13.2.

B. Straight Tenckhoff catheter.
   1. The straight double-cuff Silastic catheter developed by Tenckhoff and Schechter is the second most widely-used catheter worldwide.
   2. Tenckhoff recommended a curved, arch-shaped tunnel with both the intraperitoneal and external segments directed caudally.
   3. May be implanted with trocar or surgically; does not require a laparotomy for removal.

C. Curled or coiled catheter.
   1. Modification of the straight Tenckhoff catheter with a coiled intraperitoneal segment to prevent catheter migration.
   2. Most widely used catheter worldwide.
   3. May be inserted with a trocar or surgically; does not require laparotomy for removal.
   4. Advantages.
      a. The coiled catheter does not become malpositioned as frequently as the straight Tenckhoff.
      b. Decreased infusion pain.

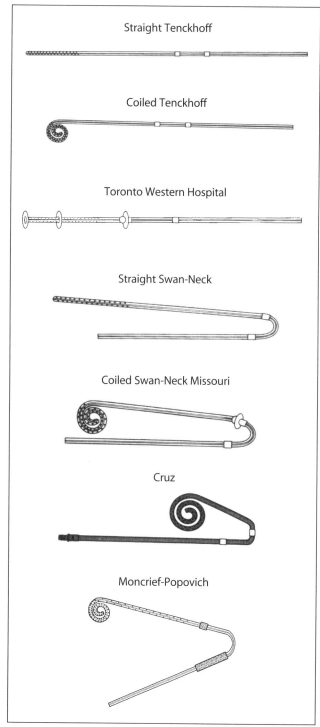

Straight Tenckhoff

Coiled Tenckhoff

Toronto Western Hospital

Straight Swan-Neck

Coiled Swan-Neck Missouri

Cruz

Moncrief-Popovich

Figure 13.2. Chronic peritoneal dialysis catheters. From top: Double-cuff Tenckhoff catheter with straight intraperitoneal segment; double-cuff Tenckhoff catheter with coiled intraperitoneal segment; Toronto Western Hospital catheter with preperitoneal flange and bead and intraperitoneal discs; swan-neck catheter with straight intraperitoneal segment; swan-neck Missouri catheter with preperitoneal flange and bead and coiled intraperitoneal segment; Cruz catheter with coiled intraperitoneal segment; Moncrief-Popovich catheter with wider tunnel angle and longer subcutaneous cuff.

c. Decreased incidence of pain from catheter tip pressure against organs.

D. The Toronto Western Hospital (TWH) catheter is a straight double-cuff catheter with two perpendicular discs around the distal segment. The purposes of the discs are to hold omentum and bowel away from the catheter and to retain the catheter position in the pelvis.
   1. TWH catheter has a 1 cm Dacron disc or flange on the base of the peritoneal cuff and a silicone bead 1 mm below the disc. This forms a groove in which the surgeon tightly ties the peritoneum.
   2. TWH catheters must be implanted and removed surgically.
   3. Advantages.
      a. Fewer drain problems.
      b. A lower incidence of malposition.
      c. A lower incidence of pericatheter leaks.
   4. Catheter survival is similar to that of Tenckhoff catheters.

E. Swan-neck catheters.
   1. The straight Tenckhoff and coiled Tenckhoff catheters have been modified by curving the subcutaneous tunnel segment at a 170° arc angle to form a "swan-neck" in the tunnel segment.
   2. The purpose of the permanently curved tunnel segment is to avoid the problems that occur when the catheter gradually straightens due to "shape memory" (catheters moving out of the pelvis, and subcutaneous cuffs pushing out through the exit site).
   3. A stencil should be used to mark the insertion and exit sites so that the catheter is implanted in a similarly shaped tunnel.
   4. The swan-neck Missouri catheter has adapted the preperitoneal disc and bead from the TWH catheter, but placed them at an angle for a tighter seal. It must be surgically implanted. Because of the curved tunnel and slanted flange, catheters are specific for the right or left side.
   5. Advantages.
      a. Decreased incidence of early drainage failure due to catheter migration.
      b. Lower incidence of cuff extrusion.
      c. Lower incidence of pericatheter leaks in swan-neck Missouri catheters.
      d. Catheter survival may be somewhat improved.

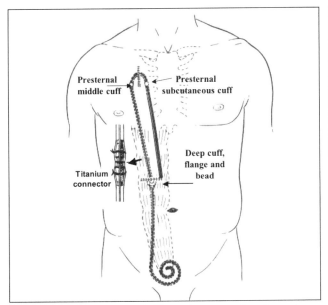

Figure 13.3. Swan-neck Missouri presternal peritoneal dialysis catheter.

Source: Twardowski, Z.J., Prowant, B.F., Pickett, B., Nichols, W.K., Nolph, K.D., & Khanna, R. (1996). Four-year experience with swan neck presternal peritoneal dialysis catheter. *American Journal of Kidney Diseases, 27*(1), 99-105. Used with permission.

F. Presternal catheter.
1. This catheter is a modification of the swan-neck Missouri catheter with the exit site located in the parasternal area of the chest (see Figure 13.3).
2. The catheter has two sections joined by a titanium connector at the time of implantation: the lower section includes the coiled intra-peritoneal segment, the deep cuff and part of the tunnel segment. The upper section includes the rest of the tunnel section with an arch-shaped segment between two cuffs and the external segment.
3. Rationale for the presternal catheter.
   a. The chest wall is subject to far less motion than the abdomen, facilitating healing.
   b. The catheter exit is farther away from abdominal ostomies, gastrostomy tubes, and diapers in infants, reducing the risk of cross-contamination.
   c. There is less subcutaneous fat in the presternal or parasternal area than the abdomen. The presternal catheter has been recommended for patients with body mass index > 35.
   d. Patients may take tub baths.
4. Has been implanted surgically, by laparoscopy, percutaneously or using the Moncrief-Popovich method. However, implantation is more difficult than that of abdominal catheters.

5. Longer length causes a somewhat slower flow rate.
6. There is a slight risk of disconnection in the tunnel, but this is extremely rare in adults. It is more of a risk in growing infants and children.
7. Survival is similar to that of swan-neck abdominal catheters.

G. Cruz catheter.
1. This double-cuff catheter has a "pail handle" configuration in the tunnel segment. This is formed by two 90-degree bends, one just outside the exit and one behind the subcutaneous cuff.
2. The pail-handle design helps to ensure caudal direction of both the coiled intraperitoneal segment and the exit site.
3. Made of polyurethane, which is radiopaque.
4. The catheter material is damaged by polyethylene glycol, mupirocin ointment, and alcohol. There have been reports of catheter cracking and breaking. There has also been a report of cuffs becoming loose after several years.
5. The catheter wall is thinner, and the diameter of the inner lumen is larger than standard silicone catheters, which provides faster inflow and outflow rates.
6. Theoretically, other advantages of this catheter would be similar to those listed for swan-neck catheters above.

H. The Moncrief-Popovich catheter.
1. A double-cuff, swan-neck catheter with an elongated subcutaneous cuff (2.5 cm), tapered at either end.
2. When this catheter is implanted, the external segment is completely buried under the skin in the subcutaneous tunnel. The external segment is brought out through a surgical incision 3–5 weeks later.
3. The major theoretical advantage is decreased catheter-related infections. Other outcomes are similar to other swan-neck catheters.

I. The T-fluted (Ash Advantage) catheter.
1. Has a T-shaped design, so that the intraperi-toneal segment, which is at a right angle to the external segment, lies against the abdominal wall.
2. The intraperitoneal segment has grooves or flutes along the entire length to channel the dialysis fluid as it infuses and drains.
3. These catheters have a somewhat shorter drain time and lower residual intraperitoneal volume compared to Tenckhoff catheters.

Table 13.3

Characteristics of Catheters Implanted in 2004

	U.S. – Adults	U.S. – Pediatrics	Worldwide Adults
Tenckhoff	59%	58%	65%
Swan-neck	36%	42%	26%
Cruz	5%	0	4%
Moncrief-Popovich	1%	0	1.5%
Double-cuff	94%	56%	94%
Coiled IP segment	95%	100%	70%
Surgically implanted	76%	67%	72%

Data from a 2005 survey of 63 PD programs

Source: Negoi, D., Prowant, B.F., & Twardowski, Z.J. (2006). Current trends in the use of peritoneal dialysis (PD) catheters. *Advances in Peritoneal Dialysis, 22*, 147-152.

J. Literature reviews for evidence-based guidelines have found that no PD catheter has proven superior to the standard double-cuff Tenckhoff catheter in prevention of peritonitis.

K. A recent study suggests that the optimal catheter and exit site location for an individual patient may be determined by gender and anthropometric measurements (Crabtree, Burchette, & Siddiqi, 2005).

V. **Currently used chronic catheters** (see Table 13.3).

A. The Tenckhoff catheter is still the most widely used throughout the world, followed by swan-neck catheters.

B. More swan-neck catheters are used in pediatric than adult units, and in Europe compared to the rest of the world.

C. Almost all adult catheters are double-cuffed, in contrast to 56% of pediatric catheters.

D. Almost all catheters in the United States and the majority throughout the world have coiled intraperitoneal (IP) segments.

E. The use of swan-neck and coiled catheters has increased over the past decade.

Catheter Placement

I. **Acute catheter insertion.**

A. Minimum preparation for acute catheter insertion.
   1. Ensure that bladder is empty to decrease the risk of perforation during catheter insertion.
   2. Relieve constipation to decrease the risk of bowel perforation during catheter insertion.
   3. Remove hair with electric clippers.
   4. Obtain baseline weight and vital signs.
   5. Administer preoperative sedative/narcotic as ordered.

B. Percutaneous or bedside insertion procedure for rigid stylet (uncuffed) catheter for acute dialysis. As mentioned above, this is rarely used for patients with CKD and is mostly of historical interest.
   1. Usually performed at bedside or in a treatment room by physician with nurse circulating.
   2. Most supplies are included in the kit with the acute catheter.
   3. Staff must mask, scrub, gown, and glove.
   4. Abdomen is scrubbed with povidone-iodine and draped.
   5. Skin and subcutaneous tissues are infiltrated with local anesthetic.
   6. A small stab wound is made in the midline, 2–3 cm below the umbilicus.
   7. The stylet and catheter, or a large bore, blunt needle is inserted through the incision.

8. The patient is asked to raise the head and neck to tighten the abdominal muscles and increase the intraabdominal pressure. Then the peritoneal membrane is punctured. An audible pop may be heard, and there is markedly less resistance.
9. 2–3 L of dialysis solution is infused. This provides a cushion of fluid anterior to the mesentery and bowel, which decreases the risk of trauma or perforation while positioning the peritoneal catheter.
10. The catheter is maneuvered toward the coccyx and then advanced deep into the pelvis.
11. A small shield or device is placed at the skin exit to prevent intraperitoneal loss of the catheter.
12. If necessary, the skin is closed and/or catheter secured with sutures.
13. Antibacterial ointment is applied to the incision site.
14. Sterile dressings are applied.
15. The catheter is connected to the PD system and dialysis exchanges are initiated immediately.

C. Nursing responsibilities during percutaneous insertion procedure for rigid stylet (uncuffed) catheter for acute dialysis.
1. Gather appropriate supplies and equipment.
2. Prepare and support patient.
3. Baseline vital signs.
4. Monitor the patient.
5. Assist as a circulating nurse for bedside/treatment room procedures.
6. Warm irrigation solution (normal saline or low dextrose dialysis solution) and add medications, typically sodium heparin 1 unit per 1 mL.
7. Set up solution and tubings for manual irrigation(s) to check catheter patency.
8. Assist with catheter patency check.
   a. Connect tubing and infuse solution.
   b. Observe outflow rate and drain volume.
   c. Check for dialysate leaks.
9. In and out exchanges may be continued until dialysate is no longer grossly bloody.
10. If catheter will not be used immediately, lock with heparinized solution before catheter is capped.
11. May assist with final dressings.
12. Ensure that catheter is secured to prevent accidental removal or intraperitoneal loss.

II. Chronic catheter implantation.

A. Management before chronic catheter implantation.
1. Nasal cultures may be obtained to determine if patient is a *S. aureus* carrier.
2. Treating *S. aureus* carriers has been shown to reduce infections by two thirds.
   a. Nasal application of mupirocin prior to catheter implantation reduces the risk of exit site/tunnel infection (evidence-based).
   b. Oral rifampin has also been shown to eradicate *S. aureus* nasal carriage.
3. Patient education topics.
   a. Type of catheter and insertion site.
   b. Prophylactic treatment for *S. aureus* carriers.
   c. The catheter and insertion procedure.
   d. What to expect during the recovery period.
   e. Postoperative exit site care.
   f. Catheter break-in procedures.
4. The peritoneal dialysis staff may be responsible for determining and marking the optimal site for chronic catheter placement independently or in collaboration with the physician or surgeon.
   a. Evaluate catheter position with patient in both supine and upright positions.
   b. Consider catheter type and insertion technique.
   c. Avoid skin folds and scars.
   d. Avoid the belt line.
   e. Consider ability of patient to see and reach the proposed catheter exit site for routine catheter care.
   f. A stencil should be used to place markings for swan-neck catheters.
   g. Presternal catheter exit sites should not be placed directly over the sternum in patients who may require open-heart surgical procedures.
5. Patient should bathe or shower using an antibacterial soap or disinfectant on the morning of the procedure.
6. Remove hair with electric clippers.
7. Prophylactic antibiotic should be given before surgery so that the drug is in the tissues during the surgical procedure. This is an evidence-based recommendation and reduces early peritonitis but not exit or tunnel infections.
   a. A first-generation cephalosporin has been advocated (evidence-based).
   b. Although the use of vancomycin has been discouraged because of the potential for development of resistant organisms, at least

one study has shown that it may be more effective than a cephalosporin in preventing early peritonitis (Gadallah et al., 2000), so the 2005 International Society for Peritoneal Dialysis (ISPD) guidelines state that "each program must consider using vancomycin for prophylaxis for catheter placement, carefully weighing the potential benefit versus the risk of use of vancomycin in hastening resistant organisms."

8. Ensure that bladder is empty to decrease the risk of perforation during catheter insertion.
9. Relieve constipation to decrease the risk of bowel perforation during catheter insertion.
10. Obtain baseline weight and vital signs.
11. Administer preoperative sedative/narcotic as ordered.

B. Common elements of catheter implantation procedures.
   1. Procedure should be performed by an experienced clinician.
   2. Placement in the operating room under sterile conditions is preferred.
   3. General anesthesia should be avoided when possible.
   4. Sedation is typically used in addition to local anesthesia.
   5. The catheter should be immersed in sterile saline, and cuffs thoroughly soaked and gently squeezed to remove air.
   6. Catheter should be flushed prior to implantation to remove any particulate matter.
   7. The peritoneal incision should be either lateral or paramedian.
   8. The intraperitoneal segment is directed between the parietal and visceral peritoneum with tip toward the pelvis, to the right or left of the bladder.
   9. The left side is preferred because migration is more likely on the right side due to upward direction of peristalsis.
   10. The deep cuff should be within the medial or lateral border of the rectus sheath abutting the preperitoneal fascia. This reduces the incidence of pericatheter leaks and hernias.
   11. Catheter patency is tested after the intraperitoneal segment has been placed and/or after creation of the subcutaneous tunnel, before the wound is closed.
   12. Nonreactive, absorbable sutures are recommended.
   13. The exit site of a catheter placed in an arched or curved tunnel should be directed downward.
   14. The subcutaneous cuff should be located approximately 2 cm from the skin exit.
   15. If a straight tunnel is used, it is recommended that the catheter should exit laterally.
   16. Sutures should not be used at the exit site. The stab wound should be only slightly larger than the catheter.
   17. The incision and exit site should be covered with separate, absorbent, sterile dressings.

C. Insertion techniques for chronic PD catheters.
   1. No method has been uniformly shown to be superior in uncomplicated patients. Successful outcomes are related more to the experience of the operator than to procedure or catheter design. High risk patients and those with prior abdominal surgeries may benefit from visual inspection of the peritoneum during catheter placement.
   2. Surgical placement by open dissection (mini-laparotomy) is most widely used. This technique is required for Toronto Western Hospital, swan-neck Missouri, and presternal catheters, as these all have a flange and bead.
      a. A small skin incision is made below and lateral to the umbilicus.
      b. Tissues are dissected down to the anterior rectus sheath and a purse-string suture is placed in the posterior rectus fascia.
      c. A small incision is made into the peritoneal cavity and the catheter is placed in the pelvis using a blunt stylet.
      d. Purse string suture(s) are closed to secure the deep cuff and prevent leaks.
      e. The tunnel is created using a tunneling device.
   3. Minimally invasive surgery.
      a. Laparoscopic technique.
         (1) 1–4 minilaparotomy sites ports are surgically placed.
         (2) 10–12 mm port for 10 mm videolaparoscope.
         (3) Carbon dioxide insufflation.
         (4) A trocar is used for catheter insertion.
         (5) Purse string sutures around every peritoneal aperture.
         (6) A recent review article found a trend in diminished catheter complications versus surgical placement, but this was not statistically significant (Strippoli, Tong, Johnson, Schena, & Craig, 2004b).
      b. Mini- or microlaparoscopic technique.
         (1) A single 2 mm port is used.
         (2) Carbon dioxide is used for insufflation.

(3) Catheter is placed using a modified Seldinger technique.

(4) Catheter position visually confirmed.

(5) Outcomes similar to standard laparoscopic technique.

c. Peritoneoscopy using a minitrocar.

   (1) Uses a 2.2 mm peritoneoscope and air insufflation with local anesthesia.

   (2) Can be done at the bedside or in a treatment room, although a surgical suite is preferred.

   (3) Uses a Quill catheter guide to direct the catheter into the peritoneum. This expands to allow a cuff implantor for cuff placement.

   (4) Does not allow omentectomy or omentopexy (tacking down the omentum).

   (5) Has been reported to have decreased incidence of leaks and outflow failure and improved catheter survival.

4. "Blind" or percutaneous catheter placement, also referred to as the "bedside technique" may be used for Tenckhoff-type catheters, but is rarely used for patients with CKD and primarily of historic interest.

a. This is the least used technique for chronic catheter insertion.

b. The procedure is similar to that used for acute catheters above. It may be done using a trocar (Tenckhoff technique) or a guide wire (Seldinger technique).

c. Surgical backup should be available in case of complications.

d. Blind techniques are not recommended for obese patients or those with multiple abdominal surgeries or suspected intraabdominal adhesions.

e. This technique has an increased incidence of complications.

f. In most settings the outcomes are not as good as those obtained with laparatomy or laparoscopy.

D. Simultaneous surgical procedures can be performed at the time of catheter implantation, depending on the surgical implantation technique.

1. Pre-existing hernias can be repaired.

2. Lysis of abdominal adhesions.

3. Omentectomy, partial omentectomy, or tacking of the omentum.

4. Pelvic fixation of the catheter.

E. Evidence-based guidelines have found that no insertion technique is consistently superior in prevention of peritonitis.

F. A recent review of controlled trials found no differences between surgical laparotomy and laparoscopy for catheter insertion in the incidence of peritonitis, catheter removal, and technique failure (Strippoli et al., 2004b).

G. A recent review of controlled trials found no differences between standard implantation techniques and subcutaneous burying of the external segment in the rates of peritonitis or exit site/tunnel infection (Strippoli et al., 2004b).

Surgical Complications

I. Organ perforation.

A. Risk factors.

1. Rigid, acute catheter.

2. Blind insertion technique.

3. Abdominal adhesions.

4. Abdominal distention. This may be related to paralytic ileus, bowel obstruction, or constipation.

5. Polycystic kidney disease.

6. Bladder distention.

B. Signs and symptoms of bowel perforation.

1. Hissing sound and/or foul smell from gas release.

2. Sudden abdominal pain.

3. Inadequate drainage of dialysate.

4. Massive watery diarrhea may be seen with bowel perforation.

5. Dialysate effluent may be cloudy, odorous, or clearly fecal.

C. Diagnosis of bowel perforation.

1. Based on signs and symptoms.

2. Diagnostic dipstick of feces is positive for glucose, indicating the presence of dialysate.

D. Intervention for bowel perforation.

1. Monitor vital signs.

2. Stop peritoneal dialysis.

3. Remove catheter and rest bowel (NPO). Perforation may seal spontaneously.

4. Broad-spectrum antibiotic therapy.

5. Surgery is recommended if patient develops peritonitis, nausea, vomiting, and fever.

E. Massive voiding of dialysate is the classic sign of a bladder perforation.

F. Diagnostic dipstick of urine shows very high glucose, indicating presence of dialysate.

G. Treatment of bladder perforation.
   1. Remove catheter.
   2. Bladder drainage with Foley catheter.
   3. Reinsert peritoneal catheter.
   4. Treat with antibiotics and/or monitor for peritonitis.

II. Catheter placed preperitoneally.

A. Risk factors.
   1. Rigid, acute catheter.
   2. "Blind" or percutaneous insertion technique.

B. Assessment.
   1. Pain on inflow.
   2. Minimal or no drainage.
   3. Initially clear drainage becomes blood-tinged.

C. Intervention is catheter removal.

III. Bleeding.

A. Some blood-tinged dialysate after catheter insertion is normal. However, this usually resolves spontaneously during the first few exchanges.

B. Bleeding that does not resolve or intensifies and dialysate that is grossly bloody are abnormal.

C. Heparin, 0.5–1.0 unit/mL is added to the dialysis or irrigation solution to prevent clotting and catheter obstruction.

IV. Hemorrhage related to vessel perforation.

A. More frequent with rigid, acute catheters and blind insertion techniques. Perforation of the inferior epigastric artery may occur if blind insertion is attempted through the rectus muscle.

B. Signs and symptoms.
   1. Dialysate is red and frankly bloody.
   2. Bleeding at catheter exit site.

C. Assessment.
   1. Monitor drainage. Dialysate samples from serial exchanges may aid in evaluating whether bleeding is worsening or resolving.

   2. Dialysate samples may be sent for hematocrit.
   3. Monitor vital signs.

D. Interventions.
   1. Rapid exchanges with dialysis solution at room temperature.
   2. Local measures.
      a. Ice packs.
      b. Sand bags.
   3. Surgical repair.
   4. Replace fluid and blood losses.

V. Incisional pain.

A. Assessment.
   1. Differentiate from catheter and dialysis-related discomfort.
   2. Inspect both incision and exit site for signs of inflammation and infection.

B. Intervention.
   1. Comfort measures.
   2. Mild analgesics.

VI. Intraperitoneal loss of acute stylet catheter.

A. Risk factors.
   1. Inadequate securing of catheter at insertion.
   2. Agitated or stuporous patient may dislodge sutures or shield.

B. Assessment.
   1. Catheter may be located by palpation.
   2. Catheter may be seen on x-ray.

C. Intervention.
   1. Consider prophylactic antibiotics.
   2. Surgical retrieval of catheter.
   3. Monitor for peritonitis.

VII. Dialysate leaks. Leaks are most common when dialysis is initiated immediately after catheter implantation. For information regarding dialysate leak, see Chapter 63, *Complications Related to Intraabdominal Pressure*, II. Dialysate leaks.

Postimplantation Care for Chronic Catheters

I. Goals of postimplantation care and "catheter break-in" procedures.

A. Promote wound healing and tissue ingrowth into the catheter cuffs.

B. Maintain catheter patency.

C. Prevent early catheter complications.
   1. Dialysate leaks.
   2. Infections.

II. Avoid high intraabdominal pressure.

A. The longer the time between catheter placement and initiation of PD, the lower the risk of complications due to high intraabdominal pressure.

B. Whenever possible, ambulatory dialysis should be postponed for 10–14 days.

III. Postimplantation care and "catheter break-in" procedures.

A. Catheter irrigation (when PD is not initiated early after catheter insertion).
   1. In and out exchanges with heparinized saline or dialysis solution postoperatively until drainage is clear.
   2. Irrigation with 1000 mL heparinized saline or dialysis solution is infused and drained, typically weekly. This may be done in conjunction with weekly dressing changes.
   3. Advantages.
      a. Catheter malposition or malfunction is identified early.
      b. Relatively inexpensive.
      c. Trained patients can do the procedure independently.
   4. A disadvantage is that this requires a weekly visit to the dialysis unit for most patients.

B. Intermittent peritoneal dialysis (IPD).
   1. Dialysis may be initiated immediately after catheter implantation.
   2. Several strategies reduce intraabdominal pressure and the risk of early leaks.
      a. Low exchange volume, initially 500 mL.
      b. Dialyze with the patient in supine position.
      c. Avoid coughing and straining as these activities generate extremely high intraabdominal pressures.
      d. Avoid lifting and sudden jarring movements.
      e. Minimize physical activity during dialysis.
   3. A PD cycler is typically used for IPD.
   4. Heparin is added to all exchanges.
   5. IPD may be continued for 24–48 hours 2–3 times weekly or done nightly.
   6. Gradually increase exchange volume. Supine dialysis with full exchange volume can be achieved within a few days to a week.
   7. Advantages.
      a. Patient does not require hemodialysis access.
      b. Early documentation of catheter malfunction.
   8. Disadvantages.
      a. IPD is relatively expensive in terms of personnel time.
      b. Outpatient IPD may not be available.

Exit Site Care after Catheter Implantation

I. Goals of postimplantation care.

A. To prevent colonization during the early healing period (2–3 weeks).

B. To reduce bacteria at the exit during later healing.

C. To minimize catheter movement to promote ingrowth at the catheter cuffs.

D. To promptly diagnose complications.

II. Principles of postimplantation care procedures.

A. Recommendations for care are largely based on expert opinion, as there are insufficient studies for evidence-based guidelines.

B. Restrict postoperative dressing changes to trained staff (evidence-based).

C. Frequent dressing changes during the first 2–3 weeks are not necessary unless dressings are wet.

D. Infrequent dressing changes, e.g., weekly, decrease the risk of contamination and minimize catheter manipulation and subsequent trauma.

E. Dressing changes should be performed in a clean environment with closed doors and windows, no fans.

F. Good hand washing with disinfectant should precede care.

G. Aseptic technique, using both masks and gloves, is recommended.

H. Both nurse and patient should mask, as well as anyone else in the room.

I. A mild, nonirritating agent should be used to clean the exit and surrounding skin.

J. If strong, oxidizing agents, such as povidone-iodine and hydrogen peroxide are used to clean the skin, they should not be allowed into the wound as they damage epithelial cells and may delay healing.

K. Sterile water or saline should be used to rinse the exit. Tap water should not be used early in the postimplantation period, because it contains microorganisms.

L. The exit should be dried.

M. An absorbent, sterile dressing should be placed over the exit site (semipermeable dressings should not be used alone).

N. The catheter must be immobilized. When securing the catheter, ensure that the catheter is allowed to follow its natural direction to avoid trauma to the exit site.

O. The exit site should be evaluated at each dressing change (see exit site assessment below).

P. Showering should be avoided until the exit site is healed.

Q. The catheter exit site should not be submerged. Therefore, tub baths and swimming should be avoided.

III. Common elements of postimplantation care.

A. See Table 13.4 for distribution of common elements of postimplantation exit site care in 2005.

B. Almost all units restrict postimplantation exit site care to trained nursing staff or trained patients and caregivers.

C. Aseptic technique is used by the majority of all centers. However, it is used in significantly more pediatric than adult programs.

D. A variety of cleansing agents is used. This is likely because there is inconsistent evidence to support the benefits of a particular agent. However, there is some evidence that use of an antibacterial agent reduces the incidence of exit site infections.

E. There is also variety in the rinsing agents used.

F. Absorbent dressings are most commonly used, either alone or under semipermeable dressings.

G. Tape and adhesive dressings are most commonly used to immobilize the catheter.

IV. Trends in postimplantation exit site care in adult programs over the past decade.

A. Significantly less daily care and significantly more care at weekly intervals.

B. Significant decreases in the proportion of units using povidone-iodine and hydrogen peroxide as cleansing agents, and an increase in the use of chlorhexidine.

C. Significantly more units use absorbent dressings.

D. Units continue postimplantation dressing changes for a significantly longer time.

Progression of Exit Site Healing

I. Normal healing.

A. Exit site characteristics at 1 week.
   1. Slight tenderness in 30%.
   2. Scab almost always present.
   3. Epidermis surrounding the exit is pale pink or pink.
   4. Small amount of serosanguineous, bloody, or serous drainage around the exit in about half the patients.
   5. No swelling.
   6. Drainage inside the sinus is almost always visible, similar in character to that seen outside.
   7. No epithelium visible in the sinus.
   8. Sinus lined with white tissue, which appears hard.

B. Normal progression of healing.
   1. Exit color remains pale pink or pink.
   2. Scab size diminishes and there is no scab after 4 weeks.
   3. External drainage diminishes by 2 weeks, and is absent by 4 weeks.
   4. Drainage in the sinus diminishes, there is minimal moisture in the sinus by 3 weeks, and most sinuses are dry at 6 weeks.
   5. The sinus lining remains flat and gradually becomes plain granulation tissue.
   6. Sinus granulation tissue color gradually changes to pink, sometimes vessels become visible, and/or the surface appears mottled: partly white and partly pink. But some sinuses remain white as late as 6 weeks.
   7. Epithelium starts to enter the sinus by week 2 or 3, progresses steadily, and covers at least half of the visible sinus tract by 4–6 weeks.

Table 13.4

Distribution of Common Elements of Postimplantation Exit Site Care*

	Adults	Pediatrics	*p* Value
Exit care restricted	99%	95%	NS
Weekly frequency	61%	59%	NS
Aseptic technique (masks, sterile gloves)	60%	86%	0.031
Cleansing agent**			
Povidone-iodine	28%	36%	NS
Sodium hypochlorite	28%	14%	NS
Sterile normal saline	22%	27%	NS
Antibacterial soap	21%	18%	NS
Chlorhexidine	12%	23%	NS
Shur-clens®	8%	9%	NS
Sterile water	6%	14%	NS
Hydrogen peroxide	5%	14%	NS
Rinsing agent			
None	28%	24%	NS
Sterile saline	37%	38%	NS
Sterile water	21%	33%	NS
Tap water	14%	5%	NS
Prophylactic antibiotics to the exit site	27%	36%	NS
Type of dressing**			
Absorbent	54%	14%	< 0.001
Semipermeable	11%	23%	NS
Semipermeable over absorbent	29%	59%	0.017
Occlusive	5%	9%	NS
Type of catheter fixation**			
Tape	64%	59%	NS
Dressing	27%	46%	NS
Device	10%	9%	NS

* Data from a 2005 survey of 125 adult and 22 pediatric PD programs; NS = not significant
** Some units reported more than one practice (Prowant, 2006b; Prowant & Warady, 2006).

8. Sinus epithelium is fragile and pale pink, or occasionally white.

II. Early infection.

A. There are no signs of healing, or healing progresses normally for 2–4 weeks, then stops or regresses.

B. Progression of epithelium halts and/or epithelium regresses.

C. Sinus drainage increases and becomes purulent.

D. Sinus granulation tissue becomes slightly or frankly exuberant.

E. Note that early infection can be diagnosed by sinus characteristics alone and that the diagnosis of an early infection does not require as severe of symptoms as for diagnosis of an infection after healing is complete.

F. Risk factors for early infection.
1. Patient characteristics.
   a. *S. aureus* nasal carrier.
   b. Diabetes mellitus.
   c. Malnutrition.
   d. Obesity.
2. Catheter-related.
   a. Wound hematoma.
   b. Large or loose tunnel.
   c. Sutures at exit site.
   d. Early colonization of exit site.
   e. Excessive catheter manipulation.
3. Dialysate leak.

Chronic Exit Site Care

I. **Goals.**

A. To prevent exit site infection.

B. To identify problems promptly.

II. **Recommendations for chronic exit site care.**

A. Again, recommendations for care are based on expert opinion, as there are insufficient studies for evidence-based guidelines.

B. A multicenter study found that a patient education program based on principles of adult learning significantly reduced the incidence of exit site infections in patients on PD (Hall et al., 2004). This was replicated in a single-center study.

C. Routine exit site care is recommended daily or 3–4 times weekly, and whenever the exit becomes wet or dirty.

D. Exit care may be done in conjunction with shower or bathing. Showering is preferred. If bathing, the exit site should not be submerged in the bath water in order to prevent contamination.

E. If the patient is performing exit site care while showering, instruct to shower and shampoo as usual, but avoid the exit site. Clean the exit site at end of shower with soap and clean washcloth.

F. Elements of exit site care procedures include the following:
1. Good hand washing prior to exit site care.
2. Potable tap water may be used to clean the exit site. Boiled, cooled water, or normal saline may be used in the absence of potable tap water.

3. Cleansing agents.
   a. Antibacterial soap and water are recommended.
   b. Pure soaps are also used. However, a European multicenter study found significantly higher rates of exit infection in patients who used pure soap compared to those who used a medical disinfectant (Luzar et al., 1990).
   c. Clean washcloths may be used to clean the exit site. This is a clean procedure so sterile supplies are not necessary. Some programs recommend light colored cloths so dye does not bleed out when wet. Others recommend washing the cloths with bleach.
   d. Liquid soap is recommended. Soap should not be transferred from one container to another because of the risk of contamination.
   e. Medical disinfectants are also used.
   f. Hydrogen peroxide may be used occasionally to loosen crusts.
   g. It is critical that the cleansing agent used by an individual patient is not irritating to the skin.
4. Scabs and crusts should not be forcibly removed. They can be softened by soaking.
5. The exit site may be rinsed with potable tap water. Although bottled water has been recommended by some centers, it is not necessarily safer.
6. Boiled water, normal saline, sterile water, or a diluted hypertonic vinegar solution are options when safe tap water is not available. See Table 13.5 for the procedure for making and using vinegar solution.
7. The exit site should be patted dry with a clean washcloth or towel. Gauze may also be used. There is no reason to use sterile gauze, as this is not an aseptic procedure.
8. Prophylactic use of topical mupirocin calcium reduces the risk of *S. aureus* exit site infection and peritonitis (evidence-based). Although this was initially studied in *S. aureus* carriers, it is now widely practiced, regardless of carrier status.
   a. Mupirocin should be applied sparingly with a cotton-tipped applicator or gauze.
   b. Mupirocin calcium ointment causes structural damage to polyurethane catheters (Crabtree, 2003).
   c. Structural damage such as opacification, ballooning, and thinning at the exit have also been reported in 6% of silicone catheters studied (Khandelwal et al., 2003).
   d. Although there have been reports of

Table 13.5

Procedure for Vinegar Solution for Chronic Exit Site Care

■ To prepare solution:
- Combine 6 ounces of boiled water, 4 ounces of white vinegar and 1¾ teaspoons of table salt in a clean container.
- Shake until salt is dissolved.
- Pour solution into a clean spray bottle.
- Discard unused solution after 7 days.

■ For contaminated water, prevention of infection, or postinfection:
- Follow routine procedure for exit site cleansing.
- Rinse with tap water and pat dry.
- Spray vinegar solution on exit site and pat dry.

■ For inflamed or infected exit site, perform the following twice daily:
- Follow routine procedure for exit site cleansing.
- Saturate a gauze pad with the vinegar solution.
- Wrap around catheter or place over catheter exit site.
- Leave in place for 20 minutes.

mupirocin-resistant *S. aureus* in chronic peritoneal dialysis patients using mupirocin prophylaxis, its use is still recommended by evidence-based guidelines and expert opinion.

9. A recent multicenter study (Bernardini et al., 2005) found that gentamicin cream applied to the exit site during routine care was significantly more effective than mupirocin cream in preventing both exit site infections and peritonitis.

10. Dressings.
   a. Gauze and/or transparent semipermeable dressings are most frequently used.
   b. The use of dressings for chronic exit sites is increasing, although routine dressings are optional in many centers. At least two prospective studies have found no differences in the incidence of exit site infection between groups who wear dressings and those who do not.
   c. Dressings are indicated when the exit is likely to become dirty or irritated by clothing or external pressure, and when the exit site is inflamed or infected.
   d. Dressings may also help to secure the catheter.

G. The catheter or proximal extension tubing should be secured to avoid tension and traction as well as accidental trauma. Devices are available to secure the catheter, but have not been shown to be more effective than securing the catheter with tape and/or adhesive dressings.

III. Common elements of chronic exit site care.

A. For distribution of common elements of chronic exit site care in adult and pediatric programs in 2005, see Table 13.6.

B. Daily care with shower or bath was recommended by most programs.

C. Antibacterial soap was used by more than 80% of adult programs, but only one third of pediatric programs.

D. Adult programs were significantly more likely to use tap water for rinsing. Pediatric programs were significantly more likely not to rinse at all.

E. Both adult and pediatric programs were most likely to recommend sterile gauze for drying the exit. Adult programs were significantly more likely than pediatric programs to recommend use of a clean towel.

F. Adult units were more likely to recommend absorbent gauze dressings. Pediatric units were more likely to use a semipermeable dressing over an absorbent dressing.

G. 68% of adult centers and 69% of pediatric centers used chronic prophylactic antibiotics for *S. aureus* carriers.
   1. 43% of adult programs and 50% of pediatric programs used local antibiotics at the exit site. Mupirocin calcium ointment was most widely used, followed by gentamicin.
   2. Cyclic mupirocin ointment to the nares and cyclic oral rifampin were used less frequently, by about 25% of adult and pediatric centers.

IV. Trends in chronic exit site care in adults over the past decade.

A. More units use antibacterial soap for cleansing.

B. Fewer units in the United States use hydrogen peroxide for routine exit site care.

C. More programs in the United States require dressings.

Table 13.6

Distribution of Common Elements of Chronic Exit Site Care*

	Adults	Pediatrics	p Value
Daily care	89%	68%	< 0.019
Exit site care with shower/bath	85%	75%	NS
Cleansing agent**			
Antibacterial soap	82%	33%	< 0.001
Povidone-iodine solution	9%	24%	NS
Sodium hypochlorite	18%	14%	NS
Chlorhexidine	7%	14%	NS
Pure soap	11%	10%	NS
Routine use of hydrogen peroxide	3.2%	9.5%	NS
Rinsing agent			
Tap water	60%	14%	< 0.001
Sterile water	8%	14%	NS
Normal saline	1%	10%	NS
No rinse	29%	62%	0.006
Method of drying			
Sterile gauze	48%	67%	NS
Nonsterile gauze	11%	10%	NS
Clean towel	36%	10%	0.031
Dressings required	64%	68%	NS
Type of dressing**			
Absorbent	62%	31%	0.044
Semipermeable	11%	19%	NS
Semipermeable over absorbent	17%	44%	0.04
Occlusive	10%	6%	NS
Catheter fixaton required	89%	91%	NS
Type of catheter fixation**			
Tape	80%	70%	NS
Dressing	28%	40%	NS
Device	27%	20%	NS

* Data from a 2005 survey of 125 adult and 22 pediatric PD programs; NS = not significant
** Some units reported more than one practice (Prowant, 2006b; Prowant & Warady, 2006).

V. Evidence-based guidelines related to peritoneal dialysis access are summarized in Table 13.7.

VI. Activities to promote a healthy exit site.

Educate and encourage the patient to:
A. Wash hands before touching catheter and before exit site care.
B. Maintain good personal hygiene.
C. Keep skinfolds clean and dry.
D. Routinely examine and evaluate the exit site and catheter tunnel.
E. Keep the exit site dry.
F. Prevent tape irritation.
G. Stabilize the catheter.
 1. Minimizes catheter movement.
 2. Minimizes the risk of trauma from accidental pulling on the catheter or tubing.

Table 13.7

Summary of Evidence-Based Practice Guidelines for Peritoneal Dialysis Access

These guidelines are based on the highest level of evidence, that is, from all relevant randomized, controlled studies.

- Each center should have a dedicated team involved in implantation and care of catheters (EBPG).
- Preoperative parenteral antibiotic prophylaxis should be used preoperatively to reduce the incidence of peritonitis (CARI, EBPG).
- Catheters should preferably be implanted operatively or by laparoscopy (EBPG).
- Prophylactic therapy using mupirocin calcium ointment decreases the risk of catheter exit/tunnel infections and peritonitis (CARI).
- Use of mupirocin or gentamicin cream at the exit site is recommended to reduce the incidence of exit site infections (EBPG).

CARI = Caring for Australians with Renal Impairment (2005)
EBPG = European Best Practice Guidelines (Dombros et al., 2005)

VII. Conditions detrimental to the exit site.

A. Trauma is a significant risk factor for exit site infection.
1. Trauma has been defined as anything that breaks the integrity of the skin at the exit, the epithelium, or granulation tissue in the sinus, or a hard pull on the catheter sufficient to disrupt tissue ingrowth at the cuff.
2. Sources of trauma.
   a. Pull on the catheter.
   b. Catheter secured so tightly that there is tension on the catheter and/or pressure on the exit site.
   c. Pressure against the exit site from belts, seat belts, tight clothing, or prolonged leaning or sleeping on exit site.
   d. Accidental blunt trauma.
   e. Sensitivity or allergy to soap, disinfectant, or other agents used in exit care.
   f. Irritation or abrasion from tape or adhesives.
   g. Overly vigorous exit care, e.g., forcibly removing scab or crust.
3. Trauma that causes pain, bleeding, or deterioration of the exit site should be treated prophylactically with systemic broad-spectrum antibiotic to prevent acute infection.

B. Oil-based ointments and lotions have traditionally been discouraged.

C. Alcohol dries the skin and may damage the catheter.

D. Excessive perspiration and moisture. Frequent exit site care and dressing changes may help to keep the exit site dry.

VIII. Submerging the exit site and swimming.

A. Submerging the exit site in bathtubs, hot tubs, and whirlpools is discouraged.

B. Patients with well-healed, healthy exit sites may swim.
1. Swimming should be restricted to well-maintained chlorinated pools or clean salt water.
2. Cover the exit site with a waterproof dressing or device.
3. Exit site care should be done immediately after swimming. At this time the patient would also change into dry clothing. Some units also recommend that the cap covering the catheter or extension tubing be changed after swimming.

Exit Site Assessment

I. Characteristics of a healthy, healed exit site.

A. Features present in various combinations.
1. Surrounding skin color may be natural, darkened, light pink, or have a dark, purplish discoloration.
2. There is no external drainage.
3. Crust is absent or small.
4. The visible sinus is partly or completely covered with epithelium.
5. The visible sinus is dry, or has a small amount of clear or thick drainage.
6. There is no exuberant granulation tissue or proud flesh either externally or in the visible sinus.

B. A healthy exit site is shown in Figure 13.4.

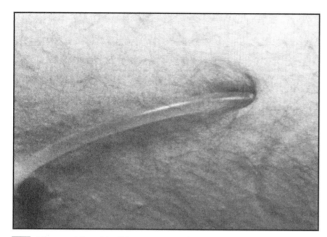

Figure 13.4. Healthy peritoneal dialysis catheter exit site.

II. Routine exit site assessment.

A. Frequency of routine assessment.
   1. With chronic exit site care, daily or 3–4 times weekly by patient or partner.
   2. At each routine clinic visit, at each peritonitis episode, and each hospitalization.
   3. Infected exits should be routinely reassessed.

B. Good lighting and magnification are essential for a good assessment.

C. Assessment parameters.
   1. Subjective.
      a. Tenderness or pain.
      b. Recent trauma.
   2. Tunnel.
      a. Palpate for induration over subcutaneous cuff.
      b. Observe for inflammation along the tunnel.
      c. Observe for hematoma along tunnel after catheter implantation.
   3. External exit site.
      a. Color and extent of discoloration.
      b. Swelling (indurated area often appears shiny with reduction or absence of skin patterning).
      c. Scab or bleeding.
         (1) Often present during healing after catheter insertion.
         (2) May result from trauma.
         (3) May signify exit site or tunnel infection. Exuberant granulation tissue bleeds easily and is often irritated by pressure from or movement of the catheter.
   d. Crust.
      (1) Crust is formed from dried, serous exudate.
      (2) A small crust or flecks of crust are frequently present in healthy exit sites.
      (3) Very large, stubborn crusts often cover exuberant granulation tissue.
   e. Drainage.
      (1) Amount and characteristics.
      (2) External drainage may not be evident until after manipulation of the catheter or pressure on the cuff or sinus track.
      (3) A clear, sticky exudate after catheter insertion may be the result of fat necrosis in the tunnel.
   4. Visible sinus.
      a. How much of the visible sinus is covered by epithelium?
      b. Epithelium appearance.
         (1) Fragile, mucosal during healing after implantation or infection.
         (2) Strong and mature in healthy exit sites.
         (3) May be macerated, e.g., in chronic cuff infections.
      c. How much of the visible sinus is covered by granulation tissue?
      d. Texture of granulation tissue.
         (1) Plain, healthy granulation tissue appears flat, firm, and dull.
         (2) Slightly exuberant granulation tissue protrudes slightly, appears shiny, some vessels may be visible.
         (3) Exuberant granulation tissue or "proud flesh" is bulging, shiny, moist, and vessels are clearly visible.
      e. Drainage amount and characteristics.
   5. Additional assessments.
      a. Inspect the catheter for wear lines and cracks or other damage.
      b. Check that the adapter is fully inserted and fits tightly.
      c. Note if cuff is visible in the sinus.
   6. Document in detail; a checklist may be useful.

Catheter-related Infections

I. Exit site infection.

A. Exit site infection is defined as inflammation of the catheter exit site with purulent drainage. A positive culture of the exit site in the absence of inflammation does not indicate infection.

B. Common responsible organisms.
 1. *Staphylococcus aureus* has been the leading cause of exit and tunnel infections.
 2. Multiple organisms are the next most common cause.
 3. *Staphylococcus epidermidis* and other gram-positive species.
 4. Pseudomonas species are the most common gram-negative organisms.
 5. Fungi.

C. Risk factors.
 1. After catheter insertion.
  a. Dialysate leak or frank bleed.
  b. Hematoma in the catheter tunnel.
  c. Early colonization of the exit site.
  d. Delayed or incomplete healing of the exit site.
  e. Excessive manipulation of the catheter or inadequate stabilization.
 2. Chronic catheter.
  a. Trauma. In one longitudinal catheter exit site study, all exit infections in previously healthy, mature exit sites were preceded by trauma.
   (1) A pull on the catheter.
   (2) Blunt trauma.
   (3) External pressure from clothing, belts, seatbelts, etc.
  b. Cuff extrusion.
  c. *Staphylococcus aureus* nasal carrier status. Patients with persistently positive nasal cultures have a threefold to fourfold risk of staphylococcal exit-site infection. It is likely that bacteria are transferred from the nares or other colonized sites to the exit site.
   (1) Protocols to control nasal carriage include oral rifampin, mupirocin ointment to the nares, and trimethoprim-sulfamethoxazole.
   (2) Topical mupirocin to the PD catheter exit site during routine care is equally effective in reducing infectious complications.
  d. Wet exit.
   (1) Due to excessive or prolonged perspiration.
   (2) Submersion.
   (3) Skin breakdown.
   (4) Dialysate leak.

D. Characteristics of an infected exit site (see Figure 13.5). The following features are present in various combinations.
 1. Exit site color may be bright pink or red.
 2. The exit site may be swollen.
 3. The exit site may be tender, sore, or painful.

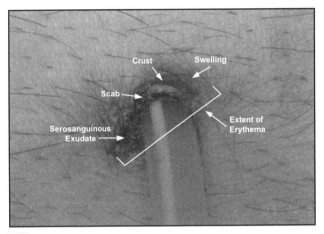

Figure 13.5. Infected peritoneal dialysis catheter exit site.

 4. There is external drainage, spontaneously, or after pressure on the sinus.
 5. External drainage is purulent or may be bloody.
 6. There may be exuberant granulation tissue or proud flesh around the exit site and/or in the visible sinus.

E. Diagnosis.
 1. Based on clinical signs and symptoms listed above. A positive skin smear alone does not indicate clinical infection as all exit sites are colonized within a few weeks after catheter insertion.
 2. Positive culture of exudate.

F. Care of the inflamed or infected exit site.
 1. Document details of exit site assessment. This can be used as a baseline to determine if therapy is effective.
 2. Increased frequency of exit site care is recommended. Daily care is most common in pediatric programs. Twice daily care is most typical in adult programs.
 3. Reassess whether cleansing agents may be irritating the exit site. Change to a milder agent if indicated.
 4. Remove scab or crust gradually, not forcibly; may need to soak with saline or liquid soap. Very large stubborn crusts sometimes form over exuberant granulation tissue (proud flesh).
 5. Keep exit site dry.
 6. Dressings are recommended.
  a. A light sterile dressing may protect against further contamination and/or irritation of the exit site.
  b. The dressing also absorbs the drainage.

7. Exuberant granulation tissue (proud flesh) may be cauterized by a physician or nurse by touching lightly with a silver nitrate stick. Cauterization should be restricted to granulation tissue only. Avoid touching adjacent epithelium.
    a. Use of a magnifying lens aids in precise cauterization.
    b. Exuberant granulation tissue becomes a gray-white or brownish color after cauterization.
    c. One application may be sufficient for an acute infection, several cauterizations, once or twice weekly, may be required for chronic infections.
8. Wet compresses (see Table 13.8) with a variety of topical disinfectants have been used alone for early infections and in conjunction with systemic antibiotic therapy for more severe infections. However, reports of efficacy have been inconsistent. Soaking solutions include hypertonic saline, normal saline, sodium hypochlorite, povidone-iodine, and hydrogen peroxide.

G. Trends in the care of infected exit sites in adult programs over the past decade.
    1. More centers recommend increased frequency of care.
    2. There is an increase in daily care and a decrease in BID care.
    3. More units are using topical soaks and topical antibiotics.

H. Therapy.
    1. There are no studies that define the best

Table 13.8

Procedure for Hypertonic Saline Soaks for Inflamed or Infected PD Catheter Exit Sites

■ To prepare solution:
  • Add 1 tbsp of salt to 1 pint of sterile water. Shake and refrigerate.
  OR
  • Boil 2 tablespoons of table salt and 1 quart of water. Pour solution into a clean, closed container. Refrigerate.

■ To apply soaks, twice or three times daily:
  • Pour solution on gauze and heat in microwave until warm to touch.
  • Wrap around catheter or place over catheter exit site.
  • Leave in place for 15–20 minutes.

---

protocol for antibiotic therapy or specify the optimal duration of treatment.
2. Topical antibiotics (e.g. mupirocin calcium, gentamicin cream or optical solution, triple antibiotic) may be useful for early or equivocal infections when there is minimal drainage.
    a. These preparations are washed away by copious drainage.
    b. Mupirocin ointment should not be used with polyurethane catheters because the poly-glycol base will degrade the polyurethane. Mupirocin cream may be used with polyurethane catheters.
3. Treatment with systemic antibiotics described below is based on published ISPD recommendations (Piraino et al., 2005), which are also available at the ISPD Web site, http://www.ispd.org.
    a. First-generation cephalosporins or penicillinase-resistant penicillins are recommended as empiric treatment for gram-positive organisms.
    b. Oral quinolones are recommended for Pseudomonas species.
    c. Vancomycin should be reserved for methicillin-resistant *S. aureus.*
    d. For refractory or severe *S. aureus* infections, rifampin may be added.
    e. Oral antibiotics are as effective as intraperitoneal therapy, except for treatment of methicillin-resistant *S. aureus.*
    f. Antibiotic treatment should be continued until the exit site appearance is healthy. A minimum of 2 weeks of systemic antibiotic therapy is recommended.
4. Chronic or recurrent infections and fungal infections require long-term antibiotic therapy.

I. Complications of exit site infection.
    1. Tunnel infection (cuff involvement).
    2. Peritonitis. As many as 20% of exit site infections are associated with subsequent peritonitis with the same organism.
    3. Exit site infection is a major reason for catheter removal and subsequent transfer to hemodialysis.

II. Subcutaneous tunnel infection.

A. Responsible organisms.
    1. Staphylococcal species are most often implicated.
    2. See organisms responsible for exit site infections (Catheter-related Infections, I. B.).

B. Risk factors.
1. Contamination during catheter insertion.
2. Delayed wound healing.
3. Early dialysate leak.
4. Exit site infection.
5. Severe trauma, such as a hard pull on the catheter.
6. External cuff extrusion.

C. Signs and symptoms.
1. Irregularity, thickening along the subcutaneous tunnel.
2. Erythema over tunnel segment.
3. Pain and tenderness along the tunnel.
4. Catheter fits loosely in tunnel.
5. Abscess over the catheter tunnel or fistula along tunnel.
6. Large amount of purulent or sanguineous drainage although the catheter exit site does not have other characteristics of an infection.
7. Simultaneous or previous exit site infection and/or peritonitis with same organism.

D. Ultrasound has been recommended as a diagnostic test. However, the sensitivity and specificity of this method are not high.

E. Treatment.
1. Systemic antibiotic therapy may be attempted; however, tunnel infections are rarely, if ever, cured.
2. When the subcutaneous cuff is infected, surgical intervention may prolong the life of the catheter.
   a. Surgical procedures that externalize (un-roof) the cuff permitting drainage and excision of granulation tissue, and shaving the external cuff from the catheter have been described. These may resolve the infection and prolong the catheter life. The wound is often left open and packed with saline-soaked gauze as a wet to dry dressing.
   b. An alternative procedure surgically removes the external catheter segment to below the subcutaneous cuff and uses a connecting device to splice a new catheter segment with cuff, which is placed in a new tunnel with a new exit site.
   c. A cuff which has completely extruded from the exit may be shaved from the catheter to avoid skin irritation, and because it is difficult to keep the cuff clean.
3. Catheter removal may be required.

F. Complications.
1. Abdominal wall cellulitis.
2. Peritonitis (discussed in Chapter 63, *Peritoneal Dialysis Complications*).
3. Catheter removal.

III. Monitoring PD catheter outcomes.

A. Catheter survival of > 80% at 1 year is considered reasonable. Survival rates of up to 90–95% at 2 years have been reported.

B. The ISPD recommends that every program monitor the incidence of catheter-related infections at least annually (Piraino et al., 2005).
1. Exit site infections.
2. Peritonitis.
3. Relapsing peritonitis.

C. Reasons for catheter removal should also be documented and evaluated.
1. Mechanical problems.
2. Exit site or tunnel infection.
3. Peritonitis.
4. Elective removal.

D. Reasons for catheter removal in the first 2 months of dialysis should be evaluated as a subgroup (Piraino et al., 2005).

Complications Related to the PD Catheter

I. Catheter malfunction.

A. Catheter malfunction is much more frequent during the first month after catheter insertion, but may occur later.

B. Unable to either drain or infuse.
1. Etiology.
   a. Kinked or clamped catheter or tubing. External pressure on catheter or tubing.
   b. Catheter has a kink or bend in subcutaneous or intraperitoneal segment.
   c. Catheter is obstructed by fibrin or blood clot.
2. Assessment and intervention.
   a. Check entire length of tubing for kinks, pressure, and closed clamps.
   b. Check that external segment of catheter is not kinked or under external pressure.
   c. Both flat plate of abdomen and lateral view x-rays are necessary to confirm or rule out internal kinks.

C. Occlusion by blood or fibrin clots.
   1. Catheter irrigation.
      a. A large syringe can be used to vigorously flush the catheter with heparinized saline or dialysis solution.
      b. If the catheter does not then drain spontaneously, attempts can be made to gently aspirate. If pressure is felt, the attempt should be abandoned so that adjacent tissue is not pulled into the catheter.
   2. Endoluminal brushes and Fogarty balloon-tipped catheters have been used to manually remove clots. Care must be taken to maintain aseptic technique and not to allow the instrument to exit the distal end of the catheter and damage the peritoneal membrane.
   3. Fibrinolysis may be effective in resolving blood or fibrin clots.
      a. Historically, streptokinase and urokinase were used. Streptokinase is no longer used due to severe allergic reactions. Urokinase 5,000 units in a volume to fill catheter and transfer set was infused and allowed to dwell for up to 2 hours before aspiration. Because urokinase was unavailable in the United States for a period of time, protocols were developed for tissue plasminogen activator (tPA).
      b. Recommendations for use of tissue plasminogen activator (tPA) in PD catheters (Zorzanello, Fleming, & Prowant, 2004).
         (1) Document the difficulty draining and/or filling.
         (2) Check the entire length of tubing and catheter for kinks, pressure on the tubing, or closed clamps.
         (3) Attempt to flush the catheter with heparinized solution.
         (4) Abdominal x-rays may be used to rule out a malpositioned catheter or an internal catheter kink.
         (5) Administer tPA, typically 1 mg/mL in sterile water in a volume sufficient to fill the catheter, and allow to dwell for 1–2 hours.
         (6) Attempt to drain by gravity, or the solution can be aspirated.
         (7) If the occlusion is resolved, flush the catheter with heparinized solution before resuming routine dialysis.

D. One-way obstruction: solution can be infused, but will not drain.
   1. Etiologies.
      a. Air lock in tubing interrupts siphon. This is unlikely with closed, nonvented systems.
      b. Constipation is the most common cause.
      c. Fibrin or blood clots surround terminal holes of catheter.
      d. Catheter placed incorrectly at insertion and has a kink or bend that allows infusion due to hydraulic pressure, but not drainage.
      e. Catheter migration out of pelvis.
         (1) Due to omental wrapping.
         (2) Due to peristalsis.
         (3) Due to poor orientation of the catheter tunnel.
         (4) Due to shape memory of a straight catheter placed in a curved or arch-shaped tunnel.
      f. Fluid is in a small, isolated area of the peritoneal cavity.
   2. Assessment and intervention.
      a. Infuse a small amount of additional dialysis solution. This will flush air bubbles out of the tubing. Flush dialysis solution into the drain bag if a Y-tubing is used.
      b. Change body position. This may relieve external pressure on the catheter or help drain fluid in an isolated area.
      c. Induce peristalsis or a bowel movement with laxatives or enemas if patient is constipated.
      d. Irrigation with a syringe containing heparinized dialysis solution or normal saline may flush fibrin or clots from the catheter and tubing.
      e. Abdominal x-rays may be used to confirm catheter position. Both abdominal flat plate and lateral x-rays may be necessary to confirm or rule out an internal catheter kink.
      f. Catheterogram using infusion of contrast media may identify loculation of fluid. This is contraindicated in patients who have a history of sensitivity to contrast media.
      g. Occasionally a catheter that has migrated out of the pelvis will spontaneously reposition itself.
         (1) Have patient assume knee-chest position in an attempt to "float" the catheter back into the pelvis.
         (2) Induce peristalsis.
         (3) Discontinue dialysis and encourage ambulation and activity.
      h. The physician or surgeon may attempt to manually reposition the catheter with a guidewire using aseptic technique. However, this is not consistently effective.
      i. Surgical repositioning or catheter replacement.
         (1) Omentectomy or partial omentectomy

may be indicated if the catheter is malpositioned due to omental wrap.

(2) Laparoscopic techniques have been used successfully to salvage malfunctioning catheters.

II. Rectal or suprapubic pain.

A. Etiology is pressure from peritoneal catheter. Intraperitoneal catheter segment may be too long, or the catheter may have been implanted too low.

B. Intervention.
1. Pain and pressure may be relieved with infusion of dialysis solution.
2. Do not drain exchanges completely. Leave a reservoir of fluid in the peritoneal cavity at the end of each exchange and between intermittent dialysis procedures to cushion the catheter. Tidal mode for nightly peritoneal dialysis may be successful.

III. Catheter cuff extrusion.

A. Etiology.
1. Placement of the external cuff too close to the skin exit.
2. Placement of a straight catheter in a curved or arch-shaped tunnel. Because of the resilience of silicone, the catheter attempts to reassume its original straight configuration after insertion. This may exert a forward force on the external cuff.
3. Tunnel is shorter than the inter-cuff catheter segment.
4. External tension, pulling on the catheter.

B. Assessment.
1. Palpation of subcutaneous cuff.
2. A portion of cuff may be visible in the sinus tract or at the skin surface.

C. Cuff extrusion is almost invariably associated with exit site inflammation and infection.

D. Intervention.
1. Vigilant daily exit site care.
2. Treat exit-site infection.
3. Surgical "un-roofing" and shaving of partially extruded cuffs may be attempted.
4. Completely extruded cuffs can be shaved from the catheter to avoid exit site irritation and because they are difficult to clean.

E. Complications.
1. Chronic exit site infection.
2. Subcutaneous tunnel infection.
3. Peritonitis.

IV. Damage to catheter.

A. Problems and risk factors.
1. Defective catheter.
2. Catheter is accidentally cut or punctured.
   a. During insertion procedure.
   b. Cut by patient or staff while removing dressings.
   c. Use of syringe and needle to obtain dialysate sample through the catheter makes a permanent puncture.
   d. Catheter nicked during cuff-shaving procedure.
3. Constant tension or bending at the adaptor site.
4. Use of cleansing agents, disinfectants, or antibiotic preparations that cause catheter deterioration.
5. Use of wrong size adapter.
6. Use of toothed hemostat to clamp catheter.

B. Signs.
1. Wear line on catheter.
2. Visible crack(s) in catheter.
3. Catheter may become brittle, and crumble, crack, or break off completely.
4. Distal segment becomes stretched and loses elasticity.
5. Dialysate leak from external catheter segment.

C. Intervention.
1. If external catheter segment is relatively long and damage is at or near the distal end, the catheter can be trimmed.
2. If there is a break in the catheter material or a dialysate leak, instruct the patient to:
   a. Stop dialysis.
   b. Clamp catheter proximal to the site of damage.
   c. Cover damaged area with a sterile dressing to prevent further contamination.
   d. Come immediately to the clinic or emergency room.
3. Procedure for trimming catheter.
   a. Clamp catheter.
   b. Disinfect catheter immediately proximal to the damaged area.
   c. With sterile scissors, cut the catheter just proximal to the damaged area.
   d. Insert a new, sterile adapter.

4. If damage is near, but > 15 mm from the exit, a Silastic catheter can be extended using a commercially available repair kit (e.g., Quinton Peri-Patch™ Repair Kit, Tyco Healthcare, Mansfield, MA).
5. Prophylactic antibiotic therapy is indicated for any catheter break or leak.

V. Adapter loose or falls out of catheter.

A. Etiology.
   1. May be caused by catheter stretching and loss of elasticity.
   2. Adapter has been used with catheter that has a larger inner lumen. This is most likely if catheter is relatively new.
   3. Confused or agitated patient.

B. Prevention. If the desired adapter is too small for the inner lumen of the catheter, an external band can be placed around the catheter to hold the adapter firmly in place (Schmidt, Craig, Prowant, & Twardowski, 1990).

C. Intervention.
   1. Instruct the patient to:
      a. Clamp the catheter.
      b. Cover the open catheter end with a sterile dressing.
      c. Come immediately to the clinic or emergency room.
   2. If catheter is stretched, disinfect the catheter proximal to the stretched area and trim the catheter as outlined above.
   3. If catheter size is the problem, disinfect the open catheter and reinsert an appropriate-size adapter.
   4. Prophylactic antibiotic therapy is indicated.

Catheter Removal

I. Indications for catheter removal.

A. Peritoneal dialysis discontinued.

B. Nonfunctioning or malfunctioning catheter; will not infuse or drain.

C. Broken, cracked, or severed catheter that cannot be repaired.

D. Unresolved dialysate leak.
   1. External.
   2. Subcutaneous.

E. Unresolved pleuroperitoneal communication.

F. Chronic or recurrent exit-site or tunnel infection that does not respond to treatment.

G. Infection of the deep (preperitoneal) catheter cuff.

H. Peritonitis.
   1. Peritonitis with concurrent chronic exit site or tunnel infection.
   2. Peritonitis that does not respond to therapy within 96 hours.
   3. Symptoms of peritonitis clear with appropriate antibiotic therapy, but recur during therapy.
   4. Consideration of catheter removal is recommended when a third episode of peritonitis is caused by the same organism(s).
   6. Fungal peritonitis.
   7. Fecal peritonitis or peritonitis with multiple gram-negative organisms.

I. Catheter-related sepsis.

J. Peritoneal membrane failure or encapsulating peritoneal sclerosis.

II. Catheter removal.

A. Removal of acute, uncuffed catheters is accomplished by simply removing the stabilizing suture and pulling out the catheter.

B. Cuffed catheters must be removed surgically.
   1. The "explant" physician or surgeon needs to know type of catheter, number of cuffs, and implant procedure.
   2. The difficulty of the removal procedure is related to the complexity of the catheter design. Catheters with more cuffs, large intraperitoneal segments, or pelvic suturing of the catheter are more difficult to remove.
   3. The surgical procedure for removing chronic peritoneal catheters has been described in detail by Ash (2002).
   4. Most catheter removal procedures use general anesthesia. However, Tenckhoff-type catheters can be removed under local anesthesia.
   5. All catheter segments including cuffs should be completely removed.

6. Caution should be taken to avoid tissue trauma, bleeding, and omental or incisional hernias.

7. The opening at the peritoneum and deep cuff is closed with sutures. The skin incision is usually sutured, but may be packed and left to heal by secondary intention in the case of cuff or tunnel infections.

C. The optimal timing of replacement of an infected chronic catheter is not known, but typically at least 3 weeks has been recommended.

III. Simultaneous catheter removal and reimplantation.

A. Originally recommended for malfunctioning or malpositioned catheters.

B. The ISPD (Gokal et al., 2000) has recommended this technique for cases of refractory or recurrent peritonitis believed due to biofilm formation (primarily coagulase negative staphylococci) and for tunnel infections (primarily *S. aureus*).

C. ISPD recommended that this approach be used only after standard antibiotic therapy when dialysate WBC is < 100/µL, and that antibiotic therapy be continued postoperatively.

D. Placement of the new catheter is done before removal of the infected catheter to reduce the risk of cross contamination.

E. Simultaneous replacement is not recommended for peritonitis episodes due to fungi, or mycobacterium, or when an intraabdominal abscess or intraabdominal source of peritonitis is suspected.

Chapter 62

Peritoneal Dialysis Therapy

Purposes

The purposes of this section are to provide a cognitive understanding of concepts and principles related to peritoneal dialysis therapy, to review principles of nursing care for patients receiving peritoneal dialysis (PD), and to summarize clinical outcomes.

Objectives

Upon completion of this chapter, the learner will be able to:
1. List in sequence three key events in the history of PD therapy.
2. Cite two absolute contraindications to PD therapy.
3. Outline the peritoneal cavity on an anatomic drawing.
4. List the sources of blood supply to the peritoneal cavity.
5. Describe the peritoneal membrane.
6. Define osmosis and diffusion as they relate to PD.
7. Define ultrafiltration as it relates to PD.
8. Discuss three factors that affect the transport of solutes in PD.
9. Discuss three factors that affect total fluid removal in peritoneal dialysis.
10. Describe the effect of lymphatic drainage on dialysis clearances and ultrafiltration.
11. List electrolytes in a typical peritoneal dialysis solution.
12. Explain why PD solutions contain dextrose.
13. Describe possible effects of PD on systemically administered drugs.

Objectives continue on next page

Objectives continued from previous page

14. Name two types of drugs frequently administered intraperitoneally to PD patients.
15. Cite two goal(s) of peritoneal catheter break-in procedures.
16. State two ways intraabdominal pressure can be minimized after catheter insertion.
17. State the primary goal of the procedure(s) for performing PD connections and exchanges.
18. State at least two reasons why the PD solution is warmed to body temperature.
19. Describe two different methods for increasing ultrafiltration during PD.
20. Differentiate continuous ambulatory peritoneal dialysis (CAPD), continuous cycling peritoneal dialysis (CCPD), and intermittent peritoneal dialysis (IPD).
21. State at least two relative advantages of continuous and intermittent PD.
22. Discuss why the double-bag Y-set is associated with lower rates of peritonitis.
23. List key components of an education program for home PD patients.
24. List key components in the follow-up and nursing management of home PD patients.
25. Explain how the dose of dialysis could be increased for a patient on CAPD, CCPD, intermittent automated peritoneal dialysis (APD), or nightly intermittent peritoneal dialysis (NIPD).
26. Cite the current NKF Dialysis Outcomes Quality Initiative (KDOQI) Clinical Practice Guidelines recommendations for adequate PD.
27. Describe four common problems or errors in collecting quantitative samples for measuring the adequacy of PD.
28. Describe the cardiovascular complications common in PD patients.
29. Identify nutritional problems common in PD patients and describe intervention strategies.
30. Discuss three strategies to preserve the peritoneal membrane.
31. Discuss the impact of patient compliance with PD on the outcomes of death and dropout.
32. Compare the dialysis access related hospitalization rates between hemodialysis and peritoneal dialysis.
33. Compare the survival of hemodialysis and PD patients.
34. List three major causes of death in PD patients.

When Level I or Level II evidence exists, treatment recommendations are identified as evidenced-based.

Historical Perspective

A. 1877 – Wegner reported peritoneal lavage in animals.

B. 1894 – Starling and Tubby described absorption from the peritoneal cavity indicating that transport through the peritoneal membrane was bidirectional.

C. 1923 – Putnam published studies of PD in dogs. Ganter described peritoneal dialysis in uremic animals and reported the first use of peritoneal dialysis for uremia in a human.

D. 1927 – Heusser and Werder reported continuous flow PD in three patients with mercury poisoning.

E. 1938 – Wear reported what was thought to be the first patient treated with PD to recover from acute renal failure. Rhodes reported first attempt to use PD in chronic renal failure.

F. 1959 – Sterile peritoneal dialysis solution became commercially available.

G. 1964 – Boen developed the first closed automated delivery system.

H. 1964 – Palmer designed a silicone catheter for chronic use.

I. 1965 – Weston and Roberts designed an acute stylet catheter.

J. 1966 – Lasker developed an automated cycler.

K. 1967 – Tenckhoff designed the silicone double-cuff catheter.

L. 1972 – Fully automated, reverse osmosis system was developed.

M. 1976 – Popovich and Moncrief described continuous ambulatory peritoneal dialysis technique.

N. 1978 – The Food and Drug Administration (FDA) approved peritoneal dialysis solution in polyvinyl bags for use in the United States.

O. 1981 – Diaz-Buxo et al. described continuous cycling peritoneal dialysis.

P. 1980s – New continuous ambulatory peritoneal dialysis (CAPD) systems, cycling machines, and catheter designs developed. Variation in dialysis prescription and regimens.

Q. 1990s – Increased emphasis on dialysis adequacy and nutrition, and individualized dialysis prescriptions. Increased use of cycler dialysis, > 30% of the United States PD dialysis population using cyclers.

R. 2000s – Improved understanding of peritoneal biocompatibility. Availability of new, more biocompatible peritoneal dialysis solutions. Approximately half of the PD population using cyclers. Renewed interest in continuous flow PD using two catheters to enhance dialysis efficiency.

Contraindications to Peritoneal Dialysis

I. **Absolute contraindications.**

A. Hypercatabolism: peritoneal dialysis unable to adequately remove uremic metabolites.

B. Patent opening between the peritoneal and pleural cavities.

C. Inadequate transfer surface area because of adhesions and scarring from:
   1. Multiple surgeries.
   2. Previous peritonitis.
   3. Sclerosing peritonitis.

II. **Relative contraindications.**

A. Chronic back pain.

B. Chronic obstructive pulmonary disease.

C. Severe diverticular disease.

D. Abdominal disease or malignancy.

E. Presence of a colostomy, ileostomy, nephrostromy, or ileal conduit.

F. Patient unable or unwilling to do home dialysis and has no suitable partner(s).

Anatomy and Physiology

I. **Description.** The peritoneum is a serous membrane that covers the abdominal organs and lines the abdominal wall (see Figure 13.6). Approximately 60% of the peritoneum is visceral peritoneum, 30% is mesenterium and omentum, and 10% is parietal peritoneum. The peritoneum is composed of thin layers of connective tissue covered with mesothelium.

II. **Size.** The peritoneal membrane is 1–2 m^2 and approximates body surface area.

III. **Nature.**

A. The dialyzing membrane consists of the vascular wall, the interstitium, the mesothelium, and adjacent fluid films.

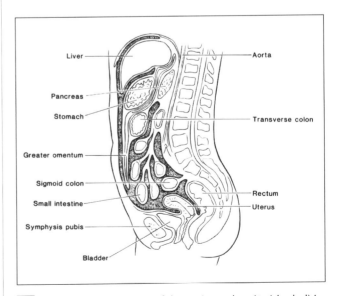

Figure 13.6. Anatomy of the peritoneal cavity (shaded) in an adult female.

B. The peritoneal membrane is continuous and closed in males.

C. In females, the ovaries and fallopian tubes open into the peritoneal cavity.

D. The peritoneal cavity normally contains about 100 mL of fluid (transudate).

IV. Blood supply.

A. The parietal peritoneum receives blood from the arteries of the abdominal wall.

B. The blood from the parietal peritoneum and abdominal wall drains into the systemic circulation.

C. The visceral peritoneum receives blood from the mesenteric and celiac arteries.

D. Blood from the visceral peritoneum converges and enters the portal vein.

E. The aorta, inferior vena cava, and the mesenteric vascular network are retroperitoneal, so prolonged exposure to dialysis fluid of a different temperature may alter core body temperature.

V. Lymph drainage.

A. Lymph drainage from the peritoneal cavity occurs through a one-way system primarily involving specialized lymph openings found in the subdiaphragmatic peritoneum.

B. Intraperitoneal fluid is absorbed by convective flow. Fluid, solutes, and large molecules, such as proteins and blood cells, are all absorbed.

C. Lymph absorption is influenced by respiratory rate, intraabdominal pressure, and posture (higher in the supine position).

D. The average lymph absorption rate in CAPD patients has been estimated to be between 1.0 and 1.5 mL/min, resulting in an average daily lymph absorption of at least 1 L.

E. Lymph drainage is returned to the venous circulation primarily via the right lymph duct and the left thoracic duct.

F. Lymph drainage from the peritoneal cavity during peritoneal dialysis results in a net decrease in ultrafiltration and solute removal.

G. The lymphatics also contribute to the host defenses of the peritoneum through the absorption of foreign substances.

Kinetics of Peritoneal Dialysis

I. **Diffusion across the peritoneal membrane** into the dialysate is the primary mechanism of waste removal in peritoneal dialysis.

A. Diffusion is defined as bidirectional movement of solutes across the peritoneal membrane from an area of higher solute concentration to an area of lower solute concentration.

B. Factors that influence solute transport.
   1. Peritoneal membrane permeability. Factors that affect membrane permeability.
      a. Infection causes inflammation, which increases solute transfer.
      b. Medications. Depending upon the drug, solute transfer may either increase or decrease.
      c. Collagen and/or vascular diseases and membrane abnormalities.
   2. Peritoneal membrane size or available membrane area (may be reduced by scarring or adhesions).
   3. Concentration gradient. The higher the concentration gradient, the more rapid the solute exchange.
   4. Solute characteristics.
      a. Size. Small molecules diffuse faster than larger molecules.
      b. Protein binding. Solutes that are protein bound have restricted transport.
      c. Water soluble substances are transferred more rapidly than lipid-soluble substances.
      d. Electrical charge. The peritoneal membrane has fixed negative charges.
   5. Peritoneal blood flow. Increased blood flow enhances clearances.
   6. Dialysis solution volume. Larger exchange volumes increase total solute removal.
   7. Dialysis solution temperature. Solutions that are cooler than body temperature slow the rate of diffusion early in the exchange until the dialysate warms to body temperature. This has a

greater effect in short dwell exchanges (as in acute dialysis or automated PD) than in long dwell exchanges.

C. Routes of solute transport.
 1. Transcellular (across cell membranes).
 2. Extracellular (through cell junctions and gaps).

D. Factors that enhance diffusion.
 1. Increased dialysis solution flow.
  a. Increased exchange volume.
  b. More exchanges.
 2. High concentration gradient.
 3. Prewarmed dialysis solution.
 4. Ultrafiltration creates a solvent drag that pulls additional solute across the membrane. This is termed convective transport, and may be associated with sieving.
 5. Sieving means that solute transfer is lower than that of water, so the solute concentration in the ultrafiltrate is lower than that in the solution which was ultrafiltered.

E. The rate of equilibration between the blood and dialysate occurs at a different rate for each solute as seen in Figure 13.7.
 1. Small molecular weight substances reach equilibrium more rapidly and are removed more efficiently than larger solutes.
 2. Sodium and potassium removal are most influenced by convective transport.

F. After an initial washout, the protein transport rate is almost constant.

G. Substances lost in the dialysate.
 1. Proteins.
 2. Amino acids.
 3. Water soluble vitamins.
 4. Electrolytes, e.g. sodium and potassium.
 5. Trace minerals.
 6. Some hormones (e.g., parathyroid hormone).
 7. Some drugs.

H. Substances absorbed from the dialysis solution into the systemic circulation include:
 1. Dextrose (100–200 g/day in CAPD with dextrose solutions).
 2. Icodextrin is absorbed when it is used as an osmotic agent.
 3. Lactate or bicarbonate.
 4. Calcium is absorbed from dialysis solutions containing 3.5 mEq/L calcium.
 5. Amino acids are absorbed when present in dialysis solutions.

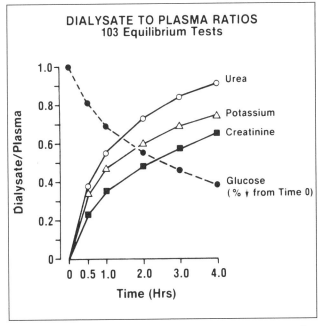

Figure 13.7. Mean dialysate to plasma ratios for multiple solutes related to dwell time; determined from 103 equilibration studies in 86 patients.

 6. Some drugs, e.g., insulin, antibiotics.

I. Removal and absorption rates vary among patients.

II. Fluid removal.

A. Fluid removal in peritoneal dialysis is a two-step process: water transport from the peritoneal capillaries to the interstitium, and transport across the peritoneal membrane into the peritoneal cavity.
 1. Both hydrostatic and colloid osmotic forces affect water transport.
 2. Transport of water across the walls of capillaries and venules is believed to occur through large and small pores and ultrasmall pores (aquaporins).
 3. Some of the aquaporins are so small that only water passes through them. Aquaporins mediate 50% of UF during a hypertonic dwell. Movement of water through the aquaporins accounts for the sodium sieving.

B. Osmosis is the movement of water across the peritoneal membrane from an area of lower solute concentration to an area of higher solute concentration.

C. Factors that influence water removal in peritoneal dialysis.
  1. Peritoneal membrane permeability and surface area.
  2. Hydrostatic pressure gradient.
  3. Colloid osmotic (oncotic) pressure. Osmotic pressure gradient depends on type of osmotic agent and concentration.
  4. Dwell time. Fluid is removed most rapidly early in the dwell when the osmotic gradient is greatest. During long dwell exchanges with dextrose solutions, after several hours, fluid will be reabsorbed from the peritoneal cavity, decreasing the total drain volume.
  5. The amount of lymphatic absorption also affects the net volume of water removed.

D. Principles of fluid removal in PD.
  1. Dextrose is added to the dialysis solution to create an osmotic gradient.
  2. Polyglucose (icodextrin) acts as a colloid osmotic agent.
  3. For dextrose solutions, the ultrafiltration rate is highest at the beginning of each exchange when the osmotic gradient is highest.
     a. Ultrafiltrate volume peaks when dialysate osmolality decreases (due to dilution and dextrose absorption) to the point where the rate of ultrafiltration is exceeded by the rate of lymphatic absorption.
     b. Reabsorption of water occurs if the dialysate is allowed to dwell past osmotic equilibrium.
     c. Use of dialysate solutions containing 1.5% (1.38 g/dL) dextrose will result in little or no fluid removal, especially with long dwell exchanges.
     d. 2.5% (2.27 g/dL), 3.5% (3.18 g/dL), and 4.25% (3.86 g/dL) dextrose solutions are more hyperosmotic and are used to increase ultrafiltration and net fluid removal.
  4. Figure 13.8 illustrates how exchange volume and dextrose concentration affect ultrafiltration in long dwell exchanges.
  5. For patients on continuous PD regimens, particularly those with high membrane permeability, shortening the exchange time, e.g., from 6 hours to 4 hours, will result in increased ultrafiltration volume.
  6. For patients on CAPD regimens who have a long overnight dwell, or NIPD/APD patients with a long daytime dwell, icodextrin solutions will maintain the osmotic gradient throughout the long dwell.
  7. Persistent use of hyperosmotic dialysis solutions

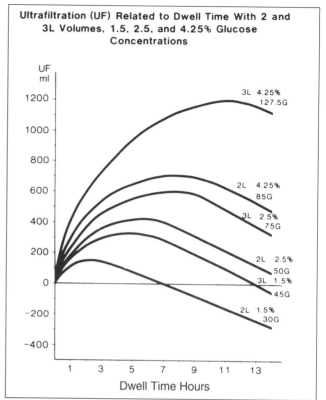

Figure 13.8. Ultrafiltration curves for 2-liter and 3-liter volumes, 2.5% and 4.25% dextrose dialysis solutions related to dwell time.

Source: Twardowski, Z.J., Khanna, R., & Nolph, K.D. (1986). Osmotic agents and ultrafiltration in peritoneal dialysis. *Nephron, 42*(2), 93-101.

may cause excessive fluid removal resulting in increased serum osmolality and/or hypovolemia, causing excessive thirst, which leads to increased fluid intake necessitating more ultrafiltration.
  8. Rapid exchanges with dialysis solutions containing ≥ 4.25% dextrose cause rapid water removal that can result in an increased serum osmolality, hypernatremia, or hypovolemic shock. Historically, the use of solutions containing 7% dextrose was associated with dialysis disequilibrium.
  9. Chronic use of hypertonic dialysis solutions results in greater exposure of the peritoneal membrane to glucose and glucose degradation products (GDPs), which may damage the membrane.

III. Drug transport.

A. Effect of systemic drugs on dialysis kinetics.
  1. Systemic vasodilators may increase clearances somewhat by augmenting blood flow to adjacent capillary beds.

2. Use of drugs that decrease abdominal blood flow will decrease clearances.

B. Effect of dialysis on drugs.
1. Factors that affect solute clearances also affect clearance of systemic drugs. Drugs that have low molecular weights, which are poorly bound to protein and are water soluble, are more readily transported across the peritoneal membrane.
2. Drugs administered intraperitoneally are transported into the systemic circulation.
3. Drugs that are removed by peritoneal dialysis may need to be given in increased frequency or dosages.
4. Drugs that are poorly removed by peritoneal dialysis and are normally excreted by the kidneys may need to be given in decreased dosages.
5. The intraperitoneal route for drug administration should be used with caution, due to the potential for deleterious effects to the peritoneal membrane.

C. Intraperitoneal insulin administration.
1. Insulin is absorbed from the peritoneal cavity and enters the systemic circulation via the hepatic portal system.
2. Peak insulin levels are reached 20–30 minutes later than with endogenous insulin, and are sustained longer.
3. Intraperitoneal insulin administration alone may be used to control serum glucose for patients on continuous forms of dialysis therapy. It is more difficult to calculate insulin dosage and control glucose for patients on continuous cycling peritoneal dialysis (CCPD) than on CAPD because most of the caloric load takes place during the day when there is only one long dwell exchange.
4. Intraperitoneal insulin may be used to provide supplemental insulin in intermittent peritoneal dialysis (IPD) or in acute dialysis with short exchanges.
5. Regular insulin is added to the dialysis solution for each CAPD exchange.
6. An increased dose of insulin is required.
   a. Insulin binds to the dialysis solution bags. However, the percentage of insulin bound to the bags does not exceed 10%.
   b. Not all of the insulin is absorbed from the dialysis solution.

IV. Individual membrane characteristics.

A. Each individual's peritoneal membrane is unique. Therefore, rates of clearance and ultrafiltration differ among patients.

B. Objective evaluation of the peritoneal membrane permeability is useful in determining the most appropriate treatment modality and in writing the dialysis prescription.

C. The KDOQI guidelines outline three methods for the assessment of individual peritoneal membrane characteristics: Peritoneal Equilibration Test (PET), Standard Peritoneal Permeability Analysis (SPA), and Peritoneal Dialysis Capacity (PDC).

D. All measurements of peritoneal transport characteristics should be obtained when the patient is clinically stable and at least 1 month after resolution of a peritonitis episode.

E. The Peritoneal Equilibration Test (PET) is a standardized diagnostic test that measures the rate of solute removal and glucose absorption in individual patients.
1. Standardized PET procedure.
   a. The exchange prior to the PET exchange must have a long dwell ($\geq$ 6 hours).
   b. Two liters 2.5% dextrose dialysis solution is allowed to dwell in the peritoneal cavity for exactly 4 hours.
   c. Dialysate samples are collected at 0, 2, and 4 hours and analyzed for creatinine and glucose.
   d. A blood sample is obtained at 2 hours for creatinine and glucose. These values are used in all calculations.
   e. The dialysate to plasma ratio for creatinine (D/P creatinine) is calculated for each sample time.
   f. The glucose over glucose at 0 dwell time (D/D0) is calculated for the 2-hour and 4-hour dwell times.
2. Faster and simpler PET procedures have been developed, but are less reliable.
   a. Four-hour PET with the initial drain and infusion done by the patient at home. Patient compliance with instructions, documentation of infusion time, and accurate timing of drain are required. There is only one 4-hour sample, so results may be more difficult to evaluate.
   b. Incenter 1-hour and 2-hour PETs using extrapolated values have been described.

3. For additional information, an unabridged PET with dialysate sampling at 0, 15, 30, 60, 120, and 240 minutes and with measurement of additional solutes (e.g., sodium, potassium, urea) can be performed (Twardowski et al., 1988).
4. Equilibration test results can be plotted on graphs representing equilibration curves from a large number of patients (see Figure 13.9).
5. The PET may be used to evaluate the patient's peritoneal membrane permeability at a single point in time, or serial studies may be used to evaluate whether changes in permeability have occurred.
6. The PET does not always provide good prediction of ultrafiltration volumes.
7. A PET using 4.25% dextrose is recommended to evaluate ultrafiltration failure.
8. Frequent errors in performing PET.
   a. Short dwell time prior to the PET exchange.
   b. Incomplete drain of prior exchange, or of PET exchange.
   c. Samples not drawn at designated times.
   d. Dialysate sample mixed with fresh dialysis solution due to improper sampling technique.
   e. Samples labeled incorrectly.
   f. Some assays use colorimetric methods to measure creatinine. These methods also read the unusually high glucose as creatinine. A correction factor (calculated for each laboratory) must be used to obtain accurate creatinine values.

F. The SPA was developed to calculate mass transfer area coefficient (MTAC) of small and middle molecular-weight solutes and to determine residual volume and ultrafiltration kinetics. This technique is often used for research purposes.
   1. 1.5% dextrose/dextran 70 solutions are used, so there is less of an osmotic gradient for ultrafiltration. There is better determination of the true diffusive MTAC characteristics of the membrane in a situation in which there is less ultrafiltration and associated convective removal of solutes.

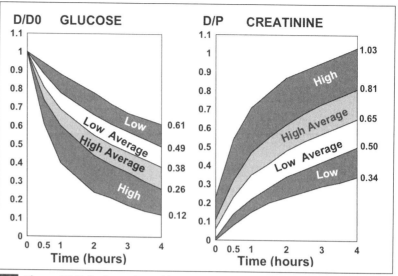

Figure 13.9. Peritoneal equilibration test curves for dialysate glucose to dialysis solution glucose at time 0 (D/D0) ratios (left) and corrected creatinine dialysate to plasma (D/P) ratios (right); determined from 103 equilibration studies in 86 patients.

2. Similar to the PET, SPA uses a single dialysis exchange and direct measurements to characterize peritoneal transport properties.

G. The PDC test establishes the MTAC and in addition, is better able to determine peritoneal fluid absorption rates and macromolecule permeability.
   1. Uses data from multiple dwells (typically 4–5) performed during a 24-hour period.
   2. Data are combined in a mathematical model to estimate peritoneal transport characteristics.

H. Interpretation of individual peritoneal membrane characteristics (based on PET).
   1. Patients with high permeability have high rates of solute transport and high rates of glucose absorption. Although clearances are good, ultrafiltration may be poor, particularly with long dwell exchanges.
      a. Initial high transport associated with a low albumin is a predictor of increased risk of death.
      b. Initial high transport not associated with low albumin, systemic inflammation, or atherosclerosis is not predictive of a poor prognosis.
   2. Patients with low permeability have low solute transport rates and slow rates of glucose absorption. Therefore, ultrafiltration is excellent, but clearances are low.

I. Companies have developed computer software to help with the evaluation and interpretation of peritoneal membrane transport.
  1. PD Adequest® developed by Baxter Healthcare Corporation (Deerfield, IL) is based on the D/P data from the standard PET.
  2. Patient On-line® developed by Fresenius Medical Care (Bad Homburg, Germany) uses the FT50 (equivalent to time D/P reaches 0.5) as the main parameter. Based on this value, all other parameters regarding small solute transport and ultrafiltration are calculated.

J. None of these tests (PET, SPA, PDC) has been shown to be clinically superior to the others and KDOQI guidelines recommend that each center should choose one of these tests and use it consistently to characterize peritoneal transport.

K. The PET is the simplest procedure to perform and has the most clinical experience related to its use.

L. Baseline peritoneal membrane transport characteristics should be established after initiating a daily PD therapy. The recommended time to perform the initial PET is at 4–6 weeks after initiation of PD, allowing ample time for healing, reducing inflammation of the peritoneal membrane, and achieving acceptable fluid balance.

M. Peritoneal membrane transport testing should be repeated when clinically indicated (e.g., loss of ultrafiltration or decrease in solute clearances).

Intraabdominal Pressure during Dialysis

I. **Peritoneal dialysis fluid** causes an increase in intraabdominal pressure proportionate to the volume of dialysis solution instilled.

II. **Increased intraabdominal pressure** is a risk factor for dialysate leak, hernias, hemorrhoids, compromised pulmonary function, and vagal stimulation leading to bradycardia.

III. **Factors that affect intraabdominal pressure.**

A. Volume of dialysis solution. Intraabdominal pressure increases as dialysis solution volume is increased.

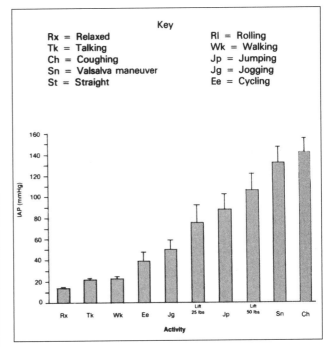

Figure 13.10. Mean ± SEM intraabdominal pressure in six upright men with 2 liters of dialysis solution in the peritoneal cavity during relaxation and various activities.

Source: Prowant, B., & Ryan, L. (1987). Intra-abdominal pressure in CAPD patients. *ANNA Journal, 14*(4), 253-257. Used with permission.

B. Body position. Intraabdominal pressure is lowest in the supine position and increases markedly in the sitting or upright positions.

C. Activity (see Figure 13.10).
  1. Coughing and the Valsalva maneuver induce extremely high intraabdominal pressures.
  2. Jumping and weight lifting also cause very high intraabdominal pressures. Because of these high pressures, it may be recommended that patients perform some exercises without fluid in the peritoneal cavity.
  3. Walking and riding a stationary bicycle are associated with lower intraabdominal pressures. Therefore, these are more appropriate exercise activities for PD patients with intraperitoneal fluid.

D. Older and obese patients tend to have higher intraabdominal pressures.

IV. **Measurement of hydrostatic intraperitoneal** pressure may be performed as an objective means of determining optimal fluid tolerance.

Table 13.9

Composition of Peritoneal Dialysis Solutions

	Standard Solution	Low Calcium Solutions	Icodextrin Solution
Sodium (mEq/L)	132.0	132.0	132.0
Calcium (mEq/L)	3.5	2.5	3.5
Magnesium (mEq/L)	0.5	0.5	0.5
Chloride (mEq/L)	96.0	95.0	96.0
Lactate (mEq/L)	40.0	40.0	40.0
pH	5.2-5.5	4.0-6.5	5.0-6.0
Osmolarity (mOsm/L)			
1.5% Dextrose	346	344	
2.5% Dextrose	396	395	
3.5% Dextrose	447	445	
4.25% Dextrose	485	483	
Icodextrin			282-286

Dialysis Solution

I. Composition.

A. Typical electrolyte concentration, pH, and osmolality of dialysis solutions commercially available in the U.S. are shown in Table 13.9.

B. Dialysis solution magnesium was lowered to 0.5 mEq/L to ameliorate the high serum magnesium levels seen in PD patients. These lower magnesium-containing solutions should be used in patients with hypoparathyroidism (evidence-based).

C. Low calcium solutions are indicated for PD patients with hypercalcemia (evidence-based).

D. Sodium lactate is added as a buffer. Bicarbonate-based solutions are available in many countries.

E. Dextrose is added to increase the osmolality to enhance ultrafiltration.
1. Most widely used osmotic agent.
2. 1.5%, 2.5%, 3.5%, and 4.25% dextrose concentrations are available.
3. Safe, effective, readily metabolized, and inexpensive.
4. Exposure of the peritoneal membrane to high glucose concentrations and glucose degradation products may contribute to both structural and functional changes in the peritoneal membrane.

F. Amino acids in dialysis solutions also act as osmotic agents.
1. Ultrafiltration is similar to 1.5% dextrose.
2. Amino acid solutions are used for only one exchange per day with a long dwell to avoid uremic symptoms and metabolic acidosis.
3. Short-term use of this solution has resulted in improvement of nitrogen balance in malnourished patients.
4. Amino acid-containing solutions should be considered in malnourished patients as part of a strategy to improve nutritional status (evidence-based).

G. 7.5% polyglucose (icodextrin)-containing solution is an alternative osmotic agent.
1. Removes fluid by colloid osmotic pressure.
2. Has a prolonged positive ultrafiltration because of the slow absorption (absorption averaged only 19% during an 8-hour exchange).
3. Indications for use of polyglucose solutions.
   a. Patients with insufficient peritoneal ultrafiltration.
      (1) Those with high transport characteristics.
      (2) Those with insufficient ultrafiltration from the long dwell exchange in either CAPD or CCPD (evidence-based).
   b. To avoid excessive exposure to glucose and GDPs.
4. Icodextrin is used for the longest dwell exchange (overnight in CAPD patients; a long daytime exchange for CCPD patients).
5. The polyglucose breaks down to maltose. Use is limited to only one exchange per day to avoid excessive accumulation of plasma maltose. Although elevated maltose and isomaltose have been documented in PD patients using one exchange with polyglucose solutions, these have not been associated with recognizable adverse effects.
6. Allergic reactions have been reported in ~ 5% of patients, primarily a skin rash that develops within the first 3 weeks of use and resolves when icodextrin is discontinued. A few patients have developed exfoliative dermatitis.

7. Maltose interferes with blood glucose monitoring results with test strips that use glucose dehydrogenase pyrroloquinoline-quinone (GDH PQQ)-based methods, yielding falsely high glucose levels. Blood glucose measurements must be done using a glucose-specific method to prevent maltose interference.
8. Outcomes.
   a. May be associated with less change in peritoneal transport over time.
   b. The use of icodextrin may improve technique survival in patients with ultrafiltration failure who might otherwise need conversion to hemodialysis.
   c. There is no difference in peritonitis rates in patients using glucose vs. icodextrin for the long dwell (evidenced-based).

H. Bicarbonate is a more physiologic buffer with a higher pH. Bicarbonate-buffered PD solutions are safe and well tolerated.
   1. Bicarbonate solutions come in double-chambered bags.
   2. Bicarbonate solutions may reduce infusion pain.
   3. Blood bicarbonate levels may increase and normalize with use of bicarbonate solutions.
   4. At the time of writing, bicarbonate solutions were not available in the United States.

I. High buffer-containing solutions should be used in patients with metabolic acidosis (evidence-based). Serum bicarbonate concentration should be monitored to avoid metabolic alkalosis.

J. Potassium is omitted from dialysis solutions because patients with kidney failure require potassium removal. Acute dialysis with rapid exchanges may lower serum potassium to normal or below normal levels. Potassium chloride is then added to dialysis solutions per physician's order to maintain serum levels within normal limits.

The Peritoneal Dialysis Process

I. Exchange or cycle.

A. An exchange or cycle is defined as the infusion, dwell, and drainage of dialysis solution. This cycle is repeated throughout the course of dialysis.

B. Infusion.
   1. Dialysis solution flows into the peritoneal cavity by gravity with a manual system and with most cycling systems.
   2. Other cyclers use a pump for solution infusion.
   3. Infusion by gravity takes approximately 10 minutes for a 2-liter volume (if catheter is patent and solution is elevated sufficiently above the level of the abdomen).
   4. Factors that affect the rate of inflow by gravity include the height of the solution, the inner diameter of the catheter and tubing, the tubing length, catheter configuration, and intraabdominal pressure.
      a. If catheter and tubing diameters are equivalent, a straight Tenckhoff catheter has the fastest infusion time.
      b. If catheter and tubing diameters are equivalent, a coiled catheter has a longer infusion time because it is longer in total length and has more curves.
      c. If catheter and tubing diameters are equivalent, a swan-neck, coiled catheter will have an even longer infusion time because of its greater length and additional curve.
      d. These differences in flow rates are not clinically significant, especially in continuous PD.

C. Dwell. The dwell or equilibration period provides time for diffusion and osmosis to take place.
   1. A typical dwell time for acute intermittent peritoneal dialysis is 30–60 minutes.
   2. In CCPD the cycler dwell time is ~1.5–2.0 hours. A single daytime exchange may last as long as 12–16 hours, or the daytime exchange may be drained after 4–6 hours, followed by a dry period or a second daytime exchange.
   3. CAPD daytime exchanges typically last 4–6 hours and the overnight exchange for 8–10 hours.

D. Drain.
   1. Dialysate typically drains from the peritoneal cavity by gravity.
   2. Some cyclers remove fluid by negative pressure.
   3. Drainage of 2 liters plus ultrafiltration takes about 10 minutes if the catheter is functioning optimally.
   4. Drain flow occurs through both the tip and side holes.
   5. Factors that affect the drain rate include the catheter position, internal or external pressure on the lines, intraabdominal pressure, catheter configuration, the tubing diameter, tubing length, and the height distance from the abdomen to the drain bag.

6. The dialysis solution drains rapidly and at a fairly constant rate during the first 7–10 minutes of the drain, and then reaches a "breakpoint" where the drain flow slows dramatically. At this point most of the final drain volume (~ 95%) has drained, and prolonging the drain time further simply prolongs the period of time in which there is no dialysis taking place.

7. In "breakpoint APD," the cycler is programmed to stop the drain at the breakpoint, based on the patient's individual drain flow profile. This increases clearances and reduces cycler alarms.

II. Warming methods.

A. When exposed to high temperature for a period of time, glucose in peritoneal dialysis solution degrades to toxic carbonyl compounds commonly know as glucose degradation products (GDPs). When there is extensive glucose degradation, the solution may have a light brown discoloration due to carmelization.

B. Therefore, PD fluids should be warmed only to body temperature, and shortly before use.

C. Regardless of the warming method used, the temperature of the solution must be monitored.
   1. Measured temperature should be approximately 37° C.
   2. Solution should be tepid to the touch.

D. Dry heating is recommended.
   1. Heating cabinet or incubator. Solutions should be warmed prior to use, but should not be left in the heater for an extended period.
   2. Heating pad.
   3. Microwave.
      a. Microwave warming results in hot spots in the solution bag, especially in the medication port. Mixing the solution after warming by inverting the bag several times will promote an even temperature distribution.
      b. Overheating can be avoided by determining the warming time required for each microwave oven by measuring the external bag temperature.
      c. Microwave exposure does not change pH or chemistries of solution.
      d. Microwave warming is not recommended by some manufacturers.
   4. Home patients may place the dialysis solution on or near a heating source, or in the sunshine.

E. Water baths are not recommended for heating peritoneal dialysis solutions because they increase the risk of contamination to the system.
   1. Water is contaminated with microorganisms.
   2. Even though the dialysis solution container is dried when it is removed from the water bath, some moisture may remain and run down to the connection.

F. Shipping and storage of PD solutions.
   1. When PD fluid is exposed to high temperatures during shipping or storage, the concentration of cytotoxic GDPs increases rapidly and doubles within a few hours. This can also occur with overheating or prolonged warming of dialysis solutions, regardless of the warming method.
   2. The concentration levels and cytotoxicity of GDPs gradually decrease when the PD fluid temperature is lowered to room temperature, and eventually return back to original levels, but the process is slow and takes up to 40 days (Erixon et al., 2005).

III. Addition of medications.

A. It is recommended that medications are added immediately before the solution will be hung and used. For cyclers, it is recommended that medications be added to each individual bag.

B. Aseptic technique is critical.

C. Disinfect multiple dose vials.
   1. 5-minute povidone-iodine soak is widely used.
   2. Sodium hypochlorite preparations are also used (e.g., Amuchina®).

D. The injection port must be disinfected as the overwrap does not guarantee sterility of the bag exterior.
   1. 5-minute povidone-iodine soak is widely used.
   2. Sodium hypochlorite is also used.

E. A 5/8-inch insulin needle will not consistently puncture the inner diaphragm of Baxter brand dialysis solution bags. A 1-inch needle is recommended.

F. Mix dialysis solution well after medication has been added.

G. Label solution container(s) with drug, dose, time, and initials.

H. Record date and time of initial use on reusable medication vials.

I. KCl comes in single dose vials without preservative. These vials should not be reused.

Acute Peritoneal Dialysis – See Chapter 12

Chronic Peritoneal Dialysis

I. **Evidence-based practice guidelines** related to delivery of peritoneal dialysis therapy are summarized in Table 13.10.

II. Types of PD therapy.

A. Intermittent peritoneal dialysis (IPD).
   1. Treatments are performed periodically, at least several times during the week. The peritoneal cavity is empty or dry between treatments.
   2. Typically performed at night with a dry day.
   3. May be done during the day, similar to CAPD exchanges, but without an overnight exchange. This is sometimes termed daily ambulatory peritoneal dialysis (DAPD). Because of the shorter dialysis time, this therapy is only sufficient for patients with residual renal function. Because of the short dwell times, it is most appropriate for patients with high transport characteristics.

B. Continuous peritoneal dialysis.
   1. The patient dialyzes 24 hours, 7 days per week. There is always dialysis solution in the peritoneal cavity except for drain and fill.
   2. In CAPD there are 3–4 daytime exchanges and a long overnight exchange. A simple cycling device may be used to perform an additional nighttime exchange.
   3. In CCPD there are 4–6 overnight exchanges and one or more long dwell daytime exchanges.

III. Technique.

A. Intermittent flow is used for almost all chronic peritoneal dialysis.
   1. Dialysis solution is first infused and then after a dwell period it is drained through the same catheter.
   2. Each fluid exchange or cycle has three distinct modes: inflow, dwell, and drain.

Table 13.10

Evidence-Based Practice Guidelines for Peritoneal Dialyis, Level I and II Recommendations

- Measurement of dialysis adequacy (KDOQI)
  - The first measurement should be performed within the first month after initiation of PD
  - Adequacy studies should be repeated every 4 months
  - If the patient has > 100 mL urine/day and renal clearances are used to determine the total weekly Kt/V_{urea}, a 24-hour urine collection for volume and clearances should be done every 2 months

- The **minimum** weekly total Kt/V_{urea} is 1.7 (KDOQI, EBPG)

- The corrected creatinine clearance target for high and high average transporters is 60 L/week; for low and low average transporters the target is 50 L/week (CARI)

- The **minimum** target for net ultrafiltration in anuric PD patients is 1.0 L/day (EBPG)

- Subjective Global Nutritional Assessment (SGA) is a valid and clinically useful measure of protein-energy nutritional status in maintenance dialysis patients (KDOQI)

- To preserve residual renal function, use angiotensin converting enzyme inhibitors (ACEs) or angiotensin receptor blockers (ARBs) in patients who require antihypertensive medications (KDOQI)

CARI = Caring for Australians with Renal Impairment (2005)
EBPG = European Best Practice Guidelines (Dombros et al., 2005).
KDOQI = Kidney Disease Outcomes Quality Initiative (National Kidney Foundation, 2006)

   3. Intermittent flow should not be confused with intermittent dialysis. It simply describes the interruption of fluid flow through the catheter during the dwell period.

B. Tidal flow (not to be confused with tidal drain mode – defined below).
   1. After the initial volume of dialysis fluid is instilled into the peritoneal cavity, at the end of each exchange only a portion of the dialysate is drained and replaced with fresh fluid.
   2. This leaves the greater portion of dialyzing fluid in constant contact with the peritoneal membrane until the dialysate is completely drained at the end of the treatment.
      a. A significant amount of solute removal continues during fill and drain times.

b. This increases the overall efficiency of the dialysis process.

3. Each tidal exchange has three distinct modes: inflow, dwell, and drain. However, the initial fill and last drain have higher volumes.

4. An example of tidal dialysis is an initial fill volume of 2 L, drain volume of 1.2 L, and a tidal infusion volume of 1 L for subsequent exchanges, with a full final drain.

C. Continuous flow is a type of intermittent PD. It is primarily a research technique aimed at enhancing dialysis efficiency.

1. The patient has two catheters. Dialysis solution is continuously infused through one catheter and drained through the other.

2. Theoretically, the constant infusion of new dialysis solution maintains a high concentration gradient facilitating diffusion, and a higher dextrose concentration enhancing ultrafiltration.

3. Dialysate mixing must occur to prevent the stream of new dialysis solution from infusing through one catheter and draining right out the other.

D. Tidal drain. At the end of a CAPD or APD exchange, dialysate is drained for a set time or a set volume. The drain phase is interrupted before complete dainage is achieved. This shortens the standard drain time by eliminating the final phase where dialysate flows slowly and there is minimal additional drain volume. Thus, what would have been additional drain time becomes additional dialysis dwell time. Only at the end of the treatment is the dialysate drained completely.

IV. Method by which the peritoneal dialysis procedure is done.

A. The basic aims of any PD delivery system should be:

1. Security – to prevent bacterial contamination.

2. Simplicity – in terms of performing the procedure (both by staff and the patient).

3. Quality – in relation to the materials used (strong and resilient, biocompatible, disposable, recyclable).

4. Convenience – in terms of patient preference, considering social background including employment, family, and patient's lifestyle.

B. Manual method. Each fluid exchange is performed manually by the patient, partner, or nurse. CAPD and DAPD are examples of PD using the manual method.

C. Automated method (sometimes referred to as automated peritoneal dialysis [APD]): exchanges or cycles are accomplished by a preset dialysis cycler. CCPD and NIPD are examples of PD treatments using an automated method. For CAPD, a small, portable cycler (automated method) may be used for an additional exchange during the night, to increase the dialysis dose.

V. Cycler.

A. Device used for automated peritoneal dialysis. Peritoneal dialysis cyclers require disposable tubing as well as prepared dialysis solution that must be attached and set up by the patient, assistant, or nurse using a specific procedure. Two types of cyclers are shown in Figures 13.11 and 13.12.

B. Warms dialysis solution.

C. Delivers dialysis solution to the patient and allows dialysate to remain in the peritoneal cavity for a preset period of time.

D. Controls are preset and determine inflow volume, dwell time, and outflow volume. The drain cycle can be controlled either by a predetermined volume or by time.

E. Generally monitors temperature, inflow and outflow rates, and inflow and outflow volumes.

F. Can be operated by the patient without assistance.

G. Requires mask, hand washing, and aseptic technique to add medications and perform connect/disconnect procedures.

H. Some cyclers can be disassembled and used for travel.

I. Some cyclers are equipped with memory chips that record details of each dialysis session (e.g., PD Link®, Baxter Healthcare Corporation, Deerfield, IL; Newton IQ®, Fresenius Medical Care North America, Lexington, MA). The patient's treatment information can easily be downloaded, so nurses can review the patient's treatment history for a period of time.

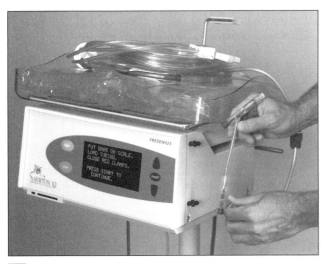

Figure 13.11. Peritoneal dialysis cycler.
Courtesy of Fresenius USA

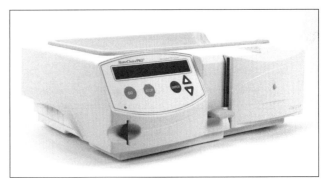

Figure 13.12. This peritoneal dialysis cycler does not depend on gravity flow, so it can be positioned at any level.
Courtesy of Baxter Healthcare Corporation

VI. Procedures.

A. An example of a procedure for initiating PD is shown in Table 13.11.

B. An example of a procedure for discontinuing PD is shown in Table 13.12.

C. An example of a procedure for changing the transfer set is shown in Table 13.13.

D. A recent study of transfer set procedures using both povidone-iodine and sodium hypochlorite reconfirmed that an external scrub or external scrub plus closed 5-minute soak does not completely disinfect the connection. Only procedures that incorporated a 5-minute open soak ensured disinfection of all surfaces (Kubey & Straka, 2005).

VII. Dialysis prescription.

A. The dialysis prescription should be individualized for each patient taking into consideration peritoneal transport rate, residual renal function, size (total body surface area), certain medical conditions, and personal preference.

B. Continuous PD therapies.
1. Continuous ambulatory peritoneal dialysis (CAPD). This continuous dialysis therapy uses manual or manual-assisted methods.
   a. Schedule.
      (1) Dialysis solution is always present in the peritoneal cavity, except for brief interruptions to drain and reinfuse fresh dialysis solution.
      (2) Dialysis takes place 24 hours, 7 days a week.
      (3) 4–5 exchanges per day.
      (4) Daytime exchanges last from 4 to 6 hours.
      (5) Overnight exchange lasts from 8 to 10 hours.
      (6) A typical pattern is to exchange the solution upon arising, at lunchtime, before or after dinner, and at bedtime.
   b. Indications.
      (1) Average or low peritoneal membrane permeability.
      (2) Preference to avoid machines or confinement to bed.
   c. Clearances are higher than those obtained with IPD because of the extremely long dwell times. Good control of fluid balance can be maintained.
   d. CAPD may be complemented with an additional exchange at night using an automated exchange device. This is indicated for patients who require additional solute clearances.
2. Continuous cycling peritoneal dialysis (CCPD). This continuous therapy uses a cycler for automated overnight dialysis, with a long dwell exchange during the day, or a single additional daytime exchange.
   a. Schedule.
      (1) 3–5 overnight cycles.
      (2) Overnight cycles last from 1.5 to 2, or even 3 hours.

Table 13.11

Example of Key Steps of a Procedure for Initiating PD

Using aseptic technique (wearing mask and sterile gloves):

1. Scrub the catheter-cap connection using a disinfectant.
2. Soak the catheter-cap connection in disinfectant.
3. Dry catheter-cap connection and remove cap.
4. Soak open catheter adapter in disinfectant.*
5. Connect sterile transfer set.
6. Connect dialysis solution system.
7. Drain any residual dialysate from the peritoneal cavity.
8. Flush PD system with dialysis solution.
9. Fill the peritoneal cavity with dialysis solution.

* Only procedures that incorporated a 5-minute open soak ensured disinfection of all surfaces (Kubey & Straka, 2005).

Table 13.12

Example of Key Steps of a Procedure for Discontinuing PD

Using aseptic technique (wearing mask and sterile gloves):

1. Scrub catheter-transfer set connection with disinfectant.
2. Soak catheter-transfer set connection in disinfectant.
3. Disconnect the transfer set from the catheter.
4. Soak open catheter adapter in disinfectant.*
5. Place cap on catheter adapter.

* Only procedures that incorporated a 5-minute open soak ensured disinfection of all surfaces (Kubey & Straka, 2005).

(3) A single, long daytime exchange lasts 12–16 hours.
   (a) Use of hypertonic solution prevents significant reabsorption, or an additional daytime exchange can be made.
   (b) Use of icodextrin should be considered for the long dwell exchange (evidence-based).
b. Indications.
   (1) High, or high average peritoneal membrane transport characteristics.
      (a) Clearances are higher than those obtained with IPD.
      (b) Better control of fluid balance can be achieved.
   (2) Patients who choose CCPD.
      (a) Preference for uninterrupted days.
      (b) School or work schedules make CAPD difficult.
      (c) Require the assistance of a partner for dialysis, e.g., children and the elderly.
      (d) Teenagers.

C. Systems for continuous therapies.
   1. Common elements: tubings are composed of polyvinyl, thermoplastic, silicone, or polypropylene materials with clamps to control fluid flow.

2. Spike or Luer-Lok® systems.
   a. These were the standard systems in North America in the 1980s.
   b. The catheter is connected to the bag via tubing with a beveled spike or Luer-Lok device, which is left in place between exchanges.
   c. During each exchange procedure, dialysate is drained from the peritoneal cavity into an empty bag. The drain bag is then disconnected and discarded. A new bag of dialysis solution is connected to the tubing and attached to the patient's catheter. Fresh dialysis solution is infused into the peritoneal cavity. The connection is covered. The empty bag is rolled up and remains attached to the patient until the next exchange procedure.
   d. This system was associated with high peritonitis rates.
3. Y-set tubings come with a drain bag on one arm of the Y and the other arm is used to attach the new solution bag. The leg of the Y is connected to the patient's catheter or transfer set.
4. Double-bag systems are Y-sets manufactured with the dialysis solution bag already attached. Double-bag or twin-bag systems are preferred for CAPD because they are more effective in preventing peritonitis (evidence-based). These are the systems most frequently used in North America and Europe. If a double-bag system is not available, any Y-set system is preferred to a spike system, because Y- and double-bag systems are more effective in preventing peritonitis (evidence-based).

Table 13.13

Example of Key Steps and Rationale for a Procedure for Changing the Transfer Set

Key Steps	Rationale
Use aseptic technique	The inner lumen of the catheter and peritoneal cavity are sterile. Use of aseptic technique reduces the risk of contamination during the procedure.
Scrub	Physically removes dirt and debris from catheter and adapter.
Closed soak	Reduces bacteria present on the outside of the tubing, catheter and adapter prior to disconnection.
Disconnect	Removes and discards old transfer set.
Open soak*	Reduces bacteria present on the adapter prior to connection of the new transfer set. (This will allow the disinfectant to come into contact with bacteria on the distal end of the adapter that may have been exposed when the connection was loose, but are not reached by the first soak if connection was later tightened.)
Connect new transfer set	Establishes a new, sterile transfer set for delivery of PD therapy.

* Only procedures that incorporated a 5-minute open soak ensured disinfection of all surfaces (Kubey & Straka, 2005).

5. Flush before fill concept.
   a. For both the Y- and double-bag systems, approximately 100 mL dialysis solution is flushed from the new dialysis solution bag to the drain bag. The patient then drains the dialysate from the peritoneal cavity. This procedure is widely referred to as "flush-before-fill."
   b. In vitro studies have shown that the flushing procedure followed by a drain was effective in eliminating *Staphylococcus epidermidis* 5 minutes after contamination. *Staphylococcus aureus* and Pseudomonas species were reduced, but not consistently eliminated.
   c. Studies consistently demonstrate lower peritonitis rates using Y systems than standard spike or Luer-Lok systems, and the standard systems should not be used (evidence-based).

D. Intermittent peritoneal dialysis (IPD). Any schedule that has a period off dialysis. Typically uses a cycling device, although it can be done manually.
   1. IPD refers to peritoneal dialysis that is done for several hours, discontinued and then repeated, either in a health care facility or at home.
   2. Exchange time on IPD is significantly shorter than in continuous dialysis. Therefore, it is ideal

for patients with very high peritoneal transport characteristics.
   3. Indications for IPD.
      a. Early use of chronic catheter (catheter break-in period).
      b. Complications related to increased intra-abdominal pressure (intraabdominal pressure is lower in the supine position), e.g., hernias and leaks.
      c. Patients in hospitals and extended care facilities, when staffing does not allow CAPD.
      d. Patients unable to achieve adequate ultrafiltration and solute clearances with CAPD, e.g., patients with high transport characteristics (evidence-based).
      e. IPD may provide adequate clearances and fluid removal for patients with significant residual renal function.
      f. Dialysis for actue renal failure.
   4. To achieve adequate clearances and fluid removal, chronic IPD is typically done 8 to 10 hours every night, this is sometimes called nightly intermittent peritoneal dialysis (NIPD). Additional time is required for patients without residual renal function.
   5. Nightly tidal peritoneal dialysis (NTPD) is another variation of IPD. This therapy uses a cycler that delivers tidal volumes.
      a. In tidal dialysis, only a portion of the full

Table 13.14

Comparison of Chronic Peritoneal Dialysis Therapies

CAPD (continuous ambulatory peritoneal dialysis)	CCPD (continuous cycling peritoneal dialysis)	NIPD (nightly intermittent peritoneal dialysis)
4–5 manual exchanges during the day; may use assist device for extra nighttime exchange(s).	Automatic cycling of exchanges overnight with a long daytime dwell.	Automatic cycling of exchanges overnight.
Solution in peritoneal cavity continuously, except for drain and fill times.	Solution in peritoneal cavity continuously, except for drain and fill times.	Dialysate is drained completely at end of dialysis; no solution in the peritoneal cavity between dialyses.
Some techniques require portable equipment, e.g., an exchange assist device.	Requires cycler; typically uses 5 liter bags.	Requires cycler; typically uses 5-liter bags.
Closed system is opened for each exchange.	Closed system opened for setup and on/off procedures.	Closed system opened for setup and on/off procedures.
Requires 20–40 minutes/exchange.	Requires ~ 45 minutes for setup and on/off procedures.	Requires ~ 45 minutes for setup and on/off procedures.
Blood chemistries stable.	Small diurnal biochemical fluctuations.	Biochemical fluctuations.
Fluid balance stable.	Diurnal fluctuations in fluid balance.	Fluid balance fluctuations.
Daytime interruptions for exchanges; sleep uninterrupted.	Sleep may be disturbed; may require an additional daytime exchange.	Sleep may be disturbed; no interruption of daytime routine.

exchange volume is drained and replaced for each exchange. For example, if a 2-liter initial fill volume is used, the cycler could be set for a 1200 mL drain volume and 1000 mL tidal fill volume.

b. Tidal volumes and dwell times must be individualized to achieve the most efficient clearances. Dwell times are shorter than in typical IPD (or CCPD).

c. Tidal peritoneal dialysis requires special equipment so that tidal volumes and cycles can be controlled.

d. Indications for tidal dialysis.

(1) Need to increase dialysis efficiency and adequacy in a patient on cycler dialysis. Weekly clearances are somewhat greater than for the equivalent time on NIPD. This is due to use of more fresh dialysis solution and greater diffusion time (due to decreased drain and fill times).

(2) Inflow or outflow pain (evidence-based).

(3) Slow drainage causing cycler alarms (evidenced-based).

e. Tidal peritoneal dialysis is more expensive because of the markedly higher volume of dialysis solution used.

E. Table 13.14 compares key elements of the three most widely used PD therapies.

Achieving Adequate Peritoneal Dialysis

I. **Residual kidney function (RKF) contributes significantly to peritoneal dialysis adequacy.**

A. PD does not deliver as much small solute clearance as hemodialysis or native kidney function. Loss of RKF cannot be entirely compensated by increasing peritoneal clearances.

B. RKF of 1 mL/min contributes around 10 L to the total weekly creatinine clearance.

C. RKF predicts survival in prospective observational studies. There is a 12% decrease in relative risk of death for every 5 L/week/1.73 m^2 increment in glomerular filtration rate (GFR) (CANUSA, 1996).

D. It is important to monitor and preserve residual kidney function (evidence-based).

E. Strategies to preserve RKF.
   1. Preferential use of angiotensin-converting enzyme inhibitors (ACEs) or angiotensin receptor blockers (ARBs) in patients who require antihypertensive medications (evidence-based).
   2. Consider use of ACE inhibitors or ARBs in normotensive patients with RKF (evidence-based).
   3. Avoid nephrotoxic drugs, e.g., nonsteroidal antiinflammatory drugs (NSAIDs), aminoglycosides (evidence-based).
   4. Avoid intravenous (IV) radiocontrast agents.
   5. Establish a protocol that outlines renal-protective strategies when IV radiocontrast agents must be used.
   6. Educate patients regarding preservation of residual kidney function.
   7. Avoid excessive fluid removal, dehydration, and hypotension.

II. Evaluating adequacy of peritoneal dialysis.

A. All patients should routinely have a careful clinical evaluation for adequacy of dialysis with special attention to signs of underdialysis. Elements of the evaluation should include:
   1. Appetite, e.g., presence of anorexia, dysguesia, nausea, vomiting.
   2. Energy and activity levels.
   3. Muscle mass, strength, and endurance.
   4. Parathesias and asthenia.
   5. Quality of sleep.
   6. Nutritional status, e.g., subjective global assessment score, prealbumin and albumin levels.
   7. Ability to achieve/maintain fluid balance and blood pressure control.
   8. Anemia and response to erythropoietic stimulating agents (ESAs).

B. Techniques for measuring PD adequacy require 24-hour urine and dialysate collections.

C. Urea kinetic modeling (Kt/V$_{urea}$).
   1. The formulas calculate the total clearance of urea (from 24-hour collections of both dialysate and urine) over a specified time, adjusted for the volume of body water estimated from sex, age, height, and weight. A formula and sample calculations are shown (see Tables 13.15 and 13.16).
   2. The National Kidney Foundation Dialysis Kidney Disease Outcomes Quality Initiative (KDOQI) guidelines recommend that urea distribution volume, the V in Kt/V$_{urea}$, should be estimated using either Watson or Hume methods using ideal or standard weight rather than actual body weight.
   3. V should not be estimated as a percentage of total body water. This method will overestimate V in obese patients, and underestimate V in underweight patients. The volume has a large impact on the results of the Kt/V$_{urea}$ equation, and inaccurate estimated volumes can result in erroneous Kt/V$_{urea}$ results in individual patients.
   4. KDOQI guidelines for PD adequacy.
      a. The original KDOQI guidelines for peritoneal dialysis adequacy were based on large observational studies in North America and Europe. These guidelines were adopted by the Health Care Financing Administration (HCFA) for clinical performance measures (CPMs).
         (1) The original recommendations were a Kt/V$_{urea}$ of ≥ 2.0 for CAPD with incremental increases for CCPD and NIPD.
         (2) The 1997 KDOQI guidelines recommended a total (dialysis + kidney) weekly corrected creatinine clearance target for high and high average transporters of 60 L/week, and 50 L/week for low and low-average transporters. This is still an evidence-based recommendation in the Australian guidelines (CARI, 2005).
      b. The most recent KDOQI guidelines are based on results of two large randomized clinical trials.
         (1) The ADEMEX study done in Mexico demonstrated that increasing Kt/V$_{urea}$ over 1.7 in this population did not lead to improved survival (Paniagua et al., 2002).
         (2) Studies in Hong Kong also found that increasing Kt/V$_{urea}$ over 1.7 did not lead

Table 13.15

Urea Clearance and Kt/V$_{urea}$ Formulas for Continuous Peritoneal Dialysis

$K = D_{urea} \times D_{volume} / P_{urea} \times t$

K = Clearance
D = Dialysate
   urea in mg/dL
   volume in mL
P = Plasma
   urea in mg/dL
t = time in minutes

Kt/V = Clearance x time/volume (TBW)

TBW* = 2.45 – 0.0952** (age) + 0.107** (Ht.) + 0.336 (Wt.)

---

*Total Body Water according to Watson formula for males.
**These numbers have been rounded in this example.

Table 13.16

Sample Kt/V$_{urea}$ Calculation

A 47-year-old Caucasian male, height 176 cm, weight 70 kg, is on CAPD with four 2 L exchanges per day.

Dialysate volume	10,000 mL
Dialysate urea nitrogen	53 mg/dL
Urine volume	950 mL
Urine urea nitrogen	408 mg/dL
Serum urea nitrogen	75 mg/dL

$$K_{dialysis} = \frac{53\ mg/dL \times 10,000\ mL}{75\ mg/dL \times 1440\ minutes}$$
$$= 4.91\ mL/min\ or\ 7.07\ L/day^*$$

$$K_{urine} = \frac{408\ mg/dL \times 950\ mL}{75\ mg/dl \times 1440\ minutes}$$
$$= 3.59\ mL/min\ or\ 5.17\ L/day^*$$

$K_{combined}$ = 8.50 mL/min or 12.24 L/day

TBW = 2.45 – 0.0952 (47) + 0.107 (176 cm) + 0.336 (70 kg)
   = 40.33 L

Kt/V = 12.24/40.33 = .30/day or 2.1/week

---

* In actual practice, only the final number would be rounded, and only to the least number of decimal places used in the entire calculation. Incorrect rounding results in error.

to improved survival in anuric patients in this patient population. Although there was a trend toward improved survival in patients with Kt/V$_{urea}$ > 2.0, this was not statistically significant.

c. Current KDOQI guidelines now recommend an **absolute minimum** Kt/V$_{urea}$ of 1.7. This minimum value must be met by all PD patients at all times, regardless of type of PD therapy or prescription (evidence-based). The best way to assure that patients meet this absolute minimum value at all times is to retain a target Kt/V$_{urea}$ of 2.0.

d. The same data used to determine Kt/V$_{urea}$ can be used for calculations of urea generation rate, protein catabolic rate, and residual kidney function.

D. Creatinine clearance.
1. Although creatinine clearance has been dropped from the KDOQI guidelines for the sake of simplicity, a total weekly creatinine clearance of 60 L for high and high average transporters and 50 L for low and low-average transporters is still recommended by the Australian guidelines (CARI, 2005).
   a. Creatinine clearance is also calculated from 24-hour collections of both dialysate and urine and is standardized using body surface

area. Creatinine clearance can be easily and inexpensively measured from the same dialysate and urine collections and blood sample as the Kt/V$_{urea}$.
   b. Creatinine diffuses more slowly than urea because of its higher molecular weight, so creatinine clearance can be used as a surrogate marker of clearance of molecules a bit larger than urea. Creatinine is both filtered in the glomerulus and secreted by the tubules, so is more readily removed when patients have residual kidney function.
2. When both Kt/V$_{urea}$ and creatinine clearance values are available and there is discordance between Kt/V$_{urea}$ and creatinine clearance values, Kt/V$_{urea}$ should be the determinant of adequacy.
3. The same data used to determine creatinine

clearances can be used for estimation of lean body mass.

E. Evaluation of fluid balance.
1. The European guidelines (Dombros et al., 2005) recommend a minimum target for net ultrafiltration in anuric PD patients of 1.0 L/day (evidence-based).
2. KDOQI guidelines state that each facility should have a program to monitor fluid balance on a monthly basis, including blood pressure, PD drain volumes, and residual kidney function (evidence-based).
3. KDOQI guidelines recommend the following strategies to optimize extracellular water and blood volume (evidence-based).
   a. Restrict dietary sodium.
   b. Restrict water intake.
   c. Use diuretics in patients with residual kidney function.
   d. Optimize peritoneal ultrafiltration and sodium removal.

F. Frequency of adequacy testing as recommended by KDOQI guidelines (evidence-based).
1. The first measurement should be performed within the first month after initiation of PD.
2. Adequacy studies should be repeated every 4 months.
3. If the patient has > 100 mL urine/day, and renal clearances are used to determine the total weekly Kt/V$_{urea}$, a 24-hour urine collection for volume and clearances should be done every 2 months.
4. In addition to the above, clinical experts recommend that repeated measurements should be done if there has been a change in residual renal function, ultrafiltration, or a change in laboratory values that could signal a change in peritoneal membrane function.
5. Clinical indications for measurement of peritoneal dialysis adequacy are listed in Table 13.17.

G. Methods of dialysate sample collection for adequacy testing.
1. Batch method.
   a. Collect all drain bags for 24 hours.
   b. Weigh or measure dialysate in each bag to determine total volume.
   c. Combine all dialysate in one container and mix well.
   d. Take sample and send to laboratory for urea and creatinine.

Table 13.17

Clinical Indications for Measurement of Peritoneal Dialysis Adequacy

- Documentation of delivered total solute clearance after a prescription change.
- Hypertension and volume-overload refractory to current therapy.
- Signs or symptoms of uremia.
- Changes in laboratory values, e.g., increasing serum creatinine, urea, or potassium.
- Failure to thrive on dialysis therapy.
- Evaluation of other undiagnosed clinical problem.

2. Aliquot method.
   a. Collect all drain bags for 24 hours.
   b. Weigh/measure each drain bag.
   c. Record the total 24-hour volume.
   d. Take at least 0.1% sample from each bag.
   e. Combine all samples and mix well.
   f. Send sample to laboratory for BUN and creatinine.

H. Problems with adequacy testing.
1. 24-hour collections for adequacy assessment are typically done by the patient at home. The dialysis done on the day of collection may not represent the dialysis that the patient routinely does. In a case where the patient frequently skips an exchange, but does dialysis as ordered on the day of collection, the clearance indices will represent what the prescribed therapy could achieve, not the amount of dialysis the patient is actually receiving.
2. The patient may make errors in performing the dialysis exactly as ordered, in saving a complete quantitative urine collection, or in bringing the collections or samples to the clinic or laboratory. Frequent errors include:
   a. Quantitative urine collection.
      (1) Not recording precise times the collection begins and ends.
      (2) Including the first voiding in the collection.
      (3) Failing to include all voidings or including partial voidings.
   b. Dialysate collection.
      (1) For continuous therapies, time is not exactly 24 hours. A longer time results in

Table 13.18

Percent of Adult PD patients with Weekly Kt/V$_{urea}$ Meeting the 2000 KDOQI Targets

	CAPD – All		CCPD – All	
Nov 94-Apr 95	23%			
Nov 96-Apr 97	36%		36%	
Oct 98-Mar 99	56%		52%	
	CAPD Hi Avg/High*	CAPD Low/Low Avg*	CCPD Hi Avg/High*	CCPD Low/Low Avg*
Oct 00-Mar 01	75%	71%	64%	53%
Oct 02-Mar 03	74%	81%	64%	58%
Oct 04-Mar 05	68%	62%	57%	60%

* Peritoneal membrane transport type by peritoneal equilibration test.
 4 hr. D/P creatinine ratio: low = 0.34-0.49; low average = 0.50-0.64; high average = 0.65-0.81; high = 0.82-1.03.

Source: Centers for Medicare & Medicaid Services. (2005). *2005 annual report, End Stage Renal Disease Clinical Performance Measures Project.* Baltimore: Department of Health and Human Services, Centers for Medicare & Medicaid Services, Office of Clinical Standards & Quality.

an increase in solute removal, somewhat overestimating clearances. A shorter time results in less solute removal, thus underestimating clearances.

(2) The patient adds an extra bag to the 24-hour collection, from the previous day or the following day.

(3) The patient does not clamp bags securely when bringing them into clinic and dialysate is lost; thus the measured 24-hour volume is less than the actual volume.

(4) Bags are not weighed or measured accurately when an aliquot is taken at home. Thus the volume measurement is inaccurate.

III. Core Indicators and Clinical Performance Measures data showed a consistent, incremental improvement in Kt/V$_{urea}$ through 2001 (see Table 13.18). The percentage of patients meeting the target began to decrease after early reports of the ADEMEX (Paniagua, 2002) and Hong Kong (Lo et al., 2003) studies, which found no statistically significant improvement in survival in patients with Kt/V$_{urea}$ > 1.7.

IV. Problems achieving targets.

A. Unless a patient has residual kidney function, it is almost impossible to achieve recommended levels of creatinine clearance.

B. Patients with low peritoneal membrane permeability will have a larger discrepancy between Kt/V$_{urea}$ and creatinine clearance than those with high membrane permeability. According to KDOQI guidelines, when there is discordance between Kt/V$_{urea}$ and creatinine clearance values, Kt/V$_{urea}$ should be the determinant of adequacy.

V. Patients at risk for inadequate dialysis.

A. Patients with no residual renal function.

B. Patients with low peritoneal membrane permeability.

C. Large patients.

D. Nonadherent patients.
  1. Although patients may meet minimum dialysis adequacy values, the adequacy collection does not represent the typical daily dialysis regimen.
  2. Assessment for nonadherence.
    a. Repeat counts of dialysis solution inventory.
    b. Monitor dialysis solution orders.
    c. Review data on computer memory cards from cycler machines.
    d. Review patient's home dialysis records.
    e. Clinical assessment for inadequate dialysis as outlined above.

E. Patients on intermittent dialysis.

VI. Methods of increasing the dose of dialysis.

A. Regardless of delivered dose, if a patient has signs and symptoms suggestive of underdialysis, or if a patient is not thriving and has no other identifiable cause other than kidney failure, consideration should be given to increasing the dialysis dose. The KDOQI guidelines list a number of indications to consider increasing the dose of dialysis. These are listed in Table 13.19.

B. CAPD.
1. Increase the exchange volume. An increase from 2.0 to 2.5 L per exchange increases clearances approximately 25%. Some patients can tolerate 3 L exchanges.
2. Increase the number of exchanges. Increasing from 4 to 5 exchanges per day increases clearances by approximately 25%.
3. Add a second night time exchange using a portable cycling device.

C. CCPD.
1. Increase the exchange volume.
   a. Larger exchange volumes are sometimes better tolerated resting in the supine position because intraabdominal pressure is lower.
   b. Increasing the exchange volume of four overnight cycles from 2.0 to 2.5 L increases clearances by 10–15%.
2. Add a second long dwell daytime exchange; this may increase Kt/V$_{urea}$ another 20%.
3. Increase the number of nocturnal cycles. Increasing from 4 to 6 cycles typically results in a 10% increase in urea clearance.
4. As cycles increase, if total time on the cycler does not also increase, the dwell time for each cycle decreases. This reduces the urea concentration in each cycle. For maximum increases in clearances, additional time on the cycler should also be added.

D. NIPD.
1. Increase exchange volume.
2. Increase the number of exchanges.
3. Increase the total time on the cycler.
4. Add a long dwell daytime exchange. In a patient with minimal RKF, a continuous (24 hr/day) PD regimen rather than intermittent PD prescription should be used to maximize middle-molecule clearance. This increases Kt/V$_{urea}$ up to 30%, depending on transport characteristics. The ISPD guidelines for solute and fluid removal (Lo et al., 2006) state that

Table 13.19

Reasons to Consider Increasing Dialysis Dose

- Evidence of volume overload
- Unexplained nausea or vomiting
- Sleep disturbances
- Restless leg syndrome
- Pruritus
- Uncontrolled hyperphosphatemia
- Hyperkalemia
- Metabolic acidosis unresponsive to oral bicarbonate therapy
- Anemia refractory to or requiring large doses of ESAs
- Uremic neuropathy
- Uremic pericarditis

ESAs = erythropoietic stimulating agents

Source: National Kidney Foundation. (2006). KDOQI clinical practice guidelines and clinical practice recommendations for 2006 updates: Hemodialysis adequacy, peritoneal dialysis adequacy, and vascular access. *American Journal of Kidney Diseases, 48*(Suppl 1), S1-322.

continuous around-the-clock dialysis is preferred to an intermittent schedule whenever possible (evidence-based).

Nursing Care of Chronic PD Patients

I. **Chronic peritoneal dialysis is almost exclusively a home dialysis therapy.** Home dialysis candidates must have an assessment of self-care abilities and suitability for home dialysis.

A. Assessment parameters.
1. Understanding of the diagnosis of CKD stage 5 disease and therapy options.
2. Cultural orientation toward health and illness.
3. Motivation for choosing home dialysis.
4. Family support for patient's decision.
5. Past experiences with self-care.
6. Level of independence in activities of daily living.
7. Premorbid roles and level of functioning.
8. Complexity of illness and degree of disability. The patient may be too ill to take the sole responsibility for dialysis.
9. Physical abilities or handicaps.
   a. Vision.
   b. Muscular strength.
   c. Fine motor coordination.

10. Family and community resources for assistance and support.
11. Is a partner required to perform some or all of the assessments or procedures?
    a. Is a partner available?
    b. Is the partner willing and motivated?
    c. Is there an alternative if the partner should be unable to perform dialysis?
12. Patient and/or partner's decision-making abilities and adherence history.
13. Physical characteristics of the home.
    a. Access to electricity and drain for automated equipment.
    b. Space for supply storage.
    c. Size and number of inhabitants. Is there an area that can be isolated for aseptic procedures?
14. Comorbid medical conditions.
15. Mental status.
    a. Mentally competent.
    b. Has intact memory and sequencing skills.
    c. Acceptance of diagnosis.
    d. Fears/perceived barriers to rehabilitation.
16. Quality of life.
17. Goals for vocational rehabilitation.

B. The National Kidney Foundation has published an outcome-driven nephrology social work assessment consisting of three components.
    1. Factors affecting adjustment to chronic kidney disease.
    2. Rehabilitation.
    3. Health-risk behavior assessment.

II. Patient education.
(Also see Section 4, Chapter 18.)

A. The patient education process is a collaborative effort among the members of the peritoneal dialysis team, which includes at least a nurse, physician, dietitian, and social worker.

B. Goals of the patient education program.
    1. To provide the patient and family members the knowledge and skills to perform PD safely in their home environment.
    2. To maintain proper nutrition.
    3. To assist the patient and family in identifying the need for and using medical and community resources.
    4. To assist the patient and family in developing skills to cope with chronic kidney disease and achieve optimum quality of life and rehabilitation.

C. Patient education is most effective when principles of adult education are incorporated.
    1. Assess learning ability and readiness to learn.
    2. Individualize goals, objectives, and plan.
    3. Differentiate what patient needs to know from total content.
    4. Objective evaluation and feedback.

D. Sample patient education outline.
    1. Normal kidney function.
    2. Chronic kidney disease.
    3. Description of the dialysis therapy and appropriate terminology.
    4. Principles of peritoneal dialysis.
    5. The peritoneal dialysis catheter.
    6. Monitoring vital signs and weight.
    7. Fluid balance.
    8. Principles of asepsis and aseptic technique.
    9. Complications of peritoneal dialysis.
    10. Problem-solving.
    11. Medications.
    12. Diet.
    13. Activities and exercise.
    14. Plan for follow-up.
        a. Clinic visits.
        b. Routine laboratory tests.
            (1) Urea and creatinine.
            (2) Potassium.
            (3) Calcium and phosphorus.
            (4) Hematocrit.
            (5) Serum albumin.
            (6) Kt/V_{urea} and creatinine clearance as markers of adequacy.
    15. Maintenance of home dialysis records.
    16. Ordering, storage, and inventory of supplies.
    17. Emergency communication system.
    18. Emergency procedures.
        a. Technical (performing dialysis procedures).
        b. Medical emergencies, e.g., chest pain.
        c. Natural disaster.
    19. Psychosocial issues.
        a. Coping with chronic kidney failure.
        b. Adjustment to dialysis therapy.
        c. Sexual concerns.
        d. Rehabilitation.
    20. Financial issues and resources.

E. Skills training.
    1. CAPD exchange procedure.
    2. Dialysis machine (cycler) procedures.
    3. Peritoneal dialysis catheter exit site care.
    4. Procedure for adding medications to the dialysis solution.
    5. Procedure for obtaining dialysate samples.

6. Procedure for managing contamination of the PD system.

III. Patient follow-up.

A. It is equally important for both patients who are in transition from training to independence and those that have been established on home PD therapy to have follow-up and monitoring.
1. Evaluate clinical status of home patients.
2. Reinforce learning and provide positive feedback regarding self-care and home dialysis.
3. Ongoing assessment of learning needs and continuing education when indicated.
4. Support adjustment to home dialysis and rehabilitation.

B. Assessment parameters.
1. Fluid balance.
2. Blood pressure.
3. Weight gains, dry weight.
4. Exit site.
5. Procedure technique.
6. Dialysis adequacy.
7. Nutrition.
8. Laboratory results.
9. Routine medications.
10. Supply and inventory.
11. Adherence to prescribed treatment.
12. Encourage routine preventive health care (e.g., mammograms) and assist in referring or scheduling, if necessary.

C. Follow-up activities.
1. Telephone calls.
2. Routine clinic visits.
3. Home visits.
4. Additional clinic visits for specific problems, e.g., peritonitis, exit site infection.
5. Education updates and review of technique procedure.
6. Individualized multidisciplinary care plan.

D. In the United States, the Centers for Medicare and Medicaid Services (CMS) require that the multidisciplinary follow-up include at least a physician, registered nurse, dietitian, and social worker.

Clinical Management Issues

I. Nonadherence has been documented as a major problem in home and self-care therapies.

A. In a study of adherence in PD patients, "noncompliance," defined as performance of < 90% of dialysis exchanges, and determined by repeated inventory of dialysis solution bags, was found in 30% of PD patients in the first 6 months of PD, and in 13% of chronic PD patients studied (Bernardini, 2000).
1. Some patients who were initially noncompliant became compliant. Others were intermittently compliant. Only a small fraction were consistently noncompliant.
2. Noncompliant patients experienced more hospital admissions and had more hospital days.
3. Noncompliant patients had a measured Kt/V_{urea} 18% lower than compliant patients.
4. Noncompliant patients were more likely to transfer to hemodialysis due to uremia.
5. Noncompliant patients were more likely to die than compliant patients.

B. Although there is a paucity of studies regarding improving adherence in PD, there is a large body of literature regarding adherence in health care settings.

II. Preserving peritoneal membrane function.

A. A small proportion of patients continue to transfer to hemodialysis due to loss of peritoneal membrane function.
1. These patients have signs and symptoms of underdialysis and fluid overload despite attempts to optimize dialysis prescription.
2. Changes in membrane function can be documented by repeat PET, SPA, or PDC tests.

B. Strategies to preserve peritoneal membrane function.
1. Prevent catheter-related infections.
   a. Prophylactic antibiotics prior to catheter insertion (evidence-based).
   b. Short course of antibiotic therapy for known contamination of the PD system.
   c. Prophylactic antibiotic therapy for dental, gastrointestinal (e.g., colonoscopy with biopsy), and other invasive procedures.
   d. Prevent exit site trauma by effectively securing the catheter.

e. Prophylactic treatment for severe exit site trauma.

f. Treat equivocal exit sites (see Chapter 61, *PD Access*).

2. Use intraperitoneal heparin any time there is fibrin or blood in the dialysate.

3. If bleeding is severe, drain dialysate and perform short exchanges until bleeding subsides.

4. Avoid introduction of disinfectants into the peritoneal cavity.

5. Use intraperitoneal medications only when absolutely necessary.

6. Reduce exposure to high dextrose solutions.

7. Avoid use of overheated dialysis solutions.

8. Rotate stock of dialysis solution to avoid using old solutions.

III. Anemia management.

A. Hemoglobin and hematocrit improve after starting PD related to both decrease in plasma volume and increase in red cell mass.

B. Although some PD patients achieve a normal hematocrit, most remain somewhat anemic.

C. Erythrocyte-stimulating agents (ESA), e.g., recombinant human erythropoietin and darbepoetin, have been shown to be safe and effective in correcting anemia in peritoneal dialysis patients.

1. In addition to the correction of anemia, other benefits of ESAs include improvements in quality of life, cognitive abilities, exercise capacity, and overall well-being.

2. Administration of ESAs.

a. Subcutaneous administration is preferred because an IV access is not readily available, and higher doses are required for intraperitoneal administration.

b. Most PD patients are taught to self-administer ESAs.

c. Adherence with treatment regimens is an important factor in determining the efficacy of ESAs in PD patients.

(1) Risk factors for nonadherence are younger age, fewer comorbidities, and longer duration of therapy (Muirhead, 2005).

(2) Darbepoetin, which is a hyperglycosylated analog of epoetin alfa, is available for the treatment of anemia. It has a prolonged serum half-life, thus allowing extended

dosing intervals that may prove beneficial in situations where patient adherence is a real concern.

D. PD patients require iron supplementation to prevent iron deficiency and maintain iron stores.

1. Targets for iron supplementation in PD patients: transferrin saturation of > 20% and serum ferritin 200–500 ng/mL.

2. The 2000 KDOQI guidelines for the treatment of anemia recommend an oral iron dose of ≥ 200 mg of elemental iron per day. Oral iron may not be sufficient to supply or replace iron needs, as iron absorption is suboptimal.

3. If oral iron fails, intravenous iron is recommended. For many patients treated with a home-based therapy, IV iron administration can present significant logistical problems.

IV. Prevention of cardiovascular complications.

A. Cardiovascular disease is the leading cause of death in the peritoneal dialysis patient population (see Chapter 63, *Peritoneal Dialysis Complications*).

B. Good blood pressure control and fluid balance are critical in preventing left ventricular hypertrophy (LVH) and congestive heart failure. LVH may regress with good control of fluid.

1. Many patients who start CAPD have a drop in blood pressure and improved blood pressure control and are able to discontinue some or all antihypertensive medications. The responsible mechanism is believed to be good control of salt and water balance.

2. Some clinicians observe that blood pressure tends to go up again after 6–12 months, but this may be a function of dietary intake and fluid balance management.

C. Some patients on low-sodium diets can become sodium depleted and will require liberalization of sodium intake.

D. Patients with diabetic autonomic neuropathy and cardiac dysfunction can develop symptomatic orthostatic hypotension.

E. CAPD patients have a more atherogenic lipoprotein profile than hemodialysis patients.

F. Several studies have shown that CAPD patients have fewer dysrhythmias than HD patients.

G. Malnutrition, inflammation, and atherosclerosis (MIA syndrome) is associated with high cardiovascular mortality and accounts for most of the premature deaths in peritoneal dialysis patients. Proper nutritional support, enhanced dialysis prescriptions, and treatment of underlying inflammation may decrease morbidity and mortality associated with MIA.

V. **For information about bone disease,** see Section 2.

VI. **Nutritional status.**

A. Protein energy malnutrition is a major problem for PD patients. Approximately half of PD patients have mild to moderate malnutrition. As many as 10% have severe malnutrition.
   1. Malnutrition is often present at the initiation of dialysis.
   2. Residual renal function is significantly lower in patients with severe malnutrition.
   3. Older adults, patients with diabetes, and patients with renal vascular disease have a higher incidence of malnutrition.
   4. Factors that contribute to malnutrition in PD patients include inadequate dialysis, comorbid illnesses, anorexia, losses of protein, amino acids and other nutrients in the dialysate, endocrine abnormalities, activation of cellular catabolic pathways, and displacement of other energy sources by glucose absorbed from the dialysate.
   5. Malnutrition is related to increased morbidity and mortality in PD patients.

B. Glucose.
   1. Glucose is absorbed from peritoneal dialysis solutions.
   2. Blood glucose and plasma insulin levels peak 45–90 minutes after infusing a hypertonic exchange. These levels remain high for a prolonged period.
   3. Isotonic solutions have minimal effects on blood glucose and insulin levels.
   4. CAPD patients have a tendency toward hyperglycemia with hyperinsulinemia. Some develop overt diabetes mellitus.
   5. Clinical implications.
      a. Constant glucose absorption can result in anorexia.
      b. There will be an increase in total caloric load if dietary intake is not modified.

c. There may be a gradual increase in dry body weight.
   6. Monitoring and intervention.
      a. Monitor number of hypertonic exchanges, dietary patterns, serum glucose, and weight gain.
      b. Avoid excessive use of hypertonic solutions by regulating sodium and fluid intake.
      c. Weight control regimen.
         (1) Avoid simple carbohydrates in diet.
         (2) Increase activity and exercise.
         (3) Restrict alcohol.
         (4) Reduce excessive fat intake.
   7. Insulin administration as ordered for diabetic patients. Careful monitoring of serum glucose.

C. Lipids.
   1. PD patients typically have an increase in serum cholesterol and triglyceride concentrations after starting dialysis therapy.
   2. PD patients have more atherogenic serum lipid profiles than patients on HD.
      a. 50–70% of PD patients have elevated triglyceride concentrations.
      b. Total cholesterol may also be high.
      c. Increased LDL-cholesterol and VLDL-cholesterol fractions and decreased HDL-cholesterol.
      d. Higher levels of apolipoprotein B.
   3. Intervention.
      a. Restrict use of hypertonic dialysis solution.
      b. Dietary modifications to reduce weight. Reduce intake of saturated fats and carbohydrates.
      c. Stop smoking.
      d. Restrict alcohol.
      e. Regular exercise program.
      f. Lipid-lowering drugs.
   4. Use of glucose polymer (icodextrin) and amino acid dialysis solutions may improve lipid profiles.

D. Proteins.
   1. Proteins and amino acids are lost in the dialysate (5–15 g/day).
   2. Total serum protein and albumin levels are often low.
   3. Abnormal plasma amino acid concentrations are similar to untreated uremia and those of hemodialysis patients.
      a. Decreased levels of essential amino acids.
      b. Increased concentration of nonessential amino acids.
   4. Intervention for low protein and amino acids.
      a. Review individual dietary prescription.

b. Increase dietary intake of proteins.

c. 50% of protein intake should be of high biologic value.

d. Nutritional supplements.

e. Amino acid supplements.

5. Amino acid supplementation via absorption from dialysis solution has been studied.

a. Amino acid solutions are used for only one exchange per day.

b. Use of amino acid solutions showed short-term improvement in protein nutrition and metabolic status.

c. BUN levels and dialysate protein losses increase.

d. 3-year study in Hong Kong found that use of amino acid solutions maintained a stable albumin and cholesterol and lowered triglycerides compared to the control group, which had decreasing albumin and cholesterol and stable or increasing triglycerides. The group receiving amino acids did not have fewer hospitalizations or better survival.

E. Nutritional assessment.

1. The KDOQI guidelines for maintenance peritoneal dialysis patients recommend routine monthly assessment of nutritional status including:

a. Serum albumin (or prealbumin) levels.

b. Estimation of dietary protein intake (such as protein equivalent of nitrogen appearance [PNA] calculated from urea kinetic modeling data).

2. Other assessment parameters.

a. Subjective global assessment (SGA). A 7-point scale modified for PD patients assesses weight change, anorexia, subcutaneous tissue, and muscle mass (evidence-based).

b. Serum creatinine, and creatinine index are valid measures of protein-energy nutritional status.

c. Serum bicarbonate should be maintained above 22 mEq/L.

d. Anthropometric measurements.

e. Dual energy x-ray absorptiometry (DEXA).

F. The KDOQI nutrition guidelines also recommend intensive nutritional counseling for every patient based on an individualized care plan.

G. See Section 8 for dietary recommendations.

Outcomes of Peritoneal Dialysis

I. **Residual kidney function.**

A. PD patients maintain residual kidney function longer than HD patients.

B. Even minimal residual kidney function contributes significantly to solute removal and dialysis adequacy.

C. Patients with no residual kidney function are at risk for poor outcomes.

1. Inadequate dialysis.

2. Increased morbidity.

3. Transfer to hemodialysis.

4. Increased mortality.

II. **Morbidity** (USRDS, 2007).

A. The USRDS data for 2005 show similar rates of hospitalization for HD vascular access infection and PD-related peritonitis.

B. PD patients averaged 1.93 hospital admissions per year in 2005.

C. PD patients averaged 15.0 hospital days/year in 2005.

D. Hospital admission rates for peritonitis have fallen over the last decade.

E. Reasons for hospital admissions are shown in Table 13.20.

III. **Patient dropout or transfer to another form of therapy.**

A. This is still greater for PD therapies than for HD.

B. Infectious complications are still the main reason for changing modality.

C. Inadequate dialysis or fluid removal is the second most frequently cited reason for transfer.

D. Catheter-related problems account for up to 15% of transfers.

E. Patient choice, malnutrition, and abdominal complications also contribute to dropout.

IV. **Transplantation.**

A. PD before transplantation may be beneficial, as a lower incidence and severity of delayed recovery

Table 13.20

**Primary Diagnosis of PD Patients Requiring
Hospital Admission, 2003-2005;
Number of Admissions per 100 Patient Years**
(USRDS, 2007)

Diagnosis	Number of Admissions per 100 Patient Years
Circulatory diseases	45.5
All "others"	42.2
Dialysis access	29.6
Digestive diseases	28.4
Respiratory diseases	9.7
Other infections	7.8
Genitourinary diseases	6.0

Table 13.21

**Primary Causes of Death in PD Patients;
Number per 1,000 Patient Years**
(USRDS, 2007)

Causes of Death	Number of Deaths per 1,000 Patient Years
Cardiovascular (acute myocardial infarction and atherosclerotic heart disease, cardiac myopathy, cardiac arrhythmia, valvular heart disease, congestive heart failure, cardiac arrest)	74.2
Other	47.4
Septicemia	24.5
Cerebrovascular disease	8.2
Malignant disease	5.4
Pulmonary infection	3.2
Other infection	4.7
Gastrointestinal hemorrhage	1.1
Other hemorrhage	1.0

of kidney function after transplantation has been reported in PD patients.

B. Transplant outcomes are similar in HD and CAPD for both adults and children.

C. Peritoneal dialysis can be used during delayed graft function after transplantation provided the peritoneal cavity remains intact during the transplant procedure.

D. The PD catheter can be left in for 3–4 months with a functioning graft. However, earlier removal after successful transplantation is advisable, because transplanted patients are at risk for catheter-related infections.

V. Survival.

A. Several large national registries have found similar adjusted survival of CAPD and HD patients for the early years of dialysis therapy.

B. USRDS data show almost identical overall survival for adult PD and HD patients beginning therapy from 1995 to 1999.

C. USRDS data show a gradual decrease in adjusted mortality for PD patients between 1996 and 2004.

D. Patients with diabetes mellitus as their primary diagnosis had the worst survival.

E. PD patients on the transplant waiting list had significantly lower mortality rates compared to those never on the transplant list.

F. Risk factors for death on PD.
1. Age > 65 years.
2. Primary cause of CKD other than glomerulonephritis.
3. Ischemic heart disease.
4. Cerebrovascular disease.
5. Peripheral vascular disease.
6. Malignancy.
7. High solute transport rate.
8. Low serum albumin.
9. Loss of residual renal function.

G. Table 13.21 lists causes of death in PD patients.

Chapter 63

Peritoneal Dialysis Complications

Purpose

The purpose of this chapter is to provide a cognitive understanding of the etiology, pathophysiology, presentation, assessment, and management of selected catheter problems, noninfectious complications of peritoneal dialysis (PD) catheter-related infections, and peritonitis.

Objectives

Upon completion of this chapter the learner will be able to:

1. State two ways intraabdominal pressure can be minimized after catheter insertion.
2. Outline assessment and intervention strategies for a catheter that will not drain and/or infuse.
3. Discuss the pathophysiologic basis, prevention, nursing assessment, and collaborative management of the following complications related to PD:
   a. Peritonitis.
   b. Pericatheter leaks.
   c. Abdominal pain.
   d. Shoulder pain.
   e. Back pain.
   f. Pneumoperitoneum.
   g. Peritoneopleural communication.
   h. Hernias.
   i. Scrotal and perineal edema.
   j. Bleeding.
   k. Decreased ultrafiltration.
   l. Encapsulating peritoneal sclerosis.
4. Differentiate eosinophilic and infectious peritonitis.
5. Discuss the effects on the peritoneal membrane of constant exposure to dialysis solutions.
6. Compare outcomes of peritoneal dialysis and hemodialysis.
7. Outline complications of peritoneal dialysis that result in transfer to hemodialysis therapy.

When Level I or Level II evidence exists, treatment recommendations are identified as evidenced-based.

Catheter-related Complications

I. Characteristics of the ideal PD catheter.

A. Provides efficient PD solution inflow and outflow.

B. No associated pain or discomfort.

C. Low incidence of malfunction.

D. Free of exit site or tunnel infections.

E. Is not the primary source of peritonitis.

II. Early catheter complications.

A. By definition occur during the first month after catheter implantation.

B. The following complications related to the catheter insertion procedure are discussed in Chapter 61, *PD Access*.
1. Organ perforation.
2. Preperitoneal catheter placement.
3. Incisional pain.
4. Postoperative bleeding.

C. Leaks may also occur early due to high intraabdominal pressure from dialysis exchanges prior to tissue ingrowth into the cuffs.
1. The risk of early leaks can be reduced by delaying ambulatory PD for 10–14 days after catheter implantation.
2. If dialysis must be initiated immediately, low volume exchanges and dialyzing with the patient in the supine position will reduce the risk of leaks (see Chapter 61, *PD Access*).

III. Catheter malfunction.

A. The catheter may not drain completely, or it may be impossible to drain or infuse.

B. External clamp or pressure on catheter or tubing.
1. Evaluation and intervention.
   a. Check entire length of tubing and external catheter for kinks and closed clamps.
   b. Check that tubing and external segment are not constricted by external pressure, e.g.,

tight waistbands or caught in bedrails or reclining chairs.
2. Intervention consists of opening or removing clamps and eliminating external pressure.

C. Internal catheter kink.
1. Catheter has a kink or bend in subcutaneous or intraperitoneal (IP) segment.
2. Typically presents as a drain problem, but may also slow infusion.
3. Both flat plate of abdomen and lateral x-rays are necessary to confirm or rule out internal kinks.
4. Surgical intervention is required.

D. Air lock.
1. Air in the tubing interrupts inflow. This is more common in vented systems.
2. Assessment. An air bubble may be seen in the tubing.
3. Intervention.
   a. Infuse additional dialysis solution. This will flush air bubbles out of the tubing. May need to squeeze the dialysis solution bag to increase pressure.
   b. Flush dialysis solution into the drain bag if a twin-bag or Y tubing is used.

E. Constipation.
1. The distended rectosigmoid colon puts pressure on the catheter.
   a. May block side holes.
   b. May displace the catheter tip.
2. This is the most common cause of impaired dialysate outflow.
3. Evaluation.
   a. History and physical examination.
   b. Abdominal x-rays show excessive stool in colon.
   c. Review medication list for drugs that may cause constipation.
4. Intervention.
   a. Stimulant laxatives or sorbitol may induce peristalsis and bowel movement.
   b. Enemas are used as a last resort (phosphate-based enemas are contraindicated).
5. Prevention.
   a. Increase dietary fiber intake.
   b. Increase daily physical activity and exercise.
   c. Avoid medications that cause constipation.
   d. Stool softeners.
   e. Maintain serum potassium within normal limits. Hypokalemia may decrease bowel motility and contribute to constipation.

F. Catheter obstruction by fibrin or blood clot.
   1. Evaluation.
      a. Patient has a history of recent catheter implantation, abdominal surgery, or abdominal trauma.
      b. Patient has obvious fibrin formation in the dialysate, or history of fibrin problems.
      c. Dialysate is bloody or blood clots are visible in the drainage.
   2. Intervention.
      a. If dialysis solution will infuse, but not drain, infuse additional dialysis solution containing heparin; the dialysis solution bag may need to be squeezed to increase pressure.
      b. Irrigation with a large syringe containing heparinized dialysis solution or normal saline may flush fibrin or clots from the catheter and tubing. Careful aseptic technique is mandatory.
      c. An embolectomy balloon catheter or similar device may be used to attempt to remove clots from the catheter. Aseptic technique is critical.
      d. Administer tissue plasminogen activator (tPA), typically 1mg/mL in sterile water in a volume sufficient to fill the catheter, and allow to dwell for 1–2 hours (see details in Chapter 61, *PD Access*).
      e. If efforts to restore patency are successful, administer heparin IP in several subsequent dialysis exchanges.

G. Catheter migration out of pelvis.
   1. Etiology.
      a. May be related to peristalsis of the ascending colon; more common with catheters placed on the right side.
      b. May be due to shape memory of a straight catheter placed in a curved tunnel.
      c. Omental wrapping.
      d. Catheter placed incorrectly at insertion.
      e. May occur when PD is delayed or interrupted.
   2. Assessment. An abdominal x-ray will document catheter migration.
   3. Intervention.
      a. Occasionally a catheter that has migrated out of the pelvis will spontaneously reposition itself.
      b. Induce peristalsis. This may move the catheter back into position, particularly if the catheter is on the left side.
      c. Encourage ambulation and activity.
      d. Have patient assume knee-chest position

during dwell with full volume of dialysis solution in an attempt to float the catheter back into the pelvis.
      e. The physician or surgeon may attempt to manually reposition the catheter with a guide wire or trocar, using aseptic procedure. This is not consistently effective.
      f. Surgical repositioning or catheter replacement. Omentectomy or partial omentectomy may be indicated.

H. Omental entrapment.
   1. Typically presents as a drain problem, but can also interfere with solution infusion.
   2. Most common in tall, thin individuals.
   3. The omentum surrounds or attaches to the catheter and pulls it up out of the pelvis.
   4. Surgical intervention is required.

I. Fluid is loculated in an isolated area of the peritoneal cavity.
   1. Adhesions are the most common cause; could also be due to catheter entrapment by omentum.
   2. Problems with drainage are more typical than impaired inflow.
   3. Peritoneography with infusion of contrast media or computerized tomography (CT) scan may identify loculation of fluid.
   4. Surgical intervention is required.

IV. Radiologic evaluation of catheter-related complications.

A. Plain x-ray (flat plate of the abdomen).
   1. Used to assess or confirm catheter malposition.
   2. Can identify distention of bowel by presence of gas and/or stool.

B. Abdominal x-ray with contrast media injected through the PD catheter (peritoneography).
   1. May show cause of catheter malfunction.
      a. Catheter kink.
      b. Catheter entrapment by omentum or loops of bowel.
   2. May show other complications.
      a. Leaks.
      b. Hernias.
      c. Adhesions.
      d. Compartmentalization of the dialysate.
   3. Is contraindicated in patients who have a history of sensitivity to contrast media.

C. CT peritoneography (CT scan of abdomen with contrast media injected through the PD catheter).
   1. Provides more detailed information about the location and dimensions of hernias, and origin and path of dialysate leak.
   2. Used to diagnosis encapsulating peritoneal sclerosis. Typical findings include increased peritoneal membrane thickness and a calcified cocoon encapsulating bowel loops. Bowel loops may be either compressed or dilated proximal to the obstruction.

D. Peritoneal scintigraphy (using radioactive isotopes injected through the peritoneal catheter) may also be used as an alternative to CT peritoneography.

E. Ultrasound studies (ultrasonography) are used to:
   1. Diagnose exit site infection with tunnel involvement.
   2. Evaluate response of tunnel infection to therapy.
   3. Evaluate etiology of relapsing or recurrent peritonitis.

V. **Damage to catheter** (see Chapter 61, *PD Access*).

VI. **Adapter loose or falls out of catheter** (see Chapter 61, *PD Access*).

VII. **Catheter cuff extrusion** (see Chapter 61, *PD Access*).

Complications Related to Intraabdominal Pressure

I. **Hernias.**

A. Reported incidence in continuous ambulatory peritoneal dialysis (CAPD) ranges from 10% to 15%. Umbilical hernias are most common.

B. Mean time to hernia development is about 1 year on dialysis; however, preexisting hernias may be diagnosed at initiation of PD therapy.

C. Etiology.
   1. Introduction of dialysis solution increases intraabdominal pressure. This may lead to hernia formation in patients with congenital or acquired defects.
   2. Increases in exchange volume further raise intraabdominal pressure.

3. Physical activity during continuous dialysis also causes additional increases in intraabdominal pressure. Lifting and straining induce very high intraabdominal pressure and may contribute to the development of hernias.
4. Coughing and the Valsalva maneuver generate the highest intraabdominal pressures (see Figure 13.10).

D. Risk factors.
   1. Patent processes vaginalis.
   2. Multiparous women.
   3. Age over 40.
   4. Previous hernia repair.
   5. Polycystic disease.
   6. Midline incision for PD catheter.

E. Common sites (see Table 13.22).

F. Assessment.
   1. Physical assessment.
      a. Painless bulges or swelling.
      b. Tender lump.
      c. Scrotal swelling.
      d. Assess for complications, such as incarceration and strangulation of the bowel.
      e. Assess for associated dialysate leaks.
   2. Diagnostic tests.
      a. Peritoneography (x-ray with contrast media).
      b. Computerized tomography with contrast.
      c. Abdominal scintigraphy.

G. Intervention.
   1. Hernia repair, which may include insertion of polypropylene mesh. A single dose of IV antibiotics preoperatively is recommended to prevent infection.

Table 13.22

Types and Locations of Hernias in Peritoneal Dialysis Patients

- Inguinal
- Umbilical
- Catheter incision site
- Other abdominal incision sites
- Catheter exit site
- Ventral
- Epigastric

2. During healing, after hernia repair, keep intraabdominal pressure low.
   a. Delay PD postoperatively or use low volume exchanges and supine dialysis to minimize intraabdominal pressure.
   b. Avoid activities that raise intraabdominal pressure, e.g., forceful coughing, straining, lifting, bending, squatting, and stair-climbing.
   c. Stool softeners or laxatives are recommended to avoid constipation.

H. Complications.
   1. Bowel incarceration and strangulation.
   2. Transmural leakage of bacteria can cause peritonitis.
   3. Early hernias at the catheter insertion site or exit site can be associated with dialysate leaks.

II. Dialysate leaks.

A. Reported incidence is from 7% to 24%.

B. Etiology.
   1. Dialysate leaks are most common prior to tissue ingrowth into the catheter cuffs after catheter implantation (see Chapter 61, *PD Access*).
   2. Leaks are more common when the deep cuff is not implanted in muscle.
   3. Catheter may have an internal hole or tear.
   4. Disruption of tissue ingrowth into a catheter cuff.
      a. Trauma.
      b. Cuff infection.

C. Sites.
   1. Dialysate leaks from catheter exit site.
   2. Extravasation into the subcutaneous tissues results in abdominal wall or genital edema.

D. Risk factors.
   1. Acute catheters may leak along catheter tract. This is more likely to occur when exit and/or tunnel is larger than the catheter diameter.
   2. Chronic catheters.
      a. Peritoneum is not closed tightly during implantation.
      b. More frequent with a midline incision than with insertion through the rectus muscle.
      c. Inadequate tissue ingrowth into catheter cuffs.
      d. Full volume dialysis exchanges immediately after catheter implantation.
      e. Early ambulatory dialysis (sooner than 10–14 days after catheter insertion).
      f. Preexisting hernia.

g. Heavy lifting, coughing or straining, bending or stooping early after catheter insertion.
3. Assessment.
   a. Document dialysis drain volumes and fluid balance.
   b. Weight gain without accompanying peripheral edema.
   c. Physical assessment.
      (1) Observe characteristics and volume of drainage from exit site.
      (2) Check for edema or asymmetry of abdominal wall.
      (3) Assess for genital edema.
      (4) Assess for increased abdominal girth.
      (5) With a subcutaneous leak, abdominal skin may be pale and have an "orange peel" appearance.
      (6) Also with a subcutaneous leak, skin indentations from elastic waistbands or catheter lying across the abdomen appear deeper and more prominent than usual.
4. Diagnostic tests.
   a. High dipstick glucose will differentiate dialysate leak from exit site exudate.
   b. CT scan with IP contrast is considered as the best diagnostic procedure to localize a leak.
5. Intervention.
   a. Exit site leak with acute catheter.
      (1) Frequent reinforcement of dressings or dressing changes using aseptic technique.
      (2) Skin can be protected with a barrier spray.
      (3) Notify physician.
         (a) Exit may be sutured.
         (b) Catheter may be removed and replaced.
   b. Exit site or subcutaneous leak with chronic catheter.
      (1) Stop PD for 14 days or longer to allow tissue ingrowth into cuff material; temporary hemodialysis therapy.
      (2) Secure the catheter and avoid further manipulation of the catheter.
      (3) If PD must be continued, decrease exchange volume, dialyze in the supine position, and avoid activities that increase intraabdominal pressure, e.g., coughing, Valsalva maneuver, straining, and lifting.
      (4) Observe for development of peritonitis, exit site or tunnel infection.
      (5) If leak persists, replacement of the catheter may be indicated.

III. Genital edema.

A. Edema of the penis or labia majora. Often associated with abdominal wall edema.

B. Risk factors.
1. High intraabdominal pressure.
2. Elderly.
3. Debilitated.
4. Malnourished.
5. Diabetes mellitus.

C. Causes.
1. May result from dialysate tracking through the soft-tissue plane from the catheter insertion site, due to a soft-tissue defect within a hernia or from a peritoneofascial defect.
2. Fluid can travel through a patent processus vaginalis to the labia or scrotum and surrounding soft tissue (see hernia, above).
3. Catheter may have an internal tear.

D. CT with contrast diagnoses more leaks than plain peritoneography.

E. Treatment.
1. The goal of conservative treatment is to lower the intraabdominal pressure.
   a. Bedrest.
   b. Supine, low volume dialysis.
   c. Cessation of PD for at least 14 days, and up to 4-6 weeks.
2. Repair or replace defective catheter.
3. Hernia repair.

IV. Gastrointestinal complications.

A. Many patients complain of anorexia, abdominal fullness, and early satiety, particularly after the initiation of PD therapy.

B. PD patients may also have symptoms of gastro-esophageal gastric reflux disease (GERD), such as "heartburn" and gastric reflux. This is likely due to the increased intraabdominal pressure from the IP fluid, although the etiology has not been well studied.

C. Delayed gastric emptying may occur in PD patients. A trial of decreased exchange volume may help determine if PD with full exchange volumes exacerbates the problem.

D. Avoiding or reducing alcohol, caffeine, spicy foods and acidic juices, and frequent small meals may reduce gastrointestinal symptoms.

E. Maintaining an upright position for at least 30–45 minutes after meals may also control symptoms.

F. PD patients have decreased fluid intake and ingest phosphate-binders and other medications which contribute to constipation. Diabetic gastroparesis may also contribute to constipation. Prevention and treatment of constipation includes increased fiber intake, either dietary or supplemental, and may require use of stool softeners and laxatives.

G. Hemorrhoids can be caused or exacerbated by PD due to increased intraabdominal pressure. Constipation can also exacerbate hemorrhoids.

V. Cardiovascular complications.

A. PD patients have cardiovascular risk factors and complications related to chronic kidney disease (CKD).

B. Many PD patients are in a state of chronic fluid overload, and this contributes to hypertension and left ventricular hypertrophy (LVH).

C. About one third of PD patients develop severe LVH. Some eventually develop overt congestive heart failure.

D. LVH increases the risk of cardiovascular morbidity and mortality.

E. Ischemic heart disease is a major cause of death in PD patients.

F. A vasovagal response (syncope) related to infusion of PD solution has been documented. The pathophysiologic mechanism is uncertain.

G. Studies have shown significant decreases in cardiac output and stroke volume after infusion of dialysis solution in some patients. This is thought to result from decreased preload related to increased intraabdominal pressure on the inferior vena cava.

H. Hyperlipidemia is exacerbated by PD therapy.
1. This is common in both men and women.
2. Dialysate protein losses include lipoproteins, especially small molecules such as high-density lipoproteins (HDL).
3. PD patients who are well nourished have increased serum cholesterol and triglyceride levels (mainly low-density lipoproteins [LDL]).
4. Increased synthesis of lipoprotein (a).

I. Interventions to lower lipid levels.
   1. Dietary modification.
   2. Pharmacologic therapy.
   3. Regular exercise.

J. Patients are susceptible to hyperglycemia and hyperinsulinemia due to the glucose load from dialysis solutions.
   1. Some patients develop type 2 diabetes mellitus.
   2. Increased insulin levels associated with insulin therapy increase the synthesis of triglycerides by the liver.
   3. Peripheral vascular disease may be exacerbated in patients with diabetes.
   4. Icodextrin and amino acid dialysis solutions aid in controlling serum glucose and triglycerides.

K. The relationship between inflammation and cardiovascular disease seen in the general population is strong in dialysis patients. 30–60% of PD patients have elevated C-reactive protein (CRP) levels.
   1. Causative factors.
      a. Decreased renal clearances of cytokines and advanced glycation end products (AGEs).
      b. Use of bioincompatible PD solutions.
      c. Comorbid medical conditions, e.g., catheter-related infections and congestive heart failure.
   2. Patients with elevated CRP are at risk for atherosclerotic events, ischemic heart disease, cerebrovascular disease, and peripheral vascular disease.

L. Homocysteine is elevated in most PD (and HD) patients. Patients with low folate levels are at increased risk of hyperhomocysteinemia. Folic acid supplementation can decrease homocysteine levels in PD patients.

M. Monitoring of cardiac hemodynamics is recommended for PD patients with LVH, cardiomyopathy, and pre-existing valvular disease.

VI. Pulmonary complications.

A. Chronic PD with 2 L IP volume results in reduction of lung volumes. These changes can persist or normalize after the first few weeks of PD.

B. Forced vital capacity decreases as IP dialysis solution volume increases.

C. Changes in patients with chronic obstructive airway disease (COPD) are no more severe. Therefore, COPD should not be an absolute contraindication to PD therapy. Exchange volume should be individualized in COPD patients.

D. PD patients have a high incidence of obstructive sleep apnea. Patients with obstructive sleep apnea have markedly more hypoxemia when they dialyze while sleeping than when they sleep without dialysate.

E. The glucose or amino acids and lactate in dialysis solutions can cause an intermediary metabolism which increases oxygen consumption and carbon dioxide excretion, similar to total parenteral nutrition.

Complications Related to Peritoneal Dialysis

I. Infusion pain.

A. This is most common during initial dialysis exchanges, but can occur later.

B. Etiology.
   1. Rapid solution infusion with "jet effect."
   2. Acidic pH of solutions.
   3. Hypertonic glucose solutions.
   4. Old or expired dialysis solutions.
   5. Catheter migration.

C. Intervention.
   1. This may resolve spontaneously over several weeks.
   2. For pain due to rapid solution infusion.
      a. Slow infusion rate.
      b. Change position.
      c. A coiled catheter will diminish or eliminate the "jet effect."
      d. Leave a reservoir of fluid at the end of drain.
   3. For pain related to acidic pH or hypertonic solutions.
      a. Avoid the use of hypertonic exchanges during early dialysis treatments.
      b. Alternate use of hypertonic exchanges.
      c. Use bicarbonate-based dialysis solutions, if available.
      d. Sodium bicarbonate can be added to the dialysis solution to raise the pH and decrease symptoms.
      e. A local anesthetic can be added to the dialysis

solution. 2% lidocaine (Xylocaine®) 3–5 mL/L of dialysis solution has been recommended.

II. Rectal or suprapubic pain.

A. Etiology.
1. Pressure or poking from peritoneal catheter.
2. IP catheter segment is too long, or catheter has been placed too low in abdomen.

B. Intervention.
1. Pain and pressure may be relieved with infusion of dialysis solution.
2. Do not drain exchanges completely. Leave a reservoir of fluid in the peritoneal cavity at the end of each exchange and between intermittent dialysis procedures to cushion the catheter.
3. May require replacement of catheter.

C. Pressure from the catheter may eventually cause erosion or laceration of an adjacent organ. Signs and symptoms would include bleeding and signs of organ perforation (see Chapter 61, *PD Access*). This would require surgical intervention.

III. Generalized abdominal pain.

A. Etiology.
1. Peritonitis.
2. Overdistention of the abdomen.
    a. Increase in exchange volume.
    b. Forget to drain prior to infusion of the next exchange.
    c. Inadequate drain times allow a gradual accumulation of residual volume and an increase in total IP volume.
    d. May be related to catheter malfunction.
3. Compartmentalization from adhesion formation. Restricting the flow to a small compartment may both cause pain and reduce dialysis efficiency.

B. Treatment.
1. Treat peritonitis (see Infectious Complications of Peritoneal Dialysis: I. Peritonitis).
2. Resolve catheter or drain problems.
3. Adhesions can be surgically lysed.

IV. Shoulder pain due to pneumoperitoneum.

A. Etiology is referred pain from the diaphragm.
1. Air in the peritoneal cavity is the most common cause.

a. Infusion of air (tubing is not primed before use).
b. Small amounts of air can accumulate over time.
c. Bowel perforation.
2. Infusion pressure from peritoneal catheter malpositioned to the subdiaphragmatic area.
3. Due to diaphragmatic irritation from initial PD exchanges.

B. Assessment.
1. Patient complaints.
2. Document recent infusion of air.
3. Assess for bowel perforation (see Chapter 61, *PD Access*).
4. Abdominal x-ray to determine catheter position or to visualize free air in the peritoneal cavity.

C. Prevention of IP air accumulation.
1. Prime new tubing.
2. Do not use vented systems.
3. With manual systems, always close clamps at completion of solution infusion.

D. Intervention to remove air is to drain dialysate with the patient in a knee-chest or Trendelenburg position after a full volume exchange.

V. Back pain.

A. Etiology and risk factors.
1. Altered spinal mechanics, especially in continuous PD.
    a. Center of gravity is moved forward.
    b. Lumbar lordosis is increased. This is further aggravated by poor posture.
2. Deconditioning.
    a. Abdominal muscle weakness.
    b. Poor posture.
    c. Poor exercise tolerance.
3. Neuromuscular diseases.
    a. Degenerative spinal bone disease.
    b. Metabolic bone disease.

B. Prevention and treatment.
1. Identify high risk patients.
2. Teach good posture and proper body mechanics.
3. Muscle strengthening exercises, e.g., pelvic tilts.
4. Decrease exchange volume.
5. Muscle relaxants and anti-inflammatory agents.
6. Transfer to nightly cycler therapy.

VI. Bleeding (hemoperitoneum).

A. Bleeding normally occurs during initial exchanges after catheter insertion or implantation. For bleeding related to surgery, see Chapter 61, *PD Access*.

B. 2 mL of blood/liter results in blood-tinged dialysate.

C. Etiology. Many sources of IP bleeding have been reported. Figure 13.13 shows a decision-making model for turbid (cloudy) or bloody dialysate.
   1. Abdominal trauma.
   2. Gynecologic.
      a. Menstruation is most common etiology. Bleeding may occur before menses.
      b. Ovulation.
      c. Ovarian cyst.
      d. Endometriosis.
   3. Polycystic kidney or liver disease.
   4. Gastrointestinal.
      a. After colonoscopy or enema.
      b. Pancreatitis.
      c. Cholecystitis.
      d. Splenic rupture.
      e. Ischemic bowel.
      f. Organ erosion or perforation.
   5. Damage to the peritoneal membrane.
      a. Peritoneal calcification.
      b. Encapsulating peritoneal sclerosis.
      c. Radiation-induced peritoneal fibrosis.
      d. Mixed connective tissue disease.
   6. Hematologic.
      a. Idiopathic thrombocytopenic purpura.
      b. Anticoagulation therapy.
   7. Neoplastic.
      a. Renal cell carcinoma.
      b. Colon cancer.
      c. Urologic cancer.
      d. Abdominal metastases.
   8. Miscellaneous.
      a. Extracorporeal lithotripsy.
      b. Leakage from extraperitoneal hematoma (e.g., posttransplant).

D. Assessment.
   1. Typically bleeding is minimal to moderate and resolves spontaneously.
   2. Observe dialysate effluent for diminishing color in subsequent exchanges.
   3. Dialysate hematocrit if bleeding is excessive.
   4. May need to rule out peritonitis.
   5. May need to rule out other acute abdominal disease.

E. Intervention.
   1. Bleeding may resolve spontaneously.
   2. Addition of heparin to the dialysis solution will prevent clotting and maintain catheter patency. If dialysis is discontinued, locking the catheter with a heparin solution may prevent clotting.
   3. Rapid exchanges with dialysis solution at room temperature may halt bleeding. It has been hypothesized that the cool solution causes vasoconstriction, leading to hemostasis.
      a. Keep patient warm.
      b. Monitor the patient's temperature.
      c. Monitor dialysate effluent for diminished bleeding in subsequent exchanges.

F. Sequelae.
   1. Bloody dialysate may provide a rich medium for bacterial growth.
   2. Hemoperitoneum causes an inflammatory reaction; excessive or prolonged bleeding may cause adhesions.

G. For hemorrhage related to vessel perforation see Chapter 61, *PD Access*.

VII. Noninfectious "peritonitis."

A. Peritoneal eosinophilia.
   1. Presentation.
      a. Turbid dialysate.
      b. Absence of abdominal pain or other symptoms of infection.
      c. Relatively low dialysate white cell count.
   2. Dialysate WBC differential shows neutrophils < 50%; eosinophils > 10%.
   3. Etiology. Thought to be an allergic response to:
      a. New peritoneal catheter.
      b. IP medications.
      c. Pneumoperitoneum.
      d. Fungal peritonitis.
   4. Therapy.
      a. Does not require antibiotic therapy.
      b. Discontinue IP medication.
      c. Resolves spontaneously in a few days or weeks.
      d. Monitor closely.

B. Aseptic peritonitis has been reported with use of icodextrin solutions.
   1. Patients present with mild abdominal symptoms and cloudy drainage.
   2. There is an increase in white blood cells with mononuclear cells predominating; cultures are negative.

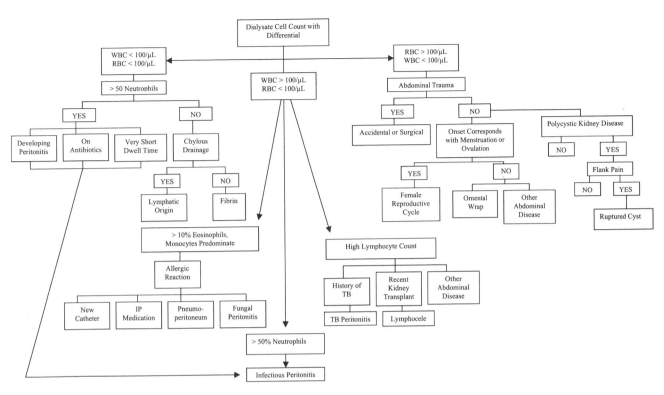

Figure 13.13. Decision-making tree for turbid peritoneal dialysis effluent in PD patients.

Adapted from Prowant B., & Schmidt, L. (1987). A decision making model and standard nursing care plan for cloudy peritoneal dialysate effluent (Abstract). *ANNA Journal, 14,*149.

3. Cloudiness may be worse in the icodextrin exchange.

4. Discontinuing icodextrin typically causes symptoms to resolve; reintroduction of icodextrin may result in reappearance of cloudy drainage.

5. The etiology of several episodes in 2001 and 2002 was believed to be contamination during the manufacturing process.

VIII. Changes in dialysate color. Some medications can cause changes in color, but not clarity, of dialysate, e.g. fluorescein eye drops cause a greenish-yellow discoloration and rifampin causes an orange discoloration.

IX. Acute hydrothorax.

A. Acute hydrothorax occurs when dialysis fluid enters the pleural cavity.

B. The pathophysiology is the presence of structural defects in the diaphragm. This is coupled with negative intrathoracic pressure and positive intraabdominal pressure, which moves dialysis solution into the pleural cavity.

C. Incidence is < 5% of PD patients.
1. More frequent in females.
2. Occurs in both adults and children.
3. Usually occurs within days or weeks of starting PD.

D. Presentation.
1. Predominantly on right side.
2. Small pleural effusions may be asymptomatic.
3. Dyspnea.
4. Worsening of shortness of breath with use of hypertonic dialysis solution.
5. Absent or diminished breath sounds; dullness to percussion.
6. Chest pain.
7. Weight gain.
8. Dialysate drains poorly and/or there is low drain volume; patient may become hypervolemic.
9. Acute respiratory failure.

E. Assessment.
1. Signs and symptoms of pleural effusion.
2. Radiologic evidence of pleural effusion.
3. Thoracentesis for relief of symptoms and/or diagnosis shows pleural fluid with composition

similar to dialysate.
  a. High glucose.
  b. Low protein.
  c. May contain D-lactate if using lactate-buffered solution.
4. Radioisotope scanning can also be used to demonstrate a peritoneal-pleural communication.
  a. Technetium-labeled macroaggregated albumin or sulfur colloid is instilled with the regular volume of dialysis solution.
  b. Patient moves around to mix solution and raise intraabdominal pressure.
  c. Subsequent scans detect isotope above the diaphragm.
5. Peritoneography with contrast media has been reported.

F. Intervention.
  1. For small effusions, PD may be continued with lower fill volume and close monitoring; discontinuing dialysis often leads to rapid resolution.
  2. If there is a massive hydrothorax with respiratory compromise, PD is discontinued and thoracentesis performed.
  3. Temporary hemodialysis for 2–4 weeks. It is possible that the peritoneo-pleural communication will reseal.

G. Correction of the defect is not uniformly successful.
  1. Pleurodesis procedures with tetracycline, bleomycin, talc, and autologous blood have been reported.
  2. Surgical repair.
  3. Instillation of fibrin glue into the drained pleural cavity.
  4. Reintroduce PD with low volumes.

X. Instillation of hot dialysis solution.

A. Etiology.
  1. Solution is overheated because of equipment error or ineffective monitoring.
  2. Solutions are microwaved for excessive time and/or solution is not well mixed after warming.

B. Assessment.
  1. Hot or burning abdominal pain.
  2. Observe for an increase in body temperature.
    a. Sweating.
    b. Flushing.

  c. Measure temperature.
  d. Check pulse rate and rhythm; cardiac dysrhythmias may occur.

C. Intervention.
  1. Drain dialysate.
  2. Monitor patient carefully until temperature returns to normal.
  3. Evaluate warming procedure and method of monitoring solution temperature.

D. It is possible to burn the peritoneal membrane with subsequent inflammation and scarring.

XI. Instillation of cold dialysis solution.

A. Etiology.
  1. Solution is not prewarmed.
  2. Warming procedure is inadequate.
  3. Equipment malfunction.

B. Assessment.
  1. Subjective complaint.
    a. Cold dialysate.
    b. Abdominal cramping.
  2. Hypothermia.
    a. Decreased body temperature.
    b. Chills.
    c. Acrocyanosis (mottled blue or purple discoloration of extremities).
    d. Possibility of cardiac dysrhythmias.

C. Intervention.
  1. Drain dialysate.
  2. Treat hypothermia.
  3. Continue PD with warm solutions.
  4. Evaluate warming procedure and method of monitoring solution temperature.
  5. Monitor patient carefully until temperature returns to normal.

XII. Hypervolemia.

A. Etiology.
  1. Inadequate fluid removal.
    a. Inadequate number of hypertonic exchanges.
    b. Exchange time is too long for selected dextrose concentrations.
    c. Inadequate sodium removal.
    d. Inaccurate dry weight.
    e. Decreased insensitive losses in chronic patients related to change in seasons; (i.e., patients do not sweat as much during fall and winter and may not decrease intake or increase UF to compensate).

f. Errors in fluid balance calculations in acute dialysis.
2. Excessive intake.
a. Increased salt and water intake in chronic patients.
b. Inadequate salt and water restrictions in acute patients.

B. Assessment.
1. Weight gain.
2. Blood pressure increased from baseline.
3. Dyspnea.
4. Peripheral edema.
5. Neck vein distention.
6. Subcutaneous edema.
7. Pulmonary edema.
8. LVH and congestive heart failure.
9. Acute dialysis flow sheet indicates patient has a positive fluid balance.

C. Intervention.
1. Increase use of hypertonic dialysis solutions. Consider use of icodextrin solution.
2. Shorten dwell times.
3. Restrict fluid intake.
4. Correct catheter malfunction.
5. For acute PD.
a. Calculate fluid balance accurately including all losses and all sources of intake.
b. Monitor vital signs and weight frequently.
c. Monitor cardiac and respiratory status.
6. Perform PET to determine if there has been a change in the peritoneal membrane function.
7. Review fluid management with patient and family.
a. Assessment of fluid balance; signs and symptoms of fluid overload.
b. Causes and management of fluid overload.

XIII. Hypovolemia.

A. Etiology.
1. Excessive fluid removal.
a. Excessive use of hypertonic solution.
b. Excessive sodium removal.
c. Inaccurate fluid balance calculations.
d. Chronic patients may experience increased insensible loss related to seasonal changes (i.e., increased sweating in summer).
2. Inadequate intake.
a. Decreased salt and water intake in chronic patients, often due to acute illness.
b. Restriction of fluid and sodium intake in acute patients.

B. Assessment.
1. Weight loss; typically under dry weight.
2. Hypotension; orthostatic hypotension.
3. Poor skin turgor.
4. Dry mucous membranes.
5. Tachycardia.
6. Patient has a negative fluid balance.

C. Intervention.
1. Discontinue use of hypertonic solutions or icodextrin solution.
2. Lengthen dwell times.
3. Replace fluid and sodium losses with bouillon or other salty liquid.
4. Review fluid management with patient and family.
a. Assessment of fluid balance; signs and symptoms of dehydration.
b. Causes and management of dehydration.
5. For acute dialysis patients:
a. Intravenous replacement may be required.
b. Calculate fluid balance accurately including all sources of intake and all losses.
c. Monitor vital signs and weight closely.

XIV. Hypokalemia.

A. An increased incidence of hypokalemia has been reported with dialysis prescriptions enhanced in an effort to meet KDOQI adequacy targets.

B. Etiology.
1. Ongoing losses and restricted or inadequate dietary intake in chronic patients.
2. Potassium wasting due to diuretic therapy.
3. Diarrhea.
4. Excessive potassium removal in acute dialysis.

C. Assessment.
1. Monitor serum chemistries.
2. Weakness.
3. Leg cramps.
4. Fatigue.
5. Dysrhythmias.
6. Constipation (a result of hypokalemia).

D. Intervention.
1. Recommended serum potassium level is > 3.5 in patients on digoxin or with history of cardiac dysrhythmias.
2. Chronic PD patients with low serum potassium should increase dietary intake.
3. If potassium supplementation is required for chronic dialysis patients, oral supplements may be used.

a. They are less expensive.

b. IP potassium administration has inherent risks of contaminating the system and irritating the peritoneal membrane.

4. For acute dialysis with short dialysis exchanges.

a. Use potassium-free dialysis solution only until potassium reaches normal limits.

b. Add KCl 2–4 mEq/L to the dialysis solution for acute dialysis patients when serum potassium normalizes. (*Note*: KCl does not routinely come in reusable vials containing bacteriostatic agents.)

c. Monitor serum potassium.

XV. Hyperkalemia.

A. Although chronic PD typically improves hyperkalemia, chronic PD patients may become hyperkalemic due to excessive potassium intake. This is related to geographic and seasonal variations, and is most commonly due to availability and increased consumption of fresh fruits and vegetables.

B. Hyperkalemia occurs because chronic PD is limited in the amount of potassium that can be removed.

C. Treatment is a combination of decreasing dietary potassium and increasing the dose of dialysis.

D. A cation-exchange resin, such as kayexalate, may be used in an emergency.

XVI. Hypernatremia.

A. Not infrequent in overnight cycler dialysis without long dwell daytime exchanges. With shorter dwell times using 132 mEq/L sodium solutions, less sodium is removed in relation to water.

B. These patients may have postdialysis hypernatremia, thirst, and an increase in blood pressure. This may result in increased fluid intake and large interdialytic weight gains.

Rare Complications

I. **Chyloperitoneum.**

A. Chylous ascites is caused by an interruption of the lymphatic drainage from the gut to the main lymphatics. Lymphatic drainage from the gut enters the peritoneal cavity and the dialysate contains intestinal chylomicrons high in triglycerides. In PD patients, this is called chyloperitoneum.

B. After a fatty meal, the dialysate has a milky white appearance; this may resolve spontaneously and recur intermittently depending on the fat content of meals.

C. Early onset may be related to a severed lymph vessel during catheter insertion.

D. Late onset has been theorized to be related to multiple peritonitis episodes resulting in adhesions that obstruct lymphatic drainage.

E. Evaluation.

1. Rule out any signs and symptoms of bacterial or fungal peritonitis; dialysate cell count should be within normal limits.

2. Assess dialysate triglyceride level; in chyloperitoneum it will be high, sometimes greater than the plasma triglyceride level.

F. Chyloperitoneum often resolves spontaneously. Temporary cessation of PD has also been recommended.

II. **Dialysis disequilibrium.** Dialysis disequilibrium can occur during the initial dialysis of uremic patients with rapid exchanges and hypertonic dialysis solutions (see Section 11, Chapter 55 for acute complications of hemodialysis).

III. **Heparin-induced thrombocytopenia.**

A. Heparin-induced thrombocytopenia (HIT) has been documented in a PD patient who had no prior heparin exposure and received 1,000 units per day IP for 7 days during treatment of peritonitis (Kaplan, Manns, & McLaughlin, 2005).

B. Patients who have transferred from HD may also be at risk for HIT if they receive IP heparin.

C. HIT should be considered in patients who present with thrombocytopenia and minor bleeding, e.g., petechiae.

IV. Peritoneal membrane changes.

A. The majority of patients on chronic PD do not have clinical evidence of changes in the peritoneal membrane characteristics.

B. Although membrane changes can occur in either direction, most individuals move toward increasing dialysate to plasma creatinine ratios and decreasing D/D0 glucose (higher membrane transport characteristics) over time.

V. UF failure.

A. Ultrafiltration (UF) failure is defined as the inability to maintain dry weight using two or more hypertonic exchanges per day. ISPD recommends basing the diagnosis of UF failure on results of a standardized 4-hour dwell.
1. < 100 mL UF from 4-hour peritoneal equilibration test with 2.5% dextrose.
2. < 400 mL UF from a 4-hour standard peritoneal permeability analysis (SPA) with 4.25% dextrose concentration.

B. The incidence of UF failure increases from 3% after 1 year to 31% after 6 years.

C. There are three etiologies of UF failure.
1. Early problems with UF, within the first 2 years of dialysis, are typically due to increased lymphatic absorption of dialysate.
2. Later loss of UF, after several years of dialysis, in combination with high peritoneal transport rates is due to loss of glucose-induced osmosis, likely due to dysfunction of the peritoneal water channels (aquaporins).
3. Loss of UF associated with loss of solute transport (formerly called Type II UF failure).
   a. Results from a decrease in effective peritoneal surface area.
   b. Etiology.
      (1) Numerous adhesions.
      (2) Encapsulating peritoneal sclerosis (EPS).

D. Assessment of UF failure.
1. Rule out excessive sodium and fluid intake.
2. Rule out loss of residual renal function as the cause of inadequate fluid removal.
3. Rule out catheter malfunction and leaks.
4. Rule out inappropriate dialysis prescription, that is, a mismatch between peritoneal membrane characteristics and prescription.
5. Rule out nonadherence with dialysis.
6. Assess peritoneal membrane function.
   a. The peritoneal equilibration test (PET) can be used. However, a modified PET using 4.25% dextrose has been recommended. This provides maximal osmotic drive and allows evaluation of sodium sieving.
   b. Other peritoneal function tests may also be used (see Chapter 62, *Peritoneal Dialysis Therapy*).

VI. Encapsulating peritoneal sclerosis (EPS).

A. EPS is a progressive inflammatory process resulting in sheets of fibrous tissue that cover, bind and constrict the viscera.

B. Classic EPS is characterized by marked sclerotic thickening of the peritoneal membrane with partial or diffuse bowel obstruction.

C. In severe cases, a thick fibrous tissue layer encapsulates the bowel like a cocoon; there are many adhesions, and the peritoneal membrane becomes thick, opaque, and has a "tanned" appearance.

D. This is one of the most serious complications of PD with the highest mortality, so it is extremely important to diagnose it in an early stage.

E. Onset may be gradual or rapid.

F. EPS is sometimes diagnosed after transfer to hemodialysis for ultrafiltration failure.

G. The cause is unknown, but various toxins and infectious etiologies have been postulated.
1. More frequent in long-term PD patients; one Japanese study found that PD duration > 8 years significantly increased the risk of EPS.
2. A high incidence of peritonitis and severe peritonitis have been proposed as contributing factors.
3. Poor biocompatibility of dialysis solutions, e.g., high dextrose concentration and low pH.
4. Toxins such as plastic particles, and disinfectants, e.g., chlorhexidine, and antibiotics, have been postulated as risk factors.
5. Use of beta blockers.
6. There may be a genetic predisposition.

H. Presentation.
1. Symptoms in early stages may be related to decreased UF and solute clearances.
2. Late presentation typically has signs and symptoms of intestinal obstruction.
   a. Recurrent cramping or colicky abdominal pain.
   b. Intermittent nausea and vomiting.
   c. Abdominal fullness and distention.
   d. Partial or complete bowel obstruction.
   e. Anorexia and weight loss, hypoalbuminemia and anemia may be seen in more advanced stages of the disease.
3. May present as recurring or nonresolving peritonitis, which may be culture negative.

I. Diagnosis.
1. Abdominal ultrasound and CT scans are the best noninvasive diagnostic tests.
2. Worsening symptoms correlate with progressive CT abnormalities.
   a. Loculated fluid collections.
   b. Peritoneal calcification.
   c. Bowel dilatation with tethering.
3. Laparoscopy or laparotomy with biopsy. The thickened, "tanned" peritoneum encasing the bowel can be readily seen.

J. Intervention.
1. Use of corticosteroids and other immuno-suppressive drugs. The use of tamoxifen in conjunction with these drugs has also been reported.
2. Good parenteral nutrition is critical for support, but is not recommended as a primary therapy.
3. Laparatomy with enterolysis for ileus or life-threatening bowel obstruction. There is a high rate of complications and postoperative mortality.

K. There has been a decrease in the incidence of EPS and incremental increases in survival; however, the mortality rate remains extremely high, both in patients who remain on PD and those who are transferred to hemodialysis.

L. Prevention.
1. Prevent peritonitis.
2. Early diagnosis and improved management of peritonitis.
3. Early catheter removal in severe peritonitis.
4. Use of biocompatible dialysis solutions.
   a. Bicarbonate buffers.

   b. Nonglucose osmotic agents.
5. Avoid IP medications whenever possible.
6. Avoid IP contamination from disinfectants and other chemicals.

Infectious Complications of Peritoneal Dialysis

I. Peritonitis.

A. Definitions.
1. The following definitions are from the International Society for Peritoneal Dialysis (ISPD) (Piraino et al., 2005).
   a. Peritonitis: inflammation of the peritoneum.
   b. Infectious peritonitis: inflammation of the peritoneum related to microorganisms.
   c. Refractory or resistant peritonitis: symptoms do not abate after 5 days of appropriate therapy.
   d. Relapsing peritonitis is now defined by as an episode that recurs within 4 weeks of the completion of antibiotic therapy for a prior episode with the same organism.
   e. Recurrent peritonitis is defined as an episode that occurs within 4 weeks of the completion of antibiotic therapy for a prior episode, but with a different organism.
   f. Reinfection or repeat infection is defined as a new peritonitis episode more than 4 weeks after completion of therapy for an earlier episode, with the same organism.
   g. Note that there are various other definitions, sometimes contradictory, related to peritonitis, particularly regarding refractory, relapsing, and recurrent episodes.
   h. Nosocomial peritonitis is peritonitis that develops in the hospital in a patient who had no infection at time of admission; this accounts for < 1% of all episodes.
2. Catheter-related peritonitis occurs in conjunction with an exit site or tunnel infection with the same organism (or there may be no growth on one culture).

B. Incidence.
1. Improved technology and connection techniques have reduced the incidence to less than 0.5 episodes per patient year or about one episode every 24–26 patient months.
2. Some programs are reporting higher rates, and

a few programs with extensive experience and expertise are reporting infections as low as one episode every 4 or 5 years. These very low rates have been associated with the use of topical antibiotic prophylaxis at the exit site and a low incidence of exit site infections.

3. The use of new, more biocompatible solutions available in Europe has lowered peritonitis rates compared to rates with traditional dialysis solutions.

C. Sequelae.
   1. Peritonitis is responsible for up to one third of hospital admissions in the PD population.
   2. Peritonitis remains the major reason for transfer to hemodialysis therapy.
   3. High peritonitis rates are associated with increased mortality.

D. Routes of contamination.
   1. Transluminal: contamination related to a break in the integrity of the closed system.
      a. Touch contamination during procedures.
      b. Skin organisms, e.g., Staphylococcal species, are most frequent.
      c. Traditionally reported as the most common route of contamination.
   2. Periluminal: along the outer surface of the catheter.
      a. Increased risk with acute catheter use, leak, or frank bleed.
      b. Increased risk with chronic catheter post-implantation before healing is complete.
      c. Staphylococcus and Pseudomonas species are most frequent.
   3. Hematogenous.
      a. Associated with transient bacteremia.
      b. May be associated with dental procedures; Streptococcal species are most frequent.
      c. Bacteremia may also occur following sigmoidoscopy or colonoscopy with biopsy.
      d. *Mycobacterium tuberculosis* peritonitis is also contracted by hematogenous contamination.
      e. Other atypical mycobacterium (e.g., *M. chelonei, M. fortuitum*).
   4. Transmural: transmigration of microorganisms across the bowel wall.
      a. Increased incidence with diverticular disease and severe vascular disease.
      b. Associated with unresolved constipation or acute treatment of constipation.
      c. May also occur with colitis, diarrhea, and gastrointestinal bleed.

   d. Enteric organisms and anaerobic organisms are seen.
   e. Multiple gram-negative organisms suggest bowel perforation.
   f. Note that gastrointestinal organisms can also be transferred by touch contamination. Good hand washing should be emphasized for patients with gastrointestinal problems.
   5. Ascending from the female reproductive tract.
      a. A rare source of peritonitis.
      b. Organisms are vaginal flora, e.g., Streptococcal and Candida species.
      c. May be associated with gynecologic procedures or intrauterine devices.

E. Compromised host defense mechanisms.
   1. Large volumes of dialysis solution in the peritoneal cavity dilute the normal macrophage concentration and humoral factors.
   2. Dialysis solution is directly toxic to macrophages, polymorphonuclear neutrophils and mesothelial cells. The low pH and high osmolality may be responsible for the toxic effects.
   3. Dialysis solution also interferes with humoral defenses.

F. Common causative microorganisms (in descending order of frequency).
   1. Gram-positive organisms, typically related to normal skin and nasal flora, are responsible for about two thirds of episodes.
      a. *Staphylococcus epidermidis* most frequent.
      b. *Staphylococcus aureus* is also common.
   2. Gram-negative organisms (Pseudomonas species, Klebsiella species, Enterobacter and Enterococcal species) are responsible for ~ 28% of episodes. Patients are more likely to be hospitalized and have worse outcomes than with gram-positive peritonitis.
      a. Water-borne organisms, such as Pseudomonas and Acinetobacter species.
      b. Gram-negative touch contamination can occur with organisms from the mouth or gastrointestinal tract.
   3. Polymicrobial peritonitis has more than one causative organism; this is seen in ~ 6% of all episodes.
   4. Mixed gram-positive and gram-negative organisms are almost always from transmural migration from the intestinal tract or bowel perforation.
   5. Anaerobic organisms (e.g., Clostridium species), primarily from the gastrointestinal tract, cause ~ 2.5% of peritonitis episodes.

Nose
Staphylococcus aureus (+)
Staphylococcus epidermidis (+)
Corynebacteria species (+, e.g., diptheroids)

Skin
Staphylococcus epidermidis (+)
Staphylococcus aureus (+)
Corynebacteria species (+, e.g.,
    Propionibacterium [an anaerobe])

Mouth and Throat
Streptococcus species (+)
Actinomycetes species (+)
Bacteroides species (- anaerobe)
Haemophilus species (-)
Neisseriae species (-)
Mycobacteria

Urethra
Peptostreptococcal species (+ anaerobe)
Bacteroides species (- anaerobe)

Intestinal Tract
Enterococcus species (+)
Enterobacter species (-), e.g., Klebsiella species,
    Proteus mirabilis, Serratia marcescens
Bacteroides species (- anaerobe)
Clostridium species (+ anaerobe)
Peptostreptococcal species (+ anaerobe)
Streptococcus species (+)
Pseudomonas species (-)
Escherichia coli (-)
Proteus species (-)
Lactobacillus species (+)
Candida species (yeast)

Vagina
Clostridium species (+ anaerobe)
Peptostreptococcal species (+ anaerobe)
Group B hemolytic streptococci (+)
Bacteroides species (- anaerobe)
Candida species (yeast)
Enterococcus species (+)

Environment (air, soil & water)
Acinetobacter species (-)
Pseudomonas species (-)

(+) = gram-positive organism
(-) = gram-negative organism

Illustration by Kristina Guardino

Figure 13.14. Microorganisms that are normal flora or pathogens in different parts of the body.

6. Yeasts, e.g., Candida species, may come from intestinal tract or vagina and cause ~ 2.5% of episodes.
7. Other unusual organisms, e.g., Mycobacterium species.
8. No growth. In almost all cases, inadequate culture techniques are believed to be responsible rather than a true sterile peritonitis.
9. Figure 13.14 shows normal flora and resident pathogens in various parts of the body.

G. Risk factors for peritonitis.
1. *Staphylococcus aureus* nasal carriage is the strongest risk factor.
2. Spiking dialysis bags is the most significant procedure-related risk factor.
3. Recurrent or chronic exit site or tunnel infections.
4. Invasive procedures not covered by prophylactic antibiotic therapy, e.g., dental, gastrointestinal, and vaginal procedures.

5. Bacteremia.
6. Children, patients with diabetes, and patients with low serum albumin have higher infection rates.
7. Immunosuppressive therapy.
8. HIV-positive patients have proportionately more gram-negative and fungal infections.
9. Catheter biofilms.
10. Depression.

H. Signs and symptoms of peritonitis.
1. Typical presentation.
    a. Turbid (cloudy) dialysate effluent (due to increase in white blood cells and fibrin).
    b. Abdominal discomfort or pain.
    c. Rebound tenderness in about half of all episodes.
2. Less frequent signs and symptoms.
    a. Fever (34–36%).
    b. Nausea (30–35%).
    c. Vomiting.

d. Chills.

e. Diarrhea.

I. Clinical course.

1. Incubation period.

a. Incubation period for touch contamination is ~ 24–48 hours.

b. Some incubation periods are very short (from 6 to 12 hours).

c. Incubation for endogenous infections (hematogenous, vaginal or gastrointestinal source) is probably shorter than for exogenous.

2. Symptoms typically decrease dramatically after initiation of appropriate antibiotic therapy and usually resolve within 1–3 days.

J. Peritonitis causes changes in peritoneal membrane structure and function.

1. Increased clearances.

2. More rapid glucose absorption resulting in earlier loss of osmotic gradient.

a. The total drain volume of long dwell exchanges is decreased.

b. Some patients will need to use higher dialysis dextrose concentrations, or icodextrin-based solution for the long dwell exchange to maintain fluid balance.

3. Increased protein losses.

4. Increased fibrin formation.

K. Diagnosis.

1. Abdominal pain.

2. Dialysate white blood cell count > 100/µL with > 50% polymorphonuclear cells (neutrophils or segmented cells).

3. Evidence of organisms on Gram stain.

4. Positive culture.

L. Recommended laboratory techniques.

1. Dialysate sample collection for culture and sensitivity.

a. At least 2-4 hour dwell time is recommended; 1-hour dwell time is the absolute minimum.

b. Dialysate must be mixed well by inverting bag several times before sampling.

c. The sample port is disinfected before sampling.

d. Sample is obtained using aseptic technique.

e. Large sample volume, 50–100 mL, reduces false negative culture results.

2. Common elements of effective culture techniques.

a. For large volume samples, the sample is centrifuged or filtered, and the sediment is cultured.

b. Blood culture bottles may be used; however, routine culture techniques may not isolate organisms.

c. There should be a protocol and time limit for transport to the laboratory and plating the specimen; this will vary amongst dialysis programs and laboratories.

d. If antibiotics have been administered, notify the laboratory, so an appropriate technique can be used to reduce false negative results.

3. If there is no growth on culture and symptoms do not abate with therapy, or symptoms recur during therapy, or the peritonitis episode relapses, special culture techniques may improve the chances of identifying the organism.

a. Fungal culture.

b. Anaerobic culture technique.

c. Acid-fast culture for mycobacterium species.

4. Gram stain.

a. Perform on spun sediment from dialysate sample.

b. Will be positive in 20–30% of samples.

c. Is of value in choosing initial antibiotic when organisms are seen.

d. Helpful in identifying fungal organisms early.

5. Dialysate cell count with differential is used to make the diagnosis.

a. Samples for cell counts are routinely obtained from the same dialysate bag as the samples for culture and Gram stain.

b. The dialysate should be mixed well prior to sampling.

c. Samples can be cytocentrofuged; this concentrates the cells for the smear.

M. Figure 13.13 is a decision model for interpreting dialysate cell counts (shown previously).

1. Occasionally in peritonitis, the WBC count is elevated, but under 100/µL, but the percentage of polymorphonuclear cells is > 50%. Reasons for this are:

a. Peritonitis is just developing.

b. Patient is already receiving antibiotics.

c. Short dwell time prior to sample collection.

d. Cell count delayed > 4 hours.

N. Negative cultures should not be greater than 20% of peritonitis episodes (Piraino et al., 2005).

1. Reasons for negative culture results at onset of clinical peritonitis are listed in Table 13.23.

2. If the negative culture rate is > 20%, continuous quality improvement efforts should include evaluation of culture methodology and interventions to improve the proportion of positive cultures.

Table 13.23

Reasons for Negative Culture Results with Clinical Peritonitis

- Patient taking antibiotics for another reason

- Patient was already receiving intraperitoneal antibiotics when sample for culture was taken

- Inadequate dwell time prior to draining sample for culture

- Inadequate sample volume

- Delay in delivering sample to laboratory

- Problems with laboratory technique

Adapted from Kelman, E., & Watson, D. (2006). Preventing and managing complications of peritoneal dialysis. In A.E. Molzahn & E. Butera (Eds.), *Contemporary nephrology nursing: Principles and practice* (2nd ed., pp. 687-709). Pitman, NJ: American Nephrology Nurses' Association.

Table 13.24

Evidence-Based Practice Guidelines for PD-Associated Peritonitis (Levels 1 and 2 Evidence)

- Prevention of Peritonitis
  - Parenteral antibiotic prophylaxis should be used preoperatively prior to catheter implantation to reduce the incidence of peritonitis (CARI, EBPG).
  - Prophylactic therapy using mupirocin calcium ointment decreases the risk of catheter exit/tunnel infections and peritonitis (CARI).
  - Disconnect systems result in lower peritonitis rates than standard spike or Luer-Lok systems, and the standard systems should not be used (CARI, ISPD).
  - Double-bag or twin-bag systems are preferred for CAPD because they are more effective in preventing peritonitis (EBPG, CARI, ISPD).
  - If double-bag systems are not available, any Y-set system is preferred to any spike system, because they are more effective in preventing peritonitis (EBPG).
  - There is no difference in peritonitis rates in patients using glucose versus icodextrin for the long dwell (CARI).

- Peritonitis is confirmed by culture and cell count of dialysate (ISPD).

- Initial treatment should be a combination of intraperitoneal antibiotics that will cover both gram-positive and gram-negative organisms (CARI, ISPD).

- Oral nystatin should be considered in conjunction with antibiotic administration to PD patients to reduce the occurrence of fungal peritonitis (CARI).

CARI = Caring for Australians with Renal Impairment (2005)
EBPG = European Best Practice Guidelines (Dombros et al., 2005).
ISPD = International Society for Peritoneal Dialysis Recommendations (Piraino et al., 2005)

O. Initial treatment described below is based on published ISPD recommendations (Piraino et al., 2005). A complete current listing of protocols is available at http://www.ispd.org. Evidence-based practice guidelines for PD-associated peritonitis are listed in Table 13.24.
   1. Antibiotic therapy is initiated prior to identification of the causative organism.
      a. The initial dose must cover both gram-positive and gram-negative organisms (Evidence-based).
      b. Gram-positive coverage.
         (1) ISPD recommends a first generation cephalosporin, such as cefazolin or cephalothin.
         (2) ISPD also recommends vancomycin as the initial drug for gram-positive coverage in programs with a high incidence of methicillin-resistant organisms; a second drug must be still used to cover gram-negative organisms.
      c. Gram-negative coverage.
         (1) A third generation cephalosporin (ceftazidime, cefepime, or carbapenem) or an aminoglycoside are recommended by ISPD.
         (2) To avoid development of resistant organisms, quinolones should be used only if local sensitivities support their use.
         (3) For patients allergic to cephalosporins, an alternative drug is aztreonam (when aminoglycosides are not used).
   2. IP administration is preferred over IV dosing for CAPD therapy, because of high local levels of antibiotic. Loading doses of antibiotics are added to dialysis solution for a long dwell exchange ($\geq$ 6 hours).
   3. ISPD dosage recommendations are for "anuric" patients. The ISPD further recommends that for patients with significant residual kidney function (> 100 mL/day urine output), the dose of antibiotic be increased by 25%.
   4. Aminoglycosides may be nephrotoxic, and

prolonged courses should be used with caution in patients with residual kidney function. Aminoglycosides also may be ototoxic, so dosing recommendations should be carefully followed.

5. Heparin 500–1000 units/L is added to the dialysis solution until effluent is clear. Heparin inhibits fibrin formation and may prevent subsequent adhesion formation.

6. In general, the recommended antibiotics are compatible in dialysis solutions and when mixed with heparin.
   a. Medications should not be mixed in the same syringe.
   b. Unless the stability of drugs in the dialysis solution has been documented, medications should be added shortly before the bag is used.
   c. Aminoglycosides should not be added to the same bag as a penicillin (e.g., ampicillin) because of chemical incompatibility.

P. For maintenance antibiotic therapy, the treatment regimen is modified based on culture results. These recommendations are also based on ISPD guidelines.
   1. Most IP antibiotics can be added either to each exchange, or to one long dwell (≥ 6 hrs) exchange daily.
   2. Most antibiotics have higher systemic absorption during peritonitis. For example, when vancomycin is given IP for an exit site infection without peritonitis, about 50% is absorbed, but during peritonitis closer to 90% is absorbed systemically.
   3. Gram-positive coverage.
      a. First generation cephalosporin.
      b. Vancomycin. *Note*: because of the increasing prevalence of vancomycin-resistant organisms, it is advisable to reserve vancomycin for organisms that are not sensitive to or do not respond to the other recommended therapies.
   4. Gram-negative coverage.
      a. Third generation cephalosporin; aztreonam is an alternative for patients with cephalosporin allergies.
      b. Aminoglycoside.
   5. Therapy is continued for 14 days in uncomplicated cases.
   6. For complicated cases including those with *S. aureus*, gram-negative, and enterococcal organisms, 21 days of therapy is recommended.

Q. Antibiotic therapy for cycler patients.

1. Whether patients on cycler therapies need to lengthen exchange times or change to CAPD to maintain optimal IP antibiotic levels is still debated.
2. Recommended antibiotic doses and duration of therapy for cycler patients are similar to recommendations for CAPD.

R. Organism-specific recommendations.
   1. Coagulase-negative staphylococcus is a common causative organism, typically transferred by touch contamination and associated with a mild form of peritonitis.
      a. Continue first-generation cephalosporin.
      b. Vancomycin is recommended for methicillin-resistant *Staphylococcus epidermidis* (MRSE).
      c. Some programs have high rates of methicillin resistance. This indicates that the organism is considered resistant to all betalactam-related antibiotics including penicillins, cephalosporins, and carbapenems. The ISPD suggests that these programs may choose to use vancomycin as empiric therapy.
   2. *Staphylococcus aureus* infections.
      a. *S. aureus* infections may be severe.
      b. *S. aureus* may be acquired by touch contamination or exit/tunnel infection. If associated with exit/tunnel infection, the peritonitis may not resolve without catheter removal.
      c. For *S. aureus* sensitive to methicillin, continue cephalosporin; oral rifampin may be added as a second synergistic drug, but should only be used for 1 week to avoid resistance. Rifampin penetrates cell membranes and biofilm, and is bacteriocidal to phagocytosed organisms.
      d. Methicillin-resistant *S. aureus* (MRSA) should be treated with vancomycin. Serum levels are dependent on the level of residual kidney function, and serum trough levels must be measured after the initial dose to determine frequency of subsequent doses.
      e. Vancomycin-resistant *S. aureus* has been reported in dialysis patients; linezolid, daptomycin or quinupristin/dalfopristin are the recommended treatment options.
   3. Streptococcal and enterococcal peritonitis may be severe and IP ampicillin is the recommended treatment. For enterococcal peritonitis, an aminoglycoside IP once daily may be added.
   4. Vancomycin-resistant enterococcus (VRE) and vancomycin-resistant *Enterococcus faecium* (VREF) have caused peritonitis in PD patients, most often after hospitalization and prior

antibiotic therapy.

5. A single gram-negative organism may be due to touch contamination, exit site infection, or from a transmural migration from the bowel, which may be related to constipation, colitis, or diverticulitis.
   a. The most common gram-negative organisms in PD peritonitis are Klebsiella species, *E. coli* and Enterobacter species.
   b. Gram-negative peritonitis has higher rates of hospitalization, catheter removal, transfer to hemodialysis, and death than gram-positive organisms.
   c. Antibiotic should be chosen based on sensitivities.

6. *Pseudomonas aeruginosa* peritonitis is often catheter related and is generally severe.
   a. Pseudomonas species should be treated with two antibiotics. Add the second drug based on sensitivities. An oral quinolone can be given.
   b. Therapy should be continued for 21 days.
   c. Catheter removal is indicated if there is a related catheter exit or tunnel infection; antibiotics should be continued for at least 2 weeks after catheter removal.

7. Multiple gram-negative organisms are often from intraabdominal pathology, e.g., diverticular disease, appendicitis. The risk of death is increased, and surgical evaluation/ intervention is recommended.
   a. The therapy of choice metronidazole. However, it is recommended that this be given in combination with ampicillin, ceftazidime or an aminoglycoside.
   b. Infection may respond to antibiotics initially, then worsen.
   c. Catheter removal is often indicated; antibiotics should be continued intravenously.

S. Fungal peritonitis is rare (≤ 3% of all episodes), but serious, and is associated with catheter removal, transfer to hemodialysis (HD) and significant mortality (~ 25% of episodes).
   1. Yeasts are the most common organisms.
   2. Risk factors.
      a. Prior antibiotic therapy.
      b. Bowel perforation.
      c. Immunosuppression.
   3. Yeast may be seen on Gram stain.
   4. Fungi can colonize silicone catheters.
   5. Catheter removal is recommended immediately upon diagnosis. Improved survival has been associated with early catheter removal.

6. Systemic chemotherapy is recommended, and two antifungal agents are commonly used.
   a. Antifungal therapy can be administered orally, intravenously or intraperitoneally. Initial therapy recommended by ISPD is amphotericin B and flucytosine. IP amphotericin B causes chemical peritonitis and abdominal pain.
   b. Based on culture and sensitivities, the amphotericin B can be replaced with other drugs.
   c. Serum concentrations must be monitored if flucytosine is continued in order to avoid bone marrow toxicity.
   d. Therapy should be continued with flucytosine and fluconazole for at least 10 days after catheter removal.

T. *Mycobacterium tuberculosis* peritonitis is uncommon.
   1. The patient typically has a positive history of tuberculosis.
   2. The peritoneum is usually a secondary site, infected by hematogenous contamination.
   3. Most patients present with fever and abdominal pain as well as turbid drainage.
   4. May be difficult to diagnosis; need smear and cultures for acid-fast organisms. The cultures take 6–8 weeks. Chances of identifying the organisms improve with centrifugation of a large volume of dialysate and performing smears and cultures on the pellet, by using liquid as well as solid culture medium, and with repeat cultures.
   5. In most cases the dialysate cell count shows a predominance of polymorphonuclear cells; however, in some cases, there is an increase in lymphocytes.
   6. Biopsy of the peritoneum or omentum may aid in diagnosis.
   7. The experts do not agree about the treatment of mycobacterium peritonitis.
      a. One strategy is to remove the catheter and continue with systemic chemotherapy; reinserting the catheter only after 6 weeks of antitubercular therapy.
      b. The other strategy is to leave the catheter in place and continue PD during therapy. This is more likely to be successful if the infection is diagnosed early and therapy is initiated promptly.
      c. Initial treatment with four drugs is recommended. Rifampin should be given intraperitoneally as long as the catheter is in place, since dialysis fluid levels are quite low

with oral administration.
d. Treatment is prolonged for a total of 12 months.

U. For all infections, repeat culture, Gram stain, and cell count with differential if no improvement.

V. Reasons peritonitis does not resolve or relapses.
1. Inappropriate drug therapy.
2. Inadequate therapy.
  a. Dosage too low.
    (1) Prescription inadequate.
    (2) Error in administering prescribed dose.
  b. Not continued long enough.
    (1) Prescription inadequate.
    (2) Antibiotic discontinued early.
3. Unresolved exit site and/or tunnel infection.
4. Ruptured viscera.
5. Intraperitoneal abscess.
6. Biofilm or colonization of catheter.

W. Catheter removal is required in up to 15% of episodes.
1. Indications.
  a. Unresolved peritonitis 3-5 days after appropriate antibiotic is initiated.
  b. Simultaneous tunnel or cuff infection.
  c. Chronic or relapsing exit site infection with the same organism(s).
  d. A third episode of peritonitis caused by the same organism occurs in a relatively short time period.
  e. Fecal peritonitis or peritonitis with multiple gram-negative organisms.
  f. Fungal peritonitis.
2. Systemic antibiotic therapy should continue after catheter removal.
3. See Chapter 61, *PD Access*, for guidelines for simultaneous catheter removal and replacement.

X. Complications of peritonitis.
1. Temporary decrease in UF capability with subsequent fluid weight gain.
2. Temporary increase in protein losses, which may contribute to compromised nutritional status.
3. Temporary decrease in clearances (due to decreased total dialysate volume due to decreased UF).
4. Catheter removal.
5. Adhesion formation.
6. Abscess formation (1%).
7. Encapsulating peritoneal sclerosis.

8. Transfer to hemodialysis therapy.
9. Death; death within 14 days of onset of peritonitis or during hospitalization for peritonitis is attributed to peritonitis.
  a. Death was the final outcome of peritonitis in 5.9% of episodes in a large single-center study (Fontán et al., 2005). Peritonitis was directly implicated in 15.2% of all mortality in PD patients.
  b. A multivariate analysis from the study above identified risk factors for death related to peritonitis.
    (1) Female gender.
    (2) Older patients.
    (3) Malnourished patients.
    (4) High serum C-reactive protein.
    (5) Low residual kidney function.

Y. Prevention of peritonitis.
1. Catheter implantation.
  a. Prophylactic intravenous antibiotics prior to catheter implantation reduce the risk of peritonitis (evidence-based).
  b. Double-cuff catheters are less likely to be removed for exit site infection.
  c. A downward directed tunnel and exit site may reduce the risk of catheter-related peritonitis.
2. Safe PD procedures.
  a. Flush-before-fill after making PD connections reduces the risk of contamination (evidence-based).
  b. The twin-bag Y-set is associated with the lowest peritonitis rates (evidence-based).
  c. Avoid manual spiking procedures, whenever possible, as these are associated with higher peritonitis rates (evidence-based).
  d. If spiking bags is required, an assist device may be used.
  e. Good hand washing with antibacterial soap and complete drying decreases the skin bacterial count by 95–99%. Skin should be completely dry before performing exchange procedures. Waterless hand sanitizer with ethyl alcohol content ≥ 62% is equally effective in the absence of visible soiling.
  f. Masks reduce the risk of contamination with nasopharyngeal organisms.
  g. Safe environment for PD exchanges or cycler procedures.
    (1) No pets in the PD room.
    (2) Close doors and windows; turn off fans.
    (3) Clean work surface.
  h. Each dialysis unit should have a protocol for

prophylactic treatment of known contamination.
  i. Effective patient training has been shown to reduce the risk of PD infections.
    (1) Based on adult learning theory and established educational principles.
    (2) Match teaching strategies to patient's perceptual style.
    (3) Require each patient to meet specific learning objectives.
    (4) Require demonstration of safe technique for all procedures.
3. Prophylactic antibiotic therapy to reduce PD catheter-related infections.
  a. Treat *Staphylococcus aureus* nasal carriers (evidence-based).
    (1) Topical mupirocin to the catheter exit site reduces the risk of *S. aureus* exit site infection and peritonitis (evidence-based). Although this was initially studied in *S. aureus* carriers, it is now widely practiced, regardless of carrier status.
    (2) Nasal mupirocin regimens and oral rifampin have also been effective in reducing *S. aureus* infections in PD patients.
  b. Applying prophylactic antibiotics at the exit site as part of routine care reduces the incidence of catheter-related infections in the PD population.
    (1) Mupirocin has been most widely studied and is most widely used.
    (2) Mupirocin ointment can degrade polyurethane, so should not be used with polyurethane catheters.
    (3) A single recent multicenter study found that found that gentamicin sulfate cream applied to the exit site during routine care was significantly more effective than mupirocin cream in preventing both exit site infections and peritonitis.
4. Prophylaxis prior to dental procedures, endoscopy, sigmoid or colonoscopy, and gynecologic procedures.
5. If cycler tubing is reused, procedures must prevent contamination ascending from the drain line.
6. Prevention of catheter-related peritonitis (see Chapter 61, *PD Access*).
  a. Prophylactic intravenous antibiotics prior to catheter implantation (evidence-based).
  b. Avoid submersion or swimming until exit site is completely healed.
  c. Prophylactic treatment of exit site trauma.
  d. Diagnose and treat exit site infections promptly.

II. Exit site and tunnel infections (see Chapter 61, *PD Access*).

III. Pancreatitis.

A. PD patients are at increased risk for developing acute pancreatitis.

B. Proposed PD-related factors.
  1. PD solutions or dialysis-related irritants.
  2. Peritonitis.
  3. Hypertriglyceridemia.

C. Elevated serum calcium is also a risk factor.

D. Signs and symptoms are similar to infectious peritonitis; however, dialysate may be clear.

E. Pancreatitis should be suspected with the following:
  1. Culture-negative peritonitis.
  2. Peritonitis fails to resolve or symptoms localize in epigastrium.
  3. Hiccoughs may be present.
  4. Bloody dialysate is seen in acute hemorrhagic pancreatitis.

F. Diagnosis.
  1. Is confirmed by serum amylase values ≥ 3 times normal; however, amylase values may be normal.
  2. Amylase should be measured in dialysate.
  3. CT scan may show an engorged, edematous pancreas or pseudocysts.
  4. The diagnosis is sometimes delayed due to co-existing infectious peritonitis.
  5. Diagnosis in some cases is made postmortem.

G. Complications.
  1. Respiratory compromise may be aggravated by further abdominal distention.
  2. Hyperglycemia.
  3. Intestinal ileus.

H. Prognosis.
  1. Mortality is high; even higher in patients with acute hemorrhagic pancreatitis.
  2. Prognosis is good if dialysate remains clear.

Transfer to HD

I. PD complications may result in transfer to hemodialysis.

A. Table 13.25 summarizes PD complications that require transfer to hemodialysis.

B. Patients who are transferred to HD early after the development of PD-related complications have better survival.

C. Reasons for not reimplanting catheters in one large program were:
1. Peritonitis (52%).
2. Death (23%).
3. Psychosocial reasons (18%).
4. Bowel perforation (5%).
5. Unable to perform PD (2%).

Table 13.25

Transfer to Hemodialysis Due to PD-Related Complications

Temporary HD
- Catheter removal due to a technical complication
  - Dialysate leak
  - Catheter malposition
  - Catheter obstruction
  - Damaged catheter that cannot be repaired
  - Internal catheter kink
- Chronic or recurrent exit or tunnel infection
- Peritonitis requiring catheter removal
  - Episode that does not respond to treatment
  - Peritonitis that relapses (same organisms) more than once
  - Peritonitis with chronic tunnel infection
  - Fungal peritonitis
- Catheter-related sepsis
- Hernias
- Erosion from tip of catheter

Permanent HD
- Adhesions with loculated pockets of fluid that do not resolve with surgical intervention
- Peritoneal membrane changes
  - Ultrafiltration failure
  - Encapsulating peritoneal sclerosis
- Organ perforation with fecal peritonitis
- Persistent back pain

References

Chapter 61

Annigeri, R., Conly, J., Vas, S.I., Dedier, H., Prakashan, K.P., Bargman, J.M., et al. (2001). Emergence of mupirocin-resistant *Staphylococcus aureus* in chronic peritoneal dialysis patients using mupirocin prophylaxis to prevent exit-site infection. *Peritoneal Dialysis International, 21*(6), 554-559.

Ash, S.R. (2002). Chronic peritoneal dialysis catheters: Procedures for placement, maintenance, and removal. *Seminars in Nephrology, 22*(3), 221-236.

Ash, S.R. (2006). Chronic peritoneal dialysis catheters: Challenges and design solutions. *International Journal of Artificial Organs, 29*(1), 85-94.

Ash, S.R., Carr, D.J., Diaz-Buxo, J.A., & Crabtree, J.H. (2005). Peritoneal access devices: Design, function and placement techniques. In A.R. Nissenson & R.N. Fine (Eds.), *Clinical dialysis* (4th ed., pp. 309-356). New York: McGraw-Hill.

Bernardini, J., Bender, F., Florio, T., Sloand, J., Palmmontalbano, L., Fried, L., et al. (2005). Randomized, double-blind trial of antibiotic exit site cream for prevention of exit site infection in peritoneal dialysis patients. *Journal American Society of Nephrology, 16*, 539-545.

Burrows-Hudson, S., & Prowant, B.F. (Eds.). (2005). *Nephrology nursing standards of practice and guidelines for care.* Pitman, NJ: American Nephrology Nurses' Association.

Caring for Australians with Renal Impairment (CARI). (2004a). *Evidence for peritonitis treatment and prophylaxis.* Retrieved June 29, 2006, from http://www.cari.org.au/dialysis_ptp_publ2004.php

Caring for Australians with Renal Impairment (CARI). (2004b). *Technique of insertion of peritoneal dialysis catheter.* Retrieved May 30, 2007, from http://www.cari.org.au/Part_4_7_Technique_of_insertion_of_PD_catheter_140904.pdf

Crabtree, J.H. (2003). Clinical biodurability of aliphatic polyether based polyurethanes as peritoneal dialysis catheters. *ASAIO Journal, 49*(3), 290-294.

Crabtree, J.H. (2006). Rescue and salvage procedures for mechanical and infectious complications of peritoneal dialysis. *International Journal of Artificial Organs, 29*(1), 67-84.

Crabtree, J.H., Burchette, R.J., & Siddiqi, N. (2005). Optimal peritoneal dialysis catheter type and exit site location: An anthropometric analysis. *ASAIO Journal, 51*(6), 743-747.

Diaz-Buxo, J.A. (2005). Access and continuous flow peritoneal dialysis (Review). *Peritoneal Dialysis International, 25*(Suppl. 3), S102-S104.

Diaz-Buxo, J.A. (2006). Complications of peritoneal dialysis catheters: Early and late. *International Journal of Artificial Organs, 29*(1), 50-58.

Dombros, N., Dratwa, M., Feriani, M., Gokal, R., Heimburger, O., Krediet, R., et al. (EBPG Expert Group on Peritoneal Dialysis). (2005). European best practice guidelines for periotoneal dialysis. *Nephrology Dialysis Transplantation, 20*(Suppl. 9), ix1-ix37.

Eklund, B., Honkanen, E., Kyllonen, L., Salmela, K., & Kala, A.R. (1997). Peritoneal dialysis: Prospective randomized comparison of single-cuff and double-cuff straight Tenckhoff catheters. *Nephrology Dialysis Transplantation, 12*(12), 2664-2666.

Flanigan, M., & Gokal, R. (2005). Peritoneal catheters and exit-site practices toward optimum peritoneal access: A review of current developments. *Peritoneal Dialysis International, 25*(2), 132-139.

Gadallah, M.F., Ramdeen, G., Mignone, J., Patel, D., Mitchell, L., & Tatro, S. (2000). Role of preoperative antibiotic prophylaxis in preventing postoperative peritonitis in newly placed peritoneal dialysis catheters. *American Journal of Kidney Diseases, 36*(5), 1014-1019.

Hall, G., Bogan, A., Dreis, S., Duffy, A., Greene, S., Kelley, K., et al. (2004). New directions in peritoneal dialysis patient training. *Nephrology Nursing Journal, 31*(2), 149-154, 159-163.

Keane, W.F., Bailie, G.R., Boeschoten, E., Gokal, R., Golper, T.A., Holmes, C.J., et al. (2000). Adult peritoneal dialysis-related peritonitis treatment recommendations: 2000 update. *Peritoneal Dialysis International, 20*(4), 396-411. Erratum in *Peritoneal Dialysis International, 20*(6), 828-829.

Khandelwal, M., Bailey, S., Izatt, S., Chu, M., Vas, S., Bargman, J., et al. (2003). Structural changes in silicon rubber peritoneal dialysis catheters in patients using mupirocin at the exit site. *International Journal of Artificial Organs, 26*(10), 913-917.

Lui, S.L., Yip, T., Tse, K.C., Lam, M.F., Lai, K.N., & Lo, W.K. (2005). Treatment of refractory *Pseudomonas aeruginosa* exit-site infection by simultaneous removal and reinsertion of peritoneal dialysis catheter. *Peritoneal Dialysis International, 25*(6), 560-563.

Luzar, M.A., Brown, C.B., Balf, D., Hill, L., Issad, B., Monnier, B., et al. (1990). Exit-site care and exit-site infection in continuous ambulatory peritoneal dialysis (CAPD): Results of a randomized multicenter trial. *Peritoneal Dialysis International, 10*(1), 25-29.

Negoi, D., Prowant, B.F., & Twardowski, Z.J. (2006). Current trends in the use of peritoneal dialysis (PD) catheters. *Advances in Peritoneal Dialysis, 22*, 147-152.

Piraino, B., Bailie, G.R., Bernardini, J., Boeschoten, E., Gupta, A.M., Holmes, C., et al. (2005). Peritoneal dialysis-related infections recommendations: 2005 update. *Peritoneal Dialysis International, 25*(2), 107-131.

Prowant, B.F. (2006a). Peritoneal dialysis access. In A.E. Molzahn & E. Butera (Eds.), *Contemporary nephrology nursing: Principles and practice* (2nd ed., pp. 661-685). Pitman, NJ: American Nephrology Nurses' Association.

Prowant, B.F. (2006b). Trends in care of the peritoneal dialysis catheter exit site post implantation in adults (abstract). *Peritoneal Dialysis International, 26*(Suppl. 2), S61.

Prowant, B.F. (2006c). Trends in chronic peritoneal dialysis (PD) catheter exit site (ES) care and antibiotic prophylaxis in adults (abstract). *Peritoneal Dialysis International, 26*(Suppl. 2), S62.

Prowant, B.F., & Twardowski, Z.J. (1996). Recommendations for exit care. *Peritoneal Dialysis International, 16*(Suppl. 3), S94-S99.

Prowant, B.F., & Warady, B.A. (2006). Pediatric peritoneal dialysis (PD) catheter exit-site (ES) care practices (abstract). *Peritoneal Dialysis International, 26*(Suppl. 2), S61.

Ronco, C., & Levin, N.W. (Eds.). (2004). Hemodialysis vascular access and peritoneal dialysis. *Contributions to Nephrology, 142.*

Schmidt, L.M., Craig, P.S., Prowant, B.F., & Twardowski, Z.J. (1990). A simple method of preventing accidental disconnection at the peritoneal catheter adapter junction. *Peritoneal Dialysis International, 10*(4), 309-310.

Strippoli, G.F., Tong, A., Johnson, D., Schena, F.P., & Craig, J.C. (2004a). Antimicrobial agents to prevent peritonitis in peritoneal dialysis: A systematic review of randomized controlled trials. *American Journal of Kidney Diseases, 44*(4), 591-603.

Strippoli, G.F., Tong, A., Johnson, D., Schena, F.P., & Craig, J.C. (2004b). Catheter-related interventions to prevent peritonitis in peritoneal dialysis: A systematic review of randomized, controlled trials. *Journal American Society of Nephrology, 15*(10), 2735-2746.

Ter Wee, P.M. (2005). Simultaneous removal and reinsertion of peritoneal dialysis catheters: Do we know why and when? *Peritoneal Dialysis International, 25,* 545-546.

Twardowski, Z.J. (2006). History of peritoneal access development. *International Journal of Artificial Organs, 29*(1), 2-40.

Twardowski, Z.J., & Nichols, W.K. (2000). Peritoneal dialysis access and exit-site care including surgical aspects. In R. Gokal, R. Khanna, R.T. Krediet, & K.D. Nolph (Eds.), *Textbook of peritoneal dialysis* (2nd ed., pp. 307-361). Boston: Kluwer Academic Publishers.

Twardowski, Z.J., & Prowant, B.F. (1996a). Classification of normal and diseased exit sites. *Peritoneal Dialysis International, 16*(Suppl. 3), S32-S50.

Twardowski, Z.J., & Prowant, B.F. (1996b). Exit-site healing post catheter implantation. *Peritoneal Dialysis International, 16*(Suppl. 3), S51-S70.

Twardowski, Z.J., Prowant, B.F., Pickett, B., Nichols, W.K., Nolph, K.D., & Khanna, R. (1996). Four-year experience with swan neck presternal peritoneal dialysis catheter. *American Journal of Kidney Diseases, 27*(1), 99-105.

Verger, C. (2004). Maintenance of functioning PD access and management of complications (review). *Contributions to Nephrology, 142,* 410-421.

Zorzanello, M.M., Fleming, W.J., & Prowant, B.F. (2004). Use of tissue plasminogen activator in peritoneal dialysis catheters: A literature review and one center's experience. *Nephrology Nursing Journal, 31*(5), 534-537. Comment in *Nephrology Nursing Journal, 31*(6), 695.

Chapter 62

Bernardini, J., Nagy, M., & Piraino, B. (2000). Pattern of noncompliance with dialysis exchanges in peritoneal dialysis patients. *American Journal of Kidney Diseases, 35*(6), 1104-1110.

Blake, P., Burkart, J.M., Churchill, D.N., Daugirdas, J., Depner, T., Hamburger, R.J., et al. (1996). Recommended clinical practices for maximizing peritoneal dialysis clearances. *Peritoneal Dialysis International, 16*(5), 448-456.

Brunkhorst, R.R. (2005). Individualized PD prescription: APD versus CAPD. *Peritoneal Dialysis International, 25*(Suppl. 3), S92-S94.

Burkart, J.M., Schreiber, M., Korbet, S.M., Churchill, D.N., Hamburger, R.J., Moran, J., et al. (1996). Solute clearance approach to adequacy of peritoneal dialysis. *Peritoneal Dialysis International, 16*(5), 457-470.

Burrows-Hudson, S., & Prowant, B.F. (Eds.). (2005). *Nephrology nursing standards of practice and guidelines for care.* Pitman, NJ: American Nephrology Nurses' Association.

CANADA-USA (CANUSA) Peritoneal Dialysis Study Group. (1996). Adequacy of dialysis and nutrition in continuous peritoneal dialysis: Association with clinical outcomes. *Journal of the American Society of Nephrology, 7*(2), 198-207.

Caring for Australians with Renal Impairment (CARI). (2005). *Dialysis adequacy* (PD). Retrieved June 29, 2006, from http://www.cari.org.au/dialysis_adequacy_published.php

Centers for Medicare & Medicaid Services. (2005, December). *2005 annual report, End Stage Renal Disease Clinical Performance Measures Project.* Baltimore: Department of Health and Human Services, Centers for Medicare & Medicaid Services, Office of Clinical Standards and Quality.

Churchill, D.N. (2005). Impact of peritoneal dialysis dose guidelines on clinical outcomes. *Peritoneal Dialysis International, 25*(Suppl. 3), S95-S98.

Daugirdas, J.T., Blake, P.G., & Ing, T.S. (Eds.). (2006). *Handbook of dialysis* (4th ed.). Philadelphia: Lippincott Williams & Wilkins.

Diaz-Buxo, J.A. (2005). Clinical use of peritoneal dialysis. In A.R. Nissenson & R.N. Fine (Eds.), *Clinical dialysis* (4th ed., pp. 421-489). New York: McGraw Hill.

Dombros, N., Dratwa, M., Feriani, M., Gokal, R., Heimburger, O., Krediet, R., et al. (EBPG Expert Group on Peritoneal Dialysis). (2005). European best practice guidelines for peritoneal dialysis. *Nephrology Dialysis Transplantation, 20*(Suppl. 9), ix1-ix37.

Enia, G., Sicuso, C., Alati, G., & Zoccali, C. (1993). Subjective global assessment of nutrition in dialysis patients. *Nephrology Dialysis & Transplant, 8*(10), 1094-1098.

Erixon, M., Wieslander, A., Lindén, T., Carlsson, O., Forsbäck, G., Svensson, E., et al. (2005). Take care in how you store your PD fluids: Actual temperature determines the balance between reactive and non-reactive GDPs. *Peritoneal Dialysis International, 25*(6), 583-590.

Foley, R.N., Parfrey, P.S., Harnett, J.D., Kent, G.M., Murray, D.C., & Barre, P.E. (1996). Impact of hypertension on cardiomyopathy, morbidity and mortality in end-stage renal disease. *Kidney International, 49*(5), 1379-1385.

Gahl, G.M., & Jorres, A. (2000). Nightly intermittent peritoneal dialysis: Targets and prescriptions (review). *Peritoneal Dialysis International, 20*(Suppl. 2), S89-S92.

Gokal, R., & Harty, J. (1996). Are there limits for CAPD? Adequacy and nutritional considerations. *Peritoneal Dialysis International, 16*(5), 437-441.

Gokal, R., Khanna, R., Krediet, R.T., & Nolph, K.D. (Eds.). (2000). *Textbook of peritoneal dialysis* (2nd ed.). Dordrecht: Kluwer Academic Publishers.

Harty, J., & Gokal, R. (1996). The impact of peritoneal permeability and residual renal function on PD prescription (review). *Peritoneal Dialysis International, 16*(Suppl. 1), S47-S52.

Kagan, A., & Rapoport, J. (2005). The role of peritoneal dialysis in the treatment of refractory heart failure. *Nephrology Dialysis Transplantation, 20*(Suppl. 7), vii28-vii31.

Kubey, W., & Straka, P. (2005). Comparison of disinfection efficacy of four PD transfer set change procedures (abstract). *Peritoneal Dialysis International, 25*(Suppl. 1), S9.

Li, F.K., Chan, L.Y., Woo, J.C., Ho, S.K., Lo, W.K., Lai, K.N., et al. (2003). A 3-year, prospective, randomized, controlled study on amino acid dialysate in patients on CAPD. *American Journal of Kidney Diseases, 42*(1), 173-183.

Lo, W.K., Bargman, J.M., Burkart, J., Krediet, R.T., Pollock, C., Kawanishi, H., & et al., for the ISPD Adequacy of Peritoneal Dialysis Working Group. (2006). Guideline on targets for solute and fluid removal in adult patients on chronic peritoneal dialysis. *Peritoneal Dialysis International, 26*(5), 520-522.

Lo, W.K., Ho, Y.W., Li, C.S., Wong, K.S., Chan, T.M., Yu, A.W., et al. (2003). Effect of Kt/V on survival and clinical outcome in CAPD patients in a randomized prospective study. *Kidney International, 64*(2), 649-656.

Lo, W.K., Tong, K.L., Li, C.S., Chang, T.M., Wong, A.K.M., Ho, Y.W., et al. (2001). Relationship between adequacy of dialysis and nutritional status, and their impact on patient survival on CAPD in Hong Kong. *Peritoneal Dialysis International, 21*, 441-447.

McIntyre, C.S. (2007). Update on peritoneal dialysis solutions. *Kidney International, 71*, 486-490.

Muirhead, N. (2005). Erythropoietic agents in peritoneal dialysis. *Peritoneal Dialysis International, 25*(6), 547-550.

National Kidney Foundation (NKF). (2000). Clinical practice guidelines for nutrition in chronic renal failure. *American Journal of Kidney Diseases, 35*(6, Suppl. 2), S1-S140. Erratum in *American Journal of Kidney Diseases, 38*(4), 917.

National Kidney Foundation (NKF). (2006a). KDOQI clinical practice guidelines and clinical practice recommendations for 2006. Update: Peritoneal dialysis adequacy. *American Journal of Kidney Diseases, 48*(Suppl. 1), S91-175.

National Kidney Foundation. (2006b). KDOQI clinical practice guidelines and clinical practice recommendations for 2006 updates: Hemodialysis adequacy, peritoneal dialysis adequacy, and vascular access. *American Journal of Kidney Diseases, 48*(Suppl. 1), S1-322.

Nissenson, A.R., & Fine, R.N. (Eds.). (2005). *Clinical dialysis* (4th ed.). New York: McGraw Hill.

Paniagua, R., Amato, D., Vonesh, E., Correa-Rotter, R., Ramos, A., Moran, J., et al., for the Mexican Nephrology Collaborative Study Group. (2002). Effects of increased peritoneal clearances on mortality rates in peritoneal dialysis: ADEMEX, a prospective, randomized, controlled trial. *Journal American Society of Nephrology, 13*, 1307-1320.

Povlsen, J.V., & Ivarsen P. (2005). Assisted automated peritoneal dialysis (AAPD) for the functionally dependent and elderly patient. *Peritoneal Dialysis International, 25*(Suppl. 3), S60-S63.

Prowant, B., & Ryan, L. (1987). Intra-abdominal pressure in CAPD patients. *ANNA Journal, 14*(4), 253-257.

Rodby, R.A., & Firanek, C.A. (2003). Aliquot versus batch sampling methods for measurements of peritoneal dialysis adequacy in patients receiving CAPD. *Peritoneal Dialysis International, 23*(1), 87-89.

Rusthoven, E., van der Vlugt, M.E., van Lingen-van Bueren, L.J.,

van Schaijk, T.C., Willems, H.L., Monnens, L.A., et al. (2005). Evaluation of intraperitoneal pressure and the effect of different osmotic agents on intraperitoneal pressure in children. *Peritoneal Dialysis International, 25*(4), 352-356.

Sitter, T., & Sauter, M. (2005). Impact of glucose in peritoneal dialysis: Saint or sinner? *Peritoneal Dialysis International, 25*(5), 415-425.

Szeto, C.C., Chow, K.M., Lam, C.W., Cheung, R., Kwan, B.C., Chung, K.Y., et al. (2005). Peritoneal albumin excretion is a strong predictor of cardiovascular events in peritoneal dialysis patients: A prospective cohort study. *Peritoneal Dialysis International, 25*(5), 445-452.

Twardowski, Z.J. (2005). Physiology of peritoneal dialysis. In A.R. Nissenson & R.N. Fine (Eds.), *Clinical dialysis* (4th ed., pp. 357-384). New York: McGraw-Hill.

Twardowski, Z.J., Khanna, R., & Nolph, K.D. (1986). Osmotic agents and ultrafiltration in peritoneal dialysis. *Nephron, 42*(2), 93-101.

Twardowski, Z.J., Nolph, K.D., Khanna, R., Prowant, B.F., Ryan, L.P., Moore, H.L., et al. (1987). Peritoneal equilibration test. *Peritoneal Dialysis Bulletin, 7*(3), 138-147.

U.S. Renal Data System (USRDS). (2007). *USRDS 2007 annual data report: Atlas of end-stage renal disease in the United States.* Bethesda, MD: National Institutes of Health, National Institute of Diabetes and Digestive and Kidney Disease.

Witowski, J., & Jorres, A. (2005). Effects of peritoneal dialysis solutions on the peritoneal membrane: Clinical consequences. *Peritoneal Dialysis International, 25*(Suppl. 3), S31-S34.

Chapter 63

Bargman, J.M. (2000). Non-infectious complications of peritoneal dialysis. In R. Gokal, R. Khanna, R.T. Krediet, & K.D. Nolph (Eds.), *Textbook of peritoneal dialysis* (2nd ed., pp. 609-646). Boston: Kluwer Academic Publishers.

Bonifati, C., Pansini, F., Torres, D.D., Navaneethan, S.D., Craig, J.C., & Strippoli, G.F.M. (2006). Antimicrobial agents and catheter-related interventions to prevent peritonitis in peritoneal dialysis: Using evidence in the context of clinical practice. *International Journal of Artificial Organs, 29*(1), 41-49.

Caring for Australians with Renal Impairment (CARI). (2004a). *Evidence for peritonitis treatment and prophylaxis.* Retrieved June 29, 2006, from http://www.cari.org.au/dialysis_ptp_publ2004.php

Caring for Australians with Renal Impairment (CARI). (2004b). *Treatment of peritoneal dialysis-associated peritonitis in adults.* Retrieved June 29, 2006, from http://www.cari.org.au/Part_4_13_Treatment_of_PD_associated_peritonitis_in_adults.pdf

Chin, A.I., & Yeun, J.Y. (2006). Encapsulating peritoneal sclerosis: An unpredictable and devastating complication of peritoneal dialysis. *American Journal of Kidney Diseases, 47*(4), 697-712.

Chow, K.M., Szeto, C.C., Leung, C.B., Kwan, B.C.H., Law, M.C., & Li, P.K.T. (2005). A risk analysis of continuous ambulatory peritoneal dialysis-related peritonitis. *Peritoneal Dialysis International, 25*, 374-379.

Crabtree, J.H. (2006a). Hernia repair without delay in initiating or continuing peritoneal dialysis. *Peritoneal Dialysis International, 26*, 178-182.

Crabtree, J.H. (2006b). Rescue and salvage procedures for mechanical and infectious complications of peritoneal dialysis. *International Journal of Artificial Organs, 29*(1), 67-84.

Dell'Aquila, R., Rodighiero, M.P., Bonello, M., & Ronco, C. (2004). Conditions leading to catheter removal or substitution. *Contributions to Nephrology, 142*, 435-446.

Diaz-Buxo, J.A. (2005). Clinical use of peritoneal dialysis. In A.R. Nissenson & R.N. Fine (Eds.), *Clinical dialysis* (4th ed., pp. 421-489). New York: McGraw Hill.

Diaz-Buxo, J.A. (2006). Complications of peritoneal dialysis catheters: Early and late. *International Journal of Artificial Organs, 29*(1), 50-58.

Dombros, N., Dratwa, M., Feriani, M., Gokal, R., Heimburger, O., Krediet, R., et al. (EBPG Expert Group on Peritoneal Dialysis). (2005). European best practice guidelines for periotoneal dialysis. *Nephrology Dialysis Transplantation, 20*(Suppl. 9), ix1-ix37.

Fontán, M.P., Rodríquez-Carmona, A., García-Naveiro, R., Rosales, M., Villaverde, P., & Valdés, F. (2005). Peritonitis-related mortality in patients undergoing chronic peritoneal dialysis. *Peritoneal Dialysis International, 25*, 274-284.

Fried, L.F., & Piraino, B.M. (2005). Infections in peritoneal dialysis. In A.R. Nissenson & R.N. Fine (Eds.), *Clinical dialysis* (4th ed., pp. 491-513). New York: McGraw Hill.

García-Ureña, M.Á., Rodríguez, C.R., Ruiz, V.V., Hernández, F.J.C., Fernández-Ruiz, E., Gallego, J.M.V., et al. (2006). Prevalence and management of hernias in peritoneal dialysis patients. *Peritoneal Dialysis International, 26*, 198-202.

Goffin, E. (2006). Aseptic peritonitis and icodextrin. *Peritoneal Dialysis International, 26*, 314-316.

Hall, G., Bogan, A., Dreis, S., Duffy, A., Greene, S., Kelley, K., et al. (2004). New directions in peritoneal dialysis patient training. *Nephrology Nursing Journal, 31*(2), 149-154, 159-163.

Kaplan, G.G., Manns, B., & McLaughlin, K. (2005). Heparin induced thrombocytopaenia secondary to intraperitoneal heparin exposure. *Nephrology Dialysis Transplantation, 20*, 2561-2562.

Kawaguchi, Y., Saito, A., Kawanishi, H., Nakayama, M., Miyazaki, M., Nakamoto, H., et al. (2005). Recommendations on the management of encapsulating peritoneal sclerosis in Japan, 2005: Diagnosis, predictive markers, treatment and preventive measures. *Peritoneal Dialysis International, 25*(Suppl. 4), S83-S95.

Kawanishi, H., & Moriishi, M. (2005). Epidemiology of encapsulating peritoneal sclerosis in Japan. *Peritoneal Dialysis International, 25*(Suppl. 4), S14-S18.

Kawanishi, H., Watanabe, H., Moriishi, M., & Tsuchiya, S. (2005). Successful surgical management of encapsulating peritoneal sclerosis. *Peritoneal Dialysis International, 25*(Suppl. 4), S39-S47.

Keane, W.F., Bailie, G.R., Boeschoten, E., Gokal, R., Golper, T.A., Holmes, C.J., et al. (2000). Adult peritoneal dialysis-related peritonitis treatment recommendations: 2000 update. *Peritoneal Dialysis International, 20*(4), 396-411. Erratum in *Peritoneal Dialysis International, 20*(6), 828-829.

Piraino, B. (2006). Peritoneal dialysis infections recommendations (review). *Contributions to Nephrology, 150*, 181-186.

Piraino, B., Bailie, G.R., Bernardini, J., Boeschoten, E., Gupta, A., Holmes, C., et al. (2005). Peritoneal dialysis-related infections recommendations: 2005 update. *Peritoneal Dialysis International, 25*(2), 107-131.

Prowant B., & Schmidt, L. (1987). A decision making model and standard nursing care plan for cloudy peritoneal dialysate effluent (abstract). *ANNA Journal, 14*, 149.

Salzer, W. (2005). Antimicrobial-resistant gram-positive bacteria in PD peritonitis and the newer antibiotics used to treat them. *Peritoneal Dialysis International, 25*, 313-319.

Scanziani, R., Pozzi, M., Pisano, L., Barbone, G.S., Dozio, B., Rovere, G., et al. (2006). Imaging work-up for peritoneal access care and peritoneal dialysis complications. *International Journal of Artificial Organs, 29*(1), 142-152.

Strippoli, G.F.M., Tong, A., Johnson, D., Schena, F.P., & Craig, J.C. (2004a). Antimicrobial agents to prevent peritonitis in peritoneal dialysis: A systematic review of randomized controlled trials. *American Journal of Kidney Diseases, 44*(4), 591-603.

Strippoli, G.F.M., Tong, A., Johnson, D., Schena, F.P., & Craig, J.C. (2004b). Catheter-related interventions to prevent peritonitis in peritoneal dialysis: A systematic review of randomized, controlled trials. *Journal American Society of Nephrology, 15*, 2735-2746.

Troidle, L., & Finkelstein, F. (2006). Treatment and outcome of CPD-associated peritonitis (review). *Annals of Clinical Microbiology and Antimicrobials, 5*(6).

Troidle, L., Gorban-Brennan, N., & Finkelstein, F.O. (2005). Outcome of patients on chronic peritoneal dialysis undergoing peritoneal catheter removal because of peritonitis. *Advances in Peritoneal Dialysis, 21*, 98-101.

Yasuda, G., Shibata, K., Takizawa, T., Ikeda, Y., Tokita, Y., Umemura, S., et al. (2002). Prevalence of constipation in continuous ambulatory peritoneal dialysis patients and comparison with hemodialysis patients. *American Journal of Kidney Diseases, 39*(6), 1292-1299.

Zorzanello, M.M., Fleming, W.J., & Prowant, B.F. (2004). Use of tissue plasminogen activator in peritoneal dialysis catheters: A literature review and one center's experience. *Nephrology Nursing Journal, 31*(5), 534-537. Comment in *Nephrology Nursing Journal, 31*(6), 695.

Suggested Readings

Burrows-Hudson, S., & Prowant, B.F. (Eds.). (2005). *Nephrology Nursing standards of practice and guidelines for care*. Pitman, NJ: American Nephrology Nurses' Association.

Davies, S.J., Phillips, L., Griffiths, A.M., Russell, L.H., Naish, P.F., & Russell, G.I. (1998). What really happens to people on long-term peritoneal dialysis? (Review). *Kidney International, 54*(6), 2207-2217.

Hall, G., Bogan, A., Dreis, S., Duffy, A., Greene, S., Kelley, K., et al. (2004). New directions in peritoneal dialysis patient training. *Nephrology Nursing Journal, 31*(2), 149-154, 159-163.

Kelman, E., & Watson, D. (2006). Preventing and managing complications of peritoneal dialysis. In A.E. Molzahn & E. Butera (Eds.), *Contemporary nephrology nursing: Principles and practice* (2nd ed., pp. 687-709). Pitman, NJ: American Nephrology Nurses' Association.

Kelman, E., & Watson, D. (2006). Technical aspects of peritoneal dialysis. *Contributions to Nephrology, 150*.

Molzahn, A., & Butera, E. (Eds.). (2006). *Contemporary nephrology nursing: Principles and practice* (2nd ed.). Pitman, NJ: American Nephrology Nurses' Association.

Section 14

Choosing Home Therapies

Section Editor
Karen E. Schardin, BSN, RN, CNN

Authors
Connie Anderson, MBA, BSN

M. Kay Deck, BS, RN

Maria Luongo, MSN, BA, RN

Karen E. Schardin, BSN, RN, CNN

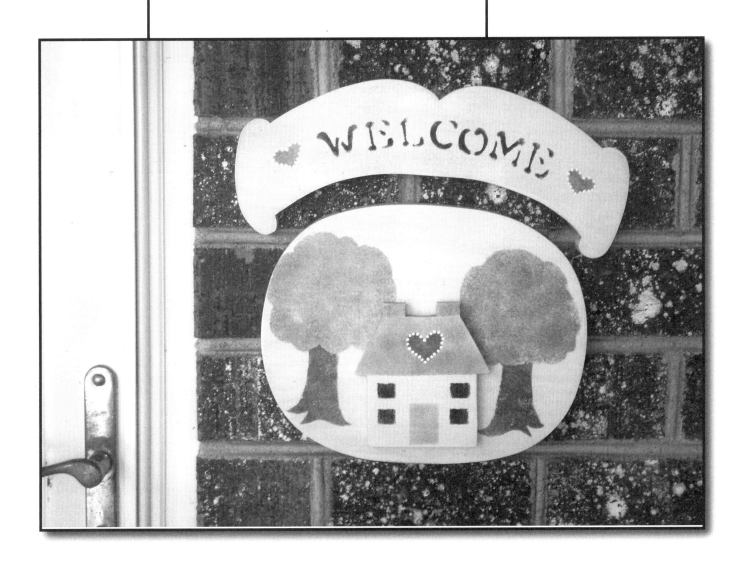

About the Authors

Karen E. Schardin, BSN, RN, CNN, Section Editor and Author, is Director of Clinical Field Services at NxStage Medical, Inc., in Carson City, Nevada.

Connie Anderson, MBA, BSN, is Vice President of Clinical Services at Northwest Kidney Centers in Seattle, Washington.

M. Kay Deck, BS, RN, is Director of Nursing and Education at NxStage Medical, Inc., in Lawrence, Massachusetts.

Maria Luongo, MSN, BA, RN, is CAPD Nurse Manager at Massachusetts General Hospital in Boston, Massachusetts.

Choosing Home Therapies

Section 14

Choosing Home Therapies

Introduction

The patient with later stages of chronic kidney disease has the option to select home dialysis as his or her modality of kidney replacement therapy. The process of educating the patient and family about dialysis options should ideally occur as part of chronic kidney disease management but may occur later in the patient's health care experience. Key to the successful implementation of home dialysis is the patient's motivation to assume self-care responsibility and the support, facilitation and management of this process by the home training nurse.

Chapter 64

Overview of Home Dialysis

Purpose

The purpose of this chapter is to provide an overview of home dialysis to assure the following patient outcomes: (1) The patient and/or family will receive information regarding all available modalities that are appropriate enabling an informed decision regarding treatment and setting; (2) The patient and/or family will be able to perform dialysis safely and effectively while achieving and maintaining a reasonable fluid balance; (3) The patient and/or family will identify, report, and participate in the management of dialysis-related problems (Burrows-Hudson & Prowant, 2005).

Objectives

Upon completion of this chapter, the learner will be able to:
1. Identify the clinical advantages to patients on home dialysis therapies.
2. Identify the necessary components that are required for a successful home dialysis program.
3. Identify the training requirements necessary to assure patients are safe and competent to perform home dialysis.
4. Explain the role of the nursing staff in managing and monitoring patients at home.

I. **Home dialysis – A treatment option.**

A. Hemodialysis was the first treatment option available for home dialysis therapy. It took almost 10 more years before peritoneal dialysis caught on as a mainstream home therapy.

B. In 1973 when the Medicare End Stage Renal Disease (ESRD) Program became available to ESRD patients, 40% of the 11,000 dialysis patients were on home hemodialysis. Following Medicare's payments for treatment, the number of home patients has decreased dramatically with only 0.4% on home hemodialysis and 11% on some form of peritoneal therapy, continuous ambulatory peritoneal dialysis (CAPD) or continuous cycling peritoneal dialysis (CCPD). Virtually no patients are at home on intermittent peritoneal dialysis (IPD).

II. **Home dialysis – Its beginning and its history.**

During the period of 1960–1970, home hemodialysis accounted for a large proportion of patients treated with dialysis. Who was the first to do home hemodialysis remains controversial as many programs were being initiated simultaneously.

Hemodialysis was not the only form of home therapy. Peritoneal dialysis as a home treatment option emerged in the 1970s and for many patients became the treatment of choice. This was due to the simplicity of performing the treatment and the ability to dialyze at home without an assistant.

A. In 1960, Belding Scribner and colleagues from the University of Washington developed the Teflon arteriovenous shunt, an access that made long-term intermittent hemodialysis dialysis possible for the treatment of ESRD. In 1961 equipment such as the Kiil dialyzer was developed and used for ongoing dialysis treatments.

B. As developments with hemodialysis continued during the 1960s, Drs. Fred Boen and Henry Tenckhoff of Seattle were working on methods of providing peritoneal dialysis as a therapy for ESRD patients.
   1. A closed peritoneal dialysis fluid supply system was initiated to reduce the risk of peritonitis.
   2. Tenckhoff developed the first indwelling peritoneal catheter which became the industry standard for long term peritoneal dialysis.

C. The 1960s were the time during which the medical, social, financial, and ethical problems were discussed associated with the treatment of patients with ESRD.
   1. In 1962 there were no funding sources to cover the cost of dialysis treatments, and the demand for treatment far exceeded the available financial resources.
   2. The financial burden of ESRD treatment led directly to the development of home hemodialysis in the United States.

D. During the 1960s, the University of Washington trained and supported 52 patients, their families and physicians on home hemodialysis. These persons came from all over the United States, Chile, Malaysia, Philippines, and the Sudan.

E. The early beginning of home dialysis.
   1. In 1961, the first patient treated on home hemodialysis was in Japan dialyzing on a coil dialyzer that was immersed in an electric washing machine.
   2. A committee in Seattle was mandated to ration the resources of hemodialysis based on selected criteria and was forced to deny a 15-year-old girl access to treatment. That denial began home hemodialysis in the United States.
   3. In 1963, home hemodialysis was being performed in India on a wealthy Madras businessman.
   4. Between 1963 and 1964, John Merrill in Boston began a home dialysis program with a nurse performing the treatments in the patient's home using twin-coil dialyzers.
   5. In 1964, Dr. Scribner, in conjunction with Les Babb, built an automated hemodialysis proportioning machine. It was used by the first home hemodialysis patient in Seattle.
   6. Also in 1964 in London, Stanley Sheldon and colleagues initiated the first overnight home hemodialysis (10–12 hours) using a setup similar to that used in Seattle.
   7. In 1966, Kolff began a home hemodialysis program at the Cleveland Clinic.
   8. It took until 1970 before home IPD became possible for selected patients; it was not widely used as a therapy.
   9. In 1972, Tenckhoff developed a system for in-line peritoneal dialysate using reverse osmosis and an ultraviolet light to sterilize the fluid.
   10. In Bologna, Italy, in 1972, the concept of short daily hemodialysis treatments was introduced as a potential home therapy by Dr. Bonomini.

11. In 1976, Drs. Popovich and Moncrief in Austin, Texas, developed the technique known as CAPD. CAPD is a home peritoneal dialysis method of self-treatment that requires no automated equipment.
12. In 1981, Diaz-Buxo initiated CCPD as another form of self-therapy done at home during the night.
13. In 1994, nocturnal home hemodialysis began in Toronto, Canada.
14. In 1997, Lynchberg Nephrology Dialysis in Virginia began a nightly home hemodialysis program patterned after the Toronto program.
15. Beginning in 2000, innovative changes to home hemodialysis equipment have allowed patients in the United States opportunities to select a variety of therapies for home treatment (i.e., standard 3 three treatments per week, short daily, or long nocturnal dialysis).

III. Home dialysis – Its decline and resurgence.

A. Since 1980, the number of patients in the United States selecting home dialysis as a treatment option declined. This decline was related to numerous causes.
    1. Increase in the number of dialysis facilities providing in-center treatment; care is readily available in local communities.
    2. Increase in patients' age and number of co-morbidities.
    3. Financial reimbursement to units and physicians is better for in-center therapy as compared to home dialysis.
    4. Some patients are less independent and have less desire to take responsibility for their own treatments.
    5. In-center treatments allow patients to socialize with other patients and lessen their feelings of isolation.
    6. Home dialysis assistants, either family members or others, are not as readily available due to changes in the work force.
    7. Nephrologists have less experience with home dialysis because so few programs in the United States are available. Therefore, they may not promote home dialysis as a viable option to their patients.
    8. Some of the important dialysis related medications are not available to home patients.
    9. The infrastructure necessary for a successful home program is costly and many dialysis facilities do not want to incur the additional costs.

B. Since the year 2000, the focus in the nephrology community has been on the revival of home dialysis.
    1. New, innovative, and easy-to-operate equipment can offer patients a variety of home dialysis therapies will help revive home hemodialysis.
        a. Short daily treatment (SDHD).
        b. Slow nocturnal dialysis (SNHD).
        c. Daily nocturnal dialysis (DNHD).
    2. Since 2005, increased payments have given physicians incentives to have patients on home dialysis.

IV. Benefits of home dialysis.

The benefits of home dialysis are many and varied. Benefits include clinical advantages, better patient outcomes, and personal benefits for the home dialysis patients. Most advantages are experienced with SDHD, SNHD, DHND, CAPD, or CCPD home treatments.

A. Clinical advantages and better patient outcomes include:
    1. More frequent dialysis is an efficient means for removing waste products. Predialytic serum urea and creatinine levels are near normal and remain steady during the week.
    2. The relative risk of death is less for home patients.
    3. Blood pressure and fluid control are improved.
    4. Acid-base balance is improved.
    5. Increased appetite improves the patient's nutritional state.
    6. The intradialytic complications of hypotension, cramps, nausea, or vomiting are lessened.
    7. Achieving the dry weight becomes a reality.
    8. The dose and/or number of medications can be reduced.
    9. The number of hospitalizations is decreased.

B. Personal benefits.
    1. Increased rehabilitation and ability to work.
    2. Flexible dialysis schedules.
    3. Improved sexual functioning.
    4. Increased energy, endurance, strength, and feeling of well-being.
    5. Improved family and social relationships.
    6. Increased independence.
    7. Better knowledge about illness and its treatment.

V. Requirements of a home program.

The Medicare Conditions of Coverage provide guidance through regulations on the necessary requirements for an organization to establish and maintain a home dialysis program for either peritoneal or hemodialysis. A successful home program has many integrated segments that are centered around patient education, support, and follow-up.

A. Conditions of coverage requirements for a home program.
1. Multidisciplinary team for care planning processes.
2. Qualified personnel to provide the self-dialysis training.
3. Competency with medication management and administration.
4. Social service and nutritional support.
5. Surveillance of the patient's home adaptation.
6. Installation and maintenance of equipment.
7. Monitoring of laboratory and treatment results.
8. Monitoring water quality when used with hemodialysis.
9. Oversight of supplies.

B. Additional requirements.
1. Policies and procedures specific to each type of home dialysis therapy that clearly define program expectations and patient's responsibilities.
2. On-call nursing, technical, and medical support.
3. Follow-up clinics.
4. Environment conducive to learning.
5. Variety of teaching methods and materials geared to patient learning.
6. Appropriate and usable dialysis access.
7. Home surveys to assure that storage space and plumbing and electrical supplies are adequate.
8. Home hemodialysis assistants identified.
9. Ability to provide "back-up" dialysis in a facility.
10. Early identification of suitable candidates for home dialysis.
11. Trainers skilled in adult education teaching methods.
12. Tools to objectively measure patient's/helper's skills and competency to perform dialysis treatments.
13. Communication methods to reach patients at home for changes to procedures.
14. Local water and power companies should be informed when there are persons on home therapies so they can be placed on a priority for reinstatement of services during water and power failures.

VI. Patient selection.

The main objective in patient selection is to accurately assess a patient's motivation to learn and ability to provide safe and effective dialysis treatments in the home.

A. Factors involved in patient selection.
1. The patient's living circumstances and accommodations.
2. The ability of the patient and/or family to learn.
3. The level of patient and/or family anxiety regarding home dialysis.
4. The type and severity of the patient's medical condition.
5. The patient's and/or family member's motivation to learn and the patient's adherence to the treatment regimen.
6. The physician identifying and referring a patient to home therapy. The physician is a key component in a patient selecting home dialysis.
7. Availability of an assistant for hemodialysis, i.e., family member, friend, paid assistant, etc.
8. The availability of the patient and/or family to accommodate the training schedule.
9. Ability of patient and/or family member to communicate.

VII. Patient training.

The main objective of any training program for home dialysis is to assure that the patient and/or the partner are educated and understand how to perform safe, effective dialysis in the home setting without undue anxiety while achieving maximum independence.

A. Training objectives must be clearly stated and agreed to by the patient/partner.

B. One-on-one training that is tailored to the patient's learning needs seems to be the most effective method of teaching patients and partners.

C. The amount of time required to train a patient varies by modality. Both day and evening training sessions should be provided to meet patients' needs.
1. Peritoneal training may be up to 5 days.
2. Hemodialysis training may take 3–5 weeks or longer.

D. Programs must provide the necessary clinical experiences for the patient/partner to become proficient with the procedures.

E. Training manuals should contain information and procedures that are written at no higher than an eighth grade reading level.

F. Training should occur on dialysis and nondialysis days. Ancillary training for hemodialysis procedures can be done on nondialysis days, e.g., water treatment, setups, laboratory work, vital signs, aseptic technique, machine maintenance, supply ordering, record keeping, etc.

G. Multiple types of teaching methods should be employed to meet individual learning styles.

H. Repetition is the key to successful patient learning.

I. Having objective ways to assess the patient's knowledge is critical whether through tests or observational scoring data.

J. If possible, training for self-cannulation should occur while the patient is in-center, before starting formal home training.

K. Training for home hemodialysis is far more complex than for peritoneal dialysis, including the setup procedure, the procedures for initiation and termination of dialysis, and procedures for handling alarms and emergencies.

L. Training must include several dialysis sessions in the training unit that simulate the patient dialyzing at home.

VIII. Nursing roles and responsibilities.

Nurses have several roles and responsibilities in home dialysis programs. The nurse's prime responsibility is to provide the patient with complete, accurate, and understandable information to allow patient's independence in the home setting.

A. Four major nursing roles and responsibilities.
   1. Assessments: readiness for training, adherence to treatment, learning style, appropriateness of the home environment, family dynamics.
   2. Education: tailored to individual learning style, objective assessments of competency, dialysis procedures, record keeping, emergency procedures, and supply ordering.
   3. Monitoring and oversight: lab value reviews, therapy outcomes, adherence to treatment prescription, home follow-up visits, adaptation to home therapy, review of monthly logs, communication to physicians, problem lists, and care plans.
   4. Resource and support.
      a. Assistance 24 hours a day, 7 days a week.
      b. Coordination of services (technical, supplies, procedural).
      c. Communication.
      d. Ongoing patient education.

Chapter 65

Home Hemodialysis

Purpose

The purpose of this chapter is to review the use of home hemodialysis, provide a cognitive understanding of the concepts and principles related to home hemodialysis, and review principles of nursing care for patients receiving home hemodialysis.

Objectives

Upon completion of this chapter, the learner will be able to:
1. Discuss three types of home hemodialysis therapy.
2. List three benefits of daily home hemodialysis.
3. List three considerations for patient selection related to home hemodialysis.
4. Explain two reasons for partner training.
5. List four elements of a clinic visit.
6. Discuss two different systems for home hemodialysis.
7. Cite the National Kidney Foundation (NKF) Dialysis Outcomes Quality Initiative (KDOQI) Clinical Practice Guidelines for daily hemodialysis adequacy.
8. Describe two methods for obtaining post-BUN (blood urea nitrogen) samples for KT/V testing for home hemodialysis.
9. Discuss a key factor in maintaining water systems for hemodialysis in the home.
10. List three types of access used for home hemodialysis and the most frequently recommended access for use.

I. **Background information.** The resurgence of home hemodialysis brings hemodialysis procedures full circle. In the initial days of the ESRD program it was felt that patients would be able to provide their own treatments in their own home to obtain better control over their disease and personal lifestyle. The industrialization of the in-center hemodialysis shifted the focus from home hemodialysis to in-center. Now, with improvements in the knowledge of dialysis, coupled with the advances in technology, the renal industry is again interested in home hemodialysis.

II. **Basic concepts of home hemodialysis.** The purpose of this section is to define and describe concepts and principles related to home hemodialysis.

A. Concepts related to solute removal (see Section 11).

B. Concepts related to fluid removal (see Section 11).

C. Types of home hemodialysis.
   1. Intermittent hemodialysis (IHD) – conventional three-times-a-week therapy.
   2. Hemodialfiltration – currently there is no FDA approved online hemofiltration fluid equipment available in the U.S.

Significant Dates in the History of Home Hemodialysis

1961   First documented case of home hemodialysis by Nose in Japan.

1962   First free-standing outpatient dialysis facility at Seattle Artificial Kidney Center (SAKC).

1963   Sheldon performs first nocturnal treatment.

1964   First documented person to receive home hemodialysis in the United States reported by Curtis and Associates.

1966   Home hemodialysis training program developed at Seattle Artificial Kidney Center.

1969   First study of daily dialysis by DePalma and Associates in Los Angeles.

1972   Bonomini and Associates in Bologna, Italy, first used short daily hemodialysis in the home.

1973   Medicare End Stage Renal Disease Program in effect; 40% of patients on home hemodialysis.

1980   Health Care Financing Administration (HCFA) funded three multi-center studies of home hemodialysis using "paid aides."

1983   Congress introduces "composite rate" reimbursement, excluding payment for home dialysis aides.

1994   Report by Uldall and Associates of slow, overnight (nocturnal) hemodialysis.

1997   Lynchburg Nephrology Dialysis starts a nightly home hemodialysis program in the United States.

2002   Aksys – FDA approved device to be marketed for home hemodialysis.

2005   NxStage – FDA approved device to be marketed for home hemodialysis.

a. This treatment uses convection as the mechanism for uremic toxin removal.
   (1) Removes the middle molecules more efficiently.
   (2) Generally uses a high flux membrane.
b. Uses ultrapure fluid to prevent contamination of fluid delivered to the patient. Ultrapure fluids reduce the risks associated with contaminated dialysate.
   (1) Specifically designed equipment with online generation of ultrapure fluid.
   (2) May also be partially achieved through maximizing internal filtration and back filtration in the dialyzer.
c. Treatment may be done three times per week or daily.
d. Offers benefits such as correction of anemia, inflammation, oxidative stress, lipid profiles, and calcium-phosphate product.
e. May be associated with increased leakage of albumin and proteins and may compromise nutritional status. New membranes with nanocontrolled characteristics may minimize the loss of important nutrients while maximizing the benefits of middle molecule removal.
3. Daily (quotidian) hemodialysis.
   a. Generally a shortened treatment (1.5–3 hours) five to seven times per week.

b. Dialysate flow and blood flow rates may be the same as in-center (depending on equipment used).
c. Uses a high efficiency dialyzer which shows beneficial effects in controlling renal anemia and controlling cost.
d. Patients undergoing daily dialysis experience a significant increase in removal of urea, calculated at 20–40% when hemodialysis is performed six to seven times per week.
4. Nocturnal (overnight) hemodialysis.
   a. Long nightly treatments (6–8 hours); may be three to seven nights per week.
   b. Dialysate flow rate (100 mL/min) and blood flow rate (200–300 mL/min) run slower than in center rates.
   c. Home patients may have remote monitoring during therapy.
   d. Slow dialysis (6–10 hours) may allow for the equilibration of tissue and vascular compartments, which results in better clearance and decreased postdialysis rebound in solutes.
   e. Offers best control of hyperphosphatemia without phosphate binders, may require phosphate replacement in dialysate.
   f. Significant reduction in beta-2 microglobulin levels.

III. Benefits of home hemodialysis.

A. Flexibility of scheduling treatment time.
B. No transportation issues going to center for treatments.
C. Independence and convenience along with a greater sense of control over one's own health and life.
D. Improved survival rates.
E. Decreased hospitalization rates.
F. Improved opportunity for rehabilitation.
G. Improved quality of life.

IV. Benefits of daily hemodialysis.

A. Improvement in left ventricular hypertrophy.

B. Improvement in inflammatory and related biomarkers; the release of inflammatory cytokines is attenuated with the use of more biocompatible membranes.

C. Improvement in hypertension and decreased need for antihypertensive medications.
   1. This is due to improved fluid control and normalization of extracellular volume.
   2. Blood pressure medications may be decreased by half or less of previous doses.

D. Decreased fluid overload; the effects of intradialytic hypotension may be minimized.

E. Improved anemia control that may decrease medications required.

F. Improved removal of beta-2 microglobulin which may delay or prevent the progression of amyloidosis.

G. Improved hyperphosphatemia, particularly in nocturnal dialysis.
   1. May contribute to the reduction of morbidities and risk of cardiovascular incidents that are associated with elevated phosphorus and Ca X PO_4 products.
   2. There is a potential decrease in phosphate binders (particularly with nocturnal therapy).

H. Improved patient appetite and measures of nutrition.
   1. Improved albumin/prealbumin, protein intake.
   2. Increase in dry weight and lean body mass.
   3. Disappearance of anorexia and improved nutritional status is explained by:
      a. Decreased dietary restrictions.
      b. Improvement in adequacy of dialysis, cardiovascular stability, and interdialytic hydration.

I. Improved quality of life.
   1. Improved energy levels.
   2. Better rehabilitation.
   3. Decreased hospitalizations.
   4. Flexibility of treatment schedule may also improve quality of life.

J. Improved sleep patterns with a decreased prevalence or improvement in sleep apnea.

K. Decreased intradialytic symptoms resulting from improved homeostasis.
   1. Muscle cramping.
   2. Nausea and/or vomiting.
   3. Headaches.

L. Fewer postdialysis symptoms such as fatigue, cramps, "washed out" feeling, and lightheadedness.

M. Reduction in global cost of care due to reductions in costs related to hospitalizations, access complications, medications, and transportation.

V. Contraindications to home hemodialysis.

A. There are no known contraindications to daily therapy.

B. Concerns.
   1. Poorly functioning access.
   2. Marked arteriosclerosis leading to the possibility of more complications.
   3. Folic acid and vitamin B deficiencies are associated with increased homocysteine levels which may be worsened if not corrected.
   4. Blood loss associated with ineffective rinseback volume.
   5. Infection associated with increased opportunity for contamination.
   6. Need for respite care for patient and/or partner.

VI. Patient selection for home hemodialysis.

A. General considerations.
   1. Home dialysis should be discussed as an option for all patients.
   2. Early referral to nephrologists for patients with chronic kidney disease may allow for early education about modality choices.

3. Barriers to home hemodialysis.
   a. Lack of knowledge about the option.
   b. Attitude barriers, e.g., "patients should not dialyze without supervision."
   c. Fear of cannulation.
   d. Fear of failure to perform procedures appropriately.
   e. Fear of social isolation.
4. Choosing home hemodialysis requires changing knowledge, attitudes, and skills of physicians and nurses as well as patients.
5. Assessment of the patient's and partner's ability to cope with responsibilities of primary care are important to preventing therapy dropout.

B. Patient assessment.
   1. Interdisciplinary team interview is required to assess the patient's ability to perform or receive home therapy.
   2. Vascular access.
      a. The access's capability to achieve required blood flow rate for therapy.
      b. The patient's/partner's capability to perform cannulation or access catheter.
   3. Literacy.
      a. Assess patient's/partner's ability to read or memorize skills and ability to speak or read English.
      b. Assess staff's ability to teach patient/partner and provide follow-up care in native language.
   4. Vision.
      a. Assess for ability to see various size font.
      b. Assess for color blindness.
   5. Hearing.
      a. Assess for ability to hear instructions in normal conversation.
      b. Assess for ability to hear alarm sounds.
   6. Strength and energy level. Assess motor skills and ability to perform tasks required for therapy (e.g., opening and closing clamps, making connections, hanging solutions, etc.).
   7. Comorbid factors. Is the patient medically stable to dialyze at home?
   8. Adherence with current treatment plan.
      a. Ability to accommodate therapy into personal schedule.
      b. Recognize and address conflicts that may interfere with therapy.
      c. Identify reasons for nonadherence that may be either intensified by home therapy, or may be improved with patient control over schedule and therapy.
   9. Motivation for home therapy.
   10. Home visit to assess the suitability of the environment for home hemodialysis.

   a. Ability to make electrical connections.
   b. Home ownership/rental. If renting, it must be determined whether renovation required is permissible.
   c. Ability to make arrangements required for water testing and connections.

C. Partner assessment. *Note*: Some facilities do not require a partner for home hemodialysis.
   1. A partner for home hemodialysis is advised to assist with medical emergencies that may arise.
   2. A separate multidisciplinary team assessment can provide insight into a partner's motivation and willingness to provide treatments.
      a. Exploring the relationship and the ability to handle the responsibilities of hemodialysis is important.
      b. The goals are to optimize the use of support and interventional measures to avoid or identify negative effects on the partner's life.
      c. Partner burnout can be minimized by encouraging the patient to maintain primary responsibility for care when possible.
      d. Early identification and intervention may minimize the partner's burden and improve the quality of life and medical outcome of the patient.
   3. It has been reported that partners may experience comorbidities, more psychopathologic states, more physician visits, and have poorer health than counterparts.
   4. Types of partners.
      a. Spouse.
         (1) Make up 76% of home dialysis caregivers.
         (2) Women assume most responsibility for health care, including home dialysis.
      b. Family member.
      c. Friend.
      d. Paid aide with the payment made by the patient or the facility program.
      e. Staff-assisted, with some facilities providing the staff to perform the patient's treatments in the home.
      f. Assess the partner as noted previously for the patient (see B3 to B9).
      g. Assess the partner's availability for the training period and ability to participate in home treatments.
      h. Identify and assist the partner in dealing with stressors associated with home hemodialysis treatments. Most successful patient/partner relationships are found in those with a collaborative approach to home dialysis.

i. Barriers to rendering care in the home hemodialysis situation.
  (1) Fear of equipment and equipment breakdown.
  (2) Time requirement for treatment and related functions.
  (3) Complexity of home hemodialysis.
  (4) Fear of change in family relationships.
  (5) Fear of stress and demands of responsibility that may include inability to work outside the home due to home hemodialysis requirements.

VII. Patient and partner training.

A. Patient education (see Section 4 for general education principles).

B. Prior to training.
  1. Initiate a signed agreement to follow program expectations for home hemodialysis.
  2. Insure patient and partner have clear instructions about training program; e.g., start date and time, preparation and participation required, length of training days, length of training program, etc.
  3. Assess the patient's and partner's learning styles and adapt training plan and materials to meet their needs.
  4. Training regarding vascular access care and management can be completed prior to home dialysis training.
    a. Minimizes training time.
    b. Allows more flexibility in training multiple patients simultaneously.

C. Training.
  1. Use a training plan and review it with patient and partner at each session. Check off as the patient and partner demonstrate their understanding of concepts or ability to perform tasks. Table 14.1 presents suggested content for home hemodialysis training, while Table 14.2 provides a sample training agenda.
  2. Allow patient/partner to gain comfort and confidence with procedures.
  3. When teaching motor skills, master one step at a time.
    a. Teach in small sessions, building on the steps.
    b. Allow opportunities for reviewing learned skills.
  4. Training multiple patients can be done.
    a. Train one patient per shift (two patients/day).
    b. Treatment times may be increased as needed during training period.
    c. Stagger patient starts (e.g., start one patient until he/she begins to gain independence, and then start another patient.

Table 14.1

Suggested Content for Home Hemodialysis Training

- ❏ Kidney function and kidney failure
- ❏ Kidney complications
- ❏ Infection control
    Hand washing
    Personal protective equipment
- ❏ Aseptic and sterile techniques
- ❏ Access
    Types
    Initiation/discontinuation
    Management and complications
- ❏ Vital signs
    Blood pressure
    Pulse
    Temperature
    Dry weight
- ❏ Hemodialysis fundamentals
    Theory
    Equipment (dialysis and water treatment)
    Operating procedures (set up, monitoring, discontinuing, disinfection)
- ❏ Dialysis prescription (home schedule)
- ❏ Anticoagulation
- ❏ Medication administration
- ❏ Lab analysis
    Drawing labs
    Interpretation
- ❏ Nutrition and dietary considerations
- ❏ Complications
    Management of procedure complications
    Medical complications
- ❏ Treatment documentation
- ❏ Clinic visits
- ❏ Supply inventory and ordering
- ❏ Equipment maintenance
- ❏ Travel
- ❏ Back up requirements/support

Table 14.2 ———————— **Sample Training Agenda**

Day	General Theory	Equipment Theory	Skill (patient/partner)
1	Facility orientation – admission and consent forms Contact list Patient assessment Medication review Aseptic technique Universal precautions Disposal of medical waste	Training program overview	Observe treatment
2	Hemodialysis fundamentals Vital signs Dry weight Therapy prescription System setup in the home	Overview of system – components of system System requirements in the home	Observe treatment Practice taking vital signs (blood pressure, heart rate, temperature, weight)
3	Vascular access management Anticoagulation Treatment documentation	Review components of system Equipment monitoring	Observe treatment Take vital signs Document treatment on flowsheet Practice cannulation (if not experienced)
4	Administering therapy	Equipment setup for treatment	Observe setup Continue with above
5	Administering therapy	Equipment setup Treatment initiation	Set up equipment prior to treatment Observe initiation Continue with above
6	Administering therapy	Equipment setup Treatment initiation Treatment discontinuation	Initiate treatment Continue with above
7	Administering therapy Laboratory draw Laboratory analysis Nutritional assessment and review	Continue with above Lab draws	Discontinue treatment Continue with above
8	Introduction to equipment alarms and cautions	Troubleshooting overview	Observe troubleshooting demonstration Continue with above
9	Equipment troubleshooting	Air alarm Pressure alarms	Perform troubleshooting on mock system Continue with above
10	Equipment troubleshooting	Power failure – emergency rinseback Temperature alarm Blood leak	Perform troubleshooting on mock system Continue with above
11	Complications of hemodialysis Emergency kit and procedures	Manual fluid bolus Review above	Perform manual bolus and emergency take off procedures
12	Continue with above	Pretreatment procedures: Water system (if applicable) – testing procedures	Practice pretreatment procedures (if necessary) Continue to administer treatment

13	Ordering supplies
	Managing inventory
	Complications of CKD
	Dialysis medications
	Clinic visits
		Equipment maintenance:
		    Equipment disinfection
		    Water system disinfection
			Continue with above

14	General review	Final skills checklist	Administer entire treatment
15	Final review	Final troubleshooting skills test	Administer entire treatment
16	Home treatment – home visit		Administer treatment

d. Group training.
   (1) Use multiple trainers who have specific roles in the training; work from a clear and well-defined training plan.
   (2) Match the patients' skill levels and compatibility in the group.
5. Assess the patient's/partner's learning through return demonstration, discussion, oral or written exams, and observation.
   a. Document training, assessment of learning, and skill mastery.
   b. It is essential to assure that the patient and the partner retain troubleshooting skills.
6. Allow flexibility in the training plan.
   a. Ongoing evaluation of the patient's and partner's learning is necessary.
   b. Alter the training plan as soon as the need is identified.
7. Optimally, one home training nurse is assigned to train the patient and partner throughout the training process. Using multiple staff for the training is offset by having an organized, well-documented training plan and checklist to assure consistency in training.
8. The training should take place in a quiet atmosphere with minimal distractions and is usually done in a dedicated home training area.
9. The training nurse should assure that the patient and partner can demonstrate all the needed skills to perform home hemodialysis and document completion of training with a certificate of completion.

VIII. Clinical management of the home hemodialysis patient.

A. Home visits.
   1. Support from the home training nurse at the patient's first home hemodialysis treatment to observe setup and procedure will encourage the patient's and partner's confidence.
   2. Annual home visits are necessary to observe the patient in the home environment.

B. Clinic visits are usually performed monthly with the following assessments being made:
   1. Fluid status and dry weight: weight, blood pressure, shortness of breath, edema, cramping, etc.
   2. Vascular access.
      a. Treatment parameters: blood flow rates, pressure readings during treatment, etc.
      b. Site examination: swelling, redness, drainage, aneurysm, bruising, etc.

3. Laboratory review.
   a. Assure that labs are drawn correctly.
   b. Anemia parameters: Hgb, Hct, iron stores, erythropoietin stimulating agent dosage, etc.
   c. Bone metabolism and disease: serum Ca, PO_4, and PTH levels; phosphate binders, etc.
   d. Chemistries with emphasis on serum K, CO_2, albumin.
   e. Adequacy of dialysis: pre-and post-BUN, KT/V, creatinine. Compare to previous levels and treatment patient is receiving.
   f. Diabetes management if applicable: glucose records, HgA_1C, and prescribed medicine for diabetes.
   g. Cardiovascular management: lipid profiles and homocysteine levels.
4. Medication review.
   a. Verify the medications being taken, whether or not they are being taken as ordered, and if any refills are needed.
   b. If performing daily dialysis, ensure that medications are taken after treatment.
5. Treatment record review and assessment.
   a. Patient flow sheets for treatment settings and treatment completion as ordered.
   b. Symptoms or complications noted but not reported by patient/partner.
   c. Symptom or complications reported but not noted by patient/partner.
   d. Alarms noted and appropriate resolution.
   e. Dialyzer appearance at end of treatment which may indicate red cell loss and/or the need to alter heparin dosage.
   f. Overall documentation completeness.
6. Supplies and equipment.
   a. Verify appropriate use and operation.
   b. Discuss any equipment issues and equipment management.
   c. Review supply usage and inventory management.
7. Nutritional assessment.
   a. Usually done by the dietitian.
   b. May include reviews of weight, adequacy, bone metabolism and disease, anemia status, appetite, etc.
8. Psychosocial assessment.
   a. Energy level.
   b. Stress levels.
   c. Changes in relationship with partner.
   d. Financial concerns.
   e. Quality of life.

9. Skills review.
   a. The nurse assesses the patient's/partner's competence in performing dialysis procedures and troubleshooting skills.
   b. Semiannual to annual competency observation for patient's/partner's ability to perform treatments should be conducted in the training department or patient's home setting.

C. Self-care.
   1. A self-care unit/area can be used to support the home hemodialysis program.
   2. Allows patient and/or partner to gain confidence prior to going home.
      a. May be used by patient and/or partner to learn or reinforce knowledge and skills regarding care of a new or revised vascular access.
      b. Allows the patient and/or partner to have a routine vacation from the usual responsibilities.
      c. Allows the patient and/or partner respite as needed.
      d. May be used to train new or backup partners.

IX. Components of the home hemodialysis system.

A. Equipment requirements are the same as for hemodialysis in a health care facility.
   1. The NxStage machine is approved for home hemodialysis by the FDA.
      a. A small, portable system that uses volumetric balancing in a disposable cartridge.
      b. The system has no special electrical requirements and offers an option, using sterile bagged dialysate, with no water treatment system.
   2. Dialysis machines that are not approved specifically for home treatments are currently being used according to a physician's prescription.

B. Dialysate preparation using water purification system dialysate concentrate.
   1. Key component of the water treatment system is a knowledgeable user.
   2. The patient and/or partner must have a clear understanding of the water system, water testing, test results, and alarm conditions to assure safe operation.
   3. Water and dialysate should meet current Association for the Advancement of Medical Instrumentation (AAMI) Standards.

4. Equipment installation in the home must meet electrical and plumbing requirements for the equipment.
5. Maintenance will vary according to design and age of equipment. Follow manufacturer's guidelines for installation, service, and maintenance.
6. Disinfection of equipment must be done at required intervals per manufacturer's guidelines.

X. The dialysis procedure.

A. Special considerations for the home hemodialysis patient/partner (see Section 11.)
   1. The home dialysis patient and/or partner must learn the same procedures as in-center staff. In some cases additional procedures may be added to ensure safety and/or individualized care in the home environment.
   2. The treatment documentation recorded by the patient and/or partner should be reviewed at each clinic visit.
   3. Disinfection of the dialysis and water equipment must be done by either the patient and/or partner, or arrangements made with the home training facility to provide this service to comply with the manufacturer's disinfection recommendations.
   4. The patient and/or partner should have a document (using a checklist or other means) indicating that they have been observed in all treatment and equipment procedures and that they are competent to perform these treatments at home.
   5. It is recommended that the partner be present while the patient is undergoing the hemodialysis treatment at home.

B. Dialyzer reprocessing in the home (see Section 11).
   1. Reprocessing procedures must meet all of the AAMI's Recommended Practices for Reuse of Hemodialyzers.
   2. Arrangements must be made for either the appropriate equipment (AAMI standards) if reprocessing hemodialyzers in the home, or appropriate transportation procedures if dialyzers are transported to the facility for reprocessing.
   3. If reprocessed hemodialyzers are to be used, the patient and/or partner must have documentation of their competency in all procedures that they are required to perform. This includes testing for sterilants, testing for absence of

sterilants, and monitoring for complications related to dialyzer reprocessing.
4. Most facilities choose not to reprocess dialyzers for home patients.

C. Vascular access for home hemodialysis patients (see Section 12).
   1. Types of vascular accesses used for home hemodialysis.
      a. Central venous catheter (CVC).
         (1) The CVC must be able to sustain the prescribed blood flow for treatment to assure treatment adequacy.
         (2) CVCs have interlocking connectors for attachment to the patient's bloodlines. Facilities may make recommendations to patients for an additional locking device, e.g., Lock Box®, Secure Cath®, or Interlink®.
      b. Fistula.
         (1) Fistulas are the preferred dialysis access for home patients.
         (2) Fistulas have the lowest complication rates in home and daily therapies.
         (3) The patient and/or partner may use either the rotating site method or the buttonhole technique. As staff skill in training techniques improves, buttonhole technique may become the preferred method of cannulation for daily treatments.
         (4) Single needles may be used for nocturnal treatments to reduce the number of punctures. It has been considered by some to be safer in case of accidental dislodgement while sleeping.
      c. Graft.
         (1) The patient and/or partner use the rotating site method of cannulation.
         (2) Buttonhole technique is not recommended for grafts.
   2. Guidelines for vascular access.
      a. The patient or the partner must be taught cannulation technique using proper infection control practices (e.g., handwashing, cleansing of the access, and basic principles of infection prevention as outlined in KDOQI).
      b. The patient and the partner must be taught the signs and symptoms of access infection and the appropriate action to take (i.e., report the problem following the facility protocol and follow through with the treatment prescribed).

   c. Current data does not indicate that daily cannulation is harmful to fistulas or grafts.
   d. Training in cannulation techniques prior to home training may be beneficial to the home training process and in patient selection.
   e. The patient and partner must recognize the symptoms of vascular access complications, and be able to report and follow the prescribed treatment plans.

D. Adequacy of dialysis (see Section 11).
   1. The home patient's adequacy testing should meet or exceed the KDOQI Guidelines.
   2. Testing should be done monthly and be evaluated by the attending nephrologist or advanced nurse practitioner for necessary changes to the patient's dialysis prescription.
   3. The patient and/or the partner must be taught laboratory drawing procedures and know how the lab samples are transferred to the laboratory.
   4. Post-BUN samples should be drawn according to KDOQI Guidelines using either the low flow or stop flow method.
   5. KT/V is generally the accepted measure of "adequate dialysis." Other factors to be considered are creatinine, potassium, albumin, phosphorus, beta-2 microglobulin, appetite, sleep patterns, energy level, and quality of life.
   6. Standardized KT/V results of 2.0 are recommended as a minimum standard for adequacy.
   7. Minimum single pool KT/V results per treatment.
      a. 1.2 for conventional dialysis.
      b. 0.5 for short daily therapy.
   8. Physicians may have preferences for higher standards for single pool KT/V results.
   9. All patient lab results and general well-being should be considered in assessing adequate treatment.

E. Acute complications (see Section 11).
   1. The home hemodialysis patient and partner must be competent in identification and management of acute complications of hemodialysis and must be able to respond appropriately to medical emergencies.
   2. At a minimum, a partner must be able to recognize signs of a medical emergency, call for emergency assistance if needed, and treat the emergent medical symptoms.
   3. An emergency safety kit is recommended for home patients.

F. Infection control (see Sections 11 and 1).
1. The patient and partner must use appropriate infection control practices during all aspects of the home hemodialysis process to help prevent infections.
2. The patient and partner must be taught to recognize the symptoms of infections, report symptoms, and complete the prescribed treatment.

XI. Role of the home training nurse.

A. The primary role of the nurse is to teach the patient and partner to manage the patient's kidney disease and to safely and effectively perform dialysis procedures in the home.

B. The home hemodialysis training nurse must have:
1. Documented training in hemodialysis.
2. Documented training and experience in home hemodialysis training.
3. An understanding of adult learning principles.
4. The capability to assess patients for the ability to perform hemodialysis procedures in the home environment.
5. The ability to develop and execute a training plan, individualized to each patient in home training.
6. The ability to develop and implement patient selection criteria, patient schedules, and oversight of patients at home.

C. Minimum staffing for home hemodialysis programs is two nurses — one dedicated to home training and another to fill in as backup as required.

D. Having staff available on call for home patients is essential.
1. Provides optimal home services.
2. Improves patient outcomes through rapid response.
3. Prevents waste of resources.
4. Maximizes patient confidence and satisfaction.

XII. Future of home hemodialysis.

A. Home hemodialysis has shown an increase since 2002. Contributing factors include:
1. Improved mortality in home hemodialysis patients.
2. Improved clinical benefits of daily therapy.
3. New technology in home hemodialysis systems and manufacturer funding for advances in equipment and dialyzer membranes.

4. Increased interest in convective therapies.
5. Flexible dialysis prescriptions and scheduling (short daily, nocturnal, every other day, and other combinations).
6. While costs increase, particularly for daily hemodialysis, there are economic benefits for home and daily hemodialysis related to decreased hospitalization rates and lessened needs for medications.
7. Improved quality of life.
8. Patient's increased sense of independence and freedom.
9. Increased physician information and training about benefits of home hemodialysis.
10. Home hemodialysis allows one nurse to manage more patients than conventional, in-center patients.
11. Studies indicating that, if educated, more patients would choose and are capable of performing home dialysis.

B. Other considerations.
1. There is a need for improvement in vascular access outcomes, including the ability to decrease bacterial infection.
2. There is a need for improved removal of middle molecules such beta-2 microglobulin.
3. Exploring the benefits of ultrapure dialysate may lead to improvements in inflammation, maintenance of kidney function at initiation of dialysis, improvement in nutrition, and improvement in iron utilization and erythropoietin response.
4. Home dialysis, especially home daily hemodialysis, requires local and national advocacy for appropriate funding models and infrastructure to develop and promote these modalities. The federal government must have a role in understanding the benefits and costs of home and daily dialysis through the development of a tiered payment system to reflect hemodialysis dose and funding of a randomized, controlled study of the effects of short daily and nocturnal dialysis.

Chapter 66

Peritoneal Dialysis

Purpose

The purpose of this chapter is to provide an overview of the initiation of home peritoneal dialysis as a kidney replacement therapy (KRT) option. The following topics are included: interview process for prospective peritoneal dialysis candidates, individualized patient training program, initiation of peritoneal dialysis in the home setting, home management, and role of the peritoneal dialysis nurse.

Objectives

Upon completion of this chapter, the learner will be able to:
1. Define the terms, CAPD, and CCPD/APD.
2. List at least three potential candidates for peritoneal dialysis.
3. List the goals of the interview process.
4. List at least 10 of the prerequisites needed by the PD nurse to be an effective interviewer.
5. Identify the content needed for the patient's medical history.
6. Discuss three characteristics of cultural diversity.
7. Cite four actions needed to prepare the interview environment.
8. Describe six components of the interview process.
9. Discuss six actions of the interview process.
10. Identify special concerns assessed during the interview process.
11. Discuss the special needs of the geriatric patient during the interview process.
12. List five variables influenced by a language barrier.
13. Describe four issues experienced by the hearing impaired patient during the interview process.
14. Describe three issues experienced by the visually impaired patient during the interview process.
15. Identify six strategies to use when interviewing the unusually anxious patient.
16. Describe the documentation process of the interview.
17. List three locations where a patient may be trained.
18. Discuss the length and number of training sessions.
19. List the signs and symptoms of peritonitis.
20. List the signs and symptoms of an exit site infection.
21. List three clinical results a patient must record daily.
22. Describe six problem solving solutions that the patient can use in the home.
23. Describe a daily hygiene plan.
24. Identify the content of the peritoneal dialysis training sessions.
25. List the prerequisites for initiation of PD in the home.
26. Describe the inspection of the home environment.
27. List 15 activities included in the home visit.
28. Describe six features of dialysis care follow-up.
29. Discuss the role of the PD nurse as facilitator.
30. Discuss the role of the PD nurse as educator.
31. Discuss the role of the PD nurse as clinician.

I. Definition of terms.

A. Continuous ambulatory peritoneal dialysis (CAPD).
   1. Patient does 4 to 5 manual exchanges of dialysis solution exchanges through a surgically implanted catheter 7 days a week in the home setting.

B. Continuous cycled peritoneal dialysis (CCPD) or automated peritoneal dialysis (APD).
   1. Dialysis is performed by a machine during the night in the home.
   2. The night time exchanges are called cycles.
   3. The cycler does a final fill in the morning before the patient is disconnected from the machine.
   4. Some patients may need to do additional manual exchanges during the day.

II. Chronic kidney disease (CKD) management and dialysis options education (see Sections 2 and 4).

III. Contraindications for peritoneal dialysis (scc Section 13).

IV. Interviewing the potential patient for peritoneal dialysis.

A. Identifying the potential peritoneal dialysis candidate.
   1. The CKD patient who is ready to discuss dialysis options.
   2. The CKD patient who has self-selected peritoneal dialysis.
   3. The CKD patient who has uremic symptoms and must make a timely decision regarding dialysis.
   4. The hospitalized patient who must select a dialysis option before discharge. This patient may be newly diagnosed and may not have had the benefit of CKD education and disease management.
   5. The patient who is currently on hemodialysis and is experiencing vascular access issues.
   6. The patient who is currently on hemodialysis and wishes to switch treatment modality to peritoneal dialysis.
   7. The patient who has a failed transplant who must now choose a dialysis modality.
   8. The patient who is unable to assume responsibility for self-dialysis and is cared for by a spouse, family member, or caretaker.

B. The interview process.
   See Figure 14.1 for a Patient Information Sheet, and Figure 14.2 for Interview Worksheet Guidelines.
   1. The goals of the interview.
      a. Provide patient and family with information about peritoneal dialysis.
      b. Assess the patient's readiness to assume self-care responsibility.
      c. Provide a supportive environment.
      d. Identify the unique needs of each patient.
      e. Identify the individual patient needs with other members of the health care team.
   2. Prerequisites for the PD nurse interviewer.
      a. Knowledge of physical assessment.
      b. Knowledge of nursing diagnosis.
      c. Knowledge of adult education principles.
      d. Documentation skills.
      e. Appreciation of cultural diversity.
      f. Ability to individualize information.
      g. Possesses an understanding of the process of chronic disease.
      h. Possesses an understanding of CKD disease management.
      i. Knowledge of principles of peritoneal dialysis.
      j. Ability to communicate effectively.
      k. Ability to coordinate participation of other members of renal health care team.
      l. Ability to involve family members/significant others as indicated.
   3. Obtaining patient medical history.
      a. Document prior medical history.
      b. Obtain physical assessment information from primary care provider.
      c. Obtain physical assessment information from nephrologists.
      d. List current medications.
      e. List other health care providers (e.g., surgeons, specialists, consultants, etc.).
      f. List family members, significant others.
      g. Include adherence history.
      h. Include patient's current understanding of health needs.
   4. Identify patient's cultural beliefs and needs.
      a. The individual cultural needs of the patient.
      b. The patient's ethnicity.
      c. Specific cultural issues identified by the patient.
      d. The religious beliefs of the patient/family.
      e. The primary language of the patient.
      f. Arrange for interpreter if necessary.
   5. Preparation of the interview environment.
      a. Well-ventilated room.
      b. Comfortable seating.
      c. Seating for family and significant others.
      d. Appropriate lighting.

6. The interviewing process.
   a. Introduce yourself and identify your role.
   b. Explain why the interview is necessary.
   c. Include family members but establish patient as primary focus.
   d. Monitor the response of the patient and others present.
   e. Identify sensory needs hearing loss, visual problems, language barrier.
   f. Monitor the patient for fatigue or confusion.
   g. Ask one question at a time.
   h. Do not interrupt the patient.
   i. Restate question if patient seems confused.
   j. Use language the patient can understand.
   k. Validate the patient's fears/anxieties.
   l. Stop if the patient is overwhelmed.
   m. Use humor if appropriate.
   n. Be a good listener.
7. The nurse must be aware of warning signs or situations that may be predictive of future problems. Use of clinical judgment, previous experience, and professional expertise is mandated.
   a. Does the patient state that he or she cannot take self-responsibility for care?
   b. Does the patient live alone without the benefit of family/friend interaction and support?
   c. Does the patient have a documented history of nonadherence to medications and/or the plan of care?
   d. Does the patient have multiple physical/tactile impairments?
   e. Does the patient need a partner to successfully do home PD?
   f. Is there an available partner who is willing to assume responsibility?
   g. Does the patient have transportation to the dialysis unit?
   h. Does the patient express unusual concern about disruption of body image?
   i. Does the patient demonstrate an unusual level of anxiety?
   j. Do you need to stop the interview?
   k. Do you need to enlist the help of the social worker or the nephrologist?
   l. Do you need to provide additional interview time?

Patient Information Sheet

Name: _____   Date: _____

Address:_____   Home Phone Number: _____

_____   Work Phone Number:_____

_____   Email Address: _____

Nephrologist: _____

Primary Care Physician: _____

Specialty Physicians: _____

_____

_____

_____

Medical/Surgical History: _____

_____

_____

_____

_____

_____

_____

Medication List:

_____

_____

_____

_____

_____

_____

_____

_____

Allergies (medications, food, others):

_____

_____

_____

Insurance Information:

Primary:

Secondary:

Medication Coverage: ____Yes   ____No

Employment: ____Full time ____Part time ____Unemployed ____Retired

Transportation: Do you drive?   ____Yes   ____No

Family/friend drives?   ____Yes   ____No

Do you use public transportation?   ____Yes   ____No

Do you use taxis?   ____Yes   ____No

Do you use assisted transportation?   ____Yes   ____No

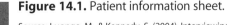

Figure 14.1. Patient information sheet.

Source: Luongo, M., & Kennedy, S. (2004). Interviewing prospective patients for peritoneal dialysis: A five-step approach. *Nephrology Nursing Journal, 31*(5), 513-520. Used with permission.

Social History

Patient age:

Marital Status: ☐ Single ☐ Married ☐ Divorced ☐ Widow/Widower

Is the patient employed? ☐ No ☐ Yes If yes, ☐ Full time ☐ Part time
     Occupation:

Is the patient retired? ☐ Yes ☐ No

Is the patient disabled? ☐ Yes ☐ No

Does the patient live: ☐ Alone ☐ With spouse ☐ With significant other
     With significant others: If yes, with whom? _____

Does the patient have children? ☐ No ☐ Yes If yes, how many? _____

Does the patient extended family? ☐ No ☐ Yes If yes, who?_____

Are family members/friends involved in the patient's life? ☐ No ☐ Yes If yes, who?_____

What are the patient's usual daily activities?

What are the patient's special interests or hobbies?

Does the patient travel nationally or internationally? ☐ No ☐ Yes If yes, where? _____

Home Environment

Where does the patient live? ☐ Apartment ☐ Home-rented ☐ Home-owned
                              ☐ Foster home ☐ Skilled nursing facility ☐ Homeless

Where will the patient do exchanges? _____ Is there sufficient privacy? ☐ Yes ☐ No

How many individuals live in the household? _____

Is there running water? ☐ Yes ☐ No Electricity? ☐ Yes ☐ No

Where will supplies be stored?_____

Are there pets in the household? ☐ Yes ☐ No

Language/Education

What is the patient's primary language? _____

What is the patient's secondary language? _____

Highest grade of school completed _____

Can the patient read English? ☐ Yes ☐ No Write English? ☐ Yes ☐ No

Read another language? ☐ Yes ☐ No Write another language? ☐ Yes ☐ No

Physical Limitations

Visual: Does the patient wear glasses? ☐ No ☐ Yes

        Have Cataracts? ☐ No ☐ Yes, Left Eye ☐ Yes, Right Eye

        Have Glaucoma? ☐ No ☐ Yes, Left Eye ☐ Yes, Right Eye

        Is the patient legally blind? ☐ No ☐ Yes

Hearing: Hard of hearing? ☐ No ☐ Yes

        Uses a hearing aid? ☐ No ☐ Yes, Left Ear ☐Yes, Right Ear

Tactile: Is the patient's sense of touch impaired? ☐ No ☐ Yes If yes, specifics _____

Extremities: Arm/leg impairments? ☐ No ☐ Yes If yes, specifics _____

        Amputations? ☐ No ☐ Yes If yes, specifics _____

        Paralyzed limbs? ☐ No ☐ Yes If yes, specifics _____

        Hand strength problems? ☐ No ☐ Yes If yes, specifics _____

Daily activities: ☐ Independent ☐ Needs assistance ☐ Dependent

Does the patient have a history of CVA? ☐ No ☐ Yes If yes, specifics _____

General Questions

     Previous experience with CKD dialysis?

     Does the patient have a family member/friend with CKD?

     Is the family member/friend on hemodialysis? PD? Transplant recipient?

     How does the patient handle stress?

     What is the most stressful situation the patient has experienced?

     How does the patient make decisions? ☐ Self directed ☐ Relies on family/spouse/other. If yes, who? _____

Financial Issues

Does the patient have: ☐ Insurance ☐ Medicare ☐ State assistance ☐ Self pay

How does the patient pay for medications? ☐ Insurance ☐ Self pay

Chronic Kidney Disease Education

Has the patient had previous CKD education? ☐ No ☐ Yes If yes, by whom? _____

What does the patient recall?

Figure 14.2. Interview worksheet guidelines, page 1 of 2.

Kidney Replacement Therapy Education and Information
Brief review of normal kidney function
Brief review of diseased kidney function
Describe symptoms of kidney failure

Hemodialysis:
Incenter hemodialysis
Home hemodialysis
Access placement:
Fistula
Graft
Catheter
Describe hemodialysis session
Role of nurse and technician
Short-term/Long-term management
Responsibilities and participation of patient

Transplantation:
Living-related donor
Living, nonrelated donor
Nonliving donor
Medical evaluation
Surgical evaluation
Waiting for transplant
Preoperative routine
Postoperative routine
Role of immunosuppression
Role of medications
Follow-up
Usual transplant clinic routine
Possible complications

Peritoneal Dialysis:
Review how PD works
Surgical evaluation
Catheter insertion routine
Postoperative catheter routine
Changes in body image
PD solution exchange demonstration
Allow patient to handle the PD tubing/equipment
Daily routine of PD
Clinic visit routine including frequency
Roles of the PD nurse, social worker, dietitian
Prevention of infection
Possible complications
Outline of the events of the first month on PD, 6 months on PD, long term
What is included in training sessions
Emergency interventions

Self-Care Issues:
Adherence to medications
Communication with health care team
Consistent follow-up care
Attendance at appointments
What is the patient's previous experience with self-care?

Figure 14.2. Interview worksheet guidelines, page 2 of 2.

Adapted from Bates, 1991; DeHaan, 2003; Prowant, 2001. Reprinted in Luongo, M., & Kennedy, S. (2004). Interviewing prospective patients for peritoneal dialysis: A five-step approach. *Nephrology Nursing Journal, 31*(5), 513-520. Used with permission.

8. The geriatric patient.
   a. Identify age-related changes in hearing, vision, and cognition.
   b. Schedule appointment early in day to diminish fatigue.
   c. May need an additional interview appointment.
   d. Provide quiet, uninterrupted environment.
   e. Sit directly in front of patient to facilitate hearing.
   f. Ask one question at a time. Repeat if necessary.
   g. Refocus the patient when necessary.
   h. Involve family in the process.
   i. Be patient.
9. The patient with language barriers.
   a. Use a professional interpreter to insure accurate communication.
   b. Instruct interpreter to translate information/response exactly as stated.
   c. The use of a family member may be uncomfortable for patient in regard to confidentiality and cultural beliefs.
   d. Family members may interject their own biases.
   e. Use of interpreter will lengthen the time of the interview.
10. The patient with a hearing impairment.
    a. Sit directly in front of patient so the patient has a clear view of your lips and facial expressions.
    b. Speak slowly.
    c. Frequently repeat information/questions.
    d. Provide written information.
11. The patient with a visual impairment.
    a. Patient may be light sensitive.
    b. Adjust lighting to avoid glare; dim lights; close shades.
    c. Written information must be in large print on nonglossy paper.
12. The unusually anxious patient.
    a. Stop the interview if necessary.
    b. Open the door to the interview room.
    c. Offer the patient some refreshments.
    d. Reschedule if necessary.
    e. Discuss anxiety with the patient's nephrologist.
    f. Enlist the help of family member if appropriate.
    g. Enlist the help of a home PD patient to provide a patient to patient experience if appropriate.
13. Documentation.
    a. Share results with other members of health care team.

b. Develop specific interview forms if appropriate.
c. Document specifics of interview and recommendations.
d. Place documentation in patient's medical record.

V. Individualized patient training program.

A. Training for the PD patient should be planned to meet the patient's individual needs.
   1. Family members and/or significant other may be included to provide support for the patient.
   2. The length of the training session should be based on the patient's ability to concentrate without feeling overwhelmed and anxious.
   3. The PD nurse not only provides the training experience, but also evaluates the patient's progress and readiness to assume responsibility for home dialysis performance.

B. Review adult learner principles (see Section 4).

C. Possible locations for training.
   1. Peritoneal dialysis unit training room.
   2. Hospital setting for hospitalized patient.
   3. Patient's home.

D. Length of training session.
   1. Determined on patient's attention span, current uremic symptoms, and ability to process information.
   2. Influenced by transportation issues and family participation.
   3. The need for an interpreter will usually increase the time needed for training.

E. Number of training sessions.
   1. Depends on the patient's ability to learn and feel comfortable with home PD procedures.
   2. Limited by reimbursement. The PD nurse must be aware of the possible restrictions and guidelines.

F. Content of training sessions.
   1. The content must be individualized for each patient.
   2. The PD nurse must be very careful in presenting information that the patient can assimilate without being overwhelmed by technical terminology and/or the amount of the information.
   3. Topics to include.
      a. Basic explanation of kidney function.

b. Theory of how PD works as a kidney replacement therapy.
c. Aseptic technique.
d. Weight and blood pressure measurement.
e. Setup of the home environment for an exchange.
f. Performing a CAPD exchange. This involves multiple demonstrations by the PD nurse and return demonstrations by the patient and/or family.
g. Addition of medications to the dialysis solution bags.
h. Technique for warming the dialysis solution bags using dry heat. Avoidance of moist heat due to danger of water borne organisms.
i. The patient is instructed not to microwave solution bags due to the danger of thermal burns and the leaching of plastics into solution creating possible chemical irritation to the peritoneal membrane.
j. Proper hand washing using antibacterial soap.
k. The use of waterless hand cleaners as an alternative means of hand washing if antibacterial soap and water are not available.
l. Wearing a face mask during exchange procedure, when adding medications to the dialysis solution bags, or when performing exit site care.
m. Problem solving in the home, including:
(1) Obstruction to flow of dialysis solution.
(2) Recognition of change in color of effluent.
(3) Presence of fibrin in effluent and appropriate use of heparin.
(4) Accidental disconnections and how to clamp the catheter and report the event to PD nurse immediately.
(5) Recognition of a tear or hole in catheter and how to clamp the catheter and report the event to PD nurse immediately.
(6) How to report a fall or tugging of catheter that may or may not result in tissue trauma.
n. Recognition of the signs and symptoms of peritonitis and seeking appropriate treatment, including:
(1) Cloudy effluent.
(2) Abdominal pain.
(3) Fever, chills.
(4) Nausea, vomiting, diarrhea.
o. Fluid balance to enhance the patient's ability to recognize the signs and symptoms of hypovolemia and hypervolemia.

p. Specific instructions/guidelines for fluid balance management.
q. The importance of recording daily weight, frequency of exchanges, dextrose percentage, and amount infused and drained.
r. Monitoring and recording daily blood pressure if able.
s. Guidelines concerning weight, blood pressure, and the appropriate use of the different dextrose concentrations.
t. Formulation of an acceptable daily dialysis routine by the PD nurse and the patient. This routine plan is based on the individual dialysis needs and lifestyle of the patient. Consideration is given to:
(1) Social and family support systems.
(2) Family members who live with the patient and their involvement in daily care.
(3) Plan for routine, low impact exercise if able.
(4) Employment status.
(5) Student status.
u. A daily hygiene plan that includes:
(1) Reminders about frequent hand washing and use of mask.
(2) Daily showers if able to stand or sit in shower stall.
(3) Use of antibacterial soap.
(4) Cleansing of exit site per facility protocol, inspecting the catheter, and appropriately securing the catheter to prevent trauma to the exit site.
(5) Applying antibacterial cream/ointment to exit site if ordered.
v. Recognition of the signs and symptoms of an exit site infection and how to seek appropriate intervention. Signs and symptoms include erythema, pain, and tenderness at the exit site or along the catheter tunnel, and/or the presence of fever.
w. Reproductive and sexual concerns.
x. Medication review to include medication's name, purpose, appropriate schedule, and route of administration.
y. Storage of supplies, maintenance of the home inventory, and ordering additional supplies.
z. How to contact nephrologist, APN, or PD nurse by telephone and/or e-mail.
aa. Identification of emergency situations and how to seek emergency help.
bb. Consultation with the social worker.
cc. Consultation with the dietitian.
dd. A copy of the unit's specific written training manual for home reference.

ee. Copies of forms to record daily dialysis progress.

4. Home dialysis is initiated when the patient and PD nurse mutually agree that the patient is ready for this responsibility.

VI. Initiation of peritoneal dialysis in the home.

A. Prerequisites for home dialysis initiation.
1. Patient has completed home training program.
2. Patient agrees to home visit.
3. Supplies are ordered and in place in the home.
4. Appropriate orders written by the nephrologist or APN.
5. PD nurse arranges home visit.
6. Family members/significant others involved as appropriate.

B. Components of the home visit.
1. A home inspection may be done prior to training program.
2. A home inspection may be done on the first day of home dialysis.
3. Consideration is given to where the patient lives (e.g., an apartment, a home that is owned, a home that is rented, a foster home, a skilled nursing facility, a shelter, or the patient may be homeless).
4. Who else lives in the home?
5. Is there running water and electricity?
6. Infection control issues are considered.
   a. Are there adequate facilities for hand washing? Review hand washing technique.
   b. Where will patient do exchanges? Is there a clean surface area? Is the area away from open windows, blowing fans, air conditioners, or heating vents?
   c. Are there pets in the home? If so, is the pet removed from the site of the dialysis exchange?
   d. Dialysis solution bags warmed by dry heat mechanism.
7. Safety issues are considered (e.g., storage of syringes and medications safely out of the reach of small children).
8. Consideration is given to supplies.
   a. Initial supplies are unpacked by patient and/or PD nurse.
   b. Initial supplies are inventoried and appropriately organized.
   c. Is there adequate storage space?
   d. Are supplies safely stored in a dry, clean area?
   e. How frequently will the patient need delivery of supplies, e.g., every 2 weeks, every 4 weeks?
   f. Who will contact the vendor for supplies — the staff of PD unit or the patient?
9. The first exchange is prepared by and performed by patient under the supervision of the PD nurse.
10. Family member/significant other may be present and participating.
11. Documentation of exchanges by patient is reviewed and reinforced.
12. The PD nurse reviews patient's individualized daily dialysis routine.
13. The PD nurse reviews the written training manual with the patient for problem solving and trouble shooting in the home.
14. The PD nurse reviews emergency contact numbers with the patient and family member/significant other.
15. The PD nurse discusses the home environment with patient and the possible need for changes to insure a safe dialysis environment.
16. The PD nurse reviews the supply of medications with patient and formulates a medication schedule for the patient if necessary.
17. The PD nurse reviews administration, storage, and documentation of erythropoietin-stimulating agents in the home environment. This is a requirement in some states.
18. The PD nurse reviews the completion of home record forms with the patient.
19. The PD nurse observes the interactions of patient with family members and/or significant others and documents appropriately.
20. The PD nurse and patient review the disposal of dialysate/effluent and used dialysis equipment.
21. The PD nurse and patient may do additional exchanges together if appropriate.
22. The PD nurse provides time for the patient's questions and concerns.
23. The PD nurse and patient discuss plans for the next PD clinic visit and review the frequency of phone call reporting.
24. The PD nurse reviews how to order supplies from the vendor and establishes an initial inventory with the patient.
25. The PD nurse documents the activities of the home visit in the patient's medical record.
26. The PD nurse shares the patient's progress with the other members of the health care team.

C. Additional home visits may be needed to evaluate unexplained clinical changes, repetitive infections, and/or changes in family unit.

VII. Management of the home peritoneal dialysis patient.

A. Home management (see Section 13).
  1. PD procedures.
  2. PD access.
  3. PD disease management.
  4. PD complications.
  5. PD adequacy.

B. Provision of dialysis care follow-up.
  1. The PD patient should be seen monthly or more frequently in the PD unit.
  2. Specific forms for the monthly visit should be developed and include:
     a. Vital signs, weight, and blood pressure.
     b. Review of current dialysis prescription.
     c. Review and list of current medications.
     d. Assessment and review of systems.
     e. Review of home record forms.
     f. Inspection and documentation of condition of PD catheter.
     g. Review of home supply inventory.
     h. Documentation of serum blood studies.
     i. Collection and documentation of PD adequacy parameters.
     j. Documentation of current plan of care.
     k. Arrangements for next follow-up appointment with nephrologists or APN and the PD unit.
  3. Other forms.
     a. Quarterly or semiannual care plans.
     b. Transplant preparation care plans.
     c. Consent forms.
     d. Problem lists.
     e. Dialysis order sheets.
     f. Assessments by social worker, dietitian, and other health care workers.
     g. Documentation of insurance information.
     h. Confidentiality release forms.
     i. Unit specific forms.

VIII. The roles of the home peritoneal dialysis nurse.

The roles of the peritoneal dialysis nurse are multi-faceted and may vary in different clinical settings. Included are the specific actions and competencies that the peritoneal dialysis nurse must use when initiating peritoneal dialysis in the home setting. These actions and competencies are not all inclusive but focus on the early education and initiation of home peritoneal dialysis.

A. In the role of a facilitator of care, the PD nurse will:
  1. Organize interview for patient and family.
  2. Plan home training program.
  3. Clarify plan with health care team.
  4. Order appropriate supplies.
  5. Plan for routine follow-up after initiation of home dialysis.
  6. Collaborate with social worker and dietitian for specific interventions.

B. In the role of an educator, the PD nurse will:
  1. Develop the content for dialysis options and interview process.
  2. Develop the content of training sessions.
  3. Coordinate educational content with the health care team.
  4. Identify patient and family learning styles.
  5. Provide written educational materials.
  6. Individualize educational reinforcement.
  7. Evaluate patient's comprehension of education material.
  8. Adjust plan to accommodate special needs and/or language barrier.
  9. Document patient's needs and accomplishments.

C. In the role of a clinician, the PD nurse will:
  1. Collaborate with the nephrologist or APN to develop an appropriate home dialysis prescription for the patient.
  2. Evaluate the effectiveness of the prescription in regard to fluid balance, blood pressure, and dialysis adequacy.
  3. Identify risks for infection.
  4. Insure infections are treated and establish follow-up interventions.
  5. Review medication program with patient.
  6. Evaluate patient's adherence with the dialysis regimen and medications.
  7. Delineate short-term and long-term disease management goals with patient and health care team.
  8. Document plan of care, patient health assessment, daily progress, and ESRD required forms.
  9. Facilitate disease management strategies.
  10. Identify peritoneal dialysis complications and intervene appropriately.
  11. Develop a relationship with the PD patient that focuses on trust and support.

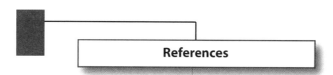

References

Anderson, C., Blagg, C.R., Kapikian, N., & Mailloux, L.U. (2001). Organizations and elements of a home hemodialysis program. In B.D. Rose (Ed.), *UpToDate in nephrology and hypertension.* Wellesley, MA.

Ayus, J.C., Mizani, M.R., Achinger, S.G., Thadhani, R., Go, A.S., & Lee, S. (2005). Effects of short daily versus conventional hemodialysis on left ventricular hypertrophy and inflammatory markers: A prospective, controlled study. *Journal of American Society of Nephrology, 16,* 2778-2788.

Babcock, D., & Miller, M. (1994). *Client education.* St. Louis: C.V. Mosby Company.

Bates, B. (1991). *A guide to physical examination.* Philadelphia: J.B. Lippincott.

Belasco, A.G., & Sesso, R. (2002). Burden and quality of life of caregivers for hemodialysis patients. *American Journal of Kidney Diseases, 39*(4), 805-812.

Blagg, C.R. (1997). The history of home dialysis: A view from Seattle. *Home Hemodialysis International, 1*(1), 1-7.

Blagg, C.R. (2000). What went wrong with home hemodialysis in the United States and what can be done now? *Hemodialysis International, 4,* 55-58.

Blagg, C.R., & Anderson, C. (2002). Home preparation and installation for home hemodialysis. In A.R. Nissenson & R.N. Fine (Eds.), *Dialysis therapy* (3rd ed., pp 87-89). Philadelphia: Hanley & Belfus, Inc.

Blogg, A.E., O'Shaughnessy, D.V., & Cairns, D.R. (1999). *Levels and predictors of distress in home hemodialysis caregivers.* Retrieved February 20, 2008, from http://eneph.com

Branson, M., & Moran, J. (2004). Supporting home dialysis therapies. The Wellbound model. *Nephrology News and Issues, 18*(3), 24-29.

Burrows-Hudson, S., & Prowant, B. (2005). *Nephrology nursing standards of practice and guidelines for care.* Pitman, NJ: American Nephrology Nurses' Association.

Campbell, D. (2001). Client education in the nephrology setting. *Dialysis and Transplantation, 30*(9), 571-574.

Daugirdas, J., Blake, P., & Ing, T. (2001). *Handbook of dialysis* (3rd ed.). Philadelphia: Lippincott Williams & Wilkins.

DeHaan, B.D. (2003). Why peritoneal dialysis should be the first treatment option. *Dialysis and Transplantation, 132*(3), 160-164.

Diaz-Buxo, J. (1996). Patient selection and the success of peritoneal dialysis. *Nephrology News and Issues, 3,* 7-19.

Diaz-Buxo, J.A., Crawford-Bonadio, T.L., St. Pierre, D., & Ingram, K.M. (2006). Establishing a successful home dialysis program. *Blood Purification, 24,* 22-27.

Fagugli, R.M., Pasini, P., Pasticci, G., Cicconi, B., & Buonocristiani, U. (2006). Effects of short daily hemodialysis and extended standard hemodialysis on blood pressure and cardiac hypertrophy: A comparative study. *Journal of Nephrology, 19*(1), 77-83.

Farina, J. (2001). Peritoneal dialysis: A case for home visits. *Nephrology Nursing Journal, 28*(4), 423-428.

Floramo, S. (2006). Use of NxStage system one for a daily home hemodialysis. *Nephrology News and Issues, 20*(11), 48-53.

Galland, R., Traeger, J., Arkouche, W., Delawari, E., & Fouque, D. (2001). Short daily hemodialysis and nutritional status. *American Journal of Kidney Diseases, 37*(1)(Suppl. 2), s95-s98.

Gokal, R., Khanna, R., Krediet, R., & Nolph, K. (2000). *Textbook of peritoneal dialysis* (2nd ed.). London: Kluwer Academic Publishers.

Goldfarb-Rumyantzev, A.S., Leypoldt, J.K., Nelson, N., Kutner, N.G., & Cheung, A.K. (2006). A crossover study of short daily haemodialysis. *Nephrology Dialysis Transplantation, 21,* 166-175.

Gropper, R. (1998). Cultural basics and chronic illness. *Advances in Renal Replacement Therapy, 5,* 128-133.

Hartwood, L., & Leitch R. (2006). Home dialysis therapies. In A.E. Molzahn & E. Butera (Eds.), *Contemporary nephrology nursing: Principles and practice* (2nd ed., pp. 607-623). Pitman, NJ: American Nephrology Nurses' Association.

Heidenheim, A.P., Leitch, R., Kortas, C., & Lindsay, R.M. (2003). Patient monitoring in the London daily/nocturnal hemodialysis study. *American Journal of Kidney Diseases, 42*(Suppl. 1), 61-65.

Henderson, L. (2000). Future developments in the treatment of end-stage renal disease: A North American perspective. *American Journal of Kidney Diseases, 35*(4)(Suppl.), S106-S116.

Hodge, M.H. (2006). Why we need the option of more dialysis. *Nephrology News and Issues, 20*(11), 76-79.

Hoenich, N.A., Levin, N.W., & Levin, R. (2006). *High quality dialyate: Its importance to the dialysis patient.* Retrieved February 20, 2008, from http://www.aami.org/publications/HH/Dialysate.Hoenich.pdf

Hoenich, N.A., Ronco, C., & Levin, R. (2006). The importance of water quality and haemodialysis fluid composition. *Blood Purification, 24,* 11-18.

Kjellstrand, C.M., & Ing, T. (2006a). *Daily hemodialysis: Dialysis for the next century.* Retrieved February 20, 2008, from http://www.aksys.com/therapy/next_century.asp

Kjellstrand, C.M., & Ing, T. (2006b). *History and revival of a superior dialysis method.* Retrieved February 20, 2008, from http://www.aksys.com/therapy/superior_method.asp

Lee, H., Manns, B., Taub, K., Gali, W.A., Dean, S., Johnson, D., & Donaldson, C. (2002). Cost analysis of ongoing care of patients with end-stage renal disease: The impact of dialysis modality and dialysis access. *American Journal of Kidney Diseases, 40*(3), 611-622.

Leitch, R., & Ouwendyk, M. (2004). Patient training and education. In R.M. Lindsay (Ed.), *Daily and nocturnal hemodialysis* (pp. 39-47). Basel, Switzerland: Kargel.

Leitch, R., Ouwendyk, M., Ferguson, E., Clement, L., Peters, K., Heidenheim, A.P., et al. (2003). Nursing issues related to patient selection, vascular access, and education in quotidian hemodialysis. *American Journal of Kidney Diseases, 42*(Suppl. 1), 55-60.

Lindsay, R.M., Leitch, R., Heidenheim, A.P., & Kortas, C., (2003). The London daily/nocturnal hemodialysis study – Study design, morbidity and mortality results. *American Journal of Kidney Diseases, 42*(Suppl. 1), 5-12.

Luongo, M., & Kennedy, S. (2004). Interviewing prospective patients for peritoneal dialysis: A five step approach. *Nephrology Nursing Journal, 31*(5), 513-520.

Marquis, B., & Huston, C. (2003). *Leadership roles and management: Functions in nursing* (4th ed.). Philadelphia: Lippincott Williams & Wilkins.

McCormick, J. (2006). Relating to teaching and learning. In A.E. Molzahn & E. Butera (Eds.), *Contemporary nephrology nursing: Principles and practice* (2nd ed., pp. 885-902). Pitman, NJ: American Nephrology Nurses' Association.

McFarlane, P.A., Bayoumi, A.M., Pierratos, A., & Redelmeier, D.A. (2003). The quality of life and cost utility of home nocturnal and conventional in-center hemodialysis. *Kidney International, 64*, 1004-1011.

McLaughlin, K., Manns, B., Mortis, G., Hons, R., & Taub, K., (2003). Why patients with ESRD do not select self-care dialysis as a treatment option. *American Journal of Kidney Diseases, 41*(2), 380-385.

Mehrabian, S., Morgan, D., Schlaeper C., Kortas, C., & Lindsay, R.M. (2003). Equipment and water treatment considerations for the provision of quotidian home hemodialysis. *American Journal of Kidney Diseases, 42*(Suppl. 1), 66-70.

Mendelssohn, D. (2004). Empowerment of patient preference in dialysis modality selection. *American Journal of Kidney Diseases, 43*(5), 930-932.

Mendelssohn, D.C., Mullaney, S.R., Jung, B., Blake, P.G., & Mehta, R.L. (2001). What do American nephrologists think about dialysis modality selection? *American Journal of Kidney Diseases, 37*(1), 22-29.

Mohr, P.E., Neumann, P.J., Franco, S.J., Marainen, J., Lockridge R., & Ting, G. (2001). The case for daily dialysis: Its impact on costs and quality of life. *American Journal of Kidney Diseases, 37*(4), 777-789.

Molzahn, A.E., & Butera, E. (2006). *Contemporary nephrology nursing: Principles and practice* (2nd ed.). Pitman, NJ: American Nephrology Nurses' Association.

National Kidney Foundation (NKF). (2000). NKF-KDOQI clinical practice guidelines for peritoneal dialysis adequacy. *American Journal of Kidney Disease, 37*(Suppl. 1), 65-136.

National Kidney Foundation (NKF). (2006). NKF-K/DOQI *clinical practice guidelines for hemodialysis adequacy: Update 2006*. Retrieved February 20, 2008, from http://www.kidney.org/professionals/kdoqi/guidelines_upHD_PD_VA/index.htm

Oberley, E., & Schatell, D.R. (1995). *Home hemodialysis and patient outcomes*. Retrieved February 20, 2008, from http://eneph.com

Payne, G. (2006). *A surveyor's perspective: Water quality for hemodialysis*. Retrieved Retrieved February 20, 2008, from http://www.ami.org/publications/HH/Water.quality.Payne.pdf

Pierratos, A., Outwendyk, M., Francoeur, R., Wallace, L., Sit, W., Vas, S., & Uldall, R. (1995). *Slow nocturnal home hemodialysis*. Retrieved February 20, 2008, from http://eneph.com

Powderly, S. (2006). Lessons learned – One facility's experience with venturing into the home hemodialysis market. *Nephrology News and Issues, 20*(11), 70-75.

Raj, D.S.C., Charra, B., Pierratos, A., & Work, J. (1999). In search of ideal hemodialysis: Is prolonged frequent dialysis the answer? *American Journal of Kidney Diseases, 34*(4), 597-610.

Robinson, K. (2001). Does pre-ESRD education make a difference? The patient's perspective. *Dialysis and Transplantation, 30*(9), 571-574.

Ronco, C., Bowry, S., & Tetta, C. (2006). Dialysis patients and cardiovascular problems: Can technology help solve the complex equation? *Blood Purification, 24*, 39-45.

Schulman, G. (2003). Nutrition in daily dialysis. *American Journal of Kidney Diseases, 41*(Suppl. 3), S112-S115.

Scribner, B.H. (1990). A personalized history of hemodialysis. *American Journal of Kidney Disease, 15*, 215.

Shetty, A., & Oreopoulos, D. (2000). Peritoneal dialysis: Its indications and contraindications. *Dialysis and Transplantation, 29*(2), 71-77.

Shurraw, S., & Zimmerman, D. (2005). Vascular access complications in daily dialysis: A systematic review of the literature. *Minerva Urologica E Nephrologie, 57*, 151-63.

Stevens, J.E. (1996). Home hemodialysis – Yes it can be learned. *Advances in Renal Replacement Therapy, 3*(2), 120-123.

Suri, R.S., & Garg, A.X. (2006). Randomized trials of frequent hemodialysis – Infinite possibilities. *Blood Purification, 24*, 123-127.

Turk, J.E., Kenley, R., Sweeney, J., & Schatell D. (2006). Giving patients the choice of home therapy, *Nephrology News and Issues, 20*(11), 14-15.

Vaslaki, L., Major, L., Berta, K., Karatson, A., Misz, M., Pethoe, F., et al. (2005). On line hemofiltration versus haemodialysis: Stable haematocrit with less erthropoetin and improvement of other relevant blood parameters. *Blood Purfication, 24*(2), 163-73.

Ward, R.A., & Ronco, C. (2006). Dialyzer and machine technologies: Application of recent advances to clinical practice. *Blood Purification, 24*, 6-10.

Section 15

Care of the Infant through Adolescent with Chronic Kidney Disease

Section Editor

Nancy G. McAfee, MN, RN, CNN

Authors

Nancy G. McAfee, MN, RN, CNN

Cindy Richards, BSN, RN, CNN

Jodi M. Smith, MD, MPH

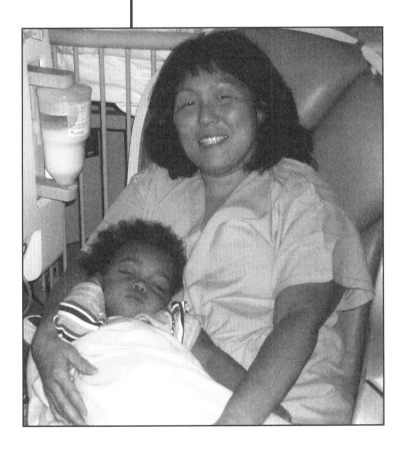

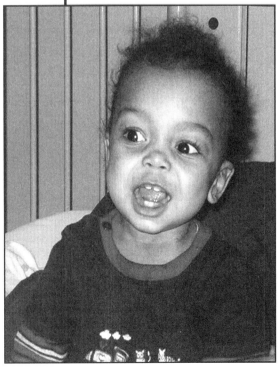

About the Authors

Nancy G. McAfee, MN, RN, CNN, Section Editor and Author, is a Dialysis Clinical Nurse Specialist at Children's Hospital & Regional Medical Center in Seattle, Washington.

Cindy Richards, BSN, RN, CNN, is a Pediatric Transplant Coordinator at Children's Hospital in Birmingham, Alabama.

Jodi M. Smith, MD, MPH, is an Assistant Professor of Pediatrics in the Division of Nephrology at the University of Washington Children's Hospital and Regional Medical Center in Seattle, Washington.

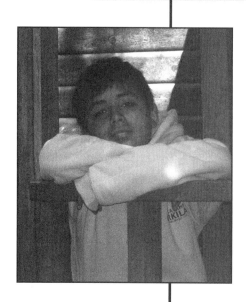

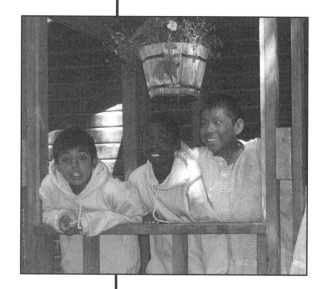

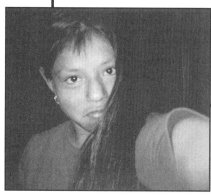

Photos by
Nancy G. McAfee

Section 15

Care of the Infant through Adolescent with Chronic Kidney Disease

Care of the Infant through Adolescent with Chronic Kidney Disease

Purpose

This section outlines the scope and challenges of caring for children from neonate through adolescence who have chronic kidney disease (CKD) stages 1-5. It differentiates their assessment and treatment from the adult care guidelines and assists in preparing and developing clinicians who treat children and adolescents with CKD.

Objectives

Upon completion of this section, the learner will be able to:
1. Discuss USRDS and NAPRTCS statistics related to pediatric CKD stage 5.
2. Recognize complications that arise from developmental failure in kidney formation.
3. Name two maturational factors limiting renal function in the developing embryo.
4. Discuss development of renal blood flow as it relates to glomerular filtration rate (GFR) after birth.
5. Discuss significance of standardized norms for comparison with other children at the same age.
6. Describe common causes of kidney disease in children.
7. Explain systemic effects of CKD on children.
8. Describe growth issues faced by children with CKD.
9. Discuss the psychosocial impact of CKD on the family.
10. Explain anticipatory guidance when working with families of chronically ill children.
11. List common causes of acute kidney failure in children.
12. Describe the effects of CKD on children.
13. Discuss specific psychosocial needs of children with CKD.
14. Describe challenges to the pediatric patient beginning PD.
15. Explain the specific needs of pediatric patients on HD.
16. Discuss a child's evaluation for transplantation.
17. List clinical issues relative to a pediatric patient beginning CRRT.
18. Describe indications for supplemental nutrition in children and identify ways of providing it.
19. Discuss renal osteodystrophy in the pediatric patient.
20. Define pediatric hypertension and management.
21. Discuss intradialytic hypotension prevention and management.
22. Assess a pediatric patient's readiness for transplantation.
23. Assess a pediatric patient's response to a hemodialysis treatment and assess dry weight.

Objectives continue on next page

Objectives, continued from previous page

24. List the most common causative organisms for peritonitis.
25. Discuss potential complications in pediatric patients on peritoneal dialysis.
26. Describe the potential cardiovascular changes seen in ESRD in pediatric patients.
27. Identify specific areas where anticipatory guidance is of benefit to the child with CKD.
28. Describe three key aspects of a transition to adult care program.

Chapter 67

Care of the Infant through Adolescent with Chronic Kidney Disease

History of Pediatric Nephrology

I. **The 1940s through 1960s.** Focused on the conservative management of CKD (e.g., dietary restrictions, diuretic therapy, electrolyte therapy, and antibacterial use).

II. **Beginning in the 1970s.**

A. Major university programs offered end-stage therapy.

B. Conservative therapy was still the most common approach.

C. Children responded differently to dialysis procedures than adults giving rise to specialized pediatric centers for the treatment of end-stage renal disease (ESRD).

III. **The 1980s brought widespread use of peritoneal dialysis (PD) modalities.**

A. Continuous ambulatory peritoneal dialysis (CAPD) programs for children were begun.

B. Automated systems allowed automated cycling peritoneal dialysis (APD) programs for infants and young children.

C. Early PD access was a hard plastic trocar that was inserted perpendicular to the abdomen and required complicated maneuvering and propping to keep it in position.

D. The hard trocar resulted in many complications including intraabdominal injury such as perforation, peritonitis, pain, and discomfort.

E. Introduction of the Tenckhoff catheter, a less rigid catheter, offered more comfort.

F. Dialysate was commercially prepared in large glass bottles that were heavy and required a warming bath to heat.

G. The development of plastic bags for dialysate made home APD possible.

IV. **The 1990s brought more changes.**

A. Smaller machines with computer technology were developed.

B. Removable data chips allowed the transport of treatment details to dialysis centers.

C. Some centers use modems to remotely download the treatment details.

V. **Hemodialysis (HD) was initially restricted to adult patients.**

A. HD blood lines were initially cut to create lower volume tubing for pediatric patients.

B. Ultrafiltration (UF) was calculated and transmembrane pressure (TMP) adjusted manually to achieve the desired goal for fluid removal.

C. Small patients required continuous weights to avoid excessive fluid loss.

D. The parallel plate dialyzer increased the extracorporeal circuit volume as venous pressure increased. In addition, it required a higher blood flow rate than most pediatric patients could tolerate.

E. Early dialysis catheters were single lumen that pulled a large volume into the extracorporeal circuit.

F. Acetate dialysate caused frequent emesis.

G. Frequent blood transfusions were required prior to the advent of erythropoetic-stimulating agents (ESA).

VI. CRRT modalities have been in use in children since the mid-1980s.

A. Early circuit attempts at continuous arterial-venous hemofiltration (CAVH) required a mean arterial pressure (MAP) of approximately 60 mmHg limiting the value for pediatric patients.

B. Pump systems made it possible to use double lumen venous lines with low speeds.

C. Volumetric systems with an integrated blood pump and UF controller made this therapy safe for children.

VII. By the end of the 1990s, the following milestones had been achieved.

A. Pediatric dialysis was recognized as a specialty with training programs worldwide.

B. Children can now safely receive care in pediatric centers and at home with a full range of treatment options available including transplantation.

ESRD

I. United States Renal Data System (USRDS) Annual Report 2006.

A. Prevalence: the number of children ages 0–19 years being treated for ESRD in 2004 was 1.5% of total ESRD population (7,272 of 472,099 patients).
   1. 1,354 pediatric patients were on hemodialysis.
   2. 957 pediatric patients were on peritoneal dialysis.
   3. 4,907 pediatric patients had functioning transplants.

B. Incidence: the number of children ages 0–19

starting therapy for ESRD.
   1. There were 1,366 children ages 0–19 in 2004.
   2. Between May 1995 and June 2004, more than 4,200 children started therapy for ESRD caused by either primary or secondary glomerulo-nephritis.
   3. Another 3,400 began treatment for ESRD caused by cystic kidney disease.

C. Preventive care measures for 4,237 pediatric patients, 0–19 years of age, initiating therapy between 2000 and 2004 included:
   1. Influenza vaccine given to 25% of the pediatric patients (HD patients 30%).
   2. Pneumococcal pneumonia vaccination administered to 8%.
   3. Hepatitis B vaccine given to 7% of total (15% of HD patients).
   4. Lipid screening performed in 50%.
   5. Serum albumin above normal range in 50%.
   6. ESA therapy begun prior to the initiation of dialysis in 39%. The mean Hb was 9.6 g/dL.

II. North American Pediatric Renal Trials and Collaborative Studies (NAPRTCS).

A. Voluntary research database collecting data on children < 21 years old.

B. 6,405 patients were registered from 113 centers (1/4/06).
   1. 4,071 patients have 12-month follow-up (FU) data.
   2. 2,817 patients have 24-month FU data.
   3. 1,028 patients have 60-month FU data.

C. There were 5,993 cases requiring dialysis initiation at age < 21 years (1/4/06).
   1. 2,131 HD.
   2. 3,858 PD.

D. There were 9,837 transplants reported in 8,990 patients.
   1. 4,380 (25%) were preemptive without an initial course of dialysis.
   2. 847 were repeat transplants.
   3. 52% were living donor transplants.

E. There were 6,405 cases of chronic renal insufficiency (CRI) registrations with NAPRTCS.

The Kidney – A Pediatric Perspective

I. Prenatal development.

A. Anatomy and physiology.
1. Urine production begins between 9 and 12 weeks of gestation, contributing to the formation of amniotic fluid.
2. The primary role of the kidneys in utero is development of amniotic fluid which is necessary for pulmonary development.
3. The primary responsibility in utero for fluid and electrolyte balance is the placenta.
4. Nephron development continues until 34 to 35 weeks gestation.
5. During the last trimester of pregnancy, there is rapid structural and functional development of the kidneys.

B. Maturational factors that limit renal function.
1. Glomerular filtration rate (GFR) is low at birth despite correction for body surface area (BSA).
2. Renal blood flow greatly increases during first week of postnatal life.
   a. At 28 weeks gestational age, the renal blood flow is 10 mL/min/m².
   b. By 35 weeks gestational age the rate is 35 mL/min/m².
3. Renal tubular immaturity leads to:
   a. Low capacity to vary sodium and water reabsorption.
   b. High fractional excretion of sodium (especially in preterm infants).
   c. Limited ability to concentrate urine.

C. Gestational history.
1. Oligohydramnios, too little amniotic fluid, suggests:
   a. Renal agenesis, which is the absence of the ureters, kidneys, and renal arteries.
   b. Renal hypoplasia (underdevelopment) or dysplasia (developmental or genetic defect with many levels of severity).
   c. Severe obstruction of urinary tract.
2. Lack of amniotic fluid around the fetus is responsible for the nonrenal features of Potter's syndrome (malformation or total absence of infant kidneys) including:
   a. Dysmorphic or altered appearance of facies.
   b. Aberrant hand and foot positioning.
   c. Pulmonary hypoplasia (incomplete development of lung tissue).
   d. Late fetal growth deficiency.

3. Polyhydramnios (too much amniotic fluid) suggests:
   a. Severe swallowing difficulties caused by neurologic disturbances or upper alimentary tract obstructive disorders.
   b. Up to 50% of patients with esophageal atresia or tracheoesophageal fistula also have renal malformations.

II. Postnatal development.

A. Development of renal blood flow (RBF).
1. Within 24 hours after birth, renal vascular resistance decreases.
2. RBF increases to 15% of the cardiac output.

B. Development of GFR.
1. RBF to the outer cortical areas increases at 36 weeks.
2. Positive pressure mechanical ventilation and CPAP can impair renal perfusion.
3. Nephron formation is complete in term infants.
4. Preterm infants will continue to develop nephrons until 36 weeks postconception age.

C. Serum creatinine concentration.
1. At birth will be equal to the mother's serum creatinine.
2. In term infants will fall to 0.4–0.5 mg/dL by 5–7 days.
3. Preterm infants may remain at 1.0–1.5 mg/dL for several weeks of life.

D. Postnatal changes in body fluid composition.
1. Total body water (TBW) normally decreases after birth related to diuresis (1–8 mL/kg/hr).
2. Diuresis (in days) depends on:
   a. The degree of excess fluid present at birth.
   b. The degree of prematurity (more premature infants have greater extracellular fluid (ECF) thus have less diuresis).
   c. Hemodynamic changes as cardiac output increases to the kidneys and pulmonary circulation opens.
   d. Decrease in circulating antidiuretic hormone (ADH) levels after delivery.

E. Tubular function.
1. The functional maturation of the nephron is age rather than body weight dependent.
2. Increase in tubular length continues until 6 months of age.
3. The reduced ability of the kidney to reabsorb sodium and water decreases its ability to concentrate urine.

4. Large amounts of electrolytes and nitrogen are retained to meet growth needs.
5. Hydrogen ion excretion is reduced for first year of life.
6. Infants less than 30 weeks of age at birth may develop hyponatremia or hypernatremia due to lower distal tubular reabsorption.
7. Infants achieve positive K+ balance within 10 days of birth if fed orally.
8. Urinary K+ may remain high if formula fed as body excretes excess K+.

Assessment of Kidney Structure and Function in CKD

I. History and physical.

A. The approach used to obtain a health history and perform a physical examination varies according to the age of the child.

B. Developmental age-appropriate care is outlined in Table 15.1.

Table 15.1

Developmental Age-Appropriate Care: Preparation/Education/Activity

Developmental Age	Nursing Interventions
0–12 months (infant)	• Support parents' ability to calm/comfort infant by providing parent(s) with adequate information and preparation to reduce their own anxiety. • Provide opportunities for the parent(s) to hold the infant.
12–24 months (toddler)	• Support parents' ability to calm/comfort toddler by providing parent(s) with adequate information and preparation to reduce their own anxiety. • Encourage parent(s) to involve toddler in developmentally appropriate scheduled activities. • Whenever safe and possible, allow toddler to handle items used in his/her care (e.g., blood pressure cuff, face mask). • Offer suggestions to parent(s) about helpful distractions during procedures. If parent(s) are unavailable, offer comfort and/or distraction as appropriate. • Stoop to the child's eye level (face-to-face) and speak softly and calmly.
2–3 years (toddler)	• Support parents ability to calm and comfort toddler by providing parent(s) with adequate information and preparation to reduce their own anxiety. • Encourage parents to use age-appropriate activity areas when available. Activity areas can include a playroom, playground, garden, library, school room, and/or teen room. • Actively involve child in treatment. Whenever safe, allow child to handle/examine equipment used in treatments/procedures. • Provide comfort and/or distraction during tests and procedures. Preparation should begin immediately preceding the event. • Give the child simple explanations of tests, procedures, using the sensory approach (i.e., what child will see, hear, taste, feel). • Provide choices whenever possible (e.g., examine eyes or ears first). • Stoop to the child's eye level (face-to-face) and speak softly and calmly
3–5 years (preschooler)	• Be honest. • Actively involve child in treatment. • Whenever safe, allow child to handle and explore medical equipment prior to use (e.g., peritoneal dialysis catheter). • Provide comfort and/or distraction during and after tests/procedures. • Use interventions that preserve the child's concept of body integrity (e.g., child-friendly bandages for venipuncture sites).

Continues on next page

Table 15.1 (continued)	Developmental Age-Appropriate Care: Preparation/Education/Activity
3–5 years (preschooler) (continued from previous page)	• Give the child short simple explanations of tests and procedures using the sensory approach (e.g., what child will see, hear, taste, feel). Ask for feedback. • Preparation should be done far enough in advance for child to process information, but not too far in advance so that child has time to fantasize — preferably a few hours before the test or procedure. • Encourage child to participate in age-appropriate activities. • Provide choices whenever possible (e.g., which ear to examine first). • Stoop to or sit at the child's eye level (face-to-face) and speak softly and calmly.
6–9 years (school-age)	• Be honest. • Encourage choices among options if possible (e.g., IV in right or left hand for the peritoneal dialysis patient receiving IV medication therapy). • Whenever safe, allow child to handle and explore medical equipment before use. • Provide comfort and/or distraction during and after tests or procedures. • Give the child developmentally appropriate explanations of tests and procedures using the sensory approach (e.g., what child will see, hear, taste, feel). Ask for feedback. • Preparation should be done far enough in advance for child to process information, but not too far in advance so that child has time to fantasize. • Encourage child to participate in age-appropriate activities. • Provide choices whenever possible (e.g., which limb for venipuncture).
9–12 years (pre-teen)	• Provide honest and accurate information about potential tests/procedures/treatments, etc. Ask for feedback about what the preteen understands. • Provide developmentally appropriate explanations using the sensory approach (e.g., what the patient will see, hear, feel, etc.). • Provide comfort and/or distraction as needed during procedures that may be uncomfortable or painful. • Encourage participation in decision making whenever possible. • Be clear about what expectations are in terms of learning/self-care/adherence. • Preparation should be done far enough in advance for child to process information. • Provide choices whenever possible (e.g., choices that lead to having some control such as you or I applying tape).
13–18 years (adolescent)	• Provide rationale for treatment. Get feedback regarding adolescent's understanding of tests/procedures/disease process and treatment plans. • Encourage adolescents to take responsibility for aspect of self-care. Provide positive reinforcement for successes. • It is important to prepare adolescent for what he/she will see, hear, feel, taste, and smell, and be expected to do.

C. Providing preventive advice or anticipatory guidance for the parents is an important component of providing care.

II. Developmental age-appropriate care (see Table 15.1).

A. Growth and development are continuous dynamic processes involving genetics, nutrition, physical, and psychological factors.

B. Privacy is important to children.
1. Adolescents have a growing need for privacy and an opportunity to discuss their growing sexuality, or lack thereof.
2. Discussions must take place about safe sexual practices and possible birth control. Many may not have a primary care provider (PCP).

C. Play therapy can facilitate trust especially for younger children.
1. Children are often able to verbalize more while involved in play.
2. Use opportunities while playing to ask questions about the child's understanding of illness, diet, therapy options, etc.

D. Child life specialists can play a vital supporting role in a dialysis clinic or unit.
   1. These trained specialists use play, biofeedback, and distraction during painful or uncomfortable procedures.
   2. Some children can learn self-calming techniques for coping.

III. Standardized norms are used for comparison to other children at same age.

A. Weight is measured and plotted on a standardized growth chart at each visit. The child should follow a standardized growth curve.

B. Height should be measured at least quarterly and plotted on a standardized growth chart (see Figures 15.1 and 15.2).

C. Head circumference is recorded routinely until age 3 years.

D. Failure to thrive or grow on dialysis may indicate an urgent need for transplantation.

E. Respiratory rate, pulse, and temperature are recorded at each visit.

F. Blood pressure (BP) (see Tables 15.2 and 15.3).
   1. Annual measurements should be recorded on all children 3 years of age and older. If there is known kidney disease, the BP should be measured at an earlier age.
   2. An appropriate size cuff is necessary to obtain an accurate reading.
      a. The cuff width should be 40% of midarm circumference.
      b. The cuff bladder should cover 80% to 100% of the arm circumference and approximately two thirds the length of upper arm.
      c. A cuff that is too small will result in a falsely elevated blood pressure reading.
   3. Measurement should be performed with a sphygmomanometer or a calibrated aneroid device with the child sitting and his or her right arm resting on a solid supporting surface at heart level.
   4. Blood pressure measurements in noncooperative, agitated children are misleading. Attempts must be made to obtain reliable resting measurements. If the child is not quiet, his/her status should be recorded with the blood pressure reading.
   5. Primary hypertension is detectable in the young, occurring in up to 5–10% of children and adolescents.
   6. Hypertension is defined as average systolic (SBP) and/or diastolic BP (DBP) that is greater than the 95th percentile for gender, age, and height on more than three occasions.
   7. Prehypertension in children is defined as average SBP or DBP levels that are greater than the 90th percentile but less than the 95th percentile.
   8. As with adults, adolescents with BP levels greater than 120/80 mm Hg should be considered prehypertensive.
   9. Elevated BP must be confirmed on repeated visits before characterizing a child as having hypertension.

IV. Health history and physical examination vary according to age of the child. Some special considerations for different age groups include the following:

A. 0–12 months (infant).
   1. Observe for potential congenital abnormalities or birth injuries.
   2. Assess for growth in terms of length, weight, and head circumference should be made frequently. The most rapid growth rate in life occurs during this time period.
   3. The development of gross and fine motor skills, language, and social interaction should be assessed and compared to normal expectations for age. Denver II is a good developmental screening tool and is available in *The Harriett Lane Handbook*, 17th ed.

B. 12–36 months (toddler).
   1. Assess growth and development frequently, as for the infant.
   2. Enormous rates of developmental change and a wide range of normal development are observed and require cautious conclusion about delayed development. This is an exploratory stage with many behavioral changes.
   3. Respect parental concern about visual and hearing acuity, eye muscle coordination, and autistic behaviors as these affect the child's long-term adaptive potential.
   4. Provide anticipatory guidance regarding:
      a. Sleeping patterns.
      b. Weaning from the bottle.
      c. Injury prevention.
      d. Dental hygiene.
      e. Toilet training and/or regression with illness or sibling birth.
      f. Separation issues.

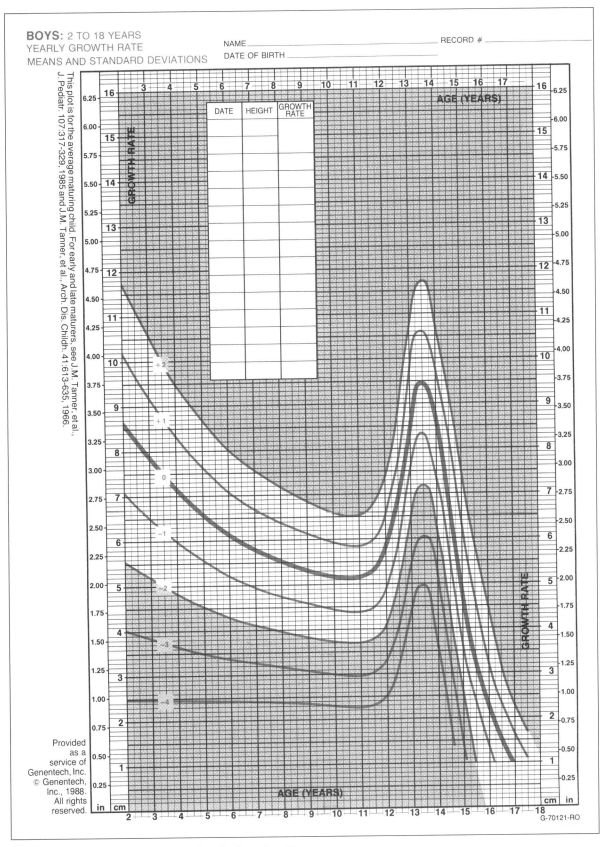

Figure 15.1. Growth velocity chart for boys 2 to 18 years.

Used with permission from Genentech, Inc.

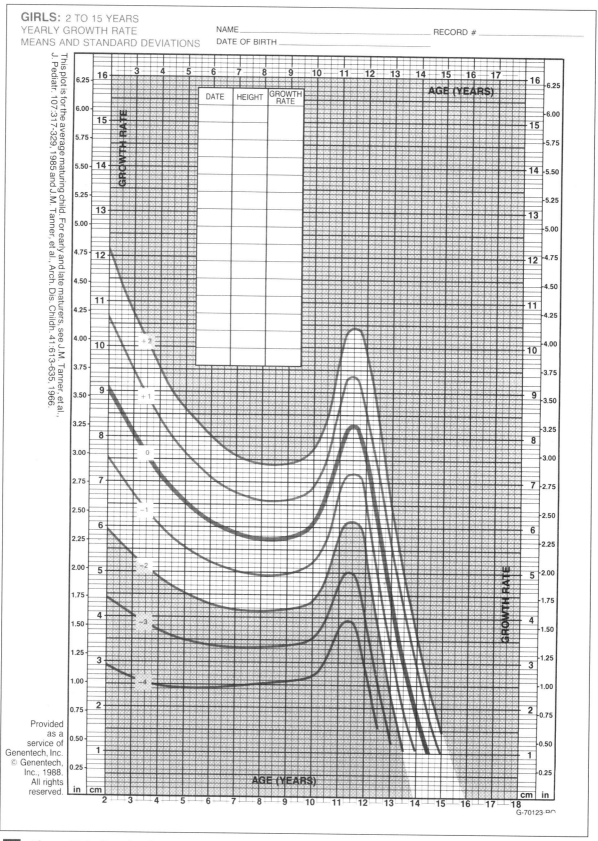

Figure 15.2. Growth velocity chart for girls 2 to 15 years.

Used with permission from Genentech, Inc.

C. 4–5 years (preschooler).
1. Survey for normal but slower growth, which continues until puberty.
2. Formal vision and hearing screening can be tested in this age group.
3. Identify delays in normal development that might be helped by early childhood intervention programs available in most school systems.
4. Investigate extremes of uncooperative behaviors toward examiner as these might indicate signs of abnormal development or environmental stresses.
5. Provide anticipatory guidance regarding:
    a. Egocentricity.
    b. Resistance to parental authority; may need to discuss setting limits and consistent discipline.
    c. Injury prevention.
    d. Vivid imagination; may need to help differentiate between imagery and lies.

D. 6–10 years (school-age).
1. Begin to elicit aspects of the medical history from the child as well as from the parent or caregiver.
2. Inquire about participation in activities that can promote physical fitness.
3. Discuss nutrition, food preferences, and appetite.
4. Assess dental health and eruption of permanent teeth.
5. The development of peer groups begins in this age group.
6. Mood changes and increasing need for privacy emerge.
7. Provide anticipatory guidance regarding:
    a. Safety.
    b. Nutrition.
    c. Substance abuse.
    d. Injury prevention.

E. 11–12 years (preteen).
1. Attempt more sophisticated information gathering from the child for history.
2. Question the patient alone about knowledge of at-risk behaviors, including smoking, alcohol and other substance abuse, and sexual activity.
3. Provide anticipatory guidance regarding:
    a. Onset of puberty.
    b. Changes in body image.
    c. Peer group interaction.

F. 13–18 years (adolescent).
1. Observe for appearance and maturation of secondary sexual characteristics. Use Tanner stages of development in evaluation of pubertal development. (Convenient tables with criteria are available in the Adolescent Medicine section of *The Harriett Lane Handbook*, 17th ed.)
2. Observe for pubertal growth spurt. Consider more frequent visits during this time frame to evaluate the effects of kidney disease as the child's growth is rapidly increasing.
3. Obtain history of onset and regularity of menses.
4. Examine for acne, scoliosis, changes in visual acuity, dental caries, and thyromegaly.
5. Question patient alone about at-risk behaviors including sexual activity and smoking, alcohol, and other substance abuse.
6. Address obesity and anorexia issues.
7. Provide anticipatory guidance regarding:
    a. Sex education.
    b. Effects of experimentation with alcohol, drugs, cigarettes, etc.
    c. Hygiene and dental care.
    d. Nutrition.
    e. Exercise.
    f. Safety issues.

V. **Physical examination by systems.**

A. General survey.
1. Alertness, awareness of surroundings, ability to cooperate, evidence of distress.
2. Symmetry, spacing, and position of facial features.
3. Positioning and posture.
4. Assessment of size for age and growth curve.

B. Skin.
1. Inspect for rashes, especially in the diaper area.
2. Pigmented, vascular, soft tissue lesions, or skin defects overlying the spine should raise suspicion of an underlying neurologic disorder.
3. Test tissue turgor and elasticity by gently pinching a fold of abdominal skin and assessing how rapidly it returns to its normal state.
4. Inspect hands and feet for skin creases and missing or fused digits.
5. Unusual bruising may be kidney related or signs of abuse.

C. Head, eyes, ears, nose, and throat (HEENT).
1. Inspect and palpate head and scalp noting symmetry of shape, bulges or swelling, dilated scalp veins, lesions, lacerations, or protuberances.
2. Palpate fontanelles and noting early closure or atypical features.

Table 15.2

Blood Pressure Levels for Boys by Age and Height Percentile

Age (Year)	BP Percentile ↓	Systolic BP (mmHg) ← Percentile of Height →							Diastolic BP (mmHg) ← Percentile of Height →						
		5th	10th	25th	50th	75th	90th	95th	5th	10th	25th	50th	75th	90th	95th
1	50th	80	81	83	85	87	88	89	34	35	36	37	38	39	39
	90th	94	95	97	99	100	102	103	49	50	51	52	53	53	54
	95th	98	99	101	103	104	106	106	54	54	55	56	57	58	58
	99th	105	106	108	110	112	113	114	61	62	63	64	65	66	66
2	50th	84	85	87	88	90	92	92	39	40	41	42	43	44	44
	90th	97	99	100	102	104	105	106	54	55	56	57	58	58	59
	95th	101	102	104	106	108	109	110	59	59	60	61	62	63	63
	99th	109	110	111	113	115	117	117	66	67	68	69	70	71	71
3	50th	86	87	89	91	93	94	95	44	44	45	46	47	48	48
	90th	100	101	103	105	107	108	109	59	59	60	61	62	63	63
	95th	104	105	107	109	110	112	113	63	63	64	65	66	67	67
	99th	111	112	114	116	118	119	120	71	71	72	73	74	75	75
4	50th	88	89	91	93	95	96	97	47	48	49	50	51	51	52
	90th	102	103	105	107	109	110	111	62	63	64	65	66	66	67
	95th	106	107	109	111	112	114	115	66	67	68	69	70	71	71
	99th	113	114	116	118	120	121	122	74	75	76	77	78	78	79
5	50th	90	91	93	95	96	98	98	50	51	52	53	54	55	55
	90th	104	105	106	108	110	111	112	65	66	67	68	69	69	70
	95th	108	109	110	112	114	115	116	69	70	71	72	73	74	74
	99th	115	116	118	120	121	123	123	77	78	79	80	81	81	82
6	50th	91	92	94	96	98	99	100	53	53	54	55	56	57	57
	90th	105	106	108	110	111	113	113	68	68	69	70	71	72	72
	95th	109	110	112	114	115	117	117	72	72	73	74	75	76	76
	99th	116	117	119	121	123	124	125	80	80	81	82	83	84	84
7	50th	92	94	95	97	99	100	101	55	55	56	57	58	59	59
	90th	106	107	109	111	113	114	115	70	70	71	72	73	74	74
	95th	110	111	113	115	117	118	119	74	74	75	76	77	78	78
	99th	117	118	120	122	124	125	126	82	82	83	84	85	86	86
8	50th	94	95	97	99	100	102	102	56	57	58	59	60	60	61
	90th	107	109	110	112	114	115	116	71	72	72	73	74	75	76
	95th	111	112	114	116	118	119	120	75	76	77	78	79	79	80
	99th	119	120	122	123	125	127	127	83	84	85	86	87	87	88
9	50th	95	96	98	100	102	103	104	57	58	59	60	61	61	62
	90th	109	110	112	114	115	117	118	72	73	74	75	76	76	77
	95th	113	114	116	118	119	121	121	76	77	78	79	80	81	81
	99th	120	121	123	125	127	128	129	84	85	86	87	88	88	89
10	50th	97	98	100	102	103	105	106	58	59	60	61	61	62	63
	90th	111	112	114	115	117	119	119	73	73	74	75	76	77	78
	95th	115	116	117	119	121	122	123	77	78	79	80	81	81	82
	99th	122	123	125	127	128	130	130	85	86	86	88	88	89	90

The Fourth Report on the Diagnosis, Evaluation, and Treatment of High Blood Pressure in Children and Adolescents

Continues on next page

Table 15.2 (continued)

Blood Pressure Levels for Boys by Age and Height Percentile

Age (Year)	BP Percentile ↓	Systolic BP (mmHg) ← Percentile of Height →							Diastolic BP (mmHg) ← Percentile of Height →						
		5th	10th	25th	50th	75th	90th	95th	5th	10th	25th	50th	75th	90th	95th
11	50th	99	100	102	104	105	107	107	59	59	60	61	62	63	63
	90th	113	114	115	117	119	120	121	74	74	75	76	77	78	78
	95th	117	118	119	121	123	124	125	78	78	79	80	81	82	82
	99th	124	125	127	129	130	132	132	86	86	87	88	89	90	90
12	50th	101	102	104	106	108	109	110	59	60	61	62	63	63	64
	90th	115	116	118	120	121	123	123	74	75	75	76	77	78	79
	95th	119	120	122	123	125	127	127	78	79	80	81	82	82	83
	99th	126	127	129	131	133	134	135	86	87	88	89	90	90	91
13	50th	104	105	106	108	110	111	112	60	60	61	62	63	64	64
	90th	117	118	120	122	124	125	126	75	75	76	77	78	79	79
	95th	121	122	124	126	128	129	130	79	79	80	81	82	83	83
	99th	128	130	131	133	135	136	137	87	87	88	89	90	91	91
14	50th	106	107	109	111	113	114	115	60	61	62	63	64	65	65
	90th	120	121	123	125	126	128	128	75	76	77	78	79	79	80
	95th	124	125	127	128	130	132	132	80	80	81	82	83	84	84
	99th	131	132	134	136	138	139	140	87	88	89	90	91	92	92
15	50th	109	110	112	113	115	117	117	61	62	63	64	65	66	66
	90th	122	124	125	127	129	130	131	76	77	78	79	80	80	81
	95th	126	127	129	131	133	134	135	81	81	82	83	84	85	85
	99th	134	135	136	138	140	142	142	88	89	90	91	92	93	93
16	50th	111	112	114	116	118	119	120	63	63	64	65	66	67	67
	90th	125	126	128	130	131	133	134	78	78	79	80	81	82	82
	95th	129	130	132	134	135	137	137	82	83	83	84	85	86	87
	99th	136	137	139	141	143	144	145	90	90	91	92	93	94	94
17	50th	114	115	116	118	120	121	122	65	66	66	67	68	69	70
	90th	127	128	130	132	134	135	136	80	80	81	82	83	84	84
	95th	131	132	134	136	138	139	140	84	85	86	87	87	88	89
	99th	139	140	141	143	145	146	147	92	93	93	94	95	96	97

BP, blood pressure

* The 90th percentile is 1.28 SD, 95th percentile is 1.645 SD, and the 99th percentile is 2.326 SD over the mean. For research purposes, the standard deviations in appendix table B–1 allow one to compute BP Z-scores and percentiles for boys with height percentiles given in table 3 (i.e., the 5th, 10th, 25th, 50th, 75th, 90th, and 95th percentiles). These height percentiles must be converted to height Z-scores given by (5% = -1.645; 10% = -1.28; 25% = -0.68; 50% = 0; 75% = 0.68; 90% = 1.28; 95% = 1.645) and then computed according to the methodology in steps 2–4 described in appendix B. For children with height percentiles other than these, follow steps 1–4 as described in appendix B.

Source: National High Blood Pressure Education Program Working Group on High Blood Pressure in Children and Adolescents. (2004). The fourth report on the diagnosis, evaluation, and treatment of high blood pressure in children and adolescents. *Pediatrics, 114*(2), 555-576. Used with permission.

Table 15.3

Blood Pressure Levels for Girls by Age and Height Percentile

Age (Year)	BP Percentile ↓	Systolic BP (mmHg) ← Percentile of Height →							Diastolic BP (mmHg) ← Percentile of Height →						
		5th	10th	25th	50th	75th	90th	95th	5th	10th	25th	50th	75th	90th	95th
1	50th	83	84	85	86	88	89	90	38	39	39	40	41	41	42
	90th	97	97	98	100	101	102	103	52	53	53	54	55	55	56
	95th	100	101	102	104	105	106	107	56	57	57	58	59	59	60
	99th	108	108	109	111	112	113	114	64	64	65	65	66	67	67
2	50th	85	85	87	88	89	91	91	43	44	44	45	46	46	47
	90th	98	99	100	101	103	104	105	57	58	58	59	60	61	61
	95th	102	103	104	105	107	108	109	61	62	62	63	64	65	65
	99th	109	110	111	112	114	115	116	69	69	70	70	71	72	72
3	50th	86	87	88	89	91	92	93	47	48	48	49	50	50	51
	90th	100	100	102	103	104	106	106	61	62	62	63	64	64	65
	95th	104	104	105	107	108	109	110	65	66	66	67	68	68	69
	99th	111	111	113	114	115	116	117	73	73	74	74	75	76	76
4	50th	88	88	90	91	92	94	94	50	50	51	52	52	53	54
	90th	101	102	103	104	106	107	108	64	64	65	66	67	67	68
	95th	105	106	107	108	110	111	112	68	68	69	70	71	71	72
	99th	112	113	114	115	117	118	119	76	76	76	77	78	79	79
5	50th	89	90	91	93	94	95	96	52	53	53	54	55	55	56
	90th	103	103	105	106	107	109	109	66	67	67	68	69	69	70
	95th	107	107	108	110	111	112	113	70	71	71	72	73	73	74
	99th	114	114	116	117	118	120	120	78	78	79	79	80	81	81
6	50th	91	92	93	94	96	97	98	54	54	55	56	56	57	58
	90th	104	105	106	108	109	110	111	68	68	69	70	70	71	72
	95th	108	109	110	111	113	114	115	72	72	73	74	74	75	76
	99th	115	116	117	119	120	121	122	80	80	80	81	82	83	83
7	50th	93	93	95	96	97	99	99	55	56	56	57	58	58	59
	90th	106	107	108	109	111	112	113	69	70	70	71	72	72	73
	95th	110	111	112	113	115	116	116	73	74	74	75	76	76	77
	99th	117	118	119	120	122	123	124	81	81	82	82	83	84	84
8	50th	95	95	96	98	99	100	101	57	57	57	58	59	60	60
	90th	108	109	110	111	113	114	114	71	71	71	72	73	74	74
	95th	112	112	114	115	116	118	118	75	75	75	76	77	78	78
	99th	119	120	121	122	123	125	125	82	82	83	83	84	85	86
9	50th	96	97	98	100	101	102	103	58	58	58	59	60	61	61
	90th	110	110	112	113	114	116	116	72	72	72	73	74	75	75
	95th	114	114	115	117	118	119	120	76	76	76	77	78	79	79
	99th	121	121	123	124	125	127	127	83	83	84	84	85	86	87
10	50th	98	99	100	102	103	104	105	59	59	59	60	61	62	62
	90th	112	112	114	115	116	118	118	73	73	73	74	75	76	76
	95th	116	116	117	119	120	121	122	77	77	77	78	79	80	80
	99th	123	123	125	126	127	129	129	84	84	85	86	86	87	88

2   The Fourth Report on the Diagnosis, Evaluation, and Treatment of High Blood Pressure in Children and Adolescents

Continues on next page

Table 15.3 (continued)

Blood Pressure Levels for Girls by Age and Height Percentile

Age (Year)	BP Percentile ↓	Systolic BP (mmHg) ← Percentile of Height →							Diastolic BP (mmHg) ← Percentile of Height →						
		5th	10th	25th	50th	75th	90th	95th	5th	10th	25th	50th	75th	90th	95th
11	50th	100	101	102	103	105	106	107	60	60	60	61	62	63	63
	90th	114	114	116	117	118	119	120	74	74	74	75	76	77	77
	95th	118	118	119	121	122	123	124	78	78	78	79	80	81	81
	99th	125	125	126	128	129	130	131	85	85	86	87	87	88	89
12	50th	102	103	104	105	107	108	109	61	61	61	62	63	64	64
	90th	116	116	117	119	120	121	122	75	75	75	76	77	78	78
	95th	119	120	121	123	124	125	126	79	79	79	80	81	82	82
	99th	127	127	128	130	131	132	133	86	86	87	88	88	89	90
13	50th	104	105	106	107	109	110	110	62	62	62	63	64	65	65
	90th	117	118	119	121	122	123	124	76	76	76	77	78	79	79
	95th	121	122	123	124	126	127	128	80	80	80	81	82	83	83
	99th	128	129	130	132	133	134	135	87	87	88	89	89	90	91
14	50th	106	106	107	109	110	111	112	63	63	63	64	65	66	66
	90th	119	120	121	122	124	125	125	77	77	77	78	79	80	80
	95th	123	123	125	126	127	129	129	81	81	81	82	83	84	84
	99th	130	131	132	133	135	136	136	88	88	89	90	90	91	92
15	50th	107	108	109	110	111	113	113	64	64	64	65	66	67	67
	90th	120	121	122	123	125	126	127	78	78	78	79	80	81	81
	95th	124	125	126	127	129	130	131	82	82	82	83	84	85	85
	99th	131	132	133	134	136	137	138	89	89	90	91	91	92	93
16	50th	108	108	110	111	112	114	114	64	64	65	66	66	67	68
	90th	121	122	123	124	126	127	128	78	78	79	80	81	81	82
	95th	125	126	127	128	130	131	132	82	82	83	84	85	85	86
	99th	132	133	134	135	137	138	139	90	90	90	91	92	93	93
17	50th	108	109	110	111	113	114	115	64	65	65	66	67	67	68
	90th	122	122	123	125	126	127	128	78	79	79	80	81	81	82
	95th	125	126	127	129	130	131	132	82	83	83	84	85	85	86
	99th	133	133	134	136	137	138	139	90	90	91	91	92	93	93

BP, blood pressure

* The 90th percentile is 1.28 SD, 95th percentile is 1.645 SD, and the 99th percentile is 2.326 SD over the mean. For research purposes, the standard deviations in appendix table B–1 allow one to compute BP Z-scores and percentiles for girls with height percentiles given in table 4 (i.e., the 5th, 10th, 25th, 50th, 75th, 90th, and 95th percentiles). These height percentiles must be converted to height Z-scores given by (5% = -1.645; 10% = -1.28; 25% = -0.68; 50% = 0; 75% = 0.68; 90% = 1.28; 95% = 1.645) and then computed according to the methodology in steps 2–4 described in appendix B. For children with height percentiles other than these, follow steps 1–4 as described in appendix B.

Source: National High Blood Pressure Education Program Working Group on High Blood Pressure in Children and Adolescents. (2004). The fourth report on the diagnosis, evaluation, and treatment of high blood pressure in children and adolescents. *Pediatrics, 114*(2), 555-576. Used with permission.

3. Texture, absence, or abundance of scalp hair may suggest an underlying problem.
4. Measure frontal occipital circumference (FOC) until age 3 years and plot on growth grid to assess for trends.
5. Inspect ears for shape, position, and alignment. Perform an exam with an otoscope.
6. Assess hearing. Gross hearing can be assessed by observing infant's or child's physical response to sound. Older children may cooperate with a whisper test.
7. Inspect eyes for size, shape, position, distance between, epicanthal folds, conjunctivae, sclerae (should be white), pupils, swelling, discharge, or excessive tearing.
8. Observe the eyes for tracking. This can also be done in infants.
9. Assess the pupil's response to light, corneal reflex, red reflex. Perform an exam with an ophthalmoscope. Younger children may not cooperate with an exam using an ophthalmoscope. However, after about age 3–4 years they can be taught to cooperate with repetitive examination.
10. Observe teeth for development and dentition.

D. Lymph nodes.
1. Examination of lymph nodes includes anterior/posterior cervical, occipital, and inguinal nodes. Attention should be given to size, mobility, tenderness, temperature, and condition of overlying skin.
2. Ages 2 to early adolescent. Superficial, enlarged, freely movable, nontender lymph nodes are easily palpable.
3. Normally supraclavicular and inguinal nodes are not palpable.

E. Musculoskeletal.
1. Inspect alignment, symmetry of size, and length of extremities. Observe for unusual masses, protuberances, and joint deformities.
2. Observe voluntary movements, flexion. Observe for unusual flacidity or spasticity of extremities.
3. Examine chest structure, spinal alignment, and structural symmetry. Inspect symmetry of gluteal folds.
4. Inspect for scoliosis, lumbar lordosis, or thoracic kyphosis.
5. Palpate bones, muscles, and joints. Assess muscle mass. Palpate to determine areas of tenderness and swelling. Examine hips for evidence of joint dislocation in infants until independently walking.

6. Observe gait. Note limp or waddle. Observe standing and sitting posture.
7. The function of joints, range of motion (ROM), bone stability, and muscle strength can be adequately evaluated by observing a child play.

F. Cardiovascular.
1. Assess chest for symmetry.
2. Palpate chest and precordium. Locate the apical pulse and the point of maximum impulse (PMI). Note any thrills, tap, or heave.
3. Auscultate each cardiac area for S1 and S2, splitting, and murmurs.
   a. Murmurs in children are frequent and require differentiation between innocent benign murmurs and pathologic murmurs.
   b. Innocent murmurs are usually soft, short, musical, midsystolic, and heard best in left second and third intercostal spaces.
   c. Pathologic murmurs may be accompanied by signs of cardiovascular disease, i.e., cyanosis or clubbing.
4. Note the rate and rhythm of the apical pulse. Normal range varies with age. Heart rate in beats per minute (bpm):
   Newborn 120–170 bpm
   1 year 80–160 bpm
   3 years 80–120 bpm
   6 years 75–115 bpm
   10 years 70–110 bpm
5. Palpate the brachial and radial pulses.
6. Inspect nails for clubbing and assess capillary refill.
7. Palpate inguinal area for femoral pulses.
8. Measure blood pressure (BP).
   a. Compare to BP standards for age (see Tables 15.2 and 15.3 on previous four pages).
   b. Single BP readings are not sufficient to diagnosis hypertension.
   c. Children with values between the 95th and 99th percentiles are classified as having significant hypertension. When above the 99th percentile, they are considered to have severe hypertension.

G. Pulmonary.
1. Inspect the chest, noting size and shape.
2. Observe the rate, rhythm, and depth of respiration. Note symmetry of chest expansion with respiration.

3. Count the respiratory rate in breaths per minute. The normal range varies with age:

Newborn	30–80 breaths per minute
1 year	20–40 breaths per minute
3 years	20–40 breaths per minute
6 years	16–22 breaths per minute
10 years	16–20 breaths per minute
17 years	12–20 breaths per minute

4. Auscultate the breath sounds. Bronchovesicular breath sounds are normally heard because a child's chest is more resonant. Note wheezes, crackles, rubs, prolonged expiration, or prolonged inspiration.

H. Abdomen.
1. Inspect shape, symmetry, configuration, umbilicus, contour, and movement with respiration. Note pulsations or distended veins.
2. Note abdominal protrusion of hernias through umbilicus or rectus abdominis muscle with straining.
3. Auscultate each quadrant for bowel sounds. Bruit or venous hums are abnormal.
4. Palpate lightly and deeply. Note size of liver, spleen, kidney, bladder, masses, or tenderness.
5. Percuss each quadrant of the abdomen.

I. Genitourinary.
1. Inspect genitalia.
   a. Females.
      (1) Inspect labia, clitoris, vaginal introitus, and urethral meatus.
      (2) Determine Tanner pubertal development stage. (Convenient tables with criteria are available in the Adolescent Medicine section of *The Harriett Lane Handbook*, 17th ed.)
   b. Males.
      (1) Observe penile length, foreskin, location of urethral meatus, scrotal anatomy, presence and location of testes, and presence of abnormal scrotal or inguinal masses.
      (2) Determine Tanner pubertal development stage. (Convenient tables with criteria are available in the Adolescent Medicine section of *The Harriett Lane Handbook*, 17th ed.)
2. Rectum.
   a. Inspect anal region and perineum for tags, dimples, redness, masses, swelling, or abscesses.
   b. Digital rectal exam is not usually performed. Deviation from expected stool pattern demands investigation.

J. Neurologic.
1. Neurologic assessment of an older child or adolescent is the same as an adult.
2. Neurologic exam of a younger child or infant.
   a. Examine on the caregiver's lap, examiner's lap, or bed.
   b. Observe degree of mental alertness and responsiveness to surroundings in young children.
   c. Sensory, motor, and cerebellar examinations require close observation of normal activity, looking for symmetric movement, muscle tone, and strength.
   d. Deep tendon reflexes can be elicited at any age.
   e. Developmental reflexes present in newborn should disappear within the first year of life: rooting, palmar grasp, Moro, and tonic neck reflexes.
   f. Observe head control, position, and movements of the head in first year of life.
   g. Evaluate grasp, arm strength, and hand control.

K. Immunization history. Obtain the immunization history and keep up to date.

L. Allergies to medications, foods, and environmental substances should be recorded.

III. Physical findings in kidney failure.

A. General.
1. Uremia may affect wakefulness and mood. The child may be irritable.
2. The presence of kidney disease or other chronic illness may be reflected in failure to thrive.

B. Vital signs.
1. Deviations from normal may be the first indication of CKD.
2. Kidney disease is most common cause of hypertension in children.
3. Urinary tract infection should be considered when there is an unexplained fever.

C. Growth.
1. Growth retardation, defined as a height below the fifth percentile for age and gender, may result from uremia, metabolic acidosis, osteodystrophy, anemia, or malnutrition associated with kidney failure.
2. Electrolyte and bicarbonate losses should be managed conservatively.
3. Bone abnormalities may result from metabolic acidosis or hyperparathyroidism.

4. Nonresponse to the administration of growth hormone may indicate a need to start renal replacement therapy (RRT).

D. Skin.
   1. Pale, sallow skin may be a sign of kidney-induced anemia.
   2. Skin excoriation and infection from scratching may indicate uremia.
   3. State of hydration is assessed by examining skin turgor and mucous membranes. Dehydration may be caused by polyuria associated with a child's inability to concentrate urine causing poor skin turgor and dry mucous membranes.
   4. Edema reflects fluid and salt retention.
   5. Vasculitic rash, such as the malar butterfly rash of lupus, may indicate an underlying systemic disorder involving the kidneys.
   6. Hypopigmented lesions on the trunk and extremities and sebaceous adenomas, similar to acne, appearing between ages 4 and 6 on nose and cheek, are associated with kidney cystic disease.
   7. Dysplastic or absent nails may predict kidney disease.

E. HEENT.
   1. Preauricular pits and/or deafness frequently occur in association with kidney anomalies such as Alport's syndrome.
   2. Watery eyes, photophobia, and cystine crystals throughout the cornea are associated with cystinosis.
   3. Cataracts and glaucoma in children are seen in Lowe's syndrome (see Kidney Diseases in Children).

F. Cardiovascular.
   1. Kidney disease is the most frequent cause of hypertension in children.
   2. Hypervolemia associated with kidney failure may result in tachycardia, gallop rhythm, and hypertension.
   3. A heart murmur may reflect a high output state related to anemia.

G. Pulmonary.
   1. Dyspnea, coughing, and an increased respiratory rate may indicate fluid overload.
   2. Rales and wheezing may also indicate kidney-induced fluid overload.

H. Abdominal.
   1. Ascites may be observed in the nephrotic syndrome.

2. Kidney enlargement may cause abdominal distention.
3. Abdominal masses may be caused by hydronephrosis, neoplasms of the kidney, or polycystic kidney disease.

I. Genitourinary.
   1. Undescended testes are associated with urinary tract anomalies, such as prune belly syndrome.
   2. Absence of a vagina in females is associated with congenital kidney anomalies.
   3. History of crying with urination or foul smelling urine may be signs of urinary tract infection (UTI).
   4. Dysuria, urgency, frequency, and hesitancy may or may not be discernible in children.

Common Causes of Kidney Disease in Children

I. Kidney diseases in children.

A. Obstruction/malformations account for 15–25% of children with CKD (USRDS, 2006).
   1. Pyelonephritis/malformations of urinary tract.
      a. Ureteropelvic junction (UPJ) or vesicoureteral junction obstruction (VUR).
         (1) Causes backflow of urine into ureters and possibly kidney pelvis during voiding.
         (2) Eagle-Barrett or prune belly syndrome (PBS) is a triad of problems including absence of abdominal muscles, urinary tract defects, and cryptorchidism.
         (3) VATER associations is a nonrandom association of anomalies, including vertebral defects, anal atresia, tracheoesophageal fistula with esophageal atresia, radial, and kidney defects.
      b. NAPRTCS cites reflux from the posterior urethral valves (PUV) as the cause of CKD in 8% of children.
      c. The outcome depends on when the malformation occurs in fetal development and the severity of the obstruction.

B. Hereditary disorders account for 15–25% of children with CKD (USRDS, 2006).
   1. Polycystic kidney disease (PKD): NAPRTCS 4%.
      a. Autosomal recessive polycystic kidney disease (ARPKD) is an inherited disorder involving cystic dilation of kidney collecting ducts and varying degrees of hepatic abnormalities consisting of biliary dysgenesis and periportal fibrosis.

b. Autosomal dominant polycystic kidney disease (ADPKD) is characterized by the presence of cysts at any point along the nephron or collecting duct. It is rarely a significant neonatal presentation but can present with same complications of ARPKD.

C. Alport's syndrome.
1. An inherited disorder characterized by progressive familial glomerulonephropathy with or without accompanying nerve deafness and ocular abnormalities.
2. Both males and females are affected. However, the disease is more severe in males.
3. Often presents with hematuria with or without proteinuria with gradual progression to kidney failure in late teens or later.

D. Congenital nephrotic syndrome.
1. Finnish type is caused by autosomal recessive inheritance of defects in the NPHS1 gene on chromosome 19, which codes for the glomerular protein nephrin.
2. The syndrome can manifest at or before birth.
3. There is massive proteinuria (1–6 g/24 hr), edema, and hypoalbuminemia.
4. Treatment is nephrectomy and institution of dialysis when unable to control proteinuria and edema.

E. Hypoplasia/dysplasia.
1. Accounts for 10–20% of children with CKD (USRDS, 2006).
2. Hypoplasia/dysplasia results in small abnormal kidneys with or without reflux.
a. The kidneys do not grow normally and involute as their function diminishes.
b. Aplastic, dysplastic, and hypoplastic kidneys make up 16%–18% of children with CKD (NAPRTCS, 2006).

IV. Glomerulonephritis accounts for 25–35% of children with CKD (USRDS, 2006).

A. Glomerulonephritis is the most common glomerular disease causing ESRD.
1. Focal segmental glomerulosclerosis (FSGS).
2. Membranoproliferative glomerulonephritis (MPGN).
3. Acute poststreptococcal glomerulonephritis (PSGN).

V. Systemic/vascular accounts for 5–15% of children with CKD (USRDS, 2006).

A. Hemolytic uremic syndrome (HUS) is characterized by hemolytic anemia, thrombocytopenia, and acute kidney failure.
1. Diarrhea positive in 90% of cases.
a. It is an acquired disease.
b. Secondary to endothelial toxicity of infectious agents, mainly *E. coli* 0157H:7.
c. It is most common in children < 3 years old.
d. The mortality rate is < 5%.
e. There is a 30% risk of kidney sequelae.
f. Rarely relapses.
g. Low risk of recurrence posttransplant.
2. Atypical HUS.
a. Is not caused by an external agent.
b. Does not usually present with diarrhea.
c. It can affect any age including newborns.
d. May be familial (either autosomal dominant or recessive).
e. It frequently has a recurrent course.
f. The kidney prognosis is poor.
g. Posttransplant recurrence is seen in 30% of cases.

B. Henoch-Schönlein purpura (HSP).
1. Typical clinical findings include a petechial and often purpuric rash, predominantly on the lower extremities.
2. Symptoms include abdominal distress with cramping pain, anorexia, and vomiting.
3. Arthralgias, frequently in lower extremity joints, are accompanied by periarticular soft tissue edema.

C. The other 0–10% of cases.
1. Acute tubular necrosis.
2. Acute tumor lysis syndrome.

Acute Kidney Injury (AKI) in Children

I. Prekidney AKI secondary to hypoperfusion of the kidneys in pediatric patients may include:

A. Volume depletion.

B. Nephrotic syndrome.

C. Sepsis.

D. Kidney vasoconstriction.

E. Hepatorenal syndrome.

F. Hypercalcemia.

G. Nonsteroidal antiinflammatory drugs (NSAIDs).

H. Altered hemodynamics within the kidney.

I. Shock.

J. Cardiac pump failure.

II. Tubulointerstitial nephritis (TIN) in pediatric patients includes:

A. Drug-induced (most common cause).
1. Antibiotics: penicillins, cephalosporins, sulfonamides, rifampin, ciprofloxacin, vancomycin, tetracyclines.
2. Diuretics: furosemide, thiazides, triamterene.
3. Nonsteroidal antiinflammatory drugs (NSAIDs): almost all agents including COX-2 inhibitors.
4. Others: acyclovir, amlodipine, captopril, ifosfamide, phenytoin.

B. Thrombus.

C. Disease.
1. Infection-related.
   a. Bacteria: streptococcus, staphylococcus, pneumococcus, salmonella, tuberculosis.
   b. Viruses: EBV, HIV, hepatitis B/C, CMV, rubella, rubeola, mumps, Hantavirus, adenovirus.
   c. Others: toxoplasmosis, mycoplasma.
2. Systemic diseases.
   a. Systemic lupus erythematosus (SLE) or lupus is a condition of chronic inflammation caused by an autoimmune disease process.
      (1) Remission rates up to 80% with corticosteroids or cytotoxic drugs.
      (2) There is significant therapy-associated toxicity.
         (a) During infections, abnormal antibodies in the blood target the tissues within the body rather than foreign infectious agents.
         (b) Bone disease can develop from use of high doses of corticosteroids.
         (c) Premature ovarian failure can occur.
         (d) Accelerated atherosclerosis is not unusual.
      (3) Medication adherence is a major difficulty due to side effects, e.g., weight gain, thinning of bones and skin, infection, diabetes, facial puffiness, cataracts.
   b. In Sjögren's syndrome, the immune system attacks and destroys moisture-producing glands (e.g., salivary glands and lacrimal glands) and the kidneys.
   c. Sarcoidosis causes a dysregulation of vitamin D production with an increase in extrarenal production.
   d. Inflammatory bowel disease: ulcerative colitis and Crohn's disease.
   e. Tubulointerstitial nephritis with uveitis.

D. Malignancy.

E. Glomerulonephritis.
1. Poststreptococcal glomerulonephritis or postinfectious glomerulonephritis.
2. Endocarditis-associated glomerulonephritis.
3. Systemic vasculitis.
4. Thrombotic microangiopathy.
   a. Hemolytic-uremic syndrome (HUS) (see previous page).
   b. Thrombotic thrombocytopenic purpura (TTP).
      (1) Affects older children and adults.
      (2) Hemolytic crises.
      (3) Central nervous system (CNS) involvement.
      (4) Frequent relapsing.
      (5) Significant morbidity.
5. Rapidly progressive glomerulonephritis.

F. Intratubular obstruction.
1. Intratubular crystal deposition such as:
   a. Tumor lysis syndrome.
   b. Ethylene glycol toxicity.
   c. Calcium oxalate deposition.
2. Medication-associated.
   a. Antivirals, such as acyclovir.
   b. Indinavir.
3. Intratubular protein deposition: multiple myeloma.

Effects of CKD on Children

I. Definition of chronic kidney disease (CKD).

A. Presence of kidney damage or decreased kidney function for at least 3 months, irrespective of underlying diagnosis.

B. Kidney damage includes any structural or functional abnormality of kidney involving pathologic, laboratory, or imaging manifestations.

C. Defined by a reduction in glomerular filtration rate (GFR) to below 60 mL/min/1.73 m2 (half of normal adult kidney function).

D. The National Kidney Foundation has defined five stages of severity, reflecting increasing degrees of kidney damage or dysfunction:
Stage 1 – Kidney Damage (normal or GFR > 90)
Stage 2 – Mild Kidney Damage (GFR < 60–89)
Stage 3 – Moderate Kidney Damage (GFR < 30–59)
Stage 4 – Severe Kidney Damage (GFR < 15–29)
Stage 5 – Kidney Failure (GFR < 15)

E. CKD staging in children is best achieved by estimating the GFR.
   1. Most common method for estimating the GFR in children is Schwartz formula, which incorporates body weight, height, and serum creatinine level: CrCl = (K X Ht) / Cr
      a. K = 0.33 LBW infants less than 1 year.
      b. K = 0.45 term infants less than 1 year.
      c. K = 0.55 in children/adolescent females.
      d. K = 0.70 in adolescent males.
   2. This method does not require a 24-hour urine collection, which is nearly impossible in children who are not toilet trained.

II. Body systems.

A. Cardiovascular.
   1. Anemia is associated with a negative impact on quality of life (QOL) in children with CKD at all stages, especially adolescents in areas of physical functioning, physical activity, and family activities.
   2. Studies of adolescents with early CKD, on dialysis, and posttransplantation show QOL is best in those with hematocrit greater than 36%.
   3. See KDOQI guideline 2006 updates (see Table 15.4) for recommendations.
      a. Operational definitions used by the KDOQI work group.
         (1) ND-CKD non-dialysis-dependent chronic kidney disease (CKD); stages 1-4 and stage 5 not on dialysis.
         (2) PD-CKD peritoneal dialysis-dependent CKD.
         (3) HD-CKD hemodialysis-dependent CKD.
      b. Identifying patients and initiating evaluation: see KDOQI Clinical Practice Recommendation (CPR) 1.1.
      c. Evaluation of anemia in CKD: see KDOQI CPR 1.2.
         (1) Children may have a need to begin erythropoietic stimulating agents (ESAs) prior to initiation of dialysis due to negative effects of low hemoglobin (Hb).
         (2) Reasons to begin ESA include growth

failure, fatigue, inattention, and decreased quality of life.
      d. Hb range KDOQI (CPR 2.1) pediatric patients should have a hemoglobin of 11–12 g/dL.
         (1) Use of ESAs (KDOQI CPR 3.1) are based on the stage of CKD, treatment regimen, pain of injection, ESA chosen (long- or short-acting), and anticipated number of injections needed.
         (2) Minimizing pain at injection site is important.
      e. Use of iron agents (KDOQI CPR 3.2), oral iron is indicated unless the patient is severally depleted or on HD when IV use is indicated.
      f. Use of pharmacologic/nonpharmacogic adjuvants (KDOQI CPR 3.3).
   4. Cardiovascular disease (CVD).
      a. Major cause of morbidity and mortality in pediatric patients on chronic dialysis, reported as either first or second most common cause according to the 2006 KDOQI Clinical Practice Guidelines Work Group for Cardiovascular Disease in Dialysis Patients (see Tables 15.5 and 15.6).
      b. Children and young adults on chronic dialysis have conventional factors leading to cardiovascular risk (hypertension, dyslipidemia, and physical inactivity).
      c. In addition, they have uremia-related risks such as anemia, volume overload, hyperhomocysteinemia, hyperparathyroidism, hypoalbuminemia, inflammation, and left ventricular hypertrophy (LVH).
      d. Inflammation is a major risk factor for cardiovascular disease.
      e. Studies suggest chronic inflammatory states may be due to chronic uremia.
      f. The increased use of central venous catheters (CVC) in children and adolescents contributes to inflammatory state.
      g. Elevations of CRP levels show the presence of chronic inflammation in many pediatric patients.
      h. Increased oxidative stress occurs in children on dialysis, independent of dialysis modality.
         (1) Children with ESRD exhibit lower trace element levels in RBC and plasma.
         (2) Oxidative stress is aggravated during every HD session.
         (3) This type of oxidative stress is associated with increased CVD in adults and likely a part of increased CVD in children with ESRD.

> # Table 15.4

KDOQI Clinical Practice Recommendations for Pediatrics

1.1 Identifying Patients and Initiating Evaluation

1.1.1 Stage and cause of CKD: In the opinion of the Work Group, Hb testing should be carried out in all patients with CKD, regardless of stage or cause.

1.1.2 Frequency of testing for anemia: In the opinion the Work Group, Hb levels should be measured at least annually.

1.1.3 Diagnosis of anemia: <u>PEDIATRIC CPR.</u> In the of opinion of the Work Group, in the pediatric patient, diagnosis of anemia should be made and further evaluation should be undertaken whenever the observed Hb concentration is less than the fifth percentile of normal when adjusted for age and sex.

1.2 Evaluation of Anemia in CKD

1.2.1 In the opinion of the Work Group, initial assessment of anemia should include the following tests:

1.2.1.1 CBC including – in addition to the Hb concentration – red blood cell indices (MCH, MCV, MCHC), white blood cell count, and differential and platelet count.

1.2.1.2 Absolute reticulocyte count.

1.2.1.3 Serum ferritin to assess iron stores.

1.2.1.4 <u>PEDIATRIC CPR.</u> In the pediatric patient, serum TSAT to assess adequacy.

2.1 Hb Range

2.1.1 Lower limit of Hb: In patients with CKD, Hb level should be 11.0 g/dL or greater.

2.1.2 Upper limit of Hb: In the opinion of the Work Group, there is insufficient evidence to recommend routinely maintaining Hb levels at 13.0 g/dL or greater in ESA-treated patients.

CPR For Pediatric 3.1 Using ESAs

3.1.1 Frequency of Hb monitoring:

3.1.1.1 In the opinion of the Work Group, frequency of Hb monitoring in patients treated with ESAs should be at least monthly.

3.1.2 ESA dosing:

3.1.2.1 In the opinion of the Work Group, the initial ESA dose and ESA dose adjustments should be determined by the patient's Hb level, the target Hb level, the observed rate of increased in the Hb level, and clinical circumstances.

3.1.2.2 In the opinion of the Work Group, ESA doses should be decreased, but not necessarily held, when a downward adjustment of Hb level is needed.

3.1.2.3 In the opinion of the Work Group, scheduled ESA doses that have been missed should be replaced at the earliest possible opportunity.

3.1.2.4 In the opinion of the Work Group, ESA administration in ESA-dependent patients should continue during hospitalization.

3.1.2.5 In the opinion of the Work Group, hypertension, vascular access occlusion, inadequate dialysis, histories of seizures or compromised nutritional status are not contraindications to ESA therapy.

3.1.3 Route of administration:

3.1.3.1 <u>PEDIATRIC CPR.</u> In the opinion of the Work Group, in the pediatric patient, the route of administration should be determined by the CKD stage, treatment setting, efficacy considerations, the class of ESA used, and the anticipated frequency and pain of administration.

3.1.3.2 In the opinion of the Work Group, convenience favors SC administration in non-HD-CKD patients.

3.1.3.3 In the opinion of the Work Group, convenience favors IV administration in patients with HD-CKD.

3.1.4 Frequency of administration:

3.1.4.1 <u>PEDIATRIC CPR.</u> In the opinion of the Work Group, in the pediatric patient, the frequency of administration should be determined by the CKD stage, treatment setting, efficacy consideration, and the class of ESA; as well, consideration should be given to the anticipated frequency of, and pain on administration of each agent and their potential effects on the child and family.

3.1.4.2 In the opinion of the Work Group, convenience favors less frequent administration, particularly in non-HD-CKD patients.

CPR for Pediatrics 3.2 Using iron agents

3.2.1 Frequency of iron status tests: In the opinion of the Work Group, iron status tests should be performed as follows:

3.2.1.1 Every month during initial ESA treatment.

3.2.1.2 At least every 3 months during stable ESA treatment or in patients with HD-CKD not treated with ESA.

3.2.2 Interpretation of iron status tests: In the opinion of the Work Group, results of iron status tests, HB level, and ESA dose should be interpreted together to guide iron therapy.

3.2.3 Targets of iron therapy: In the opinion of the Work Group, sufficient iron should be administrated to generally maintain the following indices of iron status during ESA treatment:

3.2.3.1 <u>PEDIATRIC CPR</u> HD-CKD:
- Serum ferritin > 100 ng/mL; AND
- TSAT > 20%.

3.2.3.2 ND-CKD and PKD-CKD:
- Serum ferritin > 100 ng/mL AND
- TSAT > 20%.

3.2.4 Upper level of ferritin: In the opinion of the Work Group, there is insufficient evidence to recommend routine administration of IV iron if serum ferritin is greater than 500 ng/mL. When ferritin level is greater than 500 ng/mL, decisions regarding IV iron administration should weigh ESA responsiveness, Hb and TSAT level, and the patient's clinical status.

Continues on next page

Table 15.4 (page 2 of 4) ——————— **KDOQI Clinical Practice Recommendations for Pediatrics**

3.2.5   Route of administration:
3.2.5.1 The preferred route of administration is IV in patients with HD-CKD.
3.2.5.2 In the opinion of the Work Group, the route of iron administration can be either IV or oral in patients with ND-CKD and PD-CKD.
3.2.6   Hypersensitivity reactions: In the opinion of the Work Group, resuscitative medication and personnel trained to evaluate the resuscitate anaphylaxis should be available whenever a dose of iron dextran is administered.

CPR For Pediatrics 3.3 Using Pharmacological and Nonpharmacological Adjuvants to ESA Treatment in HD-CKD
3.3.1   L-carnitine: (FULLY APPLICABLE TO CHILDREN) In the opinion of the Work Group, there is sufficient evidence to recommend the use of L-carnitine in the management of anemia in patients with CKD.
3.3.2   Vitamin C: (FULLY APPLICABLE TO CHILDREN) In the opinion of the Work Group, there is insufficient evidence to recommend the use of vitamin C (ascorbate) in the management of anemia in patients with CKD.
3.3.3   Androgens: (FULLY APPLICABLE TO CHILDREN) Androgens should not be used as an adjuvant to ESA treatment in anemic patients with CKD. (STRONG RECOMMENDATION)
Reprinted with permission from National Kidney Foundation 2006 Updates

Clinical Practice Guideline 6. Pediatric Peritoneal Dialysis
6.1   Recommended laboratory measurements for peritoneal membrane function:
6.1.1 The PET is the preferred approach to the clinical assessment of peritoneal membrane transport capacity in pediatric patients and should be performed to aid in the prescription process. (A)
6.2   Maintenance of euvolemia and normontension:
6.2.1 The frequent presence of hypertension and associated cardiac abnormalities in children receiving PD requires strict management of blood pressure, including attention to fluid status. (A)
6.3   Quality improvement programs:
6.3.1 The CQI process has shown to improve outcomes in many disciplines, including CKD stage 5. (A)
6.3.1.1 Each home training unit should establish quality improvement programs with the goal of monitoring clinical outcomes and implementing programs that result in improvements in patient care. In children, growth and school attendance/performance are clinical activities to be monitored in addition to those recommended for adult patients.
6.3.1.2 Quality improvement programs should include representatives of all disciplines involved in the care of pediatric PD patient, including physicians, nurses, social workers, dietitians, play therapists, psychologists, and teachers.

6.3.1.3 Single-center trends in pediatric clinical outcomes should be compared with national and international data.

Clinical Practice Recommendations for Guideline 6: Pediatric Peritoneal Dialysis
6.1   Dialysis initiation:
6.1.1 Dialysis initiation should be considered for the pediatric patient
6.2   Modality selection:
6.2.1 The decision regarding the selection of PD as a dialysis modality for the pediatric patient should take a variety of factors into account, including patient/family choice, patient size, medical comorbidities, and family support.
6.3   Quality improvement programs:
6.3.1 The CQI process has been shown to improve outcomes in many disciplines, including CKD stage 5. (A)
6.3.1.1 Each home training unit should establish quality improvement programs with the goal of monitoring clinical outcomes and implementing programs that result in improvements in patient care. In children, growth and school attendance/ performance are clinical activities to be monitored in addition to those recommended for adult patients.
6.3.1.2 Quality improvement programs should include representatives of all disciplines involved in the care of the pediatric PD patient, including physicians, nurses, social workers, dietitians, play therapists, psychologists, and teachers.
6.3.1.3 Single-center trends in pediatric clinical outcomes should be compared with national and international data.

6.3   **Solute clearance targets and measurements:**
6.3.1 In the absence of definitive data correlating solute removal and clinical outcome in children, current recommendations for solute clearance in pediatric patients receiving PD are as follows:
6.3.1.1 The pediatric patient's clinical status should be reviewed at least monthly, and delivery of the prescribed solute clearance should render the patient free of signs and symptoms of uremia.
6.3.1.2 All measurements of peritoneal solute clearance should be obtained when the patient is clinically stable and at least 1 month after resolution of an episode of peritonitis.
6.3.1.3 More frequent measurements of peritoneal solute clearance and RKF should be considered when clinical events are likely to have resulted in decreased clearance or when new/worsening signs or symptoms of uremia develop.
6.3.1.4 Regardless of the delivered dose of dialysis, if a patient is not doing well and has no other identifiable cause other than kidney failure, a trial of increased dialysis is indicated.
6.3.2 For patients with RKF (defined as urine $Kt/V_{urea} > 0.1/wk$):

Continues on next page

Table 15.4 (page 3 of 4) ——— KDOQI Clinical Practice Recommendations for Pediatrics

6.3.2.1 The minimal "delivered" dose of total (peritoneal and kidney) small-solute clearance should be a Kt/V$_{urea}$ of at least 1.8/wk.

6.3.2.2 Total solute clearance should be a measured within the first month after initiating dialysis and at least once every 6 months thereafter.

6.3.2.3 If the patient has FKF and residual kidney clearance is being considered as part of the patient's total weekly solute clearance determinations should be obtained at a minimum of every 3 months.

6.3.3 For patients with RKF (defined as urine Kt/V$_{urea}$ < 0.1/wk) or for those in whom RKF is unable to be measured accurately:

6.3.3.1 The minimal "delivered" dose of small-solute clearance determinations should be a peritoneal Kt/V$_{urea}$ of at least 1.8/wk.

6.3.3.2 The peritoneal solute clearance should be measured within the first month after starting dialysis and at least once every 6 months thereafter.

6.3.4 When calculating Kt/V$_{urea}$, one should estimate V or TBW by using the sex-specific nomograms based upon the following equations:
Males: TBW = 0.010 · (height · weight)$^{0.68}$ − 0.37 · weight
Females: TBW = 0.14 · (height · weight)$^{0.64}$ − 0.35 · weight

Reprinted with permission from National Kidney Foundation 2006 Updates

6.4 **Preservation of RKF:**

6.4.1 Techniques that may contribute to the preservation of RKF in pediatric patients receiving PD should be incorporated as a component of dialysis care whenever possible.

6.4.1.1 Nephrotoxic insults in those with normal or impaired kidney function should be assumed, in the absence of direct evidence, to also be nephrotoxic in patients on PD therapy who have RFK and therefore should be avoided.

6.4.1.2 Aminoglycoside antibiotics should be avoided whenever possible to minimize the risk for nephrotoxicity, as well as ototoxicity and vestibular toxicity.

6.4.1.3 "Prekidney" and "postkidney" causes of a decrease in RKF should be considered in the appropriate clinical setting.

6.4.1.4 Infections of the urinary tract should be treated promptly.

6.4.1.5 Diuretics should be used to maximize urinary salt and water excretion.

6.4.1.6 An ACE inhibitor or ARB should be considered in a PD patient who requires antihypertensive medication and had RKF.

Reprinted with permission from National Kidney Foundation 2006 Updates

6.5 **Writing the PD prescription:**

6.5.1 In addition to solute clearance, QOL, ultrafiltration/volume control, and possibly the clearance of middle molecules should be considered when writing the PD prescription.

6.5.1.1 The patient's dialysis schedule and QOL, as it relates to such issues as school and work attendance/performance should be taken into account when designing the dialysis prescription.

6.5.1.2 To optimize small-solute clearance, minimize cost, and possibly decrease the frequency of exchanges, one should first increase the instilled volume per exchange (target range, 1,000 to 1,200 mL/m^2 BSA; maximum, 1,400 mL/m^2 BSA), as tolerated by the patient, before increasing the number of exchanges per day. The volume of the supine exchange(s) should be increased first because this position has the lowest intraabdominal pressure. Objective evidence of patient tolerance may require assessment of IPP.

6.5.1.3 The patient's record of PD effluent volume from the overnight dwell of CAPD and daytime dwell of CCPD.

6.5.1.4 Factors to be considered when attempting to optimize total body volume include:
a. Dietary sodium and fluid restriction may be implemented in patients unable to maintain euvolemia/normotension with dialysis alone.
b. In patients with RKF, diuretics may be preferred over increasing the dialysate dextrose concentration to achieve euvolemia.
c. Drain volume should be optimized after the overnight dwell of CAPD and the daytime dwell(s) of CCPD to maximize solute clearance and ultrafiltration volume.
d. In patients who are hypertensive or in whom there is evidence of volume overload, ultrafiltration generally should be positive for all daytime or nighttime exchanges.
e. An effort should be made to determine the lowest possible dialysate dextrose concentration required to achieve the desired ultrafiltration volume.

6.5.1.5 To optimize middle-molecule clearance in patients who have minimal RKF, the PD prescription should preferentially include the use of CCPD with dwells 24 hr/day or CAPD. This is recommended even if small-molecule clearance is above target without the longer dwell.

6.5.1.6 The use of NIPD (e.g., no daytime dwell) can be considered in pediatric patients who are clinically well, whose combined dialysis prescription and RKF achieves or exceeds the target solute clearance, and who are without evidence of hyperphosphatemia, hyperkalemia, hypervolemia, or acidosis.

Reprinted with permission from National Kidney Foundation 2006 Updates

6.6 **Other aspects of the care of the pediatric PD patient:**

6.6.1 All children on PD therapy with anemia should follow the KDOQI Guidelines for Management of Anemia that pertain to pediatrics.

6.6.2 Management of dyslipidemias for prepubertal children on PD therapy should follow recommendations by the National Cholesterol Expert Panel in Children and Adolescents. Postpubertal children or adolescents on

Continues on next page

Table 15.4 (page 4 of 4) ———— KDOQI Clinical Practice Recommendations for Pediatrics

PD therapy should follow the pediatric recommendations provided in the KDOQI Clinical Practice Guidelines for Managing Dyslipidemia in CKD.

6.6.3 All children on PD therapy should follow the pediatric-specific recommendations provided in the KDOQI Clinical Practice Guidelines on Hypertension and Antihypertensive Agents in CKD.

6.6.4 All children on PD therapy should follow the recommendations provided in the KDOQI Clinical Practice Guidelines for Nutrition in Chronic Renal Failure.

Reprinted with permission from National Kidney Foundation 2006 Updates

Clinical Practice Guideline 8.
Pediatric Hemodialysis Prescription and Adequacy

8.1 Initiation of HD:

8.1.1 Dialysis initiation considerations for the pediatric patient should follow the adult patient guideline of a GFR less than 15 mL/ min/1.73 m². (A)

8.1.2 For pediatric patients, GFR can be estimated by using either a timed urine collection of or the Schwartz formula. (A)

8.1.3 Dialysis therapy initiation should be considered at higher estimated GFRs when the patient's clinical course is complicated by the presence of the signs and symptoms listed in Table 15.5, CPR 1 for adult patients, as well as malnutrition or growth failure for pediatric patients. Before dialysis is undertaken, these conditions should be shown to be refractory to medications and/or dietary management. (A)

Reprinted with permission from National Kidney Foundation 2006 Updates

Clinical Practice Recommendation 8:
Vascular Access in Pediatric Patients

8.1 Choice of access type:

8.1.1 Permanent access in the form of a fistula or graft is the preferred form of vascular access for most pediatric patients on maintenance HD therapy.

8.1.2 Circumstances in which a CVC may be acceptable for pediatric long-term access include lack of local surgical expertise to place permanent vascular access in small children, patient size too small to support a permanent vascular access, bridging HD for PD training or PD catheter removal for peritonitis, and expectation of expeditious kidney transplantation.

8.1.3 If surgical expertise to place permanent access does not exist in the patient's pediatric setting, efforts should be made to consult vascular access expertise among local adult-oriented surgeons to either supervise or place permanent vascular access in children.

8.1.4 Programs should evaluate their patients' expected waiting times on their local decreased-donor kidney transplant waiting lists. Serious consideration should be given to placing permanent vascular access in children greater than 20 kg in size who are expected to wait more than 1 year for a kidney transplant.

8.2 Stenosis surveillance: An AVG stenosis surveillance protocol should be established to detect venous anastomosis stenosis and direct patients for surgical revision or PTA.

8.3 Catheter sizes, anatomic sites, and configurations:

8.3.1 Catheter sizes should be matched to patient sizes with the goal of minimizing intraluminal trauma and obstruction to blood flow while allowing sufficient blood flow for adequate HD.

8.3.2 External cuffed access should be placed in the internal jugular with the distal tip placed in the right atrium.

8.3.3 The BFR of an external access should be minimally 3 to 5 mL/kg/min and should be adequate to deliver the prescribed HD dose.

8.2 Measurement of HD adequacy:

8.2.1 spKt, calculated by either formula urea kinetic modeling or the second-generation natural logarithm formula, should be used for month-to-month assessment of delivered HD dose. (B)

8.2.2 Assessment of nutrition status as an essential component of HD adequacy measurement. nPCR should be measured monthly by using either formula urea kinetic modeling or algebraic approximation. (B)

8.2.3 Principles and statements regarding slow-flow methods for postdialysis sampling and inclusion of RKF (or lack thereof) outlined in the adult guideline also pertain to pediatric patients. (B)

8.3 Prescription of adequate HD:

8.3.1 Children should receive at least the delivered dialysis dose as recommended for the adult population. (A)

8.3.2 For younger pediatric patients, prescription of higher dialysis dose and higher protein intakes at 150% of the recommended nutrient intake for age may be important. (B)

8.4 Non-dose-related components of adequacy: Accurate assessment of patient intravascular volume during the HD treatment should be provided to optimize ultrafiltration. (B)

Reprinted with permission from National Kidney Foundation 2006 Updates

Table 15.5

Cardiovascular Mortality in Pediatric CKD Stage 5

Author	Year Published	Years Data Collected	No. of Subjects	Total Deaths	% Cardiovascular Deaths
USRDS Annual	2002	1998-2000	8,549 dialysis patients	244 deaths	27%
Parekh	2002	1990-1996 (USRDS)		980 deaths	28%
Chavers	2002	1991-1996 (USRDS)	1,454 dialysis patients	107 deaths	38%
Groothoff	2002	1972-1992 (Dutch Registry)		38 deaths	45%
Honda	1999	1981-1997 (Japanese Registry)	807 PD patients	87 deaths	30%
Verrina	1999	1986-1997 (Italian Registry)	297 patients	21 deaths	57%
Reiss	1996	1969-1992	231 patients	36 deaths (26 HD+, 10PD)	14% cardiac failure 22% other cardiac
Hisano	1990	1968-1988	96 patients	28 deaths	39%
Neu	2002	1992-2001	4,546 patients	205 deaths	22%

Source: National Kidney Foundation. (2005). KDOQI clinical practice guidelines for cardiovascular disease in dialysis patients. *American Journal of Kidney Diseases, 45*(Suppl. 3), S1-S154. Used with permission.

B. Integumentary.
  1. Overall appearance of the skin may be pale or sallow.
  2. Dry or scaly skin is common as CKD worsens.
  3. Children may have bruising due to capillary fragility.
  4. Higher BUN levels cause uremic crystals to form on skin of face and chest in particular causing itching and skin breakdown.

C. Gastrointestinal.
  1. Children with CKD are particularly prone to nausea, anorexia, and/or vomiting, severely interfering with nutritional needs.
  2. As CKD progresses, a metallic aftertaste develops.
  3. Many programs place gastrostomy tubes, PEGS, MICKEYS, or feeding tubes to provide adequate nutrition in overnight drip feedings or bolus feeds.

D. Genitourinary.
  1. Evaluate and repair urinary tract abnormalities, which may include:

  a. Posterior urethral valves.
  b. Ureterovesical or ureteropelvic junction obstruction.
  c. Vesicoureteral reflux.
  d. Intermittent catheterization for neurogenic bladder.
  e. Bladder augmentation.
  f. Creation of a Mitrofanoff appendico-vesicostomy (attaches appendix between skin and bladder to provide an outlet for urinary catheterization).
  g. Removal of duplicated systems.
  2. Monitor for urinary tract infections, especially if child does not empty bladder often or catheterizes. This can be a significant source of infection.

E. Metabolic.
  1. Metabolic acidosis (serum bicarbonate (HCO_3) level < 22 mmol/L).
  a. Contributes to poor nutritional status and growth.
    (1) Decreased albumin synthesis.
    (2) Increased protein catabolism.

Table 15.6

Prevalence of Cardiovascular Risk Factors in Pediatric CKD Stage 5

Author	Year	Number of Subjects	Risk Factor Examined	Prevalence of Risk Factors
Goodman	2000	39	Coronary artery calcification	36%
Oh	2002	37	Coronary artery calcification Valvular calcification Aortic valve calcification	92% 34% 32%
Gruppen	2003	30	Aortic valve calcification	30%
Mitsfenes	2000	64 (26 HD, 38 PD)	Left ventricular hypertrophy	75% HD 68% PD

Source: National Kidney Foundation. (2005). KDOQI clinical practice guidelines for cardiovascular disease in dialysis patients. *American Journal of Kidney Diseases, 45*(Suppl. 3), S1-S154. Used with permission.

(3) Exacerbates bone disease.
(4) Increases resistance to thyroid and growth hormones.
b. Maintenance of bicarbonate level above 22 mmol/L increases appetite and decreases protein degradation and increases lean body mass.

F. Skeletal.
1. Normal bone growth is regulated by interaction of PTH, calcium, phosphorus, and vitamin D.
2. Calcium and phosphorus imbalance is caused by:
a. Increased retention of phosphorus.
b. Reduced kidney activation of vitamin D.
c. Reduced intestinal absorption of calcium.
3. There is a lack of calcitriol production.
4. Abnormal interactions, beginning in early stages of CKD, progress as the GFR declines leading to elevated parathyroid hormone (PTH) and secondary hyperparathyroidism.
5. Untreated secondary hyperparathyroidism produces renal osteodystrophy (ROD) with increased risk of bone deformities, fractures, and impaired linear growth.

III. Physical growth and sexual maturation is profoundly affected by kidney failure during childhood.

A. Abnormalities of skeletal development, with associated growth retardation, affect most CKD patients.

B. Growth failure is a major concern in childhood CKD as advances in dialysis and transplantation are able to prolong life into adulthood.

C. Factors contributing to growth failure in CKD.
1. The child's age at the onset of kidney failure.
a. CKD in first 2 years of life leads to short stature despite normal growth velocity in later childhood.
b. The greatest longitudinal growth rate occurs in first 2 years of life.
2. The etiology of the kidney disease.
3. Concomitant medications (e.g., steroids).

D. Modifiable factors.
1. Metabolic acidosis.
2. CKD mineral-bone disorder.
3. Excessive sodium and/or water loss.
4. Growth hormone/insulin-like growth factor-1 (GH/IGF-1) resistance.
5. Kidney osteodystrophy.
6. Anemia.
7. Nutrition or caloric deficiency.
a. Gastrostomy tubes, buttons, PEGS, etc.
b. Oral aversions can be helped with feeding therapy.
c. Loss of water soluble vitamins with dialysis (e.g., B's and C).
d. Metabolic imbalances.
8. Uremic growth inhibitors.
a. Malnutrition.
b. Infections and/or inflammation.
c. Elevated parathyroid hormone levels.

E. Biochemical regulators of growth.
  1. PTH.
    a. PTH stimulates bone resorption in response to hypocalcaemia.
    b. PTH increases tubular calcium reabsorption.
    c. Acidosis leads to reduction in calcium stores by stimulating osteoclast activity.
    d. Decreases kidney resorption of phosphorus.
    e. As GFR declines hyperphosphatemia results. This leads to hypocalcemia and further stimulation of the parathyroid gland.
    f. Increased bone turnover due to hyperparathyroidism results in osteitis fibrosa.
    g. Over suppression of parathyroid glands results in adynamic bone disorder.
    h. Obesity may contribute to hyperparathyroidism.
  2. Calcitriol or ergocalciferol.
    a. Increases calcium and phosphorus absorption in gut.
    b. Promotes bone mineralization.
    c. As GFR declines, levels decline leading to decreased total body calcium.
    d. Calcitonin inhibits osteoclasts but is only transiently effective.

F. Other regulators.
  1. Growth hormone.
    a. Normal levels of growth hormone (GH).
    b. Imbalance in GH-IGF-1 axis.
      (1) Pulsatile release of GH from pituitary stimulates production of IGF-1 primarily by liver.
      (2) Circulating IGF-1 is responsible for growth-promoting effects of GH, such as stimulation of longitudinal bone growth.
      (3) GH also has direct effects on some tissues like bone.
  2. Glucocorticoids are essential for osteoblast differentiation.
  3. Estrogens are necessary for epiphyseal closure in both sexes.
  4. Abnormalities in fibroblast growth factors result in abnormal phenotypes.

IV. Pubertal delays.

A. Delayed pubertal development is common in children with CKD.

B. Normal puberty is initiated by the onset of episodic nocturnal secretion of luteinizing hormone (LH) containing an increasing proportion of bioactive hormone.

C. In adolescents with CKD, secretion of LH is tonic rather than pulsatile and bioactivity of the hormone is reduced. Both phenomena may contribute to delayed sexual maturation.

D. Long-term steroid therapy has a depressant effect on hypothalamo-pituitary pulsatile secretion of growth hormone (GH), resulting in pubertal delay.

E. Sexuality is closely tied to self-concept and self-esteem.

V. Psychosocial and cognitive development.

A. Time spent on dialysis, hospital visits, admissions, illness, etc., causes considerable disruption to "normal" social activities and school attendance.

B. For many children, home dialysis programs (PD or HD) can offer increased social independence and autonomy.

C. Achievement of fewer social milestones while growing up can result in more emotional problems and decrease overall quality of life.

D. Autonomy, social, and psychosexual development is best accomplished by continuing peer-related activities despite CKD.

E. Abnormal neurocognitive development and difficulty with concentration are common.

F. Studies show marked decrease in cognitive skills as CKD progresses, making school achievement difficult.

G. Disordered psychosocial maturation.

H. Peer relationships are important for social development and self-esteem.
  1. Peer relationships and activities should be encouraged and facilitated.
  2. Interactions with peers who have similar restrictions on their lives are helpful.
  3. Adolescents with chronic illness often become marginalized by peers, rejected for being different at a time when conformity determines body image and identity.
  4. Adolescents may have difficulty developing close physical relationships with peers, further limiting development of body image, self-esteem, and independence.

Kidney Replacement Therapies in Children

I. Treatment options.

A. Patients with an estimated glomerular filtration rate < 30 mL/min/1.73 m^2 (CKD stage 4) should be educated on all modalities of kidney replacement therapy options: PD, home HD, in-center HD, transplantation, and palliative care.

B. Timely referrals allow for placement of a permanent dialysis access if necessary.

C. CKD stage 4 patients should not have forearm and upper-arm veins used for venipuncture, placement of IV catheters, subclavian catheters, or peripherally inserted central catheters (PICCs) in anticipation of the placement of permanent vascular access throughout the life span.

D. Children, like adult patients, should have a functional permanent access (PD catheter, fistula, or graft) at the initiation of dialysis therapy.

II. The Fistula First Initiative arose from CPM I calling for a primary AVF for at least 50% of adult patients initiating hemodialysis.

A. The International Pediatric Fistula First Initiative began as collaboration with ESRD Networks 9 and 10 and the Midwest Pediatric Nephrology Consortium in 2005.

B. Identified barriers to fistulae.
  1. Inadequate referral times.
  2. Lack of awareness on part of nephrologist and surgeon.
  3. Poor communication between nephrologist and surgeon.
  4. Patient and/or family resistance.

C. Additional barriers in children.
  1. Previous trauma to arm veins.
  2. Growth retardation.
  3. Obesity.
  4. Arterial/venous spasm.
  5. Kidney osteodystrophy.

D. Prevent the use of PICC lines in any patient with CKD stage 2 or greater to preserve access for later dialysis.

III. Preventive care measures.

A. Immunizations should be current in all children including those with CKD.

B. Influenza, pneumococcal pneumonia, and hepatitis B vaccinations should be given in addition to all American Academy of Pediatrics (AAP) recommended immunizations (http://www.cispimmunize.org).

C. Frequent visits for CKD care may make primary care provider (PCP) visits difficult, necessitating vaccinations be offered at the CKD visits.

D. Rising body mass index (BMI) in children entering ESRD are consistent with the general population and a major concern. In addition, the higher BMI increase the risk for disease progression.

IV. End-of-life issues.

A. Pediatric palliative care helps children and families live to their fullest potential while facing complex medical conditions.

B. Care must be child-focused, family oriented, and relationship centered.

C. Care should focus on enhancing quality of life for the child and family while relieving or preventing suffering.

D. Children do not necessarily have the same emotional barriers as adults when talking about death.

E. Discussion may require the help of trained personnel such as child life specialists, psychologists, social workers, psychiatric nurse practitioners, and art therapists, to name a few.

F. It should be an option for parents to make a choice about initiating therapy in a severely disabled child. A child with less disability can do well on kidney replacement therapy and thus not treating is rarely an option unless a severe disability is present.

Options for Therapy

I. Continuous renal replacement therapy (CRRT).

A. Indications for initiating CRRT.
  1. Acute kidney injury (AKI) or chronic kidney disease (CKD) requiring fluid management or solute management.

a. Fluid management: unstable on intermittent HD, cardiovascular instability, respiratory distress, organ transplant, cardiac surgery, diuretic intolerant, burns, volume overload, or chemotherapy.

b. Solute management: multisystem organ failure (MSOF), sepsis, catabolic state requiring daily dialysis, nutritional support, neonates with inborn errors of metabolism, trauma, pediatric patients on extracorporeal membrane oxygenation (ECMO), and/or acid-base imbalance.

2. Rhabdomyolysis.
   a. Fatty degeneration, infiltration, and destruction of muscle tissue leads to the separation and disappearance of muscle cells.
   b. Native kidneys are unable to excrete this buildup of muscle tissue, primarily due to clogging of the nephrons.
   c. Removal of this tissue is facilitated via convective clearance.
   d. Diffusion may be used to control the buildup of products of metabolism. The kidneys fail to clear these products secondary to the clogging of the nephrons.

B. Advantages of CRRT.
   1. Cardiovascular stability.
   2. Minimization of hypotensive episodes associated with delayed recovery of the kidneys.
   3. Safe, flexible fluid and electrolyte management.
   4. Minimizes the shifts in intracranial pressure due to rapid chemical clearance.
   5. CRRT is relatively simple to perform with current volumetric control machines.
   6. CRRT provides continuous toxin removal.

C. The vascular access for CRRT.
   1. The venous access can be either one double lumen catheter or two single lumen catheters. It may be possible to draw from a femoral line and return to a central line or umbilical line.
   2. The site for the catheter may be the femoral, subclavian, or jugular vein.
   3. Some centers may use a single needle option, which requires specialized equipment.

D. Pediatric issues related to CRRT.
   1. The patient's size is a unique challenge for replacement therapy options.
   2. Catheter access is difficult in the very small infant or child. Femoral lines require child to lie still while in use — not always an option.
   3. Use of AN-69 membranes requires special

techniques to avoid bradykinin release syndrome when priming circuit with blood (Brophy, 2001).

E. Nursing considerations with CRRT.
   1. Careful monitoring must be maintained for complications such as hypotension, dehydration, electrolyte and acid-base imbalances, hypothermia, bleeding, inadequate blood flow, infection, and clotted filters and/or circuits, blood leaks, and hemolysis,
   2. Access problems will limit the effectiveness of the therapy if not corrected promptly.
   3. The child should never be left alone during treatment.

II. **Peritoneal dialysis** (see Section 13 for additional information).

A. Indications for peritoneal dialysis (PD).
   1. PD is the treatment of choice for infants and small children.
   2. It is the initial modality choice in 60% of children started on dialysis (NAPRTCS, 2006).
   3. The peritoneal membrane in children is very large in relation to their body surface area.
   4. In males, the peritoneal membrane lines the abdominal cavity covering the abdominal viscera.
   5. In females, the ovaries and fallopian tubes open into the peritoneal cavity.

B. Access placement.
   1. An access is obtained in an operating room (OR) or at the patient's bedside in infant or pediatric intensive care unit (IICU/PICU).
   2. Placement in an OR allows the surgeon to perform an omentectomy at the time of placement.
   3. Laparoscopic visualization for hernias should be done with placement and corrected if found.
   4. Some units advocate insertion 2 to 6 weeks prior to the initiation of therapy to optimize healing.

C. Initial considerations.
   1. Is the gut and peritoneal membrane intact?
   2. Is the patient stable enough to tolerate the insertion of catheter?
   3. Is the respiratory status adequate to tolerate the increased fluid volume in the abdomen?
   4. Are several dialysis treatments going to be required?

D. Special needs in infants and small children.
1. The initial fluid volumes are 10–20 mL/kg to 1100 m² BSA.
2. Manual dialysis exchanges may be needed for inflow volumes less than 50 mL as in neonates and small infants.

E. Continuous cycling peritoneal dialysis (CCPD)
1. Treatment is done using a machine programmed with the prescription and cycles desired, thus the term *cycler*.
2. Settings are programmed for inflow volume and time, dwell time, outflow time, and number of cycles.
3. Cyclers maintain a running tabulation of exact volumes used and of ultrafiltrate.
4. Most cyclers require an inflow volume of at least 50 mL.
5. The automated system allows the child to receive treatment for 8–12 hours each night.
6. Older children and adolescents may require day fill(s) in addition to night treatment.
7. Some systems allow "walk away" fill(s) during the day to add to the number of cycles without requiring additional time at night. The cycler can be set up and used for one or more cycles prior to the nighttime's continuous treatment. This requires that the patient's line(s) be capped with a special sterile cap.
8. Some machines have computer programs that save data to removable chips and/or allow for modem transfer of data.

F. CAPD (continuous peritoneal ambulatory dialysis).
1. Exchanges take place during the day.
2. Technically difficult for children to perform without a caregiver present.
3. There is a higher incidence of peritonitis in children.
4. Requires caregiver to perform the treatment unless the child is older or an adolescent.
5. CAPD can used for backup in the event of power outages, natural disasters, etc.
6. It can also be used at summer camps or for trips away from home if the patient and family have been trained in the technique and child does well with longer dwell times.

G. Manual peritoneal dialysis.
1. Used in neonates or small infants when volume of fill is less than 50–100 mL/cycle.
   a. 20–40 mL/kg of dialysate is warmed to 37° C, infused over 10–15 minutes, allowed to dwell 10–20 minutes, and drained over 10–15 minutes in continuous cycles.
   b. Requires the use of a Y-set connected to a volutrol. Dialysate is connected to side of the Y with the spike. The other side with the drain bag attached is the drain.
   c. Small volume sets, such as the Dialy-Nate (www.utahmed.com), provide a closed system for manual dialysis procedures.
2. Manual dialysis is a time intensive treatment requiring the use of a timer to regulate the manual clamping and unclamping of bags.

H. Complications of PD.
1. Infection is a major complication of PD.
   a. It is the most frequent cause of hospitalization in children (USRDS, 2006).
   b. Infection is the primary reason for modality change in children and is the cited reason for 28% of the modality changes (NAPRTCS, 2006).
   c. Most commonly seen pathogens.
      (1) Gram-positive bacteria: *Staphylococcus aureus, Staphylococcus epidermidis.*
      (2) Gram-negative bacteria: *Pseudomonas, E. coli, Klebsiella.*
      (3) Fungi.
      (4) There are cases where no organism is identified in a symptomatic patient.
   d. Risk factors for infection.
      (1) Young patient age, especially when in diapers or incontinent at night.
      (2) Single cuff with an upward exit site.
      (3) Leakage, usually associated with early use or poor catheter immobilization.
      (4) Nasal carriage of *S. aureus* in child or care provider.
      (5) Prior exit/tunnel infection.
      (6) Connection contamination.
      (7) Shortened family training.
      (8) Lack of regular retraining or assessment of learning.
      (9) Environmental problem areas, e.g., fans, open windows, pets, etc.
   e. Preventive measures.
      (1) Downward directed tunnel (Bender, 2006).
      (2) Avoidance of trauma with placement.
      (3) Double cuffed catheters.
      (4) Delayed use (2–6 weeks).
      (5) Mupiricin treatment of patient and family (Cochrane, 2007).
      (6) Gentamicin treatment at exit site (Piraino, 2005).
   f. Prompt treatment of exit site and tunnel infections.

(1) Flush-before-fill, non-spike systems, APD.

(2) Prolonged training.

(3) Regular retraining of patient and care providers.

(4) Home visit assessments annually or more if indicated.

2. Mechanical problems can result from increased intraperitoneal pressure.

a. Hernias.

(1) Can be incisional, inguinal, or umbilical.

(2) Occur in 12–53% of pediatric patients on PD.

(3) The incident rate is higher in young ages.

(4) Usually require surgical correction.

b. Fluid leaks.

(1) A hydrothorax can develop secondary to the glucose peritoneal solution entering the pleura. This is often related to a diaphragmatic defect.

(2) Rare, 1–6% (2% in one pediatric series).

(3) Often modality limiting.

(4) Unilateral, usually occurring on one side of chest, more often on right side.

(5) Pleural-peritoneal diaphragmatic defect versus lymphatics.

c. Hemoperitoneum.

d. Pain.

3. Membrane-related complications of PD.

a. Ultrafiltration (UF) failure.

(1) High peritoneal solute transport with glucose absorption and dissipation of the glucose gradient needed for UF. This can occur intrinsically, secondary to recurrent peritonitis, or related to small dwell volumes. Basically what happens is that the patient absorbs the glucose, which, in turn, prevents ultrafiltration as the concentration gradient is negated.

(2) Other causes of UF failure can include increased lymphatic flow, aquaporin deficiency, loss of functional surface area, adhesions, sclerosing peritonitis, or dialysate leaks.

(3) Treatment could include shortened dwell time, increased dextrose concentration, maximized fill volume, icodextrin for long dwell times, tidal dialysis, and ultimately a modality change to hemodialysis.

b. Inadequate solute clearance.

(1) This can occur intrinsically and should be evaluated with a peritoneal equilibration test (PET).

(2) Treatment could include longer dwell times, maximized dwell volumes, longer sessions or daytime dwells on APD, and ultimately a modality change to hemodialysis.

c. Encapsulating peritoneal sclerosis.

(1) This is a rare but potentially fatal complication occurring in 1–2% of all PD pediatric patients. It is a thickening of the peritoneal membrane and vessels with calcification of the vessels and loss of mesothelial cell layer.

(2) Symptoms include loss of UF, abdominal pain, ascites, and/or intestinal obstruction.

(3) Risk factors.

(a) The amount of time treated with PD with the incidence increasing to 20% after 8 years of therapy.

(b) Recurrent bacterial peritonitis or hypertonic glucose exposure.

(c) Use of chlorhexidine or alcohol at connection sites.

(d) B-blocker therapy.

(e) Acetate dialysate.

(4) Treatment includes:

(a) Supportive therapy.

(b) Nutritional therapy.

(c) Surgery of obstruction.

(d) Immunosuppressive therapy.

(e) Changing modality to hemodialysis or transplantation.

d. Peritoneal calcification.

4. Prescription-related issues that can give rise to complications.

a. Inadequate solute clearance due to small fill volumes, too long or too short dwell times, inadequate dextrose concentration, etc.

b. Hypervolemia: need to pull excessive volumes of fluid.

c. Hypertension from inadequate UF removal.

d. Hypovolemia from vomiting, diarrhea, large urine output, etc.

(1) Longer dwell time can help.

(2) Lower glucose concentration will pull less.

(3) NG or GT feeds via pump or water.

5. Potential catheter-related complications.

a. Obstruction caused by fibrin or omentum.

b. Migration of the catheter.

c. Cuff-extrusion.

d. All generally require surgical intervention.

III. Hemodialysis (see Section 11 for additional information).

A. Indications for treatment with hemodialysis (HD).
   1. Severe fluid and/or electrolyte abnormalities.
   2. Tumor lysis.
   3. Nutritional needs.

B. Safety issues.
   1. The child must be stable enough to tolerate expected fluid shifts.
   2. The child must be carefully monitored throughout the treatment.
   3. The child must never be left unattended during the treatment.

C. Vascular access.
   1. For acute hemodialysis treatments, the access is obtained by placing a central venous catheter (CVC).
   2. If the child is small, two single lumen lines may be used.
   3. For chronic dialysis, an access (i.e., fistula or graft) should be placed early enough so that the patient initiates therapy with a permanent access. The need for a temporary CVC should be avoided.

D. The hemodialysis prescription.
   1. Using an in-center pediatric unit is ideal but not always practical due to the distance from home, finances, quality of life, etc.
   2. Another option is home hemodialysis with a caregiver providing daily, intermittent, or nocturnal treatments.

E. The dialysis procedure.
   1. Estimated blood volume (EBV).
      a. Calculation of the EBV is required and is dependent on the patient's size. The estimated blood volume can be determined by using the following formula:
      EBV = ~ 80 mL/kg
      Example: 80 (mL) x 10 (kg) = 800 mL EBV
      b. Smaller blood tubing is needed. The system should be primed with blood if more than 10% of patient's EBV will be in the circuit.
      c. When the system is primed with blood, discontinue the treatment without returning the blood in the circuit to the patient.
   2. The blood flow rate (BFR).
      a. The BFR can range from 3 to 5 mL/kg/minute. This is especially important with infants and small children.
      b. Calculate the maximum BFR using the formula: 2.5 mL x wt (kg) + 100
      Example:
      2.5(mL) x 10 (kg) +100 = 125 mL/minute
      c. Some neonatal tubing uses a smaller internal diameter requiring calculation of the blood pump speed. Refer to the specific package insert.
      d. The BFR is limited by the vascular access.
   3. Heparin use is determined by specific unit policies. One example might be:
      a. 30–50 units/kg/hour of heparin. This may be preceded with a bolus of 10–20 units/kg. Run to the end of the treatment when using a CVC. Adjust per ACT.
      b. The activated clotting time (ACT) should be > 180 seconds unless bleeding tendencies are a problem. Adjust heparin dose to keep greater than 180 seconds. Check ACT every 20–30 minutes to prevent clotting and over anticoagulation.
      c. Heparin-free dialysis.
         (1) The artificial kidney should be flushed with saline every 20–30 minutes throughout run. This volume of fluid must be added to the patient's UF goal and removed during the treatment.
         (2) Monitor the ACT every 20–30 minutes.
   4. Fluid removal during hemodialysis.
      a. The usual goal of fluid removal is < 5% of the child's predialysis weight.
      b. Accurate assessment of the patient's intravascular volume using noninvasive in-line monitoring during HD treatment optimizes ultrafiltration in children.
         (1) Targeted fluid removal should result in no more than an 8% change in blood volume in first hour of therapy.
         (2) Subsequent hours should result in no more than a 4% change per hour.
      c. Symptoms of intradialytic hypotension (e.g., yawning, headache, hypotension, tachycardia, nausea, vomiting, restlessness) should be treated promptly by decreasing the targeted ultrafiltrate rate for 5 minutes. Observe for vascular refilling.
      d. If refilling does not occur within the 5 minutes, adjust the desired target loss to reflect a new therapy goal.
      e. The estimated dry weight (EDW) needs to be adjusted often since children should be growing and gaining regularly.

F. Complications of hemodialysis.
  1. Infectious complications.
    a. Catheter, fistula or graft infection.
      (1) Catheter-related bloodstream infection (CRBSI).
      (2) Diagnosis is made when the same organism is present in peripheral and CVC cultures.
      (3) 15% of all CRBSI leads to catheter removal.
      (4) 65–75% of these infections are caused by Staphylococcus species.
      (5) Other commonly seen infectious organisms include gram-negative organisms, *Enterococcus*, *Mycobacterium*, and *Candida*.
      (6) Measures to prevent catheter-related bloodstream infections include aseptic technique, mask and gloves; limitation of access care to trained personnel; and the use of closed system positive pressure valve connectors (e.g., Tego™ – www.icumed.com/tego-connector.asp).
    b. Catheter exit site/tunnel infections.
      (1) Symptoms include erythema, tenderness, induration or purulence within 2 cm of the exit site.
      (2) Measures to prevent exit site infection include dressing changes weekly or as needed if using a transparent dressing; dressing changes every 48 hours if using an opaque dressing or gauze and tape. Catheter care is done using betadine or chlorhexidine preparations as recommended by the Centers for Disease Control (CDC).
    c. Dialysate contamination with bacteria and/or endotoxins.
      (1) Require appropriate screening be sent from the patient and the dialysate.
      (2) Positive results must be followed up with appropriate therapy and corrective actions.
  2. Noninfectious complications can include:
    a. Dialysis disequilibrium.
      (1) Etiology: thought to be due to cerebral edema that occurs secondary to the rapid decrease in plasma osmolality during the treatment and/or a change in the cerebral pH.
      (2) Prevention: this is a rare complication that may be avoided by administering mannitol to reduce the drop in plasma osmolarity early in dialysis and gentle solute removal at initiation of dialysis

therapy (Warady, 2004).
      (3) Limiting removal of blood urea nitrogen (BUN) to 30% may help prevent complications.
      (4) Symptoms: headache, nausea, and disorientation, which if untreated, may lead to blurred vision, seizure, and coma.
    b. Air embolism.
      (1) Fortunately this is now a rare occurrence since air detectors are standard on all dialysis machines. *Reminder:* Equipment malfunctions can occur at any time. Monitors and alarms can never replace the need for constant human observation and monitoring.
      (2) The source of air can be accidental disconnects, improperly connected lines, or empty intravenous bags. Discontinuing dialysis using air to rinse back the patient's blood is an extremely dangerous practice and should be discouraged.
      (3) Signs and symptoms of an infusion of air include cough, chest pain, shortness of breath, hypotension, and/or a churning sound on auscultation.
      (4) Treatment: clamp venous line, stop the blood pump, turn the patient on his/her left side with the head down, and administer 100% oxygen. A qualified physician may be able to aspirate air from the right ventricle.
    c. Hemolysis.
      (1) Etiology: overheated dialysate fluid, inadequate water treatment, hypotonic dialysate fluid, formaldehyde in the dialysate fluid, chloramines in the dialysate fluid, or an improperly occluded blood pump.
      (2) Signs and symptoms: port wine venous return, pink plasma when the blood is centrifuged.
      (3) Treatment: turn off blood pump, clamp lines, do NOT return the blood, assess the cause, change the system, transfuse if necessary, and resume dialysis for hyperkalemia.
    d. Prescription or membrane-related potential complication: intradialytic hypotension.
      (1) Symptoms: nausea and vomiting, tachycardia, restlessness, yawning, headache, and syncope.
      (2) Etiology: rapid ultrafiltration (especially if the intradialytic weight gain is excessive), delayed vascular refill, autonomic

dysfunction, paradoxical decrease in sympathetic activity, cardiac dysfunction, and decreasing extracellular fluid (ECF) osmolality.

(3) Preventive measures: avoid excessive interdialytic weight gain; longer or more frequent dialysis treatments; avoid antihypertensive drugs before dialysis if indicated and ordered; food restriction during dialysis; noninvasive volume-guided UF monitoring.

(4) Treatment: Trendelenberg position, reduce or discontinue ultrafiltration, bolus dose of normal saline or 5% albumin.

3. Access-related complications (see Section 12 for additional information).
   a. Catheter or graft thrombus.
   b. Catheter malposition and kinking.
   c. Graft or fistula stenosis.
   d. Graft or fistula steal syndrome.
   e. Inadequate blood flow.
   f. Collateral vessel development.
   g. Recirculation.
   h. All generally require surgical intervention.

Complications of Kidney Disease in Children on Chronic Dialysis

I. Bone disease.

A. Kidney bone disease occurs as result of:
   1. Acidosis.
   2. Calcium and phosphorus imbalance.
   3. Elevated levels of parathyroid hormone (PTH).
   4. Lack of calcitriol production.

B. Assessment.
   1. Left untreated results in severe kidney osteodystrophy (rickets).
   2. Increased risk of bone fractures and impaired or irregular growth.

C. Medical management.
   1. Phosphate binders.
   2. Calcium carbonate in liquid form can be given with formula as part of an enteral feeding regimen, or by bolus feeding.
   3. Calcitriol (the active form of vitamin D) helps the body absorb calcium from food and reduce the production of parathyroid hormone.

D. Nursing care.
   1. Serum phosphorus should be maintained.
      a. Adults 3.0–4.5 mg/dL (0.97–1.45 mmol/L).
      b. Children 4.5–6.5 mg/dL (1.45–2.10 mmol/L).
      c. Infants 4.3–9.3 mg/dL (1.4–3.0 mmol/L).
         (1) Phosphate binders are taken with food but not with iron supplements.
         (2) Phosphate binders enhance excretion of dietary phosphorus.

II. Anemia.

A. Definition and effect on the child (see KDOQI guidelines in Table 15.4).
   1. Anemia contributes to poor quality of life in patients with CKD.
   2. Fatigue, poor cognition, decreased energy, and activity levels.

B. Assessment and diagnosis.
   1. Assess for signs and symptoms of anemia.
      a. Angina, hypotension, tachycardia, shortness of breath.
      b. Diminished appetite and weight loss.
      c. Decreased sense of well being.
   2. Review laboratory test results.
      a. Blood urea nitrogen (BUN) and serum creatinine.
      b. Adequacy of dialysis (Kt/V_{urea}).
      c. CBC.
      d. Iron profile (serum iron, ferritin, TIBC, TSAT).
   3. Assess for the causes of anemia.
      a. Blood loss.
      b. Iron or vitamin deficiencies.
      c. Inflammation or infection.
      d. Secondary hyperparathyroidism.
      e. Medication interactions.
      f. Coexisting medical conditions.
      g. Malnutrition.
   4. Assess patient and family's understanding of:
      a. Role of kidney in anemia.
      b. Signs and symptoms of anemia.
      c. Consequences of anemia, including left ventricular hypertrophy (LVH).
      d. Signs of gastrointestinal bleeding (e.g., hematemesis, tarry stools).

C. Medical management.
   1. Administer medications needed to treat anemia.
      a. Erythropoietin-stimulating agents (ESAs).
      b. Iron supplements.
      c. Vitamins.
   2. Monitor response to therapy including:

a. Hemoglobin and hematacrit.
b. Iron profile.
c. Sense of well-being.
3. Monitor blood pressure during initiation of therapy with ESAs.

D. Nursing care.
1. Collaborate with health care provider to develop and use an anemia management protocol.
2. Encourage adherence to treatment and medication routines.
3. Teach child to self-administer ESA if appropriate to decrease perception of pain.

III. Hypertension.

A. Definition and effect on the child: optimal systolic and diastolic blood pressure should be < 95% for age, gender, and height (see BP Tables 15.2 and 15.3).

B. Assessment and diagnosis.
1. Hypertension is commonly seen in 49% of children with CKD and 50–60% of those on chronic dialysis.
2. Determination and management of BP in children should follow recommendations by The Fourth Report of the Diagnosis, Evaluation, and Treatment of High Blood Pressure in Children and Adolescents (see Tables 15.2 and 15.3).

C. Management of hypertension on dialysis requires attention to fluid status, antihypertensive medications, and intradialytic fluid accumulation by:
1. Education by dieticians reinforced regularly.
2. Limit sodium, usually no more than 2 grams per day.
3. Increased ultrafiltration (UF).
4. Longer dialysis duration.
5. More than three dialysis treatments per week or longer sessions.
6. Antihypertensives for nondialysis days.

D. Dialysis patients should have pulse pressure (PP) determined monthly before dialysis.
1. For PP greater than 60 mm Hg and systolic BP greater than 135 mm Hg, reduce by achieving ideal body weight and use antihypertensive medication for a target of PP of 40 mm Hg.

IV. Cardiovascular disease (CVD).

A. KDOQI guidelines recommend children starting dialysis be evaluated for the presence of cardiac

disease (i.e., cardiomyopathy and valvular disease).
1. Echocardiogram once patient achieves dry weight (ideally within 3 months).
2. Screen for dyslipidemias.
3. Screen for hypertension.

B. Definition and effect on the child.
1. Acute myocardial infarction, pericarditis, atherosclerotic heart disease, cardiomyopathy, cardiac arrhythmia, cardiac arrest, and/or valvular heart disease are possible effects.
2. The leading cause of death in pediatric patients on dialysis in 2006 USRDS data.
3. Accounted for 28% of deaths in dialysis patients and 27% of pediatric deaths.
4. Second leading cause of death (44/204, 22%) in North American Pediatric Trials and Cooperative Studies (NAPRTCS) registry.
5. In children age 10–19, cardiovascular mortality has increased 62% since 1991 (USRDS, 2006).

C. Assessment and diagnosis.
1. USRDS study (1991–1996): in 1454 pediatric patients, 31% developed CVD.
a. The most common cardiac event was arrhythmia 20%.
b. Vascular heart disease (VHD) in 12%.
c. Cardiomyopathy 10%.
d. Cardiac arrest 3%.
2. Arrhythmias include sinus tachycardia, premature ventricular contractions (PVC), and heart block in pediatric chronic dialysis patients.
3. Atherosclerosis (AHD) is prevalent in 10–15% of pediatric chronic dialysis patients (more common with higher serum phosphorus and calcium-phosphorus product).
4. Coronary artery calcification was associated with higher levels of C-reactive protein (CRP), plasma homocysteine, intact PTH, and higher calcium-phosphorus product.
5. Echocardiography should be used to document left ventricular hypertrophy (LVH), left ventricular dilation, and cardiomyopathy (systolic and diastolic dysfunction) at initiation of dialysis, once patient has achieved dry weight, and at 3-year intervals. LVH is a known risk factor for CVD and mortality in adults on chronic dialysis and may well contribute to CVD risk in children, too.
6. Valvular heart disease should be evaluated by echocardiography.

D. Medical management.

1. VHD should be managed following ACC/AHA guidelines.
2. Dialysis patients should have a 12-lead ECG at initiation of dialysis. They should have it repeated once they achieve dry weight (ideally within 3 months).
3. Screen for traditional CVD risk factors such as dyslipidemia and hypertension.

E. Nursing care.
   1. Onsite external automatic defibrillator and/or appropriate pediatric equipment should be kept available and in good working order.
   2. Use pediatric arrhythmia algorithm.
   3. Basic life support (BLS) and Pediatric Advanced Life Support (PALS) preferred.
   4. If there is arterial calcification in two or more sites (abdominal aorta, carotid arteries, ileofemoral axis, or femoropopliteal axis), the use of noncalcium phosphate binder is recommended.
   5. Intact PTH assay (first-generation immunoradiometric assay) should be monitored every 3 months. The targeted goal for the prevention of CVD is between 150 and 300 pg/mL (16.5–33.0 pmol/L).

V. Infection.

A. Definition and effect on the child.
   1. Infection is the second largest cause of death in pediatric patients on chronic dialysis (20%).
   2. More children have SVC than in the adult population.
   3. Infections lead to poor performance in school due to lost school days.
   4. Rates of infectious hospitalization constitute almost half of the admissions per year (USRDS, 2006).

B. Assessment and diagnosis.
   1. Monitor for temperature elevations.
   2. Monitor CRP for inflammation.
   3. Evaluate and treat suspected infections. Children with lines in place can become chronically infected.

C. Medical management.
   1. Obtain cultures and administer antibiotics. Adjust treatment based on results of culture and sensitivity reports.
   2. Evaluate for methicillin-resistant staph (MRSA).

D. Nursing care.

1. Careful questioning to ascertain possible source of infection.
2. In PD infections, a root cause analysis will determine the need for retraining.
3. Patient and family education is a vital part of any pediatric dialysis program.

Pharmacology

I. Medications specific to children (see Section 9 for additional information).

A. Growth hormone should be started when patient falls off standard growth curve.

B. Immunizations should be kept current to avoid the need for live vaccines once transplanted.

II. Emergency care.

A. Medications should be calculated for pediatric patients.

B. Appropriate BLS equipment must be on hand when caring for children.
   1. Oropharyngeal airways in sizes 00–5 for infant, child, and adult.
   2. Nasopharyngeal airways in sizes 4.5 mm–8.5 mm (18 Fr–34 Fr).
   3. Self-inflating resuscitation bag in child and adult sizes (reservoir of 450 mL for child and 1000 mL for adult).
   4. Oxygen masks for infant, child, and adult.
   5. Suction catheters 6 Fr–14 Fr.
   6. Bag-valve-mask devices in infant, child, and adult sizes.
   7. Nonrebreathing masks in pediatric and adult sizes.
   8. Automated external defibrillator able to deliver pediatric doses with arrhythmia detection algorithm on site.

III. Safety issues.

A. Tips for getting children to take their medications.
   1. Gastrostomy tubes, pegs, buttons, etc.
      a. Use a matter-of-fact approach.
      b. Expectation that this is what you do.
      c. Routine time and place for medications can help.
      d. Bribes do not work long-term and are best avoided.
   2. Fear of needles: minimizing the pain of

injection is important.
a. Ice to the injection site can help.
b. Numbing cream at the injection site.
c. Use small-gauge needles.
d. Distraction.
e. Treat injection in a matter-of-fact way without a power struggle.
f. Teach child to give self-injection; often hurts less as they distract themselves.
g. Never use the injection as a threat.

Psychosocial Issues

I. **Impact of kidney disease on child and family – changes family dynamics.**

A. Care for a child with a chronic illness involves considerable psychological and social stress.

B. Autonomy development requires attention to issues of overprotection by parents or caregivers of chronically ill children. This is made especially difficult if the parent is the caregiver "controlling" the dialysis treatments.

C. The overprotection often is a misguided attempt to compensate for the child's "suffering."

D. Parents and/or caregivers need help in understanding how to discipline and what expectations to set for the child.

E. Respite for the caregivers is to be encouraged when possible to help avoid burnout and depression.

II. **Nursing care.**

A. Autonomy development: give attention to overprotective parents and caregivers.

B. Overprotection is an attempt to compensate for the child's "suffering."

C. Parents and caregivers need anticipatory guidance in developing expectations for the child.

D. Social development and self-esteem requires peer relationships.

E. Adolescents may need support for dealing with rejection for being different at a time when conformity determines body image and identity.

F. Adolescents may need strategies for developing close relationships with peers to assist in development of body image, self-esteem, and independence.

G. Transition from childhood to adulthood is a key mediating role for adult quality of life.

H. Help with transition into adult life from family life to independent life and from school to employment.

I. School completion will assist in the transition and set expectations for an adult life.

III. **Methods to promote adherence to treatment.**

A. Factors that may influence patient adherence to therapy and/or medication regimen.
1. Misunderstanding of therapy or medication dose changes.
2. Belief that therapy and/or medications are not helpful.
3. Disorganized family structure.
4. Adolescence.
5. Complexity of therapy and/or medication regimen.
6. Body image changes.

B. Factors that help adherence.
1. Simplification of therapy and/or medication administration/dosage times.
2. Ongoing education.
3. Frequent clinic visits.
4. Behavior modification.
5. Involvement of adolescents in self-care to promote independence.
6. Planning for a future and developing life goals.
7. Counseling individual and/or family based.

IV. **Providing pediatric care.**

A. Partner with patients and families as members of the health care team.

B. Treat each family with dignity and respect.
1. Listen to patient and family perspectives and choices.
2. Incorporate patient/family knowledge, values, beliefs, and cultural backgrounds into care planning and delivery.

C. Build partnerships based on mutual respect and open communication.
1. Respect each family's uniqueness.
2. Listen carefully to understand perspectives and needs of families.

D. Share information clearly, completely, and consistently.
   1. Communicate and share information with patients/families in ways that are affirming and useful.
   2. Ensure privacy and confidentiality.
   3. Respond flexibly to family needs and negotiate differences of opinion in a timely and respectful manner.
   4. Promote and value competency and expertise each member brings to health care team.
   5. Include providers/services in family's home community/school in care team.
   6. Allow patient's/family's participation in decision making and care planning by assuring timely, complete, accurate information.

V. Patient and family education.

A. Children with ESRD need special attention paid to learning and developing skills for social and independent functioning.

B. Achieving age-specific developmental milestones is important in adjustment to adult life.

C. Whenever appropriate, children should be included in planning, implementing, and taking responsibility for their own care.

D. Education of parent and caregiver should be done at the 5–6th grade reading level.

E. The parent and caregiver may need assessment for ability to read or other cognitive dysfunction.

F. Parents need written materials for training as well as visual and verbal cues.

G. Monthly clinic visit are an opportunity to teach and reinforce prior teaching.

VI. The pediatric patient in an adult unit.

A. An adult unit must have the resources, both staff and equipment, to meet the safety needs of the pediatric patient.
   1. Pediatric patients are not just little adults. They respond differently and can be challenging.
   2. Maintaining fluid balance is a major concern.
   3. Patients must achieve dry weight or risk serious complications from LVH, chronic fluid overload, and potential cardiac complications.
   4. Crying and manipulative behaviors may hinder the staff in the process of fluid removal.

B. Transition to adult care.
   1. Transition from childhood to adulthood plays a key mediating role for later quality of life.
   2. Chronic illness may complicate the transition into adult life.
      a. From family to independent life.
      b. From school to employment.
   3. Transition programs should place expectations on the child.
   4. Independence requires that the child knows his/her medications, dialysis therapy parameters, health history, diet, and the significance of relating to care providers.
   5. Adult care providers will expect the child to be able to manage his/her own appointment and the child needs to be prepared to assume responsibility.

Pediatric Kidney Transplantation

I. Transplantation is the preferred mode of therapy for pediatric patients with CKD Stage 5 (see Section 10 for additional information).

A. Frequency of transplantation (NAPRTCS, 2005): 400–500 pediatric stage 5 CKD patients (ages 0–19) received kidney transplants annually from 1987 to 2005.

B. Frequency of dialysis initiation in pediatric CKD stage 5 patients (NAPRTCS, 2005): ranged from a high of 739 patients in 1991 to 128 patients in 2005.

II. Absolute contraindications for transplant.

A. Active or untreated malignancy.

B. Chronic HIV infection.

C. Chronic active infection with hepatitis B.

D. Severe multiorgan failure.

E. Positive current direct crossmatch.

F. Debilitating irreversible brain injury.

III. Pretransplant evaluation and preparation.

A. The cause of kidney failure is a consideration.

B. Donor source.
   1. Living donors account for 52% of transplanted kidneys; 42% of those come from parents.
   2. Deceased donors account for the other 48%.

C. Age at time of transplantation.
   1. Ages 0–1   5.3%
   2. Ages 2–5   14.9%
   3. Ages 6–12   33.7%
   4. Ages 13–17   38.4%
   5. Ages > 17   7.7%

IV. Preemptive transplant versus the need for dialysis.

A. Transplantation may be the first mode of therapy for some patients.

B. Preemptive transplants occur more frequently in children because of the parents' and patients' desire to avoid dialysis when a living donor is available.

C. Transplantation is actively promoted by pediatric nephrology centers.

D. Many centers want pediatric transplant recipients to weigh a minimum of 10 kg.

E. Morbidity is lower for children with transplantation than with dialysis therapy.

V. Patient and graft survival.

A. The living donor graft survival rate is 80% at 5 years posttransplantation.

B. The deceased donor graft survival rate is 65% at 5 years posttransplantation.

VI. Preparation for transplantation.

A. Titers and surveillance for:
   a. Tuberculosis.
   b. HIV.
   c. Hepatitis B and C.
   d. Dental infections.
   e. Skin.
   f. Sinuses.
   g. Urinary tract infections.

B. Urologic issues must be evaluated, and necessary repairs of urinary tract abnormalities must be made. These could include:
   a. Ureterovesical or ureteropelvic junction obstruction.
   b. Vesicoureteral reflux.
   c. Intermittent catheterization for neurogenic bladder.
   d. Bladder augmentation.
   e. Creation of a Mitrofanoff.
   f. Removal of duplicated systems.

C. Evaluation for cardiovascular disease (CVD) includes:
   a. Determining adequate cardiac function.
   b. Insuring that the iliac vasculature is patent.
   c. Assessing for the absence of vascular disease.
   d. Evaluating hypertension and left ventricular hypertrophy (LVH).

D. Nephrectomies may be indicated prior to transplantation in certain conditions.
   1. Polycystic kidney disease.
   2. Uncontrolled hypertension.
   3. Congenital nephrotic syndrome.
   4. Denys-Drash syndrome is a disorder with three main parts: kidney disease present at birth, Wilm's tumor, and malformation of the sexual organs.
   5. Severe reflux.
   6. High-output kidney diseases.
   7. Severe uncontrollable proteinuria.

E. Hypertension.
   1. Determine the cause and treat appropriately.
   2. Hypertension posttransplantation can cause irreversible damage to the graft.

F. Immunizations.
   1. All immunizations should be up to date for age prior to transplantation.
   2. Live virus vaccines should be administered at least 1–2 months prior to transplantation.

G. Viral surveillance and screening includes:
   1. Human immunodeficiency virus (HIV).
   2. Hepatitis B and C.
   3. Epstein-Barr virus (EBV).
   4. Cytomegalovirus (CMV).
   5. Varicella zoster virus (VZV).
   6. Measles, mumps, and rubella titers (MMR) at most centers.

H. Adequate nutrition prior to kidney transplantation is needed to:
   1. Prevent metabolic disturbances.
   2. Prevent growth retardation.
   3. Prevent malnutrition.
   4. Promote healing.

I. Neuropsychologic evaluation is needed prior to transplantation. The recipient's age determines the process for evaluation. The evaluation should include assessment for:
   1. Mental function.
   2. Neurologic abnormalities.
   3. Psychomotor delay.
   4. Seizures.
   5. Psychiatric disorders.
   6. Emotional disorders.
   7. Nonadherence.

J. The child should be malignant free for 1–2 years prior to transplantation.

K. Dental exams are required.
   1. The teeth and gums should be evaluated prior to transplantation.
   2. Needed dental work must be completed prior to transplant.
   3. The presence of infection may lead to life-threatening illness posttransplantation.
   4. Written documentation from the dentist regarding the child's dental status should be obtained.

L. Lab studies prior to transplantation.
   1. Chemistries.
   2. Hematology.
   3. Coagulation studies.
   4. Urine studies.
   5. ABO compatibility.
   6. Monthly antibody screening.
   7. Histocompatibility testing.

M. Evaluation for pulmonary disease.
   1. Asthma.
   2. Bronchopulmonary dysplasia (BPD).
   3. Tuberculosis (TB).

N. Evaluation for gastrointestinal disease.
   1. Active ulcer disease.
   2. Esophageal disease.
   3. Liver disease.
   4. Portal hypertension.

O. Evaluation for endocrine disease.
   1. Hyperparathyroidism.
   2. Diabetes.

P. Evaluation of growth and development and treatment of correctable abnormal findings.
   1. Poor or inadequate nutrition.
   2. Inadequate dialysis therapy.

   3. Anemia.
   4. Anorexia.
   5. Chronic acidosis.
   6. Need for human growth hormone therapy to maximize growth potential.

VII. **Patient and family education regarding transplant.**

A. Education of the patient and caregiver is done based on patient age and developmental stage.

B. Education of parent/caregiver should be done at 5th–6th grade reading level.

C. The parent/caregiver may need to be assessed for ability to read or other cognitive dysfunction.

D. Topics to include.
   1. Pretransplant care.
   2. Intraoperative care and risks.
   3. Postoperative care and risks.

VIII. **The transplant surgery.**

A. The location of the transplanted organ is based on the patient's size.
   1. It is usually placed in the anterior iliac fossa, extraperitoneally.
   2. In an infant or small child, the kidney may be placed intraperitoneally.

B. The blood pressure and volume status are closely monitored to keep the central venous pressure (CVP) at about 15–20 mm Hg at the time of graft reperfusion. This is necessary to maintain intravascular integrity and allograft perfusion.

IX. **The posttransplant period.**

A. Delayed graft function.
   1. Oliguria, decreased GFR, or need for dialysis in immediate postoperative period can be associated with decreased allograft survival.
   2. Acute tubular necrosis (ATN).
   3. Perfusion injury.
   4. Hyperacute rejection.

B. Surgical complications.
   1. Perfusion injury.
   2. Thrombosis.
   3. Obstruction.
   4. Bleeding.
   5. Lymphocele.

6. Urine leak.
7. Incisional problems.

C. Posttransplant care.
 1. Maintenance of circulatory function.
 2. Maintenance of pulmonary function.
 3. Maintenance of fluid and electrolyte balance.
 4. Infection prevention.
 5. Monitoring immunosuppressant therapy.
 6. Monitoring for constipation or diarrhea.
 7. Monitoring for pain.
 8. Monitoring for signs and symptoms of rejection.
 9. Education of patient and family.

D. Types of rejection.
 1. Hyperacute.
    a. Occurs within minutes up to 24 hours posttransplantation.
    b. Difficult to treat and often irreversible.
 2. Accelerated.
    a. Occurs within 3 to 5 days posttransplantation.
    b. Difficult to treat.
 3. Acute.
    a. More common in the first 6 months posttransplantation.
    b. One of leading causes of readmission posttransplantation.
 4. Chronic allograft nephropathy, also known as chronic rejection, is the most common cause of graft loss in children.

E. Infections.
 1. Bacterial infections.
    a. Pneumonia.
    b. Urinary tract infections.
 2. Viral infections.
    a. Account for 25–30% of infections in children posttransplantation.
    b. Children are five times more likely to develop primary viral infections due to lack of exposure pre transplantation, and thus lack of immunity.
    c. Viral infections.
       (1) Epstein Barr virus (EBV) is a seronegative status pretransplant is associated with a higher risk of posttransplant lympho-proliferative disease (PTLD).
       (2) Cytomegalovirus (CMV).
       (3) *Varicella zoster* virus (VZV) can be severe and have many complications including encephalitis, pneumonitis, hepatic dysfunction, and even death.
    d. Wound infections.
    e. Opportunistic infections, e.g., *Pneumocystis carinii* pneumonia (PCP).

F. Primary diseases that tend to reoccur following a transplant.
 1. Membranoproliferative glomerulonephritis.
 2. Lupus.
 3. IgA nephropathy.
 4. Membranous glomerulonephritis.
 5. Atypical HUS.
 6. FSGS.
 7. Primary hyperoxaluria: the best therapy is combined liver and kidney transplant.

G. Malignancies can return after a transplant due immunosuppressive therapy. Malignancies may include:
 1. Posttransplant lymphoproliferative disease (PTLD).
 2. Lymphoma.
 3. Skin cancers.

H. Nutrition requires close monitoring posttransplantation.
 1. Hypophosphatemia can occur due to secondary hyperparathyroidism. It may require phosphorus supplements.
 2. Hypercalcemia can also occur due to secondary hyperparathyroidism.
 3. Hypokalemia is due to pretransplant diet restrictions coupled with normal urinary output posttransplantation. It can often be treated by liberalizing the diet.
 4. Dehydration from years of fluid restriction while on renal replacement therapy (RRT).
 5. An increased appetite due to improved kidney function and the use of steroids may lead to sudden, excessive weight gains.
 6. Diabetes may develop posttransplantation due to:
    a. Tacrolimus use.
    b. Steroid use.

X. Human growth and development following transplantation.

A. Steroid usage and age at time of transplantation impact posttransplant growth. Children under the age of 6 show the best growth.

B. Improvement posttransplantation.
 1. Poor allograft function can inhibit growth.
 2. Growth can be improved by the use of growth hormone. However, it is usually started for 1–2 years posttransplantation.

C. Dental care is imperative to prevent bacterial infections.

1. Promotion of healthy teeth and gums is the goal.
2. The use of antibiotic prophylaxis is center specific.

XI. Nonadherence to medical regimen.

A. Factors influencing patient adherence.
   1. Misunderstanding of dose changes.
   2. Belief that medications are not helpful.
   3. Disorganized family structure.
   4. Adolescents need for control and lack of understanding of long-term consequences.

5. Complexity of medication regimen.
6. Body image changes.

B. Factors that can assist with patient adherence.
   1. Simplification of medication administration and dosage times.
   2. Ongoing education.
   3. Frequent clinic visits.
   4. Behavior modification.
   5. Counseling.

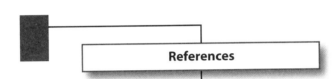

References

American Nephrology Nurses' Association (ANNA). (2007). *CKD learning module 5: Stage 5 chronic kidney disease – Pediatrics.* Pitman, NJ: Author.

American Nurses Credentialing Center (ANCC). (2002). *Pediatric nursing review manual.* Washington, DC: Institute for Research, Education, and Consultation at ANCC.

Ball, L.K. (2005). Improving arteriovenous fistula cannulation skills. *Nephrology Nursing Journal, 32*(6), 611-617.

Bender, F.H., Bernardini, J., & Piraino, B. (2006). Prevention of infectious complications in peritoneal dialysis: Best demonstrated practices. *Kidney International, 70*(Suppl. 103), S44-S54.

Biel, L., Bonadio, T., Farina, J., & Fleming, W. (2005). The peritoneal equilibration test. *Nephrology Nursing Journal, 32*(4), 452.

Boydstun, I. (2005). Chronic kidney disease in adolescents. *Adolescent Medicine Clinics, 16,* 185-199.

Brophy, P.D., Mottes, T.A., Kudelka, T.L., McBryde, K.D., Gardner, J.J., Maxvold, N.J., et al. (2001). AN-69 membrane reactions are pH-dependent and preventable. *American Journal of Kidney Diseases, 38*(1).

Burrows-Hudson, S., & Prowant, B.F. (Eds.). (2005). Continuous renal replacement therapy. *Nephrology nursing standards of practice and guidelines for care.* Pitman NJ: American Nephrology Nurses' Association.

Collins, A., Kasiske, B., Herzog, C., Chen, S., Everson, S., Constantini, E., et al. (2007). Excerpts from the United States renal data system 2006 annual data report. *American Journal of Kidney Diseases, 49*(Suppl. 1), S1-S296.

Colville, L.A., & Lee, A.H. (2006). Retrospective analysis of catheter-related infections in a hemodialysis unit. *Infection Control Hospital Epidemiology, 27,* 969-973.

Cupples, S.A., & Ohler, L. (2003). *Transplantation nursing secrets.* Philadelphia: Hanley & Belfus.

Danovitch, G.M. (2005). *Handbook of kidney transplantation.* (4th ed.). Philadelphia: Lippincott Williams & Wilkins.

Fervenza, F.C., Pattison, J., Goldsmith, D., Hartley, B., & Grande, J.P. (2004). *A color handbook of renal medicine.* New York: Thieme Medical Publishers.

Fischbach, M., Edefonti, A., Schrader, C., & Watson, A. (2005). Hemodialysis in children: General practical guidelines. *Pediatric Nephrology, 20*(8), 1054-1066.

Gerson, A., Hwang, W., Fiorenza, B.A., Barth, K., Kaskel, F., Weiss, L., et al. (2004). Anemia and health-related quality of life in adolescents with chronic kidney disease. *American Journal of Kidney Diseases, 44*(6), 1012-1023.

Gilman, C., & Frauman, A. (2006). The child with kidney disease. In A.E. Molzahn & E. Butera (Eds.), *Contemporary nephrology nursing* (2nd ed., pp. 457-484). Pitman, NJ: American Nephrology Nurses' Association.

Goldstein, S.L. (2006). Pediatric acute kidney injury: It's time for real progress. *Pediatric Nephrology, 21*(7), 891-895.

Groothoff, J., Grootenhuis, M., Offringa, M., Stronks, K., Hutten G., & Heymans, H. (2005). Social consequences in adult life of end-stage renal disease in childhood. *Journal of Pediatrics, 146*(4), 512-517.

Lancaster, L.E. (Ed.). (2001). *Core curriculum for nephrology nursing* (4th ed.). Pitman, NJ: American Nephrology Nurses' Association.

McCarley, P. (2006). The KDOQI clinical practice guidelines and clinical practice recommendations for treating anemia in patients with chronic kidney disease: Implications for nurses. *Nephrology Nursing Journal, 33*(4), 423-445.

McDonald S., & Craig, J. (2004). Long-term survival of children with end-stage renal disease. *New England Journal of Medicine, 350*(26), 2654-2662.

Michael, M., Brewer, E.D., & Goldstein, S.L. (2004). Blood volume monitoring to achieve target weight in pediatric hemodialysois patients. *Pediatric Nephrology, 19,* 432-437.

Mitchell, S. (2002). Estimated dry weight (EDW): Aiming for accuracy. *Nephrology Nursing Journal, 29*(5), 421-430.

Molzahn, A.E., & Butera, E. (Eds.). (2006). *Contemporary nephrology nursing: Principles and practice* (2nd ed.). Pitman, NJ: American Nephrology Nurses' Association.

National High Blood Pressure Education Program Working Group on High Blood Pressure in Children and Adolescents. (2004). The fourth report on the diagnosis, evaluation, and treatment of high blood pressure in children and adolescents. *Pediatrics, 114*(2), 555-576.

National Kidney Foundation (NKF). (2005). KDOQI clinical practice guidelines for cardiovascular disease in dialysis patients. Am*erican Journal of Kidney Diseases, 45*(Suppl. 3), S1-S154.

National Kidney Foundation (NKF). (2006a). KDOQI clinical practice guidelines and clinical practice recommendations for 2006 updates: Hemodialysis adequacy, peritoneal dialysis adequacy, and vascular access. *American Journal of Kidney Disease, 48*(Suppl. 1), S1-S322.

National Kidney Foundation (NKF). (2006b). KDOQI clinical practice guidelines and clinical practice recommendations for anemia in chronic kidney disease. *American Journal of Kidney Disease, 47*(Suppl. 3), S1-S146.

North American Pediatric Renal Trials and Collaborative Studies (NAPRTCS). (2006). *2006 annual report* (pp. 109-145). Retrieved from https://web.emmes.com/study/ped/annlrept/annlrept2006.pdf

Onder, A.M., Chandar, J., Coakley, S., Abitbol, C., Montane, B., & Zilleruelo, G. (2006). Predictors and outcome of catheter-related bacteremia in children on chronic hemodialysis. *Journal of the International Pediatric Nephrology Association.*

Patel, H.P., Goldstein, S.L., Manahan, J.D., Smith, B., Fried, C.B., Currier, H., et al. (2007, January 31). A standard, noninvasive monitoring of hematacrit algorithm improves blood pressure control in pediatric hemodialysis patients [Electronic version]. *Clinical Journal of the American Society of Nephrology.* Retrieved January 31, 2007, from http://www.cjasn.org

Piraino, B., Bailie, G.R., Bernardini, J., Boeschoten, E., Gupta, A., Holmens, C., et al. (2005). Peritoneal dialysis-related infections recommendations: 2005 update. *Peritoneal Dialysis International, 25*, 107-131.

Purcell, W., Manias, E., Williams, A., & Walker, R. (2004). Accurate dry weight assessment: Reducing the incidence of hypertension and cardiac disease in patients on hemodialysis. *Nephrology Nursing Journal, 31*(6), 631-638.

Ramage, I., Bailie, A., Tyerman, K., McColl, J., Pollard S., & Fitzpatrick, M. (2005). Vascular access survival in children and young adults receiving long-term hemodialysis. *American Journal of Kidney Diseases, 45*, 708–715.

Reams, S.M., & Elder, V. (2003). Dry weight: To be set or not to be…that is a good question. *Nephrology Nursing Journal, 30*(2), 236-237.

Roderick, P., Willis, N., Blakeley, S., Jones, C., & Tomson, C. (2007). Correction of chronic metabolic acidosis for chronic kidney disease patients. *Cochrane Database of Systematic Reviews, 2.*

Rodriguez, H.J., Domenici, R., Drioll, A., & Goykhman, I. (2005). Assessment of dry weight by monitoring changes in blood volume during hemodialysis using Crit-Line. *Kidney International, 68*, 854-861.

Saran, R., Bragg-Gresham, J.L., Levin, N.W., Twardowski, Z.J., Wizemann, V., Saito, A., et al. (2006). Longer treatment time and slower ultrafiltration in hemodialysis: Associations with reduced mortality in the DOPPS. *Kidney International*, 1222-1228.

Schroeder, K.L., Sallustio, J.E., & Ross, E.A. (2004). Continuous haematocrit monitoring during intradialytic hypotension: precipitous decline in plasma refill rates. *Nephrology Dialysis Transplant, 3*, pp 652-656.

Seikaly, M.G., Salhab, N., & Browne, R. (2005). Patterns and time of initiation of dialysis in U.S. children. *Pediatric Nephrology, 20*(7), 982-988.

Smeltzer, S.C., & Bare, B.G. (2000). *Textbook of medical surgical nursing* (9th ed.). Philadelphia: Lippincott Williams & Wilkins.

Stam, H., Hartman, E., Deurloo, J., Groothoff, J., & Grootenhuis, M. (2006). Young adult patients with a history of pediatric disease: Impact of course of life and transition into adulthood. *Journal of Adolescent Health, 39*, 4-13.

Strippoli, G.F.M., Tong, A., Johnson, D., Schena, F.P., & Craig, J.C. (2007). Antimicrobial agents for preventing peritonitis in peritoneal dialysis patients. *Cochrane Database of Systematic Reviews, 2.*

Stuart, F.P., Abecassis, M.M., & Kaufman, D.B. (2003). *Organ transplantation* (2nd ed.). Georgetown, TX.: Landes Bioscience.

Tejani, A.H., Harmon, W.E., & Fine, R.N. (2000). *Pediatric solid organ transplantation.* Munksgaard, Copenhagen: Trykkeriet Viborg.

Twardowski, Z., Prowant, B.F, Moore, H., Lou, L., White, E., & Farris, K. (2003). Short peritoneal equilibration test: Impact of preceding dwell time. *Advances in Peritoneal Dialysis, 19*, 53-58.

United States Renal Data System (USRDS). (2006). *2006 annual data report: Atlas of end-stage renal disease in the United States.* Bethesda, MD: National Institutes of Health, National Institute of Diabetes and Digestive and Kidney Diseases.

Vimalachandra, D., Hodson, E., Willis, N., Craig, J., Cowell, C., & Knight, J. (2007). Growth hormone for children with chronic kidney disease. *Cochrane Database of Systematic Reviews, 2.*

Warady, B., Fine, R., Schaefer, F., & Alexander, S. (Eds). (2004). *Pediatric dialysis.* Boston: Kluwer Academic Publishers.

Warady, B.A., & Ho, M. (2003). Morbidity and mortality in children with anemia at initiation of dialysis. *Pediatric Nephrology, 18*(10), 1055.

White, R.B. (2004). Adherence to the dialysis prescription: Partnering with patients for improved outcomes. *Nephrology Nursing Journal, 31*(4), 432-436.

Wystrychowski, G., & Levin, N.W. (2007). Dry weight: Sine qua non of adequate dialysis. *Advances in Chronic Kidney Disease, 14*(3), e10-e16.

Section 16

Care of the Older Adult with Chronic Kidney Disease

Section Editor

Susan C. Cronin, MS, RN

Authors

Susan C. Cronin, MS, RN

Terran R. Mathers, DNS, RN

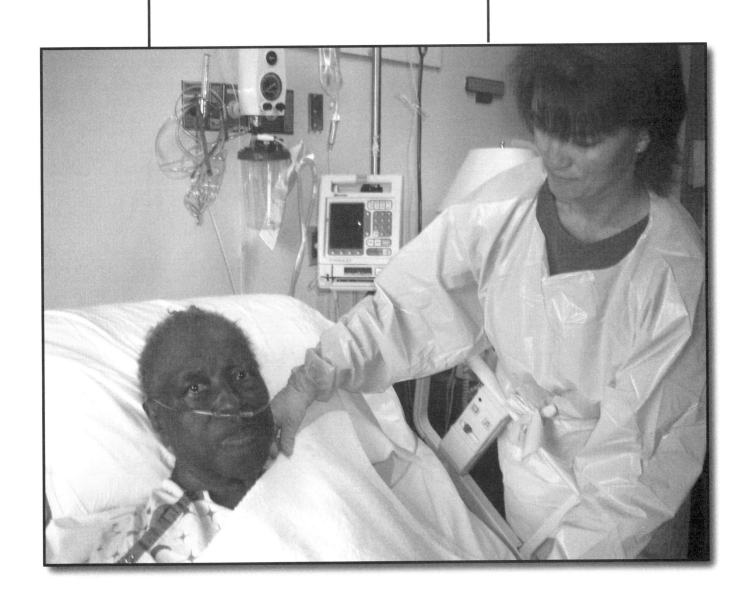

About the Authors

Susan C. Cronin, MS, RN, Section Editor and Author, is Vice President of Clinical Operations at Liberty Dialysis in Old Hickory, Tennessee.

Terran R. Mathers, DNS, RN, is an Associate Professor at Spring Hill College in Mobile, Alabama.

Section 16

Care of the Older Adult with Chronic Kidney Disease

Chapter

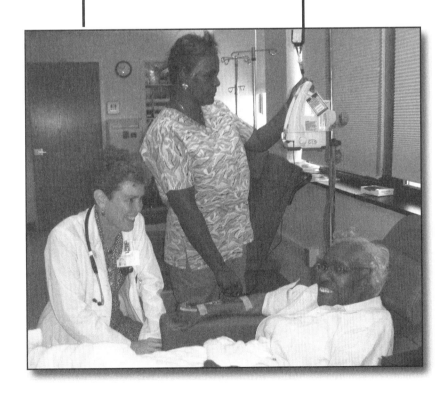

Care of the Older Adult with Chronic Kidney Disease

Purpose

The purposes of this section are to discuss alterations in anatomy, physiology, functional status, and psychosocial support systems associated with the aging process, and to develop a plan of care that will promote physical mental and psychosocial equilibrium for the older adult at the varying stages of chronic kidney disease (CKD).

Objectives

Upon completion of this section, the learner will be able to:
1. Describe the epidemiological influences contributing to the continual growth of persons over the age of 65 years.
2. Using a systems approach, identify the structural, physiologic, and functional changes occurring during the aging process.
   a. Skin and connective tissue.
   b. Cardiovascular.
   c. Respiratory.
   d. Gastrointestinal.
   e. Renal.
   f. Genitourinary.
   g. Musculoskeletal.
   h. Neurologic.
   i. Immune.
   j. Sensory.
3. Correlate structural, physiologic, and functional changes of the aging process with implications for health care.
4. Identify opportunities for preventing disease, improving quality of life, and promoting healthy aging.
5. Identify altered dynamics of renal function that predispose the older adult to CKD.
6. Identify factors contributing to the increases in CKD in the older adult population.
7. Identify risk factors that contribute to CKD in the older adult population.
8. Define the stages of CKD.
9. List the most frequent causes of acute and chronic kidney failure in the older adult.
10. Identify age-specific aspects of acute and chronic kidney failure.
11. Explore the pharmacodynamics of aging and CKD.
12. Discuss the impact of the aging process on modality selection, including in-center and home, the long-term care setting, nocturnal, transplantation, and hospice with and without therapy.

Objectives continue on next page

Objectives, continued from previous page

13. Identify factors that impact access selection and survival for the aging adult.
14. Explore the psychosocial impact of aging, chronic illness, and institutional living.
15. Identify areas of research that focus on improving quality of life and the medical and psychosocial outcomes for aging adults with CKD.

The aging of the U.S. population is one of the major public health challenges of the 21st century. With more than 70 million baby boomers in the United States poised to join the ranks of those aged 65 or over, the prevention of disease and injury is one of the few tools available to reduce the expected growth of health care and long term care costs.

Julie Louise Gerberding, MD, MPH,
Director, Centers for Disease Control and Prevention
in *The Annual CDC Report, 2006*

Aging is a natural physiologic process and part of the developmental continuum. Because aging is gradual, it is impacted by behaviors that occur far in advance of the associated outcomes. Understanding the contributing factors and overcoming society's attitude toward aging are hurdles all health care providers must face. Health care costs are increasing. Health care resources in both people and supplies are becoming more costly and limited in availability. The aging population is on the brink of a longevity revolution with an expected 70 million Americans, or one in every five people being 65 years of age or older by the year 2030 (HHS, 2005).

Amid the financial and resource constraints, caring for the vulnerable CKD population provides not only nephrology practitioners but clinicians in other areas of care with an opportunity to grow professionally by expanding their knowledge of CKD through education and experiences with aging CKD patients. As they explore opportunities for new, alternative approaches in the management and care of this population that will be resource friendly and promote disease prevention, their primary focus will be on prolongation to end stage and improved quality of life.

As we attempt to improve outcomes for CKD patients, caring for the older adult provides additional challenges. But there are rewards to be gained. Older adults bring life experiences and a unique ability to adjust to life changes based on a lifetime of adaptation. We in the clinical realm have a professional responsibility to expand our knowledge base to include information that will support high quality, safe, cost-effective care to this growing, vulnerable population.

Chapter 68

Opportunities to Improve Health and Quality of Life for the Older Adult

Poor health and loss of independence are not inevitable consequences of aging. The following approaches have proven effective in improving the health of older adults:

- Healthy lifestyles.
- Early detection of diseases.
- Immunizations.
- Injury prevention.
- Self-management techniques.

I. **Epidemiologic influences affecting longevity.**

A. Political and social factors impact the growth of the older adult population. During the depression, the birth rate was low, resulting in a leveling off of the growth of the over-65 population.
1. One hundred years ago only 3 million people (4%) in this country were over 65 (HHS, 2006).
2. During the baby boomer era (1946–1964), the birth rate exploded, with more than 76 million additions to the U.S. population (Metropolitan Life Insurance Company, 2005).

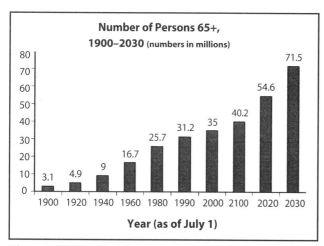

Number of Persons 65+,
1900–2030 (numbers in millions)

Year (as of July 1)

Figure 16.1. Number of persons 65+, 1900–2030 (numbers in millions).

Source: Department of Health and Human Services (HHS), Administration on Aging (AOA). Census Bureau. (2001). *A statistical profile of older Americans aged 65+, a snapshot.* Retrieved November 1, 2007, from http://www.aoa.gov/ press/fact/pdf/ss_stat_profile.pdf

B. Today the Baby Boomer cohort — not yet in the 65-years-plus population — represents 27.5% of the total U.S. population (Metropolitan Life Insurance Company, 2005).
   1. 36 million in the United States are 65 years or older (HHS, 2006).
   2. By 2030, Baby Boomers will have reached the over 65 population and will represent 20% of the total population (Metropolitan Life Insurance Company, 2005).
   3. The 85 years+ population is projected to more than double in size increasing from 4.2 million in 2000 to 8.9 million in 2030 (HHS, 2001) (see Figure 16.1).

C. As we continue to improve our understanding of disease prevention and management and continue to improve our ecologic and environmental state, we can expect life expectancy to increase (see Table 16.1).

D. Aging America is increasing the demand for health care and social services (HHS, 2006).

E. 80% of older adults have at least one chronic condition; 50% have two (HHS, 2006). Among the most frequent occurring conditions in the older adult population:
   1. Hypertension – 51%.
   2. Diagnosed arthritis – 48%.
   3. Heart disease (all types) – 31%.
   4. Cancer (any) – 21%.

Table 16.1

Epidemiologic Factors Promoting Longevity

- Decreased infant and maternal mortality
- Advances in disease prevention and management
  - Improved access to care
  - Health promotion among children and adolescents
    - Periodic physical examinations
    - Elimination of environmental hazards
    - Identification and education on social issues affecting survival
  - Immunizations across the life span
    - Primary – infant
    - Boosters – children and adolescents
    - Tetanus
    - Hepatitis vaccine
    - Flu vaccine
    - Pneumovax
  - Health screening programs supported by health maintenance programs
  - Identification and management of genetic risk factors
  - Improved public health education using a multimedia approach targeting audience of all ages
- Improved work environment through federally sponsored programs
- Better living conditions with improved sanitation
- Research focused on disease prevention and eradication

   5. Diabetes – 16%.
   6. Sinusitis – 14% (HHS, 2001).

F. 3 million older adults indicate they cannot perform basic activities of daily living (ADL) (HHS, 2006).

II. Alternative approaches to an effective health history and physical assessment of the older adult.

A. Altered function secondary to the aging process and increased incidence of disabilities requires innovative approaches to obtain accurate health histories and physical assessments of the older adult.

B. Enhance the patient's independence and maintain self-esteem.
   1. The patient should be the primary source of information.
   2. If this is not possible, the family and prior medical records may need to be alternative sources. The patient's permission should be

obtained before allowing family members or a caretaker to be present during the history and physical examination.
3. Past medical history and review of current prescribed and over-the-counter (OTC) medications should be reviewed prior to the initial encounter.

C. Interventions to facilitate an accurate history and physical assessment.
1. Creative scheduling.
   a. Choose an early appointment when an older adult is more alert.
   b. Plan for more than one visit to complete the history and physical examination.
   c. Tailor the environment to meet the needs of the older adult.
   d. Patient should remain fully clothed during the history.
   e. Environment should include a comfortable temperature, good lighting, quiet area, and no interruptions.
2. Specific approaches.
   a. Confirm that the patient has the appropriate prosthetic appliance, e.g., hearing aid, glasses, dentures.
   b. Speak directly to the patient. Face him/her and speak slowly and clearly in a low voice. Provide for language barrier by having alternate caregiver who speaks the patient's language or an interpreter preferably with clinical training.
   c. Allow extra time to answer questions. Allow time to reminisce. This may assist the interviewer with insights to the patient's concerns, coping mechanisms, adaptability, and cognitive abilities.
   d. Avoid the use of acronyms and medical terminology.

III. Alterations in normal anatomy and physiology associated with the aging process.

A. Definition of the older adult. Definitions vary and changes in the aging population are adjusting the perception and definition of "what is old" (Ham, 1997).
1. Young–old: 65–74 years.
2. Middle–old: 75–84 years.
3. Old–old: 84+ years.

B. Another categorization for two of the groups (Mathers, 2006).
1. Young–old: 50–70 years.
2. Elite–old: 100 years and above.

Table 16.2

Changes Associated with the Aging Process

Type of Change	Example
Total loss of function	Female reproductive ability
Loss of structure	Altered kidney function associated with loss of nephrons
Loss in efficiency without structure loss	Reduced conduction velocity in aging nerve fibers
Interruptions in a control system	Rise in gonadotropins in females with the reduction in feedback control of sex hormones
Increased function	Secretion of antidiuretic hormone in response to osmotic challenge

Source: Kenny, R.A. (1985). Physiology of aging. *Clinics in Geriatric Medicine*, 1(1), 44-49.

C. Whatever definition you choose to ascribe to, the aging process is physiologic not pathologic.

D. Age is not an indication of wellness or illness.

E. Aging is gradual and individual, and different systems age at different rates within an individual. Behaviors, environmental factors, and genetics may adversely affect the aging process.

F. Changes that occur are diverse in type, intensity, and effect (see Table 16.2).

G. Vulnerability to disease increases as function decreases.

H. As a person ages, incidence of chronic illness increases.

IV. Skin and connective tissue.

A. Structural changes.
1. The numbers of cells decrease over time, contributing to fewer functional cells. Red cells, hemoglobin, hematocrit, white cells, and platelets maintain normal values and functions.
2. Cellular solids and bone mass decrease.
3. Bone marrow decreases and marrow fat increases but remains adequate for hematopoiesis.
4. Cartilage loss and thinning of the vertebrae lead

to decrease in stature with loss of about 2 inches by 80 years of age.
5. Tissue elasticity throughout the body is lost.
6. Loss of dermal thickness, thin skin appearance and wrinkles develop.
7. Lean body mass is reduced.
8. Subcutaneous fat content is lost, which contributes to the inability to conserve body heat.
9. Decrease in the number and activity of melanocytes (pigment-producing cells) in the epidermis results in increased sensitivity of the skin to ultraviolet sunlight.
10. Progressive loss of melanocytes in hair bulbs and decreased number of hair follicles results in graying and thinning hair.
11. Decrease in epidermis turnover contributes in slower wound healing.
12. Subcutaneous and sweat glands decrease in number size and function, producing less oil and sweat.
13. Decreased vascular bed and responsiveness (sweating) predispose the older adult to hypothermia and hyperthermia.
14. Decreased vitamin D3 metabolism and decreased exposure to sunlight may contribute to osteoporosis and osteomalasia.

B. Functional responses to changes.
1. Reduction of intracellular fluid.
2. Decrease in subcutaneous fat content with a decline in natural insulation.
3. Lower body temperature.

C. Implications for health care.
1. Acknowledge the potential for dehydration in the presence of altered fluid dynamics.
2. Ensure adequate clothing is worn and adequate blankets are provided to ensure warmth.
3. Maintain environmental temperature between 70° F (21° C) and 75° F (24° C).
4. Be alert for infections even with normal and subnormal temperature.

V. Cardiovascular system.

A. Structural changes.
1. Heart valves become thick and rigid secondary to sclerosis, fibrosis, lipid accumulation, and calcification.
2. Aorta dilates and elongates.
3. Vessels lose elasticity and calcium deposits accumulate.
4. By age 75, 90% of the normal pacemaker cells and as much as 50% of the bundle of His cells are lost.
5. Fat accumulates around the sinus node.
6. Conducting system loses cells and fibers and becomes infiltrated with fat.

B. Physiologic response to changes.
1. Gradual loss of heart muscle efficiency and contractile strength, resulting in a decrease in cardiac output by 1% per year. Stroke volume decreases by 0.7% per year.
2. Vascular compliance decreases due to changes in the vessel walls with intima cellular proliferation and fibrosis and media elastin fragmentation and calcification.
3. Decreased elasticity in the arteries predisposes to vascular changes to the heart, kidney, and pituitary gland.
4. Resistance to peripheral blood flow increases by 1% per year.
5. Isometric contraction phase and relaxation time of the left ventricle are prolonged.
6. Intrinsic contractile function declines.
7. Excessive vagal tone.
8. Heart rate (HR) at rest and achievable maximum heart rate declines (maximum HR = [220-age]).
9. Increase in stroke volume (SV) compensates for lower HR and assists in maintaining cardiac output (CO) (CO = HR x SV).
10. In Western and developed countries, systolic blood pressure increases with a lower rate of increase in diastolic pressure.

C. Functional response to changes.
1. Chronic atrioventricular block.
2. Atrial dysrhythmias.
3. Sick sinus syndrome.
4. Bradycardia.
5. Heart rate response to stress is lower and a longer recovery time is required.
6. Reduced ability to maintain blood pressure and blood volume homeostasis.
7. Decrease in cardiac reserve, left ventricular stroke volume, left ventricular performance, cardiac output, and cardiac index.

D. Implications for health care.
1. Allow rest periods between activities to promote cardiovascular recovery.
2. Encourage patient to change position slowly, particularly from recumbent to sitting or standing.
3. Ensure blood pressure is adequate to meet circulatory demands by assessing physical and mental functions at various blood pressure levels.

VI. Respiratory system.

A. Structural changes.
1. Calcification of costal cartilage contributing to rib cage rigidity.
2. Anterior-posterior chest diameter increases.
3. Chest wall compliance decreases due to stiffening of the chest wall.
4. Thoracic inspiratory and expiratory muscles weaken.
5. Epithelial atrophy of the cilia.
6. Decreased cough reflex.
7. Dry mucous membranes.
8. Decrease in the number of alveoli as well as a decrease in strength due to loss of elasticity.

B. Physiologic response to respiratory changes.
1. Decreased lung expansion.
2. Insufficient basilar inflation.
3. Lung volumes change due to structural changes.
4. Exhalation phase is less effective.
5. Vital capacity and expiratory flow rates are reduced.
6. Residual volume and functional residual capacity increase.
7. Host defense mechanisms, including airway clearance and airway and lung immune cells, respond less vigorously.

C. Functional response to respiratory changes.
1. Less effective gas exchange.
2. Decrease in arterial PO_2 due to ventilation-perfusion mismatch.
3. Decreased ability to expel foreign or accumulated matter (decreased cough response).
4. Increased vulnerability to infection.

D. Implications for health care.
1. Encourage active respiratory activity, particularly in the bed-bound patient and endurance training for the active patient.
2. Monitor oxygen administration closely, keeping oxygen administration below 4 L/min.
3. Consider aspiration precautions for all older adult patients.
4. Advocate influenza and pneumonia immunizations.
5. Encourage smoking cessation programs.

VII. Gastrointestinal system.

A. Structural changes.
1. Mouth, teeth, and tongue.
   a. Saliva production decreased by two thirds.
   b. Salivary ptyalin is decreased.
   c. Prolonged swallowing time.
   d. Drier oral cavity.
   e. Dentin production is decreased.
   f. Shrinkage and fibrosis of root pulp.
   g. Gingavae retract.
   h. Bone density in the alveolar ridge is lost.
   i. Loss of papillae.
   j. Atrophy of the tongue.
2. Esophagus, stomach, intestines.
   a. Dilation of the esophagus.
   b. Relaxation of the lower esophageal sphincter.
   c. Esophageal motility decreases due to lower amplitude contractions after swallowing (presbyesophages).
   d. Gastric mucosa thins, acid producing parietal cells atrophy.
   e. Decreased amounts of gastric acid, e.g., hydrochloric acid, pepsin, lipase, and pancreatic enzymes.
   f. Atrophy of the small and large intestinal mucosa, reducing absorptive surface area and decreasing the ability to absorb sugar, calcium, Vitamin B12, and iron.
   g. Colonic angiodysplasia occurs (ectasia or stretching).
   h. Neural impulses to the intestines are slower and duller.
3. Liver.
   a. Decreased size.
   b. Decreased ability to regenerate damaged cells.
   c. Decreased hepatic blood flow by 0.5% to 1.5% per year.
   d. Liver decreases in size but maintains function. However, the microsomal enzyme function declines.
4. Pancreas.
   a. Ducts become dilated and distended.
   b. Entire gland may prolapse.

B. Physiologic response to changes.
1. Mouth and tongue.
   a. Breakdown of starches is inhibited secondary to decreased ptyalin.
   b. Poor swallowing associated with dry mouth.
   c. Decreased taste sensation.
2. Esophagus.
   a. Motility is decreased.
   b. Emptying is slower.
3. Stomach and intestines.
   a. Reduced motility.
   b. Decreased hunger contractions.
   c. Decreased gastric emptying.
   d. Decreased colonic peristalsis.

4. Liver.
   a. Oxidation-reduction mechanism of the cytochrome P-450 system, an enzymatic pathway resulting in active metabolites, is significantly reduced by the aging process.
   b. Altered first-pass effect. Normally, after a medication is absorbed by the stomach or intestines, it enters the portal circulation and is immediately transported to the liver, where it is taken up by the hepatic cells and metabolized. In the older adult, the first-pass effect is decreased, causing an increase in the bioavailability of the drug.

C. Functional responses to changes in the gastrointestinal tract.
   1. Tooth loss.
   2. Decreased taste sensation.
   3. Dry mouth.
   4. Prolonged swallowing.
   5. Food remains in the esophagus for an extended period of time.
   6. Fat absorption is slower, and dextrose and xylose are more difficult to absorb.
   7. Absorption of vitamin B12, vitamin D, calcium, and iron is faulty.
   8. Decreased colonic peristalsis and decreased neural impulses contribute to constipation.
   9. Less efficient cholesterol stabilization and absorption cause increased incidence of gallstones.
   10. Altered first-pass effect increases the bioavailability of some drugs.
   11. Hepatic clearance for drugs whose metabolism and excretion are dependent on the liver is altered.

D. Implications for health care.
   1. Encourage good dental care, including regular dental check-ups and flossing.
   2. Consider use of prophylactic antibiotics before dental check-ups and treatment.
   3. Encourage use of dentures and other dental appliances.
   4. Instruct patient to wet oral cavity before attempting to swallow medication.
   5. Consult a nutritionist to ensure adequate nutrition.
   6. Encourage 5–6 small meals rather than 3 larger meals.
   7. Exercise aspiration precautions for the hospitalized patient.
   8. Advise patient not to lie down for at least 1 hour following a meal.

9. Encourage patient to allow extra time for bowel movements.
10. Monitor frequency, consistency, and amount of bowel movements.
11. Be alert for symptoms of GI bleeding, including:
    a. Change in bowel habits, particularly diarrhea.
    b. Sudden decrease in hematocrit/hemoglobin.
    c. Unprecedented onset of hypotension and tachycardia.
12. Educate the patient to be alert for signs and symptoms of GI bleeding and to notify health care provider immediately.
13. Ensure age-adjusted drug doses.
14. Monitor patient very closely for adverse reaction to medications.

VIII. Renal system.

A. Structural changes.
   1. Decreased renal mass, primarily cortical losses of nephrons, glomeruli and capillaries, approximately 50–70 g by the eighth decade.
   2. Heterogeneous morphologic changes with varying degrees of atrophy, sclerosis, hypertrophy, and hyperplasia in vasculature, glomeruli, tubules, and interstitium.
   3. Renal vasculature. Sclerotic changes occur in the wall of the large renal vessels and luminal diameter decreases.
      a. Arcurate arteries: angulated and notched.
      b. Interlobal arteries: torturous and spiraling.
   4. Endothelial cells become less uniform in shape, size, and axial orientation, affecting flow and predisposing to lipid deposition.
   5. Disposition of collagen between the intima and the internal elastic lamina may replace muscular cells, leading to decreased elasticity.
   6. Hyalinization in the arteriole.
   7. Glomeruli.
      a. 33% reduction in number by the seventh decade.
      b. Mesangium expands from 6 % to 10%.
      c. Increased number of sclerotic glomeruli to 30% by the eighth decade. More pronounced in individuals with severe atherosclerosis.
      d. Decreased cortical blood flow caused by a progressive collapse and hyalinization of the glomerular tuft and abrupt termination of the arteriole.
      e. Shunt develops between the afferent and efferent arterioles, maintaining flow to the descending vasa recta that perfuse the medulla.
      f. Thickening of glomerular basement membrane.

8. Tubules and interstitium.
   a. Progressive decrease in tubular length and volume replacement by connective tissue with little inflammatory response.
   b. Prominent tubular mass in viable nephrons because of hypertrophy and hyperplasia of the tubular cells accompanied by luminal dilatation.
   c. Tubular diverticula in the vicinity of the mascula densa often contains detritus (carious matter produced by disintegration) and bacteria. May number 300 per 100 nephrons by the age of 90.
   d. Little change in connective tissue in the cortex but a noticeable increase in the medulla. Cellular contents of the medulla are increasingly replaced by intercellular material, including finely dispersed sudanophilic fat (indicative of fatty degeneration). There are also increased dispersed deposits of calcium in the medulla.

B. Physiologic response to changes.
   1. Progressive decrease in renal blood flow from 1200 mL/min to 600 mL/min by age 80, associated with fixed anatomic changes. There is a highly significant decrease in the cortical component of blood flow, with preservation of medullary flow.
   2. Paraminohippuric acid (PAH) clearance decreases from an average of 694 mL/min to 289 mL/min by the ninth decade.
   3. Creatinine clearance progressively declines 1% per year after age 40 with no change in serum creatinine levels, because creatinine generation also decreases.
   4. Glomerular filtration rate declines with age.
   5. Filtration fraction increases with age secondary to alteration in the relationship of decreased blood flow to the cortex with no change to the juxtamedullary glomeruli.
   6. Solute load per surviving nephron increases, producing solute diuresis.
   7. Diminished medullary tonicity.
   8. Impairment of renal concentrating and sodium conservation.
   9. Regulation of urine osmolality decreases with age.
   10. Decreased capacity of the cortical cells to generate ammonia from glutamine, resulting in a delayed excretion of acid load.
   11. Reduced basal plasma renin and aldosterone.

C. Functional response to changes.
   1. Age-related reduction in renal blood flow.

2. Glomerular filtration rate declines with age.
3. Diminished urine creatinine clearance.
4. Tubular maximum for PAH secretory transport and reabsorption decreases at rates closely paralleling the decreases in inulin.
5. Conservation of sodium by the kidney is impaired.
6. Maximum renal concentrating ability declines with age.
7. Decreased net acid excretion.
8. Tendency to develop hyperkalemia.
9. Decreased intestinal absorption of calcium, secondary to a reduction of vitamin D hydroxylation in the kidney.

D. Implications for health care.
   1. The glomerular filtration rate should be calculated using EITHER:
      a. Modification of Diet in Renal Disease (MDRD) (Levey et al., 2000).

      $$GFR = 186.3 \times SerumCr^{-1.154} \times age^{-0.203} \times 1.212$$
      (if patient is black), 0.742 (if female)

      b. Cockcroft-Gault formula (Hu, 2005).

      Cockcroft-Gault GFR = (140-age) x (wt in kg) x (0.85 if female) / (72 x Cr)

   2. Using the GFR, determine if the patient is in one of the stages of CKD (NFK, 1995).
      a. Stage 1. Kidney damage (normal or GFR > 90).
      b. Stage 2. Mild kidney damage (GFR < 60–89).
      c. Stage 3. Moderate kidney damage (GFR < 30–59).
      d. Stage 4. Severe kidney damage (GFR < 15–29).
      e. Stage 5. Kidney failure (GFR <15).
   3. Monitor closely drugs prescribed for patients with CKD.
   4. Medications processed through the kidneys have a narrow therapeutic to toxic ratio and should be monitored by serum levels (e.g., digoxin, aminoglycosides).
   5. Adverse drug reactions should be considered with onset of mental status changes.
   6. Patient response to combination of drugs excreted by the kidney need to be carefully monitored. These drugs may include potassium sparing diuretics, beta-adrenergic receptor antagonists, angiotensin-converting enzyme inhibitors, and nonsteroidal antiinflammatory drugs.
   7. Structural and functional changes occurring with the aging process need to be considered when evaluating kidney function in the older adult (see Table 16.3).

Table 16.3

**Structural and Functional Changes in the Kidney
Contributing to Chronic Kidney Disease in the Older Adult**

Changes	Physiologic Response
Structural Changes ■ Sclerosis of glomerular tufts and complete glomeruli ■ Sclerosis and atheromas of renal vasculature **Functional Changes** ■ Decreased renal blood flow ■ Decreased glomerular filtration ■ Altered tubular function ■ Acid-base imbalance	■ Decreased perfusion to the kidney as well as within the kidney ■ Decreased glomerular filtration ■ Inability to maintain water balance ■ Altered ability to regulate total body sodium ■ Delayed excretion of acids

8. Sodium should not be drastically reduced in the older adult. This could lead to volume contraction, and decreased blood flow to the kidneys as well as orthostatic hypotension.
9. Drugs that interfere with tubular secretion of potassium in the distal tubule necessitate close monitoring of the serum potassium in the older adult.
   a. Potassium-sparing diuretics.
   b. Adrenergic receptor antagonists.
   c. Angiotensin-converting enzyme inhibitors.
   d. Nonsteroidal antiinflammatory drugs.
10. Older adults have a defective thirst mechanism and need to be monitored closely for dehydration and hypernatremia.
11. Decreased osmoreceptor sensitivity and increased antidiuretic hormone release may predispose the older adult to water retention and hyponatremia.
12. The older adult should be monitored closely for the development of metabolic acidosis.

IX. Genitourinary system.

A. Structural changes.
   1. Bladder muscles become weak.
   2. Bladder capacity is reduced.
   3. Atrophic changes occur in most structures of the genitoreproductive system.
   4. Vaginal epithelium is thinner, drier and has less rugae.
   5. pH of vaginal secretions is altered and becomes more alkaline.
   6. Pelvic floor muscles, sacral ligaments, and other supporting structures relax.
   7. Prostatic tissue enlarges due to hyperplasia.

B. Physiologic response to changes.
   1. Increased production of urine during the night secondary to inability of the renal tubules to concentrate urine and the need to remove solute.
   2. Organ prolapse (bladder, rectum, uterus) secondary to loss of muscle tone.
   3. Urinary frequency, urgency, and nocturia.
   4. Emptying of bladder becomes more difficult and retention of large volumes of urine may occur.
   5. Micturition reflex is delayed.
   6. In males.
      a. Nocturia, urinary hesitancy, decreased urine flow, and retention are associated with prostate enlargement.
      b. Testosterone levels decline (Mayo Clinic, 2007).
      c. Erectile and ejaculatory function declines. Postejaculatory refractory period increases.
      d. Sexual response is delayed due to reduced penile sensitivity and increased threshold for tactile stimulation.
   7. In females.
      a. With menopause, rapid decline of estrogen and progesterone.
      b. Hormonal changes cause atrophic changes of uterus, vagina, external genitalia, and breasts.
      c. Sexual activity decreases, but exact role of biologic changes and sociocultural factors is unknown.

C. Implications for health care.
   1. Provide for safety and support independence for older adults when using bathroom facilities.
   2. Assist patient to urinate in upright position.
   3. Encourage the female patient to cleanse and dry

the perineal area in a front to back direction after each bowel movement.

4. Observe for signs and symptoms of urinary tract infection (urosepsis), particularly in the female patients.

5. Encourage regular health screening to include gynecologic and prostate evaluation.

6. To manage nocturia, encourage the patient to avoid diuretics, caffeine, or alcohol and decrease fluid consumption in the evening.

X. Musculoskeletal system.

A. Structural changes.
   1. Muscle fibers atrophy and decrease in number.
   2. Decreased myosin adenosine triphosphatase activity.
   3. Fibrous tissue gradually replaces muscle tissue.
   4. Decrease in muscle weight compared to total body weight.
   5. Decreased muscular strength and endurance associated with decrease in number of muscle fibers.
   6. Hyalin cartilage water content declines.
   7. Tendons shrink and harden.
   8. Bone mineral and mass are reduced.
   9. Incremental process of bone resorption without the successful formation of new bone mass leads to a gradual bone loss.
   10. Bone loss is universal, but rate is highly variable. Loss is more rapid in women after menopause than in men.
   11. Thinning discs and shortening vertebrae reduce the length of the spinal column.
   12. Cartilage surface of joints deteriorates and points and spurs form.

B. Physiologic/functional response to changes.
   1. Muscle mass, muscle strength, and muscle movements are decreased.
   2. Prolonged contraction time, latency period, and relaxation period.
   3. Decreased reflexes.
   4. Limitation of joint activity and motion.
   5. Decreased reaction time.
   6. Decreased speed of movement.

C. Implications for health care.
   1. Encourage exercise program with physical conditioning to minimize loss of muscle tone and strength.
   2. Consider judicious use of NSAIDs before exercise to minimize pain and maximize mobilization.

a. Review patient's medications to avoid combining NSAIDs with other potentially nephrotoxic drugs (e.g., ACE inhibitors).

b. Use diuretics cautiously in combination with NSAIDs.

c. Educate patient in the safe management of NSAIDs.

3. Conditions that lead to dehydration include nausea, vomiting, and diarrhea.

4. Observe for signs and symptoms of dehydration (Wikipedia, 2007).
   a. Thirst.
   b. Headache.
   c. Dry skin.
   d. Loss of appetite.
   e. Fatigue.
   f. Constipation.
   g. Reduced blood pressure.
   h. Increased heart rate.
   i. Dizziness.
   j. Fainting.

5. Interventions to mobilize the geriatric patient who is bedridden include passive range of joint motion, dangling, and standing to progressive ambulation. Muscle strengthening and conditioning therapy should also be part of the physical therapy program.

6. Suggest the use of assistive devices to promote safe ambulation.

7. Discuss home environment to determine need for modification to ensure safe ambulation and prevent falls.

8. Instruct patient in safety measures to prevent falls and fractures.

9. Encourage a diet rich in calcium and consider Vitamin D supplementation (Johnson, 2007).

XI. Neurologic system.

A. Structural changes.
   1. Decrease in brain weight.
   2. Reduction in blood flow to the brain.
   3. Reduction in nerve cells is diffuse and gradual.
   4. Moderate cortical atrophy.
   5. Gyri of the brain surface atrophy causing widening and deepening of the spaces between the gyri.
   6. Loss of neurons in the neocortex, substantia nigra, and limbic system.
   7. Dendritic changes.
   8. Reduction in cerebral blood and metabolism.
   9. Lipofuscin pigment accumulates primarily in the glial tissues.
   10. Decrease in neurotransmitters.

11. Binding sites for dopamine and serotonin decrease.
12. Peripheral nerve fibers decrease in number and size.
13. Nerve fiber conduction velocity is lower.
14. Fewer neuritic plaques.
15. Neurofibrillary tangles in hippocampal neurons (curly, twisted neuritic structures).

B. Physiologic/functional response to changes.
1. Nerve conduction velocity is slower.
2. Motor and sensory nerve conduction decreases.
3. A decrease in vibratory sensation in feet and ankles may occur.
4. Slower reflexes and a delayed response to multiple stimuli.
5. Autoregulation of blood to brain decreases with age.
6. Kinesthetic sense lessens.
7. Slowing in response to tasks and increase in time needed to recover from physical exertion.
8. Increased reaction time and increased time required in decision making.
9. Cognitive and memory changes.
10. Changes in sleep patterns occur with stages III and IV of sleep becoming less prominent. Frequent awakenings during sleep are not unusual.

C. Implications for health care.
1. Older adults need innovative teaching approaches to facilitate the learning process.
   a. Evaluate patient's readiness to learn. Pain, anxiety, or fatigue may be barriers to the learning process.
   b. Develop patient focused learning objectives.
   c. Identify the time of day that is best for the patient.
   d. Teach in a well lighted area that is free from distraction.
   e. Keep explanations simple and clear by using concrete directions and examples.
2. Allow sufficient time for the patient to recover energy levels from tasks.
3. Provide systems to promote retention of information in the form of written documentation.
   a. Give the patient written instructions, particularly when information is new.
   b. Facilitate medication management by establishing a backup documentation of all patient medications and administration instructions.
4. The home environment should be evaluated for safety.

5. Identify a care partner who will monitor the home environment and support the patient in the activities of daily living.
6. Encourage patient to gradually change position from supine to sitting to standing.
7. Altered pain response puts the older adult at risk for progression of lower extremity wounds. Extensive survey of lower extremities should be part of the routine physical assessment.
8. Ensure uninterrupted periods of sleep during nighttime hours.

XII. Immune system.

A. Structural changes.
1. Thymic involution begins at about the age of puberty with decreased serum thymic hormone activity in the older adult.
2. The number of T and B lymphocytes adapt. Novel or aberrant characteristics of T lymphocytes may appear with age.
   a. T Lymphocyte function declines.
   b. B lymphocytes produce less protective antibodies thus antibodies tend to bind with antigens less well. Response to antigen therapy may be impaired.
   c. B lymphocyte functions are regulated by T lymphocytes or their products.
   d. Age-related decreases in humoral immunity due to intrinsic defects of B lymphocytes are difficult to differentiate from those due to T lymphocyte defects (Cutler, 2007).
3. Appearance of antibodies.
4. Redistribution of lymphocytes.
5. Changes in serum immunoglobulin.

B. Physiologic/functional response to changes.
1. Alterations of T lymphocyte activities underlie much of the age-related decrease in protective immune response.
   a. Decreased response to skin tests.
   b. Production of interleukin-2 is reduced.
2. Age-associated thymus-derived lymphocyte (T lymphocyte) defects contribute to reactivation of *Mycobacterium tuberculosis* and Varicella-zoster infections.
3. Production of antiself reactive T cells.
4. Impairment in cell mediated immune responses.
5. Decreased ability to reject foreign tissue.
6. Increased laboratory autoimmune parameters, including elevation of serum complement C3 and properdin.
7. Impaired immune reactivity.

8. Increased immunoglobin A (IgA) and perhaps immunoglobin G (IgG) levels.
9. Decreased immunoglobin M (IgM) levels.
10. Diminished immunoglobin production to a challenge (vaccine or antigen) with lowered response and shortened duration.

C. Implications for health care.
1. Delayed response to common skin testing antigens (e.g., purified protein derivative tuberculin).
2. Maximal antibody response requires a larger dose of foreign antigen and is maintained for a shorter time.
3. Clinical manifestation of infection may vary in the older adult.
   a. Mental status changes frequently herald an infectious process.
   b. Temperature may be normal or subnormal.
   c. Cardinal signs of inflammation, including redness, pain, heat, swelling, and altered function may be muted.
   d. Weakness.
   e. Anorexia.
   f. Change in functional status.
4. Instruct patient to promptly seek medical attention for fever, chills, or general malaise.
5. Recommend pneumococcal, tetanus, and annual influenza vaccinations. The FDA has approved a vaccine for shingles in the adult over 60 years of age but to date there is no CDC recommendation for this vaccine.
6. Plan for outpatient procedures when possible to reduce risk of nosocomial infections.
7. Encourage older adult patients to avoid crowded and confined areas.

XIII. Sensory system.

A. Eyes.
1. Structural changes.
   a. Morphologic changes in choroids, epithelium, and retina with decreases in visual activity.
   b. Pigment accumulation.
   c. Sclerosis of pupil sphincter.
   d. Ciliary muscle atrophy.
   e. Nuclear sclerosis, causing myopia (nearsightedness) and predisposing to presbyopia (farsightedness).
   f. Increased lens size, causing myopia.
   g. Accumulation of lens fibers.
   h. Lens yellows.
   i. Increased intraocular pressure.
   j. Periorbital atrophy causing upper and lower lids to droop.
2. Physiologic/functional response to changes.
   a. Decreased rod and cone function with decreased adaptation to light and dark.
   b. Decreased speed of eye movement with difficulty in gazing upward and maintaining convergence.
   c. Distorted depth perception.
   d. Reduced accommodation causing hyperopia.
   e. Altered refractory powers.
   f. Decreased tear secretion resulting in dryness and eye discomfort as well as jeopardizing the corneal surface.
   g. Color vision may be impaired making it difficult to differentiate lower color tones: blues, greens, and violets.
3. Implications for health care.
   a. Encourage patients to see ophthalmologist at regular intervals.
   b. Maintain consistent lighting in all patient care areas.
   c. Avoid the use of greens, blues, and violets together.
   d. Make appointments for patients during daylight hours.
   e. Provide adequate handicap accesses and side rails to promote safety.
   f. Provide teaching material in large, easy-to-read print.
   g. Encourage patient to use low vision aids.

B. Hearing.
1. Structural changes.
   a. Loss of auditory neurons.
   b. Angiosclerotic calcification of inner ear membrane.
2. Physiologic/functional response to changes.
   a. Decreased tone discrimination and voice localization.
   b. Tone loss greater at high frequencies.
   c. Pitch discrimination declines.
   d. Speech discrimination declines and is worsened by background noise.
   e. Hearing loss is progressive especially at high frequencies.
3. Implications for health care.
   a. Look directly at patient when speaking and speak in a loud, low-pitched voice.
   b. Keep background noise to a minimum when conversing with patients.
   c. Encourage patient to seek audiometric evaluations and use hearing assist devices.
   d. Assess ear canal for accumulation of cerumen.

C. Smell.
1. Structural and functional changes.
   a. Decreased number of olfactory nerve fibers.
   b. Olfaction declines causing poor detection and discrimination by the eighth decade.
2. Implications for health care.
   a. Inform patient of decline is sensitivity to odors.
   b. Provide for safe environment by advising patient to install and maintain fire/smoke alarms and CO_2 monitors in the home.

D. Oral.
1. Structural and functional changes.
   a. Reduction in the integrity of epithelial and connective tissue causes a thinning of the oral mucosa and affects bone pulpal tissues.
      (1) Decrease in blood supply.
      (2) Compromised nerve innervation.
      (3) Tissue quality altered.
      (4) Calcifitic tissue changes occur.
   b. Compositional changes in saliva.
      (1) Altered sodium levels.
      (2) Increased potassium.
      (3) Decrease in secretory proteins.
   c. Reduction in taste perception. Increase in thresholds for salt and bitter tastes.
   d. Structural changes to teeth.
      (1) Erosion.
      (2) Abrasion.
      (3) Attrition.
   e. Gingival recession.
      (1) Alveolar dehiscence.
      (2) Compromised spatial position of teeth.
2. Implications for health care.
   a. Changes in eating patterns may occur. Nutritional assessment and supplementation may be necessary to ensure consumption of adequate calories, nutrients, vitamins, and minerals.
   b. Assessment for nutritional needs should include financial and psychosocial resources.
   c. Instruct patient about the use of salt and salt substitutes.
   d. Encourage daily mouth care to include brushing, flossing, or cleaning of dentures and rinsing with mouthwash.
   e. Encourage frequent evaluation and treatment by a dentist.
   f. Monitor for mouth sores and infection.
   g. Monitor for dietary intake changes related to poor fitting dentures and/or mouth sores.

E. Tactile.
1. Structural/functional changes.
   a. Reduced tactile sensation.
   b. Alteration in skin sensation of pressure or temperature changes.
2. Implications for health care.
   a. Encourage patient to change position often to prevent breaks in skin integrity.
   b. Inspect body for breaks in the skin, especially in the lower extremities.
   c. Be alert for alteration in pain response in the older adult.

XIV. Effects of aging on pharmacologic management.

A. Issues.
1. Older adults have a greater burden of acute and chronic illness.
2. Medications are a centrally important aspect of their health care.
3. Persons over age 65, while making up only 13% of the population, spend four times more on prescriptions than do persons under age 65.
4. Aging places older persons at increased risk of side effects.
5. Side effects frequently attributed to onset of a new illness or the aging process.
6. Lack of involvement of older adults in pharmacologic research and the resultant risk of under-using life-saving therapies (Pfizer, 2007).
7. Older adults often see more than one doctor.
8. Increased toxicity and adverse drug effects are due to:
   a. Age-dependent declines in GFR.
   b. Increased kidney disease in this population.
   c. Reduced tubular transport capacity.
   d. Decreased ability to acidify the urine.
   e. Drug interactions.
   f. Central nervous system changes.
   g. Double dosing, i.e., the same active ingredient in medications prescribed for different chronic diseases or the patient is prescribed the same drug under different names.

B. Nursing implications.
1. Assess for high risk medications and side effects.
2. Monitor closely for signs and symptoms of undermedication or overmedication.
3. Schedule medication for routine administration.
4. Consider significant other dispensing medication or medication dispensers with controlled distribution for the cognitively impaired.
5. Maintain the highest level of self-care, functional ability, and active participation possible (Nurse Competence in Aging, 2005).

Table 16.4

Diagnostic Parameters in the Older Adult

Test	Rationale	Adult	Older Adult	Implications
Renal Ultrasound	Renal weight decreases 20–40% between the ages of 30 and 90.	Renal length – 9 cm Abnormal – Less than 9 cm or a difference of 1.5 cm	Decrease in renal length by 2 cm	Decrease in size of kidneys in the older adults does not necessarily imply chronicity as it would in the adult.
Serum Creatinine	Decreased muscle mass and diminished production of endogenous creatinine.	Age 40–60 M 1.1–1.5 mg/dL F 1.0–.97 mg/dL	Age 60–99 M 1.5–1.20 mg/dL F 0.99–0.91 mg/dL	Serum creatinine cannot be used as a marker for kidney function in the older adult.
Creatinine Clearance	Age-related reduction in renal plasma flow and glomerular filtration rate.	140 mL/min/1.73 m^2	97 mL/min/1.73 m^2	Cockcroft and Gault formula should be used to determine Cr clearance (kidney function) in the older adult.
Urine Osmolarity	Tubular function decreases, causing less effective concentration of urine.	1,109 mOsm/kg	882 mosm/kg	Measurement of urine osmolality is of limited value in differentiating prerenal azotemia from acute tubular necrosis in the older adult.
Fractional Excretion of Sodium (FENa$^+$)	Decreased capacity to reabsorb sodium by the ascending loop of Henle.	Prerenal < 1% Intrinsic > 1%	Not reliable values	Cannot be used to differentiate between prerenal azotemia and acute tubular necrosis in the older adult.

Source: Davison, A. (1998). Renal disease in the elderly. *Nephron, 80,* 6-19; Pascual, J., Fernando, F., & Ortuno, J. (1995). The elderly patient with acute renal failure. *Journal of the American Society of Nephrology, 6*(2), 144-149.

XV. Acute and chronic kidney failure.

A. Acute kidney injury of the older adult.
1. There is an increased incidence and prevalence of acute kidney injury (AKI) with older adults.
2. Acute kidney injury is irreversible in up to 16% of elderly patients (Lameire, Van Biesen, & Vanholder, 2005).
3. Systemic diseases as well as structural and functional changes in aging kidneys contribute to AKI.
4. The presentation of AKI in the older individual is similar to that of younger patients but is more likely to be superimposed on underlying renal insufficiency (see Section 3, Acute Care).
5. The presence of other comorbid conditions may hinder the diagnosis of AKI in the older individual.
6. Diagnostic data interpretation may vary in the older population (see Table 16.4).
7. Iatrogenic factors contributing to AKI for older adults.
   a. Aggressive treatment of congestive heart contraction and decreased kidney perfusion.
   b. Salt restriction and diuretics for treatment of hypertension.
   c. Medication management leading to AKI.
      (1) Nonsteroidal antiinflammatory drugs (NSAIDs).

(2) Angiotensin-converting enzyme inhibitors (ACEI).

(3) Combinations of medications (e.g., NSAIDs, ACEI, diuretics, etc.).

8. Recovery may take longer for the older individual. However, this should not be a determinant of survival. Prompt management is recommended (Choudhury, Raj, & Levi, 2004). Death usually results from infection, GI hemorrhage, or myocardial infarction (Agrawal & Swartz, 2000).

9. Types of AKI.
   a. Prerenal failure.
   b. Intrarenal failure.
   c. Postrenal failure.

10. Prerenal failure. Causes external to the kidneys reduce renal blood flow and decrease glomerular perfusion and filtration. Accounts for 60–70% of cases of all AKI (Needham, 2005).
    a. Dehydration due to external losses of fluids with inadequate fluid replacement. Some causes may be those common to all ages, including fever, vomiting, and diarrhea. Other causes specific to the older individual may be the result of specific medications (e.g., NSAIDs, ACE inhibitors), large vessel diseases (thrombosis, embolus, dissection) (Agrawal & Swartz, 2000), or a response to the aging process (Choudhury, Raj, & Levi, 2004).
       (1) Decreased concentration of urine.
       (2) Impairment of thirst regulation.
       (3) Inability of the kidney to retain sodium.
    b. Internal redistribution of volume from intravascular to interstitial space.
       (1) Sepsis.
           (a) Decreased urine output may precede temperature spike by hours.
           (b) Absence of temperature spike is not unusual in older adults.
       (2) Hypoproteinemia.
           (a) Nephrotic syndrome.
           (b) Cirrhosis/hepatorenal failure.
           (c) Malnutrition.
           (d) Tissue injury.
               [1] Burns.
               [2] Pancreatitis.
    c. Decreased cardiac output.
       (1) Myocardial dysfunction.
       (2) Pericardial disease.

11. Intrarenal failure/causes damage renal tissue (parenchyma), resulting in nephron function impairment.
    a. Drug-induced nephropathy, caused by the alteration of intrarenal hemodynamics.

(1) ACE inhibitors.
    (a) Mechanism. Fall in blood pressure and efferent glomerular arteriolar tone that decreases transglomerular hydraulic pressure and thereby glomerular filtration rate (GFR).
    (b) Used to treat hypertension, congestive heart failure, and secondary prevention of myocardial infarction.
    (c) Risk factors.
        [1] The presence of bilateral renovascular disease.
        [2] Arterial stenosis in a solitary kidney.
        [3] Volume depletion.
        [4] Concomitant treatment with diuretics.
        [5] Low salt diet.
        [6] Cardiac failure.
        [7] Combined treatment with NSAIDs.
        [8] Presence of diabetes mellitus.
(2) Withdrawal of drug and volume repletion, if indicated, will result in renal recovery.
(3) NSAIDs.
    (a) Mechanism A. NSAIDs inhibit cyclooxygenase-mediated arachidonic acid metabolites, which, in turn, inhibit production of prostaglandins, leaving the vasoconstrictive hormones (norepinephrine and angiotensin II) unopposed. Decrease in circulating volume may result in severe renal vasoconstriction and a rapid decrease in renal blood flow and glomerular filtration rate.
    (b) Mechanism B. Immunologically mediated nephrotic syndrome. Release of lymphokines and eosinophil chemotactic factors cause a diffuse infiltration of the renal interstitium by mononuclear inflammatory cells and eosinophils, and leads to tubulitis.
    (c) Risk factors.
        [1] Heart failure.
        [2] Cirrhosis.
        [3] Nephrotic syndrome.
        [4] Volume depletion.
        [5] Combined treatment with ACE inhibitors.
    (d) Withdrawal of medication usually results in recovery of kidney function.
(4) Cyclosporine not used as it once was for

kidney transplantation (USRDS, 2006).
  (a) Mechanism. Vasoconstriction of the afferent renal arterioles caused by excessive endothelin-1 production.
  (b) Renal function improves or recovers completely after reducing the dosage or discontinuing the drug.
b. Acute tubular necrosis (ATN) (see also Section 3) responsible for 90% intrarenal AKI cases (Brady et al., 2004).
  (1) Prerenal conditions may lead to ATN if unrecognized and untreated. Causes include:
    (a) Prolonged ischemia.
    (b) Nephrotoxic agents.
      [1] ACE inhibitors.
      [2] NSAIDs.
      [3] Iodinated radiocontrast agents. Risk factors include older age, renal insufficiency as indicated by a serum creatinine > 2 mg/dL, multiple myeloma, high doses of hyperosmolar contrast agent, and two common problems seen with the older adult: diabetes mellitus and heart failure (Merck & Co., Inc., 2005a).
        [a] Renal consultation should be obtained before using a dye-dependent study in a patient with serum creatinine 2 mg/dL.
        [b] Alternative nondye diagnostic tests should be used when possible.
        [c] Hydration with $NaHCO_3$ 1 hour before and then after the contrast is given may help prevent ATN.
      [4] Chemotherapy.
      [5] Combination of nephorotoxic drugs.
  (2) Older adults have a longer recovery period and recovery may be compromised by the presence of comorbid diseases.
c. Tubulointerstitial nephritis.
  (1) A cell-mediated immune mechanism involving activated T cells that release lymphokines and eosinophil chemotactic factors.
  (2) Causes may be idiopathic or related to infection or a drug.
  (3) Clinical features.
    (a) Urinary sediment. Normal or pyuria and WBC casts.

    (b) Discrete tubular defects, such as renal tubular acidosis.
    (c) Peripheral eosinophilia.
    (d) Rash.
    (e) Fever.
  (4) Diagnosis and treatment. Medications often identified as possible causative agent in those older individuals biopsied. Discontinuation of medications will frequently result in return of kidney function (Davidson, 1998).
d. Acute glomerulonephritis (GN) (Choudhury, Raj, & Levi, 2004).
  (1) Usually results from rapidly progressive glomerulonephritis (RPGN) in the older individual.
  (2) Poststreptococcal GN for the older adult occurs in association with streptococcal infections involving the throat and skin.
  (3) Decline in renal function. Active nephritic urine sediment (hematuria, pyuria, red blood cell casts, moderate to severe proteinuria).
  (4) Renal biopsy specifies diagnosis of this disease.
e. Atheroembolic renal disease (AERD).
  (1) Occurs predominantly in elderly males with vascular disease (Medline Plus Medical Encyclopedia, 2007).
  (2) Cause. Pieces of fatty material (from arteries above the kidneys) clog the renal arteries.
    (a) There is a strong association between atrial fibrillation and atheroembolic renal disease.
    (b) May occur in conjunction with invasive angiographic procedures or as a complication of angioplasty or surgery.
  (3) Clinical features. Progresses slowly, so symptoms may not show until advanced kidney failure. Presenting symptoms may include (Medline Plus Medical Encyclopedia, 2007):
    (a) Onset of flank pain.
    (b) Blood in the urine.
    (c) Nausea and vomiting.
    (d) Foot pain, ulcers on the feet, or mottling of the toes and feet.
    (e) Abdominal pain.
    (f) Pancreatitis or hepatitis (rare).
    (g) Stroke(s) or blindness.
    (h) Uncontrolled high blood pressure.
  (4) Diagnosis. Kidney biopsy.

(5) Treatment. Medications to lower blood pressure, reduce cholesterol, and treat symptoms. Dialysis or transplantation for the kidney failure (Medline Plus Medical Encyclopedia, 2007). Surgical treatment may include angioplasty, placement of a stent, or a bypass of the occluded renal artery (Stanford University Medical Center, 2007).

(6) Prognosis depends on body's reaction to prevent fatty material from breaking off.

12. Acute obstructive uropathy.
   a. Causes in older adults (Choudhury, Raj, & Levi, 2004).
      (1) Males. Benign prostatic hyperplasia (BPH) and prostate cancer.
      (2) Females. Pelvic tumors of the uterus or cervix.
      (3) Geriatric population in general. Lymphoma, bladder carcinoma, rectal tumors.
   b. Clinical features.
      (1) Anuria associated with pelvic discomfort.
      (2) Prostatism.
      (3) Dysuria.
      (4) New onset of enuresis.
      (5) Gross hematuria.
      (6) Nausea, vomiting.
      (7) Changes in mental status.
      (8) Asterixis (involuntary jerking movements).
      (9) Manifestations associated with cause (e.g., abdominal mass associated with an enlarged bladder).
      (10) A significant number of patients are asymptomatic, and diagnosis is made during investigation for chronic renal insufficiency.
   c. Diagnosis may include urinalysis, serum chemistries, bladder catheterization (checking for obstruction), cystourethroscopy, voiding cystourethrography, abdominal ultrasonography or CT scan, retrograde pyelography, and others (Merck & Co., Inc, 2005b).
   d. Treatment consists of eliminating the obstruction by surgery, instrumentation (e.g., endoscopy, lithotripsy), or drug therapy (e.g., hormonal therapy for prostate cancer).

13. Treatment of acute kidney injury (see Section 3).
   a. Elderly patients generally become symptomatic at lower levels of blood urea nitrogen (BUN) and serum creatinine than younger patients.
   b. Symptoms. In addition to the symptoms

presented in Section 3, older individuals may present with:
      (1) Exacerbation of previously well-controlled heart failure.
      (2) Unexplained changes in mental status.
      (3) Changes in behavior.
      (4) Personality changes.
      (5) Change in sense of well being.
   c. Indications for treatment.
      (1) Pulmonary edema.
      (2) Hyperkalemia.
      (3) Severe acidemia.
      (4) Uremia.
      (5) Catabolic state.
   d. Kidney replacement therapies.
      (1) Acute hemodialysis.
      (2) Acute peritoneal dialysis.
      (3) Continuous kidney replacement. Advantages over the others include:
         (a) Improved fluid and metabolic control.
         (b) Decreased hemodynamic instability.
         (c) Enhanced possibility of removing inflammatory mediators of sepsis.
      (4) Therapeutic plasma exchange.
   e. Choice of treatment modality depends on clinical presentation of the patient as well as the patient's hemodynamic status.
   f. Osmolality and fluid shifts associated with intermittent hemodialysis are not well tolerated by older patients due to altered compensatory mechanisms associated with the aging process.
   g. Hemodynamic monitoring recommended to detect intravascular volume depletion, which further compromises perfusion to the kidney.

B. Chronic kidney disease (CKD).
   1. Incident rate. Median age of new individuals being treated for the last stage of CKD (end-stage renal disease [ESRD]) is 64.6. Ages 45–64 had the highest incident count, with those 75 years of age and above being the next largest group (USRDS, 2006) (see Figure 16.2).
   2. Prevalent rate. Median age is 58.3. Prevalent rates per million highest in the 65–74 age group (USRDS, 2006) (see Figure 16.3).
   3. Older individuals frequently do not exhibit symptoms of CKD until the glomerular filtration rate is below 10mL/min, mainly attributed to poor nutrition and decreased muscle mass associated with the aging process.
   4. Strategies to prevent or slow down progression of kidney disease.
      a. Aggressive management of hypertension.

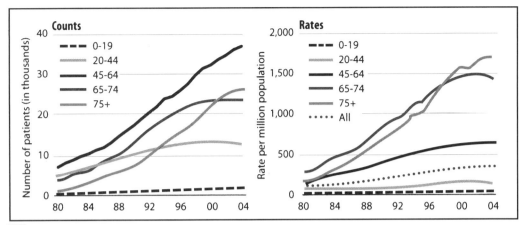

Figure 16.2. Incident counts and adjusted rates, by age.

Source: United States Renal Data System. (2006). *USRDS 2006 annual data report.* Retrieved July 25, 2007, from http://www.usrds .org/adr.htm.

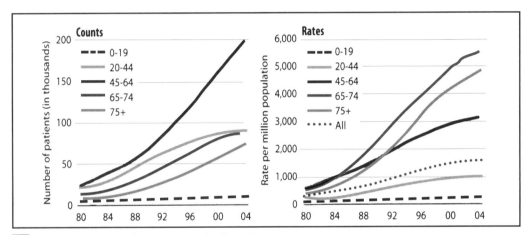

Figure 16.3. Prevalent counts and adjusted rates, by age.

Source: United States Renal Data System. (2006). *USRDS 2006 annual data report.* Retrieved July 25, 2007, from http://www.usrds .org/adr.htm.

b. Management of hyperphosphatemia.
c. Closely monitored and controlled diabetes.
d. Treatment of hyperlipidemia (NKF, 2003).
e. Although NKF (2000) recommends modification of diet to low-protein with at least 50% high biologic value of 0.6 to 0.75 g/kg/day, and high energy, this is very controversial, especially with the older individual so prone to malnutrition.
5. Causes of chronic kidney failure in the older adult.
  a. Nephrosclerosis associated with hypertensive nephropathy.
  b. Diabetic nephropathy.
  c. Tubulointerstitial disorders.
  d. Obstructive uropathy.
  e. Glomerular diseases.
  f. Polycystic disease.

6. Stages and Descriptions of CKD.
  See VIII. Renal System D.2 of this chapter.
7. Description, clinical symptoms, and treatment approaches of diseases associated with CKD outlined in part II. Alternative approaches to an effective health history and physical assessment of the older adult (earlier in this chapter).

C. Specifics of kidney replacement therapy.
  1. Early initiation of kidney replacement therapy (KRT) to reduce complications of uremia.
    a. Hypertension.
    b. Volume overload.
    c. Cardiac events.
    d. Malnutrition.
  2. Delayed KRT due to:
    a. Delayed referral from primary care health provider.

b. Overestimation of kidney function. Monitoring needed.
   (1) Regular estimation of weekly serum creatinine levels (NKF, 2002). Can be affected by:
      (a) Body weight.
      (b) Nutrition.
      (c) Sex.
      (d) Age.
      (e) Race.
   (2) Initiation of dialysis when the weekly total renal clearance (Kt/V$_{urea}$) falls below 2.0 recommended (NKF, 2002).
   (3) Cystatin C levels to detect small reductions in kidney function. More sensitive than serum creatinine. Better predictor of mortality risk in older adults (Shlipak, 2005).
3. Selection of a modality affected by:
   a. Physician preference.
   b. Patient and family preference.
   c. Functional status.
   d. Social support systems.
   e. Vascular system status.
   f. Cardiac status.
   g. Pulmonary status.
   h. Past abdominal surgeries/complications.
4. Kidney replacement therapy (KRT) options are consistent with other age groups. However, the aging process does have an impact on modality selection (will be discussed under each type below).
   a. Hemodialysis.
   b. Peritoneal dialysis.
   c. Transplantation.
   d. Conservative treatment.
5. Advantages/disadvantages of kidney replacement therapy options most commonly used by older adults (see Table 16.5).
6. Hemodialysis.
   a. In-center intermittent hemodialysis remains the primary form of KRT chosen for the older adult 65+ (USRDS, 2006).
   b. Home hemodialysis is the least used of all dialytic therapies for this age group (USRDS, 2006).
      (1) Requires another individual (who is usually the spouse) to provide physical and emotional support.
      (2) Can be a very stressful situation for both the patient and caregiver.
      (3) Caregiver may be an older individual also, and not capable or willing to take on these responsibilities.
      (4) One main advantage of home nocturnal hemodialysis for the older adult is that it is associated with restoration of impaired endothelial progenitor cells and plays a critical role in vascular repair with regards to cardiovascular disease, so common in the older adult with or without CKD.
   c. This treatment usually used for long-term care facility patients (see discussion of hemodialysis and patient care under "Nursing Home and Long-term Care" in this section).
   d. Hospice care should be considered as a supportive strategy for the CKD patient and family, especially if they have other comorbid, terminal conditions (e.g., cancer).
7. Hemodialysis complications.
   a. Hypotension.
      (1) Associated with aggressive fluid removal.
      (2) Autonomic dysfunction and decreased cardiac reserve are contributing factors.
      (3) Various approaches can be used to maintain a stable blood pressure and prevent major cardiac events (see Table 16.6).
   b. Cardiac events.
      (1) Cardiovascular disease remains the leading cause of mortality for patients 65 years of age and older who are receiving KRT (USRDS, 2006).
      (2) Causes. Hypotension, arrhythmias usually in the last hour of hemodialysis, vascular thrombosis caused by local shear stress and promote activation of hemostatic and thrombotic mechanisms (Stack & Messana, 2000).
   c. Gastrointestinal bleeding.
      (1) May go undetected. GI bleeding should be considered in the presence of an unprecedented drop in hematocrit/hemoglobin or failure of the hematocrit/hemoglobin to respond to epoetin alpha therapy.
      (2) Potential causes.
         (a) Uremic gastritis exacerbated by NSAIDs.
         (b) Angiodysplasia. Described as vascular ectasia (dilation of a tubular vessel), in the mucosa of the intestine. Usually occurs in the cecum. Bleeding may be slow or acute.
      (3) Diverticulosis with perforation associated with constipation.
      (4) Carcinoma.

Table 16.5

Comparison of Treatment Options with CKD Stage 5

Modality	Advantages	Disadvantages
In-center hemodialysis	• Limited time commitment. • Flexibility in achieving recommended clearances and fluid removal. • Less protein loss. • Provides a social support system. • Minimal learning skills required. • Minimal family involvement.	• Rapid, short treatments using some dialyzers predispose to symptoms of osmolality shift. • Increased risk of septicemia through vascular access problems or central line catheter. • Transportation to and from treatments necessary to make specific appointment times. • Increased risk of hypotension. • Heparinization may be necessary. • Added blood loss that contributes to anemia. • Specially trained personnel necessary. • Potential for self-image problems due to permanent access. • Stricter dietary and fluid restrictions.

Peritoneal dialysis	• Decreased risk of hypotension.
	• Decreased cardiovascular instability and arrhythmias.
	• Promotes consistent levels of waste product clearance.
	• No postdialysis fatigue syndrome.
	• Greater exercise tolerance.
	• No need for vascular access; uses peritoneal cavity.
	• Improved management of diabetes with intraperitoneal insulin therapy.
	• More efficient removal of B_2M and middle molecules.
	• Promotes family cohesiveness through inclusion of family members.
	• Less complicated than hemodialysis.
	• Fewer dietary restrictions.
	• Preferable for the diabetic patient.
		• Family and/or patient must have adequate intellect and motivation to learn procedure.
		• Potential for:
		  Inginal hernia.
		  Fluid leaks.
		  Vascular ischemia in lower extremities.
		  Bacterial or chemical peritonitis.
		  Exit site and tunnel infections.
		  Self-image problems with catheter placement.
		• Must have functional peritoneal membrane.
		• Social isolation.
		• Protein loss into dialysate.
		• Aggravated hyperlipidemia.
		• Contraindicated in the patient with previous abdominal trauma and surgeries.

Transplantation	• Increased survival rate over dialysis.	• Altered response to immunosuppression associated with age-related changes in the immune system.

d. Protein-energy malnutrition (PEM).
   (1) PEM occurs in 18–75% of dialysis patients (Burrowes, 2003).
   (2) Research on PEM in older adults is limited (Burrowes, 2003).
   (3) A predictor of morbidity and mortality. Related to serum albumin.
   (4) Inflammation is related to malnutrition in patients on dialysis, known as malnutrition-inflammation complex syndrome (Kalantar-Zadeh et al., 2003; Snyder & Pendergraph, 2005).
   (5) Affects iron markers. Increased serum ferritin levels and decreased TSAT levels (Kalantar-Zadeh et al., 2004; Petroff, 2005).

Table 16.6

Approaches Used to Maintain a Stable Blood Pressure

1. Frequent assessment of estimated dry weight.

2. Assess patient for presence of a pericardial effusion in the presence of unprecedented drop in blood pressure.

3. No antihypertensive medication predialysis.

4. Manage hypertension with short-acting agents.

5. Use bicarbonate dialysate.

6. Avoid removal of large amounts of fluid.

7. Use sequential ultrafiltration followed by conventional hemodialysis without fluid removal.

8. Schedule an additional treatment for fluid removal.

9. Use sodium modeling with caution.

10. Decrease bath temperature below 37° C.

11. Maintain hematocrit per NKF-DOQI guidelines.

12. Avoid large meal immediately before or during dialysis.

(6) Dialysis-related causes.
  (a) Inadequate dialysis as measured by kinetic modeling or urea with Kt/V.
  (b) Incompatible dialysis membrane causing a higher complement activation. Associated with increased amino acid release from peripheral muscle tissue consistent with increased protein catabolism.
  (c) Dialysate used for KRT.
  (d) Loss of amino acids and peptides in the dialysate.
  (e) Acidosis.
  (f) High parathyroid hormone levels.
(7) Patient-related causes.
  (a) Those changes associated with structural and functional changes in the GI tract as discussed under gastrointestinal system.
  (b) Reduction of the sensory input to the hypothalamus, which controls hunger and satiety centers.
  (c) Alterations in metabolism.
    [1] Decreased protein synthesis.
    [2] Increased protein breakdown.
  (d) Impaired ability to enhance protein synthesis I response to increased amino acids intake and decreased energy expenditure.

(e) Poverty.
(f) Disabilities leading to inability to:
  [1] Purchase food.
  [2] Prepare food.
  [3] Feed oneself.
  [4] Swallow (dysphagia).
(g) Poor dentition and/or ill-fitting dentures.
(h) Increased hospitalizations.
(i) Preexisting comorbid medical conditions.
(j) Altered senses of taste and smell.
(k) Polypharmacy.
(l) Psychosocial factors.
  [1] Lack of social support systems.
  [2] Depression.
  [3] Social isolation.
  [4] Dementia.
  [5] Finances (to purchase food).
  [6] Dependence on others.
  [7] Ethnic/cultural/religious influences.
(m) Drug-nutrient and drug-drug reactions.
(n) Inability to understand and/or read dietary changes.
(8) Treatment of PEM.
  (a) Requires a multidisciplinary approach.
  (b) Evaluation of KRT by treatment team.
  (c) Dietary consultation.
    [1] Maintain 3-day food records and dietary interviews biannually on maintenance dialysis patients (NKF, 2000).
    [2] Calculate nutrient intakes. Use to teach patients (NKF, 2000).
    [3] Identify actual nutritional intake vs. nutritional needs.
    [4] Identify need for alternative sources of nutrition.
      [a] Use of nutritional supplementation through commercially prepared products.
      [b] Consideration of alternative feeding approaches. Enteral feeding through a jejunostomy tube (J tube) reduces risk of regurgitation and subsequent aspiration.
  (d) Social service consultation (financial resources and home environment evaluation).
e. Infection.
  (1) Septicemia is another leading cause of

death in older dialysis patients, next to cardiovascular disease (USRDS, 2006).

(2) Increased risk of infection is associated with the altered immune response and the increased prevalence of malnutrition in older adults.

(3) Sources of sepsis.

   (a) Lungs in form of pneumonia associated with aspiration.

   (b) Vascular access (gram-positive).

   (c) Gastrointestinal tract (gram-negative).

   (d) Genitourinary tract (gram-negative).

(4) Clinical manifestation of infection may differ in the elderly patient. See "Implications for Health Care" under the Immune System in this chapter.

f. Dialysis-related amyloidosis (DRA).

(1) Due to the inefficiency of the kidneys, beta-2-microglobulin (a protein) builds up in the blood, forms large deposits and damages surrounding tissues (NIDDK, 2003).

(2) Common in hemodialysis patients of 5 years, especially among older adults (NIDDK, 2003). Peak occurrences in those 60–67 years of age; more common in males (Mayo, 2002).

(3) Dialyzer membranes unable to remove the protein, so deposits form in the bone, joints, and tendons. Pain and/or stiffness ensues (Copeland, 2006).

(4) Carpal tunnel syndrome most common complaint (NIDDK, 2003).

(5) Definitive confirmation. Biopsy tissue from stomach fat aspirate, oral or rectal mucosa, bone marrow, or specific organ affected, showing deposits on "Congo-red staining"(Mayo, 2002; NKF, 2003).

(6) Treatment.

   (a) Kidney transplant may stop progression.

   (b) High-flux diayzers may slow progression (NKF, 2003).

(7) Prognosis.

   (a) Mortality rare.

   (b) Significant morbidity.

   (c) Immobility seen in long-term dialysis patients (Copeland, 2006).

8. Hemodialysis: vascular access management.

a. Extensive description and review of vascular access options for hemodialysis can be found in Section 13.

b. Dialysis access procedures and complications

of dialysis access represent a major cause of morbidity, hospitalization, and cost for chronic dialysis patients.

c. The main types of vascular accesses available to the older population include the arteriovenous (AV) fistula, AV graft, and central venous catheter.

d. The success of access placement in older adults is compromised by:

(1) Vascular changes associated with the aging process.

(2) Increased number of comorbid medical conditions.

(3) Late referral patterns seen with the older adult population.

e. In April of 2004, an initiative by the Centers for Medicare and Medicaid Services was launched the use of AVF in all hemodialysis patients, older patients no exception. Use of an AVF should not be a limiting factor in older adults (Lok et al., 2005). Types of AVFs include:

(1) Forearm radiocephalic fistula connecting the radial artery to the cephalic vein. Berardinelli and Vegeto (1998) recommend end-to-end anastomosis to minimize the steal syndrome and venous hypertension in the hand. Atherosclerosis of the radial artery in older adults predisposes to poor maturation of the AV fistula in the forearm.

(2) Elbow fistula described as the anastomosis of the antecubital vein or an adjacent vein with the brachial artery. A side-to-side anastomosis is recommended to prevent peripheral ischemia.

   (a) Recommended by Berardinelli and Vegeto (1998). They report low morbidity, optimal patency rates, and minor revisions.

   (b) Miller et al. (1999) found that the adequacy rate (described as sustaining a blood flow rate of 350 mL/min) for upper arm fistulas was twice as high as compared with forearm fistulas. 54% of the elderly patients had successful upper arm AV fistulas placed as compared with a 12% lower arm successful placement.

   (c) Controversy exists regarding current recommendation by National Kidney Foundation Dialysis Outcome Quality Initiative (DOQI) guidelines (1997) recommending the initial placement of AV fistula in the lower arm and publications by Berardinelli and Vegeto (1998) and Miller et al. (1999). Their studies have concluded that the upper arm AV fistula is more efficacious in elderly patients. Research continues in this area since the 2004 initiative.

   (d) In the case of an unsuccessful maturation of an elbow fistula, placement of an AV graft above the original elbow AV fistula has been successful. The arterialized vein from the initial AV fistula is enlarged, contributing to enhanced flow through the conduit.

  f. The AV graft. A biologic, semibiologic, or synthetic graft may be implanted subcutaneously and interposed between an artery and a vein.

   (1) Alternative to an AV fistula in the absence of suitable vessels in the older adult.

   (2) Uses patient's native vessels in conjunction with a homologous saphenous vein (HSV) graft or a polytetrafluorethylene (PTFE) graft.

   (3) Major advantage. Condition of patient's vessel is not the sole determining factor for successful function and longevity. An AV graft has been successfully placed in patients with a failed AV fistula.

   (4) Disadvantages.

    (a) Thrombosis of conduit requiring multiple hospitalizations. Many older adults already have a high rate of hospitalizations due to complications of other comorbid conditions.

    (b) High rate of infection associated with the decreased immune status in the older adult population.

  g. Recommendation for improving access outcomes.

   (1) Education of health care personnel focusing on:

    (a) Maintaining the integrity of the vascular system during hospitalizations by minimizing phlebotomies in the upper extremities.

    (b) Maintaining central vein patency by judicious placement of central lines. Subclavian veins should be avoided.

   (2) Preoperative sonographic venous mapping.

   (3) Early referral to a nephrologist and consultation with a vascular surgeon.

   (4) Early placement of AV fistula.

   (5) Patient and family education regarding care of the AV fistula during maturation and after initiation of dialysis.

  h. Central line catheters.

   (1) Should be used only as an interim measure until a permanent access can be established.

   (2) Risk of infection is high, particularly in the elderly patient with a compromised immune system.

   (3) Placement of catheter should be limited to the internal jugular vein.

9. Peritoneal dialysis.

  a. The second most common dialytic therapy used by older adults, with CAPD being the most frequently chosen for ages 65+ as a new patient in 2004 (USRDS, 2006).

  b. Although physical and psychosocial considerations must be taken into account, the age range is also limited by what the local dialysis unit supports clinically.

  c. Useful for those with cardiovascular reserve.

  d. Homeostasis exhibited with blood chemistries.

  e. Technologic advances make it easier for those with sensory losses of eyesight and touch as well as manual dexterity, which decreases the rate of peritonitis.

  f. Infection rates are similar or lower in the older adult.

  g. Catheter removal associated with exit-site and tunnel infection more common in the older adult.

  h. Provides a viable alternative in the presence of multiple access failure.

10. Transplantation.

  a. Ages 65–74, 11.7% received a transplant in 2004 (USRDS, 2006).

  b. Ages 74+, 2% received a transplant in 2004 (USRDS, 2006).

  c. Elderly CKD patients transplanted have unadjusted 1-year patient survival rates that are between 15% and 40% higher than those remaining on dialysis (Stack & Messana, 2000).

  d. Barriers to transplantation in older adults.

   (1) Shortage of cadaver organs in the United States.

   (2) High rates of comorbid conditions precluding older adults from transplant.

   (3) Misconception that advanced age is a barrier to successful outcomes.

   (4) Intestinal ischemia found to be a more common complication of transplantation

in older adults, causing increased morbidity and mortality.

e. A senescent immune system in the presence of triple immunosuppressive therapy may predispose older adults to more virulent infections (Stack & Messana, 2000), but also has the potential for decreasing the incidence of graft rejection (Ponticelli, 2000).

f. Pharmacokinetic profiles of specific immune modulation agents, in particular cyclosporine, are different in elderly patients. The cytochrome P-450 microsomal enzyme system is less active among older adults, putting older adult transplant recipients at risk for cyclosporine toxicity (Stack & Messana, 2000). Currently, Tacromulis and mycophenolate mofetil are being used as baseline immunosupression for transplant patients (USRDS, 2006).

g. Approaches to improving transplantation outcomes for older adults.
   (1) Altered immune system. As discussed above, the senescent immune system may contribute to decreased graft rejection as long as the immunosuppression therapy is tailored to meet the needs of the elderly patient.
   (2) Multiple comorbid conditions can be managed by more intense pretransplant preparation.
      (a) Barium enema to determine the presence of diverticulitis.
      (b) Gallbladder ultrasound to evaluate for cholelithiasis.
      (c) Cardiac risks through the use of coronary angiography and revascularization may reduce posttransplantation cardiac events.
   (3) Continued research trials on medications posttransplant.

11. Conservative treatment.
   a. Not all patients choose to start KRT. Some choose palliative or conservative care.
   b. Some patients choose to withdraw from treatment. Causes include:
      (1) Feel as though they are a burden to others.
      (2) Quality of life concerns.
         (a) The American Nephrology Nurses' Association, in collaboration with the Renal Physicians Association and the American Society of Nephrology, developed guidelines to assist health care professionals (RPA/ASN, 2002).
         (b) Seen as a burden rather than a benefit. Neurologic and functional

status a concern (see also "End of Life Issues" in this section under Nursing Home and Long-Term Care.)
         (c) Hospice should be considered as the optimal method of patient care if dialysis is discontinued.
   c. The nurse must respect the individual's self-determination, and provide information, support, and comfort. Consideration must be given to:
      (1) Competency of the patient at the time of the decision.
      (2) Decision making without coercion.
      (3) Providing information regarding consequences of no treatment.

D. Long-term care (LTC).
   1. It is estimated that 4.5% of the older adult population lives in the LTC setting (AARP, 2004).
      a. As the population ages this percentage is expected to increase substantially.
      b. Of the end-stage renal disease (ESRD) patients living in LTC, 50% are over the age of 65 with the mean age of approximately 72 (USRDS, 2004).
      c. Diabetic patients make up 50% of this population and hypertension affects 1 out of 3 ESRD patients in this setting (USRDS, 2004).
      d. Nurses working with patients in the LTC setting will be exposed to providing care to patients with chronic kidney disease (CKD) and the complications associated with CKD.
      e. Many patients with CKD will at some time during their treatment need home health services, a short stay in a rehabilitation hospital or extended care facility.
      f. Some will require LTC in an extended care facility.
      g. For clarity, any settings requiring a lengthy stay away from home will be identified as a LTC setting.
   2. Background facts and guidelines for LTC staff.
      a. CKD diagnosis requires a team effort to care for the patient no matter what the setting. That team consists of:
         (1) Nephrologists.
         (2) Nephrology nurses (all levels).
         (3) Technicians.
         (4) Renal dietitians.
         (5) Renal social workers.
      b. When the older adult lives in the LTC setting, the support team in that setting becomes a member of the CKD team.

c. There are national guidelines developed by members of the CKD community.
   (1) The National Kidney Foundation through the Kidney Disease Outcomes Quality Initiative (NKF-DOQI). These guidelines identify the care needs of the patient with CKD.
   (2) The American Nephrology Nurses' Association (ANNA) has also developed "Standards of Clinical Practice for Nephrology Nursing" to address the care needs of this patient population.
d. Care of the older adult CKD patient living in the long-term care setting involves additional challenges for the nursing staff in that setting whether the patient requires kidney replacement (KRT)/dialysis therapy or not.
e. The complexities of care increase with the extent of CKD and the need for KRT/dialysis. In addition to the previously identified normal physiologic changes due to the aging process, there are the changes encountered with the progression of CKD.
f. Patients with CKD should be weighed daily.
   (1) Especially if on dialysis.
   (2) Essential if the patient is bed bound and cannot be weighed at the dialysis unit.
   (3) Patients should be weighed at the same time of day, on the same scale with approximately the same weight of clothing.
3. Assessment of the CKD patient.
   a. Cardiovascular complications are the greatest cause for mortality and morbidity in the older adult with CKD especially if the patient requires dialysis.
   b. Thorough assessment and observation for responses to treatment are important and include:
      (1) Listening to heart sounds.
      (2) Listening to lung sounds.
      (3) Assessing fluid status.
      (4) Checking for edema.
         (a) Edema is dependent for bed-bound patients. Check the sacral and periorbital areas.
         (b) For ambulating patients, checking lower extremities.
      (5) Checking skin turgor.
      (6) Restrictinig fluid intake.
      (7) Controlling dietary intake.
      (8) Properly administering medications.
      (9) Evaluating blood pressure.
      (10) Checking dialysis access daily.
      (11) Monitoring for changes in any of the

above and watch for side effects from therapies.
4. The hemodialysis treatment.
   a. Hemodialysis is not painful. Once the patient is stabilized, there are very few complications.
   b. There may be some complications in patients when they return from therapy to the LTC setting.
   c. Some patients complain of feeling "washed out" and want to sleep after treatment.
   d. They may complain of headache or leg cramps. Each patient reacts to the treatment differently.
   e. If the patients adhere to their physician's orders regarding medication, diet, and fluid intake, the treatment should be relatively symptom free.
   f. If the patients return to care in the LTC setting frequently experiencing hypotension, headaches, leg cramps, nausea, and vomiting, the dialysis center should be notified. The dialysis nurses can review the current dialysis prescription with the nephrologist and obtain changes in the orders as needed.
5 Fluid restrictions.
   a. Measure all PO and IV fluids including medications.
   b. Dialysis patients usually make little or no urine.
   c. Report vomiting and/or diarrhea to the dialysis unit.
6. Control dietary intake. Be aware of patient's dietary prescription. Patient may have varying dietary orders depending on each one's underlying disease.
   a. Potassium. If on low potassium diet, avoid bananas, oranges, potatoes, and salt substitute.
   b. Phosphorus. If on low phosphorus diet, avoid peanuts, beans, cheese, milk, and yogurt.
   c. Fluid. Review physician orders. Measure as part of a fluid restriction the amount of water left at the bedside.
7. Properly administer medications.
   a. Many drugs are removed by dialysis. Vitamins should be taken after the dialysis treatment.
   b. Administration of drugs should be planned around the dialysis treatments.
   c. Always administer phosphate binders as directed. DO NOT administer with iron supplements.
   d. Be sure to communicate any medication changes to the dialysis center and the nephrologist.

8. Evaluate blood pressure (BP).
   a. Evaluate the peak action time of any antihypertensive medication.
   b. Plan administration time so that the peak action does not occur during the dialysis treatment.
   c. Remember that fluid status directly affects blood pressure (increased fluid retention – increased blood pressure).
9. Monitor vascular access.
   a. Vascular access for hemodialysis is the "life-line" in the patient with ESRD.
   b. Types of access.
      (1) Arteriovenous fistula (AV fistula).
         (a) Formed by surgically joining a artery and a vein.
         (b) Fistulas are the first choice for access in all patients.
      (2) Graft.
         (a) A length of synthetic material, surgically tunneled beneath the skin, fastened on one side to an artery and on the other side a vein.
         (b) Prone to clotting and infection.
      (3) Central line catheter.
         (a) Used as a temporary access.
         (b) Placed in the internal jugular vein.
         (c) Clotting and infection are consistent problems.
   c. Maintenance of a functional vascular access is of primary concern.
      (1) The patient needs to avoid tight or heavy pressure on the access extremity.
      (2) The patient should not sleep on the access arm.
      (3) The patient should not have tight jewelry or elastic clothing at the access site.
      (4) Inspect access daily.
         (a) Check access daily for evidence of bleeding, drainage, discoloration, or pain.
         (b) Check fistulas and grafts daily for bruit ("whooshing" sound heard over access through a stethoscope) and thrill (the pulsation felt over the access by feeling with fingers).
         (c) Catheters used for dialysis usually have heparin instilled after treatment to maintain patency and should never be used to get blood samples for the lab or to give medications. They are for dialysis treatments ONLY.
10. Watch for side effects of dialysis.
   a. Evaluate for any signs of bleeding.
      (1) Large doses of heparin or some form of anticoagulation are usually used during the treatment.
      (2) Heparin, a commonly used anticoagulant, has a half-life of approximately 6 hours.
   b. Report any falls before or after a dialysis treatment to the physician and the dialysis unit.
   c. Hypotension.
   d. Unsteady gait.
   e. Seizures.
   f. Electrolyte imbalance.
   g. Always be aware of when the next dialysis treatment is due and report any side effect(s) to the unit.
11. Common side effects of dialysis.
   a. Hypotension.
      (1) Elderly patients, and patients with diabetes mellitus (DM) and heart disease may experience hypotension after dialysis.
      (2) The blood vessels may not be able to constrict and return blood to the heart which may result in very low blood pressure.
      (3) Often dialysis patients cannot compensate for the dialysis-induced fluid shift and fluid loss and may experience hypotension after their dialysis treatment.
      (4) Causes.
         (a) Removing too much fluid during dialysis.
         (b) The more fluid that is removed, the greater the chances are for hypotension.
         (c) Comorbid conditions. Heart disease and DM prevent the body from compensating for the dialysis-induced fluid loss.
         (d) Patient may be taking certain BP medications prior to dialysis.
         (e) Patient may have an infection that has not yet been identified.
      (5) Implications for health care.
         (a) Weight gains between dialysis treatments should be maintained as prescribed to minimize hypotension from dialysis-induced fluid loss.
         (b) Maintain fluid and dietary restrictions. Carefully monitor and assess patient for dehydration.
         (c) The patient should follow their prescribed fluid allotments.
         (d) Explore medications that are effective

in stimulating nerve endings in the blood vessels, allowing constriction of the vessels, which increases the blood pressure.

(e) If the patient is taking antihypertensive medications the physician may need to reevaluate and modify the dose.

(f) BP medications may need to be dispensed after dialysis instead of prior to dialysis.

(g) If patient has nausea and vomiting, report this to the dialysis staff prior to the next dialysis treatment.

(h) If patient uses nitroglycerin patches, do not put a new patch on prior to or right after dialysis.
  [1] Discuss placing the patch on the patient several hours after dialysis with the physician.
  [2] Inform the dialysis staff if the patient is wearing a nitroglycerin patch.

(i) Evaluate the medications the patient is currently taking.

(j) Maintain the patient in a good nutritional state.

(k) If hypotension is persistent, the patient should be evaluated by the nephrologist and given medication to prevent the hypotension.

  b. Nausea.
  (1) It is important to remember that many times nausea occurs as a result of hypotension.
  (2) The nausea will resolve as the BP normalizes. The nausea usually resolves in a few hours once equilibration in the body occurs.
  (3) If nausea is persistent, other causes need to be considered, so inform the dialysis team.
  (4) Causes.
    (a) Nausea may be due to:
      [1] A lowered BP.
      [2] Medications.
      [3] Uremia.
      [4] Electrolyte imbalance.
    (b) Evaluate the BP to determine if nausea is related to cardiovascular instability.
    (c) Often nausea is related to dialysis fluid shifts or losses and will resolve in a few hours or the next day.

(d) The patient may have an infection or be allergic to a medication which can cause nausea.

(e) If repeated episodes of nausea are reported to the dialysis team often dialysis treatments can be altered to prevent the nausea.

  (5) Implications for health care.
    (a) Review medications.
    (b) Review cardiac status.
    (c) Review diet.
    (d) Antiemetics may be used if needed.

  c. Headaches.
  (1) Causes.
    (a) Many times headaches are associated with the patient's sodium levels that have shifted during the treatment.
    (b) Headaches can also be associated with dialysis induced fluid loss.
  (2) Implications for health care. Headaches need to be reported to the dialysis staff for evaluation.

  d. Leg cramps.
  (1) Causes.
    (a) May be due to excessive fluid removal.
    (b) May be caused by electrolyte imbalances.
  (2) Implications for health care.
    (a) Monitor fluid intake between dialysis treatments.
    (b) Encourage use of hard candies or gum to resolve thirst.
    (c) Monitor electrolytes.

  e. Skin integrity issues.
  (1) Causes. Due to the uremic state, patients may have:
    (a) Changes in color to pale, sallow, and gray appearance.
    (b) Changes in turgor: loose, dry, and scaly.
    (c) Changes in texture.
    (d) Changes in vascularity.
    (e) Alteration in sensation.
    (f) Extreme itching.
  (2) Implications for health care.
    (a) Patient's skin should be inspected for changes in color, turgor, texture, vascularity, and sensation.
    (b) Skin care products and medications are available to use for treatment.

  f. Hypoglycemia.
  (1) Causes.
    (a) CKD often leads to poor caloric intake leading to hypoglycemia.

(b) Nausea and vomiting may also lead to hypoglycemia.

(c) 50% of stage 5 CKD patients with type 2 DM do not require antiglycemic treatment.

(d) The dialysate fluid contains glucose. Blood glucose levels taken during treatment or right after treatment may reflect the level of glucose that is in the dialysate.

(e) Blood glucose levels should normalize a few hours after treatment.

(2) Implications for health care.

(a) To prevent hypoglycemia, monitor the patient for poor appetite, which may lead to malnutrition.

(b) Evaluate the patient's need for antiglycemic medications, as the need for medication may decrease once the patient is on dialysis.

g. Blood glucose concerns.

(1) Causes.

(a) Insulin resistance is common in the nondiabetic patient with CKD. It can lead to mild hyperglycemia that would be characterized by increased thirst and weight gain.

(b) The patient may have fluctuating blood glucose levels as insulin needs change. In kidney failure there is a risk for hypoglycemia due to a reduction in the amount of insulin being catabolized in the kidneys, with higher levels of insulin remaining in circulation.

(2) Health care implications.

(a) It is important to know the patient's weight at baseline and monitor their weight daily.

(b) It is important to communicate to the patient that there may no longer be a sense of impending hypoglycemia or hyperglycemia.

(c) LTC staff needs to keep a log recording the incidence of hypoglycemia and hyperglycemia to aid in the evaluation of changes in insulin requirements.

(d) Considerations for meals must be addressed when a patient in LTC goes for treatment.

(e) It is important for the dialysis patient with diabetes to eat their meals and snacks without delay.

(f) Sending snacks and bag lunches

with the patient to dialysis can accommodate the patient's caloric requirements and prevent hypoglycemia or hyperglycemia.

12. The access site.

a. Daily care.

(1) To prevent infections and potential blood loss, the dialysis access site should never be used for IV sites or laboratory blood draws.

(2) Avoid any other puncturing of the access as the pressure within the access can lead to excessive bleeding.

(3) Check the access site and skin integrity over the entire location of the access.

(4) Monitor the bruit (using a stethoscope to listen) and the thrill (palpating the pulsation), checking for consistent quality and character.

(5) Assess the access for signs of redness, swelling, drainage, tenderness, or feeling hot to the touch.

(6) Assess a pseudoaneurysm for changes in appearance and size.

(7) Check the catheter dressing. It should always be dry and intact.

(8) Check the catheter for bleeding from the ports.

(9) Check for bleeding or drainage from the exit site.

(10) Monitor for fever.

(11) Ensure BP is not taken on access limb.

b. Potential complications.

(1) Ischemia.

(a) Check for ischemia to distal extremity due to decreased blood flow following access placement (Steal syndrome: Inadequate circulation to the extremity resulting from surgical diversion of arterial blood).

[1] Coolness.

[2] Pallor.

[3] Pain.

[4] Contractures.

(2) Infections.

(a) Exposure to nonsterile needle(s).

(b) Poor cannulation technique.

(c) Patient hygiene.

(3) Clotting of the access may be related to:

(a) Prolonged, extreme pressure over access.

(b) Patient coagulation times.

(c) Inadequate anticoagulation.

(d) If access is found to be clotted, follow LTC policy and notify dialysis facility.

(4) Bleeding. If access site bleeding occurs after the patient has returned from dialysis:

(a) Apply gentle manual pressure over the needle site for 10–20 minutes using a clean towel or gauze pad.

(b) Hemostatic agents may be used.

(c) If bleeding does not stop within 30 minutes, notify the doctor or the dialysis center.

(d) In extreme cases, transfer to the emergency room.

13. Medications and implications for LTC staff.

a. Vitamins. Vitamin D or multivitamins without minerals are used to replace vitamins lost during the hemodialysis treatment.

(1) Common names: Nephrocaps®, Nephrotabs®, folic acid.

(2) Should be taken AFTER treatment.

b. Phosphate binders to limit the gastrointestinal absorption of phosphorus and prevent renal bone disease or hyperparathyroidism.

(1) Common names: Fosrenol®, PhosLo®, Renagel®, Tums®, Oscal®.

(2) DO take with meals or snacks.

(3) DO NOT take with oral iron preparations.

c. Erythropoietin-stimulating agents (ESA) are used to treat anemia.

(1) Generally given during the dialysis treatment.

(2) Common names: Aranesp® (CKD), Epogen®, Procrit®.

d. Iron for anemia management (usually given IV during the dialysis treatment).

(1) Common names: Ferrlecit®, Venofer®, iron dextran.

(2) Oral iron preparations should be discontinued when IV iron is initiated.

e. Vitamin D to prevent and/or treat bone disease associated with kidney disease.

(1) Common names: Hectorol®, Rocaltrol®, Zemplar®.

(2) Oral vitamin D should not be dosed with oral iron preparations.

f. Antihypertensives for blood pressure management. Check with the dialysis unit to determine if these should be given prior to treatment. These drugs are often on HOLD prior to treatment.

g. Medications to AVOID.

(1) Alka-Seltzer® – high in sodium.

(2) Milk of Magnesium®/Mylanta® –

magnesium dialyzes poorly, may build up in the dialysis patient and cause neurologic problems.

(3) Aspirin (ASA) – may interfere with clotting process. (*Note*: daily doses of ASA [81 mg. PO or 325 mg PO] may be prescribed to prevent clotting of access.)

(4) Fleets enema – high in phosphorus.

14. Nutritional issues.

a. Nutrition plays a critical role in the management of the CKD patient.

b. The diet will vary depending on the type of disease, the CKD stage, as well as the type of treatment chosen.

c. Modifications are made based on age, height, weight, nutritional status, residual kidney function, type of treatment (hemodialysis or peritoneal dialysis) laboratory data, medications, and/or comorbid disease(s).

d. Dietary restrictions discussed are "generalities." Each patient's diet is individualized and needs to be reviewed before making any interventions.

e. Factors that influence nutritional status of CKD stage 5 patients.

(1) Dietary restrictions: increased needs and additional losses.

(2) Nutrients lost during the dialysis process.

(3) Dialysis procedure itself may be catabolic.

(4) Inadequate dialysis.

(5) Nausea, vomiting, anorexia (uremia), diarrhea, constipation.

(6) Difficulty chewing and/or swallowing, taste changes, bad taste in mouth.

(7) Multiple medications (food/drug/dialyzer interactions).

(8) Gastroparesis, catabolic process, acidosis.

(9) Feeling of fullness (PD), early satiety.

(10) Multiple disease states/abnormal metabolism, or comorbid conditions.

(11) Endocrine disorders.

(12) Infection, including peritonitis.

f. Implications for health care.

(1) Renal dietitian and LTC dietitian should discuss dietary prescription for patient.

(2) If patient travels from the LTC to the dialysis center during meal times, a plan should be developed to ensure patient receives adequate nutrition.

(3) Renal diet considerations.

(a) Protein: 1.0–1.2g/kg/day. 50% high biologic value.

(b) Potassium: 40–70 mEq (1500–2500 mg/day). Avoid high potassium foods and salt substitute.

(c) Sodium: 750–1000 mg/day. Avoid high sodium foods. Do not use added salt.

(d) Phosphorus: 600–1200 mg/day. Limit dairy products.

(e) Calories: > 35 kcal/kg/day.
[1] For obese patients: 25–30 kcal/kg/day.
[2] For malnutrition: 40–45 kcal/kg/day.

(f) Fluids 1–1.5 L/day plus urine output.
[1] Measure patients' output. Add to fluid limit.
[2] Example: Daily fluid limit 1000 cc.
[3] Total fluid intake allowed is 1650 cc/day.
[4] Daily urine output 650 cc.

15. Social services.
    a. Social services are provided to patients and their families and are directed at supporting and maximizing the social functioning and adjustment of the patient.
    b. Medicare regulations mandate that social work services be an integral part of patient care.
    c. The dialysis center's social worker is responsible for conducting psychosocial evaluations, recommending changes in treatment, and identifying community social agencies and other resources and assisting the patient and family in their use.
    d. Functions of the renal social worker.
       (1) Orientation of the patient to the unit and implications of kidney failure.
       (2) Informs patient of sources for financial coverage for medical costs related to KRT/dialysis.
       (3) Psychosocial evaluation.
       (4) Adjustment therapy as needed.
       (5) Reinforce "choice" of modality.
       (6) Act as a mediator in the clinic.
       (7) Grief counseling as needed.
       (8) Patient support groups.

16. Stressors in the LTC environment associated with dialysis.
    a. Stressors with dialysis can be actual or threatened.
    b. Stressors vary somewhat with those of the new admission into the LTC but exhibit many similarities.
    c. The causes may be more variant than the response.
    d. The individual who requires dialysis to survive may perceive the access surgery or the dependence on the hemodialysis machine as impacting on body image.

    e. LTC patients may feel body image is threatened by loss of control of activities of daily living (ADLs).
    f. The dual need for dialysis and housing in the LTC setting can be doubly threatening to these patients.
       (1) Stressors associated with dialysis.
           (a) Actual or threatened loss.
           (b) Distortion of body image.
           (c) Dependency on machines and medical team.
           (d) Fear of death vs. fear of living.
           (e) Patient self-concept.
           (f) Capacity to control.
           (g) Helplessness.
       (2) Implications for health care.
           (a) Explore, recognize, and identify stressors as real to the patient.
           (b) Explain all functions, programs, and procedures in clear and simplified terms.
           (c) Provide time and support to maximize self-care, especially with ADL.
           (d) Provide access to physical and occupational therapies to identify ADL needs and reinforcement to maximize self-care.
           (e) Encourage family and friends visits to be supportive and to allow for adjustment to new environment.
           (f) Encourage participation in activities provided by long-term care provider.

17. Communication between dialysis center and LTC.
    a. Treatment related communication.
       (1) Communication with the dialysis center before and after the dialysis treatment will provide the patient with consistency of care.
       (2) Notify the dialysis physician and dialysis unit of all medication changes/additions or patient problems, such as hospitalization, emergencies, access problems, or change in mentation/status.
    b. Long-term care plans reflect the choice of modality and should accompany the patient when transferred to other care facilities.
    c. Short-term care plans from both the dialysis center and the LTC should reflect continuity of care.
    d. LTC social service departments and the renal social worker should be in constant contact regarding patient issues.
    e. LTC dietitian and the renal dietitian should be in consultation regarding the renal diet

and the patient's adherence to the prescribed diet.

   f. Transportation to and from the dialysis unit is often an issue.

     (1) According to Medicare guidelines, the patient is responsible for arranging transportation. This means that the LTC facility is responsible for transportation.

     (2) Coordination with the patient's dialysis schedule is important to prevent excessive "wait times."

18. Family issues.

   a. Many older adults feel abandoned by family when long-term care placement is required.

   b. Encourage family visits that coincide with facility schedule and minimize conflicts with therapies and routine care.

19. Financial concerns.

   a. When elderly patients develop stage 5 CKD and begin dialysis treatment, they are often already eligible for Medicare.

   b. Medicare supplemental insurance premiums may be a financial factor for the stage 5 CKD patient.

   c. The dialysis center's social worker works with the patient to ensure all inquiries are addressed in a timely manner for maximum benefits.

   d. Medicare pays a portion of the costs. The social worker may be able to assist the patient in securing additional coverage.

20. Laboratory.

   a. Requirements. CKD patients who receive dialysis in-center will have monthly lab work drawn at the dialysis center. Some of the tests such as hemoglobin, hematocrit, and calcium may be drawn more frequently.

   b. Lab results for this patient population.

     (1) Serum albumin.

       (a) Reference range: 3.5–5.5 g/dL.

       (b) Minimum standard of care: > 4.0.

       (c) Plasma albumin is the principal component that maintains fluid equilibrium between the interstitial fluid and the plasma, regulating oncotic pressure.

     (2) Serum calcium.

       (a) Reference range: 9.0–11.0 mg/dL.

       (b) Standard of care: 8.4–9.5 mg/dL (KDOQI).

     (3) Phosphorus.

       (a) Reference range: 3.5–5.5 mg/dL.

       (b) Standard of care: 3.5–5.5 mg/dL (KDOQI).

       (c) As kidney failure develops, fewer nephrons are available to excrete dietary phosphorus, and plasma phosphorus rises.

       (d) Low phosphorus levels may be due to excess phosphate binding, malabsorption, diarrhea, vomiting, alcoholism, postparathyroidectomy, and diabetic ketoacidosis.

       (e) It is recommended that dietary phosphorus be restricted to 800–1000 mg/day (KDOQI). The use of phosphate-binding medications with all food intake is required to achieve this goal.

     (4) Blood urea nitrogen.

       (a) Reference range: 30–90 mg/dL.

       (b) Urea is the main nitrogenous end-product of protein metabolism. It is formed in the liver from amino acids and from ammonia compounds.

       (c) Urea is a surrogate solute currently used to measure adequacy of dialysis. It is also used to assess dietary compliance and nutritional status.

     (5) Serum creatinine.

       (a) Reference range: 3.0–12 mg/dL.

       (b) Serum creatinine is an estimate of creatinine clearance or glomerular filtration rate and is widely used because it is inexpensive and simple, and the day-to-day variation in patients with kidney disease is low.

     (6) Potassium.

       (a) Reference range: 3.5–5.5 mEq/L.

       (b) Standard of care: 3.5–5.5 mEq/L.

       (c) Symptoms of hyperkalemia include increased muscular irritability, increased contractility, arrhythmias, diarrhea, and skeletal muscle jumping. May be life-threatening.

       (d) Nondietary causes of hyperkalemia in renal patients include potassium being pushed out of cells in tissue damage as in rhabdomyolysis, reduced insulin levels, trauma, burns, tumors, massive bleeding, tissue destruction, dehydration, and potassium sparing diuretics such as:

        [1] Spironolactone (Aldactone®).

        [2] Eplerenone (Inspra®).

        [3] Triamterene (Dyrenium®).

        [4] Amiloride (Midamor®).

        [5] Angiotensin-converting enzyme

(ACE) inhibitors can also increase potassium.

(e) Symptoms of hypokalemia include lethargy, weakness in the extremities, and cardiac arrhythmias.

(f) Hypokalemia can occur with alcohol abuse, vomiting, increases in insulin, diarrhea, laxative and enema abuse, and malabsorption.

(7) Bicarbonate.

(a) Reference range: 20–27 mEq/L.

(b) Patients with stage 5 CKD have chronic metabolic acidosis as a result of the kidney's inability to excrete the hydrogen that is partly derived from protein in the diet.

(c) Dialysis corrects metabolic acidosis more directly with the use of bicarbonate-containing dialysis solution.

(8) Hemoglobin.

(a) Reference range: 10.0–17.0 g/dL (normal).

(b) Minimum standard of care > 11 g/dL to 12 g/dL (KDOQI).

(c) Hemoglobin is the oxygen-carrying compound contained in red blood cells (RBC).

(9) Hematocrit.

(a) Reference range: 30.0–40.0%.

(b) Minimum standard of care: 33.0–36.0%.

(c) Hematocrit is the percentage of red blood cell mass to the overall blood volume.

(d) Hematocrit may be high in dehydration and polycythemia. It may be low in blood loss, anemia, and inadequate dosing with ESAs.

(10) Triglycerides.

(a) Reference range: 50–160 mg/dL.

(b) Hypertriglyceridemia is found in 33–70% of patients with CKD.

(c) Heparin may increase the triglycerides.

(d) Triglycerides may also be high in liver disease, gout, pancreatitis, alcohol abuse, diabetes, peritoneal dialysis solutions, and steroid use.

(11) Glucose.

(a) Reference range: 70–126 mg/dL.

(b) Glucose levels may be high in diabetes, malignancies, burns, acute stress, use of steroids, pancreatic insufficiency, and hyperthyroidism.

(c) Glucose levels may be low in malnutrition, hyperinsulinemia, alcohol abuse, pancreatic tumors, liver failure, and pancreatic tumors.

(12) Hgb A1C.

(a) Normal range: 4.8–6.0%.

(b) Desirable range: 4–6% Nondiabetic; < 7% Diabetic.

(c) HgbA1C is a test that measures the percentage of "glycosylated hemoglobin" in the blood (when glucose in the plasma attached itself to the hemoglobin molecule). Once this glycosylation process begins, it is irreversible. The more glycosylation, the higher the values.

(d) The hemoglobin molecule has a life span of 120 days. For CKD patients, the average life span of hemoglobin has shortened to an average about 70 days. The assay reflects the average blood sugar concentration over that period of time.

c. Implications for health care.

(1) On the day that the lab work is drawn, some lab results may be out of range but would likely be corrected by that day's dialysis treatment. For example, if a patients potassium results were 6.0 mEq/dL before dialysis, the dialysis treatment would have corrected the potassium to an acceptable range for a CKD patient.

(2) Labs drawn from the extracorporeal bloodlines of a dialysis patient should be drawn from the arterial side of the extracorporeal system as close to the patient as possible.

(3) Following dialysis facility policy, lab samples are drawn prior to or at the initiation of dialysis therapy.

(a) The dialysis staff draws the lab specimen from the cannulation needle or from the extracorporeal blood lines during the initiation of dialysis treatment.

(b) *Note*: For nondialysis staff: DO NOT perform venipuncture on the limb (arm) that has the fistula or graft.

(4) Know the normal lab results for this patient population.

21. End-of-life issues.

a. Assess patient for support systems, emotional status, and perceived quality of life.

(1) A program should be in place to address the option of patients deciding to stop dialysis.

(2) The decision to either not start dialysis or end dialysis is made with the patient, family, physician, social worker, and other team members such as chaplains and/or psychiatrists.

(3) The dialysis center's social worker will explore all possible alternatives and the implications of each.

b. Research is needed.

(1) Many questions need to be answered in the determination of the direction and forum for research. Most important is that nephrology nurses have a professional responsibility to provide their patients with evidence-based practice. Research must provide the nephrology nurse with literature based on good science and focused on improved outcomes. Some areas identified are:

(a) Provide data to support earlier identification and treatment of CKD as a clinical and cost benefit for the aging population.

(b) Considering the physiologic and psychologic changes associated with the aging process, provide data to identify the best modality of therapy for the older adult in stage 5 CKD.

(2) Identify a methodology for measuring quality of life and promote implementation of programs to support patients in quality of life and end-of-life decisions.

(3) Explore alternative approaches to treatment that offer the older adult confined to the long-term care setting improved access to safe and effective therapy.

(4) Explore options for determining acuity that support improved quality and access to care.

(5) Develop and implement methods for determining and establishing the best treatment access for the older adult.

(6) Identify pathologies and explore therapies to address pathologies associated with aging that contribute to the progression of CKD and its associated morbidity and mortality.

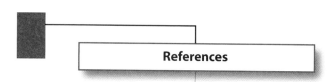

References

Agrawal, M., & Swartz, R. (2000). Acute renal failure. *American Family Physician, 61,* 2077.

Badzek, L., Hines, S.C., & Moss, A.H. (1998). Inadequate self-care knowledge among elderly hemodialysis patients: Assessing its prevalence and potential causes. *ANNA Journal, 28*(3), 293-300.

Berardinelli, L., & Vegeto, A. (1998). Lessons from 494 permanent accesses in 348 haemodialysis patients older than 65 years of age: 29 years of experiences. *Nephrology, Dialysis, & Transplantation, 13*(Suppl. 7), 73-77.

Bhatnagar, B., Maruenda, J., & Lowenthal, D.T. (1998). Ethical issues involved in dialysis for the elderly. *Geriatric Nephrology and Urology, 8*(2), 111-114.

Bonucchi, D., D'Amelio, A., Grosoli, M., Baraldi, A., & Cappelli, G. (1998). Vascularaccess for haemodialysis: From surgical procedure to integrated therapeutic approach. *Nephrology, Dialysis, & Transplantation, 13*(Suppl. 7), 78-81.

Brady, H.R., Clarkson, M.R., & Lieberthal, W. (2004). Acute renal failure. In B.M. Brenner (Ed.), *Brenner & Rector's the kidney* (7th ed., pp. 1215-1219). Philadelphia: Saunders.

Brown, E.A. (1999). Peritoneal dialysis versus hemodialysis in the elderly. *Peritoneal Dialysis International, 19,* 311-312.

Brown, V.W., & Schmitz, P.G. (1998). Acute and chronic kidney disease. *Clinics in Geriatric Medicine, 14*(2), 211-236.

Burrowes, J. (2003). Nutrition assessment and management of elderly dialysis patients. *Topics in Clinical Nutrition, 18*(4), 280.

Calkins, M. (1993). Ethical issues in the elderly ESRD patient. *ANNA Journal, 20*(5), 569-571.

Centers for Disease Control and Prevention (CDC). (2006). *Healthy aging: Preventing disease and improving quality of life among older Americans.* Retrieved November 1, 2007, from http://www.cdc.gov/nccdphp/publications/aag/aging.htm

Chou, S., & Lindeman, R. (1995). Structural and functional changes of the aging kidney. In H.R. Jacobson, G.E. Striker, & S. Klahr (Eds.), *The principles and practice of nephrology* (2nd ed., pp. 510-514). St. Louis: Mosby.

Choudhury, D., Raj, D., & Levi, M. (2004). Effect of aging on renal function and disease. In B.M. Brenner (Ed.), *Brenner & Rector's the kidney* (7th ed., pp. 2303-2341). Philadelphia: Saunders.

Copeland, S. (2006). Amyloidosis and its impact on patients with ESRD. *Nephrology Nursing Journal, 33*(1), 31-36.

Costa, P.T., Williams, T.F., & Somerfield, M. (1996). Early identification of Alzheimer's disease and related dementias. *Clinical practice guideline, quick reference guide for clinicians, No.19*. Rockville, MD: U.S. Department of Health and Human Services, Public Health Service, Agency for Health Care Policy and Research. AHCPR Publication No. 97-0703.

Cutler, R.E. (2007). *The Merck manual for healthcare professionals: Obstructive uropathy (urinary tract obstruction)*. Retrieved May 15, 2007, from http://www.merck.com/mmpe/sec17/ch229/ch229a.html

Davis, K.M., & Mathew, E. (1998). Pharmacologic management of depression in the elderly. *The Nurse Practitioner, 23*(6), 16-42.

Davison, A.M. (1998). Renal disease in the elderly. *Nephron, 124*, 126-145.

Department of Health and Human Services (HHS), Administration on Aging (AOA). (2001). *A statistical profile of older Americans aged 65+*. Retrieved November 1, 2007, from http://www.aoa.gov/press/fact/pdf/ss_stat_profile.pdf

Eliopoulos, C. (1997). Mental health problems. In C. Eliopoulos (Ed.), *Gerontological nursing* (pp. 386-411). Philadelphia: Lippincott.

Ferrans, C., & Powers, M. (1993). Quality of life of hemodialysis patients. *ANNA Journal, 20*(5), 575-581.

Gerberding, J.L. (2006). Quote from the annual CDC report (p. 1). *The Health and Economic Effects of an Aging Society*. Retrieved February 20, 2008, from www.cdc.gov/nccdphp/publications/aag/aging.htm

Gutch, C.F., Stoner, M.H., & Corea, A.L. (1999). ESRD in the elderly. In *Review of hemodialysis for nurses and dialysis personnel* (pp. 300-307). St. Louis: Mosby.

Grapsa, I., & Oreopoulos, D. (1996). Practical ethical issues of dialysis in the elderly. *Seminars in Nephrology, 16*(4), 339-352.

Hakim, R., Wingard, R., & Parker, R. (1994, November). Effect of the dialysis membrane in the treatment of patients with acute renal failure. *New England Journal of Medicine*, 1338-1342.

Ham, J. (1997). Demographics. In R.J. Ham & P.D. Sloane (Eds.), *Primary care geriatrics* (pp. 8-13). New York: Mosby.

Hirsch, B.E., & Weksler, M.E. (1991). Normal changes in host defense. In W.B. Williams & R. Berkow (Eds.), *The Merck manual of geriatrics* (pp. 877-924). Rahway, NJ: Merck Sharp & Dohme Research Laboratories.

Houser, A., Fox-Grage, W., & Gibson, M.J. (2003). *Across the states – Profiles in long term care and independent living* (7th ed.). Retrieved February 9, 2007, from http://www.research.aarp.org/health

Hu, C. (2005). *MedCalc: Glomerular filtration rate estimation*. Retrieved February 9, 2006, from http://www.medcalc.com/gfr.html

Jadoul, M. (1998). Dialysis-related amyloidosis: Importance of biocompatibility and age. *Nephrology, Dialysis, & Transplantation, 13*(Suppl. 7), 61-64.

Johnson, L.E. (2007). *The Merck manual for healthcare professionals: Vitamin D*. Retrieved July 29, 2007, from http://www.merck.com/mmpe/sec01/ch004/ch004k.html

Kalantar-Zadeh, K., Ikizler, A., Block, G., Avram, M., & Kopple, J. (2003). Malnutrition-inflammation complex syndrome in dialysis patients: Causes and consequences. *American Journal of Kidney Diseases, 42*, 864-881.

Kozak-Campbell, C., & Hughes, A. (1996). The use of functional consequences theory in acutely confused hospitalize elderly. *Journal of Gerontological Nursing, 22*(1), 27-36.

Lameire, N., Van Biesen, W., & Vanholder, R. (2005). Acute renal failure. *The Lancet, 365*(9457), 417-430.

Levey, A.S., Greene, T., Kusek, J.W., Beck, G.L., & MDRD Study Group. (2000). A simplified equation to predict glomerular filtration rate from serum creatinine (abstract). *Journal of the American Society of Nephrology, 11*, 155A.

Lok, C., Oliver, M., Su, J., Bhola, C., Hannigan, N., & Jassal, S. (2005). Arteriovenous fistula outcomes in the era of the elderly dialysis population. *Kidney International, 67*(6), 2462-2469.

Maddox, D.A., Alavi, F.K., & Zawada, E.T. Jr. (2001). The kidney and aging. In S. Massry & R. Glassock (Eds.), *Textbook of nephrology* (4th ed., pp. 1094-1105). Philadelphia: Lippincott Williams & Wilkins.

Mallick, N., & Marasi, A.E. (1999). Dialysis in the elderly, to treat or not to treat? *Nephrology, Dialysis, Transplantation, 14*, 37-39.

Mandal, A.K., Baig, M., & Koutoubi, Z. (1996). Management of acute renal failure in the elderly. *Drug and Aging, 9*(4), 226-250.

Mathers, T. (1999). Effects of psychosocial education on adaptation in elderly hemodialysis patients. *ANNA Journal, 26*(6), 587-596.

Mathers, T. (2006). The older adult with chronic kidney disease. In A.E. Molzahn & E. Butera (Eds.), *Contemporary nephrology nursing: Principles and practice* (2nd ed., pp. 501-525). Pitman, NJ: American Nephrology Nurses' Association.

Mayo Clinic. (2006). *Testosterone therapy: The answer for aging men*. Retrieved July 29, 2007, from http://www.mayoclinic.com/health/testosterone-therapy/MC00030

Mayo Reference Services. (2002). *Mayo Clinic communiqué: The laboratory diagnosis and monitoring of amyloidosis*. Rochester, MN: Author.

McCann, L. (1997). *Pocket guide to nutrition assessment of the renal patient* (2nd ed., pp. 9, 12-15). New York: National Kidney Foundation.

Medline Plus Medical Encyclopedia. (2007). *Athroembolic renal disease*. Retrieved May 30, 2007, from http://www.nlm.nih.gov/medlineplus/ency/article/000480.htm

Merck & Co., Inc. (2005a). *The Merck manual for healthcare professionals: Acute tubular necrosis (ATN)*. Retrieved May 15, 2007, from http://www.merck.com/mmpe/sec17/ch236/ch236b.html

Merck & Co., Inc. (2005b). *Merck manual of geriatrics: Infectious disease – Aging and the immune system*. Retrieved July 29, 2007, from http://www.merck.com/mrkshared/mmg/sec16/ch131/ch131c.jsp

Metropolitan Life (MetLife) Insurance Company. (2005a). *Mature Market Institute, demographic profile, the baby boomers*. New York: Author.

Metropolitan Life (MetLife) Insurance Company. (2005b). *Mature Market Institute, demographic profile, the pre-retiree population*. New York: Author.

Miller, P.E., Towani, A., Luscy, P., Deierhoi, M.H., Bailey, R., Redden, D.T., et al. (1998). Predictors of adequacy of arteriovenous fistulas in hemodialysis patients. *Kidney International, 56*, 275-280.

Morgan, B. (1990). The relationship between chronological age and perceived quality of life of hemodialysis patients. *ANNA Journal, 17*(1), 63-70.

..onal Institute of Diabetes and Digestive and Kidney Diseases (NIDDK). (2003). *Amyloidosis and kidney disease.* Retrieved June 30, 2006, from http://www.kidney.niddk.nih.gov/ku diseases/pubs/amyloidosis

National Kidney Foundation (NKF). (1995). *KDOQI guidelines: Evaluation, stratification, and classification.* Retrieved February 9, 2006, from http://www.kidney.org

National Kidney Foundation (NKF). (1997). *KDOQI clinical practice guidelines for vascular access.* Retrieved February 9, 2006, from http://www.kidney.org

National Kidney Foundation (NKF). (2000). *KDOQI clinical practice guidelines for nutrition in chronic renal failure.* Retrieved June 30, 2006, from http://www.kidney.org/ Professionals/kdoqi/guidelines_updates/doqi_nut.html

National Kidney Foundation (NKF). (2003a). *KDOQI clinical practice guidelines for bone metabolism and disease in chronic kidney disease.* Retrieved June 30, 2006, from http://www. kidney.org/professionals/kdoqi/guidelines_bone/index.htm

National Kidney Foundation (NKF). (2003b). *KDOQI clinical practice guidelines for managing dyslipidemias in chronic kidney disease: Part 3, guideline 4.* Retrieved June 30, 2006, from http://www.kidney.org/professionals/kdoqi/guidelines_lipids/ iii.htm

Needham, E. (2005). Management of acute renal failure, *American Family Physician, 72*(9), 1739-1746.

Nurse Competence in Aging. (2005). *Geriatric resources for care of older adults.* Retrieved July 29, 2007, from http://www .geronurseonline.org

Parker, J.F., Wingard, R.L., Husni, L., Ikizler, A.T., Parker, R.A., & Hakim, R.M. (1995). Effect of the membrane biocompatibility on nutritional parameters in chronic hemodialysis patients. *Kidney International, 49,* 551-556.

Pascual, J., Liano, F., & Nefrologia, S. (1995). The elderly patient with acute renal failure. *Journal of the American Society of Nephrology, 6*(2), 144-149.

Petroff, S. (2005). Evaluating traditional iron measures and exploring new options for patients on hemodialysis. *Nephrology Nursing Journal, 32*(1), 65-76.

Pfizer, Inc. (2000). *New facts about: Pharmacological management in older adults.* Retrieved July 29, 2007 from http://www.pfizer. com

Pianta, T., & Kutner, N.G. (1999). Improving physical functioning in the elderlydialysis patient: Relevance of physical therapy. *ANNA Journal, 26*(1), 11-16.

Plawecki, H., & Brewer, S. (1986). The elderly hemodialysis patient. *ANNA Journal, 13*(3), 146-149.

Ponticelli, C. (2000). Should renal transplantation be offered to older patients? *Nephrology, Dialysis, & Transplantation, 15*(3), 315-317.

Renal Physicians Association (RPA) and American Society of Nephrology (ASN). (2002). *Shared decision making in the appropriate initiation and withdrawal from dialysis: Clinical practice guidelines.* Washington, DC: Author.

Richbourg, M.J. (1997). Vision screening in older adults on dialysis: Do nephrology nurses have a role? *ANNA Journal, 24*(5), 541-549.

Schaefer, K., & Rohrich, B. (1999). The dilemma of renal replacement therapy in patients over 80 years of age. *Nephrology, Dialysis, & Transplantation, 14,* 35-36.

Shapiro, W. (1993). Renal replacement therapy in the elderly. In H.R. Jacobson, G.E. Striker, & S. Klahr (Eds.), *The principles and practice of nephrology* (2nd ed., pp. 533-541). St. Louis: Mosby.

Shlipak, M.G., Wassel Fyr, C.L., Chertow, G.M., Harris, T.B., Kritchevsky, S.B., Tylavsky, F.A., et al. (2005). Cystatin C and mortality risk in the elderly: The health, aging, and body composition study. *Journal of the American Society of Nephrology, 17*(1), 254-261.

Snyder, S., & Pendergraph, B. (2005). Detection and evaluation of chronic kidney disease. *American Family physician, 72*(9), 1723-1733.

Stack, A.G., & Messana, J.M. (2000). Renal replacement therapy in the elderly: Medical, ethical, and psychosocial considerations. *Advances in Renal Replacement Therapy, 7*(1), 52-62.

Stanford University Medical Center. (2007). *Renal vascular disease.* Retrieved May 9, 2007, from http://www.stanford hospital.com/clinicsmedServices/COE/surgicalServices/ vascularSurgery/patientEducation/renalvd

United States Renal Data System (USRDS). (2004). *USRDS 2004 annual data report.* Retrieved February 9, 2007, from http://www.usrds.org/adr_2004.htm

United States Renal Data System (USRDS). (2006). *USRDS 2006 annual data report.* Retrieved July 25, 2007, from http://www.usrds.org/adr_2006.htm

Wade-Elliott, R. (1999). Caring for the elderly with renal failure: Gastrointestinal changes. *ANNA Journal, 26*(6), 563-571.

Weil, C.M. (2000). Exploring hope in patients with end stage renal disease on chronic hemodialysis. *Nephrology Nursing Journal, 27*(2), 219-224.

Whittaker, A., & Albee, B. (1996). Factors influencing patient selection of dialysis treatment modality. *ANNA Journal, 23*(4), 369-377.

Wikipedia. (2007). *Dehydration, the signs and symptoms.* Retrieved February 9, 2007, from http://www.wikipedia.org/ wiki/Dehydration#Symptoms_and_prognosis

Youngerman-Cole, S. (2006). *Healthwise: Influenza.* Retrieved July 29, 2007, from http://www.suttersantarosa.org/health/ healthinfo/?A=C&type=info&hwid=hw122012&section=hw 122014

Section 17

Infection Control

Section Editor

Karen C. Wiseman, MSN, RN, CNN

Chapter Authors

Matthew J. Arduino, MS, DrPH

Emily Arnold, BSN, RN, CNN, CPHQ

Billie Axley, BSN, RN, CNN

Evelyn Butera, MS, RN, CNN

Geraldine Curry, BSN, RN, CNN, CPHQ

Eileen J. Peacock, MSN, RN, CNN, CIC, CPHQ

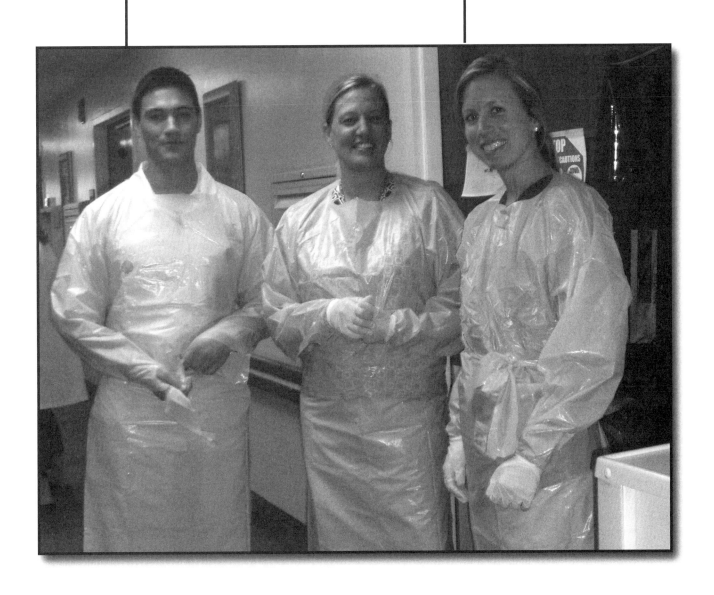

About the Authors

Karen C. Wiseman, MSN, RN, CNN, Section Editor, is Director of Policy and Regulatory Affairs at Renal Advantage, Inc., in Brentwood, Tennessee.

Matthew J. Arduino, DrPH, MS, is Lead Microbiologist at the Centers for Disease Control and Prevention in Atlanta, Georgia.

Emily Arnold, BSN, RN, CNN, CPHQ, is Post-Kidney Transplant Coordinator at UNC Hospitals, University of North Carolina, in Chapel Hill, North Carolina.

Billie Axley, BSN, RN, CNN, is Director of Quality Initiatives at Fresenius-North America (FMC-NA) in Nashville, Tennessee.

Evelyn Butera, MS, RN, CNN, is an Education/QI Specialist at Mills-Pennisula Health Services, A Sutter-Health Affiliate, in Burlingame, California.

Geraldine Curry, BSN, RN, CNN, CPHQ, is Corporate Clinical Quality Manager at Fresenius-North America (FMC-NA) in Lexington, Massachusetts.

Eileen J. Peacock, MSN, RN, CNN, CIC, CPHQ, is a Research Assistant at DaVita, Inc., in Berwyn, Pennsylvania.

The findings and conclusions in this section are those of the authors and do not necessarily represent the views of the Centers for Disease Control and Prevention or the Agency for Toxic Substances and Disease Registry.

Infection Control

Infection Control

Purpose

The purpose of this section is to provide a cognitive understanding of current concepts in infectious diseases and their implications for practice in hemodialysis centers.

Objectives

Upon completion of this section, the learner will be able to:

1. Describe the difference between exposure to tuberculosis and active disease.
2. Outline current recommendations for immunizations in patients with chronic kidney disease.
3. List the methods that decrease the risk of infections in the vascular access.
4. Identify how contamination of the delivery system fluid pathway can contribute to patient infections.
5. Explain how hepatitis B, hepatitis C, hepatitis D, and HIV are spread in the dialysis unit.
6. Describe infection control measures that should be taken with any dialysis patient.
7. List the factors that contribute to development of drug resistance.
8. Discuss the specific infection control requirements for a patient with hepatitis B.
9. Describe why persons with chronic kidney failure are predisposed to development of active tuberculosis after exposure to the bacterium.
10. List the ways that dialyzer reprocessing can contribute to bacteremia.
11. Describe how a recommendation promulgated by a professional organization may be formally adopted as a regulation.
12. Define how the CQI process may be used to address infection control issues in the dialysis unit.
13. List the reasons why patients with HIV do not require special isolation or infection control procedures.
14. Discuss the unique characteristics of the tuberculosis bacterium that make it more difficult to diagnose and treat.
15. Describe the infection control measures to be used with a patient with hepatitis delta virus (HDV).

Chapter 69

Infection Control

Overview

I.   Patients with chronic kidney disease, stage 5, are at risk of infection for a number of reasons.

A.   Impaired immune function.

B.   Presence of a vascular access to perform kidney replacement therapy.

C.   Presence of one or more additional chronic illnesses.

D.   Frequent hospitalizations, surgeries, and/or medical procedures.

E.   Provision of care in a setting where multiple patients are treated at the same time by multiple caregivers.

F.   Use of immunosuppressive medications.

II. In patients with chronic kidney disease, stage 5, infections are the second most common cause of death. A large number of hospitalizations of dialysis patients and transplant patients are due to infections.

III. In healthy individuals, inflammation is a protective mechanism that assists in removing the antigen and facilitates the healing process. Patients with CKD are known to have ongoing, micro-inflammation. Inflammation in patients with CKD is due to multiple factors.

A.   Infection.

B.   Use of bioincompatible dialyzer membranes.

C.   Backfiltration of nonsterile dialysate during the hemodialysis treatment.

D.   Periodontal disease.

E.   Ongoing uremic environment.

F.   Malnutrition.

G.   Hemolysis.

H.   Surgery.

IV. When inflammation becomes excessive or continuous, inflammatory processes no longer contribute to healing. Growth factors are inhibited and wound healing cells do not function normally. Healing is impaired and a vicious cycle of ongoing injury begins. Ongoing inflammation leads to:

A.   Loss of muscle mass and hypoalbuminemia.

B.   Cardiovascular disease.

C.   Erythropoietin resistance.

V.   Recent studies imply that cardiovascular events (such as myocardial infarction and congestive heart failure) may be influenced by infections because of increased inflammatory mediators that accompany the infections.

Bacteremia

I.   Risk factors.

A.   Kidney failure and bacteremia risk factors include:
1.   Chronic hemodialysis requiring vascular access for prolonged periods.
2.   The hemodialysis environment, which provides opportunities for transmission of infectious agents.
3.   Patients with kidney failure have higher incidence of blood stream infections (bacteremia).
   a.   Altered immune response due to kidney failure.
   b.   Impaired neutrophil function.
   c.   Frequent hospitalizations.
4.   Patient factors.
   a.   Extremes of age; older adults at greatest risk.
   b.   Chronic health problems.
      (1) Diabetes mellitus.
      (2) Disorders of the kidney.
      (3) Malnutrition.
      (4) Debilitation.
      (5) Splenectomy.
      (6) Wounds.
   c.   Immunosuppression due to:
      (1) Suppressed inflammatory response.
      (2) High level of circulating uremic toxins.
      (3) Abnormal intake of nutrients necessary for white blood cell (WBC) growth and function.
5.   Treatment factors.
   a.   Hospitalization.
   b.   Invasive procedures.
   c.   Instrumentation: artificial devices that penetrate the body.

(1) Frequency of manipulation.

(2) Site of insertion.

(3) Conditions at insertion. Portals of entry by which the infectious agent can enter the human body include disruption of the skin, the body's first line of defense. A susceptible host is one who lacks effective resistance to the infectious agent. Risk factors include:

    (a) Age of host and general health, including comorbidities.

    (b) Nutritional status.

    (c) Absent or abnormal immunoglobulins/ability of hematopoietic system to function.

(4) Skin colonization.

    (a) Number of organisms present at exposure.

    (b) Duration of exposure.

d. Catheters.

(1) Catheter colonization. A significant growth of a microorganism (> 15 colony forming units) from a catheter tip, subcutaneous segment of the catheter, or catheter hub.

(2) Duration of catheterization.

(3) Dialysis catheters are associated with a 7.6-fold increase in the relative risk of bacteremia compared to arteriovenous fistulas.

e. Immunosuppression.

(1) Suppressed inflammatory response.

(2) High level of circulating uremic toxins.

(3) Abnormal intake of nutrients necessary for WBC growth and function.

II. Causes.

A. Pathogenic organisms. Any pathogenic organism can cause bacteremia.

1. Gram-positive bacteria.

    a. Staphylococcus.

        (1) *Staphylococcus aureus.* Considered part of normal human skin flora. Colonization common in anterior nares and moist body areas. *S. aureus* causes a wide variety of infections, ranging from localized (e.g., wound infection) to disseminated disease (e.g., septicemia). Foreign bodies, such as intravascular catheters commonly lead to infection with *S. aureus.*

        (2) *Staphylococcus epidermidis.* Commonly found on skin and mucosal surfaces. This organism is a frequent cause of infection of vascular access devices. Coagulase-negative staphylococci (CNS). Eleven species of this organism, though most infections are caused by *S. epidermidis.* Infection can result from invasion from a person's endogenous strain. Foreign bodies such an intravascular catheters or prosthetic heart valves are predisposed to infection with CNS.

    b. Streptococcus.

        (1) Pneumococcus.

        (2) Enterococcus.

2. Gram-negative bacteria.

    a. *Escherichia coli.*

    b. *Klebsiella pneumonia.*

    c. Serratia.

    d. Enterobacter.

    e. Pseudomonas.

3. Fungi.

4. Viruses.

5. Mycobacteria.

B. Systemic inflammatory response syndrome (SIRS).

1. Widespread, systemic inflammatory response to invading organism(s).

2. SIRS criteria. Presence of two or more of the following:

    a. Temperature alteration.

    b. Heart rate > 90/minute.

    c. Respiratory rate > 20/min.

    d. White blood cell count alteration.

3. Causes of SIRS.

    a. Trauma/tissue injury.

    b. Pancreatitis.

    c. Radiation.

    d. Thermal injury.

    e. Infection.

        (1) Initial insult with microbial toxins.

        (2) Release of inflammatory substances.

C. Sepsis. Infection plus SIRS equals sepsis.

1. Sepsis criteria.

    a. Hypotension (functional hypovolemia).

    b. Hypoperfusion of tissues and organs.

    c. Organ dysfunction.

        (1) Oliguria.

        (2) Mental changes.

        (3) Hyperdynamic state.

            (a) Increased cardiac output.

            (b) Peripheral vasodilatation.

            (c) Decreased systemic vascular response (SVR).

2. Sepsis is a systemic response to infection, resulting in:

    a. Damage to the vascular endothelium.

    b. Microcapillary leakage occurs toward the third space.

c. Cardiac dysfunction secondary to toxins and inflammatory mediators; diminished ejection fraction.
3. Increasing incidence of sepsis is due to:
   a. Immunocompromised patients (including those with kidney disease).
   b. Resistant microorganisms.
   c. Increasing elderly population.
   d. Increased awareness of infections and their complications.
   e. Increased use of invasive procedures/lines.
4. Sepsis has been identified as one of the most common causes of death in the intensive care unit (ICU).
5. Mortality due to severe sepsis is approximately 29%.

III. Management of sepsis.

A. Management of sepsis includes:
   1. Eradication of the causative organism.
      a. Empirical intravenous antibiotics.
      b. Adjustment of antibiotics based on culture sensitivity results.
      c. Surgical management of septic source when appropriate.
   2. Hemodynamic support consists of:
      a. Administration of fluids.
      b. Use of vasoactive drugs such as:
         (1) Epinephrine hydrochloride.
         (2) Levophed®.
         (3) Vasopressin.
   3. Respiratory support.
   4. Continuous renal replacement therapy (CRRT).

B. Criteria for septic shock.
   1. Sepsis – the hypodynamic phase, including:
      a. Hypotension despite fluid resuscitation.
      b. Decreased cardiac output.
      c. Peripheral vasoconstriction.
      d. Increased systemic vascular resistance.
      e. Hypoperfusion; tissue hypoxia.
      f. Multiple organ dysfunction results in:
         (1) Oliguria.
         (2) Hepatic failure.
         (3) Mental changes.
         (4) Respiratory failure.
         (5) Disseminated intravascular coagulation (DIC).
   2. Septic shock occurs as result of bacteria and/or toxins released by bacteria circulating in the blood.
      a. Proinflammatory cytokines and other metabolites (prostaglandins) cause an increase in endothelial-derived nitric oxide.
      b. Nitric oxide causes changes in cell wall transport mechanisms. Decreases in intracellular calcium leads to vasodilatation and resistance to vasopressor agents.
      c. A primary cause of the shock is systemic vasoactive mediators released by gram-negative bacteria associated with vasodilatation, affecting almost every physiologic system.
      d. Some vessels (arterioles) remain vasoconstricted due to various inflammatory mediators (e.g., tumor necrosis factor) leading to maldistribution of blood flow.
      e. These processes affect all physiologic systems of the body.
      f. The incidence of septic shock approaches 500,000 cases annually.

IV. Interpretation of lab results.

A. Interpretation/evaluation of culture and sensitivity, CBC with differential.
   1. Identify causative agent.
      a. Using microscopy, bacterial growth is identified and classified by shape and size.
      b. Organisms are identified as gram-positive or gram-negative.
      c. Shape of organism is determined – rods vs. cocci.
   2. Organism identification by isolation from culture.
      a. Common pathogens such as Staphylococci, Streptococci, and Enterococci can be identified within 48 hours.
      b. Fungal organisms may take 10–14 days for identification.
      c. Viruses often take 2–3 weeks to grow in culture.
   3. Sensitivity reports are obtained on the isolates, based on:
      a. Minimum inhibitory concentration that will inhibit growth of an organism.
      b. Agar diffusion tests reported as resistant if growth is not altered. Reported as sensitive if growth is inhibited.
   4. White blood cell count.
      a. Provides important information concerning the inflammatory response of the patient, as well as the response to therapy.
      b. Total number of circulating leukocytes and the differential change during bacterial or viral infection.
      c. Acute bacterial infection causes a rise in the white blood cell neutrophils and increased bands (immature neutrophils).

B. When to report to physician or advanced practice nurse (APN).
   1. Consider populations at risk.
      a. Previous antibiotic therapy.
      b. Underlying chronic disease such as diabetes and kidney disease.
      c. Decreased immunity.
      d. Central venous catheter use.
      e. Over 65 years of age.
      f. Extended length of stay in health care facilities.
   2. Blood cultures.
      a. Avoid administration of antibiotics for organisms that may not be the causative agent of the infection. For example, if a single blood culture is positive for CNS and other blood cultures are negative, consider the possibility that the culture was contaminated with skin flora (*S. epidermidis*).
      b. Notify patient care providers regarding presumptive identification of Vancomycin-resistant enterococci (VRE) for implementation of appropriate isolation precautions. Vancomycin resistance is confirmed by repeating antimicrobial susceptibility testing. *Note*: Stool or rectal swab screening can detect presence of VRE due to VRE intestinal colonization prior to clinical identification.
   3. Causative agent.
      a. Organism is identified by isolation from culture.
      b. Sensitivity reports are obtained on the isolates.
   4. Complete blood count (CBC) provides:
      a. White blood cell count (WBC).
         (1) Total number of circulating leukocytes.
         (2) Differential.
      b. Red blood cell count (RBC): hematocrit/hemoglobin levels.
      c. Platelets: presence of thrombocytopenia.

Drug Resistance

I. Causes of drug resistance.

A. Repeated antibiotic therapy.

B. Misuse of antibiotics.
   1. Antibiotics should not be taken for viral infections such as a cold or flu.
   2. Antibiotics are not effective against viruses.
   3. Normal flora can be killed, allowing the multiplication of resistant bacteria.
   4. Proper collection and handling of specimens is imperative for the causative organism to be correctly identified.
      a. Avoid potential contamination of the specimen. Aseptic technique is mandatory to avoid contaminating the specimen with organisms that colonize the skin or are present on the central venous catheter hub or port.
      b. For blood cultures, specimens obtained by venipuncture are preferred over sampling from vascular catheters. Cultures drawn from central venous catheters may reflect organisms that have colonized the catheter and may not accurately reflect organisms freely circulating in the patient's blood stream.
      c. Evaluate results drawn from central venous catheters carefully. If bacterial growth is present only in the sample obtained from the central venous catheter and not from peripheral cultures, the bacteria from the central venous catheter may not be the cause of the infection and may not require treatment with antibiotics.
      d. CDC recommends treatment only for demonstrated bacteremia, and not for results obtained from catheter tips.
      e. Follow current CDC guidelines for Vancomycin use. Consider use of first generation cephalosporins when indicated.

C. Nonadherence with the prescribed treatment regimen.
   1. Failure to follow the instructions for when and how much medicine should be taken.
   2. As the person feels better may stop taking the medication before the full medication course is completed.
   3. Bacteria that have not been killed survive and develop resistance to the antibiotic.

D. Multiple-drug resistant bacteria can spread from:
   1. Person to person.
   2. Contaminated environmental surfaces/objects.
   3. Unwashed hands.

II. Methods to decrease development of antibiotic resistance.

A. Prudent use of antibiotics.

B. Patient education.
   1. When and how much medication to be taken.

2. Take all medication prescribed. Do not stop medication early.
3. Do not take medication prescribed for someone else.
4. Do not share medications with others.
5. Do not take old or outdated medication.
6. Avoid close contact when sick with a fever:
   a. Cover mouth and nose when sneezing and/or coughing.
   b. Wash hands often.
7. Be involved with own care and take an active role in decisions.
8. Remind health care team members to wash their hands.
9. If diabetic, perform regular foot checks.
10. Follow procedure for cleaning access before every cannulation.
11. Ask health care team about when to wear masks or gloves.
12. Patient and family education on hand washing and environmental cleaning at home. Additional education for patients who require wound dressing changes and/or have invasive devices such as catheters.

C. Hand hygiene. CDC continues to emphasize use of appropriate hand hygiene.
   1. Frequent hand washing.
   2. Use of waterless hand antiseptics may be appropriate if hands are not visibly soiled.
   3. It is important to set an example for proper hand hygiene for coworkers.
   4. Partner with patients to educate them on access care and infection control measures they can take. Regular and consistent patient education is critical.

D. Environmental cleaning and disinfection.
   1. Environmental cleaning with approved disinfectant.
   2. Disinfection of patient equipment.
      a. Use patient-specific equipment when possible.
      b. Adequate cleaning and disinfection of reusable equipment between patients following facility procedures.

III. Infection control precautions.

A. Isolation. Maintain isolation precautions as appropriate for infection.
   1. Patients with MRSA or VRE who do not have any uncontrolled drainage may be treated in the facility using standard and dialysis precautions defined by CDC.
   2. Patients with infective material that cannot be contained (e.g., wound drainage that is not contained by a dressing, or an incontinent patient with positive stool cultures and diarrhea that cannot be contained by adult briefs) should be treated using contact and dialysis precautions defined by CDC.
      a. Infected patients with positive cultures for VRE or MRSA whose drainage cannot be contained should be placed in a designated isolation room or area of the facility that has ready access to handwashing equipment.
      b. Infected patients may be placed in the same area as other patients with the same bacteria and antibiotic resistance (cohorted).
   3. When transferring a patient to another outpatient facility or hospital, notification of the resistant bacteria is important so appropriate precautions can be implemented.

B. Personal protective equipment (PPE).
   1. Use according to facility's infection control policies and procedures.
   2. Follow Centers for Disease Control and Prevention (CDC) recommendations and Occupational Safety and Health Administration (OSHA) standard precautions when coming into contact with any body fluids.
   3. When caring for a patient with antibiotic-resistant bacteria, a frequent change of gloves might be necessary after contact with material that could contain high concentrations of organisms (e.g., stool, wound drainage). Avoid cross-contamination via contaminated gloves (i.e., transfer of infectious material from dirty gloves to the patient or environmental surfaces).

IV. Colonization vs. infection.

A. Colonization: bacteria requires surface on which to attach.
   1. Prosthetic devices or materials can become colonized.
   2. Bacterial biofilm can form within 24 hours.
   3. Biofilm protects bacteria, allowing bacteria to grow, divide, and multiply.
      a. Resistance to antimicrobial agents is an important feature of biofilm.
      b. Biofilm is difficult to eliminate.
   4. Patient does not exhibit signs/symptoms of active infection.
   5. Strict attention to infection control practices must be followed with every patient.

B. Infection: bacterial activity.
1. Signs and symptoms of infection present.
2. Culture of bacteria from source.

V. Common resistant organisms: Gram-positive organisms.

A. Staphylococcus.
1. *Staphylococcus aureus.*
   a. MRSA – Methicillin/oxacillin-resistant *S. aureus.*
   b. CA-MRSA – Community-associated MRSA emerging as significant pathogen among patients without established risk factors for MRSA infection.
2. Common findings.
   a. Skin-to-skin contact.
   b. Compromised skin integrity.
   c. Sharing of contaminated items.
   d. Poor hygiene practices.

B. *S. epidermidis.*
1. MRSE – Methicillin/oxacillin-resistant *S. epidermidis*, coagulase-negative staphylococcus (CNS).
2. May occur after major surgical procedures involving implantation of prosthetic materials or devices (cardiac and vascular procedures).
   a. Total hip replacement.
   b. Valve replacement.

C. Streptococcus.
1. Enterococcus.
   a. VRE – Vancomycin-resistant Enterococci.
   b. Most VRE are also resistant to drugs previously used to treat infections by common disease-causing bacteria (e.g., aminoglycosides and ampicillin).
   c. Patient-to-patient transmission of the microorganisms can occur either through direct or indirect contact via:
      (1) Hands of personnel.
      (2) Contaminated patient-care equipment.
      (3) Contaminated environmental surfaces.
2. Possibility exists that vancomycin-resistant genes present in VRE can be transferred to other gram-positive microorganisms, such as *Staphylococcus aureus.*
   a. VISA – Vancomycin-intermediate *S. aureus.*
   b. VRSA - Vancomycin-resistant *S. aureus.*
   c. Researchers are concerned that *Staphylococcus aureus* may also develop resistance to Vancomycin.
   d. Resistance to vancomycin virtually eliminates

all treatment options for these common disease-causing bacteria.
   e. Decrease in new antibiotic production since 1983.

D. *Clostridium difficile.*
1. Incubation period may be 5 to10 days or 2 to 10 weeks following antibiotic treatment.
   a. Disruption in the normal enteric flora induced by antimicrobials allow *C. difficile* to overgrow and cause disease.
   b. Sudden onset diarrhea by *C. difficile* overgrowth and toxin production produces foul smelling stool containing mucus.
   c. Symptoms may include abdominal pain and distention, nausea, fever.
2. Period of communicability continues until diarrhea subsides.
3. Spread in the clinical environment is thought to be the result of ingestion of bacterial spores.
   a. Spores are stable in the environment for several months on floors, toilets and furniture in areas where patients with *C. difficile* infection have been treated.
   b. Patients with existing *C. difficile* infections are thought to be the main source of infections for other patients.
   c. Enteric precautions include isolation of infected patients, use of PPE, strict hand washing with soap and water, and "deep" cleaning of areas used by patients; restriction of patient movements in facility by treating in designated area are all used to halt spread of the organism.
4. Alcohol-based hand gels/foams not recommended as spores are resistant to alcohol.

VI. Management of patients with drug-resistant organisms.

A. Assessment of vascular access site.
1. Signs of a healthy vascular access.
   a. Surrounding skin with natural appearance.
   b. No drainage, redness, swelling, or crusting.
2. Signs of access site infection.
   a. Redness.
   b. Warmth.
   c. Swelling.
   d. Pain/tenderness.
   e. Purulent exudate.

B. Locate the source of the infection and remove source (when possible).

C. Treat the infection by initiating antibiotic therapy.
   1. Appropriate for the organism.
   2. Begin as early as possible.

D. Prevent the infection.
   1. Consistent hand washing/hand cleansing.
   2. Carefully monitor immunosuppressed patients for signs/symptoms of infection.
   3. Practice vigilant infection control.
   4. Assessment of adherence.
   5. Five most frequently cited reasons for nonadherence with therapy.
      a. Dissatisfaction with regimen.
      b. Improvement noticed prior to beginning the medication, so initiation of therapy was delayed.
      c. Improvement in symptoms after completing only part of the drug regimen.
      d. Forgetfulness in taking medications.
      e. Unwanted side effects.

E. Outbreak management.
   1. Notify identified infection control professional immediately if outbreak of resistant bacteria is suspected.
   2. Resources for developing a plan regarding the admission and discharge of patients with resolving infections and/or colonized with antimicrobial-resistant microorganisms may include local and state health departments.

Hepatitis B Virus (HBV)

I. Incidence and prevalence.

A. In the United States, approximately 1.2 million persons have chronic hepatitis B infection.

B. During 1990–2002, the incidence of reported acute hepatitis B infection in the United States declined 67%. Decline was greatest among children and adolescents indicating effective immunization practices (see Figure 17.1).

C. Risk of hepatitis B infection is 100 times that of HIV infection after a contaminated needlestick.

D. Chronically infected persons are central to the epidemiology of HBV transmission.

II. Characteristics and markers (see Figure 17.2).

A. DNA virus and member of the family Hepadnoviridae.

B. Virus has an outer covering consisting of a lipoprotein known as the surface antigen (HBsAg). Presence in the blood indicates a current infection and transmissibility.

C. Hepatitis E antigen (HBeAg) is part of the interior core antigen or HBcAG. It appears simultaneously with the HBsAg and denotes viral replication. It is thought to indicate a highly contagious state. The antibody to HBeAg indicates low viral replication, but does not confer immunity.

D. Interior core antigen (HBcAG) detected in liver tissue but not in serum. Antibodies to the core antigen (anti-HBc) appear together in the IgM class (anti-HBc-IgM), during acute hepatitis B, and the IgG class (anti-HBc-IgG), during convalescence or chronic infection. The anti-HBc does not confer immunity.

E. HBV surface antibodies (anti-HBs) appear 2 to 3 months after the onset of symptoms. Confers immunity and convalescence.

F. Many subtypes of HBV exist. Immunization or infection with one subtype provides immunity to all subtypes.

G. Vaccination is available and has been recommended for hemodialysis staff and patients since it became available in 1982.

III. Transmission. HBV is the microbe that is most efficiently transmitted in the dialysis setting.

A. Percutaneous (i.e., puncture through the skin) or permucosal (i.e., direct contact with mucous membranes) exposure to infectious blood or to body fluids that contain blood.

B. Chronically infected patients are central to the epidemiology of HBV transmission in dialysis centers. All HBsAg-positive patients are infectious and able to transmit the virus.

C. Health care workers with acute or chronic hepatitis rarely infect patients. They may continue to work when infection control measures are followed.

D. Family members of persons with acute hepatitis or chronic carriers are considered at risk.

E. HBV can be present on environmental surfaces in the absence of any visible blood and still result in transmission.

F. Virus is stable in the environment and remains viable for at least 7 days on environmental surfaces at room temperature.

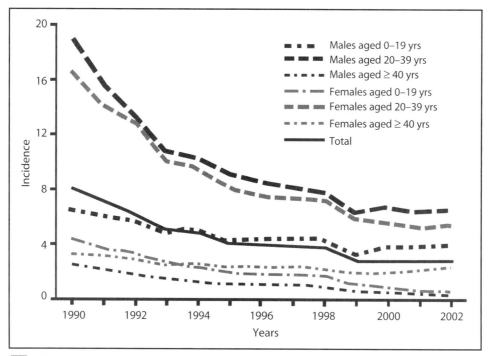

Figure 17.1. Incidence* of acute hepatitis B, by age group, sex, and year – United States, 1990–2002. (* = per 100,000 population)

Source: Centers for Disease Control and Prevention (CDC). (2004a). Incidence of acute hepatitis B – United States, 1990–2002. *MMWR, 52*(51 & 52), 1252-1254.

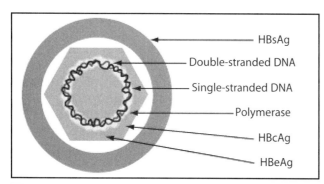

Figure 17.2. Structure of HBV.

Source: Parker, J., Dickenson, L., Wiseman, K.C., Alexander, D., & Peacock, E. (1998). Control of infectious diseases in the renal patient. In J. Parker (Ed.), *Contemporary nephrology nursing* (1st ed., p. 354). Pitman, NJ: American Nephrology Nurses' Asssociation. Used with permission.

G. Blood-contaminated surfaces that are not routinely cleaned and disinfected represent a reservoir for HBV transmission.

H. Detected in dialysis centers on clamps, scissors, dialysis machine control knobs, and doorknobs.

I. Outbreaks of HBV infection among hemodialysis patients have been caused by cross-contamination to patients via:

1. Environmental surfaces, supplies (e.g., hemostats, clamps).

2. Equipment not routinely disinfected after each use.
3. Multiple dose medication vials and intravenous solutions not used exclusively for one patient.
4. Medications for injection prepared in areas adjacent to areas where blood samples were handled.
5. Staff members who simultaneously cared for both HBV-infected and susceptible patients.

IV. Clinical features and disease outcomes.

A. Causes both acute and chronic hepatitis.

B. Incubation period 45 to 160 days.

C. Immunosuppressed adults with newly acquired infection are usually asymptomatic.

D. Clinical symptoms often insidious and include:
   1. Anorexia.
   2. Malaise.
   3. Nausea.
   4. Vomiting.
   5. Abdominal pain.
   6. Jaundice.

E. 94% to 98% of adults with normal immune status recover completely eliminating virus from the

Table 17.1

Schedule for Routine Testing for Hepatitis B Virus (HBV) and Heptatitis C Virus (HCV) Infections

Patient Status	On Admission	Monthly	Semiannual	Annual
All patients	HBsAg*			
	Anti-HBc* (total)			
	Anti-HBs*			
	Anti-HGCV, ALT**			
HBV-susceptible, including nonresponders to vaccine		HBsAg		
Anti-HBs positive (> 10 mLU/mL), anti-HBc negative				Anti-HBs
Anti-HBs and anti-HBc positive		No additional HBV testing needed		
Anti-HCV negative		ALT	Anti-HCV	
*Results of HBV testing should be known before the patient begins dialysis.				
**HBsAg = hepatitis B surface antigen; Anti-HBc = antibody to hepatitis B core antigen; Anti-HBs = antibody to hepatitis B surface antigen; Anti-HCV = antibody to hepatitis C virus; ALT = alanine aminotransferase.				

Source: Centers for Disease Control and Prevention (CDC). (2001b). Recommendations for preventing transmission of infections among chronic hemodialysis patients. *MMWR, 50*(RR05), 1-43 (Available from http://www.cdc.gov/mmwr/preview/mmwrhtml/rr5005a1.htm).

blood. They then have life time immunity from future infection.

F. Most newly acquired HBV infections in hemodialysis patients result in chronic infection and serve as ongoing source of HBV transmission.

G. Liver disease develops in two thirds of chronic carriers. Approximately 15% to 25% die prematurely from cirrhosis or liver cancer.

V. Screening and vaccination of staff.

A. Screening for HBV infection among staff is no longer considered necessary.

B. Testing for HBV markers not recommended except when required to document response to vaccination.

C. Hepatitis B vaccination recommended for all susceptible staff. Recombinant vaccines available in the United States are Recombivax HB® and Engerix-B®.

D. Test all vaccinated staff for anti-HBs 1 to 2 months after last primary vaccine series.

E. Nonresponders should receive a second series of the HBV vaccine and be retested for response. No additional doses are warranted for those who do not respond.

F. Staff not responding to the second full series of the HBV vaccine should be evaluated for HBsAg positivity and follow-up with medical evaluation and counseling.

VI. Screening and vaccination of patients.

A. Routine serologic testing (see Table 17.1).
  1. Routine serologic testing for markers of HBV infection and prompt review of the result is vital to the prevention of HBV transmission. Patients should be screened prior to or at entry to the dialysis facility (see Tables 17.2 and 17.3).
      a. HBsAg.
      b. HBsAB or Anti-HBs.
      c. Anti-HBc (total).
  2. Hepatitis B vaccination recommended for all susceptible patients.

Table 17.2

Interpretation of Serologic Test Results for Hepatitis B Virus Infection

Serologic Markers				Interpretation
HBsAg*	Total Anti-HBc[†]	IgM[§] Anti-HBc	Anti-HBs[¶]	
–	–	–	–	Susceptible, never infected
+	–	–	–	Acute infection, early incubation**
+	+	+	–	Acute infection
–	+	+	–	Acute resolving infection
–	+	–	–	Past infection, recovered and immune
+	+	–	–	Chronic infection
–	+	–	–	False positive (i.e., susceptible), past infection, or "low-level" chronic infection
–	–	–	+	Immune if titer is ≥ 10 mLU/mL

* Hepatitis B surface antigen.

[†] Antibody to hepatitis B core antigen.

[§] Immunoglobulin M.

[¶] Antibody to hepatitis B surface antigen.

** Transient HBsAg positivity (lasting ≤ 18 days) might be detected in some patients during vaccination.

Source: Centers for Disease Control and Prevention (CDC). (2001b). Recommendations for preventing transmission of infections among chronic hemodialysis patients. *MMWR, 50*(RR05), 1-43 (Available from http://www.cdc.gov/mmwr/preview/mmwrhtml/rr5005a1.htm).

B. HBV-susceptible patients (negative HBsAg and HBsAB or Anti-HBs, Anti-HBc).
  1. Vaccinate all susceptible patients with a full series of the HBV vaccine.
    a. Test for anti-HBs 1 to 2 months after last dose.
    b. If anti-HBs is < 10 mIU/mL or at a level considered susceptible, revaccinate with an additional vaccine series and retest for anti-HBs. No additional doses are warranted for those who do not respond. Consider the patient susceptible and test for HBsAg monthly.
  2. If anti-HBs is ≥ 10 mIU/mL or at a level considered as protective, consider patient immune and retest annually for antibodies.
    a. Administer booster dose if anti-HBs declines to < 10 mIU/mL or is at a level considered susceptible and continue to test annually for antibodies.
    b. Test susceptible patients monthly for HBsAg, including those who:
      (1) Have not yet received hepatitis B vaccine.
      (2) Are in the process of being vaccinated.
      (3) Have not adequately responded to vaccination.

C. HBV-immune patients.
  1. Annual anti-HBs testing of patients who are positive for anti-HBs (>10 mIU/mL, or reported as protective by the lab performing the test) and negative for anti-HBc, determines the need for booster doses of vaccine. These patients have vaccine induced immunity and may be susceptible when antibodies drop below 10 mIU/mL.
  Note: A number of new assays for hepatitis B testing have recently been licensed by the Food and Drug Administration. Many of these new assays quantify and report hepatitis results in a different manner than previous assays. CDC is aware and is in the process of developing revised guidelines. In the interim, the lab performing the testing will provide instructions for the evaluation and interpretation of hepatitis test results, based on the specific assay used by the lab.
  2. No routine follow-up testing for patients who are positive for both anti-HBs and anti-HBc. These patients have life-long immunity from a past infection and do not need to be vaccinated.

Table 17.3

Doses and Schedules of Licensed Hepatitis B Vaccines for Hemodialysis Patients and Staff Members

Group	Recombivax HB™ *			Engerix-B®		
	Dose	Volume	Schedule	Dose	Volume	Schedule
Patients aged ≥ 20 years						
Predialysis	10µg	1.0 mL	0, 1, and 6 months	20 µg	1.0 mL	0, 1, and 6 months
Dialysis-dependent	40 µg	1.0 mL	0, 1, and 6 months	40 µg	2-1.0 mL doses at one site	0, 1, 2, and 6 months
Patients aged < 20 years**	5 µg	0.5 mL	0, 1, and 6 months	10 µg	0.5 mL	0, 1, and 6 months
Staff members aged ≥ 20 years	10 µg	1.0 mL	0, 1, and 6 months	20 µg	1.0 mL	0, 1, and 6 months

* Merck & Company, Inc., West Point, Pennsylvania.
SmithKline Beecham Biologicals, Philadelphia, Pennsylvania.
Immunogenicity might depend on degree of renal insufficiency.
Special formulation.
** Doses for all persons aged > 20 years approved by the U.S. Food and Drug Administration; for hemodialysis.
Note: All doses should be administered in the deltoid by the intramuscular route.

Centers for Disease Control and Prevention (CDC). (2001b). Recommendations for preventing transmission of infections among chronic hemodialysis patients. *MMWR, 50*(RR05), 1-43 (Available from http://www.cdc.gov/mmwr/preview/mmwrhtml/rr5005a1.htm).

D. HBV-infected patients are able to transmit the virus and require additional precautions to prevent transmission.
1. Chronically infected patients (i.e., those who are HBsAg positive, total anti-HBc positive, and IgM anti-HBc negative) do not require additional HBV testing.
2. A positive HBsAg test result may be the only serologic marker initially detected in patients newly infected.
a. Repeat HBsAg testing and test for anti-HBc (including IgM anti-HBc) 1 to 2 months later.
b. Repeat HBsAg testing and test for anti-HBs 6 months later to determine clinical outcome and need for counseling, medical evaluation, and vaccination of contacts.
3. Patients who become HBsAg negative are no longer infectious.

E. Isolated Anti-HBc positive patients.
1. Patients who test positive for isolated anti-HBc

(i.e., those who are anti-HBc positive, HBsAg negative, and anti-HBs negative) should be retested for total anti-HBc, and if positive, for IgM anti-HBc.
2. If total anti-HBc is negative, the patient is considered susceptible and should be provided vaccination.
3. If total anti-HBc is positive and IgM anti-HBc is negative, follow recommendations for vaccination.
a. If anti-HBs is <10 mIU/mL even after revaccination, test for HBV DNA. If HBV DNA is negative, consider patient susceptible and test monthly for HBsAg.
b. If HBV DNA is positive, consider patient as having past infection or "low-level" chronic infection. No further testing is necessary and isolation is not necessary because HBsAg is not detectable.
c. If both total and IgM anti-HBc are positive, consider patient recently infected and test for anti-HBs in 4 to 6 months. No further routine

testing is necessary and isolation is not necessary because HBsAg is not detectable.

F. Transient HBsAg positivity lasting 18 days or less has been reported during the time the patient is receiving the vaccination series.

VII. Precautions for dialysis.

A. Preventing transmission of HBV from an infected hemodialysis patient requires infection control precautions recommended for all hemodialysis patients, routine serologic testing for markers of HBV infection, and isolation of HBsAg-positive patients during treatment.

B. Incidence of HBV infection is substantially lower in hemodialysis units where HBV infected patients are isolated.

C. Isolation practices have resulted in a 70–80% reduction in the incidence HBV infection.

D. Isolation requires a designated separate room for treatment, a dedicated machine, and dedicated equipment and supplies that will not be used by HBV-susceptible patients.

E. Staff members who are caring for HBsAg-positive patients should not care for susceptible patients at the same time.

F. If a separate room is not possible, HBsAg-positive patients should be separated from HBV-susceptible patients in an area removed from the mainstream of activity and should undergo dialysis on dedicated machines.

G. If a machine that has been used on an HBsAg-positive patient is needed for an HBV-susceptible patient, internal pathways of the machine should be disinfected using conventional protocols. External surfaces should be cleaned using a detergent germicide or a low level disinfectant.

H. HBV-infected patients should not participate in dialyzer reprocessing programs.

Hepatitis C Virus (HCV)

I. Incidence and prevalence.

A. Approximately 170 million people worldwide are infected with HCV.

B. An estimated 4.1 million of U.S. population have been infected; 3.2 million are chronically infected.

C. Number of new infections per year decreased from approximately 240,000 to 26,000 over the past 25 years. Transfusion related infections account for less than one per million units of blood.

D. Most infections are due to illegal intravenous drug use.

E. Approximately 40% to 60% of chronic liver disease is attributable to HCV.

F. There are limited incidence and prevalence data in the chronic hemodialysis population as not all dialysis units perform routine testing.
   1. Prevalence approximately 7.8%.
   2. Incidence approximately 0.34%.

II. Characteristics and markers.

A. Single-stranded RNA virus classified as a separate genus in the Flaviridae family. There are six known genotypes and more than 90 subtypes.

B. Multiple quasispecies may co-exist in a single infected individual. Infection with one genotype or subtype does not protect against reinfection or superinfection with other strains.

C. Different genotypes and subtypes have different geographic distributions. Predominant genotypes in the United States are 1a and 1b.

D. Different genotypes and subtypes are associated with different rates of disease progression, severity, and response to treatment.

E. Hepatitis C antibody (Anti-HCV) tests (enzyme immunoassays [EIAs]) and a supplemental recombinant immunoblot assay (RIBA™) detect anti-HCV in > 97% of infected persons. They do not distinguish between acute, chronic, or resolved infection.

F. Positive anti-HCV can be detected in 80% of patients within 15 weeks after exposure, in > 90% within 5 months, and in > 97% within 6 months.

G. HCV virus (RNA) can be detected in serum within 7 to 14 days after exposure and weeks before onset of ALT elevations.

H. Almost all patients develop a vigorous antibody and cell-mediated immune response that fails to clear the infection but may contribute to liver damage.

I. Anti-HCV usually persists indefinitely and does not confer immunity.

J. A vaccine is not available.

III. Transmission.

A. Most efficiently transmitted by direct percutaneous exposure to infectious blood.

B. Chronically infected person is central to the epidemiology of transmission in dialysis.

C. Number of years on dialysis is major risk factor independently associated with higher rates of HCV infection.

D. Inadequate infection control practices are associated with outbreaks of HCV in dialysis units.
1. Use of common medication carts to prepare and distribute medications at patients' stations.
2. Supply carts moved from one station to another.
3. Sharing of multiple dose medication vials, which were placed at patients' stations on top of hemodialysis machines.
4. Contaminated priming buckets that were not routinely changed or cleaned and disinfected between patients.
5. Machine surfaces not routinely cleaned and disinfected between patients.

IV. Clinical features and disease outcomes.

A. Causes both acute and chronic hepatitis.

B. Incubation period ranges from 14 to 180 days.

C. Those with newly acquired infection are asymptomatic or have a mild clinical illness; often goes unnoticed.

D. Elevated alanine aminotransferase (ALT) often precedes anti-HCV seroconversion. Characteristic feature is fluctuating ALT levels.

E. Most hemodialysis patients with newly acquired HCV infection have elevated serum ALT levels. Aspartate aminotransferase (AST) is a less specific indicator of HCV-related liver disease.

F. Up to 85% of newly infected persons develop chronic infection. Cirrhosis develops in 10% to 20% of persons who have chronic infection and hepatocellular carcinoma in 1% to 5%.

G. Liver failure from chronic hepatitis C is one of the most common causes of liver transplants in the United States.

V. Screening.

A. Routine testing of staff members is not recommended.

B. Routine ALT and anti-HCV testing of patients for monitoring transmission within centers and ensuring appropriate dialysis precautions are being followed.

C. Routine anti-HCV testing should include use of both an EIA test and confirmatory testing with a more specific assay (i.e., RIBA).

D. Use of the RT-PCR for HCV RNA as the primary screening test is not recommended.

E. Test all patients at admission for anti-HCV and ALT levels.
1. In the absence of unexplained ALT elevations, anti-HCV testing every 6 months is recommended for those testing negative for anti-HCV at the time of admission.
2. Repeat anti-HCV testing if unexplained ALT elevations are observed. Consider testing for HCV RNA if unexplained ALT elevations persist in patients who are repeatedly anti-HCV negative.

F. In the event of a seroconversion, review all other patients' routine laboratory test results to identify additional cases. Investigate potential sources for infection to determine if transmission might have occurred within the dialysis unit. Consider additional testing.

G. HCV-positive patients should receive medical evaluation.

VI. Precautions for dialysis.

A. Strict adherence to infection control precautions recommended for all hemodialysis patients.

B. Patients who are anti-HCV positive or HCV RNA positive do not have to be isolated or dialyzed separately on dedicated machines. They can participate in the dialyzer reprocessing programs.

Hepatitis Delta Virus (HDV)

I. Incidence and prevalence.

A. Global pattern of HDV infection generally corresponds to the prevalence of chronic HBV infection.

B. There is a low prevalence of HDV infection in the United States.

C. Rates less than 1% of HBsAg-positive persons in the general population.

D. Rates greater than 10% of HBsAg-positive persons with repeated percutaneous exposures (e.g., injecting drug users).

E. There is limited data on the prevalence among chronic hemodialysis patients.

II. Characteristics and markers.

A. Small circular RNA virus. Replication is defective and therefore cannot propagate in the absence of another virus.

B. Requires simultaneous infection with HBV and replicates only in hepatocytes.

C. HDV and HBV may concurrently infect an individual or superinfect a chronic HBsAg carrier.

D. Serologic course of HDV infection varies depending on whether the virus is acquired as a co-infection with HBV or as a superinfection of a person with chronic HBV infection.

E. Co-infection with HDV and HBV.
   1. Both IgM antibody to HDV (anti-HDV) and IgG anti-HDV are usually detectable during the course of co-infection.
   2. Anti-HDV generally declines to subdetectable levels after the infection resolves and there is no serologic marker that persists to indicate the patient was ever infected.
   3. Hepatitis delta antigen (HDAg) can be detected in serum in only about 25% of patients.

F. Superinfection. High titers of both IgM and IgG anti-HDV are detectable. They persist indefinitely.

G. Only a serologic test that measures total antibody to HDV is commercially available in the United States.

III. Transmission.

A. Only occurs in the presence of hepatitis B infection.

B. Transmitted by blood and blood products; percutaneous (i.e., injecting drug use) and permucosal exposure.

C. Risk factors for infection are similar to those for hepatitis B virus infection.

D. There has been only one reported case of transmission between hemodialysis patients in the United States.

E. Sexual transmission of HDV is less efficient than for HBV.

F. Perinatal HDV transmission is rare.

IV. Clinical features and disease outcomes.

A. Co-infection.
   1. Severe acute disease.
   2. Higher risk of fulminant hepatitis (2–20%) compared with those infected with HBV alone.
   3. Low risk of chronic infection.

B. Superinfection.
   1. Usually develops chronic HDV infection.
   2. Risk of severe chronic liver disease.
   3. Over 60% of patients with chronic HDV will develop cirrhosis.

C. Clinical symptoms.
   1. Anorexia.
   2. Malaise.
   3. Nausea and vomiting.
   4. Abdominal pain.
   5. Jaundice.
   6. Joint pain.

V. Screening.

A. Routine testing of hemodialysis patients is not necessary or recommended.

B. Screen for delta antibody if a patient is known to be infected with HDV, or if evidence exists of transmission of HDV in a dialysis unit.

VI. Precautions for dialysis.

A. Prevention of HBV infection will prevent HDV infection in a person susceptible to HBV.

B. Patients who are known to be infected with HDV should be isolated from all other dialysis patients, especially those who are HBsAg-positive.

Human Immunodeficiency Virus (HIV)

I. Overview.

A. According to national surveillance data, hemodialysis patients with HIV infection have increased from 0.3% in 1985 to 1.5% in 2002. Only 0.4% of these patients are reported to have AIDS.

B. There has been no reported health care-associated patient-to-patient transmission of HIV in U.S. hemodialysis centers. However, there have been cases of patient to health care worker transmissions due to needlestick injuries.

C. Occupational exposure to bloodborne pathogens from needlesticks and other sharps injuries is a problem, and it is often preventable. The Centers for Disease Control and Prevention (CDC) estimates that each year 385,000 needlesticks and other sharps-related injuries are sustained by hospital-based health care personnel. Similar injuries occur in other health care settings, such as nursing homes, clinics, emergency care services, and private homes.

D. Sharps injuries are primarily associated with occupational transmission of hepatitis B virus (HBV), hepatitis C virus (HCV), and human immunodeficiency virus (HIV), but they may be implicated in the transmission of more than 20 other pathogens.

II. General infection control measures.

A. Patients infected with HIV can be dialyzed by either hemodialysis or peritoneal dialysis.

B. Patients who are HIV-positive do not have to be isolated and can participate in a dialyzer reuse program. There is no epidemiologic evidence that dialyzer reuse in the United States has led to either an occupational or health care acquired infection with HIV. There have been a few incidents where someone has been dialyzed with a reprocessed dialyzer belonging to someone else who was HIV+. These events are rare, and to date there have been no reported seroconversions as a result of these medical errors in the United States. In addition, data from the CDC annual surveillance of dialysis-associated diseases does not suggest that reuse is a risk factor for HIV. Follow the AAMI recommended practices for reuse of hemodialyzers.

C. Infection control precautions for all dialysis patients apply. There are no special precautions for patients with HIV or AIDS. There are several reasons why no special precautions are recommended for these patients receiving care in maintenance hemodialysis centers.
   1. HIV is not efficiently transmitted in the dialysis setting.
   2. Standard infection control precautions used for the care of all hemodialysis patients are sufficient

to prevent the transmission of the virus in the dialysis setting.
   3. Transmission from the hemodialysis machine to the patient has not been observed.

D. Screening dialysis patients for HIV is not recommended for infection control purposes since these patients are not treated differently than other dialysis patients. However, patients with risk factors for HIV infection should be tested so that, if infected they can receive proper medical care and counseling on preventing the transmission of the virus.

E. The CDC has revised recommendations concerning the routine testing of certain individuals. The recommendations for HIV testing of adults, adolescents, and pregnant women in health care settings was published in September 2006. These recommendations were published to:
   1. Increase HIV screening of patients, including pregnant women, in health care settings.
   2. Foster earlier detection of HIV infection.
   3. Identify and counsel persons with unrecognized HIV infection and link them to clinical and prevention services.
   4. Further reduce perinatal transmission of HIV in the United States.

F. Per these latest CDC recommendations, diagnostic HIV testing and opt-out HIVscreening should be a part of routine clinical care in all health care settings. They also preserve the patient's option to decline HIV testing and ensure a provider-patient relationship conducive to optimal clinical and preventive care. The recommendations are intended for providers in all health care settings, including hospital emergency departments, urgent-care clinics, inpatient services, sexually transmitted disease clinics, substance abuse treatment clinics, other public health clinics, community clinics, correctional health care facilities and primary care settings. The guidelines address HIV testing in health care settings only. They do not modify existing guidelines concerning HIV counseling, testing, and referral for persons at high risk for HIV who seek or receive HIV testing in nonclinical settings.

G. The other population addressed by these recommendations is pregnant women. These guidelines reiterate the recommendation for universal HIV screening early in pregnancy, but advise simplifying the screening process to maximize opportunities for women to learn their HIV status during pregnancy. They preserve the woman's option to decline HIV testing, and ensure a provider-patient relationship conducive to optimal clinical and preventive care. All women should receive HIV screening consistent with the recommendations for adults and adolescents.

III. Occupational health measures.

A. Develop a culture of safety.
   1. Involve personnel in the planning and implementation of activities that promote a safe health care environment.
   2. Encourage reporting and removal of sharps injury hazards.
   3. Develop feedback systems to increase safety awareness.
   4. Promote individual accountability.
   5. Have an exposure control plan.

B. Use safety devices.
   1. In November of 2000 the Needlestick Safety and Prevention Act (the Act) (Pub. L. 106-430) was signed into law. This was a modification to OSHA'S Bloodborne Pathogens Standard (29 CFR 1910.1030) to set forth in greater detail the requirement for employers to identify, evaluate, and implement safer medical devices. The Act also mandated additional requirements for maintaining a sharps injury log and for the involvement of nonmanagerial health care workers in evaluating and choosing devices.
   2. One study conducted at a hemodialysis center found the use of standard arteriovenous fistula needles resulted in a needlestick injury rate of 8/58 per 100,000. The injury rate dropped to less than 1/100,000 following the introduction and use of a guarded arteriovenous fistula needle. Studies in other health care settings have also demonstrated that safety devices, when introduced with concomitant training, significantly reduce the number of needlestick injuries.

C. Actions to take after exposure.
   1. Immediately following an exposure to blood:
      a. Wash percutaneous injuries with soap and water. Flush splashes to the nose, mouth, or skin with water or irrigate eyes with clean water, saline, or sterile irrigants.
      b. Report exposure to the department, office, or individual (e.g., occupational health, infection control) responsible for managing health care worker exposures.
      c. If the source individual cannot be identified or tested, decisions regarding follow-up

should be based on the exposure risk and whether the source is likely to be infected with a bloodborne pathogen.
   2. For known sources.
      a. Test known sources for HBsAg, anti-HCV, and HIV antibody.
         (1) Consider using a rapid HIV-antibody test.
         (2) Direct virus assays (e.g., viral load assays) for routine screening of source patients are not recommended.
         (3) If the source person is not infected with a bloodborne pathogen, baseline testing or further follow-up of the exposed person is not necessary.
      b. For sources whose infection status remains unknown (e.g., the source person refuses testing), consider the source patient's medical diagnoses, clinical symptoms, and history of risk behaviors.
      c. Do not test discarded needles, used syringes, etc., for bloodborne pathogens.
   3. Unknown sources.
      a. For unknown sources, evaluate the likelihood of exposure to a source at high risk for infection.
      b. Consider likelihood of bloodborne pathogen infection among patients in the exposure setting.

IV. Management of HIV exposure.

A. Health care workers exposed to HIV should be evaluated within hours (rather than days) after their exposure and should be tested for HIV at baseline (i.e., at the time of exposure).

B. If the source person is seronegative for HIV, further follow-up of the exposed person is not necessary.

C. For purposes of considering HIV postexposure prophylaxis (PEP), the evaluation should include information about medications the exposed person might be taking and any current or underlying medical conditions or circumstances (i.e., pregnancy, breast feeding, or kidney or hepatic disease) that might influence drug selection.

D. PEP should be initiated as soon as possible, preferably within hours rather than days of exposure. For additional information regarding PEP please refer to the Updated U.S. Public Health Service Guidelines for management of Occupational exposure to HIV and recommendations for postexposure prophylaxis (see http://www.cdc.gov/mmwr/preview/mmwrhtml/rr5409al.htm).

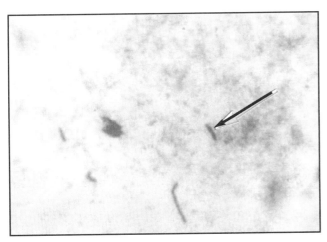

Figure 17.3. Acid fast bacteria seen on smear are tubercle bacilli.

Source: Centers for Disease Control and Prevention: Division of Tuberculosis Elimination. (2004). *Core curriculum on tuberculosis* (4th ed). Slide sets. Retrieved December 12, 2007, from http://www.cdc.gov/ tb/pubs/slidesets/core/ html/trans5_slides.htm. Used with permission.

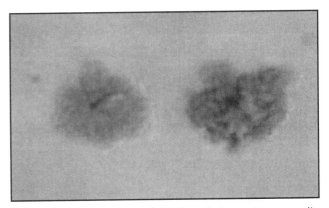

Figure 17.4. Colonies of *M. tuberculosis* growing on media.

Source: Centers for Disease Control and Prevention: Division of Tuberculosis Elimination. (2004). *Core curriculum on tuberculosis* (4th ed). Slide sets. Retrieved December 12, 2007, from http://www.cdc.gov/tb/pubs/ slidesets/core/ html/trans5_slides.htm. Used with permission.

Tuberculosis

I. General considerations.

A. Tuberculosis (TB) is a major health concern in the United States. The growth of TB globally and the presence of a large immunosuppressed population, in part due to the AIDS epidemic, contribute to the large number of TB cases.

B. Multidrug resistant strains of TB are emerging that are resistant to drugs traditionally used to treat TB. Chronic kidney disease (CKD) and diabetes mellitus are risk factors that increase the chance of developing clinical TB.

II. Etiology.

A. Tuberculosis is caused by the tubercle bacillus *Mycobacterium tuberculosis*. TB is spread primarily through respiratory means. While this disease can involve any organ, the lungs remain the primary site of infection (see Figure 17.3).

B. When respiratory droplets are released into the air, the smallest of the droplets (droplet nuclei) dry and remain airborne for indefinite periods of time and may contain one to several mycobacteria. They are the most dangerous particles because they are small enough to be inhaled and deposited in the alveoli of the susceptible host. Larger particles fall to the floor or other surfaces and are not sources of airborne transmission.

C. Infectiousness usually coincides with the number of infectious organisms in sputum, the extent of pulmonary disease and the frequency of coughing. When *M. tuberculosis* is presented to a host with a functioning immune system repeated, prolonged exposure is usually necessary for infection to occur. When the immune system is defective, infection can progress to active disease after short exposure times to small numbers of organisms.

III. Pathophysiology.

A. While *M. tuberculosis* is similar in many ways to other bacteria, there are characteristics that are important to remember when caring for patients with TB.
1. *M. tuberculosis* has a mean doubling time of 12 to 24 hours and may require weeks of growth to produce a visible colony. It can delay identification of the organism, and in some cases (e.g., drug resistant strains) can delay drug-susceptibility testing and drug therapy (see Figure 17.4).
2. The cell wall structure of *M. tuberculosis* contains an outer layer of fatty acids and waxes that are toxic to host cells and tissue and that make the bacilli insoluble in water. This cell layer contributes to its slow growth rate and also protects the organism from antimicrobial agents. The layer also prevents the body's macrophages from being able to completely destroy all the invading bacilli, contributing to the need for prolonged drug therapy.

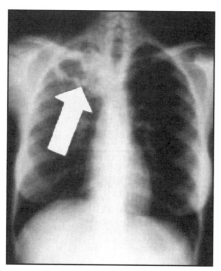

Figure 17.5. Chest x-ray of a patient with TB; arrow points to cavity in patient's right upper lobe.

Source: Centers for Disease Control and Prevention: Division of Tuberculosis Elimination. (2004). *Core curriculum on tuberculosis* (4th ed). Slide sets. Retrieved December 12, 2007, from http://www.cdc.gov/tb/pubs/slidesets/core/html/trans5_slides.htm. Used with permission.

B. Once an individual inhales tubercle bacilli into the alveoli, how the body reacts to the bacilli depends in part on host susceptibility, how many particles were inhaled, and how virulent the organisms are. The lung responds to the bacilli with inflammation and the body's normal defense mechanisms. Inflammation may lead to development of primary tubercle nodules. Cells gather around the tubercle and the outer portion becomes fibrosed. The center becomes necrotic. If the material is coughed up, it may leave a hole or cavity in the lung issue. On x-ray, these cavities are suggestive of TB (see Figure 17.5).

C. If the host has a competent immune system, multiplication and spread of the organisms are halted, usually within 2 to10 weeks. Alveolar macrophages ingest most of the bacilli, although some viable bacilli remain in the macrophages in a dormant state, and reactivation of the disease at a later time is possible. These people are considered to have TB infection or latent TB infection (LTBI). Even though they have TB, they have no signs or symptoms of the disease and are not capable of transmitting TB. These persons will have a positive reaction to a tuberculin skin test (TST). During their lifetime, these persons have a 10% risk of developing active TB. The greatest risk is within 2 years after the original infection. If the host's immune system is deficient and unable to prevent spread of the bacillus, active TB disease develops. The individual will have clinical symptoms of TB and is capable of spreading the disease to others.

D. A number of the new cases of TB are seen in older people who were infected decades earlier (LTBI), and the disease emerges when the host's immune system is weakened. Rates of TB are also increased in racial and ethnic minorities who have other risk factors for TB, such as birth in a country with high prevalence rates of TB, in individuals with HIV infection, low socioeconomic status, or exposure in congregate settings (i.e., prisons, shelters). HIV plays a key role in the resurgence of TB. HIV-positive patients have a much higher risk of developing active clinical disease after initial infection or developing disease subsequent to an earlier infection (see Table 17.4).

IV. Multidrug-resistant TB (MDR-TB).

A. There is an increased incidence of TB that is resistant to at least two of the first-line drugs used to treat TB. In the past, drug resistance was a result of inappropriate or inadequate treatment of TB, known as secondary or acquired drug resistance. Primary drug resistance occurs when only a few of the organisms present have an inherent resistance to one or more of the most commonly used antitubercular drugs. This type of MDR-TB is being spread among patients by direct exposure, particularly in areas with large populations of HIV-infected patients.

B. To prevent emergence of drug-resistant strains of TB, appropriate drug regimens must contain several different drugs to which the organism is susceptible. The dosing schedule must maintain sufficient concentrations to inhibit or kill the organisms present. Drugs must be continued long enough to ensure all organisms are eliminated. Specific drug therapy for resistant strains of TB depend on whether the organism is resistant to one or more of the drugs commonly used to treat TB. Some organisms are resistant to only one drug, while others are resistant to multiple drugs.

V. Signs and symptoms of TB.

A. Pulmonary TB should be suspected in people who complain of fever, chills, night sweats, fatigue, weight loss, decreased appetite, chest pain, prolonged and productive coughing (longer than 3 weeks), or hemoptysis.

B. Extrapulmonary TB occurs most often in people with HIV. Pulmonary TB is the most common form of TB, including those with HIV. HIV negative patients have a 10% rate of extrapulmonary TB, while those with full blown AIDS have a 70% rate of TB at sites other than the lung. Patients with HIV and impaired immune systems have a 24–45% incidence of extrapulmonary TB.

C. Patients with HIV and extrapulmonary TB demonstrate lymphatitis and miliary disease (formation of tubercles) throughout the body organs from dissemination of bacillus through the bloodstream. Symptoms include tender lymph nodes, fever, fatigue, and weight loss. People with extrapulmonary TB are usually not considered infectious unless they have an open abscess or draining lesion.

D. Anyone suspected of having TB must be immediately placed in isolation and be referred for further evaluation consisting of a physical examination, a Mantoux tuberculin skin test, chest x-ray and sputum smears and cultures.

VI. Screening for TB.

A. Screening tests in the United States are used to identify infected people who need preventive therapy and as part of the workup for those with signs or symptoms of active disease.
  1. Screen groups with disease and infection rates in excess of those in the general population.
  2. Institutional screening for staff of all health care facilities and residents of long-term care facilities.
  3. The Centers for Disease Control and Prevention (CDC) recommend all health care facilities establish a TB screening program for health care workers. The Occupational Safety and Health Administration (OSHA) mandates that employers develop and follow TB screening and control programs for staff. To assess the risk for exposure to TB in the workplace, the risk factors associated with TB must be identified. While TB can occur in any population or group, certain subpopulations have been identified as having a higher-than-average risk for TB:
    a. Close contact with infectious tuberculosis cases.
    b. Medically underserved, low-income populations, including high-risk racial and ethnic groups.
    c. Foreign-born persons from high-prevalence countries (Asia, Africa, Latin America).
    d. Older adults.

Table 17.4

Medical Conditions that Increase the Risk of Developing TB Disease Once Infection Has Occurred

- HIV Infection
- Substance abuse (especially drug injection)
- Silicosis
- Recent infection with *M. tuberculosis* within the previous 2 years
- Persons with a history of untreated or inadequately treated TB disease, including persons with chest radiograph findings with previous TB disease
- Diabetes mellitus
- Prolonged corticosteroid therapy
- Other immunosuppressive treatments (including tumor necrosis factor-alpha antagonists)
- Organ transplants
- Hematologic disorders (for example, leukemia, Hodgkin's disease)
- Other malignancies (e.g., carcinoma of the head and neck, or lung)
- Chronic kidney disease
- Intestinal bypass or gastrectomy
- Chronic malabsorption syndromes
- Being > 10% below ideal body weight

Adapted from Centers for Disease Control and Prevention. (2005b). Guidelines for preventing the transmission of *M. tuberculosis* in health-care settings. *MMWR, 54,* RR-17.

B. Tuberculin skin tests.
  1. Screening programs for TB usually consists of the Mantoux purified protein derivative tuberculin skin test (TST). Included in the group of who should be screened are people who have medical conditions that increase their risk of clinical disease when exposed to TB.
    a. Close contacts of infectious TB cases.
    b. Persons with medical conditions that increase the risk of TB.
    c. Foreign-born persons from high prevalence countries.
    d. Low-income populations, including high-risk minorities.
    e. Alcoholics and intravenous drug users.
    f. Residents of long-term care facilities (including prisons).
    g. Populations identified locally as being at increased risk for TB such as health care workers in some settings.
  2. CKD is a risk factor for TB. The CDC

recommends skin test screening in this group. Chronic kidney disease is an immuno-compromised condition with cutaneous anergy that can result in false-negative TB tests. Anergy is the absence of a reaction to a TST that can be seen in dialysis patients. Causes for anergy include infection, sarcoidosis, poor nutrition, some medications, vaccinations, and TB disease. The negative test does not exclude a diagnosis of TB disease or infection with *M. tuberculosis.* Anergy skin testing in conjunction with TST is no longer recommended routinely for *M. tuberculosis* infection.

3. The Mantoux skin test (TST) provides the most accurate results. Using a tuberculin syringe with 0.1 mL (5 units) of purified protein derivative (PPD), inject intradermally forming a wheal just under the skin. Trained staff read the test in 48 to 72 hours. Table 17.5 defines how skin tests should be read. Documentation of skin test results should include:
   a. Palpate and measure the area of induration (induration is hardness, not redness). Record all results in millimeters even if they are considered nonreactive.
   b. Interpretation of skin test results are based on risk factors of the person being tested.
   c. False-positive results to TST can be due to infections with mycobacterium other than *M. tuberculosis* or due to immunization with Bacillus Calmette-Guerin (BCG).
   d. False-negative results can occur in people recently infected with TB. It may take 2 to 10 weeks after infection to mount an immune response. People who had a negative skin test after an initial TB infection may years later manifest a positive reaction.
   e. Two-step testing is used in settings where periodic testing will occur, such as health care workers, nursing homes, and dialysis units. The first time the person is tested they are given an initial skin test. If the first test is considered negative, a second TST is given 1 to 3 weeks later. If the first and second tests are negative, then any subsequent positive skin test is more likely to be due to a recent TB infection (TB conversion).

C. QuantiFERON-TB Gold test (QFTG) is a type of blood assay for *M. tuberulosis* (BAMT).
   1. QFTG is an alternative to tuberculin skin tests (TST) and was approved by the FDA in 2005.
   2. QFTG measures the patient's immune system reaction to *M. tuberculosis* (tuberculosis antigens).

3. Blood samples must be drawn and processed within 12 hours.
4. Interpretation is less subjective than for TSTs.
5. May be less affected by BCG vaccination.
6. Conditions requiring caution in interpreting negative QuantiFERON-TB Gold test results.
   a. Human immunodeficiency virus infection or acquired immunodeficiency disease.
   b. Immunsuppressive drugs, including those used for managing organ transplants.
   c. Tumor necrosis factor (TNF).
   d. Diabetes mellitus.
   e. Silicosis.
   f. Chronic kidney disease.
   g. Certain hematologic disorders (e.g., leukemias and lymphomas).
   h. Other specific malignancies (e.g., carcinomas of the head, neck, or lung).

VII. Infectivity.

A. Infectiousness of a TB patient is directly related to the number of bacilli released into the air whenever that person coughs, talks, sings, or sneezes. Most patients are considered infectious if they:
   1. Are coughing, receiving cough-inducing or aerosol-generating procedures.
   2. Have sputum smears that show presence of acid-fast bacilli and are not receiving therapy, have just started therapy, or have poor clinical or bacteriologic response to therapy.

B. Infectiousness may persist for weeks or even months in patients with drug-resistant TB.

C. Once effective therapy is begun, patients are no longer considered infectious as long as they meet all the following criteria:
   1. They have been receiving adequate drug therapy for 2–3 weeks.
   2. They demonstrate favorable clinical response to therapy.
   3. Consecutive sputum smears collected on three separate days are negative.

VIII. Drug therapy. Antituberculosis chemotherapy is designed to kill bacilli rapidly, minimize the potential for organisms to develop drug resistance and sterilize the host's tissues. Achieving these outcomes requires multiple drug combinations being administered over a period of time. Poor follow-through with the drug regimen is one of the primary reasons for the current resurgence of TB and increases in drug resistant strains.

Table 17.5

Classification of TB Skin Test Results

An induration of 5 mm or more is considered a positive reaction in the following high risk groups. Persons should be treated for LTB1 regardless of age:	An induration of 10 mm or more is considered positive in the following persons:	An induration of 15 mm is considered positive for persons who do not have any risk factors for TB.
Persons infected with HIV.	Persons with TST or BAMT conversions.	Persons with no known factors for TB disease. HCW who are otherwise at low risk for TB disease and who received baseline testing at the beginning of employment as part of a TB screening program.
Recent contacts of a person with TB disease.	Persons born or who have lived in developing countries with high-incidence of TB disease.	
Persons with fibrotic changes on chest x-ray consistent with previous TB disease.	Persons who inject illicit drugs.	
Organ transplant recipients.	Residents and employees in congregate facilities and LTCFs (e.g., hospices, skilled nursing facilities), hospital and other health care facilities, residential settings for persons with HIV/AIDS or other immunocompromising conditions, and homeless shelters. Personnel from microbiology labs. Persons with any of the following clinical conditions that place them at high risk: • Silicosis • Diabetes mellitus • Chronic kidney failure • Certain hematologic disorders (e.g., leukemias and lymphomas) • Other specific malignancies (e.g., carcinoma of the head, neck and lung) • Unexplained weight loss of ≥ 10% of ideal body weight • Gastrectomy or jejunoileal bypass Persons living in areas with high incidence of TB disease. Children ≥ 4 years of age. Infants, children and adolescents exposed to adults with high risk for developing TB.	

Adapted from Centers for Disease Control and Prevention. (2005b). Guidelines for preventing the transmission of *M. tuberculosis* in health-care settings. *MMWR, 54,* RR-17.

Table 17.6

TB Drug Frequency Changes for Adult Patients with Reduced Renal Function and Adult Patients Receiving Hemodialysis

Drug	Change in Frequency?
Rifampin	No change
Pyrazinamide	Yes
Ethambutol	Yes
Lavofkaxacin	Yes
Cycloserine	Yes
Ethionamide	No change
p-Aminosalicylic acid	No change
Streptomycin	Yes
Capreomycin	Yes
Kanamycin	Yes
Amikacin	Yes

Adapted from Centers for Disease Control and Prevention. (2005b). Guidelines for preventing the transmission of *M. tuberculosis* in health-care settings. *MMWR, 54,* RR-17.

A. Preventive therapy is prescribed for people infected with TB (latent TB) who do not have active disease, to prevent progression to active clinical TB at a later date. Isoniazid (INH) is usually used alone for preventive therapy. Anyone taking INH should be evaluated for signs of liver disease, neurotoxicity (such as paresthesias of hands and feet), and adherence to prescribed therapy.

B. Treatment of active disease includes use of multiple drugs that the organisms are sensitive to, provision of the safest most effective therapy in the shortest time possible, and ensuring the patient adheres fully to the treatment regimen.

C. Extrapulmonary TB treatment follows the basic principles for treating pulmonary TB: a 6 to 9 month course of therapy, except for TB meningitis that requires 9 to12 months of therapy.

D. Drug-resistant TB diagnosis requires drug-susceptibility testing and prolonged treatment regimens. There have been documented reports of drug-resistant TB being spread by direct contact. It is imperative that treatment be started as soon as possible and adherence to treatment be ensured by whatever means are necessary.

IX. Chronic kidney disease (CKD) – Implications for TB.

A. Kidney disease complicates the management of TB. Antituberculosis medications may be cleared by the kidney and also by hemodialysis. Drugs cleared by the kidneys in patients with creatinine clearance less than 30 mL/minute and those receiving hemodialysis treatments are managed by changing dosing intervals (see Table 17.6).

B. Patients with CKD have additional clinical concerns such as gastroparesis that may affect absorption of TB drugs, and medications that interact with these drugs.

C. There is no data for peritoneal dialysis (PD) patients. Drug removal mechanisms differ between hemodialysis and PD, so it cannot be assumed that hemodialysis medication dosing precautions apply to PD.

D. The CDC recommends that after a known exposure to TB, immunocompromised patients should receive treatment for presumptive latent TB, regardless of skin testing results.

Vascular Access Infections

I. Overview.

Infection is the second leading cause of death in dialysis patients. Access related infections are the leading cause of infection in CKD stage 5 patients. Access infections may vary from minor infections at the needle insertion site to massive infections of the entire access, which may require graft or catheter removal. Septicemia, a life-threatening complication, increases morbidity and mortality in these patients. Access infection is a preventable complication by following standard dialysis precautions and infection control practices.

A. Infection can occur from movement of the patient's normal skin flora on or into the vascular access during cannulation or when accessing the hemodialysis catheter. Failure to follow aseptic technique or good infection control practices can also result in an access infection.

B. The primary risk factor for access infection is the type of access.

C. AV fistulas have a decreased incidence of infection compared to AV grafts or catheters.

D. Catheters have the highest incidence of infection with a rate of 0.08 to 0.7 per 100 catheter days for tunneled catheters.

E. Due to the increased risk of infection and other complications in catheters, it is recommended by NKF/DOQI guidelines that no more than 10% of patients be maintained with a permanent catheter and that 40% of prevalent patients who initiate hemodialysis have a native AV fistula constructed.

II. Types of infections and common organisms.

Note: Due to immunosuppression in patients with chronic kidney disease stage 5, these patients may not demonstrate signs and symptoms of infection normally seen in other patients. For example, a low grade temperature can be significant and a serious infection can exist with few signs or symptoms (such as little to no redness or swelling).

A. Local infection.
1. Local involving blood vessel, graft, or surrounding tissue.
2. Signs and symptoms.
a. Fever or chills.
b. Pain or tenderness of access or exit site.
c. Redness.
d. Purulent drainage from access, exit site, or catheter insertion site.
e. Induration within 2 cm of exit site.
f. Inflammation.

B. Systemic infection.
1. Systemic: sepsis from infection spilling into the blood stream.
2. Signs and symptoms.
a. Malaise.
b. Fever and chills.
c. Presence of local infection symptoms.
d. Septicemia.

C. Common organisms.
1. Gram-positive organisms (*Staphylococcus aureus*, coagulase negative staphylococci [CNS], *Staphylococcus epidermidis*).
a. The number of infections caused by *S. aureus* is higher among patients with fistulas or grafts.

b. The number of infections caused by CNS is higher among patients dialyzed with catheters.
2. Gram negative organisms (most commonly *Escherichia coli*, Pseudomonas).

III. AV fistula and graft infections.

A. Causes and risk factors.
1. Poor personal hygiene.
2. Failure to properly clean access before cannulation.
3. Failure to follow aseptic cannulation technique.
4. Cross contamination.
5. Bacterial seeding from other infected areas.
6. Noncompliance with infection control procedures.
7. Lack of hand washing.
8. Failure to recognize early signs and symptoms of infection.
9. Infection tracking/trending not included in the continuous quality improvement (CQI) process.
10. Inexperienced dialysis staff.
11. Type and location of access.

B. Prevention.
1. Teach patient proper personal hygiene.
2. Strict aseptic cannulation technique.
3. Access care and protection.
4. Train dialysis staff in infection control procedures.
5. Proper hand washing.
6. Teach patient and staff early identification of signs and symptoms of infection.
7. Track and trend infections to identify source and allow corrective action.
8. Early referral for fistula/graft access placement to minimize catheter use.
9. Improve cannulation skills (i.e., cannulation camp; mentorship program).

C. Treatment.
1. Appropriate antibiotics based on culture and sensitivity as ordered.
2. Antimicrobials at infected access site.
3. Graft or fistula removal if indicated.
4. Prophylactic antibiotics preoperatively and before dental, diagnostic or other surgical procedures.
5. Avoid cannulation of infected access.

IV. Catheter-related infections.

A. Infection is the leading cause of catheter loss. Infection in central venous catheters may occur at the exit site, at the tunnel track or systemically.

B. Intravascular catheter-related bloodstream infections lead to increased morbidity, prolonged hospital stays and increased medical costs.

C. Bacteria can spread from the patient's skin to the catheter exit site, along the exterior catheter surface or internally from external contamination of the catheter lumen or from colonization of bacteria from other infected areas.

D. Causes and risk factors.
   1. Inappropriate catheter care guidelines.
   2. Failure to access central venous catheter using aseptic technique.
   3. Catheter placement duration.
   4. Location of the catheter.
   5. Contamination of catheter connections or lumens.
   6. Internal colonization from remote sites during bacteremia.

E. Prevention.
   1. Recommendations for preventing vascular access infection have been developed by the Vascular Access Workgroup of the National Kidney Foundation – Dialysis Outcomes Quality Initiative (NKF-DOQI) in 1998. The Clinical Practice Guidelines for Vascular Access were updated most recently in 2006. These can be obtained from http://www.kidney.org/ professionals/kdoqi//guidelines.cfm.
   2. Selected recommendations for preventing hemodialysis catheter related infections.
      a. Use sterile technique during catheter insertion.
      b. Limit the use of noncuffed catheters to 3–4 weeks.
      c. Use the catheter solely for dialysis unless there is no other alternative.
      d. Restrict catheter manipulation and dressing changes to trained personnel.
      e. Replace catheter-site dressing at each dialysis treatment or if damp, loose, or soiled.
      f. Disinfect skin before catheter insertion and dressing changes.
      g. Ensure that catheter-site care products are compatible with the catheter material.
      h. Wear a surgical mask or face shield (both patient and caregiver) during connect and disconnect procedures.
      i. Use strict aseptic technique when accessing catheters or performing catheter dressing changes.
      j. Teach patient and staff early identification of signs and symptoms of infection.
      k. Track and trend infections to identify source and allow corrective action.

F. Treatment.
   1. Treat catheter infections with antibiotic therapy based on the organism isolated.
   2. Antimicrobials at infected access site.
   3. Catheter lock solutions containing antimicrobial agents used for systemic therapy.
   4. Prophylactic antibiotics preoperatively and before dental, diagnostic, or other surgical procedures.
   5. Catheter removal recommended for noncuffed catheters.
   6. Catheter removal for cuffed catheters if not responsive to treatment.
   7. Infected catheters should be exchanged as soon as possible and within 72 hours of initiating antibiotic therapy in most instances.

Infections Related to Water, Reuse, and/or Machine Contamination

Most infections related to water, reuse and/or machine contamination are caused by organisms either in the water distribution system, dialysate, or the dialysate effluent. These organisms primarily consist of gram negative bacteria frequently found in dialysis fluids and fungi. With the current state of the art and technology, virus (HBV, HCV, and HIV) transmission either through errors in reuse or contamination of machines is a rare event in the United States (see Table 17.7).

I. **Transmission of bloodborne pathogens.**

A. Reuse.
   1. No documented transmission of HBV, HCV, or HIV among facilities that reprocess hemodialyzers in the United States.
   2. Transmission of HIV has occurred in Latin America due to reuse of access needles and reuse of hemodialyzers. In both cases these devices were inadequately disinfected between uses and shared among different patients.

3. Prevention strategies for preventing the transmission of bloodborne pathogens in a reuse program include:
    a. Exclusion of HBsAg+ patients from participating in a reuse program.
    b. Follow the Association for the Advancement of Medical Instrumentation (AAMI) recommended practices for the reuse of hemodialyzers.
    c. Label and assign each patient's dialyzer with a unique identifier and place warnings on dialyzers with patients with similar names.
    d. Do not reuse access needles.

B. Machine contamination.
    1. There has been at least one outbreak of HBV at a dialysis facility associated with the failure to use external transducer protectors to protect pressure monitoring equipment in hemodialysis machines. Transducer protectors can also fail when wetted, and some have suggested this as a possible route for HCV transmission. However, there are insufficient data to suggest that this is a mechanism for HCV transmission.
    2. Contamination of frequently touched external surfaces of the hemodialysis machine can be a potential environmental reservoir for HBV and HCV. HBV can persist in an infectious state for at least 7 days while HCV has been demonstrated to persist in such a state for 24 hours.

II. Bacteremia/fungemia.

A. Reuse.
    1. Errors in dialyzer reprocessing have historically been associated with both pyrogenic reactions and bacteremia. These errors have frequently occurred in facilities performing manual or semiautomated reuse. The typical errors that have been associated with these adverse events have included:
        a. Failure to prepare dialyzer disinfectant to the correct concentration.
        b. Failure to fill the dialyzers with sufficient concentration of disinfectant.
        c. Failure to mix dialyzer disinfectant.
        d. Using disinfectant that is not compatible with the dialyzer membrane.
        e. Using water that did not meet AAMI recommended microbial and endotoxin limits.
        f. Accidentally not refilling the dialyzer with dialyzer disinfectant.
        g. Removing dialyzer header caps without

Table 17.7

Organisms Typically Associated with Infections Related to Water, Dialysate, Reuse, and/or Machine Contamination

Bacterial Pathogens

Members of the Pseudomonaceae
Pseudomonas aeruginosa, Pseudomonas putida/fluorescens
Delftia acidovorans (previously *Pseudomonas acidovorans* and *Commamonas acidovorans*)
Brevundimonas diminuta, Brevundimonas vesicularis
Burkolderia cepacia complex
Ralstonia pickettii, Ralstonia mannitolytica, Ralstonia paucula, Ralstonia gilardii
Stenotrophomonas maltophilia

Members of the Enterobacteriaceae
Enterobacter cloacae
Klebsiella pneumoniae
Serratia marcescens, Serratia liquefaciens

Nontuberculous Mycobacteria
Mycobacterium fortuitum, Mycobacterium abscessus, Mycobacterium mucogenicum

Fungi

Candida parapsilosis
Phialemonium curvatum
Fusarium spp.

---

disinfecting the O-rings, dialyzer header, and caps.
    h. Not reprocessing the dialyzer in a timely manner so that disinfectant has an appropriate contact time.
    2. Bacteremia/fungemia can be prevented by:
        a. Following AAMI recommended practice for the reuse of hemodialyzers.
        b. Reprocessing dialyzers as soon as possible after the completion of a treatment session.
        c. Preparing dialyzer disinfectant per manufacturer's labeled instructions.
        d. If manually reprocessing dialyzers, ensuring that the dialyzers use at least three compartment volumes of disinfectant to fill the blood compartment with an adequate amount of dialyzer disinfectant. Most outbreaks investigated by the Centers for Disease Control and Prevention have been associated with manual reuse.
        e. To prevent sepsis caused by header removal during dialyzer reprocessing, there are several steps that could be taken.

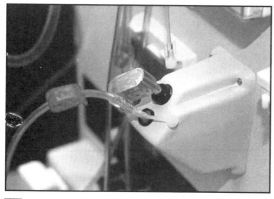

Figure 17.6. Waste handling option of COBE®
Centrysystem 3 dialysis machine.

(1) If clots cannot be removed from the
header spaces of the dialyzer consider
discarding it.
(2) If one removes the head caps from the
dialyzer, then rinse the end of the fibers
with a stream of RO water to remove
clots, and then dip the O-ring, end of the
dialyzer, and end cap in disinfectant
before reassembling the dialyzer.
(3) Use an automated process for removing
clots from the header spaces.
(4) Reevaluate heparinization protocols.

B. Machine contamination.
   1. Today with single-pass hemodialysis equipment,
      infections due to contamination of machines is
      not frequent. Patients may be infected either
      through the hands of health care workers, or by
      direct contact of the blood lines with the
      dialysate circuit as in the waste-handling option
      of the COBE® Centrysystem 3 dialysis machine
      (see Figure 17.6).
   2. There are several sources of contamination of
      the internal fluid pathways of the machine:
      water delivered to the machine, powdered
      bicarbonate concentrates that are prepared with
      treated water at the facility, and retrograde
      growth up the effluent line from the drain.
   3. Preventing bacteremia/fungemia associated
      with contaminated machines.
      a. Follow AAMI recommended practices for the
         microbial quality of water and dialysate.
      b. Disinfect water distribution system and
         hemodialysis machines at regular time
         intervals. This should be conducted at least
         monthly. Hemodialysis machines may need to
         be disinfected more frequently. Some newer

equipment allows for heat disinfection to be
performed on a daily basis.
   c. Conduct routine environmental monitoring
      of water and dialysate (e.g., microbiology and
      endotoxin testing).
   d. Perform preventive maintenance and quality
      assurance checks on equipment per
      manufacturer's recommendations.
   e. If using equipment with the ports to dispose
      of the dialyzer priming solution, follow
      manufacturer's recommendations with
      regards to preventive maintenance (routine
      changing of check valves), disinfection, and
      assessment of check valve competency.

Immunizations

I. Overview.

There is a significant opportunity for improvement in
immunization rates among dialysis patients for
influenza, hepatitis B, and pneumococcal disease. The
goal for the Centers for Medicare & Medicaid Services'
(CMS) Healthy People 2010 initiative is that 90% of
adults will be immunized against pneumococcal
disease and receive an annual influenza vaccination.
However, in 2002, only 54% of dialysis patients in the
U.S. received an influenza vaccination, and only about
12% had received a pneumococcal vaccination. Table
17.8 summarizes the goals established by the Healthy
People 2010 initiative for influenza, hepatitis B, and
pneumococcal immunizations and the most current
data on immunization rates available for adults in the
United States. Table 17.9 summarizes the most current
data available for dialysis patients. The Centers for
Disease Control and Prevention recommends all three
vaccinations for dialysis patients due to the increased
risk of infection in the CKD population.

II. Recommendations.

Table 17.10 shows a list of vaccines recommended for
persons with chronic kidney disease.

A. Hepatitis B.
   1. Each year 78,000 Americans are infected with
      hepatitis B and 5,000 die from it.
   2. Vaccination for hepatitis B is recommended for
      all pre-CKD stage 5 patients before they start
      dialysis.
   3. Vaccination is recommended for all chronic
      dialysis patients.

Table 17.8

Healthy People 2010 Goals and Current Status of Immunizations

Hepatitis B Vaccine				
Objective	Increase in hepatitis B vaccine coverage in high-risk groups	2010 Target	1995 Baseline	Opportunity to Improve
14.28a.	Long-term hemodialysis patients	90%	35%	55%
14.28c.	Occupationally exposed workers	98%	71%	27%
Influenza And Pneumococcal Vaccine				
Objective	Increase in adults vaccinated *Note*: Healthy People 2010 did not set separate ESRD goals	2010 Target	1998* Baseline (unless noted)	Opportunity to Improve
Noninstitutionalized adults aged 65 years and older				
14.29a.	Influenza vaccine	90%	64%	26%
14-29b.	Pneumococcal vaccine	90%	46%	44%
Noninstitutionalized high-risk adults aged 18 to 64 years				
14.29c.	Influenza vaccine	60%	26%	34%
14.29d.	Pneumococcal vaccine	60%	13%	47%
Institutionalized adults (persons in long-term or nursing homes)				
14-29e.	Influenza vaccine	90%	59% (1997)	31%
14-29f.	Pneumococcal vaccine	90%	25% (1997)	65%

Source: Centers for Disease Control and Prevention. (2007). *Healthy people 2010*. Retrieved August 8, 2006, from http://www.healthypeople.gov/document/html/volume1/14Immunization.htm.

4. Hepatitis B vaccines are given in a three or four dose series. Table 17.11 shows the schedules for both series.
5. Serologic testing should be performed 1-2 months after administration of the last dose of the vaccine series.
6. Patients with anti-HBs level of less than 10 mIU/mL after the vaccine series should be revaccinated followed by serologic testing.
7. Patients who do not respond to revaccination should be tested for HBsAg. If the HBsAg is positive, the patient should be considered infected and managed appropriately to prevent the spread to others. If the HBsAg is negative, the patient should be considered susceptible to infection and counseled on precautions to prevent infection.
8. Patients who have responded to the vaccine should have annual anti-HBs testing. A booster dose should be administered when anti-HBs levels are less than 10 mIU/mL.

Table 17.9

Immunization Rates for Dialysis Patients

Vaccine	USRDS 2002	NSDAD 2001
Influenza	54.0%	64.6%
Pneumococcal	12.0%	26.2%
Hepatitis B	Data not available	56.0%

B. Influenza.
1. Every year 5–20% of the population is infected with influenza, more than 200,000 people are hospitalized from complications, and 36,000 people die from the flu. People with chronic medical conditions (like chronic kidney disease) are at higher risk of developing serious flu complications such as pneumonia and bacterial infections, respiratory and cardiac ailments, Reye's syndrome, and death.
2. Inactivated influenza vaccine is recommended for all persons with impaired kidney function.

Table 17.10

Recommended Vaccinations for Persons with Chronic Kidney Disease

Vaccine	Recommended	May Use If Otherwise Indicated	Contraindicated
Anthrax		X*	
DtaP/TdapTd		X*	
Hib		X*	
Hepatitis A		X*	
Hepatitis B	X		
Influenza (TIV)	X		X
Influenza (LAIV)			
Japanese Encephalitis		X*	
MMR		X*	
Meningococcal		X*	
Pneumococcal	X	X*	
Polio (IPV)		X*	
Rabies		X*	
Rotavirus		X*	
Smallpox		X*	
Typhoid		X*	
Varicella		X*	
Yellow Fever		X*	

*No specific recommendation for this vaccine exists for patients with chronic kidney disease.

Source: Centers for Disease Control and Prevention. (2006a). *Guidelines for vaccinating kidney dialysis patients and patients with chronic kidney disease*. Retrieved June 22, 2006, from http://www.cdc.gov/nip/publications/dialysis_guide.pdf.

3. The live, attenuated influenza vaccine is not recommended for persons with impaired kidney function.
4. Vaccination for influenza is recommended annually at the beginning of the flu season (October–November).

C. Pneumococcal.
1. In 2002, approximately 65,000 people died of pneumonia; 90% of these deaths were in persons 65 years or older.
2. Complications of pneumococcal pneumonia include empyema, pericarditis, endobronchial obstruction, and death.
3. Vaccination for pneumococcal disease is recommended for persons with chronic kidney failure.

4. The pneumococcal polysaccharide vaccine (PPV) protects against 23 types of pneumococcal bacteria.
5. Revaccination every 5 years is recommended for chronic kidney failure patients over 2 years of age.

Regulations and Recommendations: What's the Difference?

Infection control practices in dialysis and kidney transplant settings are influenced by the federal end-stage renal disease (ESRD) regulations, any applicable state licensing rules, Occupational Safety and Health Agency (OSHA) regulations, and recommendations of professional associations and state and federal agencies.

I. **Regulations are mandatory requirements that must be met to practice within the "law."**

A. Implement statutes passed by legislative bodies and signed into law by the governor, for state laws, or the president, for federal laws.

B. The public can influence the content and structure of the law during the legislative process by contacting their congresspersons to educate and influence the vote.

C. Once a bill has been passed and signed into statute, the applicable state or federal agency is charged with developing regulations to implement the law.

D. Statutes are typically broad, outlining the intent of the legislature. The specifics are usually found in regulation.

E. Regulations are subject to public influence as well.

Table 17.11

Dose Schedules for Hepatitis B Vaccine

Group	Recombivax HB			Engerix B		
	Dose	Volume	Schedule	Dose	Volume	Schedule
> 20 years of age: predialysis	10 µg	1.0 mL	3 doses at 0, 1, 6 months	20 µg	1.0 mL	3 doses at 0, 1, 6 months
> 20 years of age: dialysis dependent	40 µg	1.0 mL	3 doses at 0, 1, 6 months	40 µg	Two 1.0 mL doses at one site	4 doses at 0, 1, 2, 6 months
< 20 years of age	5 µg	0.5 mL	3 doses at 0, 1, 6 months	10 µg	0.5 mL	3 doses at 0, 1, 6 months

Source: Centers for Disease Control and Prevention. (2006a). *Guidelines for vaccinating kidney dialysis patients and patients with chronic kidney disease.* Retrieved June 22, 2006, from http://www.cdc.gov/nip/ publications/dialysis_guide.pdf.

1. Proposed state and federal regulations are published for public comment before being finalized.
2. Comments received are taken into consideration in developing the final regulations.
3. Examples of current regulations: Federal regulations require ESRD facilities to prevent the transmission of infection. Essentially this requires that facilities follow the guidance issued by the Centers for Disease Control for infection control in hemodialysis facilities. These recommendations are discussed in more detail in a different section of this chapter.

II. **Recommendations are voluntary and frequently come about** as the result of critical incidents or research evidence, rather than law. Recommendations, by themselves, do not carry the weight of "law."

A. May be developed via a consensus process.

B. Professional organizations that have developed recommendations addressing infection control topics include:
   1. ANNA: *Nephrology Nursing Standards of Practice and Guidelines for Care.*
   2. National Kidney Foundation (NKF): *Kidney Disease Outcomes Quality Improvement (KDOQI) Practice Guidelines.*
   3. Association for the Advancement of Medical Instrumentation (AAMI): *Recommended Practice Dialysate for Hemodialysis.*

C. The federal agency that provides direction in the area of infection control is the Centers for Disease Control and Prevention (CDC). Their documents are designated as either "Guidelines" or "Recommendations."
   1. Recommendations are based on findings from CDC investigations of critical incidents, research or review of data and developed via expert opinion. There is an internal review process, and public comments may be solicited, but there is no requirement to incorporate such comments into the final recommendation.
   2. Guidelines are usually developed by CDC and external partners, based on evidence, and require public review and are published in the federal register for comment. Public comments have to be addressed by incorporation into the guideline or by providing a reason why the comment was not accepted. The completed document undergoes a final peer review process before being published as a guideline.

III. **Recommendations adopted as regulations.** Recommendations may sometimes be formally adopted as regulations.

A. This allows the state or federal government agency to use the work of professional organizations and other agencies, preventing the potential development of conflicting standards and reducing duplicate efforts.

B. For example, the Centers for Medicare and Medicaid Services (CMS) formally adopted the AAMI document "Reuse of Hemodialyzers" as part of the ESRD regulations, mandating that facilities that reprocess dialyzers comply with the "voluntary" guidelines that AAMI developed.

C. CDC recommendations for infection control are currently referenced in the CMS ESRD guidance to surveyors as the standard for infection control practices in dialysis. State surveyors are instructed to expect facilities to follow the CDC recommendations for standard precautions and the specific precautions related to hemodialysis.

D. The changes to the CMS's ESRD regulations proposed in 2005 included language to incorporate the CDC recommendations for infection control as regulations.

IV. **Practice guidelines and standards are more and more commonly used** as a way to organize and prioritize care delivery, and to evaluate the care delivered.

A. In this context, recommendations are sometimes used as an expected standard.

B. For example, the KDOQI guideline for dialysis adequacy is commonly used as the expected standard of care for hemodialysis and peritoneal dialysis. State surveyors are instructed to compare a facility's patient outcomes in dialysis adequacy with the KDOQI minimum targets. If the practices in the dialysis facility do not include efforts to assure each patient achieves that minimum target, those minimum targets might be included as support for the finding of a deficient practice.

C. Currently, KDOQI guidance has not been adopted as regulation. Thus, if a facility had evidence that their targets for adequacy were based on a similar scientific process, the surveyor would consider that evidence in determining whether a deficient practice existed.

CDC Recommendations for Infection Control in Hemodialysis Settings

I. **General considerations.**

A. Standard precautions are designed to protect health care workers and service users from occupational exposure to blood or other potentially infectious materials. All human blood and certain human body fluids are treated as if known to be infectious for HIV, HBV, and other bloodborne pathogens.

B. The Occupational Safety and Health Administration mandates that each employer having an employee(s) with occupational exposure establish a written Exposure Control plan designed to eliminate or minimize employee exposure. The components of the plan must include, but are not limited to:
1. Engineering and work practice controls to eliminate or minimize employee exposure (i.e., safety needles, needleless systems).
2. Personal protective equipment (PPE) (e.g., gowns, gloves, face shields).
3. Hepatitis B vaccination and postexposure evaluation and follow-up.
4. Communication of hazards to employees.

C. Standard precautions synthesize the major features of universal precautions designed to reduce the risk of transmission of bloodborne pathogens, and body substance isolation designed to reduce the risk of transmission of pathogens from moist body substances, and applies them to all patients receiving care in hospitals, regardless of their diagnosis or presumed infection status; recommended for the inpatient hospital setting.

D. In addition to standard precautions, more stringent precautions have been recommended by the CDC for the hemodialysis setting due to the increased potential for contamination with blood and pathogenic microorganisms and are the focus of this section on infection control.

II. **Recommendations for preventing transmission of infections among chronic hemodialysis patients.**

A. Published by the Centers for Disease Control and Prevention (CDC), *MMWR*, April 27, 2001, Vol. 50, No. RR-5.

B. These recommendations replace previous recommendations for the prevention of bloodborne virus infections in hemodialysis centers.

C. They provide additional recommendations for the prevention of bacterial infections in the hemodialysis setting.

D. Provides recommendations for a comprehensive infection control program.
1. Infection control precautions specifically designed to prevent transmission of bloodborne viruses and pathogenic bacteria among patients.
2. Routine serologic testing for hepatitis B and C.
3. Vaccination of susceptible patients and staff.

4. Isolation of patients who test positive for hepatitis surface antigen (HBsAg).

5. Surveillance and education.

E. Implementation of the recommendations will reduce opportunities for patient-to-patient transmission of infectious agents, directly or indirectly via contaminated devices, equipment and supplies, environmental surfaces, or hands of staff.

F. Must be carried out routinely for all patients in the hemodialysis center.

G. Includes additional measures to prevent HBV transmission.

III. Infection control precautions for all hemodialysis patients.

A. Wear gloves whenever caring for a patient or touching the patient's equipment at the dialysis station. Remove gloves and wash hands between patient or stations or more often if gloves become contaminated.

B. Wash hands after gloves are removed and between patient contacts, as well as after touching blood, body fluids, secretions, excretions, and contaminated items.

C. If hands are not visibly contaminated, a waterless antiseptic hand rub can be substituted for hand washing.

D. Items taken to a patient's dialysis station, including those placed on top of dialysis machines, should either be disposed of, dedicated for use only on a single patient, or cleaned and disinfected before being returned to a common clean area or used for other patients.

E. Unused medications or supplies (e.g., syringes, alcohol swabs) taken to the patient's station should not be returned to a common clean area or used on other patients.

F. Multiple dose vials must not be carried from station to station.

G. Common carts should not be used to prepare or distribute medications. If trays are used to distribute medications, the tray must be cleaned before using for a different patient.

H. Common supply carts that are used to store clean supplies in the treatment area should remain in a designated area at a sufficient distance from patient stations to avoid contamination with blood.

I. Residual medication from two or more vials should not be pooled into a single vial.

J. Staff members should wear gowns, face shields, eye wear, or masks when performing procedures during which exposure to blood might occur.

K. After each patient treatment, a low level disinfectant should be used to clean environmental surfaces at the dialysis station, including the bed or chair, countertops, equipment, blood pressure cuffs, clamps, external surfaces of the dialysis machine, and containers used for prime waste.

L. Blood spills must be immediately cleaned with a cloth soaked with a tuberculocidal disinfectant or a 1:100 dilution of household bleach.

M. Venous pressure transducer protectors should be changed between patients and not reused.

N. External transducer protectors that become wet should be replaced immediately and inspected.
1. If fluid is visible on the side of the transducer protector that faces the machine, qualified personnel should open the machine after the treatment is completed and check for blood contamination of the internal pressure tubing set and pressure sensing port.
2. If contamination has occurred, the machine must be taken out of service and disinfected, using either 1:100 dilution of bleach or EPA-registered tuberculocidal germicide before further use.

O. Wastes generated by the hemodialysis treatment should be considered infectious and placed in leakproof containers for disposal according to local and state regulations.

Continuous Quality Improvement and Infection Control

I. Continuous quality improvement (CQI). Assessing and improving quality is an important part of professional care. CQI has been shown to improve clinical outcomes and processes that can lead to improved morbidity, mortality, quality of life, and patient satisfaction.

II. Quality improvement plan (QIP).

A. A quality improvement plan (QIP) is a process to promote continuous quality improvement in all aspects of patient care. The plan is like a road map that leads in the right direction. The road map requires the participation of all members of the care team including patients, physicians, nurses, technicians, dietitians, social workers, vendors, housekeeping, and other customers of the dialysis unit.

B. Each dialysis unit must maintain its own specific quality improvement plan. The plan is used to identify areas for continuous monitoring that includes all areas of the organization, from the board of directors (or governing body) to staff providing patient care. The team must agree on aspects of care that need improvement and develop and adopt quality indicators. The group then collects data to determine the need for improvement. Then steps are devised and carried out to bring about change through improving the system of care. Use the indicators to measure successes.

C. Elements of a good QIP.
   1. Identify and measure key areas of care in the facility.
   2. Measure those indicators identified by CMS, KDOQI, CDC, AAMI, and OSHA.
   3. Assess facility care processes and look for areas that could be improved.
   4. Develop a system for monitoring these processes.
   5. Evaluate the changes and recommend improvements.
   6. Always monitor outcomes over time.

III. Infection control practices.

A. Key aspects of the QIP include monitoring the following infection control issues:
   1. Dialysis specific infection control precautions (CDC).
   2. Dialyzer reuse processes.
   3. Water used for dialysis and reuse.
   4. Hepatitis testing for staff and patients.
   5. Hepatitis vaccination for staff and patients.
   6. Isolation of hepatitis B patients.
   7. Influenza vaccination for patients.
   8. Tuberculosis surveillance.
   9. Pyrogenic reactions.
   10. Peritonitis exit site and peritonitis rates.
   11. Sepsis episodes.
   12. Access infection rates.
   13. Specific staff identified to monitor infection rates.

B. The facility's infection control strategies should cover the following at minimum:
   1. A written plan that is reviewed and updated as necessary.
   2. A requirement for use of personal protective equipment such as gloves, gowns, and face protection when exposure to blood or body fluids is likely.
   3. A requirement for housekeeping procedures that ensures the environment is clean and sanitary.
   4. A requirement for efficient and safe infectious waste procedures.
   5. A requirement for effective handling of blood contaminated linens and clothing.
   6. Development and implementation of an effective training program for the use of infection control practices.
   7. Maintenance of employee's training records related to infection control training.
   8. Disinfection policies and procedures for medical equipment and medical devices, including periodic bacteriologic testing of a random sample of dialysis machines.
   9. Procedures for maintaining a log of adverse patient reactions.
   10. Procedure for monthly surveillance of dialysate and water cultures.
   11. Surveillance and reporting of access infections.
   12. Disinfection of equipment.
   13. Rinsing, cleaning, disinfection, preparation, and storage of reused dialyzers.

IV. Surveillance and reporting.

A. For each indicator, data will be collected and reported in a way that allows for identification of outliers (e.g., those patients not meeting the standard or threshold set for a given indicator). An example might be the number of new tunneled catheter systemic infections in the facility. The number of infections in new catheters would be collected over a designated period of time (for example, 3 months). Compare the number of infections against other sources (sometimes referred to as *benchmarks*). In addition to a single facility's threshold (goal or standard), examples of comparative data may include the number of new tunneled catheter infections in other facilities within the organization and the 2006 KDOQI Vascular Access Infection Clinical Practice Guidelines for tunneled catheters. Using comparative data assists in identifying areas needing improvement.

B. Steps for collecting and reporting data include identification of:
1. Who is best qualified to collect the data.
2. The source or sources of the data.
3. How the data is to be collected and the frequency of collection.
4. Who will organize the data.
5. How the data will be displayed and how comparative data will be used in the report.

V. Evaluation of outcomes.

A. At regular meetings, those individuals responsible for evaluating specific outcomes report to the quality improvement team. The team will evaluate and determine whether there is an opportunity for improvement.

B. The team should record in meeting minutes the outcomes, assessments, conclusions, and recommendations for each indicator.

VI. Action steps.

A. If the evaluation of an indicator suggests a need for improvement, actions must be specified and recommendations carried out. Actions may include:
1. Knowledge issues needing in-service education and sharing of information. An example might be the technique used to cleanse and prepare catheter exit sites. Are KDOQI guidelines being used for prevention of catheter infections? Are staff following the designated procedure?
2. Behavior issues needing counseling or disciplinary action.
3. System issues requiring changes in how information is shared, staffing issues, equipment problems, and procedures. For example, does the procedure for cleansing and dressing catheters need to be changed?

B. Identify who will implement the changes and how the changes will be monitored for effectiveness.

C. Set up a pilot project. It is often better to start small than to implement a unit-wide change unless the severity of the problem indicates otherwise. Select the study group (e.g., every other new tunneled catheter patient). The study group will use a new cleaning and dressing procedure.

D. Identify what data needs to be collected and how long the data will be collected. For example, collect the number of systemic catheter infections in the patients included in the pilot study for 3 months.

VII. Assess effectiveness of pilot project.

A. Review outcome of action steps. If care and service improved and agreement is reached to change the process, write new procedures and educate all involved staff and patients as needed. For example, if the percentage of infections in the pilot study group was 3% versus 6% in the nonstudy group, a change in procedure may be warranted.

B. If care and service did not improve, further evaluation is needed to determine whether further interventions are needed. Additional data collection may be necessary to determine if the initial plan can produce change. For example, if no changes were seen in infection rates between the pilot and general group, it may mean that data needs to be collected for a longer period of time to show results. Re-examine the changes made to the current work process. Does it need revision? Are staff involved in the pilot following the new process?

VIII. Make the change.

A. If it is clear that the pilot project has produced positive change, communicate process changes to staff and patients.

B. Educate staff as needed and implement the changes unit-wide.

C. Continue collecting data over time to ensure positive outcomes.

D. Changes in policies and procedures must be approved by and adopted by the facility's governing body/organization.

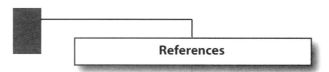

References

Adams, D., & Elliott, T. (2006). Impact of safety needle devices on occupationally acquired needlestick injuries: A four-year prospective study. *Journal of Hospital Infections, 64*, 50-55.

Alter, M.J. (n.d.). *Epidemiology of hepatitis C in dialysis units.* Retrieved August 8, 2006, from http://www.hcvadvocate.org/news/NewsUpdates_pdf/2.2_Conference_Reports/renal_agenda/Section3/alter.pdf

Alter, M.J., Favero, M.S., Miller, J.K., Coleman, P.J., & Bland, L.A. (1988). Reuse of hemodialyzers. Results of nationwide surveillance for adverse effects. *Journal of the American Medical Association, 260*(14), 2073-2076.

Alter, M.J., & Tokars, J.T. (2001). Preventing transmission of infections among chronic hemodialysis patients. *Nephrology Nursing Journal, 28*, 537-585.

Alter, M.J., Tokars, J.T., Arduibo, M.J., & Favero, M.S. (2004). Nosocomial infections associated with hemodialysis. In C.G. Mayhill (Ed.), *Hospital epidemiology and infection control* (3rd ed., pp. 1139-1160). Baltimore: Lippincott Williams & Wilkins.

American Academy of Pediatrics. (1997). Staphylococcal infections. In G. Peter (Ed.), *1997 Red book: Report of the Committee on Infectious Disease* (24th ed.). Elk Grove Village, IL: Author.

American Thoracic Society. (1994). Treatment of tuberculosis and tuberculosis infection in adults and children. *American Journal of Respiratory and Critical Care Medicine, 149*, 1359-1374.

American Thoracic Society, Centers for Disease Control and Prevention (CDC). (2003, June 20). Treatment for tuberculosis: American Thoracic Society, CDC and Infectious Diseases Society. *MMWR Recommendations and Reports, 52*(RR11).

Arduino, M.J. (1999). Proper mechanisms for assuring disinfectant concentrations for use in hemodialysis. *Nephrology News & Issues, 13*(6), 18, 23, 27.

Arnow, P.M., Garcia-Houchins, S., Neagle, M.B., Bova, J.L., Dillon, J.J., & Chou, T. (1998). An outbreak of bloodstream infections arising from hemodialysis equipment. *Journal of Infectious Diseases, 178*(3), 783-791.

Association for Professionals in Infection Control and Epidemiology, Inc. (APIC). (2005a). *Multiple drug-resistant bacteria prevention and control.* Retrieved May 26, 2006, from http://www.apic.org/AM/AMTemplate.cfm?Section=Brochures&Template=/CM/ContentDisplay.cfm&ContentFileID=2573

Association for Professionals in Infection Control and Epidemiology (APIC). (2005b). *Will antibiotics work for me when I need them?* Retrieved May 24, 2006, from http://www.apic.org/AM/Template.cfm?Section=Search&section=Brochures&template=/CM/ContentDisplay.cfm&ContentFileID=9024

Association for the Advancement of Medical Instrumentation (AAMI). (2003). *Recommended practice: Reuse of hemodialyzers,* ANSI/AAMI RD47-RD47:2002/A1:2003. Arlington, VA: Author.

Association for the Advancement of Medical Instrumentation (AAMI). (2004). *Recommended practice: Dialysate for hemodialysis,* ANSI/AAMI RD52-2004. Arlington, VA: Author.

Ball, L. (2005). Improving arteriovenous fistula cannulation skills. *Nephrology Nursing Journal, 32*(6), 611-617.

Beck-Sague, C.M., Jarvis, W.R., Bland, L.A., Arduino, M.J., Aguero, S.M., & Verosic, G. (1990). Outbreak of gram-negative bacteremia and pyrogenic reactions in a hemodialysis center. *American Journal of Nephrology, 10*(5), 397-403.

Besarab, A. (2001). Vascular access for hemodialysis. In J.T. Daugirdas, P.G. Blake, & T.S. Ing (Eds.), *Handbook of dialysis* (3rd ed., pp. 76-77). Philadelphia: Lippincott Williams & Wilkins.

Bland, L., Alter, M., Favero, M., Carson, L., & Cusick, L. (1985). Hemodialyzer reuse: Practices in the United States and implication for infection control. *Trans American Society of Artificial Internal Organs, 31*, 556-559.

Bland, L.A., Arduino, M.J., Aguero, S.M., & Favero, M.S. (1989). Recovery of bacteria from reprocessed high flux dialyzers after bacterial contamination of the header spaces and O-rings. *ASAIO Transactions, 35*(3), 314-316.

Bolan, G., Reingold, A.L., Carson, L.A., Silcox, V.A., Woodley, C.L., Hayes, P.S., et al. (1985). Infections with *Mycobacterium chelonei* in patients receiving dialysis and using processed hemodialyzers. *Journal of Infectious Disease, 152*(5), 1013-1019.

Bond, W.W., Petersen, N.J., & Favero, M.S. (1977). Viral hepatitis B: Aspects of environmental control. *Health Laboratory Science, 14*(4), 235-252.

Bridges, E.J., & Dukes, M.S. (2005). Cardiovascular aspects of septic shock. *Critical Care Nurse, 25*(2), 14-42.

Casey, K. (1993). Fighting MDR-TB. *RN, 56*, 26-30.

Centers for Disease Control and Prevention (CDC). (1985). Recommendations for preventing transmission of infection with human t-lymphotropic virus type III/lymphadenopathy-associated virus in the workplace. *MMWR, 34*(45), 682-686, 691-695.

Centers for Disease Control and Prevention (CDC). (1987). Recommendations for prevention of HIV transmission in health-care settings. *MMWR, 36*(Suppl. 2), 1S-18S.

Centers for Disease Control and Prevention (CDC). (1994). *Core curriculum on tuberculosis – What the clinician should know* (3rd ed.). Atlanta: Author.

Centers for Disease Control and Prevention (CDC). (1995). Hospital Infection Control Practices Advisory Committee: Recommendations for preventing the spread of Vancomycin resistance. *American Journal of Infection Control, 23*(2), 87.

Centers for Disease Control and Prevention (CDC). (2001a). Guidelines for the management of occupational exposures to hepatitis B, hepatitis C, and HIV and recommendations for postexposure prophylaxis. *MMWR, 50*(RR11), 1-52.

Centers for Disease Control and Prevention (CDC). (2001b). Recommendations for preventing transmission of infections among chronic hemodialysis patients. *MMWR, 50*(RR05), 1-43.

Centers for Disease Control and Prevention (CDC). (2003a). *Campaign to prevent antimicrobial resistance in health care settings: 12 steps to prevent antimicrobial resistance among dialysis patients.* Retrieved February 19, 2008, from http://www.cdc.gov/drugresistance/healthcare/dialysis/12steps_dialysis.htm

Centers for Disease Control and Prevention (CDC). (2003b). *Tips for dialysis patients to prevent antibiotic resistance.* Retrieved May 26, 2006, from http://www.cdc.gov/drugresistance/healthcare/dialysis/Tips_for_Dialysis_Patients.pdf

Centers for Disease Control and Prevention (CDC). (2004a). Incidence of acute hepatitis B – United States, 1990–2002. *MMWR, 52*(51 & 52), 1252-1254.

Centers for Disease Control and Prevention (CDC). (2004b). *Interactive core curriculum on tuberculosis: What the clinican should know.* Retrieved February 19, 2008, from http://cdc.gov/tb/webcourses/corecurr/index.htm

Centers for Disease Control and Prevention (CDC). (2004c). Tuberculosis outbreaks in prison housing units for HIV infected inmates. California 1995-1996. *MMWR, 54*, 1280.

Centers for Disease Control and Prevention (CDC). (2005a). *Community-associated MRSA information for clinicians.* Retrieved June 10, 2006, from http://www.cdc.gov/ncidod/dhqp/ar_mrsa_ca_clinicians.html

Centers for Disease Control and Prevention (CDC). (2005b). Guidelines for preventing the transmission of *M. tuberculosis* in healthcare settings. *MMWR, 54*, RR-17.

Centers for Disease Control and Prevention (CDC). (2005c). Prevention and control of influenza: Recommendations on the Advisory Committee on Immunization Practices (ACIP). *MMWR, 54*(RR-8), 1-41.

Centers for Disease Control and Prevention (CDC). (2005d). Updated U.S. public health service guidelines for the management of occupational exposures to HIV and recommendations for postexposure prophylaxis. *MMWR, 54*(RR9), 1-17.

Centers for Disease Control and Prevention (CDC). (2006a). *Guidelines for vaccinating kidney dialysis patients and patients with chronic kidney disease.* Retrieved June 22, 2006, from http://www.cdc.gov/vaccines/pubs/downloads/b_dialysis_guide.pdf

Centers for Disease Control and Prevention (CDC). (2006b). Recommendations for HIV testing of adults, adolescents and pregnant women in health-care settings. *MMWR, 55*(RR14), 1-17.

Centers for Disease Control and Prevention (CDC). (2006c). Recommendations to improve preconception health and health care – United States. *MMWR, 55*(RR06), 1-23.

Centers for Disease Control and Prevention (CDC). (2007). *Healthy people 2010.* Retrieved August 8, 2006, from http://www.healthy people.gov/

Centers for Disease Control and Prevention (CDC): Division of Tuberculosis Elimination. (2004). *Core curriculum on tuberculosis* (4th ed.). Slide sets. Retrieved December 12, 2007, from http://www.cdc.gov/tb/pubs/slidesets/core/html/trans5_slides.htm

Centers for Disease Control and Prevention (CDC), National Center for HIV, STD and TB Prevention. (2006a). *Hepatitis D virus: Slide set (1-7).* Retrieved August 8, 2006, from http://www.cdc.gov/ncidod/diseases/hepatitis/slideset/hep_d/slide_1.htm

Centers for Disease Control and Prevention, National Center for HIV, STD and TB Prevention. (2006b). *Viral hepatitis.* Retrieved August 8, 2006, from http://www.cdc.gov/ncidod/diseases/hepatitis/b/

Collins, C.H., & Kennedy, D.A. (1987). Microbiological hazards of occupational needlestick and other sharps' injuries. *Journal of Applied Bacteriology, 62*, 385-402.

Dodson, A.P., & Borriello, S.P. (1996). Clostridium difficile infection of the gut. *Journal of Clinical Pathology, 49*(7), 529-532.

Dogra, G., Herson, H., Hutchison, B., Irish, A., Heath, C., Golledge, C., et al. (2002). Prevention of tunneled hemodialysis catheter-related infections using catheter restricted filling with gentamycin and citrate. *Journal of the American Society of Nephrology, 13*, 2133-2139.

Dyer, E. (1993). Argentinian doctors accused of spreading AIDS. *British Medical Journal, 307*(6904), 584.

Favero, M.S., Deane, N., Leger, R.T., & Sosin, A.E. (1981). Effect of multiple use of dialyzers on hepatitis B incidence in patients and staff. *Journal of the Amerian Medical Association, 245*(2), 166-167.

Finelli, L., Miller, J.T., Tokars, J.I., Alter, M.J., & Arduino, M.J. (2005). National surveillance of dialysis-associated diseases in the United States, 2002. *Seminars in Dialysis, 18*(1), 52-61.

Flaherty, J.P., Garcia-Houchins, S., Chudy, R., & Arnow, P.M. (1993). An outbreak of gram-negative bacteremia traced to contaminated O-rings in reprocessed dialyzers. *Annals of Internal Medicine, 119*(11), 1072-1078.

Gordon, S.M., Oettinger, C.W., Bland, L.A., Oliver, J.C., Arduino, M.J., Aguero, S.M., et al. (1992). Pyrogenic reactions in patients receiving conventional, high-efficiency, or high-flux hemodialysis treatments with bicarbonate dialysate containing high concentrations of bacteria and endotoxin. *Journal of the American Society of Nephrology, 2*(9),1436-1444.

Hartigan, M., & White, R. (2001). Circulatory access for hemodialysis. In L.E. Lancaster (Ed.), *Core curriculum for nephrology nursing* (4th ed., pp. 313-325). Pitman, NJ: American Nephrology Nurses' Association.

Jackson, B.M., Beck-Sague, C.M., Bland, L.A., Arduino, M.J., Meyer, L., & Jarvis, W.R. (1994). Outbreak of pyrogenic reactions and gram-negative bacteremia in a hemodialysis center. *American Journal of Nephrology, 14*(2), 85-89.

Jo, H. (1993). Assessment and management of person co-infected with tuberculosis and human immunodeficiency virus. *Nurse Practitioner, 18*, 42-49.

Jochimsen, E.M., Frenette, C., Delorme, M., Arduino, M., Aguero, S., Carson, L., et al. (1998). A cluster of bloodstream infections and pyrogenic reactions among hemodialysis patients traced to dialysis machine waste-handling option units. *American Journal of Nephrology, 18*(6), 485-489.

Katsaragakis, S., Larentzakis, A., Drimousis, P., Mpantias, C., Arhontovasilis, F., & Theodorou, D. (2005). Rapid fluid removal via continuous venovenous hemodiafiltration and oxygen delivery, oxygen consumption, and outcome in septic patients with renal dysfunction. *Dialysis & Transplantation, 34*(9), 608-615, 646.

Kaysen, G., & Kumar, V. (2003). Inflammation in ESRD: Causes and potential consequences. *Journal of Renal Nutrition, 13*(2), 158-160.

Lochner, M., & Wolf, A. (2006). Human immunodeficiency virus-1 associated nephropathy (HIVAN): Epidemiology, pathogenesis, histology, diagnosis, and medical management. *Nephrology Nursing Journal, 33*, 259-267.

Lowry, P.W., Beck-Sague, C.M., Bland, L.A., Aguero, S.M., Arduino, M.J., Minuth, A.N., et al. (1990). Mycobacterium chelonae infection among patients receiving high-flux dialysis in a hemodialysis clinic in California. *Journal of Infectious Disease, 161*(1), 85-90.

Mandolfo, S., Piazza, W., & Galli, F. (2002). Central venous catheter and the hemodialysis patient. *The Journal of Vascular Access, 3*, 64-73.

Manian, F.A. (Ed.). (1997). *APIC handbook of infection control.* Washington, DC: Association for Professionals in Infection Control and Epidemiology, Inc.

McCleary, J., Caldero, K., & Adams, T. (2002). Guarded fistula needle reduces needlestick injuries in hemodialysis. *Nephrology News and Issues, 16*(6), 66-70, 72.

Miller, J., Alter, M., & Tokars, J. (1999). Protective effect of hepatitis B vaccine in chronic hemodialysis patients. *American Journal of Kidney Disease, 33*, 356-360.

Mills, E.J. (2006). Infectious disease. In S.M. Nettina (Ed.), *Lippincott manual of nursing practice* (3rd ed., pp. 1030-1048). Philadelphia: Lippincott Williams & Wilkins.

National Kidney Foundation (NKF). (2001). *KDOQI clinical practice guidelines for vascular access, 2000.* New York: Author.

National Kidney Foundation (NKF). (2006). KDOQI clinical practice guidelines for vascular access. *American Journal of Kidney Disease, 48*(Suppl. 1).

Panlilio, A.L., Cardo, D.M., Campbell, S., Srivastava, P.U., Jagger, H., Orelien, J.G., et al. (2000, March). Estimate of the annual number of percutaneous injuries in U.S. healthcare workers [Abstract S-T2-01]. *Program and abstracts of the 4th International Conference on Nosocomial and Healthcare-Associated Infections, Atlanta,* 61.

Parker, J., Dickenson, L., Wiseman, K.C., Alexander, D., & Peacock, E. (1998). Control of infectious diseases in the renal patient. In J. Parker (Ed.), *Contemporary nephrology nursing* (1st ed., p. 347-402). Pitman, NJ: American Nephrology Nurses' Association.

Peacock, E. (2006). Infections in the hemodialysis unit. In A.E. Molzahn & E. Butera (Eds.), *Contemporary nephrology nursing: Principles & practice* (2nd ed., pp. 419-453, 565-570). Pitman, NJ: American Nephrology Nurses' Association.

Pegues, D.A., Oettinger, C.W., Bland, L.A., Oliver, J.C., Arduino, M.J., Aguero, S.M., et al. (1992). A prospective study of pyrogenic reactions in hemodialysis patients using bicarbonate dialysis fluids filtered to remove bacteria and endotoxin. *Journal of the American Society of Nephrology, 3*(4), 1002-1007.

Protic, J., & Hardy, D. (1993). Resurgence of tuberculosis and emergence of multi-drug-resistant strains: Implications for health care personnel. In *Plant technology & safety management series, controlling occupational exposure to tuberculosis.* Oakbrook Terrace, IL: Joint Commission on Accreditation of Healthcare Organizations.

Rudnick, J.R., Arduino, M.J., Bland, L.A., Cusick, L., McAllister, S.K., Aguero, S.M., et al. (1995). An outbreak of pyrogenic reactions in chronic hemodialysis patients associated with hemodialyzer reuse. *Artificial Organs, 19*(4), 289-294.

Schulger, N., & Rom, W. (1994). Current approaches to the diagnosis of active pulmonary tuberculosis. *American Journal of Respiratory and Critical Care Medicine, 149*, 264-267.

Shah, C., Mittelman, M., Costerton, J., Parenteau, S., Pelak, M., Arsenault, R., et al. (2002). Antimicrobial activity of a novel catheter lock solution. *American Society for Microbiology, 46*(6), 1674-1679.

Shimokurs, G., Weber, D., Miller, W., Wurtzel, H., & Alter, M. (2006). Factors associated with personal protection equipment use and hand hygiene among hemodialysis staff. *American Journal of Infection control, 34*, 100-107.

Sohn, S., Eagan, J., Sepkowitz, K., & Zuccotti, G. (2004). Effect of implementing safety-engineered devices on percutaneous injury epidemiology. *Journal of Hospital Infections, 25*, 536-542.

Szymanski, N. (2001). Infection and inflammation in dialysis patients: Impact on laboratory parameters and anemia. *Nephrology Nursing Journal, 28*(3), 337-340.

Tokars, J.I., Alter, M.J., Arduino, M.J., & Favero, M.S. (2005). Nosocomial infections in hemodialysis units. In B.J.G. Periera, M.H. Sayegh, & P. Blake (Eds.), *Chronic kidney disease, dialysis, and transplantation: Companion to Brenner and Rector's the kidney* (2nd ed., pp. 429-450). Philadelphia: Elsevier Saunders.

Velandia, M., Fridkin, S.K., Cárdenas, V., Boshell, J., Ramirez, G., Bland, L., et al. (1995). Transmission of HIV in dialysis centre. *Lancet, 345*(8962), 1417-1422.

Wang, S.A., Levine, R.B., Carson, L.A., Arduino, M.J., Killar, T., Grillo, F.G., et al. (1999). An outbreak of gram-negative bacteremia in hemodialysis patients traced to hemodialysis machine waste drain ports. *Infection Control & Hospital Epidemiology, 20*(11), 746-751.

Welbel, S.F., Schoendorf, K., Bland, L.A., Arduino, M.J., Groves, C., Schable, B., et al. (1995). An outbreak of gram-negative bloodstream infections in chronic hemodialysis patients. *American Journal of Nephrology, 15*(1), 1-4.

World Health Organization (WHO). (2005). *AIDS epidemic update.* Retrieved August 8, 2006, from http://www.who.int/hiv/epi-update2005_en.pdf

Young, E., Contreras, G., Robert, N., Vogt, N., & Courtney, T. (2005). Incidence and influencing factors associated with exit site infections in temporary catheters for hemodialysis and apheresis. *Nephrology Nursing Journal, 32*(1), 41-49.

Zoccali, C., Mallamaci, F., & Tripepi, G. (2004). Novel cardiovascular risk factors in end-stage renal disease. *American Society of Nephrology, 15*, S77-S80.

Suggested Readings

Arduino, M.J., Tokars, J.I., Lyerla, R., & Alter, M. (2001). Preventing health-care associated transmission of bloodborne pathogens in hemodialysis facilities. *Seminars in Infection Control, 1*, 49-60.

Bayes, B., Bonal, J., & Romero, R. (1999). Sodium citrate for filling hemodialysis catheters. *Nephrology Dialysis Transplantation, 14*(10), 2532-2533.

Betjes, M., & Agteren, M. (2004). Prevention of dialysis catheter-related sepsis with a citrate-taurolidine containing lock solution. *Nephrology Dialysis Transplantation, 19*(6), 1546-1551.

El Sayed, N.M., Gomatos, P.J., Beck-Sague, C.M., Dietrich, U., von Briesen, H., Osmanov, S., et al. (2000). Epidemic transmission of human immunodeficiency virus in renal dialysis centers in Egypt. *Journal of Infectious Diseases, 181*(1), 91-97.

Favero, M.S. (2000). Role of the CDC in hemodialysis: A historical perspective. *Seminars in Dialysis, 13*(2), 64-67.

Hassan, N.F., el Ghorab, N.M., Abdel Rehim, M.S., el Sharkawy, M.S., El Sayed, N.M., Emara, K., et al. (1994). HIV infection in renal dialysis patients in Egypt. *AIDS, 8*(6), 853.

Mapes, D. (2005). Nurses' impact on the choice and longevity of vascular access. *Nephrology Nursing Journal, 32*(6), 670-673.

Marcus, R., Favero, M.S., Banerjee, S., Solomon, S.L., Bell, D.M., Jarvis, W.R., et al. (1991). Prevalence and incidence of human immunodeficiency virus among patients undergoing long-term hemodialysis. The Cooperative Dialysis Study Group. *American Journal of Medicine, 90*(5), 614-619.

Rao, T.K. (2003). Human immunodeficiency virus infection in end-stage renal disease patients. *Seminars in Dialysis, 16*(3), 233-244.

Section 18

Emergency and Disaster Preparedness

Section Editor

Norma Gomez, MBA, BSN, RN, CNN

Authors

Norma Gomez, MBA, BSN, RN, CNN

Anita Lipman, MS, BSN, RN, CNN

Debra McDillon, MSN, RN, CNN

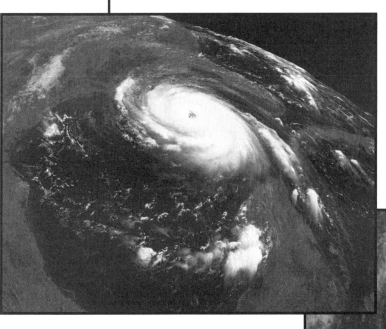

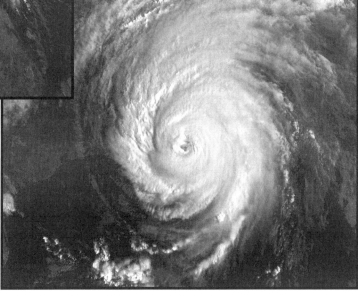

About the Authors

Norma Gomez, MBA, BSN, RN, CNN, Section Editor and Author, is Director of Education at DaVita, Inc., in Homestead, Florida.

Anita Lipman, MS, BSN, RN, CNN, is Anemia Specialist at Roche Labs in Toms River, New Jersey.

Debra McDillon, MSN, RN, CNN, is Director of Clinical Education at DaVita, Inc., in Munster, Indiana.

Title page photos from Web site (public domain): www.katrina.noaa.gov/satellite/satellite.html. Our appreciation to the National Oceanic and Atmospheric Administration (NOAA) for making the photos available.

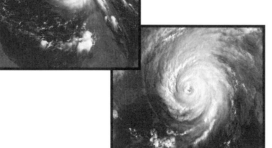

Hurricane Katrina
August 28, 2005, 11:45 a.m.

Hurricane Katrina
August 29, 2005, 10:15 a.m.

Emergency and
Disaster Preparedness

Emergency and Disaster Preparedness

Purpose

The purpose of this section is to review the different types of natural and man-made disasters, provide strategies for formulating a plan for individual facilities and to provide a general outline for developing a facility Disaster Preparedness Plan. The plan requires the collaboration of administration, clinical and technical staffs, patients, families, and community resources.

Objectives

Upon completion of this section, the learner will be able to:
1. Define the role of the nephrology nurse in disaster and emergency preparedness and response.
2. Provide strategies for training of employees, patients, and communities in disaster emergency preparedness.
3. List resources and references for further information, tools, and expert advice.
4. Identify best practices and strategies for dealing with disaster situations.

Chapter 70

General Information about Disasters

Introduction

I. **A disaster can be defined as a significant disruption** to the health and safety of a community caused by natural forces, physical failures of machinery or infrastructures, or the conduct of an individual that results in a significant disruption of health and safety of the community or the nation (ANA, 2002). Disasters, natural and otherwise, are unpredictable and occur with regularity.

II. **In the past 40 years, over 5 billion people have** been affected by over 6,000 documented natural disasters including Hurricane Katrina (2005), Asian

Tsunami (2004), Hurricane Andrew (1992), Oakland Wildfires (1991), Hurricane Hugo (1989), Loma Prieta earthquake (1989), and Hurricane Camille (1969). *Natural disasters*, along with man-made disasters, take a toll on thousands of lives and come with a cost of billions of dollars. *Man-made disasters* include occurrences such as workplace violence, school violence, chemical explosions, and terrorist attacks.

III. **Disasters do not need to be a large scale global** event. The majority will occur on a local level affecting a defined community. Specific emergency preparedness procedures should be developed for different kinds of emergencies. Each facility should assess their local area and region for potential risks of particular emergencies such as coastal areas for hurricanes and flooding. Man-made disasters such as power outages, fuel or water supply failures, chemical spills, arson, and other disasters should also be considered. Once the risks are identified, a comprehensive, systematic, emergency preparedness program should be developed that outlines concrete goals, identifiable resources, education, and communication of the plans.

IV. The federal ESRD regulations require written policies and procedures for handling emergencies that may threaten the health and safety of patients.

V. It is important to have a written disaster plan outlining the steps to be taken. The plan should be easy to understand and accessible to all personnel and patients. In addition, the plan should be evaluated and updated at least annually. Facilities should coordinate the plan with community resources: nearby units, local hospitals, and local emergency operations centers (EOC). Intrafacility agreements should exist among dialysis units that enable one unit to dialyze affected patients from another facility when that facility is no longer operational. These facilities are often called "sister" units. The physical distance between the facilities must be a consideration. If the units are close together, they may all be affected by the disaster. If they are far apart, patient transportation may be an issue. In some communities, a local hospital is identified as a command center to facilitate communication with staff and patients. Contact with the local emergency management office should be made to see how a dialysis facility fits into the overall local plan.

VI. The emergency management model created by the Federal Emergency Management Agency (FEMA) can be used as a basis for any disaster preparedness program (www.fema.gov). The model has four activity phases that are a continuous process: preparedness, response, recovery, and mitigation. This model emphasizes evaluation and applying lessons learned to future events.

A. Preparedness phase involves developing a plan to educate the workforce and other stakeholders.

B. Response phase occurs when the plan is implemented. The important components of this phase are patient management and communication.

C. Recovery phase encompasses intervention to get the community back to the pre-disaster baseline.

D. During the final mitigation stage, activities are undertaken to minimize the negative impact of the event.

VII. Included in this section is an outline of a General Disaster Plan that can be used for all types of disasters. It will use a basic three-phase process: pre-event planning, response to the event, and post-event restoration (Lettieri, 2006). Specific actions for each type of natural and man-made disaster are outlined in the various sections below. No matter what the disaster may be and what type of plan is developed, there are always communication, water, power, supplies, transportation, and safety issues to be addressed.

General Disaster Plan

I. The pre-event phase is defined by anticipation, planning, and training. The focus on this phase is to decrease risks associated with events.

A. Review possible threats to the facility. The disaster plan must address all potential threats including but not limited to:
1. Susceptibility to hurricanes, floods, tornadoes, earthquakes, wild fires, and volcanic eruptions.
2. Man-made disasters such as power outages, water main breaks, interruption in fuel and water supplies, chemical spills, arson, and bomb threats.
3. Chemical plant or nuclear power plant accidents.

B. Communication is a critical component (see Table 18.1).
1. Assess existing communication systems: cell phones, ham radios, satellite phones, toll free numbers, TV and radio public service announcements, local newspapers, and Web sites.
2. Provide an analog phone (newer phones require electricity to work).
3. Identify communication needs: purchase or rent satellite phones – training on use.
4. Identify who will have the responsibility of communicating damage of the facility before, during, and after the event, depending on type of disaster.

Table 18.1

Disaster Communications Template

Normal Status	Level I	Level II	Level III	Level IV
Normal Operations – Preparations	**Potential Threat Identified – Monitoring Phase**	**Disaster Event Identified as Threat**	**Imminent Threat**	**Post-event/Recovery**
Education — This includes patients, employees, and physicians. Includes disaster plans, personal preparedness, emergency diet, local hazards, etc.	**Monitor situation** — Monitor local news/weather, EOCs, network, etc., concerning expected conditions.	**Activate emergency team** — Team responsible for emergency coordination and preparation.	**Activate at facility level** — Team responsible for emergency coordination and preparation. Review plan and post-event procedures.	**Coordinate and respond** — Team responsible for emergency coordination and recovery.
Update contact information — Patients, employees, and physicians. Local and out-of-town.	**Education** — This includes patients, employees, and physicians. Includes disaster plans, personal preparedness, emergency diet, local hazards, etc.	**Conference calls** — Calls with primary team concerning threatened event preparation, include physicians in planning.	**Conference calls** — Calls with primary team concerning threatened event preparation, include physicians in planning.	**Conference calls** — Calls with primary team concerning event recovery, facility status, assistance needed, etc., and include physicians.
Supplies — Order and maintain 2 weeks of treatment supplies. During extreme weather "seasons," additional supplies should be on hand as physical plant allows.	**Update contact information** — Patients, employees, and physicians. Local and out-of-town.	**Post-closure signage** — Ensure signs with facility emergency contact and alternate treatment information are posted on front door.	**Update closure signage** — Ensure signs with facility emergency contact and alternate treatment information are posted on front door.	**Update closure signage** — Ensure signs with facility emergency contact and alternate treatment information are posted on front door.
Facility policy and procedures — Review policy and procedures. Ensure all employees are familiar.	**Facility policy and procedures** — Review and discuss policy and procedures. Ensure all employees are familiar.	**Communicate status to network/EOC** — Advise facility status/operational plan to network, transportation providers, and local EOC.	**Communicate status to network/EOC** — Update facility status/operational plan to network, transportation providers, and local EOC.	**Communicate status to network/EOC** — Advise facility status (damage, operations, special needs, etc.) to network, transportation providers, and local EOC.
Meetings — Schedule meetings with physicians, local EOCs, hospitals, LDOs, etc. to discuss disaster preparedness and planning.	**Inventory** — Review inventory to ensure 2 weeks of treatment supplies on hand. Update if necessary. Communicate with contracted supply vendors regarding contingency deliveries.	**Inventory** — Verify inventory includes 2 weeks of additional supplies on hand at facility. Update if necessary.	**Inventory** — Verify inventory includes 2 weeks of additional treatment supplies on hand. Make adjustments where necessary.	**Inventory** — Assess inventory of treatment supplies on hand and update if necessary. Activate appropriate contingency plans with contracted vendors for deliveries.
Local hazards — Be familiar with flood zones and evacuation areas.	**Local hazards** — Be familiar with flood zones and evacuation areas.	**Local hazards** — Be familiar with flood zones and evacuation areas.	**Local hazards** — Evaluate evacuation areas and prepare to activate plan.	**Local hazards** — Be familiar with flood zones and evacuation areas, damage areas and curfews in effect.

	Normal Status Normal Operations – Preparations	Level I Potential Threat Identified – Monitoring Phase	Level II Disaster Event Identified as Threat	Level III Imminent Threat	Level IV Post-event/Recovery
Home/Family preparedness	Encourage patients and employees to prepare their home and family for potential event.	Encourage patients and allow employees time to prepare their home and family (gas, extra money, generators, etc.).	Encourage patients and verify that employees have prepared their home and families (gas, extra money, generators, etc.). Allow additional time necessary to complete preparations.	Encourage patients and verify that employees have prepared their home and families (gas, extra money, generators, etc.). Allow additional time necessary to complete preparations.	Assess damage/status of employees, physicians, and patients and coordinate and assist where identified.
Special needs	Identify the special needs of patients, employees, and physicians.	Identify the special needs of patients, employees, and physicians.	Identify the special needs of patients, employees, and physicians.	Reassess the special needs of patients, employees, and physicians.	Identify the special needs of patients, employees, and physicians.
Communication plan / Staffing needs	Establish a call-tree, call-down, voicemail, or call system for key facility people. Identify how facility status and plans are communicated to staff and patients.	Review call-tree, call-down, voicemail, or call system for key facility people. Identify how facility status and plans are communicated to staff and patients.	Evaluate staffing needs and adjust schedules relative to threatened event.	Evaluate staffing needs and adjust schedules relative to threatened event.	Evaluate staffing needs and adjust schedules for post-event.
Physical plant	Evaluate needs to protect property and continuous operations. Agreements with local contractors, electricians, fuel, etc.	Evaluate needs to protect property and continuous operations. Agreements with local contractors, electricians, fuel, etc.	Evaluate needs to protect property and continuous operations. Agreements with local contractors, electricians, fuel, etc.	Prepare facility for event; may include boarding/shuttering, securing medical records in waterproof containers, covering machines/equipment/computers, backup data, generator, securing biohazardous waste, extra keys to key people, etc.	Evaluate facility status before allowing personnel into facility. Determine needs for reestablishing operations. Ensure water and equipment safety. Outside hazards (trees, down power lines, building damage).
Update contact information	Maintain updated contact information on patients, employees, and physicians – local and out-of-town.	Verify contact information on patients, employees, and physicians – local and out-of-town. Ask about evacuation plans.	Verify contact information on patients, employees, and physicians – local and out-of-town. Ask about evacuation plans.	Reverify contact information on patients, employees, and physicians – local and out-of-town. Ask for final evacuation plans.	Verify contact information on patients, employees, and physicians – local and out-of-town, current location (shelter, home, family, etc.).
Medical and employment records / Locate	Upon admission/employment, and in coordination with facility policies thereafter, issue patient/staff ID badges, facility emergency contact info and curfew letters and emergency contact cards.	Confirm that employees and patients can locate ID badges, facility emergency contact info, curfew letters, and emergency contact cards.	Confirm that employees and patients have located ID badges, facility emergency contact info, curfew letters, and emergency contact cards. Reissue if necessary.	Instruct employees and patients to maintain ID badges, facility emergency contact info, curfew letters, and emergency contact cards on their person at all times.	Locate and account for all of your patients, employees, and physicians – local and out-of-town (shelter, home, family, etc.). Notify network of any missing patients from your facility &/or evacuees treated at your facility.

5. Consider the facility's security system. In times of a disaster, distribute multiple keys and alarm codes to the building.

6. Consider how the patients and staff will be notified regarding status of the facility. Possible methods include:
   a. Sign on front door of clinic to inform patients and staff where to report. Provide directions.
   b. Staff member staying at facility to communicate the plan.
   c. Prearranged destination if facility not operational.
   d. Media announcements.

7. Have available a battery-operated backup radio.

8. Routinely update contact numbers for staff, patients, community resources, and vendors.
   a. If possible, before the event, determine where patients and staff will be during or after the storm: at their own home, with a relative in town, with relative out of town, shelters, etc.
   b. Inform shelters of special dietary and fluid needs of the dialysis patient as well as their priority status for transportation to a dialysis facility when travel conditions are clear.

C. Water, power, and supplies are essential considerations.

1. Identify emergency shut-off valves (electricity, gas, water, fire alarm, security, etc.).

2. There may be a "boil water advisory" issued by the community.
   a. Review water treatment components and assess ability to perform dialysis treatments.
   b. Increase testing procedures for microbial assessment.

3. Municipal water suppliers may "shock" (hyper-chlorinate) their systems to regain acceptable bacterial levels for drinking water. Review and update testing procedures for potential chlorine/chloramine breakthrough.

4. Locate emergency lighting in the patient care area, water treatment area, and along the path(s) of egress.

5. Assess the potential need for generator.
   a. Determine the size of the generator needed to run essential equipment.
   b. Implement a contract with a service to provide the correct size generator if needed post-disaster.
   c. If a facility owns a generator, develop and maintain maintenance schedules according to manufacturer's operating manual.
   d. Assess fuel needs; assume at least 2 to 3 days of fuel will be needed.
   e. Determine safe handling and storage of the fuel for a generator.
   f. Make arrangements for a contract for fuel before the event takes place.
   g. Develop a plan to protect the generator before, during, and after the disaster.
   h. Install an electrical transfer switch or automatic bus transfer (ABT) switch.

6. Keep at least 2 weeks additional inventory during times an event may occur (e.g., for hurricane season it would be in summer and fall; for winter storms it would be in winter). Remember that the reprocessing of dialyzers probably will not be performed during a disaster. Provide enough dry packs to perform treatments.

7. Put in place an agreement with a water vendor for delivery of water needs. Some facilities have agreements with local fire departments to supply water after an event.

D. Transportation for patients and staff.

1. If the facility has elevators, make an alternate plan for transporting the patients to the treatment area.

2. Contracts with local transportation companies for patient transportation prior to and after the event should be part of the facility plan.

3. Depending on the nature of the event (flooding, mudslides, iced roads) consider alternate methods for staff transportation.

4. If the disaster results in major damage or destruction to a community, pay attention to law enforcement requirements to enter the affected area. Curfews may be instituted affecting patients, staff, and physicians.

E. Hazardous waste: develop a plan for alternate disposal.

F. Include emergency standing orders in each patient's medical record regarding changes in their prescription based on a disaster.

II. Response to the threat – execution of the plan.

A. Communication is critical in this phase.
   1. Set up a command center.
   2. Place a poster in the facility door stating where patients and staff are to report.
   3. Inform patients and staff of the TV/radio stations that will announce facility closures.
   4. Advertise toll free numbers to be used at specific times postevent.
   5. Contact State Board of Nursing to assess what

tasks can be performed by an out-of-state RN or LPN in the case of a federally declared emergency. States participating in the Multistate License Pact have the advantage.

B. Implementation of the Emergency Diet Plan. If the facility does not have a 3-Day Emergency Diet Plan, refer to the National Kidney Foundation Web page (www.kidney.org). Patients should receive education on the emergency diet plan before the need to implement.

C. Triage. Before and after an event, patients may need additional treatments. If the facility was damaged, sister facilities may be dialyzing these patients. This influx of additional patients could require a change in the patient's schedule and prescribed therapy, such as decreased hours in treatment or increase in the length of time between treatments. A member of the medical team should give these orders.

III. Postevent phase – restoration.

A. Assess the facility structure before bringing patients back to dialyze.

B. Implement a process for locating patients and staff. Contact the local networks and CMS for assistance.

IV. Other issues.

A. Posttraumatic stress – emotional reactions may include feelings of shock, fear, grief, resentment, guilt, shame, helplessness, hopelessness, confusion, memory loss, interpersonal relationship issues (NCCTS, 2005). Basic objectives:
1. Enhance immediate and ongoing safety, and provide physical and emotional comfort.
2. Help survivors articulate immediate needs and concerns; gather additional information as appropriate.
3. Connect survivors as soon as possible to social support systems, including family members, friends, neighbors, and community resources.

B. Administrative issues may arise and processes may be interrupted.
1. Develop an alternative plan to deliver payroll if normal process is disrupted.
2. Identify an alternative billing process if normal process is disrupted.
3. Know your lease: Who is responsible for repairing the facility damage?

C. Provide patients with a waterproof container that contains last treatment sheet, dialysis prescription, and facility contact information.

D. Institute a form of patient identification such as an armband, name badge, or other method.

Table 18.2

Online Resources

American Association of Kidney Patients (AAKP) http://www.aakp.org/AAKP/Forms/ patientinformationsheet.pdf	Centers for Disease Control and Prevention http://www.cdc.gov http://www.pandemicflu.gov	National Council of State Boards of Nursing (NCSBN) http://www.ncsbn.org
American Hospital Association (AHA) http://www.hospitalconnect.com	Centers for Medicare and Medicaid Services (CMS) http://cms.hhs.gov	National Hurricane Center http://www.nhc.noaa.gov
American Kidney Fund (AKF) http://www.kidneyfund.org	Citizen Corps http://www.citizencorps.gov	National Kidney Foundation http://www.kidney.org
American Nephrology Nurses' Association (ANNA) http://annanurse.org	Federal Emergency Management Agency (FEMA) http://www.fema.gov	National Weather Service http://www.weather.gov
American Nurses Association (ANA) http://www.nursingworld.org	Forum of ESRD Networks http://www.esrdnetworks.org	The Weather Channel http://www.weather.com
American Red Cross http://www.redcross.org	Kidney Community Emergency Response Coalition http://www.KCERCoalition.com	United States Environmental Protection Agency http://www.epa.gov
Association of Organ Procurement Organizations (AOPO) http://www.aopo.org		United States Geological Survey http://pubs.usgs.gov http://water.usgs.gov/osw/

Chapter 71

Natural Disasters

I. Hurricanes.

A. Hurricanes are intense tropical weather systems with a well defined circulation and maximum sustained winds of 74 mph (64 knots) or higher.
1. A tropical depression is a weather system with rotating winds of 38 mph (33 knots) or less.
2. Tropical storms have sustained winds of 39-74 mph (34-63 knots).
3. Hurricanes are identified by categories and range from I to V. A category I storm has winds from 74 to 95 mph with storm surges of 4-5 feet. A category V has winds over 155 mph and storm surges higher than 18 feet.
4. The Saffir-Simpson Hurricane scale describes a hurricane's intensity.
   a. Descriptions can be found on the National Oceanic and Atmospheric Administration (NOAA) Web site (www.nhc.noaa.gov).
   b. Government and businesses use this information to estimate potential flooding and potential property damage when the hurricane makes landfall.
5. Systems are "named" according to a list developed by the National Hurricane Center.
6. In the Western Pacific, hurricanes are called *typhoons* and similar storms in the Indian Ocean are called *cyclones*.

B. Hurricane facts.
1. The United States shoreline attracts large numbers of people from Maine to Texas with an estimated 45 million people living along the hurricane-prone shoreline.
2. Hurricane season extends from the first of June to the end of November with peak months being August and September.
3. During a hurricane, homes, businesses, public buildings, roads, and power lines may be damaged by high winds and flooding. Debris can break windows and doors. Roads and bridges can be washed away by flash flooding or blocked by debris. The force of the wind alone can topple trees, remove roofs, and undermine weakened buildings. In addition, hurricanes can spawn tornadoes, which add to the destruction.

C. Hurricane warning system.
1. Very effective in providing timely warnings for people to properly prepare or move inland when a hurricane is threatening the area.
2. It is becoming more difficult to evacuate the coastal areas due to the increased population and the summer tourist seasons. People are still complacent and delay taking action, causing increased property damage and loss of life.

D. Hurricane watch.
1. During this advisory, the NOAA weather station should be closely monitored.
2. As appropriate, the staff should be allowed to leave the workplace in shifts to fuel cars and prepare homes, secure cash, home supplies, and medications.
3. Initiate facility disaster plan. Patients should be advised to begin personal preparations.

E. Hurricane warning.
1. During this advisory, monitor NOAA weather station for updates.
2. Continue following established disaster plan.
   a. Bring all outside items inside or tie down.
   b. Confirm that the facility has a battery-operated phone to continue phone service.
   c. Ensure facility has storm shutters or other approved window protection.
   d. If facility has a generator, be sure enough fuel is safely stored and is available to run the generator.

F. After the storm.
1. Everyone who must drive should do so carefully, avoiding dangling wires and flooded areas.
2. Report damaged water, sewer, and electric lines to the authorities.
3. Assess the possible presence of gas leaks.

G. Facility Action Plan.
1. Risk assessment should include the following:
   a. Facility.
      (1) Assess for potential loss of power, water, phone.
      (2) Assess potential flooding.

(3) Check roof for potential leaks or damage.

(4) Check windows for potential leaking.

b. Supplies and equipment.

   (1) Increase supply inventory during hurricane season.

   (2) Ensure equipment (including backup) is in operating order and will be secure during the storm.

   (3) Store all medical records in protective coverings and place them at least 24 inches off of the floor.

c. Community.

   (1) Assess emergency response plan, special shelters, transportation for patients and staff.

   (2) Make sure facility has a battery-operated backup radio.

d. Roles of staff members.

   (1) Chain of command procedures.

   (2) Ensure staff has time to secure their own home through flexible scheduling.

e. Education of patients.

   (1) In-center patients, peritoneal dialysis patients, and home patients should be educated on the disaster plan.

   (2) Transplant patients should be part of the transplant program's plan.

2. Communication.

a. Review and evaluate contact information to ensure it is still accurate for staff, patients, emergency contacts, community resources.

b. Perform drills to give staff hands-on preparation of what to do, to familiarize them with their roles, and to identify potential problems with the plan.

c. Keep all members of the team aware of the progress of any tropical storm or hurricane. Administrative personnel should meet when a storm is expected and make a final assessment of the plan and initiate a specific plan of action.

d. Change patient schedule to ensure all patients are dialyzed prior to the storm with an understanding they may need to go 3 days without dialysis. Notify transportation companies of schedule change.

e. Develop a communication plan in case phones are not functioning.

   (1) Include the use of cell phones, satellite phones, ham-operated radios.

   (2) Coordinate among sister facilities, local hospitals, and local, state, and federal agencies.

   (3) Develop a relationship with the local and state Emergency Operations Centers (EOC) and American Red Cross.

   (4) Use identified local radio and TV stations to get information out to the patients regarding opened and closed facilities.

3. In-center hemodialysis patients. Establish strategies to ensure transport agencies can facilitate transportation post-event.

4. Home hemodialysis patients.

a. Should keep a 2-week supply of dialysis supplies in case deliveries are delayed.

b. Must be able to perform emergency disconnect procedures in case power outage occurs during their treatment.

c. Patients should register with local water and power company for priority reinstatement of services.

d. If electrical power or water service is interrupted, they must know how to contact the dialysis staff to make alternate dialysis arrangements.

5. Peritoneal dialysis (PD) patients.

a. An electrical outage will affect continuous cycling peritoneal dialysis (CCPD) patients. These patients should possess the ability to perform manual exchanges during these times.

b. If patients are unable to perform as many exchanges as ordered, instruct them to implement the emergency diet and fluid restrictions plan.

c. Should have an emergency 5-day supply of antibiotics for peritonitis.

d. Should contact the center to report their status, when possible.

6. Transplant patients.

a. Should keep and carry with them a current list of their medications.

b. Should contact the transplant center to report their status, when possible.

7. Diabetic patients.

a. Should keep extra insulin and syringes.

b. Should keep extra batteries for glucometer.

8. Acute programs. Usually one of the staff members stays at the hospital during the storm and is then relieved post-storm.

9. All patients should:

a. Keep and carry a current list of medications.

b. Keep a 2-week supply of their medications.

c. Wear a medical information emblem.

d. Have a battery-powered AM/FM radio and flashlight with extra batteries.

e. Have a list of emergency phone numbers.

f. Prepare themselves and their household in the same ways as the general public.

H. Post-event.
 1. Assess damage and determine when treatments can resume.
 2. Curfews may be imposed.
 3. Staff and patients should have proper identification to be allowed into disaster area.

II. Tornadoes.

A. Tornadoes are violent storms that develop from powerful thunderstorms, or they can accompany tropical storms and hurricanes as the systems move onto land.
 1. Can last up to 1 hour, but most last less than 10 minutes.
 2. Appear as rotating, funnel-shaped clouds that extend from a thunderstorm to the ground.
 3. Average forward speed of a tornado is 30 mph, but winds can reach 300 mph.

B. Tornado facts.
 1. In the United States, only the National Weather Service issues tornado forecasts nationwide.
 2. Annually 1,000 tornadoes are reported across the United States, resulting in about 70 deaths each year. Most deaths are the result of flying or falling debris.
 3. Every state is at risk for tornadoes.
 4. Peak tornado seasons.
  a. Southern Plain – May to early June.
  b. Gulf Coast – early spring.
  c. Northern Plains and Upper Midwest – June and July.
  d. East of the Rocky Mountains – spring and summer months.
  e. Southern States – March through May.
  f. Northern States – late spring through early summer.
 5. Though tornadoes may move in any direction, the average tornado moves southwest to northeast.
 6. Tornadoes can occur at any time but most frequently occur between 3 and 9 p.m.

C. Tornado watch.
 1. Conditions are right for a tornado to form in the next several hours.
 2. During a tornado watch staff and patients should stay tuned to radio or television weather reports. Everyone needs to be aware of changing weather conditions.

D. Tornado warning.
 1. Indicates that a tornado has been spotted or indicated by weather radar.

2. A warning indicates imminent danger to life and property to those in the path of the storm.
3. Take immediate safety precautions.
 a. Quickly get to designated tornado-safe area. Safe areas are away from windows and glass.
 b. Cover should be taken within 1 minute of a tornado warning. Sixty-two percent of those killed by tornadoes die in the first 5 minutes after a warning is issued.
 c. Do not open windows.
 d. Do not use elevators.

E. Facility Action Plan.
 1. Devise a mechanism to receive and monitor weather reports.
 2. Know local emergency alert signals (sirens, etc.).
 3. After the tornado.
  a. All patients and staff should be accounted for.
  b. Check for injured or trapped persons.
  c. Provide first aid when appropriate.
  d. Contact authorities.
  e. Take caution for potential fires and hazards like broken electrical wires, water leaks, and gas or oil leaks. Have proper tools available to turn off these valves if necessary to do so.
 4. Evacuate patients if necessary.
 5. Patient education and preparation.
  a. Inform patients of the designated tornado safe place.
  b. Review and drill procedures for emergency discontinuation of the dialysis treatment.
  c. Instruct patients to lie face down and protect their head and dialysis access.
  d. If patients will have to miss a dialysis treatment, they should start the emergency diet plan.
  e. Patients need to inform shelter personnel about special needs such as diet and transportation issues.
 6. In-center hemodialysis patients.
  a. If patients are dialyzing in the facility, remove them from treatment using emergency disconnect protocols. Move them or help them move into the designated safe area.
  b. If moving cannot be accomplished, locate them away from windows. Place them under sturdy furniture and cover with blanket, coats, mattress, pillows, etc.
  c. Instruct patients to protect their heads and dialysis access extremities.
 7. Home hemodialysis patients.
  a. Must be able to perform emergency disconnect procedures in case power outage occurs during their treatment.

b. The patient and partner should go to safe area in lowest area of the house.

c. Protect the dialysis access and head.

d. The patient needs to get under a strong bench or heavy furniture if possible.

e. Patients residing in a mobile home must be able to get out of the mobile home quickly and take shelter in a building with a strong foundation.

f. If shelter is not available, instruct the patient to lie in a ditch or low-lying area between the tornado and mobile home.

g. Instruct patients to register with local water and power company for priority reinstatement of services.

h. Patients must know how to contact the dialysis staff to make alternate dialysis arrangements if there is a loss of power and/or water.

8. PD patients.

a. An electrical outage will affect CCPD patients. Patients should possess the ability to perform manual exchanges during these times.

b. If patients are unable to perform as many exchanges as ordered, instruct them to implement the emergency diet and fluid restrictions plan.

c. PD patients should have an emergency 5-day supply of antibiotics for peritonitis.

d. Make patients aware of emergency procedures to follow for tornadoes (see II.E.7. Home hemodialysis patients).

e. Should contact the center to report their status, when possible.

f. Instruct patients to register with local water and power company for priority reinstatement of services.

g. Inform patients of how to contact the dialysis staff so that alternate dialysis arrangements can be made if there is a loss of power and/or water.

9. Transplant patients.

a. Should keep and carry with them a current list of their medications.

b. Should contact the transplant center to report their status, when possible.

c. Should be aware of emergency procedures to follow for tornadoes (see II.E.7. Home hemodialysis patients).

10. Diabetic patients.

a. Should keep extra insulin and syringes.

b. Should keep extra batteries for glucometer.

c. Should be aware of emergency procedures to

follow for tornadoes (see II.E.7. Home hemodialysis patients).

11. All patients should:

a. Keep and carry with them a current list of medications.

b. Keep a 2-week supply of their medications.

c. Wear a medical information emblem.

d. Have a battery-powered AM/FM radio and flashlight with extra batteries.

e. Have a list of emergency phone numbers.

f. Prepare themselves and their household in the same ways as the general public.

III. Floods.

A. All floods are not alike. Some floods develop slowly, over a period of days.

1. Flash floods are usually caused by slow-moving thunderstorms or thunderstorms that move over the same area one after the other.

2. Overland flooding occurs outside a defined river or stream, such as when a levee is breached.

3. Everyone needs to be aware of flood hazards no matter where one lives, but particularly those that live in low-lying areas, near water or downstream from a dam.

4. Even very small streams, gullies, creeks, culverts, dry streambeds, or low-lying ground that appears harmless in dry weather can flood.

5. Every state is at risk from this hazard.

B. Flood facts.

1. Every year devastating floods occur throughout the United States.

a. 90% of all presidentially declared natural disasters involve flooding.

b. In the U.S., an average of 140 people lose their lives annually, and flood damage averages more than $6 billion (USGS, 2006).

c. The majority of deaths from flooding occur when people become trapped in automobiles that stall while driving through flooded areas. Nearly half of all flood fatalities are vehicle-related.

2. The principal causes of flooding in the Eastern United States and the Gulf Coast are hurricanes and storms.

3. The principal causes of floods in the Western United States are snow melts and rainstorms.

4. Flooding is the only natural disaster for which the federal government provides insurance: FEMA's National Flood Insurance Program.

Case Study: Flooding Disaster

January 9, 2000, was a cold Sunday evening. It was the kind of night when one looks forward to cuddling up with a good book to relax in preparation of a new week ahead. I was enjoying this as such when my phone rang. It was the police department in the town where the facility I managed was located. They reported that water was flowing out of the front door. With no real details to go by, I called the biomed technician who lived close to the facility, and I asked him to go assess the situation.

Within minutes, I was on the phone listening to the alarming voice of a normally calm man. I will never forget these words: "You had better get here — the unit is flooded!" I jumped in the car and raced up the Garden State Parkway headed toward the facility, not knowing what to expect.

I was not prepared for what I observed. Six inches of water covered every inch of the 11,000 square feet in our 32-station facility in New Jersey. Filth and sludge encompassed the entire floor plan. Together, the biomed technician and I discovered a huge gaping hole in the common wall that was shared between the plaza and the facility. Through the opening was a torrential flow of water. Apparently there was plumbing work completed in the utility room of this plaza that afternoon. The pipe, not tightly sealed, disconnected when the force of the water was turned on. Water burst through the wall and continued to flow until the water was discovered by the police at 9:30 in the evening.

We immediately had to make some quick decisions. First we called the grounds manager to come in to shut off the water. Within 30 minutes, people were entering the building in response to our frantic calls for help. We quickly discovered that we had no plan for such a disaster in the facility ... .and thus the adventure began.

We immediately called the housekeeping crew, and then some local staff to assist. To our pleasant surprise, the response to come in to assist was overwhelmingly positive. Someone even called his own brother to come in and video the event. The Department of Health was called due to the damage of supplies and equipment.

We all began to sweep the water out of the facility into the streets or down the drains. We soon saw the immensity of the damage with every drop. We touched base with patients to inform them of the potential delays. While everyone was disappointed, they appreciated the warning. We notified the transportation companies and anyone who could potentially be negatively affected without this knowledge.

The message quickly was sent out that we could not carry out business the next morning as scheduled. Being a large 32-station facility, with more than 185 patients, relocating each patient was a huge task. A unanimous decision to forge ahead to clean up the facility was made, and we formed a work team of several members and moved forward. For the next 10 hours we mopped and wet-vacuumed, cleaned and polished. Many supplies were discarded, while other supplies were redistributed to dry areas for the next day's work. We planned, communicated, networked, and brainstormed consistently until the facility was ready for the first patient at noon. Patients could not have been more supportive and tolerant of the delays regarding the night that was just endured.

After weeks of rebuilding and replenishing, and thousands of dollars later, the facility was back to normal, and the team spirit that was built that night is stronger than ever.

Anita Lipman

C. Flood watch.
1. A flood is possible in the area.
2. Stay alert to signs of flash flooding and be ready to evacuate on a moment's notice.
3. Flash flood watch indicates that flash flooding is a possibility in or close to the watch area.
   a. These watches are issued for flooding that is expected to occur within 6 hours after heavy rains have ended.
   b. Those in the affected area are urged to be ready to take action if a flash flood warning is issued or flooding is observed.

D. Flood warning.
1. Flooding is already occurring or will occur soon in the area.

2. Listen to local radio and TV stations for information and advice.
3. If told to evacuate, do so as soon as possible.
4. Do not drive around barricades — they are there for everyone's safety.
5. If a car stalls in rapidly rising waters, it should be abandoned immediately and the person(s) should climb to higher ground.

E. Facility Action Plan.
1. Develop a mechanism to receive and monitor weather reports.
2. Advertise the local emergency alert signals.
3. Install sump pumps with backup power.
4. A licensed electrician should raise electric components (switches, sockets, circuit breakers,

and wiring) at least 12 inches above the clinic's projected flood elevation.

5. For drains, toilets, and other sewer connections, install backflow valves or plugs to prevent floodwaters from entering.

6. Turn off all utilities at the main power switch and close the main gas valve if evacuation appears necessary.

7. After the flooding.
   a. All patients and staff should be accounted for.
   b. Evacuate patients if necessary.
   c. Patients and staff should have immunization records handy or be aware of last tetanus shot, in case of contamination during or after the flood.

8. Patient education and preparation.
   a. Instruct patients where they will go if forced to evacuate.
   b. Periodically review procedures and drills for emergency disconnect.
   c. If patients will have to miss a dialysis treatment, implement the emergency diet and fluid restriction plan.
   d. Patients need to tell shelter personnel about their special needs, such as diet and transportation to and from dialysis treatments.

9. In-center hemodialysis patients.
   a. If patients are dialyzing in the facility, stop the treatment using emergency protocols.
   b. Patients are to be moved into the designated safe area. Physical assistance is given as needed.

10. Home hemodialysis patients.
    a. Must be able to perform emergency disconnect procedures.
    b. The patient and partner should go to a safe area in highest part of the house.
    c. Should register with local water and power company for priority reinstatement of services.
    d. If electrical power or water service is interrupted, they must know how to contact the dialysis staff to make alternate dialysis arrangements.

11. PD patients.
    a. An electrical outage will affect CCPD patients. These patients should possess the ability to perform manual exchanges during these times.
    b. If patients are unable to perform as many exchanges as ordered, instruct them to implement the emergency diet and fluid restrictions plan.
    c. PD patients should have an emergency 5-day supply of antibiotics for peritonitis.
    d. Patient should be aware of emergency proce-

dures to follow for floods (see III.E.10. Home hemodialysis patients).
    e. Should contact the center to report their status, when possible.
    f. Patients should be instructed to register with local water and power company for priority reinstatement of services.
    g. Patients must know how to contact the dialysis staff so that alternate dialysis arrangements can be made if there is a loss of power and/or water.

12. Transplant patients.
    a. Patients should keep and carry a current list of their medications.
    b. Should contact the transplant center to report their status, when possible.
    c. Patient should be aware of emergency procedures to follow for floods (see III.E.10. Home hemodialysis patients).

13. Diabetic patients.
    a. Should keep extra insulin and syringes.
    b. Should keep extra batteries for glucometer.
    c. Should be aware of emergency procedures to follow for floods (see III.E.10. Home hemodialysis patients).

14. All patients should:
    a. Keep and carry with them a current list of medications.
    b. Keep a 2-week supply of their medications.
    c. Wear a medical information emblem.
    d. Have a battery-powered AM/FM radio and flashlight with extra batteries.
    e. Have a list of emergency phone numbers.
    f. Prepare themselves and their household in the same ways as the general public.

IV. Winter storms and blizzards.

A. A winter storm is defined as a storm with heavy snow and/or ice, sustained winds or wind gusts up to 35 miles per hour or greater and considerable falling or blowing snow.

B. Winter storm facts.
   1. Leading causes of death during winter storms.
      a. About 70% of the fatalities are ice- and snow-related automobile or transportation accidents.
      b. Exhaustion and heart attacks.
      c. Hypothermia, especially in the very young and elderly.
      d. Asphyxiation related to improper use of fuels with power outages.
   2. Power outages are typically caused by ice form-

ing on power lines and pulling the lines down and or breaking the poles. Outages can last 1–10 days (usually 3 days). Most local government agencies do not supply generators to homes or businesses.

C. Winter storm watch.
   1. A winter storm with heavy snow and/or ice is possible in your area.
   2. Warnings are usually issued 24–48 hours in advance of the storm.
   3. Listen to NOAA Weather radio or local stations for updated information.
   4. Prepare for a potential storm by reviewing the disaster plan and educating patients and staff of the actions to be taken in the event of a winter storm or blizzard. Make sure patients are aware of emergency diet plans if dialysis is not possible as scheduled.
   5. Changes in temperature, snowfall, and wind can occur quickly.
   6. Avoid unnecessary travel.

D. Winter storm warning.
   1. A winter storm is occurring or will soon occur.
   2. Initiate Disaster Plan.

E. Blizzard warning.
   1. Sustained winds or wind gusts up to 35 miles per hour or greater and considerable falling or blowing snow.
   2. Expected to prevail for 3 hours or longer.
   3. Visibility is reduced to less than ¼ mile.

F. Ice storm.
   1. Freezing rain or drizzle creating danger on roads, to trees and power lines.
   2. Stay indoors and dress warmly.
   3. Listen to radio or television (have battery-operated radios available).

G. Facility Action Plan.
   1. Policies and procedures to guide emergency response.
      a. Make sure there is a mechanism to receive and monitor weather reports.
      b. Because traffic accidents are the leading cause of death during winter storms, advise patients not to attempt to go out or drive until the storm is over and the roads are clear.
      c. If patients are dialyzing when a blizzard hits, have a plan for them to stay until the storm is over and the roads are clear.
      d. If patients have to miss the dialysis treatment, instruct them to begin their emergency diet and fluid restriction plan.
      e. If patients have to go to a shelter, they should notify someone from the facility.
   2. Patient education and preparation.
      a. Consider conducting educational days in the autumn related to winter storm preparedness. Include diet planning, shopping lists, shelter information, safety tips, etc.
      b. Winter storms may cause clinic closures or inability for patients to arrive for dialysis treatments.
   3. In-center dialysis patients. Review procedures patients need to follow if their regularly scheduled dialysis treatments are interrupted.
   4. Home hemodialysis patients.
      a. Should keep a 2-week supply of dialysis supplies in case deliveries are delayed.
      b. Must be able to perform emergency disconnect procedures in case power outage occurs during their treatment.
      c. Patients should register with local water and power company for priority reinstatement of services.
      d. If electrical power or water service is interrupted, they must know how to contact the dialysis staff to make alternate dialysis arrangements.
   5. PD patients.
      a. An electrical outage will affect CCPD patients. These patients should possess the ability to perform manual exchanges.
      b. If patients are unable to perform as many exchanges as ordered, instruct them to implement emergency diet and fluid restriction plan.
      c. They should keep a 2-week supply of peritoneal dialysis supplies in case delivery of supplies is delayed.
      d. PD patients should have an emergency medication 5-day supply of antibiotics for peritonitis.
   6. Transplant patients.
      a. Keep extra antirejection medication on hand in case they are unable to get to the pharmacy.
      b. Should contact the transplant center to report their status, when possible.
   7. Diabetic patients.
      a. Should keep extra insulin and syringes.
      b. Should keep extra batteries for glucometer.
   8. All patients.
      a. Keep and carry with them a current list of medications.

b. Keep a 2-week supply of their medications.
c. Wear a medical information emblem.
d. Have a battery-powered AM/FM radio and flashlight with extra batteries.
e. Have a list of emergency phone numbers.
f. Prepare themselves and their household in the same ways as the general public.

V. Earthquakes.

A. Earthquakes.
1. Occur suddenly and without warning.
2. Can seriously damage buildings, disrupt gas lines, electric and telephone service.
3. Can trigger landslides, floods, and tsunamis.
4. Aftershocks may occur for weeks after the initial earthquake.

B. Facility Action Plan.
1. Facility inspection by a structural engineer.
   a. Have a contract with an engineering firm to assess safety of building after earthquake.
   b. All storage shelves should be braced and have "lips."
   c. Use safety glass.
   d. Secure heavy equipment to the floor.
   e. Ensure dialysis machine wheels are always in the locked position except when moving.
2. Develop an evacuation plan. Designate "gathering" area after the quake away from buildings.
3. If patients are dialyzing when an earthquake occurs, instruct them to remain calm and seated until instructed otherwise by staff. Face away from any windows.
4. If patients have to miss a dialysis treatment, instruct them to begin their emergency diet and fluid restriction plan.
5. If patients have to go to a shelter, they should notify someone from the facility.
6. In-center dialysis patients.
   a. Prepare for aftershocks.
   b. Check for injuries; give first aid.
   c. Remove patients from the machine if deemed appropriate.
   d. Determine if there is any structural damage.
   e. Evacuate if deemed appropriate.
   f. Review procedures patients need to follow if their regularly scheduled dialysis treatments are interrupted.
7. Home hemodialysis patients.
   a. Patients should register with local water and power company for priority reinstatement of services.
   b. Patients must keep hemodialysis machine wheels locked at all times.
   c. Should keep a 2-week supply of dialysis supplies in case deliveries are delayed.
   d. Must be able to perform emergency disconnect procedures in case power outage occurs during their treatment.
   e. If electrical power or water service is interrupted, they must know how to contact the dialysis staff to make alternate dialysis arrangements.
8. PD patients.
   a. Ensure patients keep CCPD equipment wheels locked at all times.
   b. An electrical outage will affect CCPD patients. These patients should possess the ability to perform manual exchanges.
   c. If patients are unable to perform as many exchanges as ordered, instruct them to implement emergency diet and fluid restriction plan.
   d. They should keep a 2-week supply of peritoneal dialysis supplies in case delivery of supplies is delayed.
   e. PD patients should have an emergency medication 5-day supply of antibiotics for peritonitis.
9. Transplant patients.
   a. Should keep extra antirejection medication on hand in case they are unable to get to the pharmacy.
   b. Should contact the transplant center to report their status, when possible.
10. Diabetic patients.
    a. Should keep extra insulin and syringes.
    b. Should keep extra batteries for glucometer.
11. Acute dialysis patients. There may be increased hospital admissions and need for acute treatments due to crush injuries.
12. All patients should:
    a. Keep and carry with them a current list of medications.
    b. Keep a 2-week supply of their medications.
    c. Wear a medical information emblem.
    d. Have a battery-powered AM/FM radio and flashlight with extra batteries.
    e. Have a list of emergency phone numbers.
    f. Prepare themselves and their household in the same ways as the general public.

VI. Fires and wildfires.

A. Smoke from wildfires.
1. A mixture of gases and fine particles from burning trees and other plant materials.
2. Can hurt the eyes, irritate the respiratory system, and worsen chronic heart and lung diseases.

B. Smoke facts.
1. Can cause coughing, scratchy throat, irritated sinuses, shortness of breath, chest pain, headaches, stinging eyes, runny nose.
2. May trigger or worsen symptoms in persons who have heart or lung disease.
3. May worsen symptoms for people who have pre-existing respiratory conditions, such as respiratory allergies, asthma, and chronic obstructive pulmonary disease (COPD).
4. Symptoms of smoke inhalation.
   a. Inability to breathe normally.
   b. Cough with or without mucus.
   c. Chest discomfort.
   d. Wheezing and shortness of breath.
5. Awareness.
   a. Pay attention to local air quality reports.
   b. Listen and watch for news or health warnings about smoke.
   c. Find out if the community provides reports about the Environmental Protection Agency's Air Quality Index (AQI).
   d. Pay attention to public health messages about taking additional safety measures.
   e. Refer to visibility guides if they are available. Not every community has a monitor that measures the amount of particles that are in the air. In the western part of the United States, some communities have guidelines to help people estimate AQI based on how far they can see.
6. If persons are advised to stay indoors, keep indoor air as clean as possible.
   a. Keep windows and doors closed unless it is extremely hot outside.
   b. Run an air conditioner if available, but keep the fresh air intake closed and the filter clean to prevent outdoor smoke from getting inside.
   c. If an air conditioner is not available, and it is too warm to stay inside with the windows closed, seek shelter elsewhere.
7. Dust masks are not enough.
   a. Paper "comfort" or "dust" masks commonly found at hardware stores are designed to trap large particles, such as sawdust. These masks will not protect your lungs from smoke.
   b. For more information about effective masks, see the Respirator Fact Sheet provided by the Centers for Disease Control (CDC) National Institute for Occupational Safety and Health.

C. Facility Action Plan.
1. Perform routine life, fire, and safety inspections.

2. Maintain appropriate placement, quantity, and type of fire extinguishers.
3. Train staff in the use of fire extinguishers.
4. Develop and use policies and procedures for staff's handling and storing flammables.
5. Develop, communicate, and enforce smoking policies for patients, staff, and visitors.
6. Devise procedures for informing the Fire Department of the facility's location and determining approximate response time.
7. Institute procedures for activating the Fire Alert system.
8. Involve the staff and patients in performing emergency dialysis discontinuation drills.
   a. Drills should include evacuation procedure, use of fire extinguishers, and shut-off valves for electricity, water, gas.
   b. The drills should be evaluated and reported to supervisory personnel.
9. Learn about the history of wildfires in your area.
   a. Be aware of weather: long periods without rain increase the risk of wildfires.
   b. If considering evacuation, check the condition of the roads.
   c. Eliminate brush, trees, and other vegetation to help create a safety zone. This area should be about 30 feet from the building.
   d. Encourage patients and staff to create safety zones around their houses.

VII. Mudslides.

A. Mudslides, also known as debris flows, are a common type of fast-moving landslide that tends to flow in channels. Landslides occur when masses of rock, earth, or debris move down a slope.

B. Mudslide facts.
1. Landslide causes.
   a. Disturbances in the natural stability of a slope.
   b. Can accompany heavy rains or follow droughts, earthquakes, or volcanic eruptions.
   c. Develop when water rapidly accumulates in the ground and results in a surge of water-saturated rock, earth, and debris.
   d. Usually start on steep slopes and can be activated by natural disasters.
   e. Areas where wildfires or human modification of the land have destroyed vegetation on slopes are particularly vulnerable to landslides during and after heavy rains.
2. In the United States, landslides and debris flows result in 25 to 50 deaths each year. The health

hazards associated with landslides and mud-flows include:
   a. Rapidly moving water and debris that can lead to trauma.
   b. Broken electrical, water, gas, and sewage lines that can result in injury or illness.
   c. Disrupted roadways and railways that can endanger motorists and disrupt transport and access to health care.
   3. Some areas are more likely to experience landslides or mudflows.
   a. Areas where wildfires or human modification of the land have destroyed vegetation.
   b. Areas where landslides have occurred before.
   c. Steep slopes and areas at the bottom of slopes or canyons.
   d. Slopes that have been altered for construction of buildings and roads.
   e. Channels along a stream or river.
   f. Areas where surface runoff is directed.

C. Facility Action Plan.
   1. Learn whether landslides or debris flows have occurred previously in your area by contacting local authorities, a county geologist, county planning department, state geologic surveys, departments of natural resources, or university departments of geology.
   2. Contact local authorities about emergency and evacuation plans.
   3. During storms and rainfall, listen to the radio or watch TV for warnings about intense rainfall or for information and instructions from local officials.
   4. If landslide or debris flow danger is imminent:
   a. Quickly move away from the path of the slide. Getting out of the path of a debris flow is your best protection.
   b. Move to the nearest high ground in a direction away from the path.
   c. If rocks and debris are approaching, run for the nearest shelter and take cover (if possible, under a desk, table, or other piece of sturdy furniture).
   5. Consult a geotechnical expert (a registered professional engineer with soils engineering expertise) for advice on reducing additional landslide problems and risks. Local authorities should be able to tell you how to contact a geotechnical expert.

VIII. Volcanic eruptions.

A. Volcanoes.
   1. Spew hot, dangerous gases, ash, lava, and rock that are powerfully destructive.
   2. Volcanic eruptions may result in floods, landslides, mudslides, power outages, and wildfires.
   3. Ash.
   a. Gritty, abrasive, sometimes corrosive, and always unpleasant.
   b. Small ash particles can abrade (scratch) the front of the eye.
   c. May contain crystalline silica, a material that causes a respiratory disease called silicosis.

B. Volcano facts.
   1. The most common cause of death from a volcano is suffocation.
   2. Volcanic eruptions can result in additional threats to health, such as floods, mudslides, power outages, drinking water contamination, and wildfires.
   3. Health concerns after a volcanic eruption.
   a. Infectious disease, respiratory illness, burns, injuries from falls, and vehicle accidents related to the slippery, hazy conditions caused by ash.
   b. When warnings are heeded, the chances of adverse health effects from a volcanic eruption are very low.
   4. Volcanic gases.
   a. Most gases from a volcano quickly blow away. However, heavy gases such as carbon dioxide and hydrogen sulfide can collect in low-lying areas.
   b. The most common volcanic gas is water vapor, followed by carbon dioxide and sulfur dioxide. Sulfur dioxide can cause breathing problems in both healthy people and people with asthma and other respiratory problems.
   c. Other volcanic gases include hydrogen chloride, carbon monoxide, and hydrogen fluoride. Amounts of these gases vary widely from one volcanic eruption to the next.

C. Facility Action Plan.
   1. Close all windows, doors, and fireplace or woodstove dampers.
   2. Turn off all fans and heating and air-conditioning systems.
   3. Heed warnings, and obey instructions from local authorities. For example, stay indoors until local health officials tell you it is safe to go outside.

4. Listen to local news updates for information about air quality, drinking water, and roads.
5. Do not travel unless you have to.
   a. Driving in ash is hazardous to your health and your car.
   b. Driving will stir up more ash that can clog engines and stall vehicles.

> **Disaster preparedness is everyone's responsibility. Now is the time to take action to become prepared both at work and at home. It is never too early!**

Chapter 72

Man-made and Other Disasters

I. Terrorism.

A. Use of force or violence against persons or property in violation of the criminal laws of the United States for purposes of intimidation, coercion, or ransom (FEMA, 2006).

B. General safety guidelines.
   1. Be aware of your surroundings.
   2. Learn where emergency exits are located in the buildings you frequent.
   3. The facility should have portable battery-operated radio, flashlights with extra batteries, and a first aid kit.

II. Bomb threat.

A. Potential bombing incidents constitute a serious threat to employees, patients, assets, operations, and facilities whether the motive is found in extortion, assault, or an act of terror. This threat area has taken on relevance and is increasingly prevalent today for a number of reasons.
   1. Technology in the area of explosives and devices has advanced tremendously with the development and mass production of advanced electronics, plastics, and explosive materials.
   2. Materials necessary to construct a very powerful device are readily available from a wide variety of common sources.
   3. This information is increasingly and more readily available via "underground" publications and the Internet.

B. Following an event, the investigation and successful prosecution of bombers is very difficult as the modern weapon literally destroys most of the physical evidence that was often left by the older and more primitive devices.

C. The options available to the thoughtful attacker for effective placement of a device are numerous. Delivery can be accomplished in any of a number of ways, including:
   1. On the person of an employee, visitor, vendor, or maintenance person.
   2. Within a box, purse, briefcase, lunch box.
   3. Via a commercial carrier, private delivery service, or the U.S. mail.

D. Facility Action Plan.
   1. In any size organization, employee involvement is the key to prevention.
      a. Provide employees with awareness training on the topic of bomb threats and extortion.
      b. Develop response policies and procedures.
      c. Consult with the local law enforcement and fire officials.
   2. Bomb threats are usually received by telephone, the call is short in duration, and the caller usually refuses to answer questions.
   3. The caller relies on the person taking the message being unable to determine the veracity of the threat statement. The caller will secondly rely upon the person's inability to conduct an effective search of the facility in a very short period. If the caller can accomplish both of these objectives, the organization will be placed

into a state of confusion and panic, which is most likely the caller's intent.

4. Is it a real threat situation, or not? Evacuate or not? Each of these decisions obviously carries a very serious question of safety. You will have to determine the validity of the threat with limited information on hand, and there will not be much time.

5. Proper preplanning and training are critical to this risk management process as you will have to, in a very limited time frame:
   a. Quickly analyze the threat.
   b. Estimate the need for accurate response.
   c. Decide upon the most logical direction to take.
   d. Execute your plan.

III. Bioterrorism.

A. Bioterrorism is the intentional use of harmful, biologic substances or germs to cause widespread illness and fear. Smallpox, anthrax, botulism, nerve agents, ricin, and plague are examples of biologic agents used in bioterrorism.

B. Facility Action Plan.
   1. Check for instructions on local television, radio, and newspapers. In the event of a bioterrorism attack, it may take time to determine exactly what the illness is and how it should be treated.
   2. Be prepared to discontinue treatments.

IV. Pandemics and influenza (flu).

A. Seasonal (or common) flu is a contagious respiratory illness caused by influenza viruses. Most people have some immunity, and a vaccine is available.

B. Avian (or bird) flu is caused by influenza viruses that occur naturally among wild birds. The H5N1 variant is deadly to domestic fowl and can be transmitted from birds to humans. At the time of publication, there is no human immunity and no vaccine available.

C. Pandemic flu is a global outbreak of serious illness. Because there is little natural immunity, the disease can spread easily from person to person.
   1. An influenza pandemic occurs when a new influenza virus emerges for which there is little or no immunity in the human population, begins to cause serious illness, and then spreads easily person-to-person worldwide.
   2. The federal government, states, communities,

and industry are taking steps to prepare for and respond to an influenza pandemic outbreak.

   3. A pandemic is likely to be a prolonged and widespread outbreak that could require temporary changes in many areas of society, such as schools, work, transportation, and other public services.
   4. An informed and prepared public can take appropriate actions to decrease their risk during a pandemic.

D. Facility Action Plan.
   1. Develop a preparedness plan as you would for other public health emergencies. Review the ESRD checklist developed by the Department of Health and Human Services (DHHS) and the Centers for Disease Control (CDC) on www.pandemic.flu.gov and www.cdc.gov.
   2. Participate and promote any public health efforts in your state and community.
   3. Talk with your local public health officials. They can supply information about the signs and symptoms of a specific disease outbreak.
   4. Implement prevention and control actions recommended by your public health officials and providers.
   5. Adopt practices that encourage sick employees to stay home.
   6. Anticipate how to function with a significant portion of the workforce absent due to illness or caring for ill family members.
   7. Wash hands frequently with soap and water.
   8. Cover coughs and sneezes with tissues.
   9. Stay informed about pandemic influenza and be prepared to respond.
   10. Consult www.pandemicflu.gov frequently for updates on national and international information on pandemic influenza.

V. Chemical threat.

A. Chemical agents.
   1. Poisonous vapors, aerosols, liquids, and solids that have a toxic effect on people, animals and plants.
   2. Some chemicals may be odorless and tasteless.
   3. They can have an immediate effect (a few seconds to a few minutes) or delayed effect (2 to 48 hours).

B. Chemical facts.
   1. A chemical attack could come without warning.
   2. Signs of a chemical release include people having difficulty breathing, eye irritation, loss of

coordination, nausea, burning sensation in nose and lungs.

3. Presence of dead birds and insects may indicate a chemical agent release.

4. 1986 Emergency Planning and Community Right to Know Act (EPCRA).
   a. Communities have a "right to know" about hazardous chemicals in the area.
   b. States are mandated to have an emergency response plan for chemical emergencies.
   c. The Occupational Safety and Health Administration's (OSHA) Hazardous Waste Operations and Emergency Response Standard mandates training for staff that may take care of patients exposed to toxic chemicals.

C. Facility Action Plan.
   1. Ensure all employees have Hazard Communication Training.
   2. The disaster supply kit should include a roll of duct tape, plastic, and scissors.
   3. Identify an internal room without windows and on a high level as a safe room.
   4. If instructed to remain in the facility, close the doors and windows and turn off all ventilation. Seal windows and doors with plastic.
   5. Listen to the radio for further instruction by authorities.
   6. After the attack, use extreme caution caring for those who have been exposed. Refer them to a hospital for further treatment.

VI. Workplace violence.

A. Any act in which a person is abused, threatened, intimidated, or assaulted in his/her place of employment is considered workplace violence.

B. Examples of workplace violence.
   1. Threatening behavior – shaking fists, destroying property, throwing objects.
   2. Verbal or written threats – any expression of intent to inflict harm.
   3. Harassment – any unwelcome behavior that demeans, embarrasses, humiliates, annoys, alarms or verbally abuses a person. This includes words, gestures, intimidation, or other inappropriate behavior.
   4. Verbal abuse – swearing, insults, or condescending language.
   5. Physical attacks – hitting, shoving, pushing, or kicking.
   6. Rumors, swearing, verbal abuse, pranks,

arguments, property damage, theft, physical assaults, anger-related incidents, arson, and murder.

C. Workplace violence facts.
   1. According to the Department of Justice, 1 million individuals become victims of violent crime while working or on duty (AFSCME, 2006).
   2. Workplace violence is not limited to the traditional workplace. It can occur at off-site business-related places (conferences), at social events related to work, even threatening phone calls.
   3. Risk of violence can be greater at certain times of day, night, or year (for example, pay days, performance appraisals, late hours of the night, or early hours of the day).

D. Facility Action Plan.
   1. Review any history of violence in the workplace.
   2. Determine any risk factors associated with workplace violence. Implement preventive measures such as position of lobby entrance, position of furniture in offices, installing physical barriers between the lobby and the clinic, minimizing the number of entrances, using code cards or keys for access to certain areas in the clinic, alarm systems.
   3. Review "Decreasing Dialysis Patient Provider Conflict" toolbox from the Center for Medicare and Medicaid Services (CMS).
   4. Develop workplace policies and procedures to apply to management, employees, patients, vendors, and visitors.
      a. Provide clear examples of unacceptable behavior and their consequences.
      b. Outline the confidential process employees can use to report incidents.
      c. Outline the investigative process.
   5. Provide a confidential Employee Assistance Program (EAP) where employees can seek help.

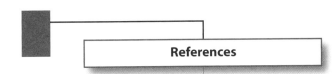

References

American Federation of State, County, and Municipal Employees (AFSCME). (n.d.). *Workplace violence fact sheet.* Retrieved April 24, 2006, from http://www.afscme.org/issues/1293.cfm

American Nurses Association (ANA). (2002). *Position statement on registered nurses' rights and responsibilities related to work release during a disaster.* Silver Spring, MD: Author.

Centers for Medicare and Medicaid Services (CMS). (2002). *Emergency preparedness for dialysis facilities.* Publication number CMS 11025. Baltimore: Author.

Centers for Medicare and Medicaid Services (CMS). (2005). *Decreasing dialysis patient provider conflict.* CMS contract #500-03-NW14 with the ESRD Network of Texas, Inc. Baltimore: Author.

Counts, C. (2001). Disaster preparedness: Is your unit ready? *Nephrology Nursing Journal, 28*(5), 491-499.

Lettieri, C. (2006). Disaster medicine: Understanding the threat and minimizing the effects [Electronic version]. *Medscape Emergency Medicine, 1*(1).

National Child Traumatic Stress Network and National Center for Posttraumatic Stress Disorder. (2005). *Psychological first aid: Field operations guide* (2nd ed.). Retrieved February 19, 2008, from http://www.ncptsd.va.gov/ncmain/ncdocs/manuals/nc_manual_psyfirstaid.html

National Hurricane Center. (n.d.). *Hurricane preparedness.* Retrieved September 7, 2006, from http://nhc.noaa.gov

National Kidney Foundation (NKF). (1998). *Planning for natural disasters: A guide for kidney patients.* New York: Author.

Renal Network, The. (1996). *Disaster planning & emergency preparedness: Guidelines & resources.* Indianapolis, IN: Author.

United States Department of the Interior. (2006). *Flood hazards – A national threat.* Retrieved October 31, 2006, from http://pubs.usgs.gov

United States Environmental Protection Agency. (1986). *Emergency planning and community right to know.* Retrieved October 31, 2006, from http://www.epa.gov

U.S. Department of Health & Human Services. (n.d.). *Pandemic flu: General information.* Retrieved October 31, 2006, from http://pandemicflu.gov/general/index.html

---

Kidney Community Emergency Response Coalition

(Web site: www.kcercoalition.com)

CMS convened a National Disaster Summit on January 19, 2006, to:
- Review disaster response in ESRD community.
- To plan for the future.
- To form a national coalition.

Nine Response Teams

1. Patient and provider tracking.
   - Developed a basic medical record and continues to work on Web-based record.
   - Established an online system to identify open versus closed facilities in disaster area.
   - Established a patient tracking process.

2. Coordination of staff and volunteers – established a database of nurses, dialysis technicians, social workers, and dietitians.

3. Physician assistance – developed tools to assist physicians prepare and respond to a disaster.

4. Patient assistance – made recommendations to update the CMS Patient Guide for Emergencies.

5. Facility operations – made recommendations to update the CMS Facility Guide for Emergencies.

6. Vendor (suppliers) services – designed Web pages to allow quick access for needed supplies during an emergency.

7. Communications – established the Kidney Care Emergency Web site and toll-free numbers.

8. Federal, state, and local agency support – developed an educational piece that was distributed to federal, state, and local emergency responders regarding the needs of individuals with kidney failure.

9. Pandemic preparedness – to develop and disseminate plans in the event of a pandemic flu.

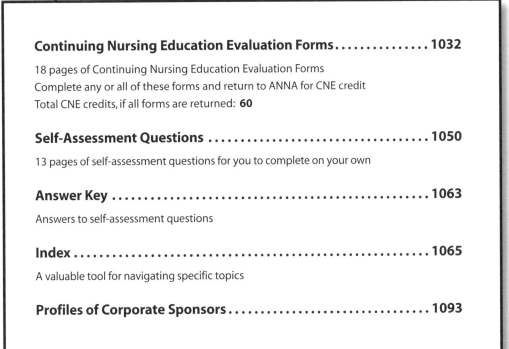

Core Curriculum for Nephrology Nursing contains 18 sections of educational content. Individual learners may apply for continuing nursing education credit by reading a section and completing the Continuing Nursing Education Evaluation Form for that section. Learners may apply for continuing nursing education credit for any or all sections.

Please photocopy this test page, complete, and return to ANNA.

You can also download it from www.annanurse.org (choose Education → CNE Activities → Publications)

Name: _____

Address: _____

City: _____ State: _____ Zip: _____

E-mail: _____ Preferred telephone: ☐ Home ☐ Work

State where licensed and license number: _____

CNE application fees are based upon the number of contact hours provided by the individual section. CNE fees per contact hour for ANNA members are as follows: 1.0-1.9 – $15; 2.0-2.9 – $20; 3.0-3.9 – $25; 4.0 and higher – $30. Fees for nonmembers are $10 higher.

CNE application fee for **Section 1** :   ANNA member $30   Nonmember $40

ANNA Member: ☐ Yes   ☐ No   ☐ Member # (if available) _____

☐ Check or money order enclosed   ☐ American Express   ☐ Visa   ☐ MasterCard

Total amount submitted: _____

Credit card number _____ Exp. Date _____

Name as it appears on the card: _____

NOTE: Your evaluation form can be processed in 1 week for an additional rush charge of $5.00.
☐ Yes, I would like this evaluation form rush processed. I have included an additional fee of $5.00 for rush processing.

INSTRUCTIONS

1. To receive continuing nursing education credit for an individual study after reading the section, complete this evaluation form.

2. Detach, photocopy, or download (www.annanurse.org) the evaluation form and send along with a check or money order payable to **American Nephrology Nurses' Assocation** to: ANNA, East Holly Avenue Box 56, Pitman, NJ 08071-0056.

3. Test returns must be postmarked by **December 31, 2012**. Upon completion of the answer/evaluation form, a certificate for **4.0** contact hour(s) will be awarded and sent to you.

This section was reviewed and formatted for contact hour credit by Sally S. Russell, MN, CMSRN, ANNA Director of Education Services.

> **CNE Application Fee for Section 1**
> **ANNA member = $30**
> **Nonmember = $40**

---

1. I verify that I have read this section and completed this education activity. _____ Date _____
Signature

2. What would be different in your practice if you applied what you have learned from this activity? (Please use additional paper if necessary.)

_____

_____

_____

_____

	Strongly disagree				Strongly agree
3. The activity met the stated objectives.					
a. Describe renal regulation of water balance.	1	2	3	4	5
b. Discuss renal regulation of solutes: electrolytes and metabolic wastes.	1	2	3	4	5
c. Outline renal regulation of acid-base balance.	1	2	3	4	5
d. List hormones secreted by the kidney and the function(s) of the hormones.	1	2	3	4	5
4. The content was current and relevant.	1	2	3	4	5
5. The content was presented clearly.	1	2	3	4	5
6. The content was covered adequately.	1	2	3	4	5

7. How would you rate your ability to apply your learning to practice?   ☐ diminished ability ☐ no change ☐ enhanced ability

Comments _____

_____

8. Time required to read the section and complete this form: _____ minutes

---

This educational activity is provided by the American Nephrology Nurses' Association (ANNA) for **4.0** contact hours.
ANNA is accredited as a provider of continuing nursing education (CNE) by the American Nurses Credentialing Center's Commission on Accreditation (ANCC-COA).
ANNA is a provider approved of continuing nursing education by the California Board of Registered Nursing, provider number CEP 00910.
This CNE offering meets the Nephrology Nursing Certification Commission's (NNCC's) continuing nursing education requirements for certification and recertification.

Chronic Kidney Disease **ANNP802**

Core Curriculum for Nephrology Nursing contains 18 sections of educational content. Individual learners may apply for continuing nursing education credit by reading a section and completing the Continuing Nursing Education Evaluation Form for that section. Learners may apply for continuing nursing education credit for any or all sections.

Please photocopy this test page, complete, and return to ANNA.

You can also download it from www.annanurse.org (choose Education → CNE Activities → Publications)

Name: _____

Address: _____

City: _____ State: _____ Zip: _____

E-mail:_____ Preferred telephone: ☐ Home ☐ Work

State where licensed and license number: _____

CNE application fees are based upon the number of contact hours provided by the individual section. CNE fees per contact hour for ANNA members are as follows: 1.0-1.9 – $15; 2.0-2.9 – $20; 3.0-3.9 – $25; 4.0 and higher – $30. Fees for nonmembers are $10 higher.

CNE application fee for **Section 2** : ANNA member $25 Nonmember $35

ANNA Member: ☐ Yes ☐ No ☐ Member # (if available) _____

☐ Check or money order enclosed ☐ American Express ☐ Visa ☐ MasterCard

Total amount submitted: _____

Credit card number _____ Exp. Date _____

Name as it appears on the card:_____

NOTE: Your evaluation form can be processed in 1 week for an additional rush charge of $5.00.
☐ Yes, I would like this evaluation form rush processed. I have included an additional fee of $5.00 for rush processing.

INSTRUCTIONS

1. To receive continuing nursing education credit for an individual study after reading the section, complete this evaluation form.

2. Detach, photocopy, or download (www.annanurse.org) the evaluation form and send along with a check or money order payable to **American Nephrology Nurses' Assocation** to: ANNA, East Holly Avenue Box 56, Pitman, NJ 08071-0056.

3. Test returns must be postmarked by **December 31, 2012.** Upon completion of the answer/evaluation form, a certificate for **3.0** contact hour(s) will be awarded and sent to you.

This section was reviewed and formatted for contact hour credit by Sally S. Russell, MN, CMSRN, ANNA Director of Education Services.

CNE Application Fee for Section 2
ANNA member = $25
Nonmember = $35

1. I verify that I have read this section and completed this education activity. _____ Date _____

Signature

2. What would be different in your practice if you applied what you have learned from this activity? (Please use additional paper if necessary.)

_____

_____

_____

	Strongly disagree				Strongly agree
3. The activity met the stated objectives.					
a. Summarize the definition and stages of chronic kidney disease.	1	2	3	4	5
b. Relate the importance of early identification and treatment of chronic kidney disease and its comorbidities.	1	2	3	4	5
c. Discuss steps used to delay the progression of CKD.	1	2	3	4	5
d. Identify the complications of CKD.	1	2	3	4	5
e. List methods of empowering the individual with CKD to make changes needed to take control of his/her own healthcare.	1	2	3	4	5
4. The content was current and relevant.	1	2	3	4	5
5. The content was presented clearly.	1	2	3	4	5
6. The content was covered adequately.	1	2	3	4	5

7. How would you rate your ability to apply your learning to practice? ☐ diminished ability ☐ no change ☐ enhanced ability

Comments _____

8. Time required to read the section and complete this form: _____ minutes

This educational activity is provided by the American Nephrology Nurses' Association (ANNA) for **3.0** contact hours.
ANNA is accredited as a provider of continuing nursing education (CNE) by the American Nurses Credentialing Center's Commission on Accreditation (ANCC-COA).
ANNA is a provider approved of continuing nursing education by the California Board of Registered Nursing, provider number CEP 00910.
This CNE offering meets the Nephrology Nursing Certification Commission's (NNCC's) continuing nursing education requirements for certification and recertification.

Core Curriculum for Nephrology Nursing contains 18 sections of educational content. Individual learners may apply for continuing nursing education credit by reading a section and completing the Continuing Nursing Education Evaluation Form for that section. Learners may apply for continuing nursing education credit for any or all sections.

Please photocopy this test page, complete, and return to ANNA.

You can also download it from www.annanurse.org (choose Education → CNE Activities → Publications)

Name: _____

Address: _____

City: _____ State: _____ Zip: _____

E-mail:_____ Preferred telephone: ☐ Home ☐ Work

State where licensed and license number: _____

CNE application fees are based upon the number of contact hours provided by the individual section. CNE fees per contact hour for ANNA members are as follows: 1.0-1.9 – $15; 2.0-2.9 – $20; 3.0-3.9 – $25; 4.0 and higher – $30. Fees for nonmembers are $10 higher.

CNE application fee for **Section 3** :   ANNA member $30   Nonmember $40

ANNA Member: ☐ Yes   ☐ No   ☐ Member # (if available) _____

☐ Check or money order enclosed   ☐ American Express   ☐ Visa   ☐ MasterCard

Total amount submitted: _____

Credit card number _____ Exp. Date _____

Name as it appears on the card: _____

NOTE: Your evaluation form can be processed in 1 week for an additional rush charge of $5.00.
☐ **Yes, I would like this evaluation form rush processed. I have included an additional fee of $5.00 for rush processing.**

INSTRUCTIONS

1. To receive continuing nursing education credit for an individual study after reading the section, complete this evaluation form.

2. Detach, photocopy, or download (www.annanurse.org) the evaluation form and send along with a check or money order payable to **American Nephrology Nurses' Association** to: ANNA, East Holly Avenue Box 56, Pitman, NJ 08071-0056.

3. Test returns must be postmarked by **December 31, 2012**. Upon completion of the answer/evaluation form, a certificate for **5.4** contact hour(s) will be awarded and sent to you.

This section was reviewed and formatted for contact hour credit by Sally S. Russell, MN, CMSRN, ANNA Director of Education Services.

> **CNE Application Fee for Section 3**
> **ANNA member = $30**
> **Nonmember = $40**

---

1. I verify that I have read this section and completed this education activity. _____ Date _____

Signature

2. What would be different in your practice if you applied what you have learned from this activity? (Please use additional paper if necessary.)

_____

_____

_____

_____

	Strongly disagree				Strongly agree
3. The activity met the stated objectives.					
a. Describe three settings and three services common to acute care nephrology.	1	2	3	4	5
b. Discuss the nephrology nurse's role in acute care program management.	1	2	3	4	5
c. Identify three challenges that the acute care nephrology nurse encounters.	1	2	3	4	5
4. The content was current and relevant.	1	2	3	4	5
5. The content was presented clearly.	1	2	3	4	5
6. The content was covered adequately.	1	2	3	4	5
7. How would you rate your ability to apply your learning to practice?	☐ diminished ability ☐ no change ☐ enhanced ability				

Comments _____

_____

8. Time required to read the section and complete this form: _____ minutes

---

This educational activity is provided by the American Nephrology Nurses' Association (ANNA) for **5.4** contact hours.
ANNA is accredited as a provider of continuing nursing education (CNE) by the American Nurses Credentialing Center's Commission on Accreditation (ANCC-COA).
ANNA is a provider approved of continuing nursing education by the California Board of Registered Nursing, provider number CEP 00910.
This CNE offering meets the Nephrology Nursing Certification Commission's (NNCC's) continuing nursing education requirements for certification and recertification.

The Individual with Kidney Disease   **ANNP804**

Core Curriculum for Nephrology Nursing contains 18 sections of educational content. Individual learners may apply for continuing nursing education credit by reading a section and completing the Continuing Nursing Education Evaluation Form for that section. Learners may apply for continuing nursing education credit for any or all sections.

Please photocopy this test page, complete, and return to ANNA.

You can also download it from www.annanurse.org (choose Education → CNE Activities → Publications)

Name: _____

Address: _____

City: _____ State: _____ Zip: _____

E-mail: _____ Preferred telephone: ☐ Home ☐ Work

State where licensed and license number: _____

CNE application fees are based upon the number of contact hours provided by the individual section. CNE fees per contact hour for ANNA members are as follows: 1.0-1.9 – $15; 2.0-2.9 – $20; 3.0-3.9 – $25; 4.0 and higher – $30. Fees for nonmembers are $10 higher.

CNE application fee for **Section 4** :   ANNA member $30   Nonmember $40

ANNA Member: ☐ Yes   ☐ No   ☐ Member # (if available) _____

☐ Check or money order enclosed   ☐ American Express   ☐ Visa   ☐ MasterCard

Total amount submitted: _____

Credit card number _____ Exp. Date _____

Name as it appears on the card: _____

NOTE: Your evaluation form can be processed in 1 week for an additional rush charge of $5.00.
☐ Yes, I would like this evaluation form rush processed. I have included an additional fee of $5.00
   for rush processing.

INSTRUCTIONS

1. To receive continuing nursing education credit for an individual study after reading the section, complete this evaluation form.

2. Detach, photocopy, or download (www.annanurse.org) the evaluation form and send along with a check or money order payable to **American Nephrology Nurses' Assocation** to: ANNA, East Holly Avenue Box 56, Pitman, NJ 08071-0056.

3. Test returns must be postmarked by **December 31, 2012**. Upon completion of the answer/evaluation form, a certificate for **4.6** contact hour(s) will be awarded and sent to you.

This section was reviewed and formatted for contact hour credit by Sally S. Russell, MN, CMSRN, ANNA Director of Education Services.

```
┌─────────────────────────────────────┐
│  CNE Application Fee for Section 4    │
│        ANNA member = $30             │
│        Nonmember = $40              │
└─────────────────────────────────────┘
```

---

1. I verify that I have read this section and
   completed this education activity. _____ Date _____
                                                    Signature

2. What would be different in your practice if you applied what you have learned from this activity? (Please use additional paper if necessary.)

   _____
   _____
   _____

	Strongly disagree				Strongly agree
3. The activity met the stated objectives.					
a. Recognize patients who are at risk for an inheritable disease or condition based on their medical history, physical exam, or laboratory findings.	1	2	3	4	5
b. Provide culturally competent services to patients with kidney disease.	1	2	3	4	5
c. Summarize three psychosocial factors to consider when a patient exhibits difficult behaviors.	1	2	3	4	5
d. Describe ways to incorporate the family in the education process.	1	2	3	4	5
e. Discuss strategies to enhance the learning of patients and family affected by CKD.	1	2	3	4	5
f. Explain Medicare benefits including eligibility, when it starts and ends, and coverage for dialysis and transplantation.	1	2	3	4	5
g. State two ways socioeconomic status can limit access to care and treatment options.	1	2	3	4	5
h. Identify the significance of low physical functioning in CKD patients.	1	2	3	4	5
i. Describe the basic ethical principles underlying initiation of dialysis.	1	2	3	4	5
j. List common symptoms seen and treatment strategies utilized at End of Life (EOL) in nephrology patients and treatment.	1	2	3	4	5
4. The content was current and relevant.	1	2	3	4	5
5. The content was presented clearly.	1	2	3	4	5
6. The content was covered adequately.	1	2	3	4	5

7. How would you rate your ability to apply your learning to practice?   ☐ diminished ability ☐ no change ☐ enhanced ability

Comments _____

8. Time required to read the section and complete this form: _____ minutes

---

This educational activity is provided by the American Nephrology Nurses' Association (ANNA) for **4.6** contact hours.
ANNA is accredited as a provider of continuing nursing education (CNE) by the American Nurses Credentialing Center's Commission on Accreditation (ANCC-COA).
ANNA is a provider approved of continuing nursing education by the California Board of Registered Nursing, provider number CEP 00910.
This CNE offering meets the Nephrology Nursing Certification Commission's (NNCC's) continuing nursing education requirements for certification and recertification.

Core Curriculum for Nephrology Nursing contains 18 sections of educational content. Individual learners may apply for continuing nursing education credit by reading a section and completing the Continuing Nursing Education Evaluation Form for that section. Learners may apply for continuing nursing education credit for any or all sections.

Please photocopy this test page, complete, and return to ANNA.

You can also download it from www.annanurse.org (choose Education → CNE Activities → Publications)

Name: _____

Address: _____

City: _____ State: _____ Zip: _____

E-mail:_____ Preferred telephone: ☐ Home ☐ Work

State where licensed and license number: _____

CNE application fees are based upon the number of contact hours provided by the individual section. CNE fees per contact hour for ANNA members are as follows: 1.0-1.9 – $15; 2.0-2.9 – $20; 3.0-3.9 – $25; 4.0 and higher – $30. Fees for nonmembers are $10 higher.

CNE application fee for **Section 5** :   ANNA member $25   Nonmember $35

ANNA Member: ☐ Yes   ☐ No   ☐ Member # (if available) _____

☐ Check or money order enclosed   ☐ American Express   ☐ Visa   ☐ MasterCard

Total amount submitted: _____

Credit card number _____ Exp. Date _____

Name as it appears on the card: _____

NOTE: Your evaluation form can be processed in 1 week for an additional rush charge of $5.00.
☐ Yes, I would like this evaluation form rush processed. I have included an additional fee of $5.00 for rush processing.

INSTRUCTIONS

1. To receive continuing nursing education credit for an individual study after reading the section, complete this evaluation form.

2. Detach, photocopy, or download (www.annanurse.org) the evaluation form and send along with a check or money order payable to **American Nephrology Nurses' Assocation** to: ANNA, East Holly Avenue Box 56, Pitman, NJ 08071-0056.

3. Test returns must be postmarked by **December 31, 2012**. Upon completion of the answer/evaluation form, a certificate for **3.4** contact hour(s) will be awarded and sent to you.

This section was reviewed and formatted for contact hour credit by Sally S. Russell, MN, CMSRN, ANNA Director of Education Services.

> **CNE Application Fee for Section 5**
> **ANNA member = $25**
> **Nonmember = $35**

---

1. I verify that I have read this section and completed this education activity. _____ Date _____
   Signature

2. What would be different in your practice if you applied what you have learned from this activity? (Please use additional paper if necessary.)

   _____
   _____
   _____

	Strongly disagree				Strongly agree
3. The activity met the stated objectives.					
a. Identify patients who are at risk or already in stages 1 and 2 of CKD.	1	2	3	4	5
b. Discuss diagnostic procedures to evaluate people who may be at risk for CKD.	1	2	3	4	5
c. Outline management strategies, both short and long term, for people with CKD stage 1 and 2.	1	2	3	4	5
d. Differentiate management plans for patients depending on their underlying pathology.	1	2	3	4	5
4. The content was current and relevant.	1	2	3	4	5
5. The content was presented clearly.	1	2	3	4	5
6. The content was covered adequately.	1	2	3	4	5
7. How would you rate your ability to apply your learning to practice?	☐ diminished ability ☐ no change ☐ enhanced ability				

Comments _____
_____

8. Time required to read the section and complete this form: _____ minutes

---

This educational activity is provided by the American Nephrology Nurses' Association (ANNA) for **3.4** contact hours.
ANNA is accredited as a provider of continuing nursing education (CNE) by the American Nurses Credentialing Center's Commission on Accreditation (ANCC-COA).
ANNA is a provider approved of continuing nursing education by the California Board of Registered Nursing, provider number CEP 00910.
This CNE offering meets the Nephrology Nursing Certification Commission's (NNCC's) continuing nursing education requirements for certification and recertification.

Evidence-Based Practice

ANNP806

Core Curriculum for Nephrology Nursing contains 18 sections of educational content. Individual learners may apply for continuing nursing education credit by reading a section and completing the Continuing Nursing Education Evaluation Form for that section. Learners may apply for continuing nursing education credit for any or all sections.

Please photocopy this test page, complete, and return to ANNA.

You can also download it from www.annanurse.org (choose Education → CNE Activities → Publications)

Name: _____

Address: _____

City: _____ State: _____ Zip: _____

E-mail: _____ Preferred telephone: ☐ Home ☐ Work

State where licensed and license number: _____

CNE application fees are based upon the number of contact hours provided by the individual section. CNE fees per contact hour for ANNA members are as follows: 1.0-1.9 – $15; 2.0-2.9 – $20; 3.0-3.9 – $25; 4.0 and higher – $30. Fees for nonmembers are $10 higher.

CNE application fee for **Section 6** : ANNA member $20 Nonmember $30

ANNA Member: ☐ Yes ☐ No ☐ Member # (if available) _____

☐ Check or money order enclosed ☐ American Express ☐ Visa ☐ MasterCard

Total amount submitted: _____

Credit card number _____ Exp. Date _____

Name as it appears on the card: _____

NOTE: Your evaluation form can be processed in 1 week for an additional rush charge of $5.00.
☐ Yes, I would like this evaluation form rush processed. I have included an additional fee of $5.00 for rush processing.

INSTRUCTIONS

1. To receive continuing nursing education credit for an individual study after reading the section, complete this evaluation form.

2. Detach, photocopy, or download (www.annanurse.org) the evaluation form and send along with a check or money order payable to **American Nephrology Nurses' Assocation** to: ANNA, East Holly Avenue Box 56, Pitman, NJ 08071-0056.

3. Test returns must be postmarked by **December 31, 2012.** Upon completion of the answer/evaluation form, a certificate for **2.8** contact hour(s) will be awarded and sent to you.

This section was reviewed and formatted for contact hour credit by Sally S. Russell, MN, CMSRN, ANNA Director of Education Services.

CNE Application Fee for Section 6
ANNA member = $20
Nonmember = $30

---

1. I verify that I have read this section and completed this education activity. _____ Date _____
Signature

2. What would be different in your practice if you applied what you have learned from this activity? (Please use additional paper if necessary.)

_____
_____
_____

	Strongly disagree				Strongly agree
3. The activity met the stated objectives.					
a. Describe the process used in establishing evidence-based practice.	1	2	3	4	5
b. Incorporate standards for care into clinical practice.	1	2	3	4	5
c. Compare KDOQI guidelines to actual clinical findings.	1	2	3	4	5
d. Identify outcomes associated with the DOPPS studies.	1	2	3	4	5
e. Describe data available on the USRDS Web site.	1	2	3	4	5
4. The content was current and relevant.	1	2	3	4	5
5. The content was presented clearly.	1	2	3	4	5
6. The content was covered adequately.	1	2	3	4	5

7. How would you rate your ability to apply your learning to practice? ☐ diminished ability ☐ no change ☐ enhanced ability

Comments _____

8. Time required to read the section and complete this form: _____ minutes

---

This educational activity is provided by the American Nephrology Nurses' Association (ANNA) for **2.8** contact hours.
ANNA is accredited as a provider of continuing nursing education (CNE) by the American Nurses Credentialing Center's Commission on Accreditation (ANCC-COA).
ANNA is a provider approved of continuing nursing education by the California Board of Registered Nursing, provider number CEP 00910.
This CNE offering meets the Nephrology Nursing Certification Commission's (NNCC's) continuing nursing education requirements for certification and recertification.

Core Curriculum for Nephrology Nursing contains 18 sections of educational content. Individual learners may apply for continuing nursing education credit by reading a section and completing the Continuing Nursing Education Evaluation Form for that section. Learners may apply for continuing nursing education credit for any or all sections.

Please photocopy this test page, complete, and return to ANNA.

You can also download it from www.annanurse.org (choose Education → CNE Activities → Publications)

Name: _____

Address: _____

City: _____ State: _____ Zip: _____

E-mail: _____ Preferred telephone: ☐ Home ☐ Work

State where licensed and license number: _____

CNE application fees are based upon the number of contact hours provided by the individual section. CNE fees per contact hour for ANNA members are as follows: 1.0-1.9 – $15; 2.0-2.9 – $20; 3.0-3.9 – $25; 4.0 and higher – $30. Fees for nonmembers are $10 higher.

CNE application fee for **Section 7** : ANNA member $20 Nonmember $30

ANNA Member: ☐ Yes ☐ No ☐ Member # (if available) _____

☐ Check or money order enclosed ☐ American Express ☐ Visa ☐ MasterCard

Total amount submitted: _____

Credit card number _____ Exp. Date _____

Name as it appears on the card: _____

NOTE: Your evaluation form can be processed in 1 week for an additional rush charge of $5.00.
☐ Yes, I would like this evaluation form rush processed. I have included an additional fee of $5.00 for rush processing.

INSTRUCTIONS

1. To receive continuing nursing education credit for an individual study after reading the section, complete this evaluation form.

2. Detach, photocopy, or download (www.annanurse.org) the evaluation form and send along with a check or money order payable to **American Nephrology Nurses' Assocation** to: ANNA, East Holly Avenue Box 56, Pitman, NJ 08071-0056.

3. Test returns must be postmarked by **December 31, 2012.** Upon completion of the answer/evaluation form, a certificate for **2.4** contact hour(s) will be awarded and sent to you.

This section was reviewed and formatted for contact hour credit by Sally S. Russell, MN, CMSRN, ANNA Director of Education Services.

CNE Application Fee for Section 7
ANNA member = $20
Nonmember = $30

1. I verify that I have read this section and completed this education activity. _____ Date _____
Signature

2. What would be different in your practice if you applied what you have learned from this activity? (Please use additional paper if necessary.)

_____

_____

_____

	Strongly disagree				Strongly agree
3. The activity met the stated objectives.					
a. Describe what constitutes advocacy.	1	2	3	4	5
b. Describe how a bill becomes a law.	1	2	3	4	5
c. Describe methods of communication with a member of Congress.	1	2	3	4	5
d. Outline the history of ANNA's advocacy over the past 3 decades.	1	2	3	4	5
e. Review the purpose and preparation for End Stage Renal Disease (ESRD) Education Week.	1	2	3	4	5
4. The content was current and relevant.	1	2	3	4	5
5. The content was presented clearly.	1	2	3	4	5
6. The content was covered adequately.	1	2	3	4	5

7. How would you rate your ability to apply your learning to practice? ☐ diminished ability ☐ no change ☐ enhanced ability

Comments _____

8. Time required to read the section and complete this form: _____ minutes

This educational activity is provided by the American Nephrology Nurses' Association (ANNA) for **2.4** contact hours.
ANNA is accredited as a provider of continuing nursing education (CNE) by the American Nurses Credentialing Center's Commission on Accreditation (ANCC-COA).
ANNA is a provider approved of continuing nursing education by the California Board of Registered Nursing, provider number CEP 00910.
This CNE offering meets the Nephrology Nursing Certification Commission's (NNCC's) continuing nursing education requirements for certification and recertification.

Core Curriculum for Nephrology Nursing contains 18 sections of educational content. Individual learners may apply for continuing nursing education credit by reading a section and completing the Continuing Nursing Education Evaluation Form for that section. Learners may apply for continuing nursing education credit for any or all sections.

Please photocopy this test page, complete, and return to ANNA.

You can also download it from www.annanurse.org (choose Education → CNE Activities → Publications)

Name: _____

Address: _____

City: _____ State: _____ Zip: _____

E-mail:_____ Preferred telephone: ☐ Home ☐ Work

State where licensed and license number: _____

CNE application fees are based upon the number of contact hours provided by the individual section. CNE fees per contact hour for ANNA members are as follows: 1.0-1.9 – $15; 2.0-2.9 – $20; 3.0-3.9 – $25; 4.0 and higher – $30. Fees for nonmembers are $10 higher.

CNE application fee for **Section 8** : ANNA member $25 Nonmember $35

ANNA Member: ☐ Yes ☐ No ☐ Member # (if available) _____

☐ Check or money order enclosed ☐ American Express ☐ Visa ☐ MasterCard

Total amount submitted: _____

Credit card number _____ Exp. Date _____

Name as it appears on the card:_____

NOTE: Your evaluation form can be processed in 1 week for an additional rush charge of $5.00.
☐ **Yes, I would like this evaluation form rush processed. I have included an additional fee of $5.00 for rush processing.**

INSTRUCTIONS

1. To receive continuing nursing education credit for an individual study after reading the section, complete this evaluation form.

2. Detach, photocopy, or download (www.annanurse.org) the evaluation form and send along with a check or money order payable to **American Nephrology Nurses' Association** to: ANNA, East Holly Avenue Box 56, Pitman, NJ 08071-0056.

3. Test returns must be postmarked by **December 31, 2012**. Upon completion of the answer/evaluation form, a certificate for **3.2** contact hour(s) will be awarded and sent to you.

This section was reviewed and formatted for contact hour credit by Sally S. Russell, MN, CMSRN, ANNA Director of Education Services.

> **CNE Application Fee for Section 8**
> **ANNA member = $25**
> **Nonmember = $35**

1. I verify that I have read this section and completed this education activity. _____ Date _____
Signature

2. What would be different in your practice if you applied what you have learned from this activity? (Please use additional paper if necessary.)

_____

_____

_____

	Strongly disagree				Strongly agree
3. The activity met the stated objectives.					
a. Perform a nutrition-focused physical examination on patients with kidney disorders.	1	2	3	4	5
b. Explain nutritional recommendations for patients receiving hemodialysis (HD) and peritoneal dialysis (PD).	1	2	3	4	5
c. Outline goals of nutritional care for geriatric patients with kidney disease.	1	2	3	4	5
d. Discuss how to meet increased nutritional needs of pregnant patients receiving dialysis or kidney transplant.	1	2	3	4	5
e. Analyze stages of behavioral change that influence patients with kidney disease to adjust to the renal nutrition regimen.	1	2	3	4	5
4. The content was current and relevant.	1	2	3	4	5
5. The content was presented clearly.	1	2	3	4	5
6. The content was covered adequately.	1	2	3	4	5
7. How would you rate your ability to apply your learning to practice?	☐ diminished ability		☐ no change		☐ enhanced ability

Comments _____

_____

8. Time required to read the section and complete this form: _____ minutes

This educational activity is provided by the American Nephrology Nurses' Association (ANNA) for **3.2** contact hours.
ANNA is accredited as a provider of continuing nursing education (CNE) by the American Nurses Credentialing Center's Commission on Accreditation (ANCC-COA).
ANNA is a provider approved of continuing nursing education by the California Board of Registered Nursing, provider number CEP 00910.
This CNE offering meets the Nephrology Nursing Certification Commission's (NNCC's) continuing nursing education requirements for certification and recertification.

Pharmacologic Aspects of Chronic Kidney Disease

ANNP809

Core Curriculum for Nephrology Nursing contains 18 sections of educational content. Individual learners may apply for continuing nursing education credit by reading a section and completing the Continuing Nursing Education Evaluation Form for that section. Learners may apply for continuing nursing education credit for any or all sections.

Please photocopy this test page, complete, and return to ANNA.

You can also download it from www.annanurse.org (choose Education → CNE Activities → Publications)

Name: _____

Address: _____

City: _____ State: _____ Zip: _____

E-mail:_____ Preferred telephone: ☐ Home ☐ Work

State where licensed and license number: _____

CNE application fees are based upon the number of contact hours provided by the individual section. CNE fees per contact hour for ANNA members are as follows: 1.0-1.9 – $15; 2.0-2.9 – $20; 3.0-3.9 – $25; 4.0 and higher – $30. Fees for nonmembers are $10 higher.

CNE application fee for **Section 9** : ANNA member – $25 Nonmember – $35

ANNA Member: ☐ Yes ☐ No ☐ Member # (if available) _____

☐ Check or money order enclosed ☐ American Express ☐ Visa ☐ MasterCard

Total amount submitted: _____

Credit card number _____ Exp. Date _____

Name as it appears on the card:_____

NOTE: Your evaluation form can be processed in 1 week for an additional rush charge of $5.00.
☐ Yes, I would like this evaluation form rush processed. I have included an additional fee of $5.00 for rush processing.

INSTRUCTIONS

1. To receive continuing nursing education credit for an individual study after reading the section, complete this evaluation form.
2. Detach, photocopy, or download (www.annanurse.org) the evaluation form and send along with a check or money order payable to **American Nephrology Nurses' Association** to: ANNA, East Holly Avenue Box 56, Pitman, NJ 08071-0056.
3. Test returns must be postmarked by **December 31, 2012.** Upon completion of the answer/evaluation form, a certificate for **3.0** contact hour(s) and **180** minutes of pharmacology content will be awarded and sent to you.

This section was reviewed and formatted for contact hour credit by Sally S. Russell, MN, CMSRN, ANNA Director of Education Services.

CNE Application Fee for Section 9
ANNA member = $25
Nonmember = $35

1. I verify that I have read this section and completed this education activity. _____ Date _____

   Signature

2. What would be different in your practice if you applied what you have learned from this activity? (Please use additional paper if necessary.)

   _____

   _____

	Strongly disagree				Strongly agree
3. The activity met the stated objectives.					
a. Describe the pharmacokinetic and pharmacodynamic changes that occur as a result of renal failure.	1	2	3	4	5
b. List the purpose, at least one example, and the major caveats or relevant facts related to the following classifications of drugs used to treat patients with renal failure: analgesics, antacids (systemic), antianemics, antidiarrheals, antiemetics, antihyperlipidemics, antihypertensives, antimicrobials, cardiotonics, cation-exchange resins, diuretics, glucocorticoids, heavy metal chelating agents, histamine H1 and H2 receptor antagonists, mineralocorticoids, phosphate binders, prokinetic agents, proton pump inhibitors, sedative-hypnotics, stool softeners, cathartics, and vitamins.	1	2	3	4	5
c. List six factors that determine the effect of dialysis on the half-life, or concentration, of a drug.	1	2	3	4	5
d. Describe the approach to determining dosing adjustments for patients with renal failure.	1	2	3	4	5
e. Identify the clinical significance of renal failure on drug activity in terms of the following areas of nursing practice: monitoring and administering medications, educating the patient, and fostering patient compliance.	1	2	3	4	5
4. The content was current and relevant.	1	2	3	4	5
5. The content was presented clearly.	1	2	3	4	5
6. The content was covered adequately.	1	2	3	4	5
7. How would you rate your ability to apply your learning to practice?	☐ diminished ability ☐ no change ☐ enhanced ability				

Comments _____

_____

8. Time required to read the section and complete this form: _____ minutes

This educational activity is provided by the American Nephrology Nurses' Association (ANNA) for **3.0** contact hours and **180** minutes of pharmacology content.
ANNA is accredited as a provider of continuing nursing education (CNE) by the American Nurses Credentialing Center's Commission on Accreditation (ANCC-COA).
ANNA is a provider approved of continuing nursing education by the California Board of Registered Nursing, provider number CEP 00910.
This CNE offering meets the Nephrology Nursing Certification Commission's (NNCC's) continuing nursing education requirements for certification and recertification.

Core Curriculum for Nephrology Nursing contains 18 sections of educational content. Individual learners may apply for continuing nursing education credit by reading a section and completing the Continuing Nursing Education Evaluation Form for that section. Learners may apply for continuing nursing education credit for any or all sections.

Please photocopy this test page, complete, and return to ANNA.

You can also download it from www.annanurse.org (choose Education → CNE Activities → Publications)

Name: _____

Address: _____

City: _____ State: _____ Zip: _____

E-mail: _____ Preferred telephone: ☐ Home ☐ Work

State where licensed and license number: _____

CNE application fees are based upon the number of contact hours provided by the individual section. CNE fees per contact hour for ANNA members are as follows: 1.0-1.9 – $15; 2.0-2.9 – $20; 3.0-3.9 – $25; 4.0 and higher – $30. Fees for nonmembers are $10 higher.

CNE application fee for **Section 10** : ANNA member $25   Nonmember $35

ANNA Member: ☐ Yes   ☐ No   ☐ Member # (if available) _____

☐ Check or money order enclosed   ☐ American Express   ☐ Visa   ☐ MasterCard

Total amount submitted: _____

Credit card number _____ Exp. Date _____

Name as it appears on the card: _____

NOTE: Your evaluation form can be processed in 1 week for an additional rush charge of $5.00.
☐ **Yes, I would like this evaluation form rush processed. I have included an additional fee of $5.00 for rush processing.**

---

1. I verify that I have read this section and completed this education activity. _____ Date _____
Signature

2. What would be different in your practice if you applied what you have learned from this activity? (Please use additional paper if necessary.)

_____

_____

_____

	Strongly disagree				Strongly agree
3. The activity met the stated objectives.					
a. Explain methods for modification of the immune system as related to organ transplantation.	1	2	3	4	5
b. Discuss criteria for living and deceased donors.	1	2	3	4	5
c. Outline the preoperative care of the renal transplant recipient.	1	2	3	4	5
d. Develop a collaborative care plan for the transplant recipient during the postoperative period.	1	2	3	4	5
e. Discuss long-term complications of kidney transplantation.	1	2	3	4	5
4. The content was current and relevant.	1	2	3	4	5
5. The content was presented clearly.	1	2	3	4	5
6. The content was covered adequately.	1	2	3	4	5
7. How would you rate your ability to apply your learning to practice?	☐ diminished ability	☐ no change		☐ enhanced ability	

Comments _____

_____

8. Time required to read the section and complete this form: _____ minutes

---

Hemodialysis   **ANNP811**

Core Curriculum for Nephrology Nursing contains 18 sections of educational content. Individual learners may apply for continuing nursing education credit by reading a section and completing the Continuing Nursing Education Evaluation Form for that section. Learners may apply for continuing nursing education credit for any or all sections.

Please photocopy this test page, complete, and return to ANNA.

You can also download it from www.annanurse.org (choose Education → CNE Activities → Publications)

Name: _____

Address: _____

City: _____ State: _____ Zip: _____

E-mail: _____ Preferred telephone: ☐ Home ☐ Work

State where licensed and license number: _____

CNE application fees are based upon the number of contact hours provided by the individual section. CNE fees per contact hour for ANNA members are as follows: 1.0-1.9 – $15; 2.0-2.9 – $20; 3.0-3.9 – $25; 4.0 and higher – $30. Fees for nonmembers are $10 higher.

CNE application fee for **Section 11** : ANNA member $30   Nonmember $40

ANNA Member: ☐ Yes   ☐ No   ☐ Member # (if available) _____

☐ Check or money order enclosed   ☐ American Express   ☐ Visa   ☐ MasterCard

Total amount submitted: _____

Credit card number _____ Exp. Date _____

Name as it appears on the card: _____

NOTE: Your evaluation form can be processed in 1 week for an additional rush charge of $5.00.
☐ **Yes, I would like this evaluation form rush processed. I have included an additional fee of $5.00 for rush processing.**

INSTRUCTIONS

1. To receive continuing nursing education credit for an individual study after reading the section, complete this evaluation form.

2. Detach, photocopy, or download (www.annanurse.org) the evaluation form and send along with a check or money order payable to **American Nephrology Nurses' Assocation** to: ANNA, East Holly Avenue Box 56, Pitman, NJ 08071-0056.

3. Test returns must be postmarked by **December 31, 2012**. Upon completion of the answer/evaluation form, a certificate for **4.2** contact hour(s) will be awarded and sent to you.

This section was reviewed and formatted for contact hour credit by Sally S. Russell, MN, CMSRN, ANNA Director of Education Services.

> **CNE Application Fee for Section 11**
> **ANNA member = $30**
> **Nonmember = $40**

1. I verify that I have read this section and completed this education activity. _____ Date _____
   Signature

2. What would be different in your practice if you applied what you have learned from this activity? (Please use additional paper if necessary.)

   _____
   _____
   _____

	Strongly disagree				Strongly agree
3. The activity met the stated objectives.					
a. Describe the principles of hemodialysis, including diffusion, osmosis, pressures, and pumps.	1	2	3	4	5
b. Outline the preparation necessary for a successful hemodialysis treatment to occur.	1	2	3	4	5
c. List the composition and function of a typical dialysate solution.	1	2	3	4	5
d. Summarize the considerations required to safely and accurately reach patient dry weight on hemodialysis.	1	2	3	4	5
e. Describe general guidelines for target values for hemodialysis adequacy.	1	2	3	4	5
4. The content was current and relevant.	1	2	3	4	5
5. The content was presented clearly.	1	2	3	4	5
6. The content was covered adequately.	1	2	3	4	5

7. How would you rate your ability to apply your learning to practice?   ☐ diminished ability ☐ no change ☐ enhanced ability

Comments _____
_____

8. Time required to read the section and complete this form: _____ minutes

This educational activity is provided by the American Nephrology Nurses' Association (ANNA) for **4.2** contact hours.
ANNA is accredited as a provider of continuing nursing education (CNE) by the American Nurses Credentialing Center's Commission on Accreditation (ANCC-COA).
ANNA is a provider approved of continuing nursing education by the California Board of Registered Nursing, provider number CEP 00910.
This CNE offering meets the Nephrology Nursing Certification Commission's (NNCC's) continuing nursing education requirements for certification and recertification.

Vascular Access for Hemodialysis

ANNP812

Core Curriculum for Nephrology Nursing contains 18 sections of educational content. Individual learners may apply for continuing nursing education credit by reading a section and completing the Continuing Nursing Education Evaluation Form for that section. Learners may apply for continuing nursing education credit for any or all sections.

Please photocopy this test page, complete, and return to ANNA.

You can also download it from www.annanurse.org (choose Education → CNE Activities → Publications)

Name: _____

Address: _____

City: _____ State: _____ Zip: _____

E-mail: _____ Preferred telephone: ☐ Home ☐ Work

State where licensed and license number: _____

CNE application fees are based upon the number of contact hours provided by the individual section. CNE fees per contact hour for ANNA members are as follows: 1.0-1.9 – $15; 2.0-2.9 – $20; 3.0-3.9 – $25; 4.0 and higher – $30. Fees for nonmembers are $10 higher.

CNE application fee for **Section 12** : ANNA member $20 Nonmember $30

ANNA Member: ☐ Yes ☐ No ☐ Member # (if available) _____

☐ Check or money order enclosed ☐ American Express ☐ Visa ☐ MasterCard

Total amount submitted: _____

Credit card number _____ Exp. Date _____

Name as it appears on the card: _____

NOTE: Your evaluation form can be processed in 1 week for an additional rush charge of $5.00.
☐ **Yes, I would like this evaluation form rush processed. I have included an additional fee of $5.00 for rush processing.**

INSTRUCTIONS

1. To receive continuing nursing education credit for an individual study after reading the section, complete this evaluation form.

2. Detach, photocopy, or download (www.annanurse.org) the evaluation form and send along with a check or money order payable to **American Nephrology Nurses' Assocation** to: ANNA, East Holly Avenue Box 56, Pitman, NJ 08071-0056.

3. Test returns must be postmarked by **December 31, 2012**. Upon completion of the answer/evaluation form, a certificate for **2.6** contact hour(s) will be awarded and sent to you.

This section was reviewed and formatted for contact hour credit by Sally S. Russell, MN, CMSRN, ANNA Director of Education Services.

> **CNE Application Fee for Section 12**
> **ANNA member = $20**
> **Nonmember = $30**

---

1. I verify that I have read this section and completed this education activity. _____ Date _____
   Signature

2. What would be different in your practice if you applied what you have learned from this activity? (Please use additional paper if necessary.)

   _____
   _____
   _____

	Strongly disagree				Strongly agree
3. The activity met the stated objectives.					
a. List the preferential order for vascular access according to the 2006 KDOQI guidelines.	1	2	3	4	5
b. State the steps for assessment for each type of vascular access.	1	2	3	4	5
c. List the possible causes and diagnoses of complications that occur with the use of vascular access.	1	2	3	4	5
d. Describe routine planning for management of the vascular access, implementation (including cannulation), and interventions for complications.	1	2	3	4	5
e. Define the ongoing evaluation by the vascular access team through continuous quality improvement.	1	2	3	4	5
4. The content was current and relevant.	1	2	3	4	5
5. The content was presented clearly.	1	2	3	4	5
6. The content was covered adequately.	1	2	3	4	5

7. How would you rate your ability to apply your learning to practice? ☐ diminished ability ☐ no change ☐ enhanced ability

Comments _____
_____

8. Time required to read the section and complete this form: _____ minutes

---

This educational activity is provided by the American Nephrology Nurses' Association (ANNA) for **2.6** contact hours.
ANNA is accredited as a provider of continuing nursing education (CNE) by the American Nurses Credentialing Center's Commission on Accreditation (ANCC-COA).
ANNA is a provider approved of continuing nursing education by the California Board of Registered Nursing, provider number CEP 00910.
This CNE offering meets the Nephrology Nursing Certification Commission's (NNCC's) continuing nursing education requirements for certification and recertification.

Section 13 ── ┌───┐ ── **4.2 Contact Hours**
│ CONTINUING NURSING EDUCATION EVALUATION FORM │
└───┘

Peritoneal Dialysis   **ANNP813**

Core Curriculum for Nephrology Nursing contains 18 sections of educational content. Individual learners may apply for continuing nursing education credit by reading a section and completing the Continuing Nursing Education Evaluation Form for that section. Learners may apply for continuing nursing education credit for any or all sections.

Please photocopy this test page, complete, and return to ANNA.

You can also download it from www.annanurse.org (choose Education → CNE Activities → Publications)

Name: _____

Address: _____

City: _____ State: _____ Zip: _____

E-mail:_____ Preferred telephone: ☐ Home ☐ Work

State where licensed and license number: _____

CNE application fees are based upon the number of contact hours provided by the individual section. CNE fees per contact hour for ANNA members are as follows: 1.0-1.9 – $15; 2.0-2.9 – $20; 3.0-3.9 – $25; 4.0 and higher – $30. Fees for nonmembers are $10 higher.

CNE application fee for **Section 13** :   ANNA member $30   Nonmember $40

ANNA Member: ☐ Yes   ☐ No   ☐ Member # (if available) _____

☐ Check or money order enclosed   ☐ American Express   ☐ Visa   ☐ MasterCard

Total amount submitted: _____

Credit card number _____ Exp. Date _____

Name as it appears on the card: _____

NOTE: Your evaluation form can be processed in 1 week for an additional rush charge of $5.00.
☐ **Yes, I would like this evaluation form rush processed. I have included an additional fee of $5.00 for rush processing.**

INSTRUCTIONS

1. To receive continuing nursing education credit for an individual study after reading the section, complete this evaluation form.

2. Detach, photocopy, or download (www.annanurse.org) the evaluation form and send along with a check or money order payable to **American Nephrology Nurses' Association** to: ANNA, East Holly Avenue Box 56, Pitman, NJ 08071-0056.

3. Test returns must be postmarked by **December 31, 2012.** Upon completion of the answer/evaluation form, a certificate for **4.2 contact hour(s)** will be awarded and sent to you.

This section was reviewed and formatted for contact hour credit by Sally S. Russell, MN, CMSRN, ANNA Director of Education Services.

┌─────────────────────────────────┐
│ **CNE Application Fee for Section 13** │
│ **ANNA member = $30** │
│ **Nonmember = $40** │
└─────────────────────────────────┘

---

1. I verify that I have read this section and completed this education activity. _____ Date _____
   Signature

2. What would be different in your practice if you applied what you have learned from this activity? (Please use additional paper if necessary.)

   _____
   _____
   _____

	Strongly disagree				Strongly agree
3. The activity met the stated objectives.					
a. Describe four components of nursing care prior to peritoneal dialysis catheter insertion.	1	2	3	4	5
b. State two ways intraabdominal pressure can be minimized after catheter insertion.	1	2	3	4	5
c. Differentiate between immediate postoperative and long-term care of the peritoneal dialysis catheter exit site.	1	2	3	4	5
d. Discuss the risk factors, pathophysiology, nursing assessment, and collaborative management of the complications related to peritoneal dialysis access.	1	2	3	4	5
e. List 5 indications for catheter removal and discuss under what circumstances simultaneous removal and reimplantation might be appropriate.	1	2	3	4	5
4. The content was current and relevant.	1	2	3	4	5
5. The content was presented clearly.	1	2	3	4	5
6. The content was covered adequately.	1	2	3	4	5

7. How would you rate your ability to apply your learning to practice?   ☐ diminished ability   ☐ no change   ☐ enhanced ability

Comments _____

8. Time required to read the section and complete this form: _____ minutes

---

This educational activity is provided by the American Nephrology Nurses' Association (ANNA) for **4.2** contact hours.
ANNA is accredited as a provider of continuing nursing education (CNE) by the American Nurses Credentialing Center's Commission on Accreditation (ANCC-COA).
ANNA is a provider approved of continuing nursing education by the California Board of Registered Nursing, provider number CEP 00910.
This CNE offering meets the Nephrology Nursing Certification Commission's (NNCC's) continuing nursing education requirements for certification and recertification.

Choosing Home Therapies   **ANNP814**

Core Curriculum for Nephrology Nursing contains 18 sections of educational content. Individual learners may apply for continuing nursing education credit by reading a section and completing the Continuing Nursing Education Evaluation Form for that section. Learners may apply for continuing nursing education credit for any or all sections.

Please photocopy this test page, complete, and return to ANNA.

You can also download it from www.annanurse.org (choose Education → CNE Activities → Publications)

Name: _____

Address: _____

City: _____ State: _____ Zip: _____

E-mail:_____ Preferred telephone: ☐ Home ☐ Work

State where licensed and license number: _____

CNE application fees are based upon the number of contact hours provided by the individual section. CNE fees per contact hour for ANNA members are as follows: 1.0-1.9 – $15; 2.0-2.9 – $20; 3.0-3.9 – $25; 4.0 and higher – $30. Fees for nonmembers are $10 higher.

CNE application fee for **Section 14** :   ANNA member $20   Nonmember $30

ANNA Member: ☐ Yes   ☐ No   ☐ Member # (if available) _____

☐ Check or money order enclosed   ☐ American Express   ☐ Visa   ☐ MasterCard

Total amount submitted: _____

Credit card number _____ Exp. Date _____

Name as it appears on the card: _____

NOTE: Your evaluation form can be processed in 1 week for an additional rush charge of $5.00.
☐ **Yes, I would like this evaluation form rush processed. I have included an additional fee of $5.00 for rush processing.**

INSTRUCTIONS

1. To receive continuing nursing education credit for an individual study after reading the section, complete this evaluation form.

2. Detach, photocopy, or download (www.annanurse.org) the evaluation form and send along with a check or money order payable to **American Nephrology Nurses' Assocation** to: ANNA, East Holly Avenue Box 56, Pitman, NJ 08071-0056.

3. Test returns must be postmarked by **December 31, 2012.** Upon completion of the answer/evaluation form, a certificate for **2.6** contact hour(s) will be awarded and sent to you.

This section was reviewed and formatted for contact hour credit by Sally S. Russell, MN, CMSRN, ANNA Director of Education Services.

> **CNE Application Fee for Section 14**
> **ANNA member = $20**
> **Nonmember = $30**

---

1. I verify that I have read this section and completed this education activity. _____ Date _____
                                                                Signature

2. What would be different in your practice if you applied what you have learned from this activity? (Please use additional paper if necessary.)

_____

_____

_____

		Strongly disagree				Strongly agree
3. The activity met the stated objectives.						
a. State the clinical advantages to patients on home dialysis therapies.		1	2	3	4	5
b. Identify the necessary components that are required for a successful home dialysis program.		1	2	3	4	5
c. Outline the training requirements necessary to assure patients are safe and competent to perform home dialysis.		1	2	3	4	5
d. Summarize the role of the nursing staff in managing and monitoring patients at home.		1	2	3	4	5
4. The content was current and relevant.		1	2	3	4	5
5. The content was presented clearly.		1	2	3	4	5
6. The content was covered adequately.		1	2	3	4	5
7. How would you rate your ability to apply your learning to practice?		☐ diminished ability	☐ no change	☐ enhanced ability		

Comments _____

8. Time required to read the section and complete this form: _____ minutes

---

This educational activity is provided by the American Nephrology Nurses' Association (ANNA) for **2.6** contact hours.
ANNA is accredited as a provider of continuing nursing education (CNE) by the American Nurses Credentialing Center's Commission on Accreditation (ANCC-COA).
ANNA is a provider approved of continuing nursing education by the California Board of Registered Nursing, provider number CEP 00910.
This CNE offering meets the Nephrology Nursing Certification Commission's (NNCC's) continuing nursing education requirements for certification and recertification.

Care of the Infant through Adolescent with Chronic Kidney Disease   **ANNP815**

Core Curriculum for Nephrology Nursing contains 18 sections of educational content. Individual learners may apply for continuing nursing education credit by reading a section and completing the Continuing Nursing Education Evaluation Form for that section. Learners may apply for continuing nursing education credit for any or all sections.

Please photocopy this test page, complete, and return to ANNA.

You can also download it from www.annanurse.org (choose Education → CNE Activities → Publications)

Name: _____

Address: _____

City: _____ State: _____ Zip: _____

E-mail:_____Preferred telephone: ☐ Home ☐ Work

State where licensed and license number: _____

CNE application fees are based upon the number of contact hours provided by the individual section. CNE fees per contact hour for ANNA members are as follows: 1.0-1.9 – $15; 2.0-2.9 – $20; 3.0-3.9 – $25; 4.0 and higher – $30. Fees for nonmembers are $10 higher.

CNE application fee for **Section 15**:   ANNA member $25   Nonmember $35

ANNA Member: ☐ Yes   ☐ No   ☐ Member # (if available) _____

☐ Check or money order enclosed   ☐ American Express   ☐ Visa   ☐ MasterCard

Total amount submitted: _____

Credit card number_____ Exp. Date _____

Name as it appears on the card:_____

NOTE: Your evaluation form can be processed in 1 week for an additional rush charge of $5.00.
☐ Yes, I would like this evaluation form rush processed. I have included an additional fee of $5.00 for rush processing.

INSTRUCTIONS

1. To receive continuing nursing education credit for an individual study after reading the section, complete this evaluation form.

2. Detach, photocopy, or download (www.annanurse.org) the evaluation form and send along with a check or money order payable to **American Nephrology Nurses' Assocation** to: ANNA, East Holly Avenue Box 56, Pitman, NJ 08071-0056.

3. Test returns must be postmarked by **December 31, 2012.** Upon completion of the answer/evaluation form, a certificate for **3.4** contact hour(s) will be awarded and sent to you.

This section was reviewed and formatted for contact hour credit by Sally S. Russell, MN, CMSRN, ANNA Director of Education Services.

┌─────────────────────────────────┐
│ **CNE Application Fee for Section 15** │
│ **ANNA member = $25** │
│ **Nonmember = $35** │
└─────────────────────────────────┘

---

1. I verify that I have read this section and completed this education activity. _____ Date _____
Signature

2. What would be different in your practice if you applied what you have learned from this activity? (Please use additional paper if necessary.)

_____
_____
_____

		Strongly disagree				Strongly agree
3. The activity met the stated objectives.						
a. Explain systemic effects of CKD on children.		1	2	3	4	5
b. Discuss specific psychosocial needs of children with CKD.		1	2	3	4	5
c. List clinical issues relative to a pediatric patient beginning CRRT.		1	2	3	4	5
d. Assess a pediatric patient's response to a hemodialysis treatment and assess dry weight.		1	2	3	4	5
e. Identify specific areas where anticipatory guidance is of benefit to the child with CKD.		1	2	3	4	5
4. The content was current and relevant.		1	2	3	4	5
5. The content was presented clearly.		1	2	3	4	5
6. The content was covered adequately.		1	2	3	4	5

7. How would you rate your ability to apply your learning to practice?   ☐ diminished ability   ☐ no change   ☐ enhanced ability

Comments _____
_____

8. Time required to read the section and complete this form: _____ minutes

---

This educational activity is provided by the American Nephrology Nurses' Association (ANNA) for **3.4** contact hours.
ANNA is accredited as a provider of continuing nursing education (CNE) by the American Nurses Credentialing Center's Commission on Accreditation (ANCC-COA).
ANNA is a provider approved of continuing nursing education by the California Board of Registered Nursing, provider number CEP 00910.
This CNE offering meets the Nephrology Nursing Certification Commission's (NNCC's) continuing nursing education requirements for certification and recertification.

Core Curriculum for Nephrology Nursing contains 18 sections of educational content. Individual learners may apply for continuing nursing education credit by reading a section and completing the Continuing Nursing Education Evaluation Form for that section. Learners may apply for continuing nursing education credit for any or all sections.

Please photocopy this test page, complete, and return to ANNA.

You can also download it from www.annanurse.org (choose Education → CNE Activities → Publications)

Name: _____

Address: _____

City: _____ State: _____ Zip: _____

E-mail: _____ Preferred telephone: ☐ Home ☐ Work

State where licensed and license number: _____

CNE application fees are based upon the number of contact hours provided by the individual section. CNE fees per contact hour for ANNA members are as follows: 1.0-1.9 – $15; 2.0-2.9 – $20; 3.0-3.9 – $25; 4.0 and higher – $30. Fees for nonmembers are $10 higher.

CNE application fee for **Section 16** : ANNA member $25 Nonmember $35

ANNA Member: ☐ Yes ☐ No ☐ Member # (if available) _____

☐ Check or money order enclosed ☐ American Express ☐ Visa ☐ MasterCard

Total amount submitted: _____

Credit card number _____ Exp. Date _____

Name as it appears on the card: _____

NOTE: Your evaluation form can be processed in 1 week for an additional rush charge of $5.00.
☐ Yes, I would like this evaluation form rush processed. I have included an additional fee of $5.00 for rush processing.

INSTRUCTIONS

1. To receive continuing nursing education credit for an individual study after reading the section, complete this evaluation form.

2. Detach, photocopy, or download (www.annanurse.org) the evaluation form and send along with a check or money order payable to **American Nephrology Nurses' Assocation** to: ANNA, East Holly Avenue Box 56, Pitman, NJ 08071-0056.

3. Test returns must be postmarked by **December 31, 2012**. Upon completion of the answer/evaluation form, a certificate for **3.0** contact hour(s) will be awarded and sent to you.

This section was reviewed and formatted for contact hour credit by Sally S. Russell, MN, CMSRN, ANNA Director of Education Services.

CNE Application Fee for Section 16
ANNA member = $25
Nonmember = $35

---

1. I verify that I have read this section and completed this education activity. _____ Date _____
Signature

2. What would be different in your practice if you applied what you have learned from this activity? (Please use additional paper if necessary.)

_____

_____

_____

	Strongly disagree				Strongly agree
3. The activity met the stated objectives.					
a. Correlate structural, physiologic, and functional changes of the aging process with implications for health care.	1	2	3	4	5
b. Identify factors contributing to the increases in CKD in the older adult population.	1	2	3	4	5
c. Identify age-specific aspects of acute and chronic kidney failure.	1	2	3	4	5
d. Explore the pharmacodynamics of aging and CKD.	1	2	3	4	5
e. Discuss the impact of the aging process on modality selection, including in-center and home, the long-term care setting, nocturnal, transplantation, and hospice with and without therapy.	1	2	3	4	5
4. The content was current and relevant.	1	2	3	4	5
5. The content was presented clearly.	1	2	3	4	5
6. The content was covered adequately.	1	2	3	4	5

7. How would you rate your ability to apply your learning to practice? ☐ diminished ability ☐ no change ☐ enhanced ability

Comments _____

_____

8. Time required to read the section and complete this form: _____ minutes

---

This educational activity is provided by the American Nephrology Nurses' Association (ANNA) for **3.0** contact hours.
ANNA is accredited as a provider of continuing nursing education (CNE) by the American Nurses Credentialing Center's Commission on Accreditation (ANCC-COA).
ANNA is a provider approved of continuing nursing education by the California Board of Registered Nursing, provider number CEP 00910.
This CNE offering meets the Nephrology Nursing Certification Commission's (NNCC's) continuing nursing education requirements for certification and recertification.

Core Curriculum for Nephrology Nursing contains 18 sections of educational content. Individual learners may apply for continuing nursing education credit by reading a section and completing the Continuing Nursing Education Evaluation Form for that section. Learners may apply for continuing nursing education credit for any or all sections.

Please photocopy this test page, complete, and return to ANNA.

You can also download it from www.annanurse.org (choose Education → CNE Activities → Publications)

Name: _____

Address: _____

City: _____ State: _____ Zip: _____

E-mail:_____ Preferred telephone: ☐ Home ☐ Work

State where licensed and license number: _____

CNE application fees are based upon the number of contact hours provided by the individual section. CNE fees per contact hour for ANNA members are as follows: 1.0-1.9 – $15; 2.0-2.9 – $20; 3.0-3.9 – $25; 4.0 and higher – $30. Fees for nonmembers are $10 higher.

CNE application fee for **Section 17** :   ANNA member $20   Nonmember $30

ANNA Member: ☐ Yes   ☐ No   ☐ Member # (if available) _____

☐ Check or money order enclosed   ☐ American Express   ☐ Visa   ☐ MasterCard

Total amount submitted: _____

Credit card number_____ Exp. Date _____

Name as it appears on the card:_____

NOTE: Your evaluation form can be processed in 1 week for an additional rush charge of $5.00.
☐ **Yes, I would like this evaluation form rush processed. I have included an additional fee of $5.00 for rush processing.**

INSTRUCTIONS
1. To receive continuing nursing education credit for an individual study after reading the section, complete this evaluation form.
2. Detach, photocopy, or download (www.annanurse.org) the evaluation form and send along with a check or money order payable to **American Nephrology Nurses' Association** to: ANNA, East Holly Avenue Box 56, Pitman, NJ 08071-0056.
3. Test returns must be postmarked by **December 31, 2012**. Upon completion of the answer/evaluation form, a certificate for **2.4** contact hour(s) will be awarded and sent to you.

This section was reviewed and formatted for contact hour credit by Sally S. Russell, MN, CMSRN, ANNA Director of Education Services.

CNE Application Fee for Section 17
ANNA member = $20
Nonmember = $30

---

1. I verify that I have read this section and completed this education activity. _____ Date _____
Signature

2. What would be different in your practice if you applied what you have learned from this activity? (Please use additional paper if necessary.)

_____

_____

_____

	Strongly disagree				Strongly agree
3. The activity met the stated objectives.					
a. Outline current recommendations for immunizations in patients with chronic kidney disease.	1	2	3	4	5
b. Identify how contamination of the delivery system fluid pathway can contribute to patient infections.	1	2	3	4	5
c. Define how hepatitis B, hepatitis C, hepatitis D, and HIV are spread in the dialysis unit.	1	2	3	4	5
d. Describe infection control measures that should be taken with any dialysis patient.	1	2	3	4	5
e. Define how the CQI process may be used to address infection control issues in the dialysis unit.	1	2	3	4	5
4. The content was current and relevant.	1	2	3	4	5
5. The content was presented clearly.	1	2	3	4	5
6. The content was covered adequately.	1	2	3	4	5

7. How would you rate your ability to apply your learning to practice?   ☐ diminished ability   ☐ no change   ☐ enhanced ability

Comments _____

_____

8. Time required to read the section and complete this form: _____ minutes

---

This educational activity is provided by the American Nephrology Nurses' Association (ANNA) for **2.4** contact hours.
ANNA is accredited as a provider of continuing nursing education (CNE) by the American Nurses Credentialing Center's Commission on Accreditation (ANCC-COA).
ANNA is a provider approved of continuing nursing education by the California Board of Registered Nursing, provider number CEP 00910.
This CNE offering meets the Nephrology Nursing Certification Commission's (NNCC's) continuing nursing education requirements for certification and recertification.

Emergency and Disaster Preparedness

ANNP818

Core Curriculum for Nephrology Nursing contains 18 sections of educational content. Individual learners may apply for continuing nursing education credit by reading a section and completing the Continuing Nursing Education Evaluation Form for that section. Learners may apply for continuing nursing education credit for any or all sections.

Please photocopy this test page, complete, and return to ANNA.

You can also download it from www.annanurse.org (choose Education → CNE Activities → Publications)

Name: _____

Address: _____

City: _____ State: _____ Zip: _____

E-mail: _____ Preferred telephone: ☐ Home ☐ Work

State where licensed and license number: _____

CNE application fees are based upon the number of contact hours provided by the individual section. CNE fees per contact hour for ANNA members are as follows: 1.0-1.9 – $15; 2.0-2.9 – $20; 3.0-3.9 – $25; 4.0 and higher – $30. Fees for nonmembers are $10 higher.

CNE application fee for **Section 18** : ANNA member $20   Nonmember $30

ANNA Member: ☐ Yes   ☐ No   ☐ Member # (if available) _____

☐ Check or money order enclosed   ☐ American Express   ☐ Visa   ☐ MasterCard

Total amount submitted: _____

Credit card number _____ Exp. Date _____

Name as it appears on the card: _____

NOTE: Your evaluation form can be processed in 1 week for an additional rush charge of $5.00.

☐ **Yes, I would like this evaluation form rush processed. I have included an additional fee of $5.00 for rush processing.**

INSTRUCTIONS

1. To receive continuing nursing education credit for an individual study after reading the section, complete this evaluation form.

2. Detach, photocopy, or download (www.annanurse.org) the evaluation form and send along with a check or money order payable to **American Nephrology Nurses' Assocation** to: ANNA, East Holly Avenue Box 56, Pitman, NJ 08071-0056.

3. Test returns must be postmarked by **December 31, 2012**. Upon completion of the answer/evaluation form, a certificate for **2.6** contact hour(s) will be awarded and sent to you.

This section was reviewed and formatted for contact hour credit by Sally S. Russell, MN, CMSRN, ANNA Director of Education Services.

> **CNE Application Fee for Section 18**
> **ANNA member = $20**
> **Nonmember = $30**

---

1. I verify that I have read this section and completed this education activity. _____ Date _____

   Signature

2. What would be different in your practice if you applied what you have learned from this activity? (Please use additional paper if necessary.)

   _____
   _____
   _____

		Strongly disagree				Strongly agree
3.	The activity met the stated objectives.					
	a. Define the role of the nephrology nurse in disaster and emergency preparedness and response.	1	2	3	4	5
	b. Provide strategies for training of employees, patients, and communities in disaster emergency preparedness.	1	2	3	4	5
	c. List resources and references for further information, tools, and expert advice.	1	2	3	4	5
	d. Identify best practices and strategies for dealing with disaster situations.	1	2	3	4	5
4.	The content was current and relevant.	1	2	3	4	5
5.	The content was presented clearly.	1	2	3	4	5
6.	The content was covered adequately.	1	2	3	4	5
7.	How would you rate your ability to apply your learning to practice?	☐ diminished ability ☐ no change ☐ enhanced ability					

Comments _____
_____

8. Time required to read the section and complete this form: _____ minutes

---

This educational activity is provided by the American Nephrology Nurses' Association (ANNA) for **2.6** contact hours.
ANNA is accredited as a provider of continuing nursing education (CNE) by the American Nurses Credentialing Center's Commission on Accreditation (ANCC-COA).
ANNA is a provider approved of continuing nursing education by the California Board of Registered Nursing, provider number CEP 00910.
This CNE offering meets the Nephrology Nursing Certification Commission's (NNCC's) continuing nursing education requirements for certification and recertification.

Self-Assessment Questions

Section 1

1. Which of the following hormones is secreted by the kidneys?
   a. Aldosterone
   b. Angiotensin
   c. Somatostatin
   d. Renin

2. The kidneys receive approximately _____%
   of the cardiac output under normal physiologic conditions.
   a. 10–15
   b. 15–20
   c. 20–25
   d. 25–30

3. When tubular filtrate enters the late distal tubule and collecting tubule, it is
   a. hypertonic.
   b. hypotonic.
   c. isotonic.
   d. None of the above

4. One etiology of intrarenal azotemia is
   a. x-ray contrast media.
   b. anaphylactic reaction.
   c. neurogenic bladder.
   d. renal artery emboli.

5. Patient problems noted in the diuretic stage of acute renal failure can include all of the following, *except:*
   a. Hypokalemia
   b. Renal hypoplasia
   c. Hyperphosphatemia
   d. Metabolic alkalosis

6. Acute poststreptococcal glomerulonephritis (APSGN)
   a. occurs primarily in the elderly.
   b. is treated with immunosuppressives.
   c. causes hypoalbuminemia.
   d. follows a streptococcal infection.

7. Malignant renal neoplasms are treated with
   a. irradiation.
   b. radical nephrectomy.
   c. chemotherapy.
   d. Both b and c

8. Blood urea creatinine (BUN) may be elevated in all of the following, *except:*
   a. Pregnancy
   b. Hypertension
   c. Fluid volume depletion
   d. GI bleed

9. Patient care following a renal angiogram includes
   a. providing education about why the test was done.
   b. assessment of pedal pulses.
   c. removing pressure dressing after 6 hours.
   d. walking patient to the bathroom immediately.

10. Creatinine clearance is
    a. the amount of blood cleared in one hour.
    b. found to increase as kidney function decreases.
    c. about 110 to 120 for a young adult.
    d. a measure of the cardiac output.

Section 2

11. The most common cause of kidney disease is
    a. diabetes mellitus (DM).
    b. hypertension (HTN).
    c. autoimmune disease.
    d. congenital disease.

12. The pathologic process associated with diabetes is
    a. autoimmune destruction of beta cells of the pancreas with subsequent insulin deficiency.
    b. abnormalities that result in resistance to insulin action.
    c. Both a and b
    d. None of the above

13. The most common cause of mortality in persons with diabetes is
    a. nephropathy or kidney failure.
    b. infection.
    c. cardiovascular disease (CVD).
    d. cerebrovascular disease.

14. Autoimmune diabetic disease is manifested by
    a. low or undetectable levels of C-peptide.
    b. ketoacidosis.
    c. little insulin secretion over time leading to the need for exogenous insulin.
    d. All of the above

15. Type 2 diabetes is characterized by
    a. relative deficiency of insulin production.
    b. decreased insulin action.
    c. increased insulin resistance.
    d. All of the above

16. Reduced GFR may be associated with an increased level of nontraditional CVD risk factors. One nontraditional risk factor is
    a. HTN.
    b. DM.
    c. infection.
    d. anemia.

17. Goals of antihypertensive therapy in patients with CKD include the desire to
    a. slow the rate of progression and reduce proteinuria.
    b. prevent the progression of cardiovascular complications.
    c. Both a and b
    d. None of the above

Section 3

18. Advantages of using a centrifugal, continuous flow device for performing TPE compared to an intermittent flow device include
    a. higher blood flow rates.
    b. smaller extracorporeal blood volume.
    c. faster treatment times compared to the intermittent flow devices.
    d. All of the above

19. For TPE procedures using a centrifuge device (e.g. COBE Spectra, Fresenius AS104), what is the name of the anticoagulant used?
    a. Heparin
    b. An anticoagulant is not needed
    c. ACD-A
    d. ACD-B

20. When using FFP or CRP as a replacement fluid, which premedications are recommended to avoid blood transfusion reactions?
    a. Zantac and an antibiotic
    b. Zofran, ASA, and an antibiotic
    c. None are needed
    d. Benadryl, SoluCortef, and/or Tylenol

21. If a patient undergoing TPE develops mild signs or symptoms of citrate toxicity, what should be done to avoid progression into a more severe citrate toxicity?
    a. Decrease the inlet flow rate and consider calcium replacement.
    b. Nothing. Just ignore the symptoms.
    c. Terminate the procedure.
    d. Give the patient Tylenol.

22. SLEDD or CRRT treatment should be initiated when
    a. the kidneys are unable to maintain the patient's fluid balance.
    b. the patient is in MSOF.
    c. the kidneys can't manage the solute load and the BUN and creatinine are rising daily.
    d. Both a and c

23. Complications that can be a result of citrate anticoagulation that require vigilant monitoring include
    a. hypocalcemia.
    b. hypernatremia.
    c. metabolic alkalosis.
    d. All of the above

24. Maintaining an effective SLEDD or CRRT program is challenging. Which of the following elements are important to a successful program?
    a. Training nephrology nurses to set up, perform, and troubleshoot all modalities
    b. Training the ICU nurses to perform the bedside patient care aspects of running these therapies
    c. Facilitating ongoing bedside collaboration and education between the nephrology nurses and ICU nurses
    d. All of the above

25. Which of the following records are important for an Acute Dialysis program to maintain and have available for inspecting agencies (CMS, JCAHO, State Health Department)?
    a. Water culture and LAL results
    b. Dialysis machine maintenance records
    c. Employee performance appraisals
    d. All of the above

26. The cause of acute tubular necrosis (ATN) in sepsis is
    a. renal hypoperfusion.
    b. ischemic injury to proximal tubule cells.
    c. ischemic injury to efferent arterioles.
    d. Both a and b

27. Infection accounts for 75% of deaths in patients with acute renal failure.
    a. True
    b. False

28. Xigris is an anti-inflammatory agent that has been proven effective in the treatment of sepsis. What medication should be avoided when a patient is being treated with Xigris?
    a. Procrit
    b. Vasopressin
    c. Heparin
    d. ACE-inhibitors

Section 4

29. Patient communication tools must include
    a. sensitivity, awareness, knowledge, and alternatives to written communication.
    b. telephones, beepers, computers, and PDAs.
    c. sensitivity, spirituality, self awareness, and self actualization.
    d. sensitivity, religious convictions, sexual awareness, and acceptance.

30. Cultural-specific health beliefs and practices affect the health and well-being of individuals of that group. Therefore, it is important for the nurse to _____ when providing care.
    a. be aware of the individual's practice patterns
    b. be aware of the individual's desire to go home
    c. be aware of the individual's marital status
    d. be aware of whether or not the individual has children

31. What action should be considered last when a dialysis patient exhibits a change in behavior?
    a. Assess the patient's mood.
    b. Warn the patient that negative behaviors will not be tolerated in the facility.
    c. Allow the patient to discuss their concerns.
    d. Assess for changes in social or family functioning.

32. Which is the most important step in working with caregivers of new dialysis patients?
    a. Clearly communicate facility policies and consequences of violations.
    b. Provide education to the caregiver.
    c. Refer the caregiver to the social worker for support.
    d. Both b and c

33. How can a patient get Medicare for ESRD at the earliest possible date?
    a. Start in-center dialysis and ask for Medicare to be backdated.
    b. Start a home dialysis training program before the third full month of dialysis.
    c. Apply for the state's Medicaid program.
    d. Contact the local senator and request help.

34. When should the nurse refer a patient to a social worker?
    a. If the patient and family are not coping well with kidney disease and treatment
    b. If the patient is not working, but may be able to work and believes he/she can't work with kidney disease
    c. If the patient is not adhering to treatment
    d. All of the above

35. Considerations for withholding treatment include all of the following, *except:*
    a. Known wishes of the patient
    b. Known wishes of the family
    c. Prior Advanced Directives
    d. Data based prognostic considerations

36. The most crucial element in the process of learning is
    a. age.
    b. gender.
    c. ability to understand language.
    d. attitude.

37. The Patient Self-Determination Act (1991) is a federal mandate that each state must address the issue of identifying care wishes of all patients on admission to acute care facilities, nursing homes, home health agencies, and hospice programs.
    a. True
    b. False

38. Patients must stop dialysis in order to be eligible for hospice benefits.
    a. True
    b. False

Section 5

39. Which of the following is correct regarding proteinuria?
    a. The first morning spot urine corresponds best to the 24 hour urine protein excretion.
    b. The mid morning spot urine corresponds best to the 24 hour urine protein excretion.
    c. Proteinuria is defined as <200mg/g in a spot urine for protein to creatinine ratio.
    d. Microalbuminuria is defined as <200mg/g in a spot urine for albumin to creatinine ratio.

40. NKF-KDOQI guidelines recommend screening for kidney disease in people at risk. The minimal parameters include
    a. blood pressure, urine protein, serum creatinine, urine sediment.
    b. blood pressure, serum creatinine, blood urea nitrogen, urine sediment.
    c. serum creatinine, urine protein, urine sediment, blood urea nitrogen.
    d. serum creatinine, blood urea nitrogen, urine sediment, urine protein.

41. The potential for malnutrition is a concern for patients with CKD stages 3 and 4. Measures to help counteract this include
    a. 0.8–1 gram/protein/kg/day.
    b. 30–35 cal/kg/day, depending on age.
    c. high biologic value protein, such as egg yolks.
    d. subjective patient reports (most accurate for determining malnutrition).

42. Which of the following medications should be avoided in CKD stages 3 and 4?
    a. Nonsteroidal anti-inflammatory drugs (e.g. ibuprofen)
    b. Biphosphonates (e.g. alendronate)
    c. Antihistamines (e.g. cetirizeine)
    d. Antibiotics (e.g. gentamicin)

43. Stage 5 CKD is defined as a GFR of less than
    a. 30 mL/min/1.73 m^2.
    b. 25 mL/min/1.73 m^2.
    c. 15 mL/min/1.73 m^2.
    d. 10 mL/min/1.73 m^2.

44. An example of a likely cause of intrinsic renal injury would be
    a. nephrolithiasis.
    b. obstruction from bladder carcinoma.
    c. nephrectomy.
    d. rhabdomyolysis.

45. Acute peritoneal dialysis, rather than hemodialysis, is used when
    a. continuous renal replacement therapy is not available.
    b. the patient is hemodynamically stable.
    c. fluid volume needs to be removed rapidly.
    d. the arteriovenous fistula needs time to mature.

46. In the long-term management of transplant recipients, it would be most important to
    a. measure antibody levels.
    b. look for signs of delayed graft function.
    c. evaluate for infection.
    d. stop all immunosuppression.

47. According to the 2006 revision of the NKF-KDOQI *Vascular Access Guidelines*
    a. all stenoses that are larger than 50% of the intraluminal diameter should be angioplastied.
    b. pediatric patients with AVG and AVF < 650mL/min/1.73 m2 should be referred for balloon angioplasty within 48 hours.
    c. a permanent access (fistula preferably) or AVG should be created at least 6 months before dialysis initiation.
    d. All of the above

48. What is the blood pressure goal for a patient with CKD and diabetes?
    a. 120/70
    b. 125/75
    c. 130/70
    d. 130/75

Section 6

49. Which of the following could be considered evidence-based practice?
    a. Use of clinical practice guidelines
    b. Explicit use of best evidence in making decisions
    c. A systematic review of multiple research studies
    d. A comparison of outcomes between groups

50. Which of the following could be considered pertinent databases to be utilized for evidence?
    a. Bibliographic databases that describe articles
    b. Systematic approaches to using pertinent literature
    c. Qualitative research databases
    d. Synopsis of recommendations for treatment

51. The first issue to consider in formulating the question for clinical practice is the need to
    a. exclude previous research.
    b. prioritize clinical issues and problems.
    c. eliminate a culture of organizational resistance.
    d. hold in-depth workshops on evidence-based practice for all staff.

52. Which of the following are standards of care?
    a. Statements used as a guide to one's practice area
    b. Summarization and synthesis of knowledge gained from research
    c. Critical assessment and evaluation of specific clinical questions
    d. Responsibilities for which its practitioners are accountable

53. Which of the following underlying principles influences nursing practice? The need to
    a. provide age-appropriate, culturally and ethnically sensitive care.
    b. realize that all patients may not need continuity of care.
    c. demonstrate that care collaboration ends upon admission to an acute care setting.
    d. educate patients only when requested.

54. Guidelines may be defined as
    a. clinical opinions of attending nephrologists.
    b. systematic statements based on scientific evidence.
    c. routine and customary care.
    d. explicit use of best evidence in making decisions.

55. Which of the following is correct regarding the NKF-KDOQI guidelines?
    a. The KDOQI are **NOT** standards of care.
    b. The KDOQI guidelines are based on expert opinion.
    c. The KDOQI guidelines are developed by nurses serving on work groups.
    d. The KDOQI guidelines improve outcomes for individuals with acute kidney injury.

56. The goal of the DOPPS was to
    a. explore practice patterns associated with improved patient outcomes.
    b. determine a means to provide cost-effective care.
    c. ascertain means to decrease the amount of dialysis required.
    d. promote adherence to the prescribed renal regimen.

57. Although there is a high mortality rate in the chronic kidney failure population, the level of health-related quality of life
    a. remains the same.
    b. lowers.
    c. increases every 5 years.
    d. decreases after 10 years.

58. Depression is considered to be
    a. a predictor of morbidity.
    b. a predictor of loss vascular access.
    c. a key quality of life indicator.
    d. difficult to assess.

Section 7

59. The purpose of position statements is to
    a. provide tools for members to become knowledgeable about health policy advocacy.
    b. represent succinct summaries of an organization's stand on an issue.
    c. formally establish a program or activity.
    d. formally approve the appropriation of funds for an authorized program or activity.

60. Which of the following is true about resolutions?
    a. They can be introduced by any member of congress.
    b. A resolution enforces a law.

    c. They are formal statements of decision or expressions of opinions.
    d. The ideas for resolutions can come from any citizen.

61. Once a bill has been passed
    a. no further input is allowed by citizens.
    b. it is referred to the appropriate regulatory agency for the development of regulations.
    c. it is referred to the appropriate regulatory agency for enactment.
    d. it goes to conference committee for final markup.

62. The most effective methods of communicating to elected officials include all of the following, *except*:
    a. Identifying yourself as a RN
    b. Expressing an appreciation for the member's time
    c. Offering assistance as a resource
    d. Providing extensive detailed information

63. All of the following are areas in which nephrology nurses can impact health policy, *except*:
    a. Participating in the Nurse Licensure Compact
    b. Obtaining a copy of a Nurse Practice Act
    c. Requesting a representative to co-sponsor a bill
    d. Voting

Section 8

64. After KRT has been initiated, protein intake should be
    a. restricted to 0.6 to 0.8 gm/kg of edema free body weight.
    b. a minimum of 1.2 gm/kg of edema free body weight.
    c. 0.8 to 1.0 gm/kg of predialysis weight.
    d. restricted to < 1.0 gm/kg/day if predialysis BUN is > 80 mg/dL.

65. Which of the following parameters can be used when assessing growth and weight gain in the pediatric patient on dialysis?
    a. Body mass index
    b. Head circumference
    c. Mid-arm circumference
    d. All of the above

66. Why are prenatal vitamins usually avoided for the pregnant patient on dialysis?
    a. They don't contain enough Vitamin C.
    b. They contain too much Vitamin A.
    c. They contain too much iron.
    d. They contain too little biotin.

67. Because there are increased calcium needs for fetal development, what is the generally recommended calcium content of the dialysate with more frequent dialysis treatments?
    a. 3.0 mEq/L
    b. 2.0 mEq/L
    c. 3.5 mEq/L
    d. 2.5 mEq/L

68. What is one consequence of inadequate amounts of energy and protein intake in older hemodialysis patients?
    a. Lower tolerance of hemodialysis
    b. The need for more time on dialysis
    c. Lower markers of functional status
    d. Lower Kt/V

69. What are 3 comorbid conditions which may affect adequate nutritional intakes in geriatric patients with CKD?
    a. Dementia, hypertension, and diabetes
    b. Dementia, poor dentition, and depression
    c. Dementia, depression, and hypertension
    d. CVA, diabetes, and hypertension

70. Why is frequent medication review especially necessary with geriatric patients?
    a. Drug interactions or inappropriate medication use can lead to confusion, memory loss and anorexia in geriatric patients.
    b. Medications must be renewed every month for patients over 65 years of age.
    c. Medications must always be titrated for elderly patients.
    d. Elderly patients have limited insurance coverage for all medications.

71. The major nutrient difference between the acute and chronic post transplant period is
    a. calories.
    b. fat.
    c. protein.
    d. phosphorus.

72. Appropriate foods to treat hypoglycemia for patients on dialysis include
    a. orange juice or apple juice.
    b. jelly beans or milk.
    c. apple juice or glucose tablets.
    d. chocolate or peanuts.

73. Protein quality for the vegetarian renal diet is determined by
    a. complementation of proteins.
    b. digestibility.
    c. amino acid content.
    d. Both b and c

Section 9

74. Which of the following organ systems is involved in drug excretion?
    a. Kidneys
    b. Lungs
    c. Intestines
    d. All of the above

75. Which of the following is a potential reason that a patient may not adhere with a medication regimen? The patient has
    a. exhibited forgetfulness about taking the medication.
    b. discontinued use of medications because of a fear of side effects.
    c. a personal dissatisfaction with the regimen.
    d. All of the above

76. Which of the following is an effect of kidney failure on drug characteristics?
    a. Absorption is decreased in kidney failure due to decreased perfusion of the organ.
    b. Distribution may be increased because of the increased fluid accumulation in kidney failure.
    c. Protein binding is increased as a result of protein accumulation in kidney failure.
    d. The half-life of most drugs is usually unchanged in kidney failure.

77. Which of the following is false regarding the effects of kidney failure on drug activity?
    a. Loading doses generally need to be reduced in kidney failure to avoid toxicity.
    b. Decreasing the maintenance dose may be necessary to reduce the potential for toxicity in kidney failure.
    c. The effects of kidney failure on the pharmacokinetics alter the dose-response curve of the drug.
    d. Increasing the dosing interval may lead to wider variations in plasma levels compared to decreasing the dose.

78. Which of the following is true regarding use of antianemic drugs in patients with kidney failure?
    a. Administration of ESA therapy can increase quality of life, but has no impact on long-term problems, such as cardiovascular disease.
    b. Adequacy of dialysis does not need to be evaluated as hematocrit rises with ESA therapy.
    c. Oral iron preparations and phosphate binders can be administered concurrently.
    d. Iron stores must be monitored periodically in patients receiving ESA therapy to ensure adequate response.

79. Which of the following is an important concept regarding the use of antihypertensives in patients with kidney failure?
    a. Aggressive dose adjustments should be made to achieve target blood pressure in patients with kidney failure.
    b. Beta-adrenergic blockers can be discontinued rapidly once a patient reaches the goal blood pressure.
    c. ACE inhibitors may be useful in slowing the progression of glomerulosclerosis in patients with kidney disease.
    d. Dihydropyridine calcium channel blockers have more antiproteinuric effects than nondi-hydropyridine calcium channel blockers.

80. Which of the following is true regarding dialyzability of drugs?
    a. Drugs that are normally primarily excreted by the kidney are usually also removed by hemodialysis.
    b. Drugs with a larger molecular weight are more likely to be removed by dialysis.
    c. Drugs that are highly protein bound are more likcly to be removed by dialysis.
    d. Drugs with a small volume of distribution are less likely to be removed by dialysis.

81. Which of the following is **NOT** part of the approach to determining the dosing adjustment in patients with kidney failure?
    a. Determining treatment goals
    b. Identifying drug interactions with other medications
    c. Estimation of creatinine clearance
    d. Adjusting the regimen based on drug response

82. Which of the following is an important concept to consider when monitoring and administering medications to patients with kidney failure?
    a. Evaluating the serum levels of medications and electrolytes as appropriate
    b. Understanding the drug characteristics of medications the patient is taking
    c. Being aware of all of the medications the patient is taking
    d. All of the above

83. Which of the following is a helpful strategy to foster adherence in patients with kidney failure?
    a. Simplify the medication regimen to fit the patient's schedule.
    b. Help the patient to understand the rational for the treatment.
    c. Provide written and verbal instructions and information regarding the medications.
    d. All of the above

Section 10

84. An autograft is transplantation of
    a. a person's own tissue.
    b. tissues between identical twins.
    c. tissues from the same species.
    d. tissues from a different species.

85. Contraindications for donating a kidney include all of the following, *except:*
    a. Current or recent malignancy
    b. Mild obesity
    c. Active infection
    d. Current substance abuse

86. Postoperative management of the kidney transplant recipient includes monitoring fluid and electrolyte balance by
    a. daily electrolyte levels.
    b. observing for hypotension.
    c. administering diuretics as prescribed.
    d. All of the above

87. Chronic rejection of a transplanted kidney
    a. occurs days to months following a transplant.
    b. is probably both T cell and B cell mediated.
    c. involves blood vessels being blocked.
    d. has no successful treatment.

88. Pancreas transplantation is performed to treat
    a. type 1 diabetes.
    b. type 2 diabetes.
    c. renal transplant patients.
    d. Both a and c

89. Simultaneous pancreas-kidney transplants
    a. improve outcome if done early in the course of renal failure.
    b. decrease the risk of immunosuppression.
    c. offer greatest 1-year graft survival.
    d. jeopardize the kidney's long-term function.

90. The complication most likely to occur following pancreas transplantation is
    a. arterial thrombosis.
    b. bleeding.
    c. anastamotic leak.
    d. pancreatitis.

91. The most common site for islet cell infusion for transplantation is the
    a. portal vein.
    b. subclavian vein.
    c. femoral vein.
    d. brachial vein.

92. Management of CKD prior to cardiac transplantation includes
    a. increasing the dose of ACE inhibitors.
    b. avoiding beta-blocker therapy.
    c. continual renal replacement if the patient is hemodynamically unstable.
    d. measuring the serum creatinine levels frequently.

93. Hepatorenal syndrome in liver failure patients may occur because of
    a. renal vasoconstriction.
    b. a decrease in blood volume.
    c. decreased sympathetic nervous system stimulation.
    d. decreased function of the renin-angiotensin system.

Section 11

94. Which substance is **NOT** usually contained in dialysate?
    a. Glucose
    b. Potassium
    c. Bicarbonate
    d. Citric acid

95. If breakthrough of chloramines or chlorine is detected or in the water exiting the first carbon tank, then the next action taken should be to
    a. test after the second carbon tank for chloramine and chlorine breakthrough.
    b. stop all hemodialysis treatments and divert patients to another facility.
    c. take no further action at this time and retest in 2 hours.
    d. Both a and b

96. Chronic inflammation is believed to be from long-term exposure to low levels of
    a. Endotoxin
    b. Magnesium
    c. Potassium
    d. Pure water

97. Potential causes of a hypotensive episode during hemodialysis include
    a. hypoxemia.
    b. medications.
    c. eating.
    d. All of the above

98. The most common cause of intradialytic morbidities is
    a. too much fluid removed.
    b. rate of decrease in blood volume.
    c. reduced peripheral vascular resistance.
    d. Both b and c

99. Hemolysis during dialysis is related to exposure of the patient's blood to
    a. chloramines and nitrosamines.
    b. formaldehyde.
    c. high dialysate temperature.
    d. All of the above

100. If the patient is receiving a digitalis derivative, the nurse should be certain that
    a. the dialysate potassium is 0.
    b. the dialysate potassium is 2 mmol or greater.
    c. the digitalis derivative is not given on dialysis days.
    d. the digitalis derivative dose is increased on dialysis days.

101. Minimal changes in Hct and blood volume may be acceptable if the patient
    a. is getting near his Hct threshold and the UFR is in minimum.
    b. has a large urinary output and the UFR is in minimum.
    c. has diarrhea or a small weight gain and the UFR is in minimum.
    d. All of the above

102. Patients who have a pyrogenic reaction, which can emanate from inadequately reprocessed hemodialyzers, exhibit which of the following symptoms?
    a. Malaise, positive blood cultures
    b. Chest pain, shortness of breath, access pain
    c. Fever, chills, rigors, nausea and vomiting, body aches, hypotension
    d. Bright red or dark blood in the extracorporeal circuit

103. According to the Centers for Disease Control and Prevention (CDC)
    a. patients with hepatitis B may participate in a reuse program.
    b. patients who are HIV positive or have AIDS may participate in a reuse program.
    c. patients who have tuberculosis may participate in a reuse program.
    d. Both b and c

Section 12

104. Patient evaluation for long-term access placement must include
    a. history of any previous surgery.
    b. determining the patient's dominant arm.
    c. history of bleeding disorders.
    d. All of the above

105. Early complications of arteriovenous fistulas include observing for
    a. edema in the opposite extremity.
    b. a nonmaturing outflow vein.
    c. steal syndrome.
    d. pseudoaneurysms.

106. An advantage of arteriovenous grafts is
    a. they are technically easier to cannulate.
    b. they have the lowest rate of thrombosis.
    c. they are associated with increased survival rates.
    d. they can utilize the buttonhole technique.

107. Central venous catheters
    a. are interposed between an artery and a vein.
    b. provide a vessel for cannulation.
    c. are reinforced to prevent collapse.
    d. become infected easily.

108. Assessments of arteriovenous fistulas and arteriovenous grafts should be made for
    a. neck and facial edema.
    b. catheter occlusion.
    c. increased sensation in the arm.
    d. pulses in the access extremity.

109. Assessment related to percutaneous catheters should exhibit
    a. an absence of respiratory distress.
    b. a reddened exit site.
    c. an inability to withdraw anticoagulants.
    d. an inability to push saline.

110. For all health care facilities, the Centers for Disease Control and Prevention (CDC) recommends _____ seconds of vigorous handwashing prior to cannulating an AVG or AVF.
    a. 10
    b. 15
    c. 20
    d. 25

111. When choosing the sites prior to cannulation, 50% of the discernible vessel should be reserved for the _____ site, and the remainder for the _____ site.
    a. arterial...venous
    b. venous...arterial

112. Buttonhole cannulation is repeated cannulation into the same puncture site. The scar tissue tunnel tract allows the needle to
    a. pass through to the inflow vessel.
    b. make a different path each time.
    c. pass through to the outflow vessel.
    d. None of the above

113. The primary access failure rate should include which of the following?
    a. Forearm straight grafts – 25%
    b. Forearm loop grafts – 30%
    c. Upper arm grafts – 15%
    d. Tunneled catheters – 5%

Section 13

114. Patients having a chronic peritoneal dialysis catheter implanted need to be taught
    a. postoperative exit site care.
    b. how to determine where the catheter should be placed.
    c. what kidney failure is.
    d. about all the different types of catheters available.

115. Following peritoneal dialysis catheter implantation, a patient is instructed that
    a. the exit site will always be tender.
    b. baggy clothes will have to be worn.
    c. the catheter will need to be changed monthly.
    d. well-healed, healthy exit sites make swimming possible.

116. Characteristics of an infected exit site may include all of the following, *except:*
    a. Tender or painful area
    b. Purulent drainage
    c. Color at site that is pale
    d. Edema

117. Factors that influence solute transport across the peritoneal membrane include all of the following, *except:*
    a. Peritoneal membrane size
    b. Time of day
    c. Peritoneal blood flow
    d. Dialysis solution volume

118. The peritoneal dialysis cycle is
    a. infusion, dwell, and drainage.
    b. drainage, dwell, and infusion.
    c. dwell, infusion, and drainage.
    d. infusion, drainage, and dwell.

119. Warming methods are problematic for peritoneal dialysis because
    a. it is difficult to get them warm enough.
    b. the correct methods are different for each person.
    c. people like different temperatures.
    d. the glucose may degrade to toxic carbonyl compounds.

120. Continuous cycling peritoneal dialysis (CCPD) uses which of the following schedules?
    a. Every other day for 4–6 hours
    b. 4 times throughout the day
    c. 3–5 overnight cycles
    d. Twice a week

121. Dialysate leaks are most common when
    a. the deep cuff is implanted in muscle.
    b. the catheters are intact.
    c. proper care has not been given to the exit site.
    d. the tissue has not grown into the cuff.

122. Cardiovascular complications of peritoneal dialysis include
    a. hyperlipidemia.
    b. increases in cardiac output.
    c. hypoglycemia.
    d. right ventricular hypertrophy.

123. Electrolyte disturbances that occur with peritoneal dialysis may include
    a. hypokalemia.
    b. hypernatremia.
    c. hyperkalemia.
    d. All of the above

Section 14

124. Which of the following is **NOT** a goal when interviewing the prospective peritoneal dialysis patient?
    a. To provide education information for patient and family
    b. To assess the patient's readiness for self care
    c. To provide a supportive environment
    d. To start immediate training

125. The environment for the interview is very important to facilitate learning and to diminish anxiety. All of the following should be in place, *except:*
    a. Appropriate seating for patient and others
    b. Background music playing
    c. Well ventilated room
    d. Nonglare lighting

126. Which of the following is **NOT** true when interviewing a patient with a language barrier?
    a. Instruct the interpreter to translate information/response exactly as stated.
    b. The use of an interpreter will lengthen the interview.
    c. Family members may interject their own biases.
    d. The utilization of the family to interpret is the optimal choice.

127. When training the peritoneal dialysis patient, the nurse should
    a. individualize the training as much as possible.
    b. include the family members when possible.
    c. document each training session.
    d. All of the above

128. Problem-solving techniques that are taught to the home peritoneal dialysis patient include
    a. what to do when obstruction of dialysate flow occurs.
    b. recognizing change in color of effluent.
    c. what to do when any tubing is disconnected.
    d. All of the above

129. A daily hygiene program at home should include all of the following, *except:*
    a. A daily shower if possible
    b. Inspection and cleansing of the exit site
    c. Use of perfumed soaps and lotions at the exit site
    d. Careful hand washing before each exchange

130. As part of the health care team, the _____ instructs the peritoneal dialysis patient about adequate protein intake.
    a. social worker
    b. occupational therapist
    c. dietitian
    d. psychiatrist

131. In initiating home peritoneal dialysis and providing home care management, the peritoneal dialysis nurse must be able to
    a. provide appropriate education for the patient and family.
    b. coordinate the members of the health care team.
    c. establish a relationship with the patient and family.
    d. All of the above

Section 15

132. Renal tubular immaturity leads to
    a. decreased capacity to vary sodium and water reabsorption.
    b. increased ability to concentrate urine.
    c. decreased excretion of sodium.
    d. kidney transplant.

133. HUS is most commonly caused by
    a. staphylococcus infection.
    b. E. coli infection.
    c. pseudomonas infection.
    d. streptococcus infection.

134. CKD staging in children is best achieved by
    a. obtaining a 24 hour creatinine clearance test.
    b. estimating the GFR using a formula that incorporates height, weight, and creatinine.
    c. using the creatinine and BUN as the markers.
    d. using height and weight as the markers.

135. Administration of ESAs in children are
    a. given subcutaneously on a weekly basis and dose adjusted to reach target range.
    b. given IV monthly until target is reached, then titrated.
    c. determined by treatment setting, class of ESA and anticipated frequency and pain.
    d. held until the hemoglobin is less than 10.0 g/dL to avoid pain of the injections as long as possible.

136. In a patient with HUS, which of the following is **NOT** appropriate care?
    a. Hemodialysis
    b. Peritoneal dialysis
    c. Antibiotic therapy
    d. Transfusion of red blood cells

137. Important aspects in preparing children for kidney transplantation include the need to
    a. control or improve renal osteodystrophy.
    b. correct anemia with blood transfusions.
    c. perform native nephrectromies.
    d. hold immunizations until after transplantation.

138. Accurate assessment of patient intravascular volume using noninvasive in-line monitoring during the HD treatment
    a. is a substitute for continuous arterial blood pressure monitoring.
    b. may be particularly helpful in correcting anemia in patients weighing less than 35 kg.
    c. may optimize ultrafiltration in pediatric patients.
    d. is a substitute for ECG monitoring.

139. Growth hormone should be started
    a. on all children with CKD to optimize growth potential.
    b. on all children starting dialysis.
    c. when patient falls off standard growth curve.
    d. Both a and b

140. CRRT is a therapy used for
    a. daily hemodialysis when the patient is fluid overloaded.
    b. acutely ill children who are unstable.
    c. home dialysis on the very small child or infant.
    d. adults only.

141. Circumstances in which a CVC may be acceptable for pediatric long-term access include
    a. lack of local surgical expertise to place a permanent vascular access.
    b. patient size being too small to support a permanent vascular access.
    c. expectation of expeditious kidney transplant.
    d. All of the above

Section 16

142. Three million older adults indicate they cannot perform basic activities of daily living (ADL).
    a. True
    b. False

143. Important aspects of interviewing an older adult include
    a. face the patient when talking with him or her.
    b. avoid acronyms and medical terminology.
    c. allow extra time for answers.
    d. All of the above

144. Structural changes in the cardiovascular system in the older adult include
    a. heart valves become flaccid and weak.
    b. aorta narrows.
    c. vessels lose elasticity and calcium deposits accumulate.
    d. conducting system experiences increase in cells and fibers.

145. Structural changes in the respiratory system of the older adult include
    a. chest diameter increases.
    b. chest wall compliance increases.
    c. cough reflex increased.
    d. moist mucous membranes.

146. Physiologic responses to changes in the GI system for the older adult include
    a. improved swallowing.
    b. taste sensitivity increased.
    c. increased motility of the lower tract.
    d. slower metabolism in the liver.

147. Physiologic response to changes in the renal system in the older adult include
    a. progressive decrease in renal blood flow.
    b. decreased ability to clear substances.
    c. solute load for nephrons increases.
    d. All of the above

148. Which of the following medications is processed through the kidneys and has a narrow therapeutic to toxic ratio?
    a. Digoxin
    b. Aminoglycosides
    c. Beta blockers
    d. Both a and b

149. Structural changes in the genitourinary system for the older adult may include
    a. weakened bladder muscles.
    b. increased bladder capacity.
    c. vaginal pH more alkalotic.
    d. prostatic tissues shrink due to hypoplasia.

150. Implications for health care with changes in the musculoskeletal system of the older adult are to
    a. encourage exercise to improve muscle tone and strength.
    b. caution about symptoms of dehydration.
    c. provide for a safe environment with mobilization.
    d. All of the above

151. Physiologic and functional response to changes in hearing as part of the sensory system of the older adult include
    a. decreased tone and voice localization.
    b. tone loss is greater at lower frequencies.
    c. pitch discrimination improves.
    d. Both a and b

Section 17

152. One of the factors that contributes to the development of drug-resistant organisms is
    a. nonadherence to handwashing procedures.
    b. completing the full course of antibiotics as prescribed.
    c. prescribing antibiotics based on culture and sensitivity reports.
    d. use of antibiotics to treat viral infections.

153. Outbreaks of hepatitis C in dialysis centers have been due to
    a. reuse of hemodialyzers on patients with hepatitis C.
    b. inadequate use of standard infection control procedures.
    c. contamination of the internal fluid pathway of the dialysis machine.
    d. failure to vaccinate patients for hepatitis C in a timely manner.

154. Mary Smith has just been released from the hospital, and her discharge summary indicates that she is colonized with MRSA. Colonization means that Mrs. Smith
    a. is actively infected with MRSA.
    b. has no signs or symptoms of active infection.
    c. is **NOT** able to spread MRSA to others.
    d. will not progress to active infection.

155. Patients with chronic kidney disease should receive a booster dose of hepatitis B vaccine when their hepatitis B antibody titers (anti-HBs) drop to
    a. < 15 mIU/mL.
    b. < 5 mIU/mL.
    c. < 10 mIU/mL.
    d. < 20 mIU/mL.

156. The route of transmission of tuberculosis is most commonly through
    a. contact with infected blood.
    b. inhalation of the organism into the lungs.
    c. ingestion of the organism through the fecal/oral route.
    d. touching objects and surfaces contaminated with TB.

157. The vascular access with the lowest incidence of infection is the
    a. AV graft.
    b. central venous catheter.
    c. AV fistula.
    d. None of the above

158. To prevent infections related to the dialysis unit's water, the water system should be disinfected
    a. daily.
    b. weekly.
    c. monthly.
    d. yearly.

159. The Centers for Disease Control and Prevention (CDC) recommends that persons with chronic kidney disease receive which vaccines?
    a. Hepatitis A, hepatitis B, and influenza
    b. Influenza, hepatitis B, and pneumococcal
    c. Hepatitis B, influenza, and whooping cough
    d. Pneumococcal, MMR, and influenza

160. To prevent infection, multiple dose medication vials must be kept
    a. on the patient's dialysis machine.
    b. on a designated medication cart that moves between patient stations.
    c. in the pocket of the nurse's scrub jacket.
    d. in a centralized area designated for medication preparation.

161. After each dialysis treatment, all reusable supplies and equipment are
    a. discarded and not reused.
    b. disinfected before use on another patient.
    c. used as long as there is no visible contamination.
    d. used for no more than three times before being discarded.

162. The Quality Improvement team in the dialysis center should include
    a. all members of the health care team.
    b. only the persons involved in addressing each specific problem.
    c. just the center's governing body.
    d. only the nurse manager and medical director.

Section 18

163. An example of a natural disaster is
    a. war.
    b. bioterrorism.
    c. nuclear accident.
    d. volcanic eruption.

164. The key to effective disaster management is
    a. risk assessment.
    b. post-disaster mitigation.
    c. pre-disaster planning and preparation.
    d. All of the above

165. What action should you **NOT** take during an earthquake?
    a. Face away from the windows.
    b. Start immediate termination procedures.
    c. Keep machine wheels locked at all times.
    d. Have patients protect their head and access.

166. Tornados generally last
    a. 10 minutes.
    b. 20 minutes.
    c. 1 hour.
    d. 2 hours or more.

167. The leading cause of death in a winter storm is
    a. heart attack.
    b. hypothermia.
    c. asphyxiation.
    d. ice and snow related automobile accidents.

168. Bioterrorism includes all of the following, *except:*
    a. Ricin
    b. Anthrax
    c. Asian flu
    d. Small pox

169. Which of the following questions is appropriate to ask to determine if the facility is ready to respond to a disaster?
    a. Do you perform disaster drills?
    b. Do you have a written disaster plan?
    c. How do you communicate to your staff and patients when the facility is closed?
    d. All of the above

170. The pre-event phase is focused on
    a. implementation of the plan.
    b. anticipation, planning, and training.
    c. minimizing the negative impact of the event.
    d. risk assessment, communication, and mitigation.

171. Which of the following must be assessed prior to using a generator as part of the disaster plan?
    a. Maintenance log
    b. Size of generator needed
    c. Fuel and fuel storage availability
    d. All of the above

172. The most common health concern after a volcanic eruption is
    a. infectious disease.
    b. respiratory illness.
    c. injuries from falls.
    d. All of the above

Answer Key

Section 1
1. d
2. c
3. b
4. a
5. b
6. d
7. d
8. a
9. b
10. c

Section 2
11. a
12. c
13. c
14. d
15. d
16. d
17. c

Section 3
18. d
19. c
20. d
21. a
22. d
23. d
24. d
25. d
26. d
27. a
28. c

Section 4
29. a
30. a
31. b
32. b
33. b
34. d
35. b

36. c
37. a
38. b

Section 5
39. a
40. a
41. b
42. a
43. c
44. d
45. a
46. c
47. d
48. b

Section 6
49. b
50. a
51. b
52. d
53. a
54. b
55. a
56. a
57. b
58. c

Section 7
59. b
60. c
61. b
62. d
63. a

Section 8
64. b
65. d
66. b
67. d
68. c
69. b

70. a
71. c
72. c
73. d

Section 9
74. d
75. d
76. b
77. a
78. d
79. c
80. a
81. b
82. d
83. d

Section 10
84. a
85. b
86. d
87. a
88. d
89. b
90. c
91. a
92. c
93. b

Section 11
94. d
95. a
96. a
97. d
98. d
99. d
100. b
101. d
102. c
103. d

Section 12
104. d
105. b
106. a
107. c
108. d
109. a
110. b
111. a
112. c
113. d

Section 13
114. a
115. d
116. c
117. b
118. a
119. d
120. c
121. d
122. a
123. d

Section 14
124. d
125. b
126. d
127. d
128. d
129. c
130. c
131. d

Section 15
132. a
133. b
134. b
135. c
136. c
137. a
138. c

139. c
140. b
141. d

Section 16
142. a
143. d
144. c
145. a
146. d
147. d
148. d
149. a
150. d
151. a

Section 17
152. d
153. b
154. b
155. c
156. b
157. c
158. c
159. b
160. d
161. b
162. a

Section 18
163. d
164. d
165. b
166. a
167. d
168. c
169. d
170. b
171. d
172. d

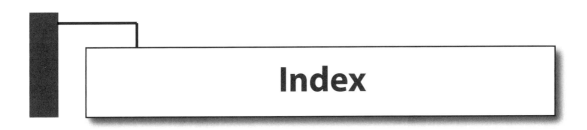

Index

Page numbers followed by f indicate figures.
Page numbers followed by t indicate tables.

Antifungal agents, 588, 589t, 599t
   in peritonitis, 844
Antigen, 621
Antigen-presenting cells, 621, 622
Antihistamines, 592, 596t
Antihyperlipidemic agents, 455t, 455–456, 583–584, 596t
Antihypertensive therapy, 104, 107, 584–588
   benefits of, 104, 104t, 112
   in children, 920
   in dialysis, 178, 596t
   in older adults, 960
   in pregnancy, 552
Antiinflammatory agents
   in dialysis, 596t
   in older adults, acute kidney injury from, 174, 946, 947
   precautions in chronic kidney disease, 423
Antilymphocyte globulin in kidney transplantation, 624, 627t
Antineoplastic agents, 599t
Antipsychotic agents, 599t
Antituberculosis agents, 987, 990–992
   in dialysis, 599t, 992, 992t
   resistance to, 987, 988, 992
Antiviral agents, 589, 599t
Anuria in acute kidney injury, 527
Anxiety
   in chronic kidney disease, 348, 356–357
   in plasma exchange, 294t
Aortic stenosis, angiography in, 83f
APACHE II (Acute Physiology and Chronic Health Evaluation II) Score, 145
Apheresis, 279–280
Aplasia, renal, 45
Apoptosis, 319, 325
Appetite
   in dialysis, 531
   in older adults, 541
Aquaporins, 26, 799
Arachidonic acid, 16, 17f
Arcuate arteries, 6, 6f
Arginine in dialysis, 531
Arm circumference measurements in nutrition assessment, 526
Arrhythmias
   in children, 920, 921
   drug therapy in, 596t
   in hemodialysis, 182, 182f, 712–713
      potassium serum levels affecting, 201, 202f
   in plasma exchange, 295t
Arterial blood pressure, mean, 186t
   in autoregulation of renal blood flow, 15, 17
Arteriovenous fistula
   for dialysis access, 486–491, 741–745
      in acute care setting, 435
      advantages and disadvantages of, 743
      cannulation procedure, 754–760
      in children, 913
      complications of, 743–745, 747, 760, 761
      definition of, 741
      facility differences in, 489, 489f
      failure to mature, 446, 447t

flow measurement in, 754, 754t
      in home therapy, 869
      indications for, 742
      infections of, 993
      locations of, 741, 742f
      maturation of, 753, 753t
      nursing process in, 752–762
      in older adults, 953–954, 957
      prevalence of, 487t, 488f, 491
      quality improvement process in, 761–762
      recirculation measurement in, 754, 756t
      role of advanced practice nurse in, 446
      in stage 3 and 4 CKD, 425
      static pressure measurement in, 754, 755t
      surgical techniques in, 741, 742f
      survival and failure rates in, 490
   for plasma exchange access, 290
   traumatic, 747–748
   Web site resources on, 127
Arteriovenous grafts
   for dialysis access, 486–491, 745–748
      in acute care setting, 435
      advantages and disadvantages of, 746
      cannulation procedure, 754–760
      complications of, 744–745, 746–748, 760–761, 761
      definition of, 745
      facility differences in, 489, 489f
      flow measurement in, 754, 754t
      in home therapy, 869
      indications for, 745
      infections of, 993
      locations of, 746, 746f
      nursing process in, 752–762
      in older adults, 953, 954, 957
      prevalence of, 487t, 488f
      quality improvement process in, 761–762
      role of advanced practice nurse in, 446
      in stage 3 and 4 CKD, 425
      static pressure measurement in, 754, 755t
      survival and failure rates in, 490
      types of, 745
   for plasma exchange access, 290
Arteriovenous hemodiafiltration, continuous (CAVHDF), 231, 232–233, 251, 256
Arteriovenous hemodialysis, continuous (CAVHD), 231, 232–233, 251, 256
Arteriovenous hemofiltration, continuous (CAVH), 231, 232–233, 233f, 251, 256
Ascites, 181, 652
Aseptic technique in peritoneal dialysis catheterization, 781, 782, 783t
Asian culture, 341, 343
Aspirin intoxication, 169–170, 171t
Assimilation process, 339
Association for the Advancement of Medical Instrumentation infection control recommendations, 999
Atheroembolic renal disease in older adults, 175, 947–948
Atherosclerosis
   in children, 920–921
   with malnutrition and inflammation in peritoneal dialysis, 821

in older adults, 175, 947–948
   renal artery stenosis in, 54
ATN-ISS (Acute Tubular Necrosis Individual Severity Score), 145–146
Atrial fibrillation, renal perfusion in, 647
Atrial natriuretic peptide, 17, 18f, 147
Atrophy, muscular, in dialysis, 384–386
Atropine, 188t
   and diphenoxylate in diarrhea, 582
Auscultation, in physical assessment of kidneys, 64
Autoantibodies, 82
Autografts, 612
Autoimmune disorders in diabetes mellitus, 102
Automated peritoneal dialysis, 424, 808
Autonomy issues, 394, 396
   in acute care settings, 143
   for children, 922
   in end-of-life care, 399
   in genetic testing, 326
Autosomes, 315, 319f
   dominant disorders, 323, 323f
   recessive disorders, 323–324, 324f
AV Fistula First, 127
Avian flu, emergency management plans on, 1027
Ayurvedic therapy, 560
Azathioprine in kidney transplantation, 624, 625t
Azotemia, 34, 144
   in chronic renal disease, 96
   intrarenal, 36–40
   postrenal, 40–41
   prerenal, 34–36, 35t
      differentiated from acute tubular necrosis, 39–40

B

B lymphocytes, 281t, 621, 942
Bacillus Calmette-Guerin vaccine, 990
Back pain in peritoneal dialysis, 831
Bacteremia, 166t, 971–974, 995–996
Bacteria
   colonization by, 975
   in hemodialysis water supply, 682, 683
   in urine, 79–80
      in pregnancy, 60
Bacterial infections, 588, 589t, 971–977
Base, 27
Basic life support, pediatric, 921
Basiliximab in kidney transplantation, 628t, 629
Basophils, 281t
Beck Depression Inventory Fast Screen, 355
Behavior changes
   assessment of, 349
   in chronic kidney disease, 347, 348
   in education of patient and family, 365–366
   ethical issues in, 396
   facilitation of, 351
   in nutrition interventions, 558–559
Benchmarks in infection control quality improvement, 1002
Beneficence principle, 143, 326, 394, 399

Capillaries, glomerular, 6
CapWiz Legislative Action Center, 503, 513–514
Carbohydrates, dietary, 554
    in chronic kidney disease, 414
    in diabetes mellitus, 536, 537, 538, 539t
    in kidney transplant recipients, 533t
Carbon adsorption process in water treatment, 684
Carbon dioxide in acid-base balance, 27, 28, 29, 30
    in hemodialysis, 190
Carbonic acid, 27, 28
Carbonic anhydrase, 28, 29
Cardiac arrest in hemodialysis, 713
Cardiac output
    diminished, acute injury in, 34
    in hemodialysis, 183, 185f, 186t, 697–698, 699
        and hypotension, 704
    renal fraction of, 6
Cardiomyopathy in left ventricular hypertrophy, 113
Cardiopulmonary resuscitation, advance directives on, 395, 399
Cardiotonic agents, 590, 599t
Cardiovascular system, 104–106
    in children, 900, 902
        and chronic kidney disease, 905, 910, 910t, 911t
        and dialysis, 920–921
        and kidney transplantation, 924
    in chronic kidney disease, 104–106, 111–115
        and anemia, 106, 108t, 113–114
        in children, 905, 910, 910t, 911t
        delaying progression of disorders in, 107–111, 108t, 529
        and heart failure, 590
        and lipid disorders, 96, 114
        pathophysiology in, 104, 105f
        risk factors affecting, 105t, 105–106, 111, 427t
        stage 1 and 2, 414
        stage 3 and 4, 418
        stage 5, 426, 427t
    cultural differences in disorders of, 340
    in diabetes mellitus, 102, 452
        and pancreas transplantation, 643
    examination of
        in children, 900
        in kidney transplantation, 614
        in nutrition assessment, 526
        in pancreas transplantation, 632
    exercise benefits for, 384, 385t, 386
    in hemodialysis, 182–184, 386, 950
    in hypertension, 104, 111–112
    in kidney transplant recipient, 443
        pediatric, 924
        postoperative management of, 618, 620
        preoperative assessment of, 614
    in lipid disorders, 96, 114, 494
    and mineral metabolism, 480, 481, 482t
    in older adults, 936
        hemodialysis affecting, 950
    in pancreas transplantation, 632, 643
    in peritoneal dialysis, 820–821, 829–830

pharmacokinetics in disorders of, 573t
Care planning
    for end-of-life care, 397–399
    patient-centered, 352
    role of caregivers in, 354
Caregiver stress, 348–349, 353, 354
Carnitine deficiency in hemodialysis, 705, 707
Casts, urinary, 75t, 78, 79–81
Catabolism, 530
    in acute kidney injury, 159–160, 528
    in dialysis, 483t, 484t, 675, 675f, 676–677, 680–681
Cathartics, 594–595
Catheterization, 487–488
    bacteremia in, 972
    central venous. See Central venous catheterization
    in hemodialysis
        arteriovenous fistula and graft cannulation in, 754–760
        central venous catheters in, 748–751
        in children, 918, 919
        complications of, 436, 752f, 760–761, 761, 918, 919
        in home therapy, 869
        infections in, 447, 448t
        nursing process in, 752–762
        patient consent to, 308
        quality improvement process in, 761–762
    locking solutions in, 759
    outcomes in, 491
    patient consent to, 308
    in peritoneal dialysis, 768–795
        acute, 434, 771–772, 772f, 776–777
        catheter break-in procedures in, 781
        in children, 916
        chronic, 772–776, 774f, 777–779
        complications of, 229–230, 779–780, 783–784, 788–794, 825–827, 916
        damage to catheter in, 793–794
        evidence-based guidelines on, 786, 787t
        exit site care in, 438–439, 781–790
        extrusion of catheter cuff in, 793
        fixation methods for catheters in, 783t, 786f
        historical aspects of, 769–771, 772t
        infections in, 438–439, 783–784, 788–791
        irrigation of catheter in, 781
        malfunction of catheter in, 791–793, 825–826
        migration of catheter in, 826
        obstruction of catheter in, 826
        outcomes in, 791
        placement technique, 229, 776–779
        postimplantation care in, 781–788
        radiologic evaluation of catheter in, 826–827
        rectal or suprapubic pain in, 793, 831
        removal of catheter in, 794–795
        in stage 3 and 4 CKD, 425
        temporary, in emergency, 229–230
    in plasma exchange, 289–290, 292–293
    prevalence of, 487t, 488f
    pulmonary artery, in hemodynamic monitoring, 183–184, 183f–184f, 185f, 186t

    in SLEDD/CRRT, 251–262
    survival and failure rates in, 490
    tunneled catheters in, 488, 488f, 491, 749, 761
Cation-exchange resins in chronic kidney disease and hyperkalemia, 590
CAVH (continuous arteriovenous hemofiltration), 231, 232–233, 233f, 251, 256
CAVHD (continuous arteriovenous hemodialysis), 231, 232–233, 251, 256
CAVHDF (continuous arteriovenous hemodiafiltration), 231, 232–233, 251, 256
Cells, 318, 322f
    age-related changes in, 325
    composition and structure of, 322f
    division of, 318–319, 323f
Centers for Disease Control and Prevention infection control recommendations, 999, 1000–1001
Centers for Medicare and Medicaid Services, 127
    infection control recommendations, 999–1000
Central venous catheterization, 487–488, 490, 491, 748–751
    advantages and disadvantages of, 750
    arteriovenous fistula and grafts after, 490
    complications of, 751, 752f, 760–761
        infections in, 994
        in plasma exchange, 290
    definition of, 748
    in home hemodialysis, 869
    KDOQI guidelines on, 491
    locations of, 748f, 749–750, 750f
    in older adults, 953, 954, 957
    outcomes in, 491
    patient instructions on, 306–307
    in plasma exchange, 289–290, 293
    prevalence of, 487–488
    types of, 488, 488f, 491, 749, 749f
Central venous pressure monitoring, 183, 184, 186t
Centrifugation systems in plasma exchange, 280–281
    combined with filtration system, 282
Cerebrospinal fluid, pH of, 29
Change process
    in empowerment of patients, 123–124
    in evidence-based practice, 466–467, 468t
    facilitation of, 351
    motivational interviewing in, 124
    in nutrition-related behaviors, 558–559
    in patient-centered care planning, 352
    transtheoretical model of, 123
CHD (continuous hemodialysis), 233
Chelating agents, 592
    in aluminum toxicity, 592, 715
    in iron toxicity, 592
Chemical exposures, emergency management plan on, 1027–1028
Chemoreceptors in acid-base balance, 29
Chest examination in nutrition assessment, 525–526
Chest pain in hemodialysis, 709
Children, 541–551, 886–927

Clinical Nurse Specialist, 444
Clostridial infections, drug-resistant, 976
Coagulation disorders, 115
    in hemodialysis, 192, 209–210
    in kidney transplantation, preoperative
        assessment of, 616–617
COBRA (Consolidated Omnibus Budget
    Reconciliation Act), 374–375
Cochrane Collaboration, 464, 465
Cockcroft-Gault formula, 83, 98, 601, 939
Codons, 317, 321f
Cognitive function, 349
    in children with chronic kidney disease, 912
Colic, renal, 74
Collaborative management, 122, 126
    in continuous renal replacement therapies,
        269–270, 270f, 278
Collecting system
    anatomy of, 6
    in fluid and electrolyte regulation, 19t, 22–24
Colloids in acute kidney injury, 147
Colonization compared to infection, 975–976
Color
    of dialysate, 833
    of urine, 74, 75t
Column systems in plasma exchange, 282–283
Columns, renal, anatomy of, 5–6, 6f
Communication
    in acute care settings, 140–141
    on adverse events and medical errors, 396
    cultural diversity in, 342, 343, 345
    with elected officials on policies, 514–516
    in emergency and disaster events, 1011,
        1012t–1013t, 1014–1015
    in family, 350
    first language of patient used in, 368
    in genetic counseling, 337
    between long-term care facility and dialysis
        center, 961–962
    on nutrition with patients and family, 558,
        560
    therapeutic, in nurse-patient relationship,
        351
Compensation process in acid-base balance, 28
Competency
    cultural, 338, 339, 359
    in decisional capacity, 396
Complement components, 82
Complementary and alternative medicine, 344
Compliance with therapy. See Adherence with
    therapy
Computerized axial tomography, 85
    in peritoneal dialysis complications, 827
Conation, 349
Concordance between patient and clinician, 122
Conductivity of dialysate
    in hemodialysis, 212, 673–674
        and ultrafiltration, 208–209
    in SLEDD/CRRT, 239
Confidentiality issues in genetic testing, 326–
    327, 332
Congenital disorders
    acute kidney injury in, 35t, 40
    chronic kidney disorders in, 44–45

family history of, 334
Congo red dye test in amyloidosis, 58
Congress
    budget process in, 508, 512
    legislative process in, 506–508, 507f
Consent to procedures, 396
    in end-of-life care, 400
    in genetic testing, 326, 327
    release form on, 308
Constipation
    in dialysis, 531, 825
    in older adults, 541
    stool softeners and cathartics in, 594–595
Contamination
    of dialysate, 918
    of equipment in dialysis, 995, 996
    of water supply in hemodialysis, 682, 682t
Continuous arteriovenous hemodiafiltration
    (CAVHDF), 231, 232–233, 251, 256
Continuous arteriovenous hemodialysis
    (CAVHD), 231, 232–233, 251, 256
Continuous arteriovenous hemofiltration
    (CAVH), 231, 232–233, 233f, 251, 256
Continuous hemodialysis (CHD), 233
Continuous peritoneal dialysis, 807, 809–811, 812t
    ambulatory, 424, 809, 812t, 817, 872
        daily checklist on, 217f
        orders for, 223f
        in stage 3 and 4 CKD, 424
    in children, 915
    cycling, 809–810, 812t, 817, 872
        orders for, 224f–225f
    daily checklist on, 217f
    equipment in, 810–811
Continuous renal replacement therapies
    in acute care setting, 134, 135, 231–278,
        439–440
    anticoagulation in, 267–269
        with Fresenius 2008K system, 240, 240f,
            241, 242f, 243f–246f
        with Prisma system, 251, 252f–257f
    bedside inservice checklist on, 248f, 251,
        258f, 272
    in children. See Children, continuous renal
        replacement therapies in
    collaboration of staff in, 269–270, 270f, 278
    dialysis solutions in, 265–267
    education and training of nurses on, 270–
        272, 277
    equipment and system components in, 238f,
        238–269
        alarms of, 276
        training of nurses on, 271
    historical aspects of, 231–232
    in ICU environment. See Intensive care units,
        SLEDD/CRRT in
    indications for, 235, 278
    initiation of, 273–274
    maintenance of treatment in, 274
    medication clearance in, 237–238
    nursing care interventions in, 269–277
    nutrition in, 277, 528–529
    priming of circuit in, 263
    program selection and development, 277–278

progress record on, 249f
    replacement solutions in, 263–265
    termination of, 275, 276f
    therapeutic effects of, 235–238
    treatment overview in, 272–273
    troubleshooting during, 275–276
    types of, 232–233
    vascular access for, 251–262
Continuous ultrafiltration, slow (SCUF), 231,
    232, 250, 256
Continuous venovenous hemodiafiltration
    (CVVHDF), 232, 233, 234f, 256
    with Fresenius 2008K system, 242
    with Prisma system, 250
Continuous venovenous hemodialysis
    (CVVHD), 232, 233, 234f, 256
    with Fresenius 2008K system, 242
    with Prisma system, 250
Continuous venovenous hemofiltration
    (CVVH), 232, 233, 233f, 256
    with Fresenius 2008K system, 242
    with Prisma system, 250
Contrast agents
    adverse reactions to, 84, 85–86
        in older adults, 947
    in antegrade pyelography, 86
    in computed tomography, 85
    precautions in chronic kidney disease, 109
    in retrograde pyelography, 86
Control sense, loss of, 357
    adherence with therapy in, 359
    empowerment strategies in, 122–125
Convection in SLEDD/CRRT, 236, 236f
COPD, peritoneal dialysis in, 830
Coping styles, 347–348, 358
    of children, 353
    cultural diversity in, 340–341
    in family, 353–354
    spirituality in, 360
Cortex, renal, anatomy of, 5, 6f
Cortical collecting tubule in fluid and electrolyte
    regulation, 19t, 22–24
Corticosteroid therapy
    in chronic kidney disease, 591–592
    in kidney transplantation, 623, 626t–627t
    in plasma exchange, 297
Cost issues. See Financial issues
Costovertebral angle, 64
Counseling
    on exercise and physical activity, 388
    genetic, 336–337
    in grief, 402
Countercurrent multiplying and exchange
    mechanism, 22, 23f, 24–26, 154
Cramps in hemodialysis, 708–709
Creatinine
    secretion into proximal tubule, 22
    serum levels of, 81, 82, 83
        in acute kidney injury, 34, 39t, 40, 173t
        in chronic kidney disease, 96
        in hemodialysis, 191
        as nutritional indicator, 483t, 484t, 484–
            485
        in older adults, 962

sieving coefficient, 237t
urinary, 77, 82–83
Creatinine clearance, 82–83
in acute kidney injury, 34, 39t, 40, 173t
calculation of, 82–83, 98, 601
and glomerular filtration rate, 82, 98
in peritoneal dialysis, 814–815
Crepitus, mediastinal, 189
Crossmatching in kidney transplantation, 621
CRRT. *See* Continuous renal replacement
therapies
Cruz catheters in peritoneal dialysis, 774f, 775,
776t
Cryoglobulinemia, plasma exchange in, 283
Cryoprecipitate-reduced plasma, 285–286
Crystalloids in acute kidney injury, 147
Crystals in urine, 75t, 79, 79f
Cultural issues, 338–345
in acute care settings, 142–143
assessment of, 339, 341–342
in chronic kidney disease risk, 340
in communication, 342, 343, 345
in coping styles, 340–341
definitions of, 338, 339
in education of patient and family, 367
in end-of-life care, 345, 400
in evidence-based treatment, 340
in health beliefs, 339, 343–344, 345
imposition of, 338
in nutrition, 344, 559–561
organizational, 396
resources on, 345
in spirituality and religion, 341, 344–345,
359–360
terminology related to, 338–339
CVVH (continuous venovenous
hemofiltration), 232, 233, 233f, 256
with Fresenius 2008K system, 242
with Prisma system, 250
CVVHD (continuous venovenous
hemodialysis), 232, 233, 234f, 256
with Fresenius 2008K system, 242
with Prisma system, 250
CVVHDF (continuous venovenous
hemodiafiltration), 232, 233, 234f,
256
with Fresenius 2008K system, 242
with Prisma system, 250
Cyanocobalamin, 582
Cycler device in peritoneal dialysis, 808, 809f
Cycling peritoneal dialysis, continuous, 809–810,
812t, 817, 872
orders for, 224f–225f
Cyclophosphamide in kidney transplantation,
625t
Cyclosporine
in heart transplantation, 648, 649, 650, 650t
in kidney transplantation, 624, 625t
in older adults, acute kidney injury from,
174, 946–947
Cylindruria, 79
Cystatin C, 81, 98
Cystic kidney disorders, 45–46
acquired, 46, 329

medullary, 46, 329
polycystic, 45–46, 328–329
in children, 46, 902–903
Cytapheresis, definition of, 279

D

Daclizumab in kidney transplantation, 628t, 629
Daily dialysis
in home, 862, 863
nutrition in, 530–531
slow extended, 231–278. *See also* Slow
extended daily dialysis (SLEDD)
Daily living activities, physical activity levels in,
383
Darbepoetin alfa in anemia, 419, 581
Databases
on guidelines in evidence-based practice,
466, 466t
types of, 465
Decision making
ethical issues in, 394–396
in nursing process, 469
by patient and family, 395
in advance care planning, 397–399
capacity and competency in, 396
in preparation for kidney replacement
therapy, 125
Deionization in water treatment, 685–686
Dementia in older adults, 541
Dendritic cells, 621
Denial, as coping mechanism in chronic kidney
disease, 347, 353
Dental assessment in potential kidney transplant
recipient, 615
Dependency issues in chronic kidney disease,
348
Depression, 348, 354–356
education of patient and family in, 355, 356,
369
in end-of-life care, 402
in older adults, 355, 541
and quality of life in hemodialysis, 354–355,
493f, 493–494
spirituality in, 360
Developmental kidney disorders, 44–45
Dextrose in dialysis solutions, 799, 800, 804, 804t
in CRRT, 266t
in hemodialysis, 209t
in peritoneal dialysis, 220
Diabetes insipidus, nephrogenic, 58, 59–60
Diabetes mellitus, 102–103
and chronic kidney disease, 95, 102–103
classification of, 101t
delaying progression of, 107, 108t, 529
ethnic differences in, 102–103, 103t
medication management in, 538
nutrition in, 536–540
risk for, 95
role of advanced practice nurse in, 449–
453
stage 1 and 2, 413, 414
stage 3 and 4, 417–418
stage 5, 429

emergency and disaster management plans
on, 1017, 1019, 1021, 1022, 1023
ethnic and cultural differences in, 102–103,
103t, 340
gastroparesis in, 452, 537–538
glucose blood levels in, 449–450
and chronic kidney disease, 102, 103, 107,
529
control guidelines, 107
importance of, 536
and kidney transplantation, 532
monitoring of, 125, 537
and nephropathy, 53, 54
and peritoneal dialysis, 821
recommendations on, 537
hemodialysis in, 449
hyperkalemia in, 453
hypertension in, 53–54, 103, 104, 453
infections in, 453
insulin therapy in, 450t
islet cell transplantation in, 644–645
kidney transplantation in, 443, 532, 534, 617
long-term complications in, 102
nephropathy in, 52–54, 102–103, 631, 641
microalbuminuria in, 53, 77
neuropathy in, 102, 452, 631, 641
nutrition in, 452–453, 536–540
and kidney transplantation, 532, 534
oral medications in, 451t
pancreas transplantation in, 629–643
peritoneal dialysis in, 449, 821
proteinuria in, 53, 77, 99, 103
reimbursement for supplies and training in,
539, 540
self-management training in, 538–539
types of, 102, 630–631
Dialysance in hemodialysis, 664–665
Dialysate
color changes, 833
contamination of, 918
in hemodialysis
in acute care setting, 194–206, 433
composition of, 193, 193t, 194–206, 671–
672, 673–674
delivery system for, 668–671, 670f
and dialysis disequilibrium syndrome,
193, 193t
flow rate of, 194, 212, 427, 674
in home, 868
in home therapy, 868
temperature of, 674, 703, 705, 707
in peritoneal dialysis
in acute care setting, 434
composition of, 220, 226, 804t, 804–805
leakage of, 828
temperature of, 834
in SLEDD/CRRT, 265–267
Dialysis
in acute kidney injury, 147, 176
aluminum toxicity in, 592, 593, 714–715
anemia in, 477–480, 705, 820, 919–920
in children, 887–888, 905, 914–921
compared to preemptive transplant, 924
delivered dose in, 485

exit site care in, 785
nutrition in, 546–549
specification sheet on, 264f
delivered dose of, 485–486
depression in, 354–355, 493f, 493–494
Dialysis Outcomes and Practice Patterns
Study (DOPPS) on, 473–494
dialyzability of drugs in, 596, 598t–600t
drug dosage and frequency in, 596–597
encephalopathy in, 714–715
ethical issues in, 395
exercise and physical functioning in, 381–
393
financial issues in, 370, 371–372
hemodialysis, 660–729. *See also*
Hemodialysis
in home, 856–879. *See also* Home dialysis
hypertension management in, 584
infections in
in hemodialysis, 970–1003. *See also*
Infections, in hemodialysis
in peritoneal dialysis, 788–791, 838–846.
See also Infections, in peritoneal
dialysis
in reprocessing and reuse, 725–726, 994,
995–996
iron toxicity in, 592
mineral metabolism in, 480t, 480–481, 481t,
482t
muscle atrophy in, 384–386
nutrition in. *See* Nutrition, in dialysis
in older adults, 540, 950–954
in home, 876, 950
in long-term care setting, 955–964
nutrition in, 540, 960–961
physical functioning in, 383–384
peritoneal, 767–847. *See also* Peritoneal
dialysis
in pregnancy, 61, 121, 552
preparation for, 125, 126
reprocessing and reuse in, 725–729
infections related to, 994, 995–996
slow extended daily, 231–278. *See also* Slow
extended daily dialysis (SLEDD)
valvular calcification in, 115t
vascular access for, 486–491, 738–762
infections in, 992–994
patient instructions on, 306–307
release form on, 308
in stage 3 and 4 CKD, 425
Dialysis disequilibrium syndrome, 710, 836, 918
in acute care setting, 192–194, 230
osmolality in, 193, 193t, 710
prevention of, 193–194, 195t, 230, 710
signs and symptoms in, 193t, 230, 710
Dialysis facilities
advance care planning in, 397
communication with acute care facilities,
141–142
data collection in DOPPS, 475, 475t
emergency and disaster events affecting,
1010–1029
exercise programs in, 386–388, 392
Dialysis Outcomes and Practice Patterns Study
(DOPPS), 473–494

case mix and mortality outcomes in, 475–
476, 476t
on clinical practice patterns, 477–491
facility-level data collection in, 475, 475t
geographic distribution of target samples in,
473, 474f
on health-related quality of life, 492–494
on medications, 494
research design in, 473–475, 474f, 475t
statistical analysis in, 475, 475t
Dialysis Outcomes Quality Initiative (DOQI),
472
Dialyzer membrane reaction, 194, 715–716
Dialyzers
in hemodialysis. *See* Hemodialyzers
reprocessing and reuse of, 725–729
infections related to, 994, 995–996
in SLEDD/CRRT, 262, 263
Diarrhea
drug therapy in, 582
in older adults, 541
Diet. *See* Nutrition
Diffusion, 13t
across peritoneal membrane, 798–799, 799f
in hemodialysis, 662–663
in SLEDD/CRRT, 236f, 236–237
Digoxin, 178, 188t, 418
Diphenhydramine hydrochloride in plasma
exchange, 297
Diphenoxylate and atropine in diarrhea, 582
Dipstick test in proteinuria, 77, 77t, 99
Disability benefits, 377–378
Disaster and emergency events, 1010–1029. *See
also* Emergency and disaster events
Discharge planning
in kidney transplantation, 620–621
in pancreas transplantation, 641
in peritoneal dialysis, 216
Disequilibrium in dialysis, 710, 836, 918
in acute care setting, 192–194, 230
osmolality in, 193, 193t, 710
prevention of, 193–194, 195t, 230, 710
signs and symptoms in, 193t, 230, 710
Distal tubules, 10
early part of, 10, 19t, 22
in fluid and electrolyte regulation, 19t, 22
late part of, 10, 19t, 22–24
intercalated cells in, 29–30
Distribution of drugs, 571t, 571–572, 577
volume of, 571, 596
Diuretic agents
in chronic kidney disease, 417, 590–591
in dialysis, 178–179, 599t
effect on kidney function, 647
Diuretic stage of acute kidney injury, 42–43,
161–162, 527
Dizziness in hemodialysis, 716
DNA, 314, 314f
in cell division, 318–319
in gene expression, 317, 321f
tests in analysis of, 325–328, 332
Do not resuscitate orders, 395, 399
Dobutamine, 179t, 188t
Documentation and record keeping
in acute care settings, 139

in hemodialysis, 210–211, 304
in peritoneal dialysis, 218–219, 220f, 227,
228t
in SLEDD/CRRT, 241, 249f, 251, 258f–
261f, 271–272
on hemodialysis water supply, 687
on hemodialyzer reprocessing and reuse, 726
Donors
in kidney transplantation, 441, 609–612
deceased, 609, 610–612
living, 441, 609–610
shortage of, 352
in pancreas transplantation, 633–634
Dopamine, 147, 179t, 188t
DOPPS (Dialysis Outcomes and Practice
Patterns Study), 473–494
Dose-response curve in drug therapy, 575, 576f,
578
Doxercalciferol, 421–422, 595
Dressings in peritoneal dialysis catheterization,
781, 782, 783t, 785, 786t
in exit site infection, 789
Droperidol in nausea and vomiting, 582, 583
Drug-induced disorders, 169–172
in acute kidney injury, 42
in children, 904
from nephrotoxic agents. *See* Nephrotoxic
agents
in older adults, 174, 541, 944
acute kidney injury in, 945–946, 947
Drug resistance, 974–977
in tuberculosis, 987, 988
Drug therapy, 568–602
abbreviations avoided in, 602
absorption of drugs in, 569–571, 570t, 576–
577
in acute care setting, 439
adherence with, 576, 602
affecting microorganism resistance, 974
chronic kidney disease affecting, 578
in cardiovascular disease, 107
in children, 921–922
classification of agents in, 579–595
clearance of drugs in, 237–238, 572–574
cost of, 375–376
in diabetes mellitus, 451t, 538
and dialysis, 596–597, 598t–600t, 800–801
in acute care setting, 178–179, 226
administration of drugs in, 226, 806–807
fluid balance assessment in, 693
outcomes in, 490–491, 494
in stage 5 CKD, 427–428
distribution of drugs in, 571t, 571–572, 577,
596
dose-response curve in, 575, 576f, 578
drug effects in, 575, 578
drug interactions in, 575–576
education of patients on, 602
error prevention in, 601–602
excretion of drugs in, 572, 577
half-life of drugs in, 574, 577, 578f
hemodynamic responses to, 188t
in lipid disorders, 455t, 455–456, 494, 583–
584, 596t
look-alike/sound-alike drugs in, 601

mechanism of action in, 575, 578
metabolism of drugs in, 572, 577
monitoring of, 597–602
in older adults, 174, 541, 939, 940, 944
   acute kidney injury from, 945–946, 947
   dialysis affecting, 960
   in long-term care setting, 956–957, 960
organ system dysfunction affecting, 573t
pharmacodynamics in, 569, 575–576, 578
pharmacogenetics and pharmacogenomics
   in, 330–332
pharmacokinetics in, 569–578
in plasma exchange, 287, 288, 289, 293–297
precautions in chronic kidney disease, 423
resistance to, 974–977
   in tuberculosis, 987, 988, 992
safe administration of, 601–602
steady state concentration in, 574, 577–578
therapeutic index in, 575–576, 578
time course of action in, 574f, 574–575, 577–578
in tuberculosis, 987, 990–992, 992t
   and dialysis, 599t, 992, 992t
   resistance to, 987, 988, 992
Dry weight, 526, 692
   estimated in hemodialysis, 702–704
   ideal, obtained in hematocrit-based blood volume monitoring, 717–724
Dual energy x-ray absorptiometry (DEXA) in nutrition assessment, 526
Dyslipidemia. See Lipid disorders
Dysplasia, renal, 45, 903

E

Earthquakes, emergency management in, 1023
Economic issues. See Financial issues
Ectopic kidneys, 45, 45f
Edema
   in hemodialysis, 181, 746
   in peritoneal dialysis, 829
   pulmonary, 187t
   severity grading, 181, 181t
Education of patient and family, 122–125, 361–369
   in acute kidney injury, 43, 161, 302–303
   benefits of, 351
   in central venous catheterization, 306–307
   characteristics of adult learners in, 362–365
   cultural sensitivity in, 367
   in depression, 355, 356, 369
   in diabetes mellitus, 538–539
   on drug therapy, 602
     and antibiotic resistance, 974–975
   in emergency management, 1021, 1022
   enhancement of learning in, 369
   evaluation of, 366–367, 368t
   in family-centered approach, 368–369
   first language of patient used in, 368
   on genetics, 330, 331t, 333
   in hemodialysis
     in acute care settings, 212–213, 214, 302–303
     on fluid balance, 693, 694–695

in home, 859–860, 865t–866t, 865–867, 870
   and hypotension, 707
   sample brochure for, 302–303
   on vascular access, 213, 761–762
in kidney transplantation, 351, 441, 613, 620–621
   in children, 925
on nutrition, 558–559
in older adult patients, 942
in pancreas transplantation, 641, 642t, 643t
in pediatric patients, 890t–891t, 923
   age-appropriate activities in, 890t–891t
   in kidney transplantation, 925
in peritoneal dialysis, 777, 786, 818–819
   in home, 859–860, 876–878, 879
principles of learning in, 362
retention of learning in, 368
in stage 1 and 2 CKD, 415
in stage 3 and 4 CKD, 416, 424–425
teaching activities in, 365–367, 367t
teaching-learning process in, 361–362
theories of learning in, 362, 363t, 364t
Education of personnel
   on chronic kidney disease stage 3 and 4, 425–426
   on genetics and genomics, 332, 333
   on hemodialyzer reprocessing and reuse, 726
   on SLEDD/CRRT, 270–272, 277
Effective filtration pressure, 14, 14f
Efferent arterioles, 6, 6f, 8f, 9, 15
Eicosanoids, 16, 17f, 32
Elderly, 540–541, 932–964. See also Older adults
Elections
   and communication with elected officials on policies, 514–516
   participation in, 513
Electrical power supply in emergency and disaster events, 1014
Electrocardiography, potassium serum levels affecting, 202f
Electrolyte balance
   in liver disease, 652–653
   regulation of, 17–22, 19t
   in urine, 76–77
Embolism
   air, 294t, 712, 918
   atheroembolic, in older adults, 175, 947–948
   pulmonary, 187t
Embryonic and fetal development, 11–12, 889
Emergency and disaster events, 1010–1029
   communication in, 1011, 1012t–1013t, 1014–1015
   federal regulations on, 1011
   in flu pandemic, 1017
   natural disasters, 1016–1026
   nutrition in, 1015
   planning for, 1011–1014
   posttraumatic stress in, 1015
   recovery and restoration phase in, 1011, 1015
   response to, 1011, 1014–1015
   in terrorism and violence, 1026–1028
   triage in, 1015
   Web site resources on, 1015, 1027, 1029

Emergency Medical Treatment and Labor Act, 143, 144t
Employment
   group health plans in, 371, 373, 377
   and socioeconomic status, 376–377
Empowerment strategies in chronic kidney disease, 122–125
Encapsulating peritoneal sclerosis in peritoneal dialysis, 837–838, 916
Encephalopathy in dialysis, 714–715
End-of-life care, 397–402
   in acute care settings, 143
   advance directives on, 395, 397, 399
   allow a natural death (AND) orders in, 399
   assisted suicide in, 400
   for children, 398, 913
   cultural diversity in, 345, 400
   decision making in, 395
   do not resuscitate orders in, 395, 399
   ethical issues in, 394–395, 396, 399–400
   financial issues in, 400, 401
   futile interventions in, 394–395, 400
   for older adults, 964
   palliative care in, 399–402
   planning for, 397–399
   symptoms in, 401–402
   Web site resources on, 402
   withholding and withdrawal of treatment in, 394–395
End-stage kidney disease
   in children, 888
   financial issues in, 371, 372
   infection control in, 998–1000
   kidney transplantation in, 609, 612
     and pancreas transplantation, 631
   mortality rates in, 473, 475–476
   physical activity levels in, 383, 387, 391
   psychosocial issues in, 346–359
   spirituality in, 360
   Web site resources on, 127
End-stage liver disease, 650–652
Endocrine system assessment in potential kidney transplant recipient, 615
Endothelin, 16, 32
Endothelium-derived relaxing factor, 32
Endotoxins
   in hemodialysis water supply, 682, 683
   in hemodialyzer reprocessing and reuse, 725–726, 727, 728
Energy therapies, 344
Enteral nutrition
   in children, 549–551
   in diabetes mellitus, 538, 539t
Enterococcal infections
   drug-resistant, 976
   in peritoneal dialysis, 839, 843–844
Environmental factors
   in aging process, 325
   interaction with genetic factors, 330
   in mutations, 319
   in risk for chronic kidney disease, 96, 330
Enzymes, 320t
Eosinophiluria, 79

three compartment model on, 696, 697f
and ultrafiltration, 207–208, 692, 694, 697
in hypervolemia. *See* Hypervolemia
in hypovolemia. *See* Hypovolemia
in kidney transplantation, 618–619
in liver disease, 650–652, 651f, 652f
nephron functions in regulation of, 17–24, 19t
in peritoneal dialysis, 815, 834–835
in plasma exchange, 287, 288, 289, 291–292
and recommended daily fluid intake, 558
in SLEDD/CRRT, 235–236
and urine concentration, 24–27, 26–27
Fluid intake, 558
in children, 545t, 547t, 550t
in dialysis, 531, 693, 694
in kidney transplantation, 533t
in older adults, 540, 961
Folic acid, 494, 582
Food-borne infections in kidney transplant recipients, 532–534
Foot processes of glomerular capillary membrane, 8, 8f
Fresenius 2008K SLEDD and CRRT system, 238f, 238–241
anticoagulation orders for, 243f–246f
bedside inservice checklist on, 248f
Friction rub, pleural, 189
Fungal infections, 166t, 995–996
in peritoneal dialysis, 840, 844
Fungemia, 166t, 995–996
Furosemide, 188t
Fused kidneys, 45
Futile interventions, 394–395, 400

G

Gadolinium in magnetic resonance imaging, adverse reactions to, 85
Gagne's hierarchy of learning, 362, 364t
Gastric acid secretion, 592–593, 594
Gastrointestinal system
in children, 543–544, 910
in diabetes mellitus, 452, 537–538
drug therapy in disorders of
histamine H2 receptor antagonists in, 592–593
pharmacokinetics in, 573t
prokinetic agents in, 593–594
stool softeners and cathartics in, 594–595
in hemodialysis, 189
in older adults, 950
in kidney transplant recipient, preoperative assessment of, 615
in older adults, 541, 937–938
in hemodialysis, 950
in peritoneal dialysis, 829
perforation in catheter insertion, 779–780
protein-energy malnutrition in disorders of, 535
Gastroparesis
in diabetes mellitus, 452, 537–538

prokinetic agents in, 593–594
Gender differences
in coping styles, 341
in urethra anatomy, 11
Genes, 314–315, 317f
expression of, 317, 321f
variable, 324
mapping of, 315
mutation of, 319–320
regulation of, 317–318
Genetics, 312–337
and aging process, 325
in complex or multifactorial disorders, 321–322
counseling on, 336–337
definition of, 314
education of patient and family on, 330, 331t, 333
historical aspects of, 313
interaction with environmental factors, 330
in kidney diseases, 328–330
in pharmacogenetics and pharmacogenomics, 330–332
responsibilities of nurses related to, 332–333
tests in analysis of, 325–328, 332
Web site resources on, 331t
Genital examination in children, 901, 902
Genome, 322–323
Genomic Applications in Practice and Prevention (EGAPP), 327
Genomics
application to nursing practice, 333–334
definition of, 314
responsibilities of nurses related to, 332–333
Genotypes in pharmacogenetics, 332
Geriatric Depression Scale, 355
Geriatric patients, 540–541. *See also* Older adults
Germicides in hemodialyzer reprocessing and reuse, 725, 728–729
Glomerular capillaries
anatomy of, 6, 8f, 8–9
hydrostatic pressure in, 13–14
Glomerular filtrate
composition of, 14–15
excretion of, 24
reabsorption of, 17, 24
Glomerular filtration, 13–17
membrane structure and function in, 8f, 8–9
net or effective filtration pressure in, 14, 14f
Glomerular filtration rate, 13t, 15
autoregulation of, 15–17
in cardiovascular disease and CKD, 104–105
in diagnosis of CKD, 43, 95, 95t
estimation of, 82–83, 98
in children, 905
monitoring of, 106
in older adults, 939
in pregnancy, 60
in stages of CKD, 44, 44t, 96–98, 100t, 100–101
Glomerulonephritis, 49–51, 151–152
in children, 903, 904
in Goodpasture syndrome, 49, 50–51
and hepatitis C, 654

in older adults, 175, 947
pregnancy in, 61
Glomerulosclerosis in diabetes mellitus, 103
Glomerulus, 8
age-related changes in, 938
blood flow regulation in, 15–17
diseases of, 49–51, 151–152
terms describing, 50t
in fluid and electrolyte regulation, 19t
Glucocorticoid therapy
in chronic kidney disease, 591–592
in kidney transplantation, 623, 626t–627t
in plasma exchange, 297
Glucose
blood levels of
in diabetes mellitus. *See* Diabetes mellitus, glucose blood levels in
in hemodialysis, 191
in older adults, 959, 963
in peritoneal dialysis, 830
cotransport with sodium, 20f, 21
in dialysate, 193, 193t, 433
in hemodialysis, 671
in peritoneal dialysis, 821, 830
reabsorption of, 20f, 21
sieving coefficient, 237t
tubular load of, 21, 21f
tubular transport maximum, 21
in urine, 21, 21f, 75t, 76
Goodpasture syndrome, 49, 50–51, 164–165, 165f
Gout, 58
Government
communication with elected officials in, 514–516
federal, 506–512. *See also* Federal government
health insurance programs, 370, 371–375
learning opportunities for nurses in, 516
regulations on infection control practices, 998–999
requesting official proclamation from, 514
state, 512–513. *See also* State governments
Granular casts in urine, 75t, 80f, 80–81
Granulocytes, 282t
Grief
in chronic kidney disease, 347, 357
counseling for, 402
Growth, of children, 542, 543, 544
in kidney failure, 901–902, 911–912
in kidney transplantation, 925, 926–927
rate of, 892, 893f–894f
Growth hormone
secretion in children, 912
therapy in children, 543
Guided imagery techniques in anxiety, 356–357
Guidelines and standards for care, 469–471. *See also* Standards and guidelines for care
Guilt feelings of parents, 353
Guyton curve in hemodialysis, 695f, 695–696, 719, 719f

H

Half-life of drugs, 574, 577, 578f
Hand hygiene in infection control, 219, 975, 1001
Hardness of water supply in hemodialysis, 683–684
Head examination in nutrition assessment, 524–525
Headache in dialysis, 958
Healing of wounds
  in dialysis, 531, 782–783
  in kidney transplantation, 619
  in older adults, 540
Health beliefs
  of children, 352–353
  cultural diversity in, 339, 343–344, 345
  in family, 350
Health care proxy, 399
Health care workers
  in acute care settings, 138–139, 142–143
    team approach of, 136–137, 144
  cultural diversity in attitudes toward, 342
  education of. See Education of personnel
  expectations for physical functioning of patients, 389–390, 391f
  hepatitis B virus infection in, 977, 979
  HIV exposure in, 985, 986
  immunizations in, 997t
  in kidney transplantation, team approach of, 352, 612
  needlestick injuries in, 985, 986
  professional integrity of, 394
  in SLEDD/CRRT, collaboration of, 269–270, 270f
  standard precautions for infection control in, 220, 1000
  tuberculosis screening in, 989
Health history, 64, 65t–73t
Health insurance, 371–376
Health Insurance Portability and Accountability Act (HIPAA), 375
Health policy, 499–516
  advocacy in, 502–505
  learning opportunities for nurses in, 516
  political processes in, 506–516
Health Policy Committee of ANNA, 504
Health Policy Workshop of ANNA, 516
Health-related quality of life in hemodialysis, 492f–493f, 492–494
Health Savings Accounts, 374
Healthy People 2010, 128
Hearing, age-related changes in, 943
Heart disorders, 112–113
  and acute kidney injury, 34, 35t, 42
  in children, 920–921
  and chronic kidney disease, 114, 115, 115t, 647–648
  in hemodialysis, 712–713
  in plasma exchange, 295t
Heart failure, 113
  and chronic kidney disease, 647–648
    cardiotonic agents in, 590
  in hemodialysis, 745

hemodynamic monitoring in, 187t
  in hypertension, 104t, 112
  in plasma exchange, 295t
Heart rate in hemodialysis, 182, 211
Heart sounds in hemodialysis, 182
Heart transplantation, 61–62, 145, 647–650
  nephrotoxicity of calcineurin inhibitors in, 648, 649, 650t
Height measurements in children
  growth charts on, 892, 893f–894f
  in nutrition assessment, 542
HELLP syndrome, 134, 135, 168–169
Hematocrit
  and blood flow rate, 232, 232f
  in hemodialysis, 191
    in blood volume monitoring, 703–704, 706–707, 717–724
  in older adults, 963
Hematuria, 74
Hemodiafiltration, 861–862
  continuous arteriovenous (CAVHDF), 231, 232–233, 251, 256
  continuous venovenous (CVVHDF), 232, 233, 234f, 242, 250, 256
Hemodialysis, 126, 660–729
  in acute care settings, 176–214, 433–434, 435
    assessment prior to, 176–192
    complications of, 436–437
    education of patient and family in, 212–213, 214, 302–303
    flowsheet on, 304
    indications for, 432
    intradialytic assessment and interventions in, 210–213
    orders for, 305
    posthemodialysis assessment and evaluation in, 213–214
    prescription of, 433–434
    treatment plan in, 192–210
  adequacy of, 676, 678
    in acute care setting, 192
    in home therapy, 869
    in stage 5 CKD, 428
  advanced practice nurse role in, 426–430
    in vascular access care, 445–448
  air embolism in, 712, 918
  anemia in, 477–479, 705
  anticoagulant therapy in, 209–210, 212, 427, 434, 690–692
  arterial pressure in
    postpump or predialyzer, 672–673
    prepump, 672
  blood leak detection in, 674
  blood pressure in, 211, 212, 213, 697–700, 704–707
    relationship to blood volume, 698–699, 700f
    time lag phenomenon in, 699–700
  in children, 887–888, 905, 917–919
    delivered dose in, 485
    nutrition in, 546–548
    specification sheet on, 264f
  clearance rate in, 664, 664f
  complications of, 704–716

  in acute care settings, 436–437
  in children, 918–919
  in home therapy, 869–870
  infections, 970–1003. See also Infections, in hemodialysis
  in older adults, 950–953
  in stage 5 CKD, 428
continuous arteriovenous (CVAHD), 231, 232–233, 251, 256
continuous (CHD), 233
continuous venovenous (CVVHD), 232, 233, 234f, 242, 250, 256
daily
  in home, 862, 863
  nutrition in, 530–531
delivered dose of, 485–486, 676, 678
depression in, 354–355, 493f, 493–494
in diabetes mellitus, 449
dialysance in, 664–665
dialysate in. See Dialysate, in hemodialysis
Dialysis Outcomes and Practice Patterns Study (DOPPS) on, 473–494
dialyzer membrane reactions in, 194, 715–716
diffusion in, 662–663
discontinuation of, 689–690
disequilibrium syndrome in, 192–194
and drug therapy
  dosage and frequency in, 596–597, 598t–600t
  drug dialyzability in, 596, 598t–600t
  fluid balance assessment in, 693
  outcomes in, 490–491, 494
  in stage 5 CKD, 427–428
dry weight in, 692
  estimated, 702–704
  ideal, obtained in hematocrit-based blood volume monitoring, 717–724
duration of treatment in, 427, 433, 679, 679f
education of patients in. See Education of patient and family, in hemodialysis
emergency and disaster management plans on, 1016–1026
equipment and components in, 212, 665–672
  diagram of, 666f
  preparation of, 687–688
  reprocessing and reuse of, 725–729, 994–995
exercise and physical functioning in, 382, 383–387
fluid balance in. See Fluid balance, in hemodialysis
Guyton curve in, 695f, 695–696, 719, 719f
hemolysis in, 710–712, 918
historical aspects of, 661–662, 739
  in home therapy, 857–858, 862
in home, 862–870
  clinical management of, 867–868
  education of patients in, 859–860, 865t–866t, 865–867, 870
  emergency and disaster management plan on, 1017, 1018–1019
  indications for, 863–865

treatment of, 155
Inulin, in glomerular filtration rate
  measurement, 98
Iothalamate, in glomerular filtration rate
  measurement, 98
Iron
  deficiency of, 419–420, 580, 581–582
  supplemental, 419, 557–558
    in children, 548, 549
    in chronic kidney disease, 113–114, 428,
      580, 581–582
    in peritoneal dialysis, 820
    in pregnancy, 552, 553
  total binding capacity, 581
  toxicity in dialysis, 592
Ischemia
  of extremity, in dialysis in older adults, 959
  renal
    acute tubular necrosis in, 36–38, 37f, 150,
      152–153, 166, 167f, 432
    duration of, 152
    pain in, 74
    in scleroderma, 57–58
Islet cell transplantation, 644–645
Isografts, 612
Isolation precautions in infection control, 975
  in hepatitis B virus, 982
  history of, in hemodialysis patient, 177
  in tuberculosis, 989

J

Joint Commission on Accreditation of Health
  Care Organizations (JCAHO), 128
Jugular vein catheterization for hemodialysis
  access, 749–750
Justice and ethical issues
  in acute care settings, 143
  in genetic testing, 326
Juxtaglomerular complex or apparatus, 9f, 10–
  11, 15f, 15–16
Juxtamedullary nephrons, 5, 7, 7f, 8, 10
  countercurrent multiplying and exchange
    mechanism of, 22, 23f, 24–26

K

Kayexalate in hyperkalemia, 201–202
KDOQI. See Kidney Disease Outcomes Quality
  Initiative (KDOQI) guidelines
Ketones in urine, 75t, 76
Kidney Care Partners, 504–505
Kidney Community Emergency Response
  Coalition, 1029
Kidney Disease: Improving Global Outcomes
  (KDIGO), 128
Kidney Disease Awareness Education Week, 504,
  514
Kidney Disease Outcomes Quality Initiative
  (KDOQI) guidelines, 472–473
  on anemia, 113, 114, 477–480, 820
  on classification of chronic kidney disease
    stages, 96, 100t, 100–101
  components of, 472
  currently available, 472–473

on definition of chronic kidney disease, 95,
  95t
development of, 472
on dialysis dose, 485–486, 676, 678, 679
in DOPPS study, 477–491
on exercise, 388
on hemodialysis adequacy, 676, 678, 679
on hemodialysis vascular access, 486–491,
  994
on infection control practices, 994, 999, 1000
on mineral metabolism, 480–481
on nutrition, 482–485, 822
on pediatric patients, 905, 906t–909t
on peritoneal dialysis adequacy, 813–814,
  815, 816, 816t
Kidney Disease Quality of Life, 355
  Short Form, 355, 492, 493, 494
Kidney Exercise Demonstration Project, 383,
  384, 385f, 392
Kidney replacement therapy (KRT), 125–126
  in children, 913–921
  continuous. See Continuous renal
    replacement therapies
  ethical issues in, 394–395
  and heart transplantation, 648, 650
  hemodialysis in. See Hemodialysis
  kidney transplantation in. See Kidney
    transplantation
  and liver transplantation, 655
  nutrition in, 527, 528–529
    and protein-energy malnutrition, 534
  in older adults, 949–955
    in long-term care setting, 955–964
  peritoneal dialysis in. See Peritoneal dialysis
Kidney transplantation, 608–628
  acute care in, 436
  bone disorders in, 443, 534, 620
  in children, 923–927
    nutrition in, 549, 550t, 924, 926
  classification of chronic kidney disease in,
    101t
  complications of, 619–620, 925–926
  contraindications to, 613, 923
  delayed graft function in, 619
  in diabetes mellitus, 443, 532, 534, 617
  discharge planning in, 620–621
  donors in, 441, 609–612
    deceased, 609, 610–612
    living, 441, 609–610
    shortage of, 352
  education of patients in, 351, 441, 613, 620–
    621, 925
  emergency and disaster management plans
    on, 1019, 1021, 1022
  evaluation of candidates for, 441, 612, 613–
    617
    pediatric, 924–925
  exercise and physical functioning in, 381
  financial issues in, 370, 371, 621
    Medicare benefits in, 372
  graft rupture in, 619
  historical aspects of, 609
  immunosuppressant therapy in, 623–629
    in older adults, 955
    and pancreas transplantation, 638

long-term management in, 442–443
nutrition in, 531–534
  in children, 549, 550t, 924, 926
  and food safety issues, 532–534
  in pregnancy, 553
  and protein-energy malnutrition, 535
  in older adults, 951t, 954–955
operative procedure in, 618, 618f
  in children, 925
  with pancreas transplantation, 636–637
organ sharing and distribution network in,
  612
and pancreas transplantation, 631–632, 634–
  635
  operative procedure in, 636–637
perioperative care in, 441–442
peritoneal dialysis prior to, 822–823
postoperative management in, 442, 618–621
  in children, 925–927
in pregnancy, 553
pregnancy after, 61, 121, 620
preparation for, 126, 442
  in children, 924–925
  in immediate preoperative care, 617–618
proteinuria in, 99
referral for, 351–352, 612, 617
rehabilitation in, 621
rejection in. See Rejection, in kidney
  transplantation
role of advanced practice nurse in, 440–445
in stage 3 and 4 CKD, 424
survival statistics in, 609, 924
team approach to, 352, 612
terminology related to, 612, 621

L

Labeling of hemodialyzers, 727
Lactate
  in CRRT dialysis solutions, 266t
  in peritoneal dialysis solutions, 804, 804t, 830
Laparoscopy, peritoneal dialysis catheter
  insertion in, 778–779
Laplace theorem, 699
Laxatives, 594–595
Lead poisoning, 330
Learning
  Gagne's hierarchy of, 362, 364t
  levels of, 367t
  need assessment for, 365
  principles of, 362
  process of, 361–362
  readiness for, 365
  retention of, 368
  strategies enhancing, 369
  theories of, 362, 363t, 364t
Leg cramps in dialysis, in older adults, 958
Legislation
  on acute care settings, 143, 143t, 144t
  and advocacy on health policy issues, 502–505
  Americans with Disabilities Act (ADA), 375
  Consolidated Omnibus Budget
    Reconciliation Act (COBRA), 374–
    375
  on health insurance benefits, 374–375

with impact on kidney patients, 509t–511t
on infection control practices, 998–999
on organ donation and transplant
procedures, 612
Patient Self-Determination Act (PSDA), 143,
143t, 397
proposal and enactment of, 506–508
of state governments, 513
terminology related to, 506
Legislative Committee of ANNA, 503, 504
Leukapheresis, 279
Leukocyte esterase in urine, 75t, 78–79
Leukocytes
count in hemodialysis, 191
in urine, 75t, 78f, 78–79, 80, 80f
Leukotrienes, 16, 17f
Libido in chronic kidney disease, 120, 121
Life Options Kidney Rehabilitation Advisory
Council, 387
Lifestyle factors
in chronic kidney disease, 96, 108t, 109
cultural diversity in, 341
in hypertension, 112, 112t
in psychosocial impact of chronic disease,
346–347
Lipid disorders, 96, 114
cardiovascular disease in, 96, 114, 494
delaying progression of, 108t
drug therapy in, 455t, 455–456, 494, 583–
584, 596t
in hemodialysis, 494
in kidney transplant recipients, 443, 456, 532,
534
in peritoneal dialysis, 821, 829–830
role of advanced practice nurse in, 454–456
signs and symptoms of, 454
in stage 3 and 4 CKD, 418
in stage 5 CKD, 429
Lipoprotein levels, 454
Lithiasis. See Calculi
Lithium carbonate toxicity, 172
Liver disease
end-stage, 650–652
in HELLP syndrome, 168–169
in hepatitis B, 977–982
in hepatitis C, 982–983
in hepatorenal syndrome, 653–654
pharmacokinetics in, 573t
sodium and water retention in, 650–652,
651f, 652f
toxic acute tubular necrosis in, 38
Liver transplantation, 61–62, 650–655
Living will, 399
Location of kidneys, 5
ectopic, 45, 45f
Locking solutions for catheters, 759
Loin pain-hematuria syndrome, 73
Long-term care setting, 955–964
immunizations in, 997t
nutritional status in, 540, 541, 956
Loop of Henle
active diluting segment of, 10, 22, 25
anatomy of, 9f, 9–10
ascending limb, 9, 19t, 22, 25

descending limb, 9, 19t, 22, 25
in fluid and electrolyte regulation, 19t, 22,
23f
Loperamide in diarrhea, 582
Losartan, pharmacogenetics of, 332
Lower extremity
cramps in dialysis, 958
examination in nutrition assessment, 526
Lungs
examination in nutrition assessment, 525–
526
transplantation of, 61
tuberculosis of, 987, 988, 988f, 989
Lupus erythematosus, 55–57
nephritis in, 55–57, 57t, 904
plasma exchange in, 283
pregnancy in, 61
Lymphatic system
anatomy of, 7
in children, 900
peritoneal, 798
staging of involvement in kidney cancer, 47,
48t
Lymphocytes
age-related changes in, 942
B cells, 281t, 621, 942
size of, 282t
specific gravity of, 281t
T cells, 281t, 621, 622, 942

M

Macroalbuminuria in diabetic nephropathy, 103
Macrophages, 621
Macula densa, 15–16
Magnesium
in dialysis solutions, 433, 804, 804t
in CRRT, 266t
in hemodialysis, 671
dietary, in kidney transplant recipients, 532
reabsorption of, 21, 22
serum levels in hemodialysis, 191, 206
Magnetic resonance imaging, 85
angiography technique, 84
Malnutrition, 534–535
in acute kidney injury, 527
in chronic kidney disease, 523
in hemodialysis, 951–952
in kidney transplant recipients, 531–532
in older adults, 540, 951–952
in peritoneal dialysis, 821
protein-energy. See Protein-energy
malnutrition
Manipulative therapies, 344
Mannitol in hemodialysis and ultrafiltration,
209t
Mantoux tuberculin skin test, 989–990
Medicaid, 372
Medical errors, 601–602
in abbreviation use, 602
ethical issues in, 396
Medicare, 370, 371–372, 374–375, 377
drug coverage in, 375–376
hospice benefits in, 401

Medigap insurance plans, 372, 374
Medulla, renal, 5–6, 6f
cystic disease of, 46, 329
Medullary collecting duct in fluid and electrolyte
regulation, 19t, 24
Meiosis, 318, 323f
Membrane filtration in plasma exchange, 281–
282
Membrane reactions in hemodialysis, 194, 715–
716, 725
Memory in learning process, 364, 368
Mendelian inheritance, 323–324, 323f–325f
Mercury poisoning, 330
Mesonephros, 11
Messenger RNA, 317, 321f
Meta-analysis, 465
Metabolism
acids produced in, 27
and bone disorders in chronic kidney
disease, 108t, 115–118
in children with chronic kidney disease, 910–
911
of drugs, 572
chronic kidney disease affecting, 577
in kidney transplant recipients, 619, 620
mineral, 108t, 115–118, 529
in dialysis, 480t, 480–481, 481t, 482t
in pancreas transplant recipients, 640, 641
in protein-energy malnutrition, 535
Metamyelocytes, 281t
Metanephros, 11
Metastasis
of kidney cancer, 47, 48t
to kidneys, 47
Methanol poisoning, 171–172
Methylprednisolone
in chronic kidney disease, 591–592
in kidney transplantation, 623, 627t
Microalbuminuria, 77, 98, 99
in cardiovascular disease, 105
in diabetic nephropathy, 53, 77, 103
testing for, 99, 107
Microarray technology, 327f, 327–328
Micturition, 32
age-related changes in, 940
Military health benefits, 373
Mineralocorticoids in chronic kidney disease,
593
Minerals, 556–558
metabolism of
and bone disorders in chronic kidney
disease, 108t, 115–118, 529
in dialysis, 480t, 480–481, 481t, 482t
supplemental, in children, 545t, 547t, 549,
550t
Missouri swan-neck catheter in peritoneal
dialysis, 774, 774f, 775, 775f, 778
Mistrust, cultural diversity in, 342
Mitosis, 318, 323f
Modification of Diet in Renal Disease (MDRD)
creatinine clearance formula, 83
glomerular filtration rate equation, 98, 601,
939
on protein in chronic kidney disease, 422, 529

Moncrief-Popovich catheters in peritoneal
dialysis, 774f, 775, 776t
Monitoring
in hemodialysis, 182–184, 186t–187t, 672–
674, 689
in plasma exchange, 290–293
Monoclonal antibody in kidney transplantation,
627t, 629
Monocytes, 281t
Monosomy syndromes, 321
Mood changes, 348, 349
Morphine, 188t
Mortality
and end-of-life care. See End-of-life care
in peritoneal dialysis, 823, 823t
in stage 5 CKD, 399
Motivational interviewing, 124
Mouth
age-related changes in, 937, 938, 944
examination of
in nutrition assessment, 525
in potential kidney transplant recipient,
615
Mudslides, emergency management plan on,
1024–1025
Multidisciplinary team in acute care settings,
136–137, 144
Multiple organ dysfunction syndrome, 166t
in sepsis, 166, 973
Muromonab in kidney transplantation, 629
Muscle atrophy in dialysis, benefits of exercise in,
384–386
Muscle cramps in hemodialysis, 708–709
Mutations, 319–320, 327–328
Mycobacterial infections, tuberculosis in. See
Tuberculosis
Mycophenolate mofetil in kidney
transplantation, 623–624, 628t
Mycophenolic acid in kidney transplantation,
623–624, 628t
Myelocytes, 281t
Myocardial infarction
in children, 920
in hypertension, 104t, 112
Myoglobin in urine, 78

N

National Council of State Boards of Nursing,
513
National Kidney Foundation Kidney Disease
Outcomes Quality Initiative
guidelines. See Kidney Disease
Outcomes Quality Initiative
(KDOQI) guidelines
Native Americans
culture of, 343, 344, 345
health insurance plan for, 373
Natural disasters, 1016–1026
Nausea
antiemetics in, 582–583
in dialysis, 716
in older adults, 958
in plasma exchange, 296t
Neck examination in nutrition assessment, 525

Necrosis, acute tubular. See Tubular necrosis,
acute
Needle phobia, 752
Needlestick injuries in health care workers, 985,
986
HIV prophylaxis in, 986
standard precautions in, 1000
Neoplasms. See Tumors
Nephralgia, 73–74
Nephrectomy
medical, in chronic kidney disease, 417
radical, in renal neoplasms, 47
Nephritis
acute interstitial, 151, 164
hereditary (Alport's syndrome), 329, 903
in lupus erythematosus, 55–57, 904
tubulointerstitial
in children, 904
in older adults, 175, 947
Nephrocalcinosis, 59
Nephrology Nurses Week, 505
Nephrology nursing standards and guidelines,
470–471, 471t
Nephrons
acute tubular necrosis of, 36–40. See also
Tubular necrosis, acute
cortical, 5, 7, 7f, 10
embryonic and fetal development of, 11–12
functions of, 12, 19t
in fluid and electrolyte balance, 17–24,
19t
hypertrophy in chronic kidney disease, 96
juxtamedullary, 5, 7, 7f, 8, 10
countercurrent multiplying and
exchange mechanism of, 22, 23f, 24–
26
structure and function of, 7f–10f, 7–11
tubular component in, 7, 9f, 9–10
vascular component in, 7, 8–9
Nephropathy
chronic allograft, in kidney transplantation,
619–620, 623
diabetic, 52–54, 102–103, 631
microalbuminuria in, 53, 77
pancreas transplantation in, 641
drug-induced, in older adults, 946
familial juvenile hyperuricemic, 329
HIV-associated, 58–59
hypertensive, 54
membranous, and hepatitis C, 654
Nephrophthisis, familial juvenile, 329
Nephrosclerosis, 54
Nephrostomogram, 86
Nephrotic syndrome, 51, 903
Nephrotoxic agents, 34, 35t, 43, 169–172
avoidance of, 107–109, 147, 160
in immunosuppressive therapy, 62
in heart transplantation, 648–649, 650
in liver transplantation, 654–655
intrarenal injury from, 36, 37f, 38, 153–154
in older adults, 945–946, 947
SLEDD/CRRT in exposure to, 235
tubular necrosis from, 37f, 38, 150–151, 153–
154, 433
Net filtration pressure, 14, 14f

Neurologic system
age-related changes in, 941–942
examination of
in children, 901
in hemodialysis, 190
in kidney transplantation, preoperative,
615
in pancreas transplantation,
preoperative, 632–633
of kidneys, anatomy of, 7
in micturition, 32
Neuromuscular blocking agents in hemodialysis,
179
Neuropathy
in diabetes mellitus, 102, 452, 631
pancreas transplantation in, 641
kidney pain in, 73
Neutrophils, 281t
Nicotinic acid in hyperlipidemia, 455t, 456, 584
Night therapy
hemodialysis in, 126
in home, 862
nutrition in, 530–531
in older adults, 950
peritoneal dialysis in, intermittent, 811–812,
812t, 817
Nitric oxide, 16
Nitrites in urine, 75t, 76, 78
Nitroglycerin, 188t
Nociceptors, 73
Nocturnal therapy. See Night therapy
Nonmalificence principle, 143, 394, 399
in genetic testing, 326
Norepinephrine, 16, 179t, 188t
North American Pediatric Renal Trials and
Collaborative Studies, 888
Nose examination in nutrition assessment, 525
Nucleotides, 314, 315f
Nurse in Washington Internship, 516
Nurse Licensure Compact (NLC), 513
Nurse-patient relationship, 350–351
Nurse practice acts, 513
Nurse Practitioners, 444–445
Nurses, advanced practice, role of. See Advanced
practice nurse role
Nursing process
standards and guidelines for care in, 469–471
steps in, 469
Nutrition, 519–561
in acute kidney injury, 147, 159–160, 432,
527–529
behavior modification in, 558–559
in bone disorders, 118, 529
in cardiovascular disease, 108t, 112t
in children, 541–551, 911
age-related changes in, 543–544, 545t,
547t
in kidney transplantation, 549, 550t, 926
in conservative management of CKD, 529
cultural diversity in, 344, 559–561
in depression, 355
in diabetes mellitus, 452–453, 536–540
and kidney transplantation, 532, 534
in dialysis, 482–485, 528, 530–531, 705, 707,
821–822

in children, 546–549

common problems in, 531

and diabetes mellitus, 538

in home, 867

and hypoxemia, 698, 698f

in older adults, 540, 960–961

and outcomes, 482–485

in pregnancy, 552

and protein-energy malnutrition, 535

screening and assessment of, 523–524

vitamins in, 494, 528

education strategies on, 558–559

in emergency and disaster events, 1015

in hyperkalemia, 119

important nutrients in, 553–558

KDOQI guidelines on, 482–485, 822

in kidney transplantation, 531–534

in children, 549, 550t, 926

food safety issues in, 532–534

in pregnancy, 553

and protein-energy malnutrition, 535

and malnutrition, 534–535. *See also*
Malnutrition

in older adults. *See* Older adults, nutrition in

parenteral, 386, 551

in pregnancy, 552–553

protein in. *See* Protein, dietary

screening and assessment, 523–526

in children, 542–543, 551

malnutrition indicators in, 523, 524, 535

self-care in, 125

in SLEDD/CRRT, 277

in stage 1 and 2 CKD, 414–415

in stage 3 and 4 CKD, 417, 422–423

in stage 5 CKD, 430, 435

O

Obesity

and chronic kidney disease, 95, 96, 422

in kidney transplant recipients, 532, 534, 617, 620

weight reduction surgery in, 532

Obstructive pulmonary disorders, chronic,
peritoneal dialysis in, 830

Obstructive urinary disorders

acute, 40–41, 155–156

in children, 902, 904

chronic, 52

in older adults, 175, 948

pain in, 74

Occupational exposures

HIV prophylaxis in, 986

immunizations in, 997t

in needlestick injuries, 985, 986, 1000

standard precautions for infection control in, 1000

to tuberculosis, 989

Odor of urine, 74

OKT3 in kidney transplantation, 627t, 629

Older adults, 540–541, 932–964

acute kidney injury in, 172–175, 945–948

atheroembolic kidney disease in, 175, 947–948

chronic kidney disease in, 932–964

epidemiology of, 948, 949f

evaluation of, 413

definition of, 935

depression in, 355, 541

diagnostic parameters in, 945t

drug therapy in, 174, 541, 939, 940, 944

acute kidney injury from, 945–946, 947

dialysis affecting, 960

in long-term care setting, 956–957, 960

exercise and physical functioning in, 382, 383–384

glomerulonephritis in, 175, 947

health insurance plans for, 374

hemodialysis in, 950–954

compared to other treatment options, 951t

in long-term care setting, 956, 957

nutrition in, 540

immunizations in, 997t

kidney transplantation in, 954–955

compared to other treatment options, 951t

in long-term care settings, 955–964

nutritional status of, 540, 541

nephritis in, 164, 175, 947

normal changes in aging process, 935t, 935–944

nutrition in, 540–541

in chronic kidney disease, 949, 956, 960–961

gastrointestinal changes affecting, 937, 938

in long-term care setting, 540, 541, 956, 960–961

and protein-energy malnutrition, 951–952

sensory changes affecting, 944

obstructive urinary disorders in, 175, 948

peritoneal dialysis in, 951t, 954

in home, 876

population trends in, 933–934, 934f, 934t

sepsis in, 174, 952–953

tubular necrosis in, acute, 174–175, 947

Oligohydramnios, 889

Oligonucleotide testing, allele-specific, 328

Oliguria

in acute kidney injury, 34, 38, 144, 153, 157–161, 527

clinical course of, 41–42

SLEDD/CRRT in, 235

Organ Procurement and Transplant Network, 612

Organizational culture, 396

Osmolality, 13t, 24

of blood

compared to urine osmolality, 76

in dialysis disequilibrium syndrome, 193, 193t

of extracellular fluid, 26, 27

of glomerular filtrate, 24, 26, 27

osmoreceptor response to, 26

of renal interstitial fluid, 24–25

of urine, 27, 75t, 76

in acute kidney injury, 38, 39, 39t

compared to blood osmolality, 76

Osmolarity, 13t

in acute kidney injury, 173t

Osmole (Osm), 13t

Osmoreceptors, 24, 25–26, 27

Osmosis, 13t

in hemodialysis, 665

in peritoneal dialysis, 799

reverse, in water treatment, 684–685, 685f

Osmotic agents in hemodialysis and
ultrafiltration, 208, 209t

Osmotic demyelination syndrome in
hemodialysis, 198

Osmotic (oncotic) pressure, colloidal, 13t, 14

in peritoneal dialysis, 800

Osteodystrophy, renal, 430

Osteomalacia in chronic kidney disease, 117

Osteoporosis in kidney transplant recipient, 443, 620

Oxygen

arterial saturation, 186t

in hemodialysis, 184, 700–701, 708, 723

inspired fraction, 184, 189t

mixed venous saturation, 186t

in hemodialysis, 700, 701–702, 723

supplemental, in hemodialysis, 708

uptake measurement in exercise testing, 381, 382

P

Pain, 64, 73–74

assessment of, 64, 73

in end-of-life care, 401

in nephralgia, 73–74

neurologic pathways in, 73

in peritoneal dialysis, 830–831

catheter-related, 229, 793, 831

rectal or suprapubic pain in, 793, 831

referred, 74

in renal colic, 74

Palliative care, 125–126, 399–402

definition of, 401

pediatric, 398, 913

Palpation

of bladder, 64

of kidneys, 64

Pancreas transplantation, 629–643

complications of, 637, 637t

contraindications to, 633

donors in, 633–634

drainage options in, 636

education of patients in, 641, 642t, 643t

historical aspects of, 630

islet cell, 644–645

and kidney transplantation, 631–632, 634–635

operative procedure in, 636–637

long-term benefits of, 641–643

organ procurement process in, 633–634

postoperative management in, 639–641

preoperative assessment in, 632–633

rejection of, 638t, 638–639, 639t

Supplemental Security Income, 377
Suprapubic pain from peritoneal dialysis
    catheter, 793, 831
Surgery
    history of, in hemodialysis patient, 177
    transplantation. *See* Transplantation
Swan-Ganz catheters in hemodynamic
        monitoring, 183–184, 183f–184f
Swan-neck catheters in peritoneal dialysis, 774,
        774f, 776, 776t
Swimming, peritoneal dialysis catheter exit site
        care in, 787
Sympathetic nervous system in blood pressure
        regulation, 16, 585
Sympatholytics in hypertension, 584, 585–586

T

T lymphocytes, 281t, 621, 622, 942
Tacrolimus
    in heart transplantation, 648, 649, 650t
        interaction with other drugs, 649, 650,
            650t
    in kidney transplantation, 624, 626t
    in older adults, acute kidney injury from, 174
Tamm-Horsfall protein, 79, 80
Team approach
    in acute care settings, 136–137, 144
    in kidney transplantation, 352, 612
Temperature
    of body
        in hemodialysis, 180–181, 213, 709–710
        in nutrition assessment, 524
    of dialysate, 834
        in hemodialysis, 674, 703
        in peritoneal dialysis, 834
        in SLEDD/CRRT, 239, 267
    of hemodialysis water supply, 683
Tenckhoff catheters in peritoneal dialysis, 773,
        774f, 776, 776t
    insertion of, 779
Terrorism and violence, emergency management
        plans on, 1026–1028
Therapeutic index of drugs, 575–576, 578
Therapeutic plasma exchange (TPE). *See* Plasma
        exchange, therapeutic (TPE)
Thirst in dialysis, 531
Thrombocytapheresis, 279
Thrombocytopenia
    in HELLP syndrome, 168–169
    heparin-induced
        in hemodialysis, 210, 692
        in peritoneal dialysis, 836–837
    thrombotic, and purpura, 904
        and hemolytic uremic syndrome, 166–
            168, 168t
        plasma exchange in, 283
        variations of, 168
Thrombosis
    in hemodialysis, 744, 748, 752f, 760
    in kidney transplantation, 619
    in pancreas transplantation, 637, 640
Thrombotic thrombocytopenic purpura, 904
    and hemolytic uremic syndrome, 166–168,
        168t

plasma exchange in, 283
    variations of, 168
Thromboxane, 16, 17f
Thymoglobulin in kidney transplantation, 624,
        627t
Thyroid disorders, pharmacokinetics in, 573t
Tidal drain in peritoneal dialysis, 808
Tidal flow in peritoneal dialysis, 807–808
Tidal peritoneal dialysis, nightly, 811–812, 812t
TNM staging of kidney cancer, 47, 48t
Tornadoes, emergency management plan in,
        1018–1019
Toronto Western Hospital catheter in peritoneal
        dialysis, 774, 774f, 778
Training
    of patient and family. *See* Education of
        patient and family
    of personnel. *See* Education of personnel
Transfer RNA, 317, 321f
Transferrin saturation, 419, 581
Translocation, 321
Transmembrane pressure
    in hemodialysis, 212, 665, 674
    in SLEDD/CRRT, 236, 236f
Transplantation, 61–62
    of heart, 61–62, 145, 647–650
    islet cell, 644–645
    of kidney, 608–628. *See also* Kidney
        transplantation
    of liver, 61–62, 650–655
    of pancreas, 629–643. *See also* Pancreas
        transplantation
    terminology related to, 612
Transport maximum, tubular, 12, 13t, 21
Transportation issues in emergency and disaster
        events, 1014
Transporter proteins, 320t, 332
Transtheoretical model of intentional change,
        123
Trauma
    peritoneal dialysis catheter exit site infection
        in, 787, 789
    and posttraumatic stress in emergency and
        disaster events, 1015
Triage in emergency and disaster events, 1015
TRICARE military health plan, 373
Triceps skinfold thickness in nutrition
        assessment, 526
Triglyceride levels, 454, 963
Trisomy syndromes, 321
Trust, cultural diversity in, 342
Tuberculin skin test, 988, 989–990, 991t
Tuberculosis, 987–992
    in chronic kidney disease, 989–990, 992
    etiology of, 987, 987f
    infectivity in, 987, 990
    pathophysiology in, 987–988
    peritonitis in, 844–845
    renal, 49
        pregnancy in, 61
    risk factors for, 987, 988, 989t
        chronic kidney disease as, 989–990
    screening for, 989–990
    signs and symptoms in, 988–989
    treatment of, 987, 990–992

adherence with, 990
    in dialysis, 599t, 992, 992t
    drug resistance in, 987, 988, 992
Tubular necrosis, acute, 36–40, 37f, 150–151,
        432–433
    differentiated from prerenal azotemia, 39–40
    ischemic, 36–38, 37f, 150, 152–153, 432
    in kidney transplantation, 619
    manifestations of, 162
    in older adults, 174–175, 947
    pathophysiology of, 36–38, 37f, 151f
    in sepsis, 166, 167f
    SLEDD/CRRT in, 235
    toxic, 37f, 38, 150–151, 153–154, 433
Tubules
    acute necrosis of, 36–40. *See also* Tubular
        necrosis, acute
    age-related changes in, 939
    chronic disorders of, 46–47
    distal. *See* Distal tubules
    proximal
        anatomy of, 9, 9f
        in fluid and electrolyte regulation, 17–22,
            19t
        reabsorption in, 10f, 12, 13t, 17–22
            of bicarbonate, 29, 30f
            obligatory, of water, 22
        secretion of, 10f, 12, 13t
        transport maximum, 12, 13t, 21
Tubuloglomerular feedback, 15–16
Tubulointerstitial injury, malnutrition in, 527
Tumor lysis syndrome, 235
Tumors
    cell division and cell cycle in, 319, 325
    cultural differences in risk for, 340
    of kidney, 47–48, 48t
    screening for, in potential kidney transplant
        recipient, 615

U

Ultrafiltration
    in hemodialysis, 207–209, 212, 434, 665, 686
        conductivity profiling in, 208–209
        estimated dry weight in, 692, 702–704
        fluid balance in, 207–208, 692, 694, 697
        hematocrit-based blood volume
            monitoring in, 718–724
        hypotension in, 704–705, 706
        isolated or sequential, 703, 706
    in peritoneal dialysis
        in acute care setting, 219
        in children, 916
        failure of, 837, 916
        rate of, 800, 800f
    in SLEDD/CRRT, 235–236
        filtration fraction in, 236
    slow continuous (SCUF), 231, 232, 250, 256
Ultrasound studies, 84–85
    in acute kidney injury, 173t
    in peritoneal dialysis complications, 827
Ultraviolet irradiation in water treatment, 686
United Network for Organ Sharing
    in kidney transplantation, 609, 612
    in pancreas transplantation, 630

Sponsorships

ANNA thanks the following companies for their sponsorship of this book.
See their company profiles on the following pages.

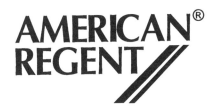

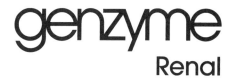

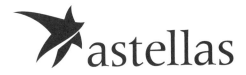

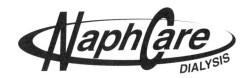

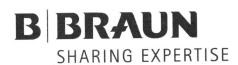

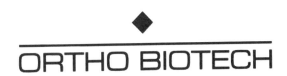

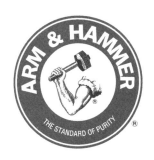

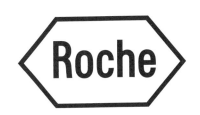

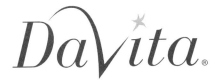

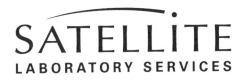

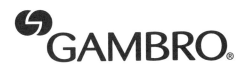

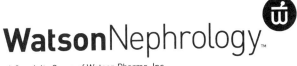

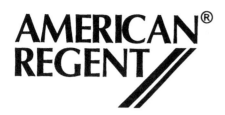

American Regent, Inc.
One Luitpold Drive
PO Box 9001
Shirley, NY 11967

Telephone: 800-645-1706 or 631-924-4000
Web sites: www.americanregent.com
www.venofer.com

American Regent, "Your IV Iron Company," is the manufacturer and distributor of Venofer® (iron sucrose injection, USP), the #1 selling IV iron in the U.S.[1] Venofer® is available in 100mg/5mL and 200mg/10mL single-dose vials (preservative free). Venofer® is covered nationally by CMS/Medicare and has been assigned a permanent national HCPCS Code "J1756" for services provided on or after January 1, 2003.

American Regent continues its commitment to the renal community with quality services provided by a highly trained and knowledgeable field Sales Force and a Clinical Support Team of Nephrology Specialists. Some of these services include Facility-Based In-services and CE Presentations, Facility-Based Iron Management Review, Patient Education Programs, Professional Speakers Bureau, Resource Center for Clinical Inquiries, a Reimbursement Hotline, a Patient Assistance Program, and Regional Iron and Anemia Workshops. For additional information, visit our Web sites at www.american regent.com and www.venofer.com.

[1] Based on IMS Health, National Sales Perspectives™ – 3rd Quarter 2007 Results (October 2007)

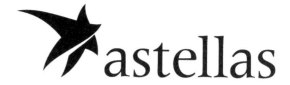

Astellas Pharma US, Inc.
Three Parkway North
Deerfield, IL 60015

Telephone: 847-317-8800
Web site: www.astellas.com/us

Astellas is a recognized leader in transplantation and has been committed to the field of immunology for more than 20 years. Dedicated to supporting the advancement of care for patients, Astellas continues to build upon its legacy and leadership in transplantation by investing in ongoing clinical research, new product development, and patient education.

Astellas has developed the Transplant Experience program to provide a resource for transplant recipients and caregivers throughout every stage of the transplant experience – pretransplant, the first year after transplant, and beyond. The program includes tools, tips, and advice from experts in transplantation, including physicians and nurses, and also provides peer-to-peer information from transplant recipients. For more information about organ donation and transplantation, visit www.TransplantExperience.com.

Astellas Pharma US, Inc., located in Deerfield, Illinois, is a U.S. affiliate of Tokyo-based Astellas Pharma Inc. Astellas is a pharmaceutical company dedicated to improving the health of people around the world through the provision of innovative and reliable pharmaceutical products. The organization is committed to becoming a global category leader in focused areas by combining outstanding R&D and marketing capabilities. In the U.S., Astellas markets products in the areas of Immunology, Urology, Anti-Infectives, Cardiovascular and Dermatology. For more information about Astellas Pharma US, Inc., please visit our Web site at www.astellas.com/us.

B|BRAUN
SHARING EXPERTISE

B. Braun Medical Inc.
824 Twelfth Avenue
Bethlehem, PA 18018

Telephone: 800-848-2066
Web site: www.bbraunusa.com

B. Braun Medical Inc. has been a leader in providing the dialysis community with innovative products for more than 30 years. The Renal Therapies Division (RTD) of B. Braun provides equipment and related disposable products to treat chronic renal failure through hemodialysis, and acute kidney failure through continuous renal replacement therapy (CRRT). The Dialog® Plus Hemodialysis System incorporates the latest in state-of-the-art dialysis technology. For continuous renal replacement therapy (CRRT), the B. Braun Diapact® CRRT System allows the user to perform a wide range of high flow intermittent or continuous renal replacement and plasma therapies.

In early 2008, the Renal Therapies Division will be offering the B. Braun Diacap @ Polysulfone® Low and High Flux dialyzers. This dialyzer is a further development of the proven polysulfone technology continuing B. Braun's commitment to the development of new techniques and innovations for dialysis and renal replacement therapy that will continue to improve patient care, and offer more ways to meet the challenging demands of nephrology.

The Renal Therapies Division (RTD) of B. Braun offers a full line of high quality products for hemodialysis and continuous renal replacement therapy supported by the RTD team of clinical nurses, field service personnel, customer service, and 24/7 technical assistance. For more information, contact the Renal Therapies Division at 800-848-2066 or email: rtd@bbraun.com.

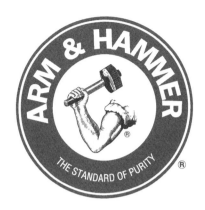

Church & Dwight Co., Inc.
469 North Harrison Street
Princeton, NJ 08543-5297

Telephone: 800-221-0453
Web site: www.ahperformance.com

Church & Dwight Co., Inc. is the maker of ARM & HAMMER® brand sodium bicarbonate. Our ARM & HAMMER® brand dialysis grade sodium bicarbonate, developed specifically for use in kidney dialysis, is used in more bicarb based dialysate than any other brand in North America. This superior product is available in dialysis concentrates produced by our "Partners in Quality Care," a unique alliance between Church & Dwight and the nation's leaders in dialysis products and services.

Through our Partners in Quality Care, Church & Dwight also supports your efforts by making available practical, straightforward educational materials for both patients and staff. These include easy-to-follow patient education pamphlets in both English and Spanish: *A Guide to Managing Fluid Intake, A Guide to Taking Control of Your Life on Dialysis*, and *Hemodialysis: Step by Step*. For dialysis facility staff, we offer a handbook entitled *Sodium Bicarbonate Mixing Considerations* as well as two educational self-study programs accredited by ANNA: *ESRD Care of the Diabetic Patient* and *Acid-Base Balance in Hemodialysis Patients with End Stage Renal Disease*. All of these resources are available at no charge to dialysis clinics upon request.

To receive educational resources for patients and professionals, contact Christi Schofield at cschofield@ki-lipton.com or 267-893-5677.

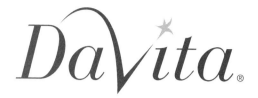

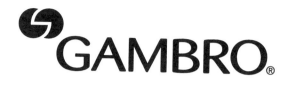

DaVita
601 Hawaii Street
El Segundo, CA 90245

Telephone: 866-400-2266
Web site: www.davita.com/careers

Changing the Face of Kidney Care

DaVita strives to provide comprehensive care by focusing on superior clinical outcomes and quality of life for our patients.

DaVita is the largest independent provider of dialysis services in the U.S. dedicated to treating patients suffering from chronic kidney failure. We have over 30,000 teammates serving approximately 103,000 patients nationwide, over one-third of the dialysis community. These teammates work in over 1,300 outpatient dialysis facilities and over 700 hospital acute units, located in 43 states and the District of Columbia.

At DaVita we believe a company can also be a community, and with dedicated individuals, we can make a difference in the way healthcare is practiced. Even though we are a member of the FORTUNE 500®, our real pride comes in the way of consistently achieving clinical care outcomes which surpass national averages, and having fun while we do it. Come see for yourself how committed we are to our shared vision of becoming the greatest kidney care company the world has ever seen.

To learn more about nephrology nursing, please go to www.davita.com.

To learn more about our DaVita Village and the career path opportunities that await you, please go to www.davita.com/careers/.

Gambro
14143 Denver West Parkway
Lakewood, CO 80401

Telephone: 800-525-2623
Web site: www.gambro.com

Gambro is a global medical technology company and a leader in developing, manufacturing, and supplying products, therapies, and services for In-center Care, Peritoneal Dialysis, Renal Intensive Care, and Hepatic Care.

Gambro was founded in 1964 and has more than 8,000 employees, production facilities in 11 countries, sales subsidiaries in more than 40, and sales in more than 100 countries.

genzyme
Renal

Genzyme Renal
500 Kendall Street
Cambridge, MA 02142

Telephone: 800-847-0069
Web site: www.genzyme.com

Genzyme, a global health care company, delivers innovative biotechnology products and services in therapeutics, surgery and diagnostic areas. Genzyme is the manufacturer of Renvela® (sevelamer carbonate), Renagel® (sevelamer hydrochloride), and Hectorol® (doxercalciferol). Genzyme is a leader in health care awareness and education for renal care specialists and patients worldwide.

For more information visit www.genzyme.com or call 1.800.847.0069.

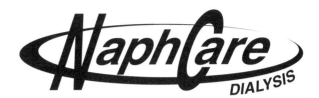

NaphCare, Inc.
950 22nd Street North
Suite 825
Birmingham, AL 35203

Telephone: 800-834-2420
Web site: www.naphcare.com

NaphCare, Inc. was founded in 1989 and has since enjoyed steady growth in the correctional healthcare industry. NaphCare provides a diverse range of services to the correctional industry, ranging from comprehensive healthcare (medical, mental health, dental, and pharmacy), developing provider-networks, and complete on-site dialysis and nephrology services.

NaphCare provides on-site chronic and acute dialysis and nephrology-related services to correctional facilities across the country. In 2007 alone, we performed over 50,000 dialysis treatments and provided nephrology-related services for almost 4000 Chronic Kidney Disease patients. Our clients include State Departments of Corrections, Federal Bureau of Prisons, and local county jails.

Our Mission
Our Mission is to be the provider of choice for Dialysis and Nephrology Services to the Correctional Industry.

Products and Services
✓ Complete On-Site Dialysis and Nephrology Services
✓ Comprehensive Correctional Healthcare Services
✓ Provider Networking (Federal Bureau of Prisons)
✓ Electronic Medical Management System – TechCare™

Based in Birmingham, Alabama NaphCare employs more than 500 dedicated health care professionals in 19 states. Please contact us if you are interested in hearing more about the services we provide, or would like to hear more about Correctional Nephrology Nursing opportunities in your area.

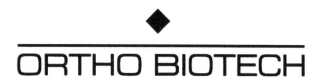

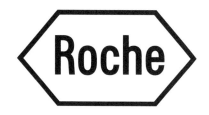

Ortho Biotech Products, L.P.
430 Route 22 East
PO Box 6914
Bridgewater, NJ 08807-0914

Telephone: 908-541-4000
Web site: www.orthobiotech.com

Ortho Biotech Products, L.P. is a leading bio-pharmaceutical company devoted to helping improve the lives of patients with cancer and with anemia due to multiple causes, including chronic kidney disease. Since it was founded in 1990, Ortho Biotech and its worldwide affiliates have earned a global reputation for researching, manufacturing, and marketing innovative products that enhance patients' health.

Located in Bridgewater, N.J., Ortho Biotech is an established market leader in anemia management. The company also markets treatments for recurrent ovarian cancer, rejection of transplanted organs, and other serious illnesses.

For more information, visit www.orthobiotech.com.

Roche
340 Kingsland Street
Nutley, NJ 07110

Web site: www.rocheusa.com
www.roche.us

About Roche

Hoffmann-La Roche Inc. (Roche), based in Nutley, N.J., is the U.S. pharmaceuticals head-quarters of the Roche Group, one of the world's leading research-oriented healthcare groups with core businesses in pharmaceuticals and diagnostics. For more than 100 years in the U.S., Roche has been committed to developing innovative products and services that address prevention, diagnosis and treatment of diseases, thus enhancing people's health and quality of life. An employer of choice, in 2007 Roche was named Top Company of the Year by *Med Ad News*, one of the Top 20 Employers (*Science*) and ranked the No. 1 Company to Sell For (*Selling Power*). In previous years, Roche has been named as a Top Company for Older Workers (AARP) and one of the Best Companies to Work For in America (*Fortune*). For additional information about the U.S. pharmaceuticals business, visit our websites: http://www.rocheusa.com or www.roche.us.

All trademarks used or mentioned in this release are protected by law.

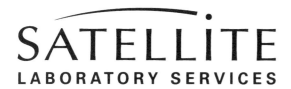